Encyclopedia of Clinical Child and Pediatric Psychology

Encyclopedia of Clinical Child and Pediatric Psychology

Edited by

Thomas H. Ollendick

Virginia Polytechnic Institute and State University
Blacksburg, Virginia

and

Carolyn S. Schroeder

University of Kansas
Lawrence, Kansas

Kluwer Academic/Plenum Publishers
New York   Boston   Dordrecht   London   Moscow

Library of Congress Cataloging-in-Publication Data

Encyclopedia of clinical child and pediatric psychology/edited by Thomas H. Ollendick,
  Carolyn S. Schroeder.
      p.   cm.
    Includes index.
    ISBN 0-306-47490-5
      1. Clinical child psychology—Encyclopedias.   2. Child development—Encyclopedias.   3.
  Child psychology—Encyclopedias.   I. Ollendick, Thomas H.   II. Schroeder, Carolyn S.

  RJ503.3.E53 2003
  618.92′89′003—dc21

                                                                          2003046115

ISBN 0-306-47490-5

©2003 Kluwer Academic/Plenum Publishers, New York
233 Spring Street, New York, New York 10013

http://www.wkap.nl/

10   9   8   7   6   5   4   3   2   1

A C.I.P. record for this book is available from the Library of Congress

Permissions for books published in Europe: *permissions@wkap.nl*
Permissions for books published in the United States of America: *permissions@wkap.com*

Printed in the United States of America

ADVISORY BOARD

Preface

The *Encyclopedia of Clinical Child and Pediatric Psychology* is intended to be an authoritative and comprehensive resource that provides up-to-date information on a broad array of problems and issues related to children, adolescents, and their families as defined by the fields of clinical child and pediatric psychology. It is designed to be of particular interest and use to laypersons, parents and grandparents, and undergraduate and graduate students in training, as well as diverse medical and mental health professionals who live with and/or work with young persons but who have limited information on a particular topics. Inasmuch as the scope of clinical child and pediatric psychology is extensive, a range of topics is included that cover typical and atypical development, physical and mental health problems and disorders, assessment and treatment methods, and professional issues such as training and ethics. For those interested in further information a list of readings is included for each topic or entry. The topics are listed in alphabetical order to aid in the quick retrieval of information and the Index is extensive in its cross-listing of topics. We hope the Encyclopedia will be most beneficial to those who, for whatever reason, desire to obtain brief, authoritative, and up-to-date information on a particular topic or issue affecting children and their development, whether that development be characterized as typical or atypical.

A brief comment on the disciplines of Clinical Child Psychology and Pediatric Psychology is in order. Clinical child psychology is a specialty of professional psychology that attempts to integrate basic tenets of clinical psychology, developmental psychology, child psychopathology, and child and family development. Clinical child psychologists conduct scientific research and provide psychological services to infants, toddlers, children, adolescents, and their families with a focus on understanding, preventing, diagnosing and treating psychological, cognitive, emotional, developmental, behavioral, and family problems of children. Of particular importance to clinical child psychologists is an understanding of the basic psychological needs of children and the social contexts that influence child development and adjustment. Thus, typical and atypical development and the impact of life stresses are of concern for the clinical child psychologist.

The specialty of pediatric psychology, like clinical child psychology, is interested in the psychological needs of children but the focus is on the psychosocial aspects of illness. In addition to child and family development, the knowledge base includes the biological, cognitive, affective, and social bases of health and disease. Pediatric psychologists engage in scientific research on how children's experiences and behavior are affected by physical illness, injury, and disability, and how their behavior in turn affects children's health. Pediatric psychologists, thus, work closely with other allied health professionals and their services include helping children and families deal with health issues through prevention and treatment. As a result, pediatric psychologists are found in health care settings such as children's hospitals, developmental clinics, pediatric or medical group practices, as well as in traditional clinical child or academic arenas.

Both of these disciplines are enjoined by their interest in infants, toddlers, children, adolescents, and their families. As such, they frequently complement one another, and many pediatric and clinical child psychologists work along side one another, as well as a host of other professionals, for the benefit and welfare of those they serve. Clinical child and pediatric psychology are emerging, exciting, and energetic fields of study and we are most pleased to be intimately associated with them. Although much remains to be learned, a lot has been learned in the last few decades—enough to warrant encyclopedic coverage.

In a comprehensive project such as this, many persons are to be acknowledged. Among the foremost are our distinguished Advisory Board and our equally distinguished list of contributors. Quite obviously, without them, up-to-date and scholarly treatment of topics and issues could hardly have been possible. We would also like to acknowledge Mariclaire Cloutier, Publishing Director, Behavioral Sciences, at Kluwer Academic/Plenum Publishers, for her commitment to this project and her encouragement to us to undertake it. Equally so, we thank Siiri Lelumees, Child Psychology Editor at Kluwer Academic/Plenum Publishers, for her editorial direction and encouragement. In addition, we would like to give thanks to the many youngsters and their families who have, perhaps unknowingly and unwittingly, served as the real impetus and reinforcement for undertaking this project.

Finally, we would like to thank our respective friends and mates, Mary (THO) and Steve (CSS) who tolerated, encouraged, and supported us during this long and seemingly endless process. They were real troopers! We also wish to thank our children, Laurie K. Perryman and Kathleen M. Smith (THO), and Mark S. Schroeder and Matthew E. Schroeder (CSS), as well as our children's children, Braden T. Perryman and Ethan R. Perryman (THO) and Zoe Margaret Schroeder (CSS). We have learned much from them as well. And, should our adult children read this Preface, we look forward to thanking more of our grandchildren in the future! Without them, life would be less meaningful and enjoyable for us. To our "grand" children, we dedicate this effort.

THOMAS H. OLLENDICK
CAROLYN S. SCHROEDER

Aa

Abuse

See: Child Maltreatment; Psychological Maltreatment

Academic Achievement

DEFINITION

Academic achievement is defined as the knowledge and skills that an individual learns through direct instruction. Achievement tests measure what a person has learned, whereas aptitude tests (including tests of intelligence) assess a person's potential for learning.

Academic achievement tests are used for a variety of purposes. In educational settings, achievement tests are often used to place students in appropriate grade levels, screen students for academic difficulties, and monitor the academic progress of students in a school or a school district. Achievement tests such as The Stanford Achievement Test and the Iowa Test of Basic Skills are administered annually by many schools to children in all grades across the United States. A student's score on the test or the average score for a particular school can be compared to the national or state averages for the year that the test was given.

Individually administered achievement tests are typically administered by school or clinical psychologists as part of a comprehensive psychoeducational evaluation of a child having academic difficulties. Academic achievement tests play less of a role in clinical evaluations.

TYPES OF ACHIEVEMENT TESTS

There are three types of individually administered achievement tests: screening tests, comprehensive tests, and single-subject tests. Screening tests typically cover only three areas of achievement: reading, mathematics, and spelling, and have only one subtest measuring each area. Comprehensive tests also cover these three subject areas but have two or more subtests in each subject area, each of which measures different aspects of the subject area. Comprehensive achievement tests typically include other skills areas such as listening comprehension and oral and written language skills. Single-subject tests consist of several subtests measuring different skills within one subject area.

STANDARDIZATION

Most tests of academic achievement are standardized using a large group of people (usually 4,000 or more) that closely reflect the demographic characteristics of the population according to the most recent census data at the time the test was developed. For most tests, sampling is stratified within each age group by gender (roughly equal number of males and females at each age/grade level tested), geographic region (usually West, South, Northeast, and North Central), race/ethnicity (whites, African Americans, Asians, and Hispanics), and level of education of the parent (or individual if an adult is being tested).

SCORES ON ACHIEVEMENT TESTS

Raw scores on achievement tests can be converted into a variety of score types. The most commonly used score is a standard score which has a mean of 100 and standard deviation of 15. Scores on academic achievement tests follow a normal distribution or a bell-shaped curve. Generally speaking, standard scores between 85 and 115 are considered average, scores above 115 are above average, and scores below 85 are below average. To compare individuals of the same age, age-based standard scores should be used. When individuals are compared against others in their grade, grade-based standard scores should be used.

Age- and grade-equivalent scores are useful for communicating test results to parents because the general public understands the meaning of these scores. If the mean raw score for 8-year-old children on a spelling test is 25, then any child who obtains a score of 25 has an age-equivalent score of 8 years. Similarly, if the mean score for third graders on a spelling test is 25, then a child obtaining a score of 25 is said to have a grade-equivalent score of third grade for spelling. However, there are many pitfalls associated with the use of age- or grade-equivalent scores. Age or grade equivalents are not equally spaced through the scale, thus the difference between fifth and sixth grade-equivalent scores may not be the same as the difference between tenth and eleventh grade-equivalent scores. Grade scores are sometimes misleading because a child who obtains a grade equivalent of 4.0 is not functioning like a child in Grade 4. He or she only shares the same number of test items correct with the average child in Grade 4. Thus, age- and grade-equivalent scores should be viewed with caution.

Percentile ranks are also used to interpret achievement scores and tell how a child's score ranks in comparison to a reference group, usually the standardization sample. For example, if a child scores at the 70th percentile, this means that the child scored at or above 70 percent of the children in the standardization sample.

RELIABILITY AND VALIDITY

The reliability and validity estimates for most standardized achievement tests are quite good. The reliability coefficients for subtest and composite scores are quite acceptable, and achievement tests correlate well with other measures of academic achievement and intelligence. Achievement scores at a young age are typically less reliable than at an older age. Scores on

achievement tests in kindergarten or first grade are very dependent upon prior academic exposure, readiness for learning, maturity, and other factors. Thus, a child could score in the superior range in kindergarten, yet by Grade 1 or 2, score only in the average range. All of the mainstream measures of achievement appear to be measuring the same achievement constructs across racial, ethnic, and gender lines and thus do not appear to be biased against any particular group.

WHAT DO THE TESTS MEASURE?

There are a number of different types of screening tests that can be used as a quick or brief assessment of academic achievement in reading, mathematics, and spelling. The reading subtest is designed to measure an individual's ability to recognize letters and pronounce words. The spelling subtest measures an individual's ability to copy marks resembling letters and to write words dictated to the child. The arithmetic subtest of many screener tests requires the respondent to count, solve word problems, and simple (e.g., $2 + 2 = \_\_$) to complex (e.g., $\log_b 81 = 4$, $b = \_\_$) computations.

There are many comprehensive academic achievement tests that are frequently used. Most comprehensive achievement tests assess the broad areas of reading, written language, oral language, and mathematics. The individual receives a score for each subtest given and related subtests are combined to form a Composite or a Broad Cluster score for a given area. Typically, the reading cluster consists of scores from subtests that measure skills such as the ability to read letters and words of increasing difficulty, the speed with which an individual can read simple words (reading fluency), and passage comprehension which is defined as the ability to read sentences and demonstrate understanding of what is read (e.g., touch your nose). Written Language Cluster scores typically include subtests that measure an individual's ability to write sentences incorporating designated words, to write a brief story describing some action taking place in one or more pictures, and to spell. Oral Language Clusters usually assess an individual's expressive vocabulary including giving directions, generating a story, and recalling details from a passage. The Mathematics Cluster typically includes an assessment of skills such as counting, reading number symbols, solving simple word problems to more complex tasks such as solving single- and multistep word problems, interpreting graphs, and solving problems related to statistics and probability. In addition to obtaining scores for each cluster area, a total achievement score that reflects a person's overall performance across the various clusters can be obtained for most comprehensive measures of achievement.

CLINICAL UTILITY

Screening tests are just that—screening measures to indicate potential problems, and the results should not be used for clinical or educational decisions. Low scores on any one area of a screening test are often used as a decision to refer the child for more comprehensive testing. Scores on comprehensive measures of achievement are often useful for diagnostic purposes. For example, low scores on all of the oral subtests might indicate a hearing problem. When administered in conjunction with other cognitive or intelligence measures (e.g., IQ tests), comprehensive achievement tests can help to determine if a child has a learning disability. A child who scores significantly below average in the mathematics cluster subtests, but who scores within the average range on an intelligence test, might be diagnosed with a learning disability in math.

Single-subject achievement tests are almost always used for diagnostic purposes. These tests are given when the individual has demonstrated difficulties in a particular academic area. Diagnostic tests provide information about specific weaknesses/strengths in a particular skill area. For example, the problems a child in Grade 4 is having in math might be caused by a failure to adequately learn the prerequisite skills in addition and subtraction when regrouping numbers is required (e.g., subtracting 15 from 32). This kind of detailed information is generally not available on more comprehensive tests.

CONCLUSIONS

Academic achievement tests are among the most sound and objective measures of knowledge and performance available. They are useful for assessing an individual's strengths and weaknesses in specific subject areas and they can provide educators with information about how a student is progressing in the classroom. However, scores on an achievement test do not necessarily translate into academic performance in the classroom. A student can score quite high on achievement tests and yet be failing in one or more subject areas. It is important to note that no one test is a valid measure of a child's academic skills, intellectual ability, or learning style. It is, therefore, necessary to interpret any academic achievement score within the broader context of a student's life including his or her

psychosocial history, motivation, intelligence, and test-taking skills.

To find out more about measures of achievement, the reader is referred to Jerome Sattler (2001). Chapters 19 and 20 of Sattler's book discuss issues related to the assessment of culturally and linguistically diverse children. Additional references on this topic are provided in these chapters.

See also: Intellectual Assessment; Learning Disorders; School Age Assessment; Underachievement; Validity

Further Reading

Sattler, J. M. (2001). *Assessment of children: Cognitive applications* (4th ed.). San Diego: Jerome M. Sattler.
www.apa.org/science/testing.html

Laura Stoppelbein
Jean Spruill

Accidental (Unintentional) Injuries

BACKGROUND

Unintentional injuries are a major threat to the health of children and adolescents in the United States. Despite the low base-rate of serious injuries among children, they are more vulnerable to accidental or unintentional injuries than to any other threat in their environment. Each year between 20–25 percent of all children sustain an injury requiring medical attention, missed school, and/or bed rest.

Unintentional injuries are the leading cause of death for individuals between the ages of 1 and 21. In the general population, approximately one in every 17 deaths in the United States is the result of an injury. Of these deaths, 67 percent are categorized as unintentional. For children under the age of 15, motor vehicle accidents, drownings, burns (and other fire-related injuries), and suffocations account for the majority of deaths due to unintentional injury. Adolescents are particularly at risk for injuries. Injuries kill more adolescents than all diseases combined, with adolescent males at a greater risk of being involved in a fatal injury than their female counterparts across all types of injury. For adolescents aged 15 and older, motor vehicle accidents, poisonings, drowning, and injuries from other land transport devices are responsible for the majority of injuries.

TYPES OF INJURIES

Motor Vehicle

Injuries that occur while the child is a passenger in a motor vehicle are the most common type of injuries among children from age one to adulthood. Although these injuries have been reduced in recent years due to the enactment of laws mandating the use of child safety seats, many children are still injured each year in motor vehicle collisions. Motor vehicle accidents are also a major threat to adolescents. The risk of a motor vehicle crash is particularly high during the first year that a teenager is learning to drive. In 1998, the death rate for male adolescent drivers was more than twice as high as it was for female adolescent drivers. Several reasons have been proposed for this high level of risk among adolescents, including lack of driving experience, low rates of safety belt usage, a higher risk of driving after drinking alcohol, and higher levels of nighttime driving among adolescents.

Drowning

Drowning is the second leading cause of injury-related death in children between the ages of 1 and 14. The majority of drowning victims are male, and among children aged 5–19 years, a disproportionate number of drownings occur in African American children. Most drownings involving children under the age of 5 years occur in swimming pools. Other water hazards include bathtubs and buckets of liquid, as well as open water, such as rivers and lakes.

Fire

Fire-related burns are also a major concern. Each year in the United States, over 400,000 residential fires occur and account for approximately 3,600 deaths and 18,600 injuries. Of these injuries and deaths, children under the age of 5, older adults, and people in lower income brackets are the most likely to be affected. The majority of residential fires occur during the winter months and are started by either cooking or smoking. Most fatal residential fires occur in homes that do not have a working smoke detector. Fireworks pose another burn threat for children. Over 40 percent of individuals who are injured from fireworks are children under age 14. Males suffer fireworks-related injuries three times more often than females, with boys between the ages of 5–14 being the most likely to sustain this type of injury. Over half of all fireworks-related injuries are burns, however, contusions and lacerations may also occur. Firecrackers, bottle rockets, and sparklers account for the majority of these injuries.

Suffocation

Suffocation is the fourth leading cause of death for children under the age of 15. In 1997, nearly 700 children aged 14 and under died from airway obstruction injuries (i.e., suffocation, choking, and strangulation). Of these children, nearly 80 percent were under the age of 5. Common causes of suffocation include ingestion of small objects, becoming tangled in strings or ribbons, entering confined spaces with limited amounts of air (e.g., a car trunk, an abandoned refrigerator), and placing plastic objects (e.g., plastic bags, balloons) over the nose and mouth.

Poisoning

Although fewer injury-related deaths are attributed to poisoning, they are a significant health threat to children. Every year, approximately 900,000 visits to the emergency room occur because of ingestion of a poisonous substance. The majority of poisonings involve children under the age of 6. Common household items, such as cleaning agents, plants, and medications, are implicated in most instances of poisoning.

Pedestrian Injuries

Children are also at a high risk for pedestrian injuries. Pedestrian injuries are the second leading cause of motor vehicle-related deaths, ranking second to motor vehicle occupant injuries. In 1998, 25 percent of children between the ages of 5 and 9 who were killed in traffic crashes were pedestrians. This type of injury is the fifth leading cause of death among children aged 1–4.

Playground Equipment

Injuries that occur while children are playing on playground equipment are very common and account for about 200,000 emergency room visits annually. Most of these types of injuries occur in public playgrounds, and 35 percent of them are severe. Children usually sustain these injuries by falling off of the playground equipment (e.g., slides, monkey bars). Relatedly, in recreational injuries, an estimated 140,000 children are treated in emergency rooms each year for head injuries sustained while riding a bicycle. Only 25 percent of children aged 4–14 wear helmets when bicycling. This rate drops to near zero for adolescent bicycle-riders. In 1991, costs associated with bicycle-related head injury or death were estimated to exceed $3 billion.

Firearms

Unintentional shootings account for 20 percent of all firearm-related fatalities among children aged 14 and under. In 1997, over 2,500 children under the age of 14 sustained nonfatal firearm-related injuries. The death rate due to unintentional firearm injuries among children under the age of 15 in the United States is nine times higher than the rates in 25 other industrialized countries combined. The possession of a firearm in the home (especially if it is kept unlocked and loaded) is associated with an increased risk of unintentional firearm injuries among children.

The importance of injuries as a threat to the health and development of children became more apparent as contagious diseases decreased over time. There is an increasing role for clinical child and pediatric psychologists in the examination of injury events, causes, and characteristics, and in the control or prevention of childhood injuries. The Centers for Disease Control and Prevention has the responsibility for recording epidemiological data on injuries and in the development and evaluation of effective control strategies.

See also: Injury Prevention; Safety and Prevention

Further Reading

Centers for Disease Control and Prevention (CDC), National Center for Health Statistics (NCHS). (1999, June). Deaths: Final data for 1997. *National Vital Statistics Reports 47* (19).
CDC. (1999). Childhood injury fact sheet. Retrieved on April 13, 2002 at http://www.cdc.gov/ncipc/factsheets/childh.htm.
CDC, NCHS. (2001). *Healthy people 2000: Final review.* Hyattsville, MD: Public Health Service.
CDC. (2002). About CDC. Retrieved on April 13, 2002 at http://www.cdc.gov/aboutcdc.htm.

SUNNYE E. MAYES
KERI J. BROWN
MICHAEL C. ROBERTS

Acquired Heart Disease

See: Cardiovascular Disease

Acromegaly

See: Gigantism and Acromegaly

Acute Stress Disorder

Acute Stress Disorder (ASD) was introduced into the 4th edition of the American Psychiatric Association's *Diagnostic and Statistical Manual of Mental Disorders (DSM-IV)*. ASD is similar to Posttraumatic Stress Disorder (PTSD) in that it represents a specific pattern of symptoms or reactions in response to traumatic events. However, it differs from PTSD in that it reflects reactions that occur in the first month (2–28 days) following a traumatic event and emphasizes symptoms of dissociation.

Specifically, in *DSM-IV*, ASD is described as a set of symptoms that develop following exposure to an unusually severe stressor or event that causes or is capable of causing death, injury, or threat to the physical integrity of oneself or another person; the individual's reaction must include intense fear, helplessness, or horror; the disturbance must last for 2 days to 4 weeks and must occur within 4 weeks of the traumatic event. One salient feature of ASD is that, either during or after the traumatic event, three or more *dissociative symptoms* will be present. Such symptoms include: a subjective sense of numbing, detachment, or absence of emotional responsiveness; reduced awareness of one's surroundings (e.g., "being in a daze"); derealization (i.e., the experience of unreality or loss of reality); depersonalization (i.e., the experience of loss of one's identity as a person); and dissociative amnesia (i.e., inability to recall important aspects of the trauma). The other symptom clusters of ASD are similar to those for PTSD, including: *reexperiencing the event* (as through flashbacks, recurrent thoughts and images, a sense of reliving the event, or distress when exposed to reminders of the event), *avoidance* (of thoughts, feelings, conversations, places, people, or activities that arouse recollections of the event), and *marked anxiety or increased arousal* (e.g., difficulty sleeping or concentrating; irritability; exaggerated startle response; motor restlessness). In addition, the disturbance must result in clinically significant impairment in everyday functioning (e.g., problems with school, family, friends, etc.) that impairs the individual's ability to pursue necessary tasks (e.g., obtaining necessary assistance, mobilizing personal resources). Finally, the disturbance must not be due to the direct physiological effects of a substance (e.g., medication, drugs) or a general medical condition.

The diagnosis of ASD was intended to help identify, early on, individuals who would later develop PTSD, so that appropriate treatment and preventive measures could be implemented. However, Bryant (2000) notes that the diagnosis has had a mixed reception. Concerns include that it has limited empirical support, it may pathologize transient stress reactions in traumatized individuals, and its primary function is to predict another diagnosis (PTSD).

Little research has examined ASD in adults and children. Available evidence suggests that clinical and sub-clinical levels of ASD predict later PTSD in adult trauma victims (e.g., motor vehicle accident victims, assault victims, typhoon survivors). However, a substantial percentage of adult trauma victims who eventually develop PTSD do not show evidence of ASD early on, so the ASD diagnosis misses many adults who subsequently develop PTSD.

Existing studies of ASD in children have been conducted primarily in pediatric patients treated in emergency medical settings for burns or injuries. Daviss, Mooney, Racusin, Ford, Fleischer, and McHugo (2000) assessed 54 youth (7–17 years) who were hospitalized for injuries, the majority of whom (93 percent) met the initial criteria for ASD (i.e., exposure to an event that is capable of causing death, injury, or threat to physical integrity). However, only 7 percent of the youth met criteria for ASD; another 22 percent had significant but subclinical levels of ASD. These authors also found substantial discrepancies in parents' and nurses' reports of ASD symptoms in the children. In a follow-up of these youth (one month or more later), Daviss and associates found that ASD symptoms were relatively weak predictors of subsequent PTSD symptoms in the youth compared to acute parental distress and preexisting child psychopathology. Moreover, only the ASD symptom cluster for hyperarousal/anxiety correlated significantly with PTSD symptoms; the ASD dissociative symptom cluster was unrelated to PTSD symptoms. These findings do not support the theoretical linkage between early dissociative symptoms and later PTSD in children. Further investigation of the validity and utility of the ASD diagnosis in children is needed.

See also: Accidental (Unintentional) Injuries; Burns, Pediatric; Child Maltreatment; Exposure to Violence; Posttraumatic Stress Disorder

Further Reading

American Psychiatric Association (1994). *Diagnostic and statistical manual of mental disorders, 4th Edition (DSM-IV)*. Washington, DC: Author.

Bryant, R. A. (2000). Acute Stress Disorder. *PTSD Research Quarterly, 11*, 1–8. Available online through the National Center for Post-Traumatic Stress Disorder.

Daviss, W. B., Mooney, D., Racusin, R., Ford, J., Fleischer, A., & McHugo, G. J. (2000). Predicting posttraumatic stress after hospitalization for pediatric injury. *Journal of the American Academy of Child and Adolescent Psychiatry, 39*, 576–583.

National Center for Post-Traumatic Stress Disorder. http://www.ncptsd.org.

ANNETTE M. LA GRECA

Acute Subdural Hematomas

See: Traumatic Brain Injury

Adaptive Behavior Assessment

DEFINITION

Adaptive behavior is comprised of a loosely defined set of skills associated with personal dependence and social competence. The assessment of adaptive behavior is based upon a comparison with the skill levels of same-age peers within a specified cultural context.

Adaptive behavior is presumed to be multidimensional. While the number of domains and their labels vary across assessment instruments, the content of adaptive behavior items generally falls into five broad categories: (1) motor/physical; (2) self-help/independence; (3) interpersonal/social; (4) responsibility/vocational; and (5) cognitive/communication. Adaptive behavior assessment also traditionally includes a measure of challenging behaviors such as aggression and self-stimulation. Many instruments include a separate subscale made up of a list of problem behaviors commonly seen in children and adolescents.

Adaptive behavior and intelligence are related constructs. Deficits in adaptive behavior and intelligence constitute the primary criteria in definitions of mental retardation. Adaptive behavior assessment instruments typically include items that reflect, or depend upon, cognitive functioning. However, empirical studies demonstrate that adaptive behavior and intelligence are clearly distinct constructs with only a modest overlap or correlation between them.

ASSESSMENT INSTRUMENTS

Structured adaptive behavior assessment was introduced by Edgar Doll in 1935 with the development of the Vineland Social Maturity Scale; many varied

Table 1. Adaptive Behavior Assessment Instruments

	AAMR adaptive behavior scales	Scales of independent behavior-revised	Vineland adaptive behavior scales
Publisher	Pro-Ed (1993)	The Riverside Publishing Co. (1997)	American Guidance Service, Inc. (1984)
Age range	3 months to 60+ years	3 months to 80+ years	Birth to 19 years
Method of administration	Questionnaire	Questionnaire or structured interview	Structured interview
Domains	Communication, self-care, home-living, social skills, community use, self-direction, health and safety, functional academics, leisure, and work	Motor skills, social interaction and communication skills, personal living skills, community living skills, problem behaviors	Communication, daily living skills, socialization, motor skills, maladaptive behavior

instruments have appeared in the intervening years. Common contemporary adaptive behavior assessment instruments (see Table 1) include: the American Association on Mental Retardation (AAMR) Adaptive Behavior Scales (ABS) including the Residential and Community scale and the School scale; the Scales of Independent Behavior-Revised (SIB-R); and the Vineland Adaptive Behavior Scales (VABS).

A recent reorganization of the items from the AAMR ABS has been published as the Assessment of Adaptive Areas scale (AAA). The AAA uses the original standardization sample for the ABS and provides a score for each of the adaptive skill areas included in the 1992 AAMR definition of mental retardation.

ISSUES IN ADAPTIVE BEHAVIOR ASSESSMENT

The criterion of adaptive behavior deficits was added to the definition of mental retardation (MR) in part to respond to criticism regarding the impact of cultural differences on IQ scores. However, cultural context is also essential in the determination of expected adaptive behavior skills. An individual's level of adaptive skills is meaningful only in the context of the expectations and demands of the cultural environment. Thus, concerns about cultural differences continue to plague adaptive behavior assessment instruments as well.

An individual's adaptive behavior skill level is generally understood to reflect typical performance in daily life rather than maximum performance. This assumption is commonly incorporated into the wording of adaptive behavior items by emphasizing what the individual *does* rather than what he or she *can do*.

While definitions of adaptive behavior generally imply that the construct possesses trait characteristics (i.e., consistency across time and setting), considerable evidence suggests that measures of adaptive behavior are substantially affected by the method of measurement, the setting in which the behaviors are assessed, and the content of the items. The extent to which level of adaptive behavior should be viewed as an individual trait remains in question.

CLINICAL APPLICATIONS

The assessment of adaptive behavior most often contributes to a decision regarding the diagnosis of mental retardation and to subsequent determinations regarding eligibility for support services, legal competence, and eligibility for participation in research protocols. Adaptive behavior levels may also be used to clarify an individual's level of impairment and the intensity of supports that are required. Adaptive behavior assessment can assist in the development of goals and objectives for individualized education programs and other interventions by identifying areas of strength and weakness and specific skills that require remediation. Finally, regular assessment of adaptive behavior can contribute to the monitoring of progress as an individual moves through an intervention program.

See also: Cognitive Development; Mental Retardation; Intellectual Assessment; Developmental Issues in Assessment for Treatment

Further Reading

Meyers, C. E., Nihira, K., & Zetlin, A. (1979). The measurement of adaptive behavior. In N. R. Ellis (Ed.), *Handbook of mental deficiency, psychological theory and research.* (2nd ed., pp. 431–481). Hillsdale, NJ: Erlbaum.

Reschly, D. J. (1982). Assessing mild mental retardation: The influence of adaptive behavior, socioeconomic status, and prospects for nonbiased assessment. In C. R. Reynolds & T. B. Gutkin (Eds.), *The handbook of school psychology* (pp. 209–250). New York: Wiley-Interscience.

Widaman, K. F., & McGrew, K. S., (1996). The structure of adaptive behavior. In J. W. Jacobson & J. A. Mulick (Eds.), *Manual of diagnosis and professional practice in mental retardation* (pp. 97–110). Washington, DC: American Psychological Association.

DONALD P. OSWALD
CARLA A. DISALVO

Adherence

See: Treatment Adherence

Adjustment Disorders

DEFINITION AND CLINICAL PRESENTATION

According to *DSM-IV*, Adjustment Disorder is defined as the appearance of clinically significant emotional and/or behavioral symptoms in response to an identifiable stressor(s) that occur within three months of the onset of the stressor(s); and the emotional/behavioral response is not merely an exacerbation of an existing Axis I or Axis II disorder. Further, the individual's response appears to be in excess of what one would normally expect, given the nature of the stressor(s), and is characterized by substantial impairment in social or academic/occupational functioning. Importantly, symptoms are expected to dissipate with the termination of the stressor(s) and/or its consequences. Although there is no typical clinical presentation of Adjustment Disorder in children and adolescents, recent advances in formal diagnostic schemes (e.g., *DSM-IV*) have contributed to a more comprehensive picture of the disorder.

Adjustment Disorder is categorized into six subtypes that allow clinicians to more precisely classify the disorder according to predominant symptom clusters: (1) *Adjustment Disorder with Depressed Mood* subtype is analogous to what used to be known as "reactive depression," in that depressed mood is the primary presenting problem and a specific stressor can be identified as the precipitant; (2) *Adjustment*

Disorder with Anxiety subtype is characterized by major symptoms of worry and nervousness. It should not be confused with Axis I Anxiety Disorders, which involves panic, generalized anxiety, and motor tension in the absence of an identifiable antecedent stressor; (3) *Adjustment Disorder with Mixed Anxiety and Depression* subtype is used when it is difficult to discern the primary emotional disturbance associated with the disorder and/or when individuals present with a combination of both anxiety and depression; (4) *Adjustment Disorder with Disturbance of Conduct* subtype is commonly seen in adolescence and involves behavior which violates the rights of others or age-appropriate social norms and rules (e.g., truancy, fighting, vandalism, reckless driving). The key distinction between this subtype and Axis I Conduct Disorder is that Adjustment Disorder with Disturbance of Conduct is much shorter in duration and can be linked to identifiable environmental stressors; (5) *Adjustment Disorder with Mixed Disturbance of Emotions and Conduct* subtype is used when the predominant symptoms represent a combination of both emotional difficulties (i.e., anxiety and depression) and conduct problems; and (6) *Adjustment Disorder, Unspecified* subtype is infrequently used, but is applied to classify maladaptive responses that do not fit into one of the specific subtypes (e.g., physical complaints, social withdrawal). The most common presentation of Adjustment Disorders in children and adolescents is one of the mixed subtypes. As a rule, females are more likely to be classified in the Adjustment Disorder with Depressed Mood subtype, whereas males are more likely to be seen in the Adjustment Disorder with Mixed Disturbance of Emotions and Conduct subtype.

Despite refinement in diagnostic taxonomy, Adjustment Disorder remains a controversial diagnostic category largely because of the perceived lack of specificity in its parameters and its seemingly all-encompassing nature. Furthermore, there is little evidence to suggest that subtyping according to predominant symptom complex has predictive validity in terms of treatment. Nevertheless, many clinicians consider Adjustment Disorder to be a distinct, albeit transitional diagnostic label, in that the degree of symptomatology in Adjustment Disorder exists somewhere between the less severe problem-level diagnoses (i.e., V Codes) and the more severe major mental disorders (e.g., Axis I Major Depressive Disorder). Still others suggest that Adjustment Disorder is retained in diagnostic nomenclature because it represents a less pathological and less stigmatizing label for children.

INCIDENCE

Adjustment Disorder is one of the most frequently diagnosed conditions in children and adolescents. Indeed, some have suggested that the high rate of Adjustment Disorder diagnosis in this population may be due in part to the inclusive nature of the disorder. Trends in incidence rates of Adjustment Disorder diagnosis accurately reflect these concerns. To illustrate, early estimates of the disorder from the 1970s and 1980s that utilized less refined diagnostic criteria indicated incidence rates ranging from 16 to 42 percent, depending on the population studied (e.g., general population, inpatient, etc.). More current estimates place incidence rates around 2–8 percent for the general population of children and adolescents, although rates as high as 34 percent have been observed in special populations, such as psychiatric emergency service admissions.

CORRELATES

Even though Adjustment Disorder is considered largely a *subthreshold* diagnosis, it can be accompanied by significant morbidity. Suicidal behavior is one of the more serious sequelae associated with Adjustment Disorder. Estimates vary, but evidence indicates that suicide attempts are observed in approximately 25 percent of adolescents with Adjustment Disorder, particularly when impulsivity is part of the clinical presentation. It should be noted that significant life stressors, such as hospitalization, bereavement following loss of a family member, chronic illness, and divorce often precede Adjustment Disorder. However, there is ample evidence to suggest that Adjustment Disorder and suicidal behavior frequently occur subsequent to events of lesser magnitude. The most common precipitants associated with the manifestation of Adjustment Disorder (and even suicidal behavior) include school problems, problems with parents, peer rejection, substance use, and problems with boyfriends/girlfriends. Furthermore, data indicate that a significant minority of adolescents with Adjustment Disorder later develop more severe diagnoses, such as antisocial personality disorder, bipolar disorder, and drug abuse. Chronicity of behavioral symptoms accompanying Adjustment Disorder diagnosis has been identified as a reliable indicator of more severe complications later on in life.

ASSESSMENT

Adjustment Disorders are typically diagnosed through clinical interviews and/or by use of interview checklists that follow *DSM-IV* diagnostic taxonomy. For research purposes, others have implemented a variety of structured and semistructured interview schedules designed for use with children and adolescents. The key differential diagnostic consideration in clinical assessment hinges on the identification of a perceived proximal stressor in the environment that precipitates the manifestation of behavioral/emotional symptoms. Importantly, the utilization of different assessment methods serves as an additional factor impeding the establishment of more reliable diagnostic parameters and accurate incidence estimates of Adjustment Disorder.

TREATMENT

Not unlike psychotherapeutic treatments for other stress-related reactions, treatment of Adjustment Disorder is best approached from a therapeutic stance that attempts to first remove or minimize the precipitant stressors. If this is not possible, cognitive behavioral approaches should be utilized that assist children and adolescents in identifying and modifying the precipitant stressor(s) in an attempt to reinterpret and/or neutralize the impact of the stressor on the child's life. Often encouraging children to simply verbalize their fears or apprehensions surrounding the stressors can substantially minimize their impact. Systematic relaxation and guided imagery techniques have also proven to be effective in minimizing fear and anxiety reactions to stressors. Attempts should also be made to engage parents in treatment so that a supportive home environment is established. In the case of older adolescents, writing assignments that provide the opportunity for expression of emotions about the immediate stressor can prove to be beneficial in a matter of weeks. In the case of Adjustment Disorders that involve high degrees of both emotional impairment (i.e., depression) and impulsivity, medication (antidepressants/anxiolytics), and/or hospitalization may be indicated to protect against suicidal behavior.

PROGNOSIS

As with most aspects of Adjustment Disorder, prognostic estimates vary greatly. As a general rule, children and adolescents with Adjustment Disorder fair more poorly than adults with the disorder. This may be due to the sheer number of stressful events that youth must navigate in the process of growing up. Alternatively, it could suggest that youth simply have developed fewer adequate coping mechanisms to handle the significant stressors in their ever-changing environment. In either case, recovery rates of Adjustment Disorder vary from 30 to 97 percent, depending on the nature of the stressor(s) encountered (severity, chronicity) and on the population examined. There is some suggestion that children and adolescents who are older at the time of symptom onset and who present with predominantly the depressed subtype demonstrate faster recovery time and have fewer hospital readmissions. As noted previously, the chronicity of behavioral symptoms, not the number and types of symptoms, is the best prognostic indicator of future outcome. A number of authors have indicated that although recovery rates from Adjustment Disorders are encouraging, recovery often takes more than 6 months, which exceeds the 6-month duration parameter established in the diagnostic criteria.

See also: Classification and Diagnosis; Cognitive-Behavior Therapy for Children; Developmental Issues in Assessment for Treatment; Interviewing

Further Reading

American Psychiatric Association. (1994). *Diagnostic and statistical manual of mental disorders* (4th ed.). Washington, DC: Author.

Despland, J., Monod, L., & Ferrero, F. (1995). Clinical relevance of adjustment disorder in *DSM-III-R* and *DSM-IV*. *Comprehensive Psychiatry, 46*, 454–460.

Kovacs, M., Gatsonis, C., Pollock, M., & Parrone, P. (1994). A controlled prospective study of *DSM-III* adjustment disorder in childhood. *Archives of General Psychiatry, 51*, 535–541.

Newcorn, J., & Strain, J. (1992). Adjustment disorder in children and adolescents. *Journal of the American Academy of Child and Adolescent Psychiatry, 31*, 318–327.

Strain, J., Smith, G., Hammer, J., McKenzie, D., Blumenfield, M., Muskin, P., Newstadt, G., Wallack, J., Wilner, A., & Schleifer, S. (1998). Adjustment disorder: A multi-site study of its utilization and interventions in the consultation-liaison psychiatry setting. *General Hospital Psychiatry, 20*, 139–149.

JOHN M. CHANEY
JANELLE L. WAGNER
LARRY L. MULLINS

Adolescence

DEFINITION

Adolescence refers to a transition period during the lifespan between childhood and adulthood. The age of onset and conclusion vary between genders with girls entering and exiting adolescence at an earlier age than boys. Adolescence is marked by changes in physical development, cognitive development, social and self-concept development, and individual ecology.

PHYSICAL DEVELOPMENT

Adolescent physical development is marked by two significant changes: a growth spurt and puberty (i.e., sexual maturation). Both the timing and rate of these changes show much individual variation, and can be influenced by a variety of biological and environmental factors. Both the onset of puberty and the growth spurt are dependent upon the maturation of the hypothalamic–pituitary–gonadal axis of the neuroendocrine system of the brain.

Growth Spurt

During the growth spurt, adolescents begin to grow taller and heavier and begin to take on adult appearances. The age of onset of this growth spurt in North American and European children range from about 9–10 years in girls and 10–12 years in boys, and the age at which these children reach maximal growth stature is 13–15 years in girls and 14–17 years in boys. Girls on average tend to be taller and heavier than boys as their growth spurt tends to occur earlier than boys', but boys eventually catch up and exceed girls in body size. In addition to growing taller and heavier, girls begin to develop broader hips and boys begin to develop broader shoulders. With this change in physical stature comes a change in physical performance. Strength, motor, and aerobic performance increase linearly with age, with the performance of boys on average being greater than that of girls.

Sexual Maturation

Sexual maturation occurs at roughly the same time as the growth spurt. During sexual maturation, secondary sex characteristics, which include breast development, genital development, widening of the hips, appearance of pubic hair, and changes in voice, are developed. Another sign of sexual maturation is menarche (i.e., the onset of menstrual period) for girls. Menarche usually begins 2 to 3 years after the onset of breast development, with an average age of onset of 12–13, but there is widespread variation in age of onset, and a trend toward earlier onsets. Menstrual periods may remain irregular and be marked by a lack of ovulation for several years after menarche. Puberty is considered early if it occurs prior to age 8 in girls and age 9 in boys; it is considered delayed if there are no signs by age 13 in girls and 14 in boys.

SEXUAL BEHAVIOR

During sexual maturation, higher and more variable sex hormones are present, and these heightened hormones seem to enhance sexual motivation. In addition, as adolescents begin to mature sexually and begin to look more like adults, changes in behavior and role expectations also occur. One of these changes is the social relationship between boys and girls, with the relationship often becoming more emotionally and sexually intimate. Sexual intimacy between teens is becoming more common and seems to have increased over the last several decades, and seems to gradually increase as adolescents go through school transitions.

COGNITIVE DEVELOPMENT

Adolescence is also marked by cognitive maturation. As children enter adolescence, they are leaving concrete operations and entering the final stage of Piaget's (1970) cognitive development, formal operations. At this stage in cognitive development, thinking becomes more rational, systematic, and abstract. The adolescent is able to think about hypothetical situations, and is able to imagine hypothetical alternatives to realities. This indicates that the adolescent is now able to see inconsistencies and flaws in the real world, which makes them more prone to question authority.

Piaget suggested that during this period of formal operations, adolescents can become more egocentric than they were during younger years. Elkind (1967) identified two forms of egocentrism that he believes to be present during adolescence. The first is "imaginary audience," which describes the idea that adolescents believe that their thoughts, feelings, and beliefs are unique only to themselves. Some studies have suggested that the egocentrism of adolescence is more linked to the development of social perspective taking skills than to the formal operations stage of cognitive development.

SOCIAL AND SELF-CONCEPT DEVELOPMENT

Social relationships also change during adolescence. Part of this change in social relationships comes from adolescents' attempts to attain a stable self-identity; that is Erikson's famed "identity crisis" (1963). During the identity crisis, adolescents are trying to figure out who they are in relation to others and who and what they want to become. In order to resolve this identity crisis, adolescents tend to become independent of their parents and associate more with peers (1963) of different groups or cliques. Therefore, peers become an important source of support during the adolescent period, and strongly influence who the adolescent will become. Erikson theorized that during this process some loss of self-esteem can occur as the adolescent begins to seek an identity. However, most teens show an increase in self-esteem over the course of adolescence.

Another part of the change in social relationships comes from the ability to take on new social perspectives. Adolescents go through two stages of social perspective taking. The first stage, *mutual role taking*, occurs at 10–12 years of age, in which teens develop the ability to consider their own and another person's perspective and recognize that the other person can do the same. The second stage, at 12–15 years of age, is *societal role taking*, during which teens become capable of comparing another person's perspective with that of a social system. During these stages, an adolescent's friendships begin to change to emphasize intimacy, loyalty, and emotional support.

CLINICAL CONCERNS

Nutritional Deficits

Sexual maturation and the growth spurt are subject to biological and environmental factors. Nutritional deficiencies associated with chronic illness can delay linear growth and pubertal onset. In addition, anorexia nervosa, bulimia nervosa, and obesity can also result in pubertal delay.

Sexually Transmitted Diseases and Adolescent Pregnancy

As adolescents go through social transitions, the perceived benefits of engaging in sexual activities are increased and the perceived costs are decreased. Adolescents may have the view that they are not susceptible to the consequences of risky behavior, such as engaging in unprotected intercourse and having intercourse with multiple partners. These risky behaviors can lead to a number of consequences that include the contraction of sexually transmitted diseases (STDs) and pregnancy.

Juvenile Delinquency and Substance Abuse

Adolescents who get into trouble with the law by being truant from school, running away from home, or by committing a more serious offense (e.g., stealing) are considered juvenile delinquents. One predictor of juvenile delinquency is low parental supervision and control. In addition, peer groups can have an influence on an adolescents' delinquent behavior.

Substance abuse is another problem that can lead to juvenile delinquency. Almost all adolescents have been exposed to illicit drugs. However, for some adolescents, drug experimentation can lead to substance abuse, which can lead to interference with school and home obligations and social interactions, can become dangerous if used in potentially hazardous situations, and can result in legal problems.

Other Clinical Concerns and Interventions

Some of the other clinical concerns associated with adolescence include depression, suicide, dropping out of school, gang membership, eating disorders, conduct disorders, and dysfunctional familial interactions. Interventions for these and other clinical concerns can range from the use of individual, group, and family therapy to day treatment programs and, when appropriate, psychotropic medications.

See also: Adolescent Health; Adolescent Pregnancy; Adolescent Sexuality; Day Treatment; Family Intervention; Multisystemic Therapy

Further Reading

Centers for Disease Control. (1995). Trends in sexual risk behavior among high school students—United States, 1990, 1991, and 1993. *Morbidity and Mortality Weekly Report, 44*, 124–132.

Crooks, R., & Baur, K. (Eds.). (1996). *Our sexuality* (6th ed.). New York: Brooks/Cole.

Elkind, D. (1967). Egocentrism in adolescence. *Child Development, 38*, 1025–1033.

Erikson, E. H. (1963). *Childhood and society* (2nd ed.). New York: Norton.

Piaget, J. (1970). Piaget's theory. In P. H. Mussen (Ed.), *Carmichael's manual of child psychology* (3rd ed., pp. 703–732). New York: J Wiley.

Shaffer, D. R. (Ed.). (1998). *Developmental psychology: Childhood and adolescence* (5th ed.). Pacific Grove: Brooks/Cole.

CHRISTA J. ANDERSON
JOHN COLOMBO

Adolescent Abortion

DEFINITION

Abortion is defined as a termination of pregnancy before the fetus can live outside the mother's body. Spontaneous abortion, also known as miscarriage, involves the spontaneous and natural loss of the fetus. In an induced abortion, the pregnancy is terminated either surgically or medically. Most induced abortions are performed in the first trimester to minimize health risks. Less than 9 percent of abortions are performed between 14 and 24 weeks, and only in situations where the health of a fetus or mother is at risk would an abortion be performed after 6 months.

INCIDENCE

Each year, in the United States, approximately one million adolescents will become pregnant. Of these pregnancies, almost 78 percent of them will be unintended and the majority will be unwanted. Although the teen pregnancy rate in our country has continued to decline since 1991, the United States still has the highest teen birth rate in the developed world—a reported 48.5 births per 1,000 females ages 15–19 in the year 2000. Fifty-five percent of teen pregnancies result in live births, 14 percent end in miscarriages, and it is estimated that 31 percent are terminated through abortion.

LEGAL ISSUES

Abortion continues to generate controversy about adolescents' rights to make decisions versus parental rights to be involved in their adolescents' choices. Even though abortion was made legal in 1973, our society maintains barriers for adolescents to access abortions. In addition, there is discomfort about providing information and access regarding ways to avoid an unintended pregnancy to the sexually experienced adolescent. Many state governments have restricted an adolescent's ability to seek an abortion unless their parents have been notified and/or parental consent is obtained. State requirements range from parental consent to parental notification to having no specific stipulations. The development of legislation regarding adolescents and abortion has stemmed from the following assumptions: (1) adolescents are at greater risk for the medical, emotional, and psychological complications of abortion; and (2) adolescents do not have the cognitive abilities to make a rational decision about the benefits and risks of abortion.

Despite this controversy, most adolescents (as many as 55 percent) voluntarily share information regarding their abortion with their parents. Information sharing increases as an adolescent's age decreases. According to one study, 75 percent of adolescents 15 and younger told their parents about their abortion. It appears that teens who choose not to disclose information to their parents are afraid of their parents' response. They feel their parents may retaliate in a negative fashion or physically abuse them, especially if they live in unstable and abusive households.

PSYCHOLOGICAL OUTCOMES

Research describing postabortion emotional and psychological consequences on adolescents is limited, but indicates that it is typically a nontraumatic but stressful experience. For most teens, an unintended pregnancy causes distress and it is difficult to untangle the impact of an abortion for a young person above and beyond the impact of a pregnancy. However, there is no evidence that the decision to have an abortion causes psychopathology in adolescents. The choice to have an abortion, for some teens, is related to a period of growth and maturity in their development. The positive impact of an abortion on a teen's mental health includes increased self-esteem, sense of control in their life, maturity level, and freedom. It has been suggested that since the majority of teen pregnancies are unplanned, teens may experience a sense of relief after the abortion as they no longer have to worry about the consequences of an unwanted pregnancy such as parenting a child.

Even though a vast majority of the research details positive psychological outcomes for teens, those adolescents with poor emotional well-being prior to the pregnancy may have more difficulty adapting. These adolescents report negative emotions including depression, high anxiety, and low self-esteem after an abortion. The most consistent finding with postabortion adjustment is preabortion (baseline) emotional state. Other predictors such as age, ethnic group, race, religion, level of education, or living situation do not appear to be related to the psychological outcome. If an adolescent functions effectively before the abortion, she will most likely continue to function effectively after the abortion.

The support of significant others, especially adults, has been found to be important in helping adolescents make the best decision for them. Studies suggest that adolescents benefit when parents are involved in the decision-making process, but parents should be included only if they can remain neutral and supportive of their daughter. Educating an adolescent about all available options (childbearing and parenting, adoption, and abortion) may assist her in determining which choice she would feel comfortable with and would be right for her at that time. Planned Parenthood has fact sheets on adolescent pregnancy, abortion, and women's health that can be accessed through their Web page.

See also: Adolescent Parenting; Adolescent Pregnancy; Adolescent Sexuality; Sexually Transmitted Diseases in Adolescents; Sexuality Education

Further Reading

Adler, N. E., & Tschann, J. M. (1993). The abortion debate: Psychological issues for adult women and adolescents. In S. M. Matteo (Ed.), *American women in the nineties: Today's critical issues* (pp. 193–212). Boston: Northeastern University Press.
The Alan Guttmacher Institute. Facts in brief—Teen sex and pregnancy. Retrieved March 20, 2002, from http://www.agi-usa.org/pubs/fb_teen_sex.html
Planned Parenthood. Retrieved March 20, 2002, from http://www.plannedparenthood.org/
Pope, L. M., Adler, N. E., & Tshcann, J. M. (2001). Postabortion psychological adjustment: Are minors at increased risk? *Journal of Adolescent Health, 29,* 2–11.

VERONICA M. RAMIREZ
SUSAN L. ROSENTHAL

Adolescent Assessment

Assessment of adolescents typically refers to youth aged 13–18 years. Assessments during the adolescent age range provide information about learning abilities and disabilities, need for educational interventions or accommodations, vocational interests and aptitude, social and emotional functioning, and behavioral functioning. The scope of the assessment depends upon the specific referral question(s) or types of problems suspected, and also the purpose for which the information will be used (e.g., to assist with planning psychotherapy interventions, to provide career guidance, to assist with documentation of disabilities for the purpose of special accommodations on college entrance exams, etc.).

DEVELOPMENTAL TASKS DURING ADOLESCENCE

During the adolescent age range, young people undergo rapid physical changes and have numerous developmental tasks to accomplish on their path to adulthood. The onset of puberty in early adolescence heralds the beginning of rapid skeletal growth and sexual maturation. Physically, girls often reach the peak of their growth spurt at the beginning of the adolescent age range (i.e., 12 years) and complete their growth by about 15 years. In contrast, boys may reach their physical growth peak at around 14 years and continue growing until about 17 years. Brain growth and maturation continues through midadolescence in boys and girls. The frontal lobes—the executive center of the brain—are the last areas to develop. Maturation of this area of the brain provides a neurological basis for a higher level of thinking and planning ability during the adolescent years than was possible in younger years. Specifically, adolescents begin to think abstractly, become more adept at using reasoning and problem-solving skills, learn to evaluate their performance critically and modify their behavior accordingly, and have the capacity to plan for the future. Cognitively, they enter the age of formal operational thought, described by Piaget as more abstract, logical, and idealistic than thought processes of younger children. Adolescents are no longer bound to their concrete experiences as the basis for their thought; they now can think and reason hypothetically. Egocentric thinking is also characteristic of adolescents, and can be manifest by their attention-seeking behavior and desire to be noticed. Adolescents may be preoccupied with themselves and assume that others are equally interested in them. This type of thinking may stem from their newly acquired ability to "step outside of themselves" and think abstractly about who they are and the persona they want to present to others.

Socially and emotionally, adolescents begin to seek autonomy and independence from adult authority, increase their peer group affiliations and interactions, and become interested in heterosexual relationships. As Erikson (1968) wrote, adolescents experiment with various roles and identities drawn from their environment, and work toward the goal of developing their individual identity. This process may include decisions about their educational and vocational goals, sexual orientation, the peer group with which they will affiliate, and moral and ethical issues (e.g., whether or not to use drugs, whether or not to have intercourse, etc.). Often, early adolescence is a time when youth strive to be like others in their chosen peer group, whereas in late adolescence there usually is an evolution toward an independent identity. Most developmental researchers agree that identity development begins, but does not end, in adolescence. The process of identity formation may extend for many years, and a healthy identity is one that is adaptable, flexible, and open to changes across the lifespan.

COMMON REASONS FOR REFERRAL

Several types of problems may emerge and provide a reason for referral during adolescence. Given the many physiological, psychological, and cognitive changes during this age range, adjustment problems may emerge as adolescents attempt to cope with the stressors they encounter during the teen years. Behavioral or emotional problems are the most frequent reason for referral, and an assessment can help clarify the nature and severity of the problem. Cohen and colleagues (1993), who studied the prevalence of conduct and emotional problems in boys and girls through the teen years, reported that conduct problems overall were more prevalent than emotional problems in this age group (14 vs. 2 percent, respectively). In the teen years, conduct problems were more prevalent among boys than girls, but emotional problems were more prevalent among girls than boys. Anxiety disorders occurred more often than depression among both girls and boys. Other researchers have found that certain problems in early to midchildhood are associated with a higher risk of conduct problems in adolescence. For example, children with Oppositional Defiant Disorder (ODD) who are not successfully treated will often develop conduct problems by adolescence, and conduct problems may predispose them to antisocial personality disorder in adulthood. Attention-Deficit/Hyperactivity Disorder (ADHD), once thought to remit during adolescence, is now known to persist in most cases where younger children have the disorder. It is common for disorders to be comorbid, or co-occur, during adolescence. For example, conduct disorder is often associated with other behavioral or mood disorders, such as ADHD, depression, or anxiety. Adolescence is a time when body image is very important, and eating disorders such as anorexia nervosa or bulimia may emerge. Substance abuse may also be a cause for concern, especially as it is often comorbid with other behavioral or emotional disorders. Finally, late adolescence is the time when one may see the onset of schizophrenia symptoms. The prevalence of schizophrenia is about 1 percent of the adult population, but prevalence data are not reliable for children and adolescents under the age of 18 years. Adolescents who show disturbance in their thought processes, impaired judgment and reality testing, delusions, or hallucinations will need to be assessed to determine if they have a psychotic disorder.

In addition to behavioral and emotional problems, adolescents may also struggle with the cumulative effects of learning problems and/or ADHD that interfere with their academic achievement and place them at great risk for school failure and/or dropping out. This problem is compounded by a tendency for public schools to reduce special education services during junior high and high school years. Assessment is important to document whether the adolescent continues to need an individualized educational program, including special accommodations in the classroom, to address the impact of their disability on their achievement. This is especially important if the adolescent is preparing to take college entrance exams, and needs documentation of his/her learning disability in order to request special accommodations on the exams.

Children with mental retardation and other severe disabilities will need assistance with daily living skills and adaptive functioning to prepare them for whatever level of independent functioning is possible for them after high school graduation. In fact, all children who receive special education services must receive "transition services" from the public schools to help them prepare for either vocational choices or higher education following high school.

PROFESSIONALS WHO CONDUCT ADOLESCENT ASSESSMENTS

Inasmuch as many of the same professionals who work with school-aged children also work with adolescents, see the entry on School Age Assessments as well. Psychologists can evaluate an adolescent's cognitive or intellectual functioning, adaptive functioning, academic achievement, and to some extent, their language and motor skills as they relate to school functioning. Psychologists can also assess behavioral and social/emotional functioning, though many other professionals may be involved in assessment and treatment of adolescents, depending upon the presenting problem. Many emotional disorders are amenable to pharmacological treatment, and child psychiatrists will add an important dimension to the assessment team in these cases. Adolescents with substance dependence or abuse will often be treated by specialists in substance abuse treatment. Those with eating disorders will need medical assessment and treatment in addition to psychological services. For treatment of serious behavioral and emotional disorders that cause significant functional impairment, inpatient psychiatric treatment is sometimes warranted for the adolescent. Often, the evaluation and treatment in such settings will include a team of professionals who provide both individual and milieu therapy from a number of perspectives to address the adolescent's problems.

ASSESSMENT APPROACHES WITH ADOLESCENTS

Social/Emotional Functioning

Assessment approaches with adolescents who have behavioral, social, or emotional problems typically include a detailed clinical interview with the adolescent about the nature and the degree of functional impairment caused by their symptoms. Often, adolescents will complete self-report behavioral questionnaires that provide indices of the nature and severity of their symptoms compared to normative groups of their peers, or in other cases, groups of individuals with diagnosed psychiatric disorders. The Minnesota Multiphasic Personality Inventory—Adolescent (MMPI-A) is an example of the latter type of measure. Other age-normed and empirically derived behavioral scales include the Behavior Assessment System for Children (BASC), the Child Behavior Checklist (CBCL), and the Conners Questionnaires. These scales allow the adolescent to endorse symptoms of both internalizing (e.g., anxiety, depressive, somatization, withdrawal) as well as externalizing (e.g., aggression, conduct, hyperactivity) problems. These scales also tap social and adaptive problems, and the BASC assesses the adolescent's attitude toward school and parents. The BASC, CBCL, and Conners Questionnaires have the advantage of including parent and teacher versions as well; thus, they provide age-normed, cross-informant ratings of an adolescent's behavior across different environments. In addition to these broadband scales, there are more narrowband scales that focus on a specific set of symptoms. Scales such as the Reynolds Adolescent Depression Inventory, Brown Attention Deficit Disorder Scale—Adolescent, the Revised Children's Manifest Anxiety Scale, the Multidimensional Anxiety Scale for Children, or the Beck Youth Inventories (which measure self-esteem, anger, anxiety, depression, etc.) target specific symptoms of concern and provide detailed information that can assist in formulating a diagnosis.

Assessment methods will also typically include a clinical interview with parents or other caretaking adults to obtain information about the nature, frequency, and severity of current behavioral or emotional symptoms. Often factors in the adolescent's medical, developmental, educational, or family history will provide clues as to the nature of the current problem. A family history of certain types of psychiatric disorders in first or second degree relatives can suggest possible genetic etiologies to the adolescent's presenting problems. In other cases, factors such as a prior history of child abuse or neglect, marital discord, parental adjustment problems, high family stress, loss of or separation from a parental figure, or economic disadvantage can add risk to the adolescent's social/emotional adjustment. However, it is just as important for an assessment to focus on the positive, or protective, factors in an adolescent's environment that may balance the risks and provide a means for the adolescent to adapt to or overcome the adversity in their lives. The presence of several protective factors can improve the adolescent's prognosis for a positive response to intervention.

Finally, projective assessment methods may provide information about the integrity of the adolescent's thought processes, predominant mood, and relationships. Methods such as projective storytelling, sentence completion, or inkblot analyses elicit the adolescent's responses in a less structured manner than behavioral questionnaires. The psychologist who conducts the evaluation will choose from among these various approaches to obtain the most appropriate types of information regarding an adolescent's social/emotional functioning. Ideally, the evaluation should provide important information about differential diagnosis and intervention approaches that could benefit the adolescent and family. Interventions may be done in outpatient, inpatient, or day treatment settings, depending upon the nature and severity of the problems. At times, the focus of treatment is the adolescent; at other times it is the family. Often, adolescent interventions can occur in a group setting with peers as well (e.g., groups that work on social skills). The advancement of psychotherapy research in recent years has led to many empirically validated, developmentally appropriate, and culturally appropriate approaches to treatment for common social, behavioral, and emotional problems in the adolescent years. Weisz and Weiss (1993) reviewed the literature on outcome of psychotherapy in over 200 studies of about 11,000 children and adolescents, and found that approximately 75 percent of the cases reported improvement in their symptoms following psychotherapy compared to untreated controls, and these improvements were maintained over time.

Cognitive and Academic Abilities

Typically, learning problems will have been identified long before the adolescent years, although occasionally adolescents will present during junior high or high school because the compensation methods they have been using in earlier grades are no longer effective. Students with mild learning disabilities or ADHD may find that the academic demands of the higher grades exceed their ability to keep up with the pace. At this time, it is important to seek an assessment that will clarify the nature of their difficulties and provide information about appropriate interventions. Cognitive measures commonly used with adolescents include the Wechsler Intelligence Scale of Children—3rd edition (WISC-III) through age 16 years 11 months, the Wechsler Adult Intelligence Scale—3rd edition (WAIS-III) beginning at

17 years, the Stanford–Binet Intelligence Scale—4th edition, Kaufman Adult Intelligence Test, and the Woodcock–Johnson—3rd edition Tests of *Cognitive Abilities*. Measures such as the Leiter International Performance Scale—Revised are useful for adolescents who have hearing impairment or severe language deficits that would prevent them from using language or understanding verbal instructions. For adolescents who do not use English as their first language, it is required by law that the cognitive testing be administered in their first language. A translator may be used to assist with the testing in these cases. Measures of academic achievement are the same as those listed for assessment of school age children. Many of the tests revised within the past few years now have excellent normative data for adolescents and young adults that will facilitate an accurate evaluation of adolescent learning strengths and weaknesses.

Assessment of Attention and Activity Level

ADHD typically is diagnosed during the early school age years, but the symptoms may persist into the adolescent years. Often, problems with organization of materials, attention to detail in academic work, or losing track of due dates for assignments will bring an adolescent to the attention of a psychologist for assessment. These persistent symptoms of ADHD have a negative impact on academic achievement, and sometimes are associated with the development of secondary behavioral and/or emotional problems. Additional detail on assessment of ADHD is provided in another entry in this encyclopedia.

See also: Attention-Deficit/Hyperactivity Disorder; Conduct Disorder; Learning Disorders; School Age Assessment; Underachievement

Further Reading

Carr, A. (1999). *The handbook of child and adolescent clinical psychology: A contextual approach*. New York: Routledge.

Cohen, P., Cohen, J., Kasen, S., Velez, C., Hartmark, C., Johnson, J., Rojas, M., Brook, J., & Streuning, E. (1993). An epidemiological study of disorders in late childhood and adolescence—1. Age- and gender-specific prevalence. *Journal of Child Psychology and Psychiatry, 34,* 851–867.

Erikson, E. H. (1968). *Identity: Youth and crisis*. New York: Norton.

Santrock, J. W. (1995). *Life-span development*. Dubuque, Iowa: William C. Brown Communications, Inc.

Sattler, J. M. (2001). *Assessment of children: Behavioral and clinical applications* (4th ed.). San Diego, CA: Jerome M. Sattler.

Weisz, J., & Weiss, B. (1993). *Effects of psychotherapy with children and adolescents*. London: Sage.

JAN L. CULBERTSON

Adolescent Health

DESCRIPTION

Adolescence is defined as the time period from 11 to 21 years and is often characterized as consisting of three stages—early (11–14 years), middle (15–18 years), and late (18–21 years). The growth and development of adolescents across these three stages can be divided into three related areas—biological growth (puberty), cognitive maturation, and psychosocial development.

Puberty is marked by sexual maturation and physical growth. During this time, there is an increase in hormone production, which leads to the development of secondary sexual characteristics (e.g., pubic hair) and reproductive capability. Both genders have a period of accelerated growth, which is often called a "growth spurt." Cognitive maturation is characterized by the adolescents' new ability to think more hypothetically and abstractly, which includes problem solving and negotiation. Abstract thinking abilities usually begin around 14 years of age. Psychosocial development involves developing a sense of identity and increased ability to have and maintain intimate friendships and relationships. It is important to note that an adolescent's development across the areas of biological growth, cognitive maturation, and psychosocial development do not occur simultaneously. For example, an adolescent may be sexually mature, but not have advanced thinking abilities.

RISK-TAKING BEHAVIOR

Most adolescents progress through puberty and accomplish the tasks of adolescent development with minimal disruption. In fact, despite popular notions, "storm and stress" is not the norm for most adolescents. Only a small percentage of adolescents actually experience moderate or severe psychological symptomatology that impairs functioning. However, adolescents may engage in risk-taking behavior.

Risk-taking behaviors can be defined as behaviors that are not part of a psychiatric disorder, such as an eating disorder, or part of environmental factors, such as poverty, but which have potential health-related consequences. Adolescents may not be seeking the thrill of risks when engaging in these behaviors; instead, the behavior may be part of "growing up." For example, a developmental task of adolescence is the establishment of intimate relationships. A decision to have intercourse

as part of a dating relationship could lead to the acquisition of a sexually transmitted disease (STD).

There are several variables and factors that seem to affect whether or not an adolescent engages in risky behaviors. Low self-esteem, impulsivity, deviance, and inadequate social skills have been linked to increased engagement in risk behaviors. Adolescents who have parents who set developmentally appropriate limits and supervision, are warm and firm, and are open to independent beliefs are less likely to conform to peer norms and engage in risk-taking behavior.

MORBIDITIES/MORTALITIES

The major morbidities/mortalities of adolescence are psychosocial in nature (see Figure 1). Unintentional injuries and accidents continue to be the largest cause of death in adolescents in the United States. Furthermore, the nonfatal injuries resulting from automobile accidents account for the largest number of hospital days among adolescents. One out of every five adolescents has received injury-related care in emergency rooms.

Homicide resulting from violence is the second leading cause of death in adolescents in the United States. Approximately, 18 percent of all deaths in adolescents are a result of homicide. Nationally, 4 percent of adolescents are treated by a doctor or nurse for injuries sustained during a physical fight.

With regard to substance use, drug-related deaths account for approximately 18 percent of the deaths that occur in the 12–24-year-old age group. Some experimentation during adolescence may be normative; almost 55 percent of teenagers have tried an illegal drug before they leave high school. In addition, most individuals addicted to tobacco began experimentation

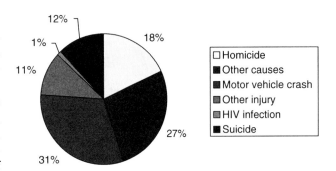

Figure 1. Major causes of mortality in adolescents, ages 10–24, United States, 1999.
Source: Centers for Disease Control. (2000, June 9). Youth risk behavior surveillance. Retrieved April 7, 2002 from http://www.cdc.gov/mmwr/preview/mmwrhtml/ ss4905a1.htm

during their adolescent years believing that they could remain nonaddicted social smokers.

An important part of adolescent development is learning to manage sexual feelings and behaviors. For adolescents who choose to be sexually active, sexually transmitted diseases (STDs) represent a significant risk. Each year, approximately 3 million teens are infected with an STD, and it is estimated that approximately 1 percent of adolescents will die of complications from AIDS.

Risk behaviors do not occur in isolation. Adolescents who engage in one risk behavior are more likely to engage in other risk behaviors. For example, the use of alcohol and other substances increases the likelihood of traffic-related accidents, risky sexual behavior, and involvement in delinquent behaviors.

CHRONIC HEALTH CONDITIONS

Chronic health conditions are illnesses or impairments that are expected to last for an extended period of time and require medical attention and care that is above and beyond what is normally expected for an individual of the same age. Currently between 10–20 million American children and adolescents have some type of chronic health condition or impairment. Examples of chronic illnesses which affect adolescents are: juvenile rheumatoid arthritis, asthma, cystic fibrosis, diabetes, spina bifida, hemophilia, seizure disorders, neuromuscular disease, and AIDS. At least 10 percent of children with chronic conditions have a condition that is severe enough to impact their daily lives.

Chronic illnesses can impact the process of mastering the developmental tasks of adolescence. Several developmental tasks (e.g., re-negotiation of parent–adolescent relationships, establishment of intimacy with others, development of a sense of identity, and transitions into adult roles) may be impacted when an adolescent has a chronic health condition. The presence of a chronic condition has many potential effects including the delay of biological maturation, limitations in opportunities to interact with peers and the world, and changes in the ways others (both peers and family) view and relate to the adolescent. For example, an adolescent with Juvenile Rheumatoid Arthritis who is taking prednisone may experience distorted facial features, which may impact her sense of body image. In addition, this same adolescent may be unable to attend school during flares of the illness, thus, limiting her academic and social progression. The parents may become involved in insuring that the adolescent takes her medicine and does her exercises, which impacts the adolescent's ability to establish independence. On the other hand, chronic illnesses can serve as a protective factor for adolescents. Most children with chronic illnesses engage in less risk-taking behaviors than their healthy peers.

SUMMARY

In general, most adolescents do not engage in life-altering risk-taking behavior, and those with chronic conditions are remarkably resilient. However, for all adolescents it is important to monitor their progression as they mature physically, develop advanced cognitive skills, and form new relationships with parents, peers, and romantic partners.

See also: Accidental (Unintentional) Injuries; Adolescent Sexuality; Cognitive Development; Emotional Development; High Risk Kids; HIV; Risk and Protective factors; Sexual Development; Social Development in Adolescence; Social Development in Childhood; Substance Abuse

Further Reading

American Academy of Pediatrics. (1993). Psychosocial risks of chronic health conditions in Childhood and adolescence (RE9338) [Electronic version]. *Pediatrics, 93*(6), 876–878.

Center for Disease Control. (2000, June 9). Youth risk behavior surveillance. Retrieved April 7, 2002 from http://www.cdc.gov/mmwr/preview/mmwrhtml/ss4905a1.htm

Irwin, C. E., Igra, V., Eyte, S., & Millstein, S. (1997). Risk-taking behavior in adolescents: The paradigm. *Annals New York Academy of Sciences, 817*, 1–35.

National Institute on Drug Abuse. (2001). Monitoring the future national survey results on adolescent drug use: Overview of key findings. Retrieved April 10, 2002 from http://www.monitoringthefuture.org/pubs/monographs/overview2001.pdf

Steinberg, L. (1999). *Adolescence* (5th ed.), Boston, MA: McGraw-Hill.

MARY B. SHORT
SUSAN L. ROSENTHAL

Adolescent Parenting

DESCRIPTION

Adolescent pregnancy is a topic of national concern because it can have long-lasting negative consequences for young parents and their children. Young women who begin their childbearing as adolescents are often unprepared for the tasks of parenting, have relatively high rates of depression, are less likely to complete high school, and are more likely to require public assistance, compared to women who do not begin childbearing until adulthood. In addition, children of adolescent parents have an increased risk of being maltreated, experiencing behavioral and developmental problems, and repeating the pattern of adolescent parenthood.

INCIDENCE

The United States has one of the highest adolescent birth rates in the industrialized world. Despite a steady decline over the past decade, approximately 500,000 adolescents give birth annually, representing 12.5 percent of the infants born in the United States. Although the decline has occurred among all racial and ethnic groups, African-American adolescents have experienced a greater decline (26 percent), compared to Caucasian (19 percent) and Hispanic (12 percent) adolescents. Nevertheless, the birth rate among African-American adolescents aged 15–19 is approximately 2.5 times the rate among Caucasian adolescents (84 vs. 33 per 1,000). In some low-income, minority communities, adolescent parenthood is part of the normative life course and may make sense given the limited educational and employment opportunities available to youth.

RISK AND PROTECTIVE FACTORS

Social Support

The demands of parenthood are often incompatible with the developmental tasks of adolescence. Competent parenting requires patience, empathy, and maturity. Adolescents, who are striving for their own identity, may focus on themselves, rather than on their child's needs.

Social support has the potential to ameliorate adolescent parenting, particularly when adolescents are young, immature, and need assistance. Although support and family involvement are generally viewed as positive, they can also be sources of strain and stress. When family members provide unwanted or conflicting advice, model inappropriate parenting techniques, or take over parental duties, adolescents do not gain parenting skills and experience. High levels of support may foster dependence and interfere with the

development of the maturity and autonomy that young mothers require for adulthood. The optimal level of support enables adolescents to negotiate the tasks of adolescence such as completing their education and preparing for adulthood, while gaining parenting skills and caring for their child.

Multigenerational Households

Adolescent parenting has to be examined within the changing family patterns in the United States. In the past, adolescents who became pregnant often married and lived with the father of their child. However, current trends indicate that the vast majority (79 percent) of adolescents who give birth are single. Rather than marrying and setting up independent households, most adolescent mothers live in their family of origin and share caregiving with their mother (the baby's grandmother). Grandmothers are often viewed as providing support, nurturance, and sociological, financial, and legal stability. This two-generational pattern of family caregiving has captured the attention of policymakers, as illustrated in the Personal Responsibility and Work Opportunity Reconciliation Act of 1996, which requires adolescent mothers to live with a guardian in order to receive financial assistance.

Despite the enthusiasm of policymakers, the data on multigenerational households present a mixed picture. Grandmothers are often instrumental in the early phases of adolescent parenting, providing guidance and care for the child, and enabling the mother to continue her education. Children raised with both a mother and a grandmother in the household, rather than by a single parent, have better social and cognitive outcome during childhood, fewer behavior problems, and less deviant behavior during adolescence. On the other hand, studies of multigenerational households have documented tensions related to role transitions and childrearing responsibilities. Adolescent mothers in multigenerational households have been described as less nurturant during play and feeding than adolescent mothers living independently, perhaps because when grandmothers are in the home, young mothers defer to them and do not gain the skills of parenting. Prolonged mother–grandmother co-residence (5 years or more) is associated with a lack of economic success among adolescent mothers and behavioral and academic problems among their children. For many young mothers, leaving home is a rite of passage that occurs after they have completed their education, formed a stable partnership, and are ready for the autonomy and independence associated with raising their child. As they approach adulthood, the most competent mothers leave their family of origin to set up an independent household, leaving the least competent mothers in multigenerational households.

Fathers

Recent attention has been directed to the fathers of infants born to adolescent mothers, many of whom are adolescents themselves. Fathers are often excluded from multigenerational households. Grandmothers, who often serve as gatekeepers, may not welcome fathers, particularly those who lack education or employment skills and do not contribute financially. Fathers who feel welcomed by the child's maternal grandmother may be more involved in their child's care, thereby gaining the skills of fatherhood.

In communities where fathers do not live with their partner and children, there may be less dependence on fathers and fewer expectations for them to fill typical paternal roles. Thus, it is not surprising that approximately one third of the fathers of babies born to adolescent mothers lose touch with them within 5 years after delivery.

Adolescent fathers are often unprepared for parenting and have limited knowledge about child development. Yet adolescent mothers who report a positive relationship with their baby's father feel better about themselves and their competence as mothers, provide a more child-focused childrearing environment, and are more likely to retain custody of their children. There is also evidence that children benefit from direct involvement with their father, through better language and developmental skills; the benefits of positive father involvement are not necessarily dependent on whether the parents live together or separately. Thus, paternal involvement may be an important protective factor for children of adolescent mothers.

Outcomes

Despite the stigma that has been associated with adolescent parenting in the past, there are many examples of successful outcomes. For example, children of adolescent parents are most likely to stay in school and avoid the pattern of adolescent pregnancy when their mothers complete their own education, form a stable partner relationship, and support themselves without requiring public assistance. The variability among adolescent parents points to the need to move away from negative stereotypes and to examine how programs can

be developed that capitalize on individuals' strengths and enable them to accomplish the tasks of adolescence and learn to care for their children.

See also: Adolescent Pregnancy; Adolescent Sexuality; Parenting Practices; Risk and Protective Factors

Further Reading

Black, M. M., Papas, M. A., Hussey, J. M., Hunter, W., Dubowitz, H., Kotch, J. B., English, D., & Schneider, M. (2002). Behavior and development among preschool children born to adolescent mothers: Risk and three-generation households. *Pediatrics, 109* (4), 573–580.

Leadbeater, B. J., & Way, N. (2001). *Growing up fast: Transitions to early adulthood of inner-city adolescent mothers.* Mahwah, NJ: Erlbaum.

Moore, K. A., Manlove, J., Terry-Humen, E., Williams, S., Papillo, A. R., & Scarpa, J. (2001). *Fact at a glance 2001.* Child Trends. http://www.childtrends.org/factlink.asp.

U.S. House of Representatives. (1996). *Personal responsibility and work opportunity reconciliation act of 1996.* Conference report H.R. 3734. Report No. 104-725. Washington, DC: U.S. Government Printing Office.

MAUREEN M. BLACK
WENDY M. STEVENSON

Adolescent Pregnancy

DEFINITION

Adolescent pregnancy includes live births, legally induced abortions, and estimated fetal losses (i.e., spontaneous abortions and stillbirths) among females aged 19 or younger.

PREVALENCE

The United States continues to have one of the highest teen pregnancy rates among developed nations with 800,000–900,000 adolescents 19 years of age or younger becoming pregnant each year. Overall, 54 percent of adolescent pregnancies result in birth, 32 percent are aborted, and 13 percent end in miscarriage. According to the Centers for Disease Control (CDC), there has been a decline in pregnancy rates among females aged 15–19 years. The decline has been attributed to stable rates of sexual experience and activity among this age group and to the increased use of condoms. Increased use of long-acting hormonal methods introduced in the early 1990s also has been associated with this decline.

PREVENTION OF ADOLESCENT PREGNANCY ISSUES

Adolescents are exposed to the positive aspects of sexuality without comparable exposure to information on responsible sexual behavior, contraception, and access to confidential care. In addition, while many adults may view adolescent pregnancy as a negative life event, not all adolescents hold this opinion. Furthermore, the earlier the age at which adolescents engage in sexual activity, the greater the risk for a teenage pregnancy. Unfortunately, parents are often uncomfortable with teenage sexual behavior and unable to initiate necessary conversations about either abstinence or contraception.

The design of effective adolescent pregnancy prevention programs depends on an understanding of adolescent beliefs about sexuality, their sexual knowledge, and how these impact on their decision-making. For some adolescents, for example, their reluctance to acknowledge their sexual behavior impairs proper contraceptive use. Adolescents also may deny their own risk of pregnancy or hold misconceptions such as believing that only frequent sexual activity can lead to pregnancy, that they are infertile, or that they will not get pregnant because they have not gotten pregnant yet. Many adolescent girls express statements such as, "I never thought I could get pregnant," or "I have had sex so many times without protection and I never got pregnant." In addition, adolescents often are unaware of the time in their menstrual cycle of greatest risk for fertility or of the impact of irregular cycles on ovulation.

OUTCOMES OF TEENAGE PREGNANCY AND CHILDBEARING

Children of adolescent mothers who had limited prenatal care often have poor outcomes, including low birth weight. Adolescents may receive inadequate prenatal care because they are unaware of available services, lack health insurance, have negative attitudes toward health care providers, or perceive early prenatal care as unimportant. Other risk factors for negative neonatal outcomes that are commonly seen among pregnant adolescents include poor nutrition, substance use, and genital infections. Many special programs have been developed in the United States to help prepare pregnant teenagers for delivery, motherhood, and future family planning. Such programs include multidisciplinary teams and provide education on nutrition, postpartum care, and use of contraceptives. In general,

adolescent-only clinics have demonstrated positive effects on birth weight, timing of prenatal care, and number of prenatal care visits.

The adolescent who decides to continue her pregnancy may be emotionally and cognitively unprepared to cope with the demands of the pregnancy and/or caring for a baby. Many younger adolescents lack abstract thinking and may be unable to connect the pregnancy with the responsibility of motherhood. Furthermore, as adolescents attempt to establish an identity and fit in with peers, they are likely to have difficulty identifying with the motherhood role. Thus, becoming pregnant and a parent during the adolescent years can be disruptive to the process of attaining the adult skills and the sense of identity necessary to be an independent and successful contributor to society. Many parenting adolescents find it difficult to complete a high school education, to become financially secure adults, and to establish safe and stable households for themselves and their children. A key factor contributing to these negative outcomes is rapid repeat childbearing, that is, giving birth to a second child within 24 months of the first birth. However, not all adolescent parents experience these negative consequences. Adolescents benefit from supportive parents, health care providers, and other adults who are available to assist them with pregnancy and motherhood.

See also: Adolescent Abortion; Adolescent Health; Adolescent Parenting; Adolescent Sexuality; Sexuality Education; Sexually Transmitted Diseases in Adolescents

Further Reading

Apfel, N., & Seitz, V. (1996). African American adolescent mothers, their families, and their daughters: A longitudinal perspective over twelve years. In B. J. R. Leadbetter, and N. Way (Eds.), *Urban girls resisting stereotypes creating identities.* New York: New York University Press.

Centers for Disease Control. (1998). National and state specific pregnancy rates among adolescents—United States, 1992–1995. *Morbidity and Mortality Weekly Report, 47,* 497–504.

Darroch, J. E., & Singh, S. (1999). Why is teenage pregnancy declining? The roles of abstinence, sexual activity and contraceptive use. New York: The Alan Guttmacher Institute.

Emans, S. J., Smith, V. A. M., & Laufer, M. R. (1998). Teenage pregnancy. In S. J. Emans, M. R. Laufer, & D. P. Goldstein (Eds.), *Pediatric and adolescent gynecology* (pp. 675–713). New York: Lippincott-Raven.

Hamburg, B. A., & Dixon, S. L.(1992). Adolescent sexuality, pregnancy, and child rearing: developmental perspectives. In M. K. Rosenheim & M. F. Testa (Eds.), *Early parenting and coming of age in the 1990s* (pp. 17–33). New Brunswick, NJ: Rutgers University Press.

LISA C. MILLS
SUSAN L. ROSENTHAL

Adolescent Sex Offenders

DEFINITION

Adolescent sex offenders (ASO) are defined as adolescents from 13 to 17 who commit illegal sexual behavior as defined by the sex crime statutes of their jurisdictions. ASOs commit a wide range of illegal sexual behaviors, ranging from limited exploratory behaviors committed largely out of curiosity to repeated aggressive assaults. While some illegal sexual behavior by ASOs is limited, such as touching a child over the clothes, other ASOs have extensive, aggressive sexual behavior including forced anal or vaginal intercourse.

PREVALENCE

ASOs commit a substantial number of sex crimes, including 17 percent of all arrests for sex crimes, and approximately one third of all sex offenses against children. Sexual offenses against young children are committed more often by boys between the ages of 12 and 15 than by any other age group. Younger adolescents rarely commit sex offenses against adults, although the risk of offending against adults increases steadily after an adolescent reaches age 16. Females under the age of 18 account for 8 percent of arrests for sex offenses.

CHARACTERISTICS

The characteristics of adolescent sex offenders are very diverse:

1. Some are otherwise well-functioning youth with limited behavioral or psychological problems.
2. Some are youth with multiple nonsexual behavior problems or prior nonsexual juvenile offenses.
3. Some are youth with major psychiatric disorders.
4. Some come from well-functioning families; others come from highly chaotic or abusive backgrounds.

Contrary to common assumption, most adolescent sex offenders have not been victims of childhood sexual abuse. The self-reported rates of sexual victimization of ASO range from 20 to 55 percent. Several studies have shown higher rates of self-reported physical abuse than sexual abuse.

Adolescent sex offenders are significantly different from adult sex offenders in several ways:

1. Adolescent sex offenders are considered to be more responsive to treatment than adult offenders and do not appear to continue re-offending into adulthood, especially when provided with appropriate treatment.
2. Adolescent sex offenders have fewer number of victims than adult offenders and, on average, engage in less serious and aggressive behaviors.
3. Most adolescents do not have deviant sexual arousal and/or deviant sexual fantasies that many adult sex offenders have.
4. Very few adolescents are sexual predators or pedophiles; they do not meet the diagnostic criteria for paraphilia as defined in the *Diagnostic and Statistical Manual of Mental Disorders* of the American Psychiatric Association.
5. Few adolescents appear to have the same habitual, long-term tendencies to commit sexual offenses as some adult offenders.
6. Across a number of treatment research studies following ASOs for several years, the overall sexual recidivism rate is consistently low, generally under 10 percent.
7. Rates for sexual re-offenses are substantially lower than rates of recidivism for other non-sexual delinquent behavior, suggesting that many ASOs have more general behavior problems rather than specifically sexual problems.

ASSESSMENT

Clinical assessment of ASOs should focus on the youngster's history of sexual and nonsexual behavior, family environment, and social ecology. Clinicians should obtain multisource information on the behavior involved in the sexual offense(s), prior delinquent behavior, social functioning, school functioning, drug or alcohol use, history of abuse or neglect, attitude toward the offense, sexual behavior history and sexual interests, access to potential victims, and the caregiver's ability to provide supervision and willingness to be involved in treatment.

There is no test or scientifically validated system that can reliably determine if an adolescent has committed a sex offense or will commit such an act in the future. In general, mental health professionals overestimate the risk of recidivism in ASOs.

TREATMENT

Adolescent sex offenders are treated in several settings: outpatient, community-based programs; group homes; inpatient psychiatric hospitals; residential centers; and incarcerated facilities. Many ASOs are successfully treated in short-term group treatment programs that meet weekly for 1–1.5 hr for 8–28 months. Most ASOs can safely remain in the community during treatment, although some will need more secure placement. Decisions about placement in residential or incarcerated settings should depend on the extent of comorbid disorders, availability of adequate adult involvement and supervision, and the ASOs self-control and attitude. The possible negative effects of out-of-home placement, such as increased risk of socialization into a delinquent lifestyle, negative peer influences, weakening of family ties, absence of parental involvement in treatment, and disruption of normal adolescent social development should be considered. ASOs, like other youth, should never be placed out-of-home simply on the basis of a "better-safe-than-sorry" rationale.

Adolescent sex offenders are typically treated in group therapy, and topics that are covered include sex education, legal versus illegal sexual behavior, victim empathy, relapse prevention, social skills training, and reducing other delinquent behavior. Many treatment programs have educational groups for the parents or caregivers of the adolescents. Other approaches take an ecological approach and provide services in homes, schools, and neighborhoods. Two random assignment studies have supported the effectiveness of Multi-Systemic Therapy (MST), a short-term intensive ecological approach designed primarily for highly delinquent youth, but no random assignment studies have been conducted testing other approaches.

PROGNOSIS

Most studies report that the recidivism rate for ASOs who receive treatment is around 10 percent. Studies suggest that rates of sexual re-offense (5–14 percent) are substantially lower than the rates for other delinquent behavior (8–58 percent). Adolescent offenders against children tend to have slightly lower sexual recidivism rates than adolescents who rape other teens. There is limited evidence to support the assumption that the majority of ASOs will become adult sex offenders.

See also: Multisystemic Therapy; Sexual Behavior Problems; Sexuality Education

Further Reading

Becker, J. (1998). What we know about the characteristics and treatment of adolescents who have committed sexual offenses. *Child Maltreatment*, 3(4), 317–329.
Bonner, B. L., Marx, B. P., Thompson, J. M., & Michaelson, P. (1998). Assessment of adolescent sexual offenders. *Child Maltreatment*, 3(4), 374–383.
Chaffin, M., Letrourneau, E., & Silovsky, J. F. (2002). Adults, adolescents, and children who sexually abuse children: A developmental perspective. In J. E. B. Myers, L. Berliner, J. Briere, C. T. Hendrix, C. Jenny, & T. A. Reid (Eds.), *The APSAC handbook on child maltreatment* (2nd ed., pp. 205–232). Thousand Oaks, CA: Sage.
Hanson, R. K., Gordon, A., Harris, A. U. R., Marques, J. K., Murphy, W., Quinsey, V. L., & Seto, M. C. (2002). First report of the collaborative outcome data project on the effectiveness of psychological treatment of sex offenders. *Sexual Abuse: A Journal of Research and Treatment*, 14, 169–194.

MARK CHAFFIN
BARBARA L. BONNER

Adolescent Sexuality

DEFINITION

Adolescence is the time period in which much of the foundation for the development of healthy sexuality is created. The onset of puberty is not simply a biological event. The development of secondary sexual characteristics increases adolescents' body awareness and sexual feelings and behaviors. The timing of puberty also plays a role in adolescents' sense of sexual self. For example, early developing girls are more likely to have a negative body image, engage in problem behaviors, and are more vulnerable to depression. This impact of the timing of puberty likely is related to both hormonal changes and changes in the way peers and adults relate to a sexually mature adolescent girl.

During this time of change, there are several developmental tasks that adolescents need to accomplish in order to become healthy sexual adults. Adolescents need to manage feelings of sexual arousal and experience positive feelings about their body and its physical changes. An additional goal for an adolescent is to develop healthy sexual and romantic relationships, that is, collaboration focused on mutual interests and reciprocity, a commitment to the relationship, and the sharing of private and personal communication.

SEXUAL DECISION-MAKING

During adolescence, many teens are faced with decisions as to what sexual behaviors to engage in and with whom. These decisions are influenced by many factors including family relationships and values, cultural expectations, and opportunity. Gender also plays an important role in cultural expectations; the American culture portrays sexual desire as important and appropriate for boys and as almost nonexistent for girls. Unfortunately, society tends to focus the attention on coital behaviors rather than noncoital behaviors, and on the negative outcomes (pregnancy and sexually transmitted diseases [STDs]) of sexuality rather than on pleasure.

Parent–adolescent relationships play an important role in helping adolescents make healthy sexual decisions. Parent–adolescent discussions regarding sexuality have been related to less risky behavior, less conformity to peer norms, and a greater belief that parents are the best source of information about sex. Greater parental supervision also leads to less risky sexual behavior. Finally, adolescents with peers who are sexually experienced are more likely to be sexually experienced themselves.

Another factor in sexual decision-making is the adolescent's level of cognitive maturation. A young adolescent may have difficulty anticipating the potential risks in a situation, such as being alone with someone to whom she is attracted. In addition, the lack of hypothetical reasoning may lead the adolescent to underestimate the risk of acquiring an STD or becoming pregnant.

PREVALENCE OF SEXUAL BEHAVIORS

Little has been documented about adolescent sexual behaviors other than intercourse, but "virginal" and sexually experienced teens do engage in a range of behaviors. For example, a 1992 study of Los Angeles teens, found that 29 percent of "virgin" teens engaged in heterosexual masturbation of a partner and 31 percent had experienced masturbation by a partner in the past year. Further of these "virginal" teens, 11 percent of males and 8 percent of females engaged in fellatio with ejaculation, and 9 percent of males and 12 percent of females engaged in cunnilingus. Approximately 1 percent engaged in anal sex. Being sexually experienced does not necessarily mean that a teen is currently sexually active. For example, the Center for Disease Control reports that between 64 percent and 66 percent of students will have had sexual intercourse by the time they are 18; on the other hand, only 36 percent of adolescents report having sexual intercourse within the last 3 months.

Adolescents who begin having sex at an earlier age tend to have more sexual partners, and approximately 16 percent of sexually experienced adolescents have had four or more partners by the time they are 18 years old. About 58 percent of teenagers report using a condom the last time they had intercourse.

During adolescence, some teenagers engage in sexual behaviors with teens of the same gender. Adolescents who describe themselves as heterosexual may have engaged in homosexual behavior and those adolescents who describe themselves as gay or lesbian may not have engaged in any same-gender sexual behavior. Thus, there is not a direct link between behavior and sexual orientation. Adolescents need support to explore their sexual orientation and to separate behaviors and identity.

PREVENTION PROGRAMS

Evaluations of prevention programs have indicated that programs that focus on delaying sexual initiation but also provide information about contraception have the best outcomes (abstinence plus programs). Successful programs:

- focus on the reduction of sexual behaviors that lead to unintended pregnancy/HIV/STDs
- use behavioral goals and teaching methods which are appropriate to age, sexual experience, and culture of the participants
- are based on theoretical approaches (e.g., behavioral change theories)
- allow sufficient time
- provide accurate information about risks of unprotected sex
- use varied teaching methods
- directly address social pressures on sexual behavior
- provide models and opportunities to practice skills
- have leaders with adequate training.

Participants in programs with these guidelines delay their sexual initiation, and the sexually experienced participants have fewer sexual partners and are more likely to use condoms. Furthermore, these programs have not resulted in an increase in the number of teens who are sexually experienced or an increase in the frequency with which sexually experienced teens have intercourse. Providing adequate supervision, support, and education can help adolescents make healthy sexual decisions.

See also: HIV; Identity Development; Pediatric Human Immunodeficiency Virus-1 (HIV); Sexual Orientation: Homosexuality; Sexually Transmitted Diseases in Adolescents

Further Reading

Blythe, M. J., & Rosenthal, S. L. (2000). Female adolescent sexuality: Promoting healthy sexual development. *Obstetrics and Gynecology Clinics of North America, 27*(1), 125–141.

Brooks-Gunn, J., & Paikoff, R. (1997). Sexuality and developmental transitions during adolescence. In J. Schulenberg, J. L. Maggs, & K. Hurrelmann (Eds.), *Health risks and developmental transitions during adolescence* (pp. 190–219). New York: Cambridge University Press.

Centers for Disease Control. (2000, June 9). Youth risk behavior surveillance. Retrieved April 7, 2002 from http://www.cdc.gov/mmwr/preview/mmwrhtml/ss4905a1.htm

The Center for Health and Health Care in Schools. Problem behavior prevention and school-based health centers: Program and prospects. Retrieved March 20, 2002, from http://www.healthinschools.org/sbhcs/papers/uiexec.asp

Kirby, D. (1997). *No easy answers: Research findings on programs to reduce teen pregnancy (Summary).* Washington, DC: The National Campaign to Prevent Teenage Pregnancy.

National Center for Chronic Disease Prevention and Health Promotion. Adolescent and school health: Programs that work. Retrieved March 20, 2002, from http://www.cdc.gov/nccdphp/dash/rtc

Schuster, M. A., Bell, R. C., & Kanouse, D. E. (1996). The sexual practices of adolescent virgins: Genital sexual activities of high school students who have never had vaginal intercourse. *American Journal of Public Health, 86*(11), 1570–1576.

MARY B. SHORT
SUSAN L. ROSENTHAL

Adoption

DEFINITION

Adoption is the act of legally assuming parental rights and responsibilities of another person, typically a child under the age of 18. Once a child is legally adopted, the adoptive parents take on the same responsibilities to the child as the birth parents would, and the child assumes all rights of a child born into a family. Adoption may occur when the birth parents are unable, unwilling, or legally prohibited from caring for the child and should be based on the long-term welfare of the child. Three parties are involved in the process of adoption: the adopted child, the birth parents, and the adoptive parents. These parties are often referred to as the adoption triad.

There are several different types of adoption. One distinction made in adoption procedures is whether the adoption is public or private. Public adoptions place children from the child welfare system in permanent homes by public, government-operated agencies, or by private agencies contracted by a public agency. In contrast, private agency adoptions are conducted by a nonprofit or for-profit agency, which may be licensed by the state in which it operates. Similarly, in an independent or nonagency adoption, birth parents directly place their children in adoptive homes through the services of a licensed or unlicensed facilitator, certified medical doctor, member of the clergy, or attorney.

Another distinction made in adoption procedures is based on the postadoption relationship between the adoption triad. In *traditional adoption* (also known as anonymous adoption, confidential adoption, or classic adoption) the identities of the birth parents and adoptive parents are unknown to each other. An *open adoption* refers to an adoption in which the birth parents exchange specific identifying information with the adopting parents in order to have contact in the future. A *cooperative adoption* is similar to an open adoption except that the birth parents may have an active and continued role in the child's life, including visitation. Cooperative adoptions may include birth parents assisting in major decisions regarding the child.

EPIDEMIOLOGY

Adoption statistics were collected by the National Center for Social Statistics from 1957 through 1975, when individual states voluntarily reported data on all finalized adoptions. Since that time, the federal government has had no system in place to collect comprehensive data on adoption. Some of the most recent data have been collected by the National Center for State Courts funded by the Children's Bureau's Adoption Information Improvement Project from 1990 to 1995. Their data are obtained from review of court records, bureaus of vital statistics, and social service agencies. These statistics indicate that throughout the 1990s, approximately 120,000 children were adopted each year. It is estimated that 1,000,000 children in the United States live with adoptive parents and that approximately 2 percent of the population is adopted. About half (52 percent) of adoptions are by nonrelatives and 48 percent are by relatives, including stepparents.

In 1997, the passage of the Adoption and Safe Families Act created a renewed interest in adoption data collection. The Adoption and Foster Care Analysis and Reporting System (AFCARS) now requires states to collect case-specific data on all adopted children who were placed by the state child welfare agency or by private agencies under contract with the public child welfare agency. Additionally, AFCARS requires reporting data for adopted children in foster care for whom the state child welfare agency has responsibility for placement, care, or supervision. States are encouraged to report all other finalized adoptions.

There has been a shift in the characteristics of adopted children. Early on, the majority of adoptions were of Caucasian infant children; however, over time, the number of these children placed for adoption has declined dramatically. It is hypothesized that this phenomenon is due to the increased use of birth control and the legalization of abortion. As a result, parents looking to adopt children have shifted their focus to *transracial* adoptions, intercountry adoptions, and adoption of *special needs* children (e.g., older children, children with emotional problems).

PROCEDURE

The first step in the adoption process is the identification of a child being placed for adoption and a match with potential adoptive parents who appear able to meet the child's needs. The adoption process generally begins with an evaluation and counseling of the prospective adoptive parents (i.e., home study), which may occur before or after placement and is typically performed by a licensed social worker or caseworker. This information is provided to the judge who either approves or disapproves the request for adoption. Once the request is approved, the adoption is valid and the adopted child has the same rights as a child born into a family and the birth parents' parental rights are legally terminated. If the birth parents revoke their consent to the adoption, they may petition the court for a legal hearing where they must provide compelling reasons as to why the adoption should be invalidated; however, very few adoptions are invalidated.

Depending on the agency used in the adoption, the process may be very costly. Domestic public agency adoptions (e.g., special needs children) range from zero to $2,500. Domestic private agency adoptions may cost from $4,000 to upward of $30,000. Domestic independent adoptions range from $8,000 to $30,000 and above. Domestic adoption costs typically include agency fees (e.g., adoptive parents' home study), medical fees (e.g., child's birth), and attorney fees. Intercountry adoptions facilitated by a private agency or conducted independently result in costs of $7,000–$25,000. Intercountry adoption costs vary considerably depending on the foreign country involved. Some costs include

Immigration and Naturalization Services or State Department fees, translation services, escort services (i.e., individual transporting of the child to the United States), travel fees, foreign agency fees, and other US agency costs similar to domestic adoptions.

The adoption process is complex and does not end once the adoption is approved or validated. Typically, there is an adjustment period that takes place and other issues related to the adoption often arise. In some cases, the adoptive parents and the adopted child may find their new relationship disappointing due to high expectations by both parties. Similarly, adoptive parents may have difficulty deciding when and how to tell children they are adopted. Studies have suggested that when children are told about the adoption around preschool age, they generally have a positive reaction and parents feel comfortable discussing the adoption from that point on. Furthermore, it is critical that the adoptive parents be the ones to tell children that they are adopted lest they receive the information from someone else. In general, it is expected that an open, honest explanation to the child is the most beneficial. If adoptive families will be encounter difficulties broaching these subjects, it may be helpful for the family to seek counseling services, which are often available through the adoption agency.

IMPORTANT ADOPTION ISSUES

Outcomes

Again, comprehensive data on adoption outcomes are somewhat lacking. In general, it has been found that the younger the child is at the age of adoption, the more successful the adoption will be. Overall, it is estimated that 3 percent of adoptions result in discontinuation whereas 11–14 percent of special needs adoptions are discontinued. Adoption outcomes have been considered good to excellent in 70 percent of cases, unclear in 20 percent, and bad in 10 percent.

Transracial Adoption

In transracial adoption, adoptive parents of one race adopt a child of another race. In practice, these adoptions are typically Caucasian parents adopting children of color. Transracial adoptions elicit some degree of controversy. Some individuals oppose transracial adoptions stating that it may be psychologically damaging to the child, particularly in relation to racial identity and ethnicity. Others argue that empirical evidence suggests that these children have outcomes similar to other adopted children and do not appear to exhibit difficulties with school, self-esteem, or self-concept. However, some studies have suggested that Black children adopted by Caucasian parents are less likely to identify themselves as Black and more likely to identify themselves as *mixed* than Black children raised in same-race adoptive households.

Intercountry Adoption

Intercountry adoption in the United States dates from the end of World War II and appears to coincide with the decline of infants available for adoption within the United States. In general, children adopted from foreign countries are infants or are very young. Research suggests that children adopted from foreign countries do as well as those adopted within the United States; however, little is known about how these children are perceived in the United States. Recently, there has been a push for regulation and control of intercountry adoption directing it toward a more child-centered activity.

See also: Foster Care; Parent–Child Interaction Therapy; Termination of Parental Rights

Further Reading

Adamec, C., & Pierce, W. L. (1991). *The encyclopedia of adoption.* New York: Facts on File.
Adoption.com Web site (n.d.). Retrieved May 15, 2002, from http://www.adoption.com.
National Adoption Information Clearinghouse Web site (n.d.) Retrieved May 18, 2002, from http://www.calib.com/naic.
Pertman, A. (2000). Adoption nation: How the adoption revolution is transforming America. New York: Basic Books.
Treseliotis, J., Shireman, J., & Hundleby, M. (1997). *Adoption: Theory, policy and practice.* London: Cassell.

LISA M. WARE
CHERYL B. MCNEIL

Advertisement

See: Television and Children: Advertising

Aggression

DEFINITION

A variety of definitions of aggression have been offered, with most converging on a common element of behavior that is intended to harm others. By itself, aggression does not constitute a diagnosis in any of the common classification systems; however, it occurs as part of the clinical picture in a number of disorders, either as a primary symptom (e.g., in conduct disorder) or as a commonly associated problem (e.g., among children with developmental delays). Recent research has distinguished between subtypes of aggressive behavior. Perhaps the most prominent distinction is between aggression that is primarily in reaction to provocation and is impulsive or retaliatory in intention (labeled as hostile or reactive aggression) versus aggressive behavior that is planned and designed to achieve some specific outcome (called instrumental or proactive aggression). Although the subtypes have different correlates (e.g., reactive–hostile aggression is more likely than instrumental–proactive aggression to be associated with impulsivity and faulty social cognitive processes), the two types of behavior are highly related. Recently, attention has focused on a distinction between overt aggression (harm or threat of harm by means of physical injury or damage to property) and relational aggression (harm though hurtful manipulation of peer relationships). Relational aggression appears particularly important in understanding the phenomenon of aggression among girls, and when definitions of aggression focus on only overt or physical aggression, much relationally aggressive behavior that is hurtful to girls is overlooked.

PREVALENCE/INCIDENCE

Although estimates of the prevalence of aggression vary depending on the definition employed and characteristics of the sample, all reports agree that aggressive behavior among children is relatively common, and that for a small group of youth it presents a serious and major mental health concern. For example, mothers report that a quarter of 30-month-old children have physically attacked others, and over one-third of high school students report engaging in physical fights. Against this backdrop of overall rates of aggression, there is a small group of children (approximately 5 percent) who are highly aggressive at an early age and whose aggression persists over time. In contrast, for most children, physical aggression shows decline with age from early to middle childhood. Although overt and physical aggression are more common in boys than girls, relational aggression is more frequent in girls.

CORRELATES

At the community level, aggression in children is related to violence and a lack of resources in the community. At the family level, childhood aggression is commonly associated with parental aggression, harsh and inconsistent parenting, poor parent–child attachment, marital conflict, and family social disadvantage. Aggression among siblings, particularly if paired with problems in parenting, is often related to child aggression in other contexts, and high levels of sibling conflict may provide a training ground for the development of aggression. At the child level, although aggression may be associated with biological factors (e.g., arousal), situational and psychological factors are critical. For example, aggression is related to both deficits and distortions in the processing of social information. In particular, aggressive children are more likely to attend to aggressive cues in interactions, to attribute ambiguous peer behaviors to hostile intentions, and to generate and value more aggressive solutions to social problems. Not surprisingly, aggression is linked to peer rejection and aggressive children often congregate together, although the quality of these friendships is poor. Aggressive children often are involved in bullying other children, particularly those who lack social competence or assertiveness skills. Finally, research has consistently demonstrated an association between aggressive behavior and exposure to television violence.

ASSESSMENT

As with all childhood disorders, adequate assessment of aggression requires gathering information from multiple informants and across multiple settings. In particular, assessment should focus, not only on the child's behavior and characteristics, but also on the social context that surrounds the behavior. Assessment of both antecedents to aggression (e.g., bullying from peers, modeling of aggression in the home) and the consequences of the behavior (e.g., instrumental gains) are critical in understanding the aggression and in planning treatment. Given that many forms of aggression are not overt and may be easily overlooked by adults, the perspective of peers is often invaluable in assessing child aggression. A number of well-validated questionnaires with extensive normative bases have been developed to gather parent, teacher, and child self-reports of aggressive behavior. Observations and peer ratings or nominations also are useful.

TREATMENT

Efforts at prevention of childhood aggression, using community or school-based services to reach at-risk families of young children have demonstrated some success, although a lack of community resources may limit the overall impact of these programs. As noted above, parenting difficulties often are part of the clinical presentation of child aggression, and behavioral parent training is a recommended and useful treatment. Similarly, the social information processing difficulties that characterize children with aggression have spurred the development of successful social or problem-solving skills and anger management training treatments for elementary-school aged children. Not infrequently, these forms of parent and child training are combined to enhance treatment outcome. Pharmacological treatments have limited utility in managing childhood aggression, and treatments based on the idea of catharsis or release of "pent-up" aggressive behavior do not appear particularly useful.

PROGNOSIS

Aggressive behavior has the unfortunate distinction of being one of the most stable of child characteristics. Children who display frequent, intense, and varied types of aggressive behavior in multiple settings are at significant risk for a host of problems in adolescence and adulthood, including criminality, substance abuse, and academic under-achievement. When the aggressive behavior is accompanied by peer rejection, attention-deficit/hyperactivity disorder (ADHD), low intelligence, or family factors such as teen parenthood, the risk for poor child outcome is even higher. In contrast, a positive parent–child relationship, positive parenting style, higher child intelligence, and prosocial peer interactions are factors that protect against the development or continuation of aggression.

See also: Anger; Bullies; Conduct Disorder; Oppositional Defiant Disorder; Temper Tantrums

Further Reading

Crick, N. R., Nelson, D. A., Morales, J. R., Cullerton-Sen, C., Casas, J. F., & Hickman, S. E. (2001). Relational victimization in childhood and adolescence: I hurt you through the grapevine. In J. Juvonen & S. Graham (Eds.), *Peer harassment in school: The plight of the vulnerable and victimized* (pp. 196–214). New York: Guilford Press.

Dodge, K. A. (2002). Mediation, moderation, and mechanisms in how parenting affects children's aggressive behavior. In J. G. Borkowski & S. L. Ramey (Eds.), *Parenting and the child's world: Influences on academic, intellectual, and social-emotional development. Monographs in parenting* (pp. 215–229). Mahwah, NJ: Lawrence Erlbaum.

Lochman, J. E., Whidby, J. M., & FitzGerald, D. P. (2000). Cognitive-behavioral assessment and treatment with aggressive children. In P. C. Kendall (Ed.), *Child and adolescent therapy: Cognitive-behavioral procedures* (2nd ed., pp. 31–87). New York: Guilford Press.

Tremblay, R. E. (2000). The development of aggressive behaviour during childhood: What have we learned in the past century? *International Journal of Behavioral Development, 2*, 129–141.

Vitiello, B., & Stoff, D. M. (1997). Subtypes of aggression and their relevance to child psychiatry. *Journal of the American Academy of Child and Adolescent Psychiatry, 36*, 307–315.

http://www.nncc.org/Child.Dev/aggression.html

CHARLOTTE JOHNSTON
CARLA M. SEIPP

Agoraphobia

See: Panic Attacks/Panic Disorder (FAS)

Alcohol-Related Neurodevelopmental Disorder

See: Fetal Alcohol Syndrome

Alliance

See: Treatment alliance

Alpha-Adrenergic Agents

See: Pharmacological Interventions

Anger

DEFINITION

Anger can be defined as a response to a perceived offense or threat against an individual. The perceived threat can vary greatly from actual physical threats to threatening one's pride. Because anger is an emotion that can trigger sympathetic fight–flight arousal, it can be an emotion that individuals have difficulty controlling.

As noted by Lochman and colleagues (1997, 2001), intense uncontrolled feelings of anger have been associated with externalizing behavior problems such as aggression and Conduct Disorder.

SOCIAL–COGNITIVE CORRELATES

The emergence of anger has been documented in early infancy, and variations in the facial expression and cognitive "experience" of anger are apparent developmentally throughout childhood. Most of the previous research on social–cognitive experiences in childhood has focused on angry, rage-filled aggression as influenced by a hostile attributional bias. The hostile attributional bias can be defined as an individual's tendency to misperceive an ambiguous situation as threatening, when in reality it is not. For instance, a child with the hostile attributional bias might perceive a threat in a situation in which a peer "accidentally" bumps into him. In this situation, the threat may be misperceived because the child believes that the peer purposely or intentionally bumped into him. The hostile attributional bias occurs because angry aggressive children experience difficulties in processing or encoding ambiguous or neutral cues. Therefore, their perception of the ambiguous situation becomes biased and they attend to more hostile cues in others, as suggested by Dodge and colleagues (1990) and Lochman and colleagues (1997, 2001).

However, it is not entirely clear whether the hostile attributional bias results from biological encoding processes in the brain that predispose how information is processed, or if aggressive children have actually learned schemas for the behavior of others that lead to the attending and recall of hostile cues. To gain a better understanding of the underlying causes of aggression in children, several conceptual models have been proposed to account for the cue-encoding or schema factors that result in the hostile attributional bias.

Anger occurring during everyday interactions can be conceptualized as a mediator between the hostile attributional bias and the aggressive action taken, or as a stimulus for both. Anger can arise before or during social interactions, and can impair, or flood, social information processing in at least two ways. First, the initial perception of threat in a situation can trigger anger and a physiological response. Physiological responses such as increased heart rate serve to heighten the sympathetic nervous system and prepare for fight or flight. A vicious circle is then enacted as the increased physiological reactivity reinforces the likelihood that the initial hostile attributional bias will recur and escalate. Second, prior feelings of anger, left over from conflicts even hours or days earlier, can alter subsequent cue-encoding and lead to the aggressive child's cognitive processing of the stimulus.

Another model of the effects of anger focuses more on preexisting schemas, which are cognitive–emotional beliefs stored in memory. Schemas can influence sound information processing especially through their priming effects on hostile attributional biases. Schemas involve prior learned expectations about the hostility of peers and being treated (un)fairly by peers, which can be instantaneously evoked by certain cues, and then interfere with information processing. These preexisting schemas are consistently recalled in similar situations, create expectations that are relatively impervious to disconfirmation, and provide social goals for action (such as a need to be dominant and in control). This is especially true if the schema is strongly held. As schemas are invoked, anger can be triggered which can then affect physiological arousal.

PHYSIOLOGICAL CORRELATES

Physiological responsiveness to emotional arousal has been repeatedly found and associated with anger in particular. These physiological patterns seem to vary as a function of the appraisals or emotional reactions the individual relates to the stimulus, as well as to the behavioral response the stimulus elicits. Research on heart rate by Raine and colleagues (1997) has traditionally produced the most robust findings, with angry, aggressive children tending to have lower resting heart rates and higher heart rate reactivity to anger-provoking stimuli. Blood pressure has also been associated with anger. Elevated resting blood pressure levels and high reactivity to stress have been paralleled to an angry, hostile, "Type A" temperament in adults as well as children, as noted by Pine and associates (1996).

ASSESSMENT

Behavior rating scales are one of the most frequently utilized assessment methods in any clinical evaluation and can be particularly useful in the assessment of angry aggression. The ease of administration as well as the ability to obtain information from multiple informants provides clinicians with a broad behavior profile. Commonly used rating scales include the Behavior Assessment System for Children and the Child Behavior Checklist. Behavior rating scales such as the Spielberger State Trait Anger Inventory target the expression of anger as more of a stable personality trait and current state feelings of

anger specifically. As anger can be influenced by social–cognitive misperceptions discussed earlier, an evaluation of attributional style, cue encoding biases, and problem-solving abilities is an important component of clinical assessment of anger. Measurements assessing cue encoding deficiencies including the hostile attributional bias as well as other social–cognitive processes typically use children's responses to hypothetical vignettes describing peer provocation, conflicts with authority figures, and associating positive outcomes to the use of aggression. Structured interviews also are valuable assessment instruments, as they can provide more detailed information about the presence of anger than behavioral rating scales or hypothetical vignettes. Examples of structured interviews commonly used include the Diagnostic Interview Schedule for Children and the Child Assessment Schedule. Direct observation and sociometric ratings of behavior through peer ratings are two alternative assessment procedures that may provide a more complete picture of the presence of anger and aggression in everyday settings such as school.

TREATMENT

There are four main types of cognitive–behavioral interventions that benefit uncontrolled anger and social–cognitive deficits. The first involves child cognitive–behavioral interventions that focus on children's dysfunctional social–cognitive processes and poor self-regulation. These forms of cognitive–behavioral intervention address anger management training, attribution retraining, and social problem-solving training. Second, parent behavior modification is focused on changing parent interaction with the child in order to regulate or decrease aggressive behavior. Interventions can also be school based with school behavior modification. In this type of intervention, teachers are taught how to decrease aggressive child behavior through their interactions with the child similar to the parent intervention. Finally, multicomponent cognitive–behavioral interventions focus on the child, parent, and school all in one intervention, and have been generally found to produce the strongest positive effects in empirical outcome research.

See also: Aggression; Cognitive-Behavior Therapy; Conduct Disorder; Rage

Further Reading

Dodge, K. A., Price, J. M., Bachorowski, J., & Newman, J. P. (1990). Hostile attributional biases in severely aggressive adolescents. *Journal of Abnormal Psychology, 99*, 385–392.

Lochman, J. E., Dane, H. E., Magee, T. N., Ellis, M., Pardini, D. A., & Clanton, N. R. (2001). Disruptive behavior disorders: assessment and intervention. In B. Vance & A. Pumareiga (Eds.), *The clinical assessment of children and youth behavior: Interfacing intervention with assessment* (pp. 231–262). New York: Wiley.

Lochman, J. E., Dunn, S. E., & Wagner, E. E. (1997). Anger. In G. Bear, K. Minke, & A. Thomas (Eds.), *Children's needs, II* (pp. 149–160). Washington, DC: National Association of School Psychology.

Pine, D. S., Wasserman, G., Coplan, J., Staghezza-Jaramillo, B., Davies, M., Fried, J., Greenhill, L., & Shaffer, D. (1996). Cardiac profile and disruptive behavior in boys at risk for delinquency. *Psychosomatic Medicine, 58,* 342–353.

Raine, A., Reynolds, C. Venables, P. H., & Mednick, S. A. (1997). Biosocial bases of aggressive behavior in childhood. In A. Raine, P. A. Brennan, D. P. Farrington, & S. A. Mednick (Eds.), *Biosocial bases of violence* (pp. 107–126). New York: Plenum Press.

HEATHER MCELROY
JOHN E. LOCHMAN
NANCY PHILLIPS

Anorexia Nervosa

DEFINITION

Anorexia nervosa is a psychiatric disorder with significant medical consequences. The fourth edition of the *Diagnostic and Statistical Manual of Mental Disorders* (1994) published by the American Psychiatric Association provides diagnostic criteria for this disorder. These include; refusal to maintain weight above 85 percent of expected weight for height or failure to make expected weight gains during the adolescent growth period, an undue influence of body shape on self-evaluation, an intense fear of becoming fat even though underweight, and the absence of three consecutive menstrual cycles in women who have passed menarche. Technically, the diagnostic category entitled Eating Disorder Not Otherwise Specified can be utilized when making a diagnosis if all components are present except the missed menstrual periods; however, these patients are really considered to have anorexia nervosa as the nature of the disorder and the prognosis is similar. This is a frequent occurrence in younger adolescents whose weight loss has postponed the onset of menarche. Recently, there has been a decreased emphasis on the need for the patient to report feelings of being "fat." It is not uncommon to have a patient whose weight loss results from a stated desire to simply change eating habits to a more healthy eating style rather than a change of eating style based on feeling overweight.

INCIDENCE/PREVALENCE

A generally accepted incidence rate for anorexia nervosa is one in every 200 American females between the ages of 12 and 18. Age of onset is usually in the teenage years with some suggestion of a bimodal distribution describing an increased age of onset in early adolescence and in late adolescence. In certain high-risk populations, specifically private girls' schools and upper socioeconomic status communities, the rate has been estimated to be as high as 1 in 100 females. It is estimated that between 5 and 10 percent of all patients with anorexia nervosa are males, and it is felt that the disorder, when it occurs in males, is very similar to that occurring in females.

ETIOLOGY

Anorexia nervosa is thought to have multiple possible causes. Prominent among the probable causes is cultural factors. The disorder occurs primarily in Western, industrialized nations. In the American culture over the last 20–30 years, there has been increased emphasis on the thin female body as the ideal. It has been shown that females as young as 11 and 12 report feeling that they should be thinner, and 60 percent report that they have already been on a diet. Developmental factors have also been implicated in the etiology of anorexia nervosa. The rapid weight increase and body shape changes that occur in early adolescence are thought to trigger concerns about body shape and possible avoidance of physical maturity. Research has suggested the etiological factors in late adolescent onset of anorexia nervosa are more related to social, emotional, and family factors. The personality of the patient with anorexia nervosa is also thought to be a contributing factor. Patients are described as rather inflexible in their thinking with a concrete cognitive style. Patients with anorexia nervosa tend to be achievement oriented, self-disciplined, and often show symptoms similar to obsessive-compulsive disorder. Lack of a positive self-image, fear of loss of control, and perfectionism have also been used to characterize persons with anorexia nervosa. In summary, the current theories of the etiology of anorexia nervosa speculate on cultural, personality, and family factors, including possible genetic predisposition, as multiple determinants of anorexia nervosa.

ASSESSMENT

The assessment of anorexia nervosa is accomplished by interview, by medical/nutritional evaluation, and by the use of self-report measures. The assessment interview should focus on the history of weight loss, the patient's current attitude about body shape and weight as well as nutritional beliefs, personality style and current exercise or sports activities, and school performance. Medical and nutritional assessments are used to determine the patient's current health condition. Patients who are medically compromised usually require inpatient treatment initially. There are a number of self-report questionnaire instruments measuring eating disorder related attitudes and beliefs (e.g., Eating Assessment Test, Eating Disorders Inventory—2) that are useful in assessing a patient's belief system and for research. These instruments by themselves, however, cannot be used for diagnosis as they have a very high false positive rate.

TREATMENT

Following the historical recognition and description of the disorder, most therapeutic interventions for anorexia nervosa were based on psychodynamic theory. More recently, standard practice divides the treatment of anorexia nervosa into two major components. The first of these is refeeding, the process in which the patient is restored to a normal healthy weight. Refeeding is usually accomplished through hospitalization and forced weight gain utilizing behavioral methodologies. The purpose of hospitalization is for weight gain and not necessarily for psychotherapy, and it is becoming increasingly common to utilize hospitalization on a medical unit as opposed as a psychiatric unit. Treatment guidelines published by the American Psychiatric Association in 2000 purposed specific medical criteria be used in the decision to hospitalize for weight gain. The emphasis on refeeding arises from the realization that patients who are medically compromised are unable to benefit from psychotherapeutic interventions. In addition, until a patient is restored to a normal healthy weight, they are resistant to treatment and oftentimes resent being forced into a psychotherapeutic relationship before they are ready. The second major component of treatment for patients with anorexia nervosa is psychotherapy. A number of different approaches have been used and in the ideal situation should be tailored to the specific needs of the patient or family. Cognitive behavioral approaches are utilized to address distortions in thinking with regard to nutrition, body shape, and health. Interpersonal and supportive psychotherapy has also been utilized in a more traditional model. Group psychotherapy is contraindicated for patients with anorexia nervosa until they have reached a normal weight and have come to the realization that they truly do have the disorder. Group psychotherapy for patients with anorexia nervosa is better utilized for prevention of relapse rather than as initial treatment. The use of psychopharmacologic agents in the treatment of anorexia nervosa is questionable. Patients with anorexia nervosa often present as depressed; however, it is recommended that an assessment of the patient's depression is withheld until weight is restored. The side effects of malnutrition can often give the impression of depression, and the need for antidepressant medication should be assessed only following weight restoration.

PROGNOSIS

In general, the literature suggests that about one third of patients with anorexia nervosa will fully recover. Approximately one third will have an intermediate recovery involving periodic relapses with periods of normal functioning, and one third will continue to have serious interruptions in life adjustments based on the disorder. It has been estimated that between 10 and 15 percent of patients with anorexia nervosa will die from the disorder. Early, aggressive intervention is necessary in order to improve outcome.

See also: Bulimia Nervosa; Eating Disorders; Feeding Disorders; Growth Disorders

Further Reading

Attie, I., & Brooks-Gunn, J. (1989). Development of eating problems in adolescent girls: A longitudinal study. *Developmental Psychology, 25,* 70-79.

Comerci, G. D. (1993). Special problems in the adolescent: Eating disorders. In F. D. Burg, J. R. Inglefinger, & E. R. Ward (Eds.), *Gellis & Kagan's current pediatric therapy* (pp. 818-826). Philadelphia: W. B. Saunders.

Hsu, L. K. G. (1990). *Eating disorders.* New York: Guilford.

Linscheid, T. R., & Butz, C. (in press). Anorexia nervosa and bulimia nervosa. In M. C. Roberts (Ed.), *Handbook of Pediatric Psychology* (3rd ed.). New York: Guilford.

THOMAS R. LINSCHEID

Anticonvulsants

See: Pharmacological Interventions; Epilepsy

Antidepressants

See: Pharmacological Interventions

Antisocial Behavior

DEFINITION/CLINICAL PRESENTATION

Antisocial behavior does not constitute a particular diagnostic category; instead, the term is used to refer to a broad range of behaviors that represent violations of social rules. Antisocial behaviors encompass acts such as aggression or violence, bullying, theft, fire-setting, lying, or truancy. Based on arrest records, the most common delinquent acts include arson, vandalism, thefts/burglaries, assaults, rapes, and status offense (running away, curfew violation). Youth with antisocial behavior also may be described using legal terms such as juvenile delinquents or young offenders (these terms vary across jurisdictions), or as having Oppositional Defiant Disorder (ODD) or Conduct Disorder (CD) (diagnostic categories within the *Diagnostic and Statistical Manual of Mental Disorders, Fourth Edition* [*DSM-IV*]).

PREVALENCE

Given the lack of a standard definition, it is difficult to estimate the prevalence of antisocial behavior among youth. Studies of inner-city youth in the United States estimate that 10 percent of 11–12-year-old children have contact with police, and 7–9 percent of boys and 3 percent of girls have committed assaults or robberies. Antisocial behaviors, particularly criminal or delinquent acts, tend to increase throughout the teen years, and it is important to note that, among antisocial youth, a relatively small number of chronic, serious offenders are responsible for a disproportionately large amount of crime. Antisocial behavior is more common among boys than girls (by a ratio of approximately 3 to 1), although this gender disparity may be narrowing. Finally, although the number of children arrested for antisocial acts has increased over the past 10 years, self-reported rates of delinquency appear relatively stable.

CORRELATES

Antisocial behavior is consistently associated with social disadvantage at both the community and family levels. At the community level, antisocial behavior is more prevalent in neighborhoods that are socially disadvantaged, dangerous, and have high numbers of deviant peers and a tolerance for deviant behavior. Child antisocial behavior is also intimately linked to inconsistent, harsh, and coercive parenting, and to poor parent–child attachment. These parenting difficulties, especially in a child with a difficult temperament, increase the risk for antisocial behavior, particularly among boys. In addition, parents of children with antisocial behavior are often characterized by high rates of depression, antisocial behavior, substance abuse, marital conflict, and life stress. Youth with antisocial behavior are more likely to experience early parenthood, academic and attentional difficulties, substance abuse problems, internalized problems such as depression and suicide, and may be victims of crime. Antisocial behavior in combination with Attention-Deficit/Hyperactivity Disorder (ADHD) appears as a particular risk factor for longer lasting and more severe antisocial behavior.

ASSESSMENT

Reflecting the strong associations between antisocial child behavior and community and family disadvantage, an emphasis must be placed on assessing the child's antisocial behavior in context, particularly in the context of the family. Multiple methods of assessment, including interviews, rating scales, and observations, and multiple informants, including parents, teachers, and the child, all typically are needed to provide a comprehensive picture of the nature and severity of the child's behavior.

TREATMENT

Several family-based interventions have been evaluated and have shown positive results in reducing child antisocial behavior, maintaining such improvements over time, and in improving other areas of family life (e.g., sibling conflict or parental functioning). One such intervention, parent management training, focuses on changing parenting behaviors such as ineffective commands and harsh punishment that promote or maintain deviant child behaviors. A second effective treatment, multisystemic therapy recognizes the contributions of family, school, peers, and neighbors to child antisocial behavior, and focuses on altering the interactions between the child and each of these systems. This treatment is useful even with severely impaired youth and has demonstrated a positive impact on rates of arrest and recidivism for adolescents up to 5 years later. In contrast to these interventions, psychodynamic therapy, relationship therapy, and play therapy have not been shown to be effective in changing rates of antisocial behavior. Effective school-based interventions have focused on behaviors such as bullying, social skills, and conflict resolution. The core components of such programs typically attempt to increase parental awareness and involvement with their child, to promote classroom rules and structure, and to provide skills training and feedback for appropriate and inappropriate behavior. One caution in using group interventions with antisocial children is that placing antisocial adolescents together in poorly structured group treatments may actually increase antisocial behavior. Finally, children with antisocial behavior often require several types of services across a range of settings. As a result, there is a need to integrate the multiple services provided and to evaluate these "wraparound" service programs.

PROGNOSIS

Children whose antisocial behavior begins in childhood frequently have a more serious, violent, and chronic course than those with adolescent-limited antisocial behavior. Not surprisingly, these children's antisocial behavior is typically first apparent in the home setting, and then spreads to school and community settings. Evidence suggests that 25–50 percent of children with disruptive behavior proceed to more serious delinquent acts, and about 40–60 percent of delinquent youth continue their antisocial behaviors and become chronic offenders. In addition to the early onset of antisocial behavior, impulsivity, difficult temperament, peer problems, and low intelligence or academic difficulties are child-level predictors of continued antisocial behavior. Within the family, inappropriate parenting, poverty, parental psychological problems, and parental substance abuse are among the predictors of continued antisocial behavior. Finally, living in a disadvantaged community surrounded by deviant peers is also predictive of continued problems.

See also: Bullies; Conduct Disorder; Delinquent Behavior; Oppositional Defiant Disorder; Parent Training

Further Reading

Espiritu, R. C., Huizinga, D., Crawford, A., & Loeber, R. (2001). Epidemiology of self-reported delinquency. In R. Loeber & D. P. Farrington (Eds.), *Child delinquents: Development, interventions, and service needs* (pp. 47–66). Thousand Oaks, CA: Sage.
Kazdin, A. E. (2000). Treatments for aggressive and antisocial children. *Child and Adolescent Psychiatric Clinics of North America, 9*, 841–858.
Loeber, R., & Farrington, D. P. (2000). Young children who commit crime: epidemiology, developmental origins, risk factors, early interventions, and policy implications. *Development and Psychopathology, 12*, 737–762.
Shaw, D. S., Bell, R. Q., & Gilliom, M. (2000). A truly early starter model of antisocial behavior revisited. *Clinical Child and Family Psychology Review, 3*, 155–172.

CHARLOTTE JOHNSTON
DOUGLAS SCOULAR

Anxiety Disorders

DESCRIPTION/CLINICAL PRESENTATION

According to the 4th edition of the *Diagnostic and Statistical Manual of Mental Disorders* (*DSM-IV*), with the exception of separation anxiety disorder, which is the only anxiety disorder specific to childhood, the same criteria are applied for diagnosing anxiety disorders in adults and children. For all anxiety disorders, symptoms must be present for a specific time period (at least 4 weeks for separation anxiety disorder; 6 months for all other anxiety disorders), be age-inappropriate, and interfere in functioning. *DSM-IV* anxiety disorders include separation anxiety disorder, social phobia, specific phobia, generalized anxiety disorder, agoraphobia, panic disorder with and without agoraphobia, obsessive-compulsive disorder, posttraumatic stress disorder, acute stress disorder, anxiety disorder due to a general medical condition, substance-induced anxiety disorder, and anxiety disorder not otherwise specified. Common features shared across anxiety disorders include: (1) avoidance of feared objects, situations or events *or* enduring such objects, situations, events with severe distress; (2) maladaptive thoughts or cognitions, typically regarding harm or injury to oneself or loved one; and (3) physiological arousal or reactions (e.g., palpitations, sweating, irritability).

PREVALENCE AND CORRELATES

Prevalence and correlates of anxiety disorders in children vary depending on the specific type of anxiety disorder (see sections on specific anxiety disorders in this volume). Generally, the prevalence of different anxiety disorders in child and adolescent samples ranges from 3 to 13 percent in community samples, and 6 to

16 percent in clinic samples. As noted by Messer and Beidel (1994), children with anxiety disorders tend to have high trait anxiety, temperaments that are less flexible and more rigid, and have less physical and cognitive self-confidence than children without any disorder. Also, the family environments of children with anxiety disorders tend to promote less independence for the child.

ASSESSMENT

A variety of semistructured (e.g., Anxiety Disorders Interview Schedule for *DSM-IV*: Child and Parent Versions) and structured (e.g., Diagnostic Interview Schedule for Children) diagnostic interviews are available for assessing anxiety disorders in children and adolescents. In addition, there are measures that assess symptoms of general anxiety, such as the Revised Children's Manifest Anxiety Scale and the State-Trait Anxiety Inventory for Children. Self-rating scales that contain subscales to assess more specific anxiety disorders are the Multidimensional Anxiety Scale for Children and the Screen for Anxiety and Related Emotional Disorders. These assessment tools are frequently used in the initial assessment for different anxiety disorders, as well as in the continued monitoring of treatment response. When assessing specific anxiety disorders, it is important to thoroughly assess for the presence of comorbid psychiatric disorders including other anxiety, mood, and externalizing disorders.

TREATMENT

Silverman and Berman (2001) reported that considerable evidence has been accumulated demonstrating the efficacy of exposure-based cognitive behavior therapy for reducing childhood anxiety disorders. Cognitive behavior therapy has been found to be efficacious in treating anxiety disorders in children, whether delivered using an individual child format, a format that involves increased parental involvement, and a format that involves increased peer group involvement. Overall, results from these studies indicate positive treatment gains for up to one year posttreatment. In addition, a follow-up study conducted by Barrett and colleagues showed that positive treatment gains were maintained for up to 7 years posttreatment.

The pharmacological literature on the treatment of childhood anxiety disorders is in its infancy when compared to the literature on exposure-based cognitive behavior therapy, as noted by Stock and associates

(2001). Birmaher and colleagues examined the efficacy of the antidepressant fluoxetine (Prozac) in 21 children with separation anxiety disorder, social phobia, and overanxious disorder; 81 percent of the children displayed moderate to marked improvement of their anxiety symptoms and no side effects were reported by any of the children. Because research is so sparse, pharmacological interventions have been recommended with only the more difficult or "resistant" cases, rather than the frontline approach to be used with all cases.

See also: Behavioral Diaries; Cognitive–Behavioral Play Therapy; Generalized Anxiety Disorder; Parent Training; Problem-Solving Training; Separation Anxiety Disorder; Social Phobia

Further Reading

Messer, S. C., & Beidel, D. C. (1994). Psychosocial correlates of childhood anxiety disorders. *Journal of the American Academy of Child and Adolescent Psychiatry, 33,* 975–983.
Silverman, W. K., & Berman, S. L. (2001). Psychosocial interventions for anxiety disorders in children: Status and future directions. In W. K Silverman & P. D. A. Treffers (Eds.), *Anxiety disorders in children and adolescents: Research, assessment and intervention* (pp. 313–334). Cambridge, UK: Cambridge University Press.
Stock, S. L., Werry, J. S., & McClellan, J. M. (2001). Pharmacological treatment of paediatric anxiety. In W. K Silverman & P. D. A. Treffers (Eds.), *Anxiety disorders in children and adolescents: Research, assessment and intervention* (pp. 355–367). Cambridge, UK: Cambridge University Press.

WENDY K. SILVERMAN
LISSETTE M. SAAVEDRA

Anxiolytics

See: Pharmacological Interventions

Aplastic Anemia

See: Bone Marrow Failure and Primary Immunodeficiency

Applied Behavior Analysis

Applied behavior analysis has been defined as the science in which procedures derived from the principles of behavior are systematically applied to improve socially significant behavior to a meaningful degree and to demonstrate experimentally that the procedures employed were responsible for the improvement in that behavior (Baer, Wolf, & Risley, 1968).

The principles of behavior referred to are essentially those of operant conditioning. Central to operant conditioning is the fact that human behavior is affected by the events that precede it (antecedents) and those that follow it (consequences). The likelihood that a particular behavior will be exhibited again in the presence of the prevailing antecedent events depends on the consequences of that behavior. If the behavior is followed by reinforcement, it is more likely to occur again. If it is not followed by reinforcement, or if it is followed by punishment, it is less likely to occur again.

The procedures of applied behavior analysis involve the identification of the antecedents and consequences that are currently associated with a particular behavior, and then systematically changing those antecedents and consequences to change the behavior. These procedures can be used to increase the occurrence of behaviors that are not occurring enough (or not occurring at all), as well as to decrease the occurrence of (or elimination of) behaviors that are occurring too much.

The stage of identifying the existing antecedents and consequences of a behavior is referred to as conducting a functional assessment of the behavior. A detailed and accurate functional assessment is necessary for the development of a successful applied behavior analysis intervention.

In the definition of applied behavior analysis, the reference to experimental demonstration that the procedures employed were responsible for the change in behavior is an important aspect of applied behavior analysis. Evaluation of outcome is integral to the approach and enables it to readily contribute to the search for empirically supported treatments.

In the field of autism, the acronym ABA is often used to refer to a behaviorally based approach to teaching children with autism. While this approach, also called discrete trial training, does have its roots in applied behavior analysis, it is a narrow application of the principles of applied behavior analysis.

See also: Behavior Modification; Functional Analysis; Positive Reinforcement

Further Reading

Baer, D. M., Wolf, M. M., & Risley, T. (1968). Current dimensions of applied behavior analysis. *Journal of Applied Behavior Analysis, 1,* 91–97.

Grant, L., & Evans, A. (1994). *Principles of behavior.* New York: Harper Collins.
Hudson, A. (1998). Applied behavior analysis. In A. Bellack, M. Hersen (Series Eds.), & T. Ollendick (Vol. Ed.), *Comprehensive clinical psychology (Vol. 5). Children and adolescents: Clinical formulation and treatment* (pp. 107–129). New York: Pergamon.
The Association for Behavior Analysis. http://www.wmich.edu/aba
The Cambridge Centre for Behavioral Studies. http://www.behavior.org

ALAN HUDSON

Arrhythmia

See: Cardiovascular Disease

Asperger's Disorder

DEFINITION

Asperger's Disorder is a Pervasive Developmental Disorder that is characterized by (1) qualitative impairments in social interaction; (2) restricted patterns of behavior or interests; and (3) average language and cognitive development. Significant impairment in functional activities must also be present for a diagnosis. Asperger's Disorder occurs in approximately 8 per 10,000 births. The diagnostic boundary between Asperger's Disorder and high-functioning autism is hazy, and there is debate as to whether the two disorders are in fact distinct. Like most other Pervasive Developmental Disorders, the etiology of Asperger's Disorder is thought to be neurobiological. As yet, there are no medical tests for Asperger's Disorder, and diagnosis is based on behavioral assessment and developmental history. The diagnosis is often made after the age of 5 years, when cognitive abilities can be assessed more reliably and impaired peer relationships become more apparent. Children with Asperger's Disorder may function fairly well in structured interactions with responsive adults, but may demonstrate more social difficulty with children their own age.

SYMPTOM PRESENTATION

Symptoms of Asperger's Disorder are similar to those seen in children with autism who have average to above average intelligence. Qualitative impairments in *social*

Table 1. Selected Educational Intervention Strategies for Youth with Asperger's Disorder

Strategy	Description
Social skills training	Adult-directed, small group intervention in which role playing, problem solving, immediate feedback, and group discussions are used to promote interpersonal problem solving, affective understanding, and perspective taking
Peer buddy system	Peers are trained in how to provide positive support, coaching, and feedback to individuals with Asperger's Disorder to improve their interaction skills and increase their repertoire of socially appropriate behavior
Peer education	Teacher-directed activities geared toward teaching peers to appreciate diversity and providing specific strategies for interacting with children with different styles
Building on strengths	Provision of classroom activities in which the individual with Asperger's Disorder is encouraged to share his/her special interests and skills with peers (e.g., provide tutoring in math, lead a small group focusing on the Civil War) to promote respect and understanding
Self-monitoring	Adult-directed instruction in which the individual with Asperger's Disorder is taught cognitive–behavioral strategies for recognizing, monitoring, and rewarding increases in his/her appropriate behaviors and decreases in his/her inappropriate behaviors

functioning are characterized by poor social reciprocity, or difficulty modifying their behavior in response to situational demands or the behavior of others. Thus, their social style is often described as one-sided, rigid, awkward, and/or intrusive. Many individuals with Asperger's Disorder have difficulty interpreting nonverbal cues (such as gestures, facial expressions) and lack social-emotional understanding and empathy (i.e., the ability to take the perspective of another, or to put oneself in another's shoes). Deficits in social cognition, problem solving, and judgment are marked in comparison to overall cognitive functioning. In spite of adequate vocabulary and language development, their social use of language (i.e., pragmatics) is often impaired. For example, their discourse tends to be pedantic and limited to their own interests, and their ability to initiate and sustain a back-and-forth conversation is impaired. As a result of these characteristics, most individuals with Asperger's Disorder have difficulty making and keeping friends.

The *restricted range of interests* observed in persons with Asperger's Disorder usually involves an extreme interest in one particular subject which is unusual either in intensity or content (e.g., the Civil War; alternative fuel sources). This interest often occupies a large amount of the individual's free time and may become socially intrusive, as the individual may persist in discussing this favorite topic regardless of the listener's interest. Individuals with Asperger's Disorder may also develop behavioral rituals and routines, insist that others participate in their enactment, and/or become highly distressed if their routines or expectations are violated.

TREATMENT

Because children with Asperger's Disorder function at relatively high cognitive levels, their educational needs are often overlooked. Both educational and behavioral treatments are essential for promoting optimal functioning for persons with Asperger's Disorder. Treatment approaches designed for high functioning children with autism are often appropriate for children with Asperger's Disorder. Individualized educational plans, home–school collaboration, and access to appropriate therapies when needed (e.g., social skills intervention, behavioral self-monitoring) are essential for promoting gains in academic areas as well as social and communicative functioning. Children with Asperger's Disorder may recognize that they are different from their peers, which may contribute to increased vulnerability to anxiety and depression. As a result, treatment for these symptoms—through psychotherapy, medication, or a combination of both—is important for many older children, adolescents, and adults with Asperger's Disorder. Provision of vocational supports is also important, as deficits in social interaction and social judgment can impede successful adaptation to many work environments. Table 1 presents some selected intervention strategies designed to promote adaptive functioning for persons with Asperger's Disorder.

OUTCOME

Studies suggest that individuals with Asperger's Disorder may experience a better outcome than individuals with other autism spectrum disorders. They are more likely to get married, become employed, and live independently than persons with autism. However, they may also be at increased risk for other psychiatric conditions, such as anxiety, mood disorders, and obsessive–compulsive disorder.

See also: Autistic Disorder; Cognitive-Behavior Therapy; Pervasive Developmental Disorders; Speech and Language Assessment

Further Reading

American Psychiatric Association. (2000). *Diagnostic and statistical manual of mental disorders* (4th ed., text revision). Washington, DC: Author.

Cohen, D., & Volkmar, F. R. (1997). *Handbook of autism and other pervasive developmental disorders* (2nd ed.). New York: John Wiley & Sons.

Committee on Educational Interventions for Children with Autism. (2001). *Educating children with autism.* Washington, DC: National Academy Press.

WENDY L. STONE
SUSAN L. HEPBURN

Assessment

See: Screening Instruments

Assessment of Global Functioning

Global functioning typically refers to a clinician's judgment of a youth's overall level of functioning in performing various roles and day-to-day activities, as would be observed in school, at home, and in interactions with others in general. Assessment of global functioning is considered so important that it was incorporated in the multiaxial system of the American Psychiatric Association's *Diagnostic and Statistical Manual of Mental Disorders (DSM-IV)* as Axis V, or more specifically, as Global Assessment of Functioning (GAF). The GAF was derived from the Global Assessment Scale (GAS), authored by Jean Endicott and colleagues in 1976, which was in turn derived from the Health-Sickness Rating Scale developed by Lester Luborsky in 1962. The clinician is instructed to consider psychological, social, and occupational functioning on a hypothetical continuum of mental health illness in assigning the youth a score from 1 to 100, using 10 anchor descriptions. A higher score indicates better functioning. The clinician rates the youth's lowest level of functioning during a time period that is specified by the clinician (e.g., last month, last year).

The 10 anchor descriptions consist primarily of symptom descriptions with some examples of impaired functioning. For the most part, functioning is measured by the lack of impairment (e.g., the anchor for a score 90 begins with "absence of minimal symptoms"). David Shaffer and colleagues modified the anchor descriptions in 1983 to reflect examples pertinent to children, with this adaptation referred to as the Children's Global Assessment Scale (CGAS). There is no training for scoring the CGAS or GAF. It is assumed that they can be readily used by professionals who have had formal educational and clinical experience in working with a variety of childhood psychiatric disorders.

In the narrative introduction to *DSM-IV*, impairment in functioning is stipulated as a criterion for receiving a diagnosis. In order to meet the criteria for a disorder, the individual must have impairment in one or more important areas of functioning or experience significant distress. In general, impairment is not defined in the diagnostic criteria, although for some diagnoses, a vague statement is included about the disturbance causing clinically significant impairment in social, academic, or occupational functioning.

A diagnosis consists of a constellation of symptoms, whereas impairment reflects the consequences or effects of symptoms on day-to-day functioning. Level of functioning is regarded as a more rigorous criterion for need for treatment than the presence of a set of symptoms. Epidemiological research, in which community rather than clinical samples are studied, has confirmed the need to incorporate the requirement of impairment when trying to identify youths in need of services. Without this requirement, the proportion of youths meeting criteria for diagnosis has consistently been inordinately high. Epidemiological studies have also demonstrated that even when youths did not meet diagnostic criteria for any common diagnosis, youths with functional impairment were as likely to receive specialty mental health services as were youths that had both a diagnosis and impairment.

In fact, when the Center for Mental Health Services (CMHS) of the Substance Abuse and Mental Health Services Administration operationalized the definition of Serious Emotional Disturbance (SED), they required the presence of diagnosis and functional impairment which substantially interferes with or limits the child's role or functioning in family, school, or community activities. In applying for federal block grant funds from CMHS, each state must demonstrate that they are meeting the needs of youths with SED. In addition, this operationalized definition of SED is used to determine prevalence rates for the purpose of identifying the mental health needs of children at a national and state level.

Various measures, which yield a global score or a total score reflecting on functioning, have been widely used and include the CGAS, Columbia Impairment Scale (CIS) developed by Hector Bird and colleagues (1996), and the Child and Adolescent Functional Assessment Scale (CAFAS) authored by Kay Hodges (2000). The CGAS yields one numeric value; the CIS generates a total score from 13 items; and the CAFAS generates a total sum based on scores for 8 subscales assessing various domains of functioning.

The CGAS has typically been used in research published in the psychiatric literature, such as medication studies. The CIS was developed for epidemiological studies in the hope that parents and youths could complete the measure. However, parents tend to score their children as healthier than they are, as judged by nonclinician raters who scored the CGAS after detailed interviews with the child and parent. As a result, the nonclinician CGAS has been recommended over the CIS as a measure of impairment in epidemiological studies. The version for the youth is not recommended because of consistently poor psychometric properties (i.e., its reliability and validity). The CAFAS is widely used to evaluate outcome in applied clinical settings and in clinical research.

The CAFAS consists of a set of behavioral descriptions (e.g., expelled from school, bullies peers) which are grouped into levels of impairment (e.g., severe, moderate, etc.) for each domain (e.g., school, home, etc.). According to an annual survey on how the states are evaluating their children's services conducted by the Georgetown University National Technical Assistance Center for Children's Mental Health, the CAFAS is used by approximately 25 states. In addition, the 67 System of Care Initiative sites awarded grants by the CMHS use the CAFAS as an outcome measure. There is considerable evidence of criterion-related and predictive validity of the CAFAS.

In addition to the role of identifying need for treatment, measures of global level of functioning, according to *DSM-IV*, are useful in measuring the impact of treatment, in predicting the outcome of treatment, and in planning treatment. While no rationale or justification is given for these assertions in *DSM-IV*, the empirical literature does support them. Numerous studies have used the CGAS and the CAFAS to demonstrate the impact of intervention on improvement in functioning. Global measures of functioning are commonly used as quality assurance or performance indicators to monitor quality of care and to ensure accountability of providers. In fact, functioning has come to be viewed as an important criterion for assessing treatment outcome because it ensures that clinically meaningful and significant change has taken place. Showing change in symptom counts is not considered sufficient for demonstrating efficacy for an evidence-based treatment. To

be considered efficacious, the treatment should demonstrate an impact on the child's everyday functioning in the real world. There is evidence to suggest that impacting functioning is more difficult to accomplish than reducing symptoms, based on the findings of a community sample study, which examined the relationship between service dose and outcome.

The assertion that the level of functioning at the onset of treatment is a prognostic indicator of eventual outcome also has empirical support. A higher level of impairment is associated with poorer response to psychotherapy. In addition, in a community study in which youths were evaluated 5–7 years after their initial assessment, the findings indicated that the likelihood of having a diagnosis and functional impairment in adolescents was much higher for those with a diagnosis and impairment as a child, as compared to healthy children.

It makes intuitive sense that global functioning would be useful in treatment planning because the score would have implications for level of care decisions and for documenting the need for more intensive or costly treatments. In fact, studies using the CAFAS have shown that a higher degree of impairment at intake means that the individual is much more likely to need a stronger intervention. Higher impairment on the CAFAS has been shown to correspond to a more intensive level of care, more restrictive or therapeutic placement, and more serious psychiatric disorders. Also, prediction studies have shown that higher impairment on the CAFAS at intake was significantly related to more restrictive care, higher cost, more bed days, and more days of services at 6 and 12 months post intake, more restrictive living arrangement and higher number of days in out-of-family care at 6 months, significantly greater likelihood of contact with the law and poor school attendance at 6 months post intake, and significantly greater likelihood of recidivism during the year after discharge from a juvenile justice residential placement. The assertions that global functioning is important in identifying need for service, in treatment planning, in assessing the impact of treatment, and in predicting the response to treatment are thus supported by the literature.

See also: Behavior Rating Scales; Classification and Diagnosis; Clinical Utility; Risk Assessment and Risk Management

Further Reading

Bird, H. R., Andrews, H., Schwab-Stone, M., Goodman, S., Dulcan, M., Richters, J., Rubio-Stipec, M., Moore, R. E., Chiang, P., Hoven, C., Canino, G., Fisher, P., & Gould, M. S. (1996). Global measures of impairment for epidemiologic and clinical use with children and adolescents. *International Journal of Methods in Psychiatric Research, 6,* 295–307.

Hodges, K., & Kim, C. S. (2000). Psychometric study of the Child and Adolescent Functional Assessment Scale: prediction of contact with the law and poor school attendance. *Journal of Abnormal Child Psychology, 28*(3), 287–297.

Manteuffel, B., & Stephens, R. L. (2002). Overview of the national evaluation of the comprehensive community mental health services for children and their families program and summary of current findings. *Children's Services: Social Policy, Research, and Practice, 5*(1), 3–20.

KAY HODGES

Assessment of Parent–Child Interactions

RATIONALE FOR THE ASSESSMENT OF PARENT–CHILD INTERACTIONS

Assessment of the parent–child relation is critical to diagnosis and treatment of children's behavior problems. Both internalizing (i.e., anxiety, depression) and externalizing (i.e., conduct problems) behavior disorders have their origins, at least in part, in early parent–child interactions, and many of the symptoms of behavior disorders are maintained and exacerbated by interactions between the parent and child. However, most studies examining the relation between parent–child interactions and specific childhood disorders to date have focused on the externalizing disorders of childhood.

These studies have shown differences in the interaction patterns of families of children with significant behavior problems and families of children who have not been referred for behavior problems. Specifically, referred children are less likely to comply with their parents' commands than nonreferred children and are more likely to whine, yell, and issue countercommands in response to their parent's commands. Mothers of referred children give more commands to their child, more often repeat commands before the child has sufficient opportunity to comply, and engage in more negative verbal behavior toward their child than mothers of nonreferred children. A strong and consistent correlation between negative parenting behaviors and problematic child outcomes has been shown in many studies. For this reason, the promotion of optimal parenting styles and parent–child interactions is often the focus of treatments for children with significant behavior problems, making the assessment of parent–child interactions essential for treatment planning.

DIRECT OBSERVATION

Observations of parent–child transactions are invaluable for revealing the nature and the quality of the parent–child relationship. Several observational systems exist for assessing interactions between family members of children with conduct problems. Direct behavioral observation measures are considered the hallmark of behavioral assessment because they provide the most objective description of target behaviors, such as noncompliance to parental commands and the effectiveness of parents' responses. When a family is observed either in the home or clinic, major child-rearing dimensions that require intervention can be determined, including both physical negative behaviors and verbal negative behaviors such as criticism. Qualitative aspects of the interaction can also be evaluated, including parents' tone of voice, use of age-appropriate language, and degree of warmth.

The Dyadic Parent–Child Interaction Coding System-II (DPICS-II) is a widely used system that allows for easy and efficient direct observation of parent–child interactions in a standardized laboratory setting using a reliable and valid method. The system contains 25 categories that may be coded for both parent and child behavior during an interaction. The parent–child dyad is typically observed from behind a one-way mirror while they play with a standard set of toys selected to encourage positive, interactive play. The dyad is observed during three standard DPICS situations to allow assessment of the quality of their social interactions in situations that differ both in the amount of parental control required and the demand placed on the child for compliance.

Designed for both research and clinical purposes, the DPICS-II coding system was intended to provide practicing clinicians with a manageable and practical way to measure pretreatment and posttreatment changes as well as ongoing treatment progress. Simultaneously, the DPICS-II was intended to provide researchers with a reliable and valid system to measure the interactive behaviors with sufficient detail and specificity to advance our knowledge of the assessment and treatment of children with behavior problems. Further, by allowing coding of the same behaviors for parents and children, it is possible for clinicians and researchers to use the DPICS-II to describe behaviors within the interaction that may elicit or maintain the children's behavior problems and assess changes in these behaviors during and after treatment.

Since its development, the system has been used both clinically and in research to describe parent–child interactions. In addition to distinguishing dyads with and without disruptive behavior disorders, the coding system has been used by Webster–Stratton to distinguish parent–child interactions of mothers of neglected children from children with behavior problems and normal control children, and to distinguish abusive from nonabusive families. The system has also been employed as a measure of pretreatment to posttreatment changes for children with behavior problems.

Q-SORTS AND RATING SCALES

Additional methods of assessment of parent–child interactions include Q-sorts and parent rating scales. The Attachment Q-set developed by Walters and Deane (1985) is a measure of a child's attachment-related behaviors in the behavioral dimensions of security, dependency, and sociability. The Q-set consists of 90 behaviorally descriptive items that are sorted by a parent into nine piles or stacks according to the extent to which they are characteristic or uncharacteristic of the child. The Q-set has demonstrated a significant relationship with observations of home behavior and laboratory-based classifications of attachment security using the Strange Situation. Dimensions of parent–child interactions can also be assessed through parent-completed questionnaires, such as the Parent–Child Relations Questionnaire (PCR) developed by Roe and Siegleman (1963). The PCR is a 5-point, 130-item questionnaire that generates scores for 6 subscales that reflect a parents' affectionate behaviors and 4 subscales that reflect either rewarding or punishing behaviors.

The transactional nature of a child's presenting problems makes the assessment of parent–child interactions critical to determining the appropriate course of treatment. Whether direct observation, Q-sorts, rating scales, or a combination of methods are utilized, the information that is gathered from the assessment assists in determining the frequency, intensity, and duration of the child's behavior problems across settings and with different parents, and provides information on the parent behavioral antecedent and consequent behaviors that may be serving to maintain the child's behavior problems. This information can identify the target behaviors within both members of the dyad that require change and can provide a baseline against which to assess the changes that occur with treatment.

See also: Aggression; Behavior Rating Scales; Behavioral Observation; Disruptive Behavior Disorders; Parent–Child Interaction Therapy

Further Reading

Eyberg, S. M., Bessmer, J., Newcomb, K., Edwards, D., & Robinson, E. (1994). *Dyadic parent–child interaction coding system II: A manual.* Social and Behavioral Sciences Documents (Ms. No. 2897). San Rafael, CA: Select Press.
Roe, A., & Siegleman, M. (1963). A parent–child relations questionnaire. *Child Development, 34,* 355–369.
Waters, E., & Deane, K. (1985). Defining and assessing individual differences in attachment relationships: Q-methodology and the organization of behavior in infancy and early childhood. In I. Bretherton, & E. Waters (Eds.), *Growing points of attachment theory and research* (pp. 41–65). *Monographs of the Society for Research in Child Development, 50*(1–2, Serial No. 209).

JANE G. QUERIDO
SHEILA M. EYBERG

Asthma

DEFINITION

Asthma is a chronic inflammatory disorder of the airways that is characterized by wheezing, tightness in the chest, shortness of breath, and coughing. The pathophysiology of asthma implicates both airway obstruction (e.g., edema leading to mucus formation, narrowing of bronchioles, contraction of smooth muscle) and inflammation (e.g., airway hyperresponsiveness to various stimuli). Asthma is a reactive airway disease that is "intermittent," in that attacks generally occur episodically, varying in intensity from mild to status asthmaticus (i.e., sudden, continuous asthma attack). It is also "reversible" in that airways return to their previous condition spontaneously or following treatment.

INCIDENCE

Asthma is the most common chronic illness of children in the United States, affecting approximately 4.8 million children aged 18 years and younger. The most common age of diagnosis is between 5 and 13 years; however, recent research suggests that prevalence rates in children younger than 4 years old has increased by 160 percent in the last two decades. Asthma has been found to be more common in boys than girls in early childhood; however, the incidence equalizes in adolescence and then changes course by increasing in adulthood for females. Pediatric asthma differentially affects minority children and children of low socioeconomic status living in inner cities. For example, African American and Hispanic children are three times more likely to be hospitalized or die from asthma compared to Caucasian children.

PSYCHOLOGICAL CORRELATES

One of the major challenges of managing asthma is adhering to the daily treatment regimen. Rates of adherence range from 30 to 70 percent for medications and metered-dose inhalers and are a major cause of the morbidity associated with asthma. Asthma has been found to be the leading cause of absenteeism for school-age children, accounting for 10.1 million lost days each year. These absences from school, coupled with reduced participation in sports and extracurricular activities, may be associated with increased levels of anxiety and depression in children with pediatric asthma. Furthermore, children with asthma are also reported to have slightly higher rates of learning disorders but similar rates of grade failures, suspensions, and IQ and achievement scores compared to healthy children. Although medications, such as theophylline and corticosteroids, have been implicated in problems with cognitive functioning, the evidence to date is mixed. Recent evidence using quality of life measures has suggested that asthma has a significant impact on both the child and parent's daily functioning.

ETIOLOGY

Both genetic and environmental factors have been implicated in the etiology of asthma. When one parent has been diagnosed with asthma or hay fever/allergies, there is a 50 percent risk of the child developing asthma. Environmental factors include living in an urban setting, exposure to allergens (e.g., dust mites, molds, fungus, pet dander, cockroach droppings) and irritants (e.g., cold air, sudden changes in temperature, cigarette smoke, chemicals), stress, viral infections, and exercise.

ASSESSMENT

The diagnosis of asthma is based on the patient's medical history (e.g., symptoms, history of wheezing, allergies, and familial history), physician examination of the upper respiratory tract, chest, and skin; x-rays of the lungs, pulmonary function tests, peak flow tests, and bronchial provocation testing. An asthma diagnosis can be established using medical history, day and night

symptoms, as well as evidence of airway obstruction that is reversible in nature (e.g., FEV_1 percent predicted increases after the use of short-acting inhaled beta$_2$-agonists). Asthma severity has been classified into four distinct groups using the criteria above: mild intermittent, mild persistent, moderate persistent, and severe persistent.

TREATMENT

Treatment for asthma requires three primary components: (1) education about the physiological aspects of asthma, common triggers, and skills training for treatment; (2) preventive therapies to control airway inflammation and hyperresponsiveness, and (3) short-term therapies in the event of an acute attack. Education is a key component of asthma treatment, since children need to be able to accurately detect symptoms of asthma and utilize the correct medication as symptoms occur. Furthermore, the role of adherence to the medical treatment should be emphasized. Preventative therapies include the use of long-term medications, such as corticosteroids, cromolyn sodium, theophylline, leukotriene modifiers, or long-acting beta$_2$-agonist, as well as avoidance of environmental triggers. For emergencies and acute attacks, patients can be given short-acting inhaled beta$_2$-agonists, anticholinergics, or short-term systemic corticosteroids. These quick-acting medications are utilized to provide prompt relief of bronchoconstriction and associated symptoms, such as coughing and wheezing.

PROGNOSIS

Though it is often commonly assumed that children will "outgrow" asthma, approximately 75 percent of children with asthma will continue to have the disease in adulthood. Furthermore, pediatric asthma is associated with significant morbidity and mortality. The morbidity associated with asthma is more common and includes increased utilization of emergency rooms, hospitalizations, increased financial costs, school absenteeism, limitations in activities, comorbid conditions (e.g., allergies, hay fever) and disruptions to family and caregiver routines. Although asthma deaths are rare among children, 246 children between the ages of 0 and 17 died in 1998 as a result of asthma complications. However, the advent of new treatments and intensive interventions focusing on adherence and education show promise for the future.

See also: Adherence; Anxiety Disorders; Depressive Disorder; Learning Disorders; Quality of Life

Further Reading

Bender, B., Wamboldt, F. S., O'Conner, S. L., Rand, C., Szefler, S., Milgrom, H., & Wamboldt, M. Z. (2000). Measurement of children's asthma medication adherence by self-report, mother report, canister weight, and Doser CT. *Annals of Allergy, Asthma, and Immunology, 85*, 416–421.

Bender, B. G. (1999). Learning disorders associated with asthma and allergies. *School Psychology Review, 28*(2), 204–214.

Claudio, L., Tulton, L., Doucette, J., & Landrigan, P. J. (1999). Socioeconomic factors and asthma hospitalization rates in New York City. *Journal of Asthma, 36*(4), 343–350.

Myers, T. R. (2000). Pediatric asthma epidemiology: incidence, morbidity, and mortality. *Respiratory Care Clinics of North America, 6*(1), 1–14.

Homa, D. M., Mannion, D. M., & Lara, M. (2000). Asthma mortality in US Hispanics of Mexican, Puerto Rican, and Cuban heritage, 1990–1995. *American Journal of Respiratory and Critical Care Medicine, 161*, 504–509.

ALEXANDRA L. QUITTNER
AVANI C. MODI
MELISSA A. DAVIS

Attachment

DEFINITION AND ADAPTIVE SIGNIFICANCE

First popularized by John Bowlby, the term "attachment" refers to the relationship an infant or child has with its caregiver(s). From an ethological perspective, a positive attachment between caregiver and infant is extremely important for the infant's survival in that the attachment motivates the child to maintain proximity with his/her caregiver(s), and thus avoid starvation, exposure, or predation. As such, the predisposition to form an attachment can be seen as an adaptive trait that raises the probability of the infant's survival to reproductive age.

Relationships are typically considered to be bidirectional, although the term attachment has been used traditionally to refer to the child's attachment to the caregiver, whereas the caregiver's emotional tie to the infant has been characterized as "bonding."

DETERMINANTS OF ATTACHMENT

The formation of an emotional bond between an infant and his or her primary caregiver(s) develops gradually over the course of the first year of life, as the infant learns that his or her needs will (or will not) be consistently met and as a result develops expectations about adult behavior relative to his or her signals. Thus, the responsiveness of the caregiver is an important factor in the formation of positive attachments. Researchers have found that those caregivers who responded promptly when the infant was in distress were sensitive to their primary needs (e.g., feeding and changing diapers), adapted their caregiving to the temperament and changing needs of the infant, and, in general, were more affectionate and playful. They tended to be more securely attached than those caregivers who were less responsive in these ways.

DEVELOPMENT OF ATTACHMENT

At birth, infants exhibit a preference for their mothers' voices, and this is soon followed by a preference for their mothers' faces. However, despite these preferences, infants will exhibit favorable responses to a variety of social and nonsocial stimuli. From approximately 2–7 months, infants are fairly indiscriminate in their "attachments." They prefer people over other lifelike stimuli (e.g., puppets) and respond to attention from almost anyone with positive emotional responses (e.g., smiles and coos). It is not until around 7–10 months that infants express specific attachments to their primary caregiver(s). These specific attachments are denoted by several coincidental developments, as at these ages, infants commonly begin to exhibit a fear of strangers, and a fear of separation from their caregivers (although this tends to decrease during the second year). Furthermore, around this time infants begin to locomote (e.g., crawl or scoot), and this gives them more control over their environment and helps them maintain proximity to the preferred caregiver and avoid strangers. By the end of the first year, the attachment figure is the infant's main source of comfort and is used as a secure base from which the infant ventures out to explore the world.

INDIVIDUAL DIFFERENCES IN ATTACHMENT

The standard means of measuring the quality of infant–caregiver attachments is the Strange Situation Paradigm developed by Mary Ainsworth. This procedure is used to assess the quality and strength of infants' attachment to their caregiver by exposing them to situations in which they are alone with their mother (used to see how well infants use their mother as a secure base from which to explore the rest of the room), separated from their mother and introduced to a stranger with and without the mother present (used to see how infants respond to being separated and to encountering a stranger), and reunited with their mother (to see how infants respond once their mother returns and how well they are soothed).

Based on infants' reactions to this procedure, Ainsworth and her colleagues were able to classify infants into one of three categories: secure, ambivalent/resistant, or avoidant. Infants who are securely attached will explore while the mother is present, will become mildly distressed when the mother leaves, will be happy and seek physical contact on the mother's return. In the presence of a stranger, securely attached infants explore less, will interact with the stranger in the presence of the mother, show no increase in distress when the stranger leaves (i.e., baby is alone), and are indifferent upon the return of the stranger. Infants classified as ambivalent stay close to the mother at all times and explore the room very little. They become very distressed when the mother leaves. However, on her return they are ambivalent; choosing to remain close but resisting physical contact with the mother. Furthermore, ambivalent infants tend to be withdrawn when a stranger is present and avoid or ignore them even in the presence of their mother. Infants classified as avoidant show little distress when the mother leaves the room and ignore or avoid her upon her return; they tend to treat strangers in the same manner.

CLINICAL RELEVANCE

Researchers have found that children who were securely attached as infants tend to be better problem solvers as toddlers and tend to be more socially outgoing and responsive as toddlers and children (are more likely to be leaders in their peer group, initiate play, and were more sensitive to the feelings of other children) than insecurely attached children (i.e., those classified as ambivalent or avoidant). Furthermore, insecurely attached infants tend to be at a higher risk for behavior problems later in childhood. Thus, understanding the strength and quality of the child–caregiver relationship may help clinicians in their diagnosis as well as in the structuring of potential interventions.

It is important to understand that attachment relationships are not necessarily stable over time and can fluctuate as a function of parental or environmental circumstances. Thus, securely attached infants may become insecure if the parents become less able to meet their needs because of divorce, onset of mental health problems, birth of a new baby, or other life stresses. Likewise, insecure infants may become more secure if their environments become more stable. The instability seen in some children's attachment status may explain the inconsistency in research which links quality of attachment to the development of mental health problems later in life. Moreover, environments that predispose children to insecure attachments also typically contain a wide range of other risk factors, so it is not always possible to determine whether adverse effects are due to poor quality attachment or other factors. It is, however, reasonable to consider disordered attachment, especially at extreme levels, as a risk factor for the development of problems later in life.

See also: Cognitive Development; Developmental Milestones; Emotional Development; Motor Development; Parenting Practices; Risk and Protective Factors

Further Reading

Shaffer, D. R. (2002). *Developmental psychology: Childhood and adolescence* (6th ed.). Belmont, CA: Wadsworth.

Vasta, R., Haith, M. M., & Miller, S. A. (1998). *Child psychology: The modern science* (3rd ed.). New York: Wiley.

D. JILL SHADDY
JOHN COLOMBO

Attention-Deficit/ Hyperactivity Disorder

DESCRIPTION/CLINICAL PRESENTATION

Attention-Deficit/Hyperactivity Disorder (ADHD) is defined by developmentally inappropriate levels of inattention and/or hyperactivity and impulsivity that are persistent and pervasive. Diagnostic guidelines for ADHD are provided in the *Diagnostic and Statistical Manual of Mental Disorders, Fourth Edition* (DSM-IV) published by the American Psychiatric Association. Symptoms of ADHD are divided into two core clusters: inattention (e.g., distractible, cannot concentrate), and hyperactivity–impulsivity (e.g., runs or climbs about, fidgets). Subtypes of ADHD are specified depending on whether the child has a significant level of symptoms in either or both clusters. Thus, children may fit criteria for inattentive type, hyperactive–impulsive type, or combined type (if criteria for both clusters are met). In addition, there must be evidence that the symptoms occur in more than one situation, began before age 7, have been present for at least 6 months, and cause impairment.

The majority of children diagnosed with ADHD meet the combined type criteria (about 65 percent), with about 30 percent meeting the inattentive type criteria, and only 5 percent meeting the hyperactive–impulsive type criteria. Some research has suggested that girls are more likely to have the inattentive type, although currently this is subject to debate. Children with ADHD present differently depending on their subtype of ADHD. Children with the inattentive subtype are often described by parents and teachers as "daydreamers," or likely to wander off. Those with the hyperactive–impulsive type are described as constantly active, having low frustration tolerance, and being loud. These symptoms generally decrease and change over the course of development. For example, a child who is constantly "on the go" may be less active as an adolescent, although he/she may still have subjective feelings of restlessness.

INCIDENCE/PREVALENCE

A general consensus is that 3–5 percent of children meet diagnostic criteria for ADHD. ADHD has been studied and found all over the world (e.g., United States, Canada, Britain, New Zealand, Puerto Rico, Germany, China, India, and Holland). By definition, the onset of ADHD is in childhood (recall that symptoms must be present before age 7 for a diagnosis to be made), but symptoms may persist into adolescence and adulthood. The prevalence of ADHD decreases with age, which some experts argue is because the criteria for ADHD were designed for children and are limited in appropriateness for adolescents and adults (e.g., excessive running and climbing is appropriate to describe activity levels in children, but may not be appropriate for adults). More boys are affected than girls, with gender ratios varying from 4:1 to 9:1 in samples of children who are referred to clinics for ADHD symptoms and from 2:1 to 3:1 in epidemiological or community-based samples. The difference in gender ratios between clinic-referred and community samples indicates that girls with ADHD may be less likely to be referred for treatment than boys with ADHD.

CORRELATES

ADHD is associated with family, academic, and psychosocial problems. Children with ADHD are more likely to have problems in their relationships with parents (e.g., more conflict, less family cohesion), teachers (e.g., negative interactions), and peers (e.g., rejection, dislike). These social difficulties are particularly apparent among children who have both ADHD and co-occurring conduct problems. Educational difficulties are widely prevalent; for example, children with ADHD are more likely to require special education and grade retention, and up to one third of these children have a learning disability. Psychosocial problems are also a concern. About 35 percent of children with ADHD have significant problems with aggressive, oppositional, and argumentative behaviors. In addition, approximately 30 percent of children with ADHD have an anxiety and/or depressive disorder.

It is important to note that the types of problems experienced differ somewhat depending on the subtype of ADHD. Children with the inattentive type appear to have more difficulties with academic performance and may have more anxiety, whereas children with the hyperactive–impulsive or combined subtype are more likely to have behavior problems such as oppositional-defiant and conduct disorders and aggression with peers, and may have more speech and language and family discord problems. Gender also impacts the type of associated problems. Girls with ADHD are less likely to have oppositional-defiant or conduct disorders or to be aggressive than boys.

ASSESSMENT

Assessment of ADHD requires gathering of information from both parents and teachers, and often the child. A clinical interview will elicit information such as symptom presentation, developmental history, and level of impairment or functioning in social, academic, and family domains. For more formal diagnostic purposes, structured interviews such as the Diagnostic Interview Schedule for Children Version 4 that assess diagnostic criteria as outlined in the *DSM-IV* are recommended. Given the need for evidence of a developmentally inappropriate level of symptoms that occur across situations, assessments rely heavily on standardized rating scales completed by parents and teachers. Several ratings scales have been developed for this purpose, including the Conners' Parent and Teacher Rating Scales (2001) and the ADHD Rating Scale developed by DuPaul and colleagues. These scales can also be helpful in assessing the effects of medication treatment for ADHD. Psychoeducational testing may be conducted to assess the child's academic functioning, although such testing is not necessarily informative for diagnosis. Similarly, computerized tests of attention, although useful in research, have not yet demonstrated sufficient sensitivity and specificity to be used in diagnosing individual children.

TREATMENT

The results of a recent large treatment study for ADHD, conducted in several cities in the United States and Canada by the Multimodal Treatment Study of Children with Attention-Deficit/Hyperactivity Disorder Cooperative Group, indicate that carefully titrated and monitored stimulant medication is superior to the usual treatment offered in the community and to psychosocial treatment in reducing ADHD symptoms. However, the psychosocial treatment did have some effect and a combination of medication and psychosocial treatment was best for reducing oppositional behavior and problems with anxiety or depression, and for improving social skills and parent–child interactions. Expert consensus guidelines put forth by Conners and colleagues (2001) recommend a preliminary trial of psychosocial treatment (e.g., parent training, classroom behavior management) for younger children, those with milder ADHD symptoms, or those with co-occurring anxiety problems, and a combination of psychosocial and medication treatment for most other children. A variety of other treatments, including special diets or supplements and biofeedback training, are widely marketed but have little or no evidence to indicate that they are beneficial.

PROGNOSIS

Although historically it was believed that children outgrew the symptoms of ADHD, recent evidence shows that this is not the case for many children. Anywhere from 30 to 80 percent of children with ADHD have symptoms that persist into adolescence and adulthood. In addition to the continuation of ADHD symptoms, children with ADHD are at risk for academic or occupational underachievement, antisocial behavior, and substance abuse in adolescence and early adulthood. However, with the exception of academic problems, most other risks appear to be primarily associated with the oppositional or conduct problems that may co-occur with ADHD, rather than the ADHD symptoms per se. Recent studies indicate that treatment of the ADHD with stimulant medication during childhood may lower the risk for negative outcomes in adolescents and adults.

See also: Disruptive Behavior Disorders; Learning Disorders; Oppositional Defiant Disorder; Parent Training; Summer Treatment Programs

Further Reading

American Psychiatric Association. (1994). *Diagnostic and statistical manual of mental disorders* (4th ed.). New York: Author.
Barkley, R. A. (1998). *Attention-deficit hyperactivity disorder: A handbook for diagnosis and treatment* (2nd ed.). New York: Guilford.
Conners, D. K., March, J. S., Frances, A., Wells, K. C., & Ross, R. (2001). Expert consensus guideline series: Treatment of attention/deficit-hyperactivity disorder. *Journal of Attention Disorders,* 4(Supp. 1).
The MTA Cooperative Group. (1999). A 14-month randomized clinical trail of treatment strategies for attention-deficit/hyperactivity disorder. *Archives of General Psychiatry, 56,* 1073–1086.
Weiss, M., Hechtman, L. T., & Weiss, G. (1999). *ADHD in adulthood: A guide to current theory, diagnosis, and treatment.* Baltimore: Johns Hopkins University Press.
www.chadd.org

CHARLOTTE JOHNSTON
JENEVA OHAN

Attrition

See: Treatment Attrition

Auditory Comprehension Deficit

See: Central Auditory Processing Disorder

Autistic Disorder

DEFINITION

Autistic disorder, or autism, is a pervasive developmental disorder that is characterized by a triad of behavioral features: deficits in social relating and reciprocity, impaired language and communication skills, and a restricted range of interests and activities. Autism occurs in approximately 17 per 10,000 births, and is 4–5 times more common in males than females. This disorder is not specific to any socioeconomic level, ethnicity, or geographic area, and can be found worldwide in all social classes. The etiology of autism is organic, though no single pathologic event has been identified that is uniquely or universally associated with autism. Autism can co-occur with a variety of other neurobiological disorders, such as tuberous sclerosis, phenylketonuria, fragile X syndrome, and neurofibromatosis. In addition, approximately 25 percent of individuals with autism develop seizure disorder in their lifetimes.

SYMPTOM PRESENTATION

Symptoms of autism are highly influenced by developmental processes, and therefore change in character over time. There is also significant individual variability in symptom presentation as a function of developmental level (see Table 1). Approximately 75 percent of individuals with autism function intellectually within the range of mental retardation; however, some individuals with autism have average or above average cognitive ability.

Qualitative *social impairments* represent a core feature of autism and may be evident in several domains. Limited social responsiveness, affective expression, and use of nonverbal social-communicative behaviors (e.g., eye contact, facial expression, and gestures) often characterize individuals with autism. These impairments are best conceptualized as a failure to develop reciprocal social relationships rather than a deliberate withdrawal from others. Individuals with autism can and do form social attachments and demonstrate affectionate behavior, though the quality of their interactions may be described as "one-sided" and "on their own terms" rather than flexible or reciprocal. Social impairments lead to a diminished capacity for peer relationships and impede vocational success for many adults with autism.

Qualitative impairments in *communicative functioning* can be expressed in a delay in or lack of development of spoken language, impaired language understanding, deficits in the use of nonverbal forms of communication, and the presence of unusual language features that may include repetitive or stereotyped speech. Language delays are present in almost all young children with autism, and are often accompanied

Table 1. Behavioral Features of Autism at Different Developmental Levels: Comparisons to Nonautistic Peers

| Feature | Developmental level | |
	Preschool and younger	School age and older
Social behavior	*Less likely to*: respond to social bids (e.g., "hard to reach"), smile responsively, look at others during interactions, engage in reciprocal back-and-forth play, show interest in other children, imitate others, direct facial expressions to others *More likely to*: focus attention on nonsocial activities/interests	*Less likely to*: initiate social bids in a socially appropriate way, understand the emotions and perspectives of others, sustain flexible, back-and-forth interactions with others, seek interactions with peers of own age *More likely to*: initiate social interactions only in relation to own interests
Language/communication	*Less likely to*: meet language milestones on time, use gestures (such as pointing, shaking head) to communicate, use eye contact during communicative acts, communicate to direct another person's attention, follow simple directions, respond to name *More likely to*: communicate by manipulating another person's hand, obtain desired objects on their own instead of communicating their needs to others	*Less likely to*: coordinate verbal and nonverbal behaviors in a flexible and spontaneous manner, use communication for social purposes (e.g., to chat), initiate and sustain conversations in a reciprocal manner, communicate for a variety of reasons *More likely to*: demonstrate literal language understanding and use, show unusual prosody (e.g., rate of speech, inflection), talk exclusively about specific areas of personal interest
Restricted activities and interests	*Less likely to*: demonstrate a broad repertoire of play activities, engage in simple doll play (e.g., feeding) *More likely to*: engage in repetitive play activities (e.g., lining up toys), focus attention on parts of objects instead of the whole object, demonstrate repetitive motor behaviors	*Less likely to*: engage in a broad range of age-appropriate interactive play/leisure activities, engage in imaginary or symbolic play, respond flexibly to transitions or changes in routines *More likely to*: insist on enactment of routines or rituals, develop an intense special interest (e.g., naval aircraft)

by a failure to communicate nonverbally through gestures or facial expressions. About 50 percent fail to acquire functional or meaningful spoken language, and must be taught to communicate using other methods, such as picture systems or augmentative devices that allow them to communicate. In those who acquire spoken language, features such as echolalia (i.e., repeating phrases heard elsewhere), concrete or overly literal language, unusual rhythm or pitch, and limited conversational skills are often present. Difficulty acquiring language is often accompanied by impoverished symbolic and imaginative play.

Restricted interests and repetitive activities may take the form of repetitive motor activities (e.g., hand-flapping or jumping), overly-focused interests (e.g., train timetables; weather in state capitals), and/or rigid adherence to routines and rituals (e.g., driving a certain route to school, eating dinner at exactly 6:00). Preoccupation with parts of objects (e.g., the wheels of a toy car) or with sensory-based repetitive play (e.g., spinning or lining up objects) are also seen. Repetitive behaviors and insistence on sameness can interfere with learning new skills and can also pose behavioral challenges to parents and teachers.

TREATMENT/OUTCOME

Individualized educational and behavioral treatments are essential for promoting optimal functioning for persons with autism. Recent research suggests that specialized early intervention can be extremely effective in promoting significant gains in social, communicative, and cognitive functioning. Intervention in the school years usually requires implementation of educational modifications (e.g., visual supports, positive routines) that capitalize on the strengths and learning styles of children with autism. Collateral therapies, such as speech-language therapy and occupational therapy are often needed. Some children with autism require intensive educational interventions involving 1:1 instruction in a highly structured environment; others benefit from being fully included in classrooms for typically developing children, with only a minimum of special educational supports. Psychopharmacological intervention targeting symptoms such as anxiety, obsessive–compulsive behaviors, attention, mood swings, or sleep disorders can sometimes be a helpful adjunct to educational and behavioral interventions. Psychotherapy aimed toward reducing anxiety or compulsive behaviors may be of benefit to older children functioning at higher cognitive levels.

Long-term outcome for individuals with autism is variable. Studies have consistently demonstrated that cognitive functioning and the acquisition of functional language by 5 years are predictive of more optimal outcomes in adulthood. Because autism is a neurobiological condition, the goals of treatment are not to "cure" the disorder, but rather to help individuals achieve optimal social, behavioral, and adaptive functioning.

See also: Asperger's Disorder; Fragile X Syndrome; Pervasive Developmental Disorder—Not Otherwise Specified; Pervasive Developmental Disorders

Further Reading

American Psychiatric Association. (2000). *Diagnostic and statistical manual of mental disorders* (4th ed., text revision). Washington, DC: Author.

Cohen, D., & Volkmar, F. R. (1997). *Handbook of autism and other pervasive developmental disorders* (2nd ed.). New York: John Wiley & Sons.

Committee on Educational Interventions for Children with Autism. (2001). *Educating children with autism*. Washington, DC: National Academy Press.

WENDY L. STONE
SUSAN L. HEPBURN

Avoidant Disorder

See: Social Phobia

Bb

Bacterial Infections

See: Pediatric Infectious Diseases

Bed Wetting

See: Enuresis

Behavior and Functional Analysis

DEFINITION

Behavior analysis refers to the process of analyzing children's behavior in terms of fundamental learning principles. Basically, there are three types of learning: (1) classical conditioning, which refers to a form of learning in which a once neutral stimulus comes to evoke an involuntary response, (2) operant conditioning, which is concerned with learning that occurs as a result of the positive or negative consequences of behavior, and (3) modeling, which pertains to the process of learning behavior through observing others. In clinical practice, behavioral analysis is part of an operant-based assessment in which a problematic target behavior and the observable antecedent and consequent environmental events that are thought to be

relevant to the target behavior are examined. Following this assessment, which is also known as a *functional analysis*, treatment focuses on altering or rearranging the antecedent and consequent stimuli that elicit or reinforce the problematic behavior.

METHOD

Behavior analysts employ a variety of assessment techniques or methods to gather information about maladaptive behaviors and the personal or environmental factors that may maintain or exacerbate them, including direct observation, self-reports, structured interviews, and, at times, psychophysiological recordings. The information is typically arranged in schematic models. The so-called antecedents–behavior–consequences (ABC) model developed by Stuart (1970) is basic but can be very useful for understanding children's behavior. In the case of Jenny, a 6-year old child with severe behavior problems, the ABC model shows that Jenny's difficult behavior at home is maintained, for the greater part, by her mother's responses (see Figure 1). More specifically, mother reinforces the oppositional behavior by giving Jenny an ice cream cone. It is interesting to note that mother's behavior, in turn, is also reinforced as Jenny stops with yelling and crying as soon as she gets her ice cream.

In a variation of the ABC model, the B component is split into three response systems: a physiological system, a cognitive system, and a behavioral system, as suggested by Lang (1968). In particular, in the case of anxiety, this model is commonly used as it nicely covers the various dimensions of this type of problem, respectively autonomic sensations (e.g., tachycardia, increased

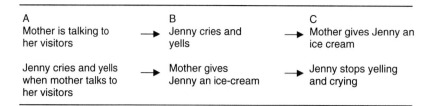

Figure 1. Example of a Functional Analysis according to the ABC Model.

respiration), catastrophic thoughts (e.g., "I am going to die"), and avoidance or escape behavior.

The more complex SORKC model suggested by Kanfer and Phillips (1970) attempts to incorporate information regarding the individual whose behavior is assessed. The acronym SORKC summarizes the components that should be assessed in order to get a full picture of a child's problem behavior: S refers to the stimulus that elicits the target behavior, O refers to the biological condition of the organism, R refers to the target behavior, K refers to the contingency relations between the target behavior and its consequences, and finally C refers to the consequences of the target behavior. Ollendick and Cerny (1981) have applied this model specifically to children and adolescents.

CLINICAL APPLICATION

For behavior therapists, the functional analysis is the hallmark of therapy. Many believe that a thorough analysis of the problem behavior yields the optimal starting point for the intervention. It should be borne in mind, however, that the functional analysis is frequently conducted by means of an informal, subjective, and unsystematic process of unknown reliability. Many of the controlling variables in a functional analysis are hypothetical constructs for which no objective test has been made in order to determine whether these variables actually control the target behavior. Moreover, the clinical utility of the functional analysis has yet to be empirically substantiated. In particular, it remains to be seen whether a functional analysis indeed increases the effectiveness of the intervention.

See also: Behavior Modification; Behavior Therapy; Cognitive-Behavior Therapy; Parent Training

Further Reading

Kanfer, F. H., & Phillips, J. S. (1970). *Learning foundations of behavior therapy.* New York: Wiley.

Lang, P. J. (1968). Fear reduction and fear behavior: Problems in treating a construct. In J. M. Schlien (Ed.), *Research in psychotherapy* (Vol. 3). Washington, DC: American Psychological Association.

Ollendick, T. H., & Cerny, J. A. (1981). *Clinical behavior therapy with children.* New York: Plenum.

Stuart, R. B. (1970). Situational versus self-control in the treatment of problematic behaviors. In R. D. Rubin (Ed.), *Advances in behavior therapy.* New York: Academic Press.

PETER MURIS

Behavior Contracts

Behavior contracts have their origins in applied behavior analysis. A behavior contract is a formal agreement, usually written, that specifies the behaviors that are required of the child and the reinforcement that will be delivered contingent on the occurrence of the desirable behavior. Often the contract will also specify inappropriate behavior and the consequences that will be delivered contingent on that behavior.

When developing a behavior contract, it is important to describe the desirable (or undesirable) behavior in specific terms. This is done in order to prevent future disputes arising regarding whether or not a particular behavior actually occurred. Equally important is for the other party to adhere to the contract. Reinforcement or punishment must be delivered promptly and be contingent on the behavior described in the contract.

Behavior contracts have been used in school settings with children who have behavior problems. Reinforcement for desirable behaviors such as prompt attendance at class and completion of work is specified, along with the punishment for behaviors such as hitting other children. One important variation of school-based contracts involves the specification of reinforcers delivered at home contingent on desirable behaviors at school. The advantage of such a contract is that reinforcers available at home are often more powerful than those available at school, for example access to television and pocket money. This is frequently referred to as a "home-school" report card.

Behavior contracts involve the establishment of rule governed behavior in the child, as they assist the child to learn to follow rules that state desired behaviors and their consequences. Technically speaking these are command rules, as the clinician controls the reinforcement that follows behavior. This is in contrast to the advice rules involved in problem solving training where the clinician does not control the consequences associated with various problem solutions, but merely provides advice about them.

See also: Applied Behavior Analysis; Parent Training; Positive Reinforcement; Rule Governed Behavior

Further Reading

Grant, L., & Evans, A. (1994). *Principles of behavior.* New York: HarperCollins.

Hudson, A. (1998). Applied behavior analysis. In A. Bellack, M. Hersen (Series Ed.), & T. Ollendick (Vol. Ed.), *Comprehensive clinical psychology (Vol. 5). Children and adolescents: Clinical formulation and treatment* (pp. 107–129). New York: Pergamon.

Kaminer, Y. (2000). Contingency management reinforcement procedures for adolescent substance abuse. *Journal of the American Academy of Child and Adolescent Psychiatry, 39,* 1324–1326.

Schoen, S. F., & James, D. A. (1991). If at first you don't succeed ... *Journal of Instructional Psychology, 18,* 273–277.

Smith, S. E. (1994). Parent-initiated contracts: An intervention for school related behaviors. *Elementary School Guidance and Counselling, 28,* 182–187.

SOPHIA XENOS
ALAN HUDSON

Behavior Modification

The procedures used in behavior modification are based on the principles of operant conditioning. Central to operant conditioning is the fact that human behavior is affected by the events that precede it (antecedents) and those that follow it (consequences). The likelihood that a particular behavior will be exhibited again in the presence of the prevailing antecedent events depends on the consequences of that behavior. If the behavior is followed by reinforcement, it is more likely to occur again. If it is not followed by reinforcement, or if it is followed by punishment, it is less likely to occur again. Behavior modification procedures typically involve the use of reinforcement or punishment to change behaviors.

The term behavior modification is sometimes used interchangeably with the term applied behavior analysis, however many authors consider that there is a difference between the two, with the former referring to an earlier and less well-developed set of procedures than the latter. Applied behavior analysis involves the identification of the antecedents and consequences that are currently associated with a particular behavior, and then systematically changing those antecedents and consequences to change the behavior. Behavior modification, on the other hand, is less concerned with identifying the antecedents and consequences that currently maintain the behavior. In contrast, it relies on the introduction of reinforcement or punishment that will be more powerful than any existing consequences, and hence overcome the effects of those consequences. Its focus is upon changing the behavior, not necessarily understanding the conditions under which it occurs.

Applied behavior analysis procedures are generally preferred to traditional behavior modification procedures as they are more likely to be effective and typically are less intrusive. Take, for example, a child who calls out in class to get the teacher's attention. A traditional behavior modification approach might involve following the calling out with a punishment such as being kept in at lunch time. An applied behavior analysis approach would recognize that the purpose of calling out was to get the teacher's attention. It would then teach the child an appropriate way of achieving this, such as by putting up his hand, and then provide reinforcement for doing so.

See also: Applied Behavior Analysis; Positive Reinforcement; Token Economies

Further Reading

Grant, L., & Evans, A. (1994). *Principles of behavior.* New York: HarperCollins.

Hudson, A. (1998). Applied behavior analysis. In A. Bellack, M. Hersen (Series Eds.), & T. Ollendick (Vol. Ed.), *Comprehensive clinical psychology (Vol. 5). Children and adolescents: Clinical formulation and treatment* (pp. 107–129). New York: Pergamon.

Mace, F. C. (1994). The significance and future of functional analysis methodologies. *Journal of Applied Behavior Analysis, 27,* 385–392.

Martin, G., & Pear, J. (1996). *Behavior modification: What it is and how to do it* (5th ed.). Englewood Cliffs, NJ: Prentice Hall.

ALAN HUDSON

Behavior Rating Scales

DEFINITION

Most behavior rating scales measure children's levels of emotional or behavioral problems; they require someone who has a close relationship with the child (e.g., parent, teacher) to report the frequency or intensity of selected behaviors. Such rating scales can be employed as part of the diagnostic process or as an index to evaluate treatment outcomes. A big advantage of behavior rating scales is that they are quick and easy to administer. For this reason, it is not surprising that pediatricians, clinical child psychologists, and school psychologists frequently include these scales in their assessment batteries.

CHILD BEHAVIOR CHECKLIST (CBCL)

One of the most frequently used behavior rating scales for measuring emotional and behavioral symptoms in children and adolescents is the Child Behavior Checklist (CBCL) developed by Achenbach (1991). The CBCL can be employed in youths between 4 and 18 years of age; it contains 118 items that measure psychopathological symptoms and 20 items that measure social competence. Parents are asked to indicate on 3-point scales the extent to which each item applies to their child: 0 = "not," 1 = "sometimes," or 2 = "often." The CBCL assesses two broad domains of psychopathology: one is externalizing, which reflects behavioral problems, and the other is internalizing, which refers to emotional problems. In addition, items can be grouped into eight so-called narrow-band scales: withdrawn, somatic complaints, anxious-depressed, social problems, thought problems, attention problems, delinquent behavior, and aggressive behavior. There are also versions of this checklist available for completion by teachers youths aged 11–18 years.

The CBCL covers a broad range of behavioral and emotional symptoms that are particularly relevant when assessing children and adolescents in clinical settings. Yet, for screening or research purposes, this questionnaire seems less useful as it is quite long and contains many items that are not relevant to the majority of children. Moreover, researchers have had difficulties replicating the eight syndrome dimensions of the CBCL and to relate them to current conceptualizations of child psychopathology.

STRENGTHS AND DIFFICULTIES QUESTIONNAIRE (SDQ)

The Strengths and Difficulties Questionnaire (SDQ) developed by Goodman (2001) contains 25 items, some positive and others negative, of which respondents are asked to indicate on a 3-point scale (0 = "not true," 1 = "somewhat true," 2 = "certainly true") how much they apply to the child being evaluated. The SDQ covers the most important current domains of child psychopathology (i.e., emotional symptoms, conduct problems, hyperactivity-inattention, and peer problems) as well as personal strengths (i.e., prosocial behavior) and can be completed by parents, teachers, and youths aged 11–16 years. The extended version of the SDQ also includes a brief impact supplement that asks the respondent whether the child has a problem, and if so, to what extent this problem causes distress, social impairment, and burden. The psychometric properties of the SDQ are satisfactory and there is good evidence indicating that it can be employed as an effective screen for child problems in community samples.

OTHER SCALES

A brief search in the literature reveals that there are many other scales for rating children's behavior. Commonly used are the Rutter Questionnaire, the Devereux Elementary School Behavior Rating Scales, Conners' Teacher Rating Scale, the Behavioral Problem Checklist, the Walker Problem Behavior Identification Checklist, and the Behavior Evaluation Scale.

RELIABILITY AND VALIDITY

Like other standardized assessment instruments, behavior rating scales should display sound psychometric properties. Thus, these scales should be reliable in terms of their internal consistency and test–retest stability. Furthermore, it seems particularly important that behavior rating scales be able to differentiate between children with and without the pertinent behavior problems and that they be sensitive to measuring treatment outcomes.

CLINICAL APPLICATION

As mentioned earlier, behavior rating scales provide information about children's (problematic) behavior in a time-efficient way. It should be borne in mind, however, that behavior ratings depend greatly upon who completes the scale and the situation in which the behavior occurs: Parents, teachers, and professionals may all disagree in rating a particular child, because they evaluate the behavior differently and encounter the child in different settings. For example, Achenbach and his colleagues (1987) demonstrated that, while agreement within categories of informants (parents, teachers) was reasonably high, agreement between informants in different categories was low. For example, the mean correlation between parents was 0.59, whereas the mean correlation between parents and teachers was only 0.27. This finding underlines the fact that it is frequently necessary to administer rating scales to various informants in order to get a more complete picture of a child's behavior.

See also: Assessment; Child Self-Reports; Developmental Issues in Assessment for Treatment; Psychometric Properties of Tests

Further Reading

Achenbach, T. M. (1991). *Manual for the Child Behavior Checklist 4–18 and 1991 profile.* Burlington, VT: University of Vermont, Department of Psychiatry.

Achenbach, T. M., McConaughy, S. H., & Howell, C. T. (1987). Child/adolescent behavioral and emotional problems: Implications of cross-informant correlations for situational specificity. *Psychological Bulletin, 101*, 213–232.

Goodman, R. (2001). Psychometric properties of the Strengths and Difficulties Questionnaire. *Journal of the American Academy of Child and Adolescent Psychiatry, 40*, 1337–1345.

Vance, H. B. (1998). *Psychological assessment of children: Best practices for school and clinical settings.* New York: Wiley.

PETER MURIS

Behavior Therapy

DEFINITION

The application of behavioral principles to the problems of children and their families has a long and rich tradition. This is a tradition that began in the early 20th century with the treatment of childhood fears and phobias, and that has continued into the 21st century to include the treatment of a wide range of pediatric and clinical child psychology problems. Nearly every problem reviewed in this Encyclopedia has been addressed, at one time or another, with behavior therapy. It is

a therapeutic medium that has enjoyed wide application and considerable empirical support.

Some authors define behavior therapy by the behavioral techniques employed in treatment (e.g., relaxation training, systematic desensitization, exposure/response prevention), whereas others define it as a system of intervention closely wedded to the basic principles of learning theory (e.g., classical conditioning, operant conditioning, vicarious conditioning—modeling). Still, others simply define it as a methodological approach to behavior change. In 1981, Ollendick and Cerny integrated these various definitions and put forth the following definition or description of behavior therapy as applied to children: "The essence of child behavior therapy, then, is that it represents a conceptual perspective of child behavior, that is, a model of behavior, that is based on empirical methodology and that focuses on the psychological problems of children and their families. Child behavior therapy rests firmly on common principles, models, and procedures of *behavioral psychology*, and specializes in the application of those models and procedures to the problems of children and their families" (p. 3). This definition remains applicable today.

A primary assumption of behavior therapy is that the proper subject matter is behavior itself rather than some hypothetical, underlying, intrapsychic process that is not available to scientific scrutiny. Within this approach, behavior is broadly defined as any measurable or observable change in a person. Historically, behavior therapists proposed three major classes or modalities of behavior: motor responses, physiological responses, and cognitive responses. Motor responses consist of overt behaviors such as walking, talking, eating, crying, and refusing to do what is requested. It is these responses to which most laypersons refer when describing "behavior." Physiological responses are those behaviors that occur internally as a function of changes in nervous system activity. Respiration, blood flow, heart rate, perspiration, and changes in electrical activity of the brain are major examples of physiological responses. Although most of these responses are not directly observable, changes in this response system are measurable with electronic or mechanical recording equipment. The third major class of behavior is cognitive. Cognitive activity includes thinking, imagining, perceiving, dreaming, and so on. Because cognitive responses are internal, private events, they are the most difficult to measure or observe independent of self-report. Still, they are measurable and important dimensions of child behavior.

In recent years, behavior therapists have also begun to study affective (i.e., emotional) responses as a fourth major class of behavior. Although many aspects of emotional responding can be captured through the motoric, physiological, and cognitive processes associated with such responding, the "quality" or experience of the emotional response might not be fully captured (e.g., how a person "feels" may be as important as what he or she thinks and what he or she does). Thus, these days all four of these response classes are included in the proper study of behavior therapy.

METHOD AND CLINICAL APPLICATION

A variety of behavioral treatment procedures have been developed over the years and most of them have been described elsewhere in this volume. Notable procedures include systematic desensitization, relaxation training, exposure/response prevention, social skills training, modeling, and parent training.

Behavior therapy procedures are closely aligned with procedures described elsewhere in this volume under the entries of cognitive-behavior therapy and operant conditioning. The primary difference in these modalities, at least historically, is that cognitive-behavior therapy tended to emphasize the cognitive response class of behavior, whereas the operant conditioning approach tended to emphasize the motoric response class of behavior. In contrast, behavior therapy from the onset emphasized multiple ways of responding, incorporating elements of all four classes of response. However, it should be noted that these were and are relative emphases only, as all three of these behavioral approaches address the four primary classes of behavior (motoric, physiological, cognitive, and affective), just in varying degrees. As a result, these three behavioral interventions are interdependent ones and not easily differentiated. The primary juncture between these approaches is their affinity to principles of behavioral psychology, adoption of an empirical methodology, and their pursuit of evidence-based practice.

EFFECTIVENESS

In general, behavior therapy interventions have been found to be a highly effective set of procedures for the treatment of most common behavioral and emotional problems of children and adolescents, as well as useful in work with children presenting with pediatric problems such as headache and recurrent abdominal pain. Principles of behavior therapy have also been found to be useful in the management of other disorders such as cancer and diabetes. In recent reviews of psychosocial treatment procedures with children and adolescents, Kendall (2000) and Schroeder and Gordon (2002) identified behavior therapy procedures as highly effective. Moreover, Ollendick and March (2003) recently noted that these procedures are as effective as pharmacological approaches in the treatment of most childhood disorders. Thus, collectively, these procedures enjoy considerable empirical support for their use.

See also: Child Psychotherapy; Cognitive-Behavior Therapy for Children; Evidence-Based Treatments; Measurement of Behavior Change; Operant Conditioning

Further Reading

Kendall, P. C. (Ed.). (2000). *Child and adolescent therapy: Cognitive behavioral procedures* (2nd ed.). New York: Guilford.
Ollendick, T. H., & Cerny, J. A. (1981). *Clinical behavior therapy with children*. New York: Plenum.
Ollendick, T. H., & March, J. S. (Eds.). (2003). *Phobic and anxiety disorders in children and adolescents: A clinician's guide to effective psychosocial and pharmacological interventions*. New York: Oxford University Press.
Schroeder, C. S., & Gordon, B. (2002). *Assessment and treatment of childhood problems: A clinician's guide*. New York: Guilford.

THOMAS H. OLLENDICK
HEATHER K. BLIER-ALVAREZ
AMIE E. GRILLS

Behavioral Dentistry

Behavioral dentistry is the use of behavior theory and technology to understand, promote, and maintain oral health behavior. Oral health behaviors involve (1) developing good oral hygiene, especially at an early age, (2) obtaining periodic prophylactic treatment, and (3) obtaining restorative treatment when needed. Serious progressive dental disease can be controlled with good oral health behavior, but cavities continue to be the most prevalent disease in children in the United States. Behavioral dentistry is a response to the need for more prevention and to broaden the focus of pediatric dentistry beyond the technical precision needed to repair or remove diseased teeth to the promotion of oral health behavior.

Behavioral dentistry has long involved collaboration with psychologists to identify the role of learning in promoting and maintaining oral health behavior. This collaboration has resulted in the development of behavioral technology designed to motivate children to engage in behaviors that will prevent oral disease and maintain a clinically healthy mouth. Research has demonstrated that simply providing information, instruction, and supervision about oral health behaviors such as tooth brushing, flossing, and rinsing with topical fluoride do not reliably produce changes in oral hygiene, while contingency management programs have proven quite effective in producing reliable and somewhat durable changes in oral hygiene. Programs that have arranged for rewards to be delivered in the home environment—targeting both frequency and quality of brushing, flossing, or rinsing—have been particularly effective. Overall, using management practices that target oral hygiene in the natural environment with both corrective and positive feedback is a critical feature for success in developing important lifelong oral health habits.

Behavioral technology has also been developed to assist the dentist with the management of children's behaviors during clinic visits that can affect the successful completion of quality restorative and preventive procedures. These strategies may involve both preparing children for the visit and managing them during the visit. Preparation procedures typically involve providing sensory and/or procedural information about what to expect during a typical visit and providing an opportunity to observe a model undergoing dental treatment. The provision of information has been called the "tell-show-do" technique (e.g., telling and showing the child what to expect before doing it) and is one of the most widely used management techniques in dentistry. In addition, many pediatric dental clinics are using an "open bay" floor plan, providing the opportunity for children to both observe other children undergoing dental treatment and to be observed by others, both of which have been found to have beneficial effects on coping during treatment.

Management procedures during dental treatment typically involve various forms of distraction and contingency management. Many dental clinics attempt to divert attention and engage children in alternative activities such as watching TV, playing video games, or listening to audiotaped music or stories. These types of distractions appear to be most effective when used as rewards for cooperative, calm, coping behavior. Indeed, having at least some consequences for cooperative as well as uncooperative behavior offer the most reliable means of managing behavior once dental treatment has begun. Dentists using empirically supported management techniques rely on frequent and immediate praise, touch, and brief breaks from treatment for cooperative behavior, while using a firm voice

and redirection for uncooperative behavior. Delayed (i.e., end of treatment) consequences not tied to specific behaviors fail to teach children how to cope or improve behavior while immediate feedback, especially positive, helps establish more adaptive coping behavior.

The acceptability of the management techniques of behavioral dentistry are under close scrutiny. The techniques of behavioral dentistry are now held to the "reasonable patient" standard, which requires that the dentist discuss with the patient or parents all information that a reasonable person might consider important to deciding whether or not to consent to use of such techniques. Standards for disclosure support the patient's right to choose to refuse altogether any objectionable aspect of behavior management techniques, even if it seems unreasonable to the dentist. Although the techniques described above have all been found to be generally acceptable to parents and children, acceptability does not equate with consent. The most rigorous consent scenario is one in which the dentist provides to the parent a verbal, interpersonal description of each behavior management technique that might be used.

See also: Behavior Modification; Developmental Issues in Treatment; Pain Management; Treatment Adherence: Medical

Further Reading

Allen, K. D., Hodges, E., & Knudsen, S. (1995). Comparing four methods to inform parents about child behavior management: how to inform for consent. *Pediatric Dentistry, 17*(3), 180–186.

Kuhn, B. R., & Allen, K. D. (1994). Expanding child behavior management technology in pediatric dentistry: A behavior science perspective. *Pediatric Dentistry, 16*, 13–17.

Pinkham, J. R. (2000). Behavior management of children in the dental office. *Dental Clinics of North America, 44*(3), 471–486.

KEITH D. ALLEN

Behavioral Diaries

DEFINITION

Behavioral diaries are a form of assessment that require children to self-monitor and systematically record a wide range of target behaviors (e.g., anxious thoughts, social contacts, adherence to medication regimes, etc.).

METHODS

Occurrence of virtually any behavior of interest may be recorded through behavioral diary techniques. A distinct advantage of the behavioral diary is that it affords an opportunity for systematic recording of information regarding behaviors that might otherwise be inaccessible to the clinician or researcher. Behaviors that are particularly difficult for an outside observer to gain access include covert thoughts ("all my classmates think I am stupid") and physiological states (dizziness, stomach distress, headaches). Behaviors that occur only in a limited context (bedtime tantrums, nightmares) also are particularly well suited to diary methods.

The typical behavioral diary approach involves providing the child with a structured diary in which information is recorded in a paper-and-pencil format. However, the use of more advanced technology has become increasingly popular in data collection strategies. Clients and research participants can be telephoned on a daily or weekly basis depending on the relative frequency of the target behaviors in question. This enables the therapist or researcher to be assured that data is actually recorded in reasonable proximity to the occurrence of the behaviors. The use of on-line or web-based computer programs for data collection is on the rise and is expected to increase in use as more households are equipped with computers and internet service. Ideally, an encryption program should be used to maintain the security and privacy of data submitted through electronic means. Another technology-based diary approach is to provide children with an electronic personal digital assistant (PDA, such as the popular Palm® devices) on which a data collection program has been stored. PDAs have the advantage of being small enough to go almost anywhere with the child, thus facilitating timely data recording.

RELIABILITY/VALIDITY

Behavioral diaries hold a distinct advantage in that data may be conducted on an ongoing basis as behavior occurs, and thus may be less prone to bias than data obtained through retrospective reporting over a specified interval. Issues of selective recall are particularly problematic when working with children experiencing affective symptoms as they may unintentionally over- or under-report frequency of certain events when asked to report after a significant time delay. For instance, if a child is feeling particularly sad or lonely on the day

they present for their treatment session, they may inform the therapist that they had little social contact with peers over the previous week. However, behavioral diary methods may indicate that the child actually was approached by peers and asked to join in social activities on 4 out of 5 school days for which data was recorded. Although the idiosyncratic nature of diary development and implementation does not lend itself to standard psychometric interpretation across the literature, diary methods generally are regarded as possessing high construct validity. In terms of reliability, high interrater agreement generally has been reported for categorizations of data obtained through behavioral diary methods.

CLINICAL APPLICATIONS

Behavioral diaries are especially well suited to the area of child anxiety, given the covert nature of much of the symptom presentation. Thus, it is not surprising that this is an area in which the use of diaries has become increasingly common. Beidel and her colleagues (1991) developed a Daily Diary to assess anxious responding in children presenting with social fears. The Daily Diary asks children to record whether or not any events occurred in a given day that made the child feel anxious. For each event, children record the time, location, specific event, and their behavioral response to the event. Common events (had to read aloud in class), locations (school), responses (felt scared, but did what I was asked), and coping strategies (told myself it would be okay, everyone gets a little nervous reading aloud) are provided on the diary form as examples, as well as options for "other" responses. Additionally, children are asked to provide a rating on a 5-point scale to describe how anxious they felt (with each point on the scale accompanied by a graphic depiction of a gender neutral child figure who is smiling at one end of the continuum and appears quite distressed at the other). The Daily Diary has been developed in pictorial and standard written formats. The pictorial format is suggested for use with younger children who have limited reading and/or writing ability. Generally, moderate compliance has been found for Daily Diary completion. However, compliance rates tend to increase substantially when incentives are provided for daily completion.

Behavioral diary methods are gaining acceptance in a wide variety of pediatric settings. For example, diaries may be useful in monitoring of adherence to medical procedures (e.g., use of asthma inhalers) and wellness routines (e.g., exercise and nutritional intake). Diary data is used to obtain baseline information on adherence and to assist in the development of targeted interventions. Likewise, behavioral diaries serve as highly relevant and specific measures of treatment outcome. Diaries can be highly individualized. It is up to the professional to determine what data is most important to record for each child—and by what method. Such flexibility is a significant advantage, making behavioral diaries an important component of any comprehensive assessment package.

See also: Behavioral Observation; Behavior Rating Scales; Psychological Testing

Further Reading

Beidel, D. C., Neal, A. M., & Lederer, A. S. (1991). The feasibility and validity of a daily diary for the assessment of anxiety in children. *Behavior Therapy, 22*, 505–517.
Quittner, A. L. (2000). Improving assessment in child clinical and pediatric psychology: Establishing links to process and functional outcomes. In D. Drotar (Ed.), *Handbook of research in pediatric and clinical child psychology: Practical strategies and methods* (pp. 119–143). New York: Kluwer Academic/Plenum.

TRACY L. MORRIS

Behavioral Genetics

Behavioral Genetics is the branch of genetic science, commonly directed by medical geneticists (typically PhDs), that endeavors to identify the specific genes (genotype) that underlie individual differences in human behavior and personality (phenotype). The process can involve a number of different processes, including conducting candidate gene studies (i.e., looking specially at genes thought to be involved), conducting family-based linkage studies (i.e., studying large populations to allow novel genetic loci to be identified), conducting adoption and twin studies (i.e., comparing twins reared together with those reared apart), and conducting animal studies (i.e., using animal models with similar or related behaviors). Although twin and adoption studies consistently implicate the importance of environmental influences in the development of individual differences, high heritability estimates are believed to provide justification for molecular genetic studies aimed at identifying the specific genes and groups of genes influencing human behavior. In many cases the genetic mechanisms are thought to be complex, with susceptibility resulting from the combined actions of several genes. Recent efforts have identified

probable and multiple genetic loci underlying specific behaviors such as novelty seeking and tic disorders as well as susceptibility for behavioral syndromes such as addictive disorders (e.g., alcoholism, opioid dependence, and nicotine use), attention deficit disorder, and autism.

See also: Genetic Counseling; Parenting Practices; Risk and Protective Factors

Further Reading

Rimoin, D. L. Connor, J. M., Pyeritz, R. E., Korf, B. R. (Eds.) (2002). *Principles and practice of medical genetics* (Vol. 3). London: Churchill Livingstone.

KEITH D. ALLEN

Behavioral Observation

DEFINITION

Behavioral observation of children is the recording of their observable responses or behaviors. Observations may not only yield important information about the behavior of an individual child; they are also a crucial source of data for child research. Several famous scientists have based their theory on behavioral observations of their own children. For example, Darwin (1877) kept a daily record of the early development of his eldest son, and by comparing these data with those observed in other species, he tried to support his thesis of human evolution. Similarly, Piaget's observations of his children's development were the basis for his influential theory of cognitive development.

METHOD

Behavioral observation requires a structured set of rules for extracting information from the stream of behavior. These rules specify the target events or behaviors, the observation settings, and the observers; they also specify how the events are sampled, the dimension on which observed behavior is scored, and how the data are recorded.

An adequate definition of the target events or behaviors should be objective and should refer to directly observable components of the target behavior (e.g., counting the number of vocal tics within 1 hr, measuring the duration of a temper tantrum). Furthermore, the definition should be clear, unambiguous, and easily understood, so that any observer can accurately paraphrase it. Finally, the definition should require little or no inference, even when used across a variety of observation settings.

Behavioral observations can be conducted in naturalistic settings such as the child's home or school or in more controlled settings such as the researcher's laboratory or the clinician's office. When problems are limited to a specific environment, such as school problems or discrete phobias, or when the frequency of the behavior is relatively stable across various settings, observation in a single setting may be appropriate. However, many behaviors are susceptible to specific environmental influences, and as a result their frequency may fluctuate considerably across settings. Therefore, more representative data are usually obtained by conducting observations in multiple settings.

Observers can be categorized according to their level of participation with the observed behavior. At one extreme, there are nonparticipant (independent) observers whose only task is to collect data about the child's behavior. At the other extreme, there are self-observations conducted by the target child himself or herself. Intermediate levels of participant-observation are represented by significant others, such as parents or teachers, who are normally present in the setting where the observations take place.

Several procedures can be used to carry out systematic behavioral observations. The most accurate procedure is real-time observation. With this procedure, behavior frequency and duration are both recorded on the basis of their occurrence in an uninterrupted, natural time period. However, most behaviors cannot be observed and recorded continuously. Thus, partial records must suffice and the time in which observations are conducted must be sampled. There are various sampling procedures that can be used for this purpose. The most frequently used procedures when observing children are event sampling and time sampling. *Event sampling* is especially used when observing low-frequency behaviors. During this procedure, each occurrence of the target behavior within an observation session is registered, eventually in combination with the duration of the behavior. *Time sampling* is predominantly employed in the case of high-frequency behavior. With this procedure, an observation session is divided into brief intervals, and the observation category is scored if the relevant target behavior occurs within any part of the interval.

Frequency and duration are the most commonly used dimensions on which observed behavior is scored. Another dimension that can be employed is intensity. For example, when observing a child's physical aggression, one could add an additional dimension by which the intensity of the aggressive behavior could be scored (e.g., "other person was not hit," "other person was hit but had no observable physical damage," "other person was hit and there was physical damage").

Simple paper-and-pencil recording forms remain the most commonly used tool for collecting observation data. Video recorders can be employed when the presence of observers is disturbing or when the behaviors to be observed are so complex that repeated examination of the behavior is necessary. In some instances, computers may be helpful for analyzing videotaped behaviors.

RELIABILITY AND VALIDITY

Reliability issues are relevant to all assessment methods, including behavioral observations. Besides internal consistency and temporal stability, *interobserver agreement* is a crucial aspect of determining the reliability of behavioral observations. Interobserver agreement refers to the consistency of ratings among two or more observers who score the same behavior independently. Statistically, this type of reliability is expressed in percentage of agreement, kappa (i.e., percentage of agreement corrected for chance), or a correlation coefficient. As a rule, 80 percent agreement and 0.60 for kappa and reliability coefficients are considered as acceptable levels for interobserver reliability.

An important measurement error that may occur during the process of behavioral observation is *observer bias*. This bias is concerned with (1) observers' expectancies (e.g., observers might record how children should behave according to the hypotheses of an investigation) and (2) the information processing limitations of observers (e.g., observers have the tendency to impose patterns of regularity on otherwise complex data).

Behavioral observation often is an intrusive assessment method. The presence of an observer may represent a novel stimulus that can produce atypical responses from children. This reaction to being observed is defined as *reactivity* and should be regarded as a potential threat to the accuracy or validity of the observation. For example, children have the tendency to inhibit socially undesirable or private behaviors when they are aware of being observed, thereby significantly affecting the recording of such behaviors.

CLINICAL APPLICATIONS

Behavioral observation is a relatively laborious, time-consuming, and hence expensive assessment method. However, such observations are imperative when assessing young or mentally handicapped children, or when measuring complex behavior patterns or events that children are unwilling to report. In clinical settings, systematic observations may be helpful during the diagnostic process, as they can yield important additional information about the target behavior apart from what is reported by children themselves or by their parents. Furthermore, behavioral observations are useful when evaluating treatment progress or outcome as it becomes possible to determine the extent to which the child's behavior has actually changed.

See also: Behavior Therapy; Screening Instruments: Behavioral and Developmental; Test Bias; Reliability; Validity

Further Reading

Darwin, C. (1877). A biographical sketch of an infant. *Mind, 2,* 285–294.
Gelfand, D. M., & Hartmann, D. P. (1984). *Child behavior analysis and therapy.* New York: Pergamon.
Martin, P., & Bateson, P. (1986). *Measuring behaviour: An introductory guide.* New York: Cambridge University Press.
Piaget, J. (1954). *The construction of reality in the child.* New York: Basic Books.

PETER MURIS

Behavioral Screening

See: Screening Instruments: Behavioral and Developmental

Bereavement

DEFINITION

Bereavement describes the process that occurs when people lose someone or something significant to them. While the loss often refers to a death, genuine bereavement may also occur in situations such as a divorce, disaster, significant injury, or geographical move. The terms bereavement, grief, and mourning are often used interchangeably. In general, however, the term bereavement refers to the overall experience of loss. Grief or sorrow, the subjective state of bereavement,

characterizes the individual, personal reaction associated with the loss. Mourning, which historically referred to the psychological work of bereavement, has become a term used in the literature and by the general population to describe behaviors in response to grief (i.e., to be "in mourning"). Social, cultural, political, familial, and religious contexts often define the character of and specific behaviors associated with mourning. Examples from different cultures can include sitting shiva, waking the deceased, celebratory meals, selecting clothing or bathing the deceased, and wearing black or white.

Although no formally acknowledged diagnostic category of bereavement exists, many researchers believe that development of criteria to establish a standardized clinical description would further the understanding of this process. While bereavement and grief share some symptoms and criteria with recognized categories of psychopathology, such as depression and posttraumatic stress disorder, they do not indicate psychopathology per se.

Modifiers of the term "bereavement" often include "uncomplicated" (or "simple" or "normal"), "complicated," "traumatic," and "pathological." In uncomplicated bereavement, losses tend to follow the natural course of life with a degree of predictability (e.g., the death of an elderly or chronically ill family member). Often, the nature of the child's or families' suffering as a result of the loss in such contexts lightens or reflects a degree of relief in the changes (e.g., reduced suffering). Children and families in uncomplicated bereavement maintain social connections, reinvest in new relationships and activities, and gradually reenter life's routines. They adapt to a changed, meaningful life and do not experience persistent or incapacitating symptoms. Their coping skills in dealing with grief and mourning work effectively.

Complicated bereavement usually involves extraordinary loss (e.g., abrupt death of a sibling, sudden desertion of a marriage and family by a parent). In such situations levels of disbelief run high, and coping abilities are severely stressed. Complicated bereavement that involves traumatic grief takes on the added properties of trauma symptoms (including profound distress, fearfulness, shock, panic, and detachment) and intense longing for the lost object or person. Coping mechanisms are overwhelmed. Traumatic grief can occur in situations like the Oklahoma City federal building bombing, the events of September 11, 2001, missing children, multiple losses (fires, floods), and fatal accidents. The term "pathological" grief is often used to describe a complicated loss in which the bereft person experiences prolonged and marked emotional, social, and functional impairment (e.g., profound, recurrent hallucinatory experiences of the deceased or complete denial of the loss event). Children and families experiencing complicated bereavement should seek psychological intervention.

PRESENTATION OF BEREAVEMENT

Children and families confront loss regularly in a variety of ways. Normal life loss events such as relocation, divorce, or pets' dying, confront all children. Even childhood entertainment, such as movies (e.g., *The Lion King*) or books (e.g., the orphaned *Harry Potter*) routinely address issues of grief and loss. Such events raise questions of dealing with bereavement and create natural exposure to death and separation issues with concomitant teaching moments.

Intimate, personal loss of a loved one may also occur in childhood. The death of a family member is, inevitably, the most difficult of emotional losses for a child. Secondary losses and concurrent stressors occur as a result of a family death (e.g., change in income, possible relocation, alteration of routines, less physical and emotional availability of family members) and contribute to the child's grief response.

Children must also occasionally confront bereavement as a result of their own life-threatening or terminal illness. Grief reactions may also occur in children with handicaps or medical trauma (e.g., loss of limb, paralysis). Open communication between the child, the parents, and health care providers about the illness and its management is often imperative for the child to feel comfortable to discuss fears, anxieties, and questions.

Virtually every child in America will witness at least one disaster that involves death. Such disasters may be natural (e.g., earthquakes, floods, or tornadoes) or man-made (e.g., neighborhood violence, school shootings, or terrorist attacks). Exposure to such events occurs either directly or through the news media. Children who experience the simultaneous occurrence of tragic loss of a loved one and direct exposure to the catastrophic event are vulnerable to complicated bereavement and subsequent development of trauma symptoms. Even children not immediately affected by the event may experience adverse psychological effects from repetitive news coverage.

DEVELOPMENTAL CONSIDERATIONS

Bereavement in children correlates directly to developmental levels and efforts to make sense of or master the concept and experience of death and loss. Debate

has existed in the psychoanalytic literature as to what extent children have the capacity to understand death and to grieve; however, research over recent decades has demonstrated that even very young children experience the powerful feelings of sadness, pain, anger, and loneliness commonly associated with bereavement.

Infants experience primitive separation distress at the physical and emotional withdrawal of a nurturing caretaker. Protest, despair, and detachment are considered the classic response to separation and loss. As object permanence develops, the beginning concepts of loss can be seen in games such as "All gone." Common symptoms of loss include irritability, lethargy, and, in more severe cases, failure to thrive.

In the preschool-aged child, egocentric and prelogical thinking predominates. The child does not understand concepts of time, space, measurement, or movement and lacks comprehension of cause and effect. Magical thinking can cause the child to question the reason for the loss ("Did she die because I was mad at her?") as well as the permanency of death ("If I'm very good, maybe he'll come back."). Death is experienced in the here and now. Preschoolers seem most worried about the duration of separation from the loved one that death implies, and may view death as a form of life under changed circumstances (e.g., separation, departure, or sleep). Bereavement symptoms in young children are demonstrated in intermittent, affective shifts over brief periods of time. Asking the same questions in a repeated and unrelenting manner, in an attempt to master the finality of the loss, typifies this age group. Grief responses show a full range of feelings, including longing, sadness, anger, guilt, and blame. Common symptoms include somatic complaints (e.g., stomachaches) and regression in recently attained developmental tasks (e.g., wish to sleep with parents, loss of bladder control).

The school-aged child, with an increasing understanding of the biological functioning of the body, recognizes the permanency of death. Their thinking, however, remains literal and concrete. Concepts of death begin with visible signs (e.g., the deceased no longer breathes or moves) and progress to loss of higher function (e.g., the deceased no longer thinks). This child uses information gleaned from the media, peers, and parents to form their impressions of death and dying. School and learning problems may surface, often in relation to preoccupation with the loss. Anxiety, overt symptoms of depression, and somatic complaints such as stomachaches occur more often in this age group than in younger children.

Death becomes an abstract concept in adolescence. Theological and philosophical elements of death and loss become relevant as the teenager begins to think abstractly and symbolically. Teenagers understand complex structures and systems of the body, providing a physiological understanding of the reason for death. Responses to grief include depression, resentment, rage, mood swings, and risk-taking behaviors. Fascination with dramatic or romanticized death and suicide sometimes occurs and may find expression in copycat behavior (e.g., cluster suicides) as well as competitive behavior ("He was *my* best friend.") An increased bodily interest and narcissism may contribute to highly somatic grief responses. Such somatic symptoms may occur as the immediate perceptions described in younger children, but also may reflect more pathologically complex syndromes (e.g., eating disorders, conversion disorders).

ASSESSMENT

Not all children require intensive professional intervention during or following a loss event. However, common symptoms such as sadness, yearning, and loneliness can be distressing to the child. Parents should make adequate help available and grant children permission to, seek such assistance. Children cope best in homes where caretakers can meet the child's needs, allow honest and accurate discussion about the loss, and provide safety and consistency in life patterns. Assessment of premorbid functioning of the child and family and the influence of family and community support provides clues to adjustment and emotional security. The major goal of identifying a child at risk following a loss should focus on preventing psychopathology and maladaptive grief responses.

RISK FACTORS

No specific sign, symptom, or cluster of behaviors identifies the bereaved child or family in need of help. Duration, frequency, intensity, and severity of the presenting symptoms, however, are important variables to consider in assessing risk. Absence of any symptoms of grief, specifically an inability to discuss the loss or to express sadness and related feelings, should also be viewed with suspicion. In children, symptoms that interfere with normal activities of daily living or compromise attainment of age-appropriate developmental tasks are indications for further evaluation. Examples of behaviors that would raise a red flag include persistent physiological complaints of undetermined origin (headache, sleep disturbance); school/academic/work difficulties (declining grades, social withdrawal); or

psychological factors (persistent guilt or blame, trauma symptoms, desire to die or talk of suicide, self-abuse, severe separation distress). Also consider the conditions under which the loss occurred when evaluating risk. For example, traumatic loss, unexpected or sudden death, or multiple losses often exacerbate bereavement.

INTERVENTIONS

Numerous therapeutic interventions can allow children and families to explore behaviors and express feelings, to manage social isolation, and to foster healthy bereavement.

Psychoeducational interventions help to demystify death and dying, to explain reactions to grief, and to facilitate problem-solving. Sharing basic grief tenets (There is no right or wrong way to grieve. Everyone grieves differently.) often assists families with different coping styles or cultural beliefs. Explaining developmental differences and the need to use clear, age-appropriate language with children can assist in responding to children's questions and actions. Parents and children often need practical help and suggestions, such as how to involve the children in mourning rituals or what to do with the belongings of the deceased. Resources to offer the family might include books (both fiction and nonfiction), support groups, therapists, and community assistance.

Behavioral techniques can be useful as part of a comprehensive treatment program to manage grief reactions such as panic, sleep disturbance, or unrelenting anxiety. Traditional approaches to behavioral change, such as relaxation techniques, also help. In addition, cognitive-behavioral techniques can help children and families when obsessive ruminating over the deceased or a feeling of hopelessness occurs. Reframing, reformulating, and restructuring of worrisome or negative thoughts (e.g., "He wouldn't have died if I had gone with him that day.") have significant value. Such techniques especially help people whose sense of safety and security suffers as the result of disasters or severe traumatic loss.

The application of psychodynamic principles, which includes play therapy in young children, allows the child and family to process the loss, to deal with uncontrollable feelings, to address maladaptive defenses, and to provide insight into grief reactions. Psychodynamically oriented trauma work (e.g., empowering, creating a safe and hopeful environment, working on being a survivor and not a victim) will specifically assist those children and families who have experienced horrific loss.

Parents will often ask about the use of medication to assist in grief work. Psychopharmacological agents are not a cure and do not make the grief go away. Medication may help to relieve acute symptoms (e.g., intense hyperarousal, profound sadness, severe sleep disturbance) and to provide the emotional energy to mourn. The child and family need to understand, however, that the psychological work of grief still must occur and that this work progresses best when done in conjunction with some form of therapy.

The type of therapeutic service selected, in which to provide interventions for the bereft child, should depend upon the specific needs presented by the child and family. However, all modalities should provide a safe place for children to share feelings and where their grief will feel normal. Therapeutic services may benefit an entire family or individual members. Support or self-help groups focus on specific types of loss (e.g., death of a parent, suicide, divorce) and provide an opportunity to talk with other people who have experienced similar losses. Family counseling offers an intervention and opportunity to discuss differences in coping style and pacing of grief, where enhanced mutual support and communication grows, and where family members can share memories and say goodbye together. Couples therapy may help parents who need assistance in managing their children's grief and who struggle with marital issues related to coping with their loss. Individual treatment may help the child (or parent) who struggles with communicating needs and feelings with others or who has unique grief-related symptoms which require intensive intervention. Combinations of approaches may work well for children with evolving needs. For example, a child may participate in family therapy to deal with the loss of a sibling and also use individual treatment to address issues of personal anxiety, guilt, and ambivalence related to the death.

Children coping with a loss in the community may benefit from constructive activities that enable conversation about or activate coping with their grief. For example, sending a card or offering food to relatives of the deceased can help children learn the etiquette of behaviors and mourning rituals around bereavement. The child might perform community service or join charitable organizations, such as fund-raising in memory of the deceased. In the wake of a disaster, parents and older children can give blood or volunteer in search and recovery efforts. When a loss does not involve an actual death, such as a geographical move, empowering the child to plan a "new kids in town" party or write an essay for school or the local paper on "ways to help new kids" might help. Such activities help facilitate meaning in the loss, encourage positive remembering and memorializing, and move the child away from a sense of helplessness and hopelessness.

PROGNOSIS

Bereavement is a process that may continue for years after the loss. The belief that one must "get over" a loss has been replaced with an understanding that some form of a continuing relationship with the lost person or object is not associated with pathology and is often a great source of comfort. While acute grief symptoms subside in healthy bereavement, special occurrences (e.g., holidays, anniversaries, a song) may cause a resurfacing of the loss with accompanying bittersweet memories. Maintaining an inner representation of the deceased person or even feeling a "presence" is often a solace. An example would be a child who maintains a bond with his deceased parent as a form of reference, guidance, and support (e.g., "My mom would tell me she's proud.") "Talking" with the deceased, either through prayer, an inner dialogue, or reminiscing with friends and family can be a positive experience. The more complicated and traumatic a grief reaction, the harder it is for the child and family to recover. And with some events, such as September 11, 2001 or the suicide bombings in the Middle East, we all must actively remember.

See also: Acute Stress Disorder; Adolescence; Behavior Modification; Childhood; Child Psychotherapy; Cognitive–Behavioral Play Therapy; Cognitive-Behavior Therapy; Developmental Issues in Assessment for Treatment; Developmental Issues in Treatment; Infancy; Psychodynamic Therapy; Posttraumatic Stress Disorder

Further Reading

Gudas, L. S., & Koocher, G. P. (2001). Children with grief. In C. E. Walker & M. C. Roberts (Eds.), *Handbook of clinical child psychology* (3rd ed., pp. 1046–1056), New York: Wiley.

Melvin, D., & Lukeman, D. (2000). Bereavement: A framework for those working with children. *Clinical Child Psychology and Psychiatry, 5,* 521–539.

Stroebe, M. S., Hansson, R. O., Stroebe, W., & Schut, H. (Eds.). (2001). *Handbook of bereavement research.* Washington, DC: American Psychological Association.

LINDA SAYLOR GUDAS
GERALD P. KOOCHER

Biofeedback

DEFINITION

Biofeedback is any process in which an external device generates information to an individual about his or her physiological responses. The "bio" feedback allows the child to then regulate these responses so the response can become more adaptive. The targeted physiological response may be any response that can be measured by an external device. The most common responses targeted are muscle tension, heart rate, skin temperature, and galvanic skin response. The feedback may occur in a variety of forms, the most common being visual and auditory. The feedback may be continuous, intermittent, or provided once a threshold or criterion is crossed.

METHOD

Biofeedback should be used within a psychotherapeutic context. This means that a psychological evaluation should indicate that biofeedback is a viable treatment option for the child. Biofeedback should be used clinically only after a competent medical evaluation has been conducted to rule out health problems that may need to be treated medically. Patients coming directly to psychologists for biofeedback or other behavioral treatments of physical disorders should be referred first to a physician for a thorough medical examination.

A typical biofeedback treatment plan involves 8 to 12 sessions, 1-hr long. Initially the sessions are scheduled twice a week for the first 2 weeks and then spread out over the next 2–3 months. This schedule allows the child to learn the technique quickly and then focus on self-control and home practice for generalization.

A basic biofeedback session includes the following: (1) a review of home practice and discussion of changes that may be occurring between sessions, (2) baseline measurement of the physiological response to be targeted, (3) feedback is then given to an individual with some sort of instruction to manipulate the physiological response, (4) review of the biofeedback session with the child—and at times the parent—by comparing the baseline physiological response to the response during biofeedback, and (5) instructions for home practice.

Research studies indicate that initial feedback should be salient to the child, continuous, and given when even small changes are made. As the child learns to manipulate the response, feedback can be contingent on greater change and may be given intermittently. The clinician can experiment with a variety of forms of feedback. Many children prefer audio feedback as they can close their eyes while trying to relax.

It is important to include segments of self-control training in which the feedback is turned off and the individual is instructed to continue to manipulate the response without feedback. As the child masters the

physiological response, the therapist may also have the child image situations that might be stressful while continuing the feedback so that the child can learn to moderate her or his response during stressful situations.

Although children tend to be responsive to biofeedback, they may have greater difficulty than adults in remembering to practice outside the therapeutic setting and to record systematic changes in their symptoms. A parent can be instructed to gently remind the child to practice and record symptoms. Research also indicates that home practice is necessary for lasting changes to occur. Practicing self-control of the physiological response 10–20 min, several times a week is recommended. It is best to have the child plan out the practice schedule ahead of time and to practice earlier in the day. If the child waits until right before he goes to sleep he may fall asleep during the practice. As the child gets better at controlling the response, he or she should be encouraged to do this while continuing normal activities.

CLINICAL APPLICATIONS

A major use of biofeedback is to teach relaxation skills. A second use of biofeedback is to alter pathophysiological processes. Examples might be manipulation of temporal artery blood flow or sympathetic nervous system arousal for migraine headache, decrease flow of gastric juices for ulcers, decrease muscle tension, and increase proper posture for the chronic back pain.

Biofeedback should be considered as a therapeutic tool that can help introduce the child to therapy in a concrete and nonthreatening manner. It can be especially useful for the child who focuses on physical problems or insists his problems are not psychological. Biofeedback can also be used to increase feelings of self-efficacy and self-control. During a biofeedback session, the child can begin talking about feelings and stresses and how these may affect physical health. The child learns quickly the connection between emotions, thoughts, and physiological responses.

Biofeedback may be used when there are no viable medical alternatives if the physician determines that medication should not be used. Sometimes parents or the child do not want medication and biofeedback may become the treatment of choice. For example, a child with migraine headaches may have to use pain medication to control the pain for the rest of his or her life because there are no other medical treatments to reduce the pain. The patient may choose biofeedback to help cope and reduce the pain instead of taking pain medication, which is addictive and may have undesirable side effects.

Biofeedback has also been used in modifying behavioral problems. Two examples are hyperactivity associated with attention deficit disorder and maladaptive behaviors that are associated with mental retardation. Motor responses may be monitored using biofeedback and the child is rewarded as the problem behavior decreases.

EFFECTIVENESS

In general, children are more open and responsive to biofeedback than adults. Children are usually fascinated with the equipment, and motivation and curiosity are high. Research on nonclinical populations' response to biofeedback indicate that children between the ages of 8–12 are able to achieve greater changes in physiological responses using biofeedback than any other age group. For children with clinical problems, biofeedback may be a good alternative to medication if the medical treatment has potentially negative short- and long-term consequences for the developing child. Research evaluating the effectiveness of biofeedback with children who have headaches indicate more children improve, and to a greater degree, than adults.

Studies indicate that changes in symptoms come slowly, with most changes occurring 4–6 weeks after biofeedback therapy has begun. It is important to explain to the child and family that biofeedback does not work like most medication and that changes occur slowly and often accompany a real change in the child's behavior and attitude about the problem and how to cope with it. Also biofeedback may not eliminate the symptoms but it may reduce the intensity, frequency, and/or medication usage.

Biofeedback may be particularly useful for children, as they can cognitively understand concrete examples of what is happening in their bodies as compared to relaxation training that may be more abstract. In a culture that provides video games, robots, computers, and other hi-tech games and toys for children, they are usually attracted and eager to participate in the biofeedback session.

See also: Coping with Illness; Life Stress in Children and Adolescents; Pain Management; Relaxation Training; Self-Management

Further Reading

Andrasik, F. (1994). Twenty-five years in progress: Twenty-five more? *Biofeedback and self-regulation, 19*, 311–324.
Labbé, E. (1998). Biofeedback. In Friedman, H. A. (Ed.) *Encyclopedia of mental health*. New York: Academic Press.
Schwartz, M. S. (1995). *Biofeedback: A practitioner's guide* (2nd ed.). New York: Guilford.

ELISE E. LABBÉ

Bipolar Disorder

DESCRIPTION

Individuals with bipolar disorder experience both the "high" of mania and the "low" of depression. There are three main subtypes of bipolar disorder: Bipolar-I, Bipolar-II, and Bipolar-NOS (Not Otherwise Specified). Bipolar-I can be distinguished from the others by the presence of one or more manic or mixed episodes. A manic episode is defined by at least one week of abnormally and persistently elevated, expansive, or irritable mood. Additional symptoms may include inflated self-esteem, decreased need for sleep, pressured speech, flight of ideas, distractibility, increased motor activity, and excessive involvement in pleasurable activities. A mixed episode is defined by the presence of symptoms of both a manic and a depressive episode nearly every day for at least one week. Common symptoms include agitation, insomnia, appetite dysregulation, and suicidal thinking.

Bipolar-II involves a clinical course characterized by at least one depressive and at least one hypomanic episode. A hypomanic episode involves less severe symptoms for at least four days. While there is an observable change in the individual's functioning, the disturbance does not cause marked distress or impairment.

Bipolar-NOS is reserved for cases where the individual does not fully meet the criteria for Bipolar-I or Bipolar-II, but exhibits bipolar features. Often, individuals diagnosed with Bipolar-NOS have rapid cycling between manic and depressive symptoms, such that minimal duration criteria are not met for a manic or a depressive episode. Children with Bipolar-NOS are typically described as irritable and aggressive.

Children may be accurately assessed using the adult criteria for bipolar disorder. However, researchers have identified phenotypic differences between adult-onset and early-onset bipolar disorder. To begin with, adults usually experience mania during their initial episode, while children usually experience depression first. While adults typically experience discrete episodes of mania or depression that last 2–9 months, children usually experience longer episodes with rapid cycling (i.e., frequent changes back and forth from mania to depression) and/or mixed mania (i.e., co-occurring mania and depression). Some children with bipolar disorder cycle numerous times in a single day. One minute such a child could feel happy and giddy, the next minute, sad and withdrawn. This is referred to as ultradian cycling. By and large, childhood bipolar disorder is more of a chronic problem. Children are less likely than adults to have well periods between episodes.

ASSESSMENT

Structured diagnostic interviews that can aid in diagnosing bipolar disorder include the Diagnostic Interview Schedule for Children (DISC), Diagnostic Interview for Children and Adolescents–Revised (DICA–R), and Children's Interview for Psychiatric Syndromes (ChIPS). A semistructured interview commonly used in research on bipolar disorder is the Schedule for Affective Disorders and Schizophrenia for School-Age Children (K-SADS). The WASH-U-KSADS (Washington University K-SADS) includes additional questions regarding childhood mania. The Mania Rating Scale (MRS) is the only clinical rating scale for the severity of mania empirically tested in children. Finally, any assessment instrument should be accompanied by a clinical interview of the parent(s) and child to determine symptom onset, offset, and duration for moods; anxiety, behavior, and other disorders; as well as developmental history, family history, medical history, and social history.

DIFFERENTIAL DIAGNOSIS

It is important both to determine whether (1) symptoms of bipolar disorder can be better explained by other diagnoses and (2) what independent diagnoses may co-occur with bipolar disorder. For instance, hypersexuality may occur in children who have been sexually abused and/or in children who are manic. Similarly, children who are manic and are exhibiting very poor judgment may appear to have conduct disorder, although all their "antisocial" behavior may be confined to periods of abnormal mood. Other children with severe bipolar disorder with psychotic features may be misdiagnosed with schizophrenia. Furthermore the effects of illegal drugs or medications may mimic aspects of bipolar disorder. In diagnosing bipolar disorder, it is important to look for a constellation of co-occurring symptoms. Common comorbid conditions include Attention-Deficit/Hyperactivity Disorder (ADHD), Oppositional Defiant Disorder (ODD), Conduct Disorder, and anxiety disorders.

RISK FACTORS

Several factors are associated with the onset and/or course of childhood bipolar disorder. Twenty to forty percent of children and adolescents develop Bipolar-I within 5 years of the onset of major depression. Depressed children who experience psychomotor retardation or psychotic features are particularly at high risk. Another risk factor is a family history of bipolar disorder. Yet another is a strong family history of mood disorders (i.e., depression on the maternal and for the paternal side). In addition, family environment, social resources, and stressful life events all contribute to the course of bipolar disorder.

TREATMENT

Psychopharmacology

An essential part of treating bipolar disorder is the administration of mood stabilizers, such as Lithium® (Lithium Carbonate), Depakote® (Valproic Acid), and Tegretol® (Carbamazepine). Safety and efficacy data support their use. They are often fairly well tolerated, with mild to moderate side effects. There are limited empirical data on the newer mood stabilizers: Topamax® (Topirimate), Gabitril® (Tiagabine), Trileptal® (Oxcarbazepine), Lamictal® (Lamotrigine), and Neurontin® (Gabapentin). In general, mood stabilizers target the manic symptoms of bipolar disorder, including euphoria and irritability.

Often, children with bipolar disorder also require antipsychotic medications, such as Zyprexa® (Olanzapine), Risperdal® (Risperidone), Seroquel® (Quetiapine), Geodon® (Ziprasidone), and Clozaril® (Clozapine). These drugs help reduce hallucinations and disturbing thoughts. Children with bipolar disorder sometimes need other medications for antidepressant effects or to treat comorbid conditions. Selective Serotonin Reuptake Inhibitors (SSRIs), such as Prozac® (Fluoxetine), Zoloft® (Sertraline), Paxil® (Paroxetine), Luvox® (Fluvoxamine), and Celexa® (Citalopram) reduce depressive symptoms. Atypical antidepressants used with children include Effexor® (Venlafaxine), Remeron® (Mirtazapine), Trazodone® (Desyrel), and Wellbutrin® (Bupropion). However, all antidepressant medications are contraindicated until mania is stabilized because evidence shows that they bring about or worsen rapid cycling. In cases of comorbidity with ADHD, psychostimulants, such as Ritalin® (Methylphenidate), Concerta® (Methylphenidate HCl), Adderall® (Amphetamine), Metadate® (Methylphenidate HCl), and Dexedrine®

(Dextroamphetamine) may be used. Again, mania must first be stabilized to avoid psychostimulants triggering psychotic symptoms.

Psychotherapy

Empirical information regarding psychotherapy for bipolar disorder in children is largely nonexistent. Three types of psychotherapy are utilized in clinical practice with these children: individual, family, and group. In individual therapy, children with bipolar disorder may learn to cope and manage their symptoms better. Family therapy works on those skills, as well as addressing family communication and problem solving skills. Group therapy may be used as a medium to develop better social skills.

Finally, caregivers themselves require support services to help them cope with the burden of raising a child with bipolar disorder. Face-to-face support groups have limited availability and are not always practical for such caregivers. Hence, there is growing importance of Web sites that provide information and support. Organizations such as the Child & Adolescent Bipolar Foundation (http://www.bpkids.org) provide important resources, chat rooms, message boards, and e-mail support groups for caregivers.

In sum, children with major depression and/or a strong family history of mood disorders are at risk for bipolar disorder. Typically, children with bipolar disorder experience rapid cycling back and forth from mania to depression and/or mixed episodes. These children may be assessed using adult criteria for Bipolar-I, Bipolar-II, or Bipolar-NOS. Careful assessment procedures are necessary to rule out alternative diagnoses and to identify co-occurring disorders. Childhood bipolar disorder ought to be treated with psychopharmacology and psychotherapy in combination. However, there is little empirical information about treating bipolar disorder in children with medications, and far less information about the efficacy of psychotherapy.

See also: Cognitive-Behavior Therapy; Depressive Disorder, Major; Dysthymic Disorder; Mania; Pharmacological Interventions; Suicide

Further Reading

American Association of Child and Adolescent Psychiatry. (1997). Practice parameters for the assessment and treatment of children and adolescents with bipolar disorder. *Journal of the American Academy of Child and Adolescent Psychiatry, 36,* 157S–176S.

Geller, B., & DelBello, M. (Eds.). (2003). *Child and early adolescent bipolar disorder: Theory, assessment, and treatment.* New York: Guilford.

Geller, B., & Luby, J. (1997). Child and adolescent bipolar disorder: A review of the past 10 years. *Journal of the American Academy of Child and Adolescent Psychiatry, 36* (9), 1168–1176.

McClure, E. B., Kubiszyn, T., & Kaslow, N. J. (2002). Advances in the diagnosis and treatment of childhood mood disorders. *Professional Psychology: Research and Practice, 33*(2), 125–134.

Nottlemann, E. D., Biederman, J., Birmaher, B., Carlson, G. A., Chang, K. D., Fenton, W. S., et al. (2001). National Institute of Mental Health research roundtable on prepubertal bipolar disorder. *Journal of the American Academy of Child and Adolescent Psychiatry, 40*(8), 871–878.

Katharine D. Smith
Mary A. Fristad

Birth Weight

See: Prematurity: Birth Weight and Gestational Age

Bleeding Disorders

DEFINITION

Bleeding problems may occur because of (1) hereditary deficiencies in proteins, or factors in the coagulation pathway that lead to the prevention of bleeding (e.g., hemophilia and von Willebrand's disease) or (2) genetic or acquired disorders related to production or destruction of platelets in the bone marrow (thrombocytopenia).

INCIDENCE

Bleeding problems encompass a broad range of disorders, each with a different incidence. Readers should refer to the specific disorder for precise incidence estimates.

DIAGNOSIS

Bleeding problems may represent a primary problem associated with a hereditary disorder or failure of platelets, or may be a symptom of another problem that affects production or function of clotting factors or platelets. Besides genetics, primary coagulation or platelet abnormalities may occur following viral illness or exposure to medications or toxic substances.

Alternatively, they may be a symptom of some form of bone marrow disease, including leukemia, lymphoma, aplastic anemia, or acquired immunodeficiency disorders. Diagnosis is made on the basis of clinical symptoms, complete blood counts, bleeding times, and specialized laboratory tests for clotting factors and genetic markers.

CLINICAL SYMPTOMS

The physical symptoms of bleeding problems include easy bruising, tiny pinpoint bleeds that appear as a rash (petichae), prolonged bleeding following injury or surgery, bleeding of the mouth, nose, or other area of the body, and, in extreme cases, internal bleeding, such as in the brain, abdomen, or joints.

TREATMENT

Treatment is dependent on the underlying reason for bleeding, and may involve transfusions of platelets, replacement of clotting factor, medications, or only careful clinical monitoring. In extreme cases, bone marrow transplantation may be necessary. Alteration of activities that may increase risk of bleeding may also be part of the management plan.

PROGNOSIS

For most acute bleeding problems, the prognosis is very good; most can be effectively treated. Some bleeding problems, particularly those that are hereditary, require chronic management.

See also: Hereditary Coagulation Disorders; Platelet Abnormalities—Thrombocytopenia; Leukemia; Pediatric Human Immunodeficiency Virus-1 (HIV); Kidney, Transplantation, Pediatric; Orthopedic Disabilities; Bone Marrow Failure and Primary Immunodeficiency; Self-Management

Further Reading

Beardsley, D. S., & Nathan, D. G. (1998). Platelet abnormalities in infancy and childhood. In D. G. Nathan & S. H. Orkin (Eds.), *Nathan and Oski's hematology of infancy and childhood* (5th ed., pp. 1585–1630). Philadelphia: W.B. Saunders.
Montgomery, R. R., Gill, J. C., & Scott, J. P. (1998). Hemophilia and von Willebrand's disease. In D. G. Nathan & S. H. Orkin (Eds.), *Nathan and Oski's hematology of infancy and childhood* (5th ed., pp. 1631–1659). Philadelphia: W.B. Saunders.

F. DANIEL ARMSTRONG

Blindness

See: Visual Impairment: Low Vision and Blindness

Blood Phobia

See: Specific Phobia

Body Rocking and Head Banging

DEFINITION

Body rocking and head banging are characterized by repetitive, rhythmical movements of the child's body usually immediately before or during sleep. Body rocking is characterized by rhythmic back-and-forth movements either while the child is on all fours or while the child is sitting up. Head banging is characterized by rhythmic banging of either the forehead or the back of the head.

INCIDENCE/ETIOLOGY

Body rocking and head banging are common behaviors in children under the age of 3. Body rocking starts, on average, at about 6 months and may be accompanied by head banging or head rolling a few months later. Up to 20 percent of all infants bang their heads on purpose, although boys are three times more likely to do it than girls. These behaviors usually decrease with age, stopping by age 4 years. It is unclear why children rock their bodies or bang their heads, but some developmental experts believe that body rocking and head banging are a child's way of calming down so he or she can fall asleep. Most children who engage in these behaviors bang their head rhythmically (some also rock on all fours) as they are falling asleep, when they wake up in the middle of the night, or even while they are sleeping. Head banging can also soothe a child in pain. Infants and toddlers are more likely to bang their head when they are teething or have an ear infection. Some children bang their head during temper tantrums as a way of venting strong emotions. Ongoing head banging may also be a way for a child to get attention. The head banging and body rocking associated with certain types of blindness, autism, and mental retardation should be distinguished from these behaviors in normally developing children.

ASSESSMENT

When body rocking and head banging are persistent or causing physical damage, it is important to determine what is occurring before and after the behaviors as well as the context of the behavior.

TREATMENT

Ignoring the body rocking and head banging is the usual recommended treatment, along with protecting the child from injury by lining the sides of the crib with a soft bumper to soften the impact. It is also important to check the bolts of the crib regularly to make sure the rhythmic movement is not loosening them. It can also be helpful to have a consistent and relaxing bedtime routine to help the child calm down before bedtime. Punishment or scolding for the body rocking and head banging is not recommended.

PROGNOSIS

Rocking in babies and young toddlers generally is not a sign of any behavioral or emotional problem, and there is no need to take any precautionary steps for the baby's sake. Head banging is usually a "self-regulating" behavior so the child is unlikely to hit his or her head hard enough to cause an injury. Brain tests do not show abnormalities in these children, and the vast majority of them grow up to be healthy adults.

See also: Sleep Patterns, Normal

Further Reading

Durand, V. M. (1998). *Sleep better! A guide to improving sleep for children with special needs*. Baltimore, MD: Paul H. Brooks.
Durand, V. M., Mindell, J. A., Mapstone, E., & Gernert-Dott, P. (1998). Treatment of multiple sleep disorders in children. In C. E. Schaefer (Ed.), *Clinical handbook of sleep disorders in children* (pp. 311–333). Northvale, NJ: Jason Aronson.

Laberge, L., Tremblay, R. E., Vitaro, F., & Montplaisir, J. (2000). Development of parasomnias from childhood to early adolescence. *Pediatrics, 106*(1), 67–74.
National Sleep Foundation, 1522 K Street, NW, Suite 500, Washington, DC 20005, Phone: (202) 347-3471; Fax: (202) 347-3472; E-mail: nsf@sleepfoundation.org, http://www.sleepfoundation.org

V. MARK DURAND
KRISTIN V. CHRISTODULU

Bone and Soft Tissue Tumors

Although pediatric bone tumors (osteosarcoma and Ewing's sarcoma) and soft tissue sarcomas (rhabdomyosarcoma, neuroblastoma, retinoblastoma, Wilms' tumor) differ in terms of site, histology, prognosis, and treatment, there are many commonalties among them. They are similar in terms of coping demands placed upon the children and adolescents and their families, and in terms of the effects of surgery, radiation, and chemotherapy, as well as interruption of normal physical, psychological, and social development. Some of these effects are transitory or reversible, while others may be permanent. The psychological issues related to cancer and its treatment are similar across solid tumor malignancies and are primarily discussed in the entry on osteosarcoma.

See also: Ewing's Sarcoma; Neuroblastoma; Osteosarcoma; Retinoblastoma; Rhabdomyosarcoma; Wilms' Tumor

MARY JO KUPST
ANNE B. WARWICK

Bone Marrow Failure and Primary Immunodeficiency

DEFINITION

All blood cells are produced in the bone marrow. When the bone marrow fails or becomes ineffective in producing white blood cells, red blood cells, and/or platelets that are able to mature in the peripheral blood, then a number of clinical syndromes can occur, including anemia, platelet abnormalities, and immune system failure. The clinical syndromes and symptoms that result depend on the specific blood cell lines (white blood cells, red blood cells, and/or platelets) that are affected.

APLASTIC ANEMIA

Failure in two or more cell lines is considered aplastic anemia, which can be acquired, inherited, or congenital; its severity can also be variable. The major causes for acquired aplastic anemia include exposure to radiation, drugs, and other chemicals, viruses, immune diseases, and other disease processes (such as pre-leukemia). Genetic syndromes associated with aplastic anemia include Fanconi's anemia, Familial aplastic anemias, Schwachman–Diamond syndrome, and other nonhematologic syndromes (e.g. Down syndrome).

PRIMARY IMMUNODEFICIENCY

Clinical symptoms similar to those seen with bone marrow failure may occur when blood cell production is adequate, but the function of the blood cells is impaired. When this occurs for the T- and B-cells (white blood cells), the child is considered to have a primary immunodeficiency (e.g., SCID—Severe Combined Immunodeficiency). Immunodeficiencies may be genetic (X-linked, or autosomal recessive mutations) or acquired following a malignancy, infection, or immunosuppression.

Bone marrow failure represents a disorder at the level of blood cell production. Similar clinical features may be seen when cells are produced, but then, fail to function (e.g., chronic anemia), are destroyed once produced (e.g., some forms of thrombocytopenia), do not function properly because of genetic mutations (e.g., hemophilia), or are crowded out by overproduction of nonfunctional, abnormal blood cells (e.g., acute leukemia).

INCIDENCE

Aplastic anemia occurs in about two individuals per million each year, with about 25 percent of these related to inherited conditions. Primary immunodeficiencies (e.g., SCID, Wiscott–Aldridge Syndrome, Ataxia–Telangiectasia) have an incidence of 1 in 100,000.

DIAGNOSIS

The diagnosis of bone marrow failure includes evidence of depressed blood counts, and bone marrow aspirations and biopsies are done to determine the amount of cells present and the function of the bone marrow. The diagnosis of primary immunodeficiences are also detected by low blood counts and laboratory studies of specific markers of immune function as well as genetic studies.

CLINICAL SYMPTOMS

The clinical symptoms of bone marrow failure depend upon which blood cell lines are affected. Failure in the production of platelets will result in bruising, bleeding, or petechiae (small red spots on the skin). Failure in the production of functional red blood cells (anemia) may result in fatigue, pale appearance, and rapid heart beat (tachycardia). Failure of the white blood cells (leukocytes) may present in the form of bacterial infection, ulcers in the mouth, and fever.

The clinical symptoms of primary immunodeficiency are often evident at or shortly after birth, and may include recurrent infections, chronic diarrhea, and failure to thrive, and these may lead to malignancies such as leukemia or lymphoma.

TREATMENT

Treatment of both bone marrow failure and primary immunodeficiency may involve aggressive antibiotic support in the treatment of infections, use of immunosuppressant medications in some cases, and blood transfusion support. For many children, the best treatment option is allogeneic (from a donor) bone marrow transplantation (BMT). If this is considered an option, then the use of blood transfusions should be kept to a minimum. Repeated exposure to blood products increases the chance that the immune system will produce antibodies that ultimately reject donor blood products, including bone marrow, peripheral stem cells, and umbilical cord blood cells. Transfusions should, however, be considered in emergency situations, (e.g., severe anemia, uncontrolled bleeding) which can be life threatening.

The child with bone marrow failure or primary immunodeficiency often requires isolation (SCID is sometimes referred to as the "bubble boy syndrome"), leading to significant disruption in lifestyle. Psychosocial support in the areas of stress management, social development, participation in the educational process, and pain management can be quite helpful. Stress inoculation prior to BMT and support during and following BMT are essential components of care for these children.

PROGNOSIS

The prognosis for children with bone marrow failure or primary immunodeficiency is variable, with different degrees of severity. For severe aplastic anemia, supportive treatment of symptoms (e.g., antibiotics, transfusion) results in an overall survival rate of only approximately 30 percent at 4 years postdiagnosis. The survival rate for those undergoing BMT is 65 percent at the same point. Similarly, severe primary immunodeficiency is often fatal without BMT.

See also: Bleeding Disorders; Bone Marrow Transplantation; Failure-to-Thrive; Hereditary Coagulation Disorders; Leukemia; Lymphomas; Platelet Abnormalities—Thrombocytopenia; Relaxation Training; Self-Management; Stress Management

Further Reading

Alter, B. P., & Young, N. S. (1998). The bone marrow failure syndromes. In D. G. Nathan & S. H. Orkin (Eds.), *Nathan and Oski's hematology of infancy and childhood* (5th ed., pp. 237–335). Philadelphia: W.B. Saunders.

Bonilla, F. A., Rosen, F. S., & Geha, R. S. (1998). Primary immunodeficiency diseases. In D. G. Nathan & S. H. Orkin (Eds.), *Nathan and Oski's hematology of infancy and childhood* (5th ed., pp. 1023–1050). Philadelphia: W.B. Saunders.

Severe Combined Immunodeficiency Disease (SCID)-IL-2. http://www.icondata.com/health/pedbase/files/SEVERECO.HTM

The SCID Homepage. http://www.scid.net/

F. DANIEL ARMSTRONG

Bone Marrow Transplantation

BRIEF DESCRIPTION AND INDICATIONS

Since 1968, bone marrow transplantation (BMT) has been used to treat children and adults with cancer and other illnesses that affect the bone marrow. Bone marrow is a soft and spongy tissue that exists in the body's bones and it contains over 95 percent of the body's blood cells. Stem cells are those blood cells that produce other blood cells, and are found in the bone marrow in the breast bone, skull, hips, ribs, and spine. Historically, BMT involves extracting bone marrow surgically (i.e., via needle placed into the hip bones and/or sternum), filtering it, and infusing it into the patient. When the stem cells are collected directly from the bone marrow, the procedure is called a bone marrow transplant. In some instances, stem cells can be extracted from the bloodstream through a process called apheresis. Apheresis involves connecting the patient to a machine that extracts blood from one arm, separates the stem cells, and returns the remaining blood cells to the other arm. When stems cells are collected in this manner, the procedure is called a stem cell transplant.

Bone marrow or stem cell transplantation is necessary for some individuals who have been diagnosed as having leukemias, lymphomas, aplastic anemia, immune deficiency disorders, and some solid tumor cancers. For some patients, their illness destroys the body's bone marrow, which would eventually lead to death. For other patients, their illness can be cured only by extremely high doses of chemotherapy and/or radiation therapy. While these high doses of treatment kill cancer cells, they also kill healthy stem cells. Bone marrow or stem cell transplantation, therefore, is necessary to restore the stem cells that have been destroyed by illness and/or its treatment.

There are essentially three different types of bone marrow transplantation that are possible. An autologous transplant involves extracting the patient's own bone marrow or blood cells before high-dose treatment, freezing it, and returning it to the patient following treatment. An allogeneic transplant involves using the bone marrow or blood cells from a person who is genetically matched with the patient. This person is usually a sibling, but could be a parent, another relative, or an unrelated donor from a national or international bone marrow registry. Finally, it is possible for a patient to receive stem cells that have been harvested from an umbilical cord. It is becoming increasingly common for parents to donate umbilical cords following the birth of their child. The cord serves as a very rich source of stem cells, which can be frozen until they are needed for transplantation.

As previously indicated, bone marrow or stem cell transplants occurs after high-dose chemotherapy and/or radiation therapy. The transplant does not involve surgery, but rather is very much like a blood transfusion given through a central venous catheter into the bloodstream. The stem cells proceed into the bone marrow and start reproducing new and healthy blood cells. Following this procedure, patients are monitored in an intensive care environment to prevent and treat infections, the side effects of the chemotherapy and/or radiation, and various complications. These can include infection, excessive bleeding, nausea, vomiting, diarrhea, mouth sores, pain, fluid overload, thrombocytopenia (low platelet count), anemia (low red blood cell count), respiratory distress, extreme weakness, mental confusion, and psychological distress. Graft-versus-host disease is a potential serious complication for patients who receive an allogeneic transplant. The new transplanted cells (the graft) view the patient's tissues (the host) as foreign and attempt to destroy it. As a result of these possible complications, patients are confined to a sterile environment, take multiple antibiotics and other medications, have blood transfusions, and undergo continual laboratory testing for several weeks.

PREVALENCE

There is no central repository of all bone marrow and stem cell transplants. Nevertheless, estimates indicate that about 40,000 autologous transplants and about 19,000 allogeneic transplants have been performed in children and adults worldwide since 1970. The majority of transplants (~78 percent) use bone marrow grafts, about 20 percent use peripheral blood cells, and about 2 percent use umbilical cord blood cells. Over the last five years, the number of bone marrow transplants has gradually declined, while the number of stem cell transplants has gradually risen. Children and adolescent comprise about 15 percent and 35 percent of the recipients of autologous and allogeneic transplants, respectively.

PSYCHOLOGICAL CONSIDERATIONS

Pediatric psychologists are generally involved in the psychological evaluation of children and families at the time they are being considered for BMT. The nature and extent of these evaluations vary by transplant program, but generally include an assessment of child development, adherence history, quality of life, psychological adaptation and coping, and family resources. In addition to assessment-based services, psychological interventions are developed and implemented as needed to enhance both pre- and posttransplant health outcomes.

Research on the psychological impact of the combination of high-dose therapy and pediatric BMT suggests that children can experience considerable stress, pain, emotional discomfort, and cognitive impairment. Furthermore, elevated levels of parent and family stress have been reported in this population as well.

See also: Childhood Cancers; Coping with Illness; Medical Hospitalization; Parenting the Chronically Ill Child; Preparation for Medical Procedures

Further Reading

Bishop, M. M., Welsh, H., Coons, M., & Wingard, J. R. (2001). Blood and marrow transplantation. In J. R. Rodrigue (Ed.), *Biopsychosocial perspectives on transplantation* (pp. 19–38). New York, NY: Kluwer Academic/Plenum.

BMTnet Home Page. http://www.bmtnet.org/home/index.asp (Accessed July 2002).

Cool, V. A. (1996). Long-term neuropsychological risks in pediatric bone marrow transplant: What do we know? *Bone Marrow Transplantation, 18* (Suppl 3), S45–S49.

Vannatta, K., Zeller, M., Noll, R. B., & Koontz, K. (1998). Social functioning of children surviving bone marrow transplantation. *Journal of Pediatric Psychology, 23*, 169–178.

JAMES R. RODRIGUE
STEPHANIE TOY

Brain Contusions

See: Traumatic Brain Injury

Brain Injury

See: Traumatic Brain Injury

Breath-Holding Spells

DEFINITION/CLINICAL PRESENTATION

Breath-holding spells (BHS) are common in healthy, otherwise normal infants and young children, have a dramatic presentation, and are often terrifying for parents to observe. Although use of the participle "holding" in BHS suggests a voluntary action, BHS are actually involuntarily and reflexive. BHS occur while the child is awake and engaging in active respiration, typically last from 2–20 seconds (but can last as long as a minute or more), and are described as simple or severe, depending on the progress of the event. Those that progress from distress (typically indicated by crying) silent respiration to a change in skin color are said to be simple and those that progress further to loss of consciousness and/or actual seizures are said to be severe. BHS are also distinguished by the differential changes in skin color that accompany them. Cyanotic BHS, the most common type, is characterized by rapidly occurring bluish or purplish discoloration of the skin, and pallid BHS is characterized by paleness or deficiency in skin color. Although crying occurs in both types, it is more prominent in cyanotic than in pallid BHS. A typical BHS episode involves an environmental event that is distressing for the child, followed by crying that diminishes to quietness accompanied by change in color (cyanotic or pallid) and ending with the child being disoriented but conscious (simple) or unconscious (severe).

INCIDENCE AND FREQUENCY

Estimates of severe BHS incidence range as high as 4.6 percent for young children and as high as 27 percent for simple BHS. Afflicted children exhibit the cyanotic type in 54–62 percent of cases, pallid type in 19–22 percent, both types in 12 percent, and an indeterminate type in the remaining 12 percent. Age of onset is generally between 3 and 18 months of age, although as many as 10 percent of cases begin before 3 months and a similar percentage begin after 18 months. Frequency ranges from several times a day to as low as once a year, with the majority of children exhibiting several episodes per week. Peak frequency is in the second year and gradually but continuously diminishes thereafter. The average age of cessation is 3 years and BHS is rare after age 8.

CORRELATES

Approximately 20–30 percent of breathholders have a family member who exhibited BHS during childhood. There are no well documented differences between genders, and studies attempting to detect significant behavioral or psychological differences between breathholders and controls have been unsuccessful.

ETIOLOGY

The majority of research on the etiology of BHS is on physiological (over-) response to environmental events. The findings suggest that dysregulation of the autonomic nervous system is a primary underlying condition for BHS in general. Precipitating events for pallid versus cyanotic BHS differ, however. Pallid BHS events are precipitated abruptly, usually by events involving pain or fear (e.g., falling, banging head). Such events (over) stimulate the vagal nerve which leads to bradycardia (slowed heart rate) or asystole (temporary cessation of heart contractions) and syncope (faintness).

Pallid events can also be induced in the laboratory via application of ocular pressure (e.g., using fingers to apply pressure to a child's closed eyes). Cyanotic BHS occur less abruptly and is typically the culminating part of an emotional (usually angry) reaction to upsetting events (e.g., discipline, loss of toy). The child cries, exhibits expiratory apnea, changes color (purple or blue), and sometimes loses consciousness. The underlying physiology is less well-established but factors known to lead to cyanoses and syncope, such as increased cerebral and thoracic pressure (from a grunt-like response) and temporary pulmonary malfunctions (e.g., ventilation–perfusion mismatches) are thought to be involved. Although both types of BHS are involuntary, their occurrence and the behavioral patterns associated with them can be influenced by environmental conditioning processes (e.g., increased crying due to sympathetic parental response).

ASSESSMENT

Parent interviews are used to obtain a detailed history of BHS and to inform diagnosis. The interviews usually include questions pertaining to changes in skin color, alteration in body tone, frequency and duration of loss of consciousness or seizures, and the social events preceding and following BHS. Videotaped documentation of BHS can be used to supplement parental verbal report. Physical examinations that include checks for anatomical or functional airway abnormalities are also used, especially with children who have frequent cyanotic BHS. Lab testing is used with frequent BHS accompanied by loss of consciousness. BHS lab tests include the electrocardiogram (EKG) to check for heart-related problems in both types of BHS and the electroencephalogram (EEG) to examine the characteristic sequence of changes exhibited during the pallid type and to rule out the possibility of epilepsy. Lastly, blood tests can rule out faintness due to anemia.

TREATMENT

In most cases treatment primarily involves demystification about the phenomenon and reassurance about its nonpathological nature and nonharmful outcome. Demystification should include a layperson's account of how interrupted breathing patterns can lead to loss of consciousness. Parents are also instructed that a diagnosis should not lead to dramatic changes in the way the child is treated or attended to with two exceptions. First, if parents have been overly solicitous toward the child, either prior to or following BHS, this should be remedied. Second, if parents have surrendered some of their authority to the child in an attempt to minimize upset, this too should be corrected. Additionally, if the child is known to be anemic, physician-guided treatment with iron supplements can decrease the frequency of BHS.

When BHS occur, caregivers should place the child in a lateral, supine position and guard against head injury and aspiration until recovery occurs. If necessary, the oral airway should be cleared. These preventive maneuvers should be conducted with, and the overall approach to the child marked by, emotional neutrality. Although pharmacotherapy is rarely beneficial for patients with cyanotic BHS, patients with severe and frequent pallid BHS may benefit from medication that slows parasympathetic activity.

PROGNOSIS

Although reports of serious health consequences following BHS are rare, BHS are almost always frightening to encounter. Generally, however, the scientific literature provides a very optimistic prognosis. Long-term negative effects for cyanotic BHS have not been reported. Long-term effects for pallid BHS are isolated to an increased risk for faintness episodes (e.g., at the sight of blood) in adolescence and adulthood.

See also: Behavior Modification; Childhood; Interviewing; Positive Reinforcement

Further Reading

Blum, N. J. (2002). Breath holding spells. In F. D. Burg, J. R. Ingelfinger, R. A. Polin, and A. A. Gershon (Eds.), *Current pediatric therapy* (17th ed., pp. 380–381). Philadelphia: Saunders.

Breningstall, G. N. (1996). Breath-holding spells. *Pediatric Neurology, 14*, 91–97.

DiMario, F. J. (1992). Breath-holding spells in children. *American Journal of Diseases of Children, 146*, 125–131.

STEPHANIE SPEAR
PATRICK C. FRIMAN

Bruxism

DEFINITION

Bruxism is the habit of repetitively clenching and grinding the teeth without awareness that one is doing it. It most often occurs at night during sleep, but it may also occur during the day.

INCIDENCE/ETIOLOGY

Bruxism can occur at any age and is very common in children; over 50 percent of normal infants and 15 percent of children between 3–17 years engage in this behavior. While bruxism is typically associated with stress, it may also be triggered by abnormal occlusion (the way the upper and lower teeth fit together), or crooked or missing teeth.

ASSESSMENT

Symptoms of bruxism include: dull headaches; sore and tired facial muscles; earaches; sensitive teeth; and locking, popping, and clicking of the jaw. During a dental examination, a dentist may recognize damage resulting from bruxism, including: enamel loss from the chewing surfaces of teeth; flattened tooth surfaces; loosened teeth; and fractured teeth and fillings.

TREATMENT

In persistent and severe cases of bruxism, it is treated by placing a removable, custom-fitted plastic appliance called a night guard between the upper and lower teeth. Although the clenching and grinding behavior may continue, the teeth wear away the plastic instead of each other. In some cases, abnormal occlusion may be adjusted and high spots removed so that the teeth fit together in a more comfortable position. Missing teeth may be replaced and crooked teeth may be straightened with orthodontic treatment to eliminate possible underlying causes of bruxism. Biofeedback and stress management have also been found to be helpful in treating headaches and jaw pain resulting from bruxism.

PROGNOSIS

Bruxism may cause permanent damage to teeth and chronic jaw pain unless properly diagnosed and promptly treated.

See also: Behavioral Dentistry; Normal; Sleep Patterns; Stress Management

Further Reading

Laberge, L., Tremblay, R. E., Vitaro, F., & Montplaisir, J. (2000). Development of parasomnias from childhood to early adolescence. *Pediatrics, 106* (1), 67–74.

Lofland, K. R., Cassisi, J. E., & Drabman, R. S. (1995). Nocturnal bruxism in children. In C. E. Schaefer (Ed.), *Clinical handbook of sleep disorders in children* (pp. 203–222). Northvale, NJ: Jason Aronson.

Mindell, J. A. (1996). Treatment of child and adolescent sleep disorders. *Child & Adolescent Psychiatric Clinics of North America, 5*(3), 741–751

National Sleep Foundation, 1522 K Street, NW, Suite 500, Washington, DC 20005; Phone: (202) 347-3471; Fax: (202) 347-3472; E-mail: nsf@sleepfoundation.org; http://www.sleepfoundation.org

V. MARK DURAND
KRISTIN V. CHRISTODULU

Bulimia Nervosa

DEFINITION

Bulimia nervosa is a psychiatric disorder with diagnostic criteria described in the fourth edition of the *Diagnostic and Statistical Manual of Mental Disorders* published by the American Psychiatric Association. The disorder is best described as recurrent episodes of binge eating followed by purging to prevent weight gain. Bingeing episodes involve the consumption of large quantities of food in a brief amount of time with a feeling of lack of control over eating. Binges need to occur at least twice a week for three months in order to meet diagnostic criteria. Purging may be accomplished by a variety of methods. There are two subtypes of bulimia nervosa defined by method of purging; purging subtype involves self-induced vomiting or laxative or diuretic abuse, nonpurging subtype involves purging by excessive calorie restriction and exercise. Unlike anorexia nervosa, the goal of purging is not weight loss; rather it is to prevent weight gain. Patients with bulimia nervosa place undue emphasis on body shape and weight for self-evaluation.

INCIDENCE/PREVALENCE

Early studies utilizing self-report measures estimated the prevalence of bulimia nervosa to be as high as 12–19 percent for high school and college age females. Utilizing stricter diagnostic criteria, later studies have suggested rates in the 2–4.5 percent range. Onset is generally in high school and the disorder often continues during the college years. Most patients with bulimia are of the purging subtype.

ETIOLOGY

Speculation as to the etiology of bulimia nervosa has focused on personality traits, the continuum of bulimia nervosa with normal eating and exercise practices, and the comorbidity of the disorder with other emotional and addictive disorders. Individuals with bulimia nervosa tend to have impulsive and socially outgoing personality styles. They are susceptible to mood swings and have difficulty maintaining goal-directed behaviors. This type of personality is also said to explain the increased incidence of other addictions in patients with bulimia, especially alcoholism. It has been estimated that 60 percent of bulimia nervosa patients have a comorbid Axis 1 diagnosis, with major depression the most common. While sexual abuse has been reported to occur at a higher than normal rate in patients with eating disorders, it is particularly significant in the history of patients with bulimia nervosa. In addition, there is evidence that patients with bulimia nervosa experience early onset puberty and early sexual experiences. Low self-esteem is frequently found in individuals with a diagnosis of bulimia nervosa.

ASSESSMENT

The assessment of bulimia nervosa is accomplished by interview, by medical/nutritional evaluation, and by the use of self-report measures. The assessment interview should focus on the history of the binge–purge cycle, the method(s) of purging, the patient's state of mind and feelings during the binge, and the location and frequency of purging. In addition, it is important to assess the patient's current attitude about body shape and weight, personality style, and comorbid addictions or emotional disorders. Medical and nutritional assessments are used to determine the patient's current health status. Patients who are medically compromised usually require inpatient treatment initially, but this is much less common in bulimia nervosa than in anorexia nervosa. There are a number of self-report questionnaire instruments for measuring eating-disorder-related attitudes and beliefs (e.g., Eating Disorders Inventory-2) that are useful in assessing a patient's belief system and for research. These instruments by themselves, however, cannot be used for diagnosis as they have a very high false positive rate.

TREATMENT

Bulimia nervosa can be successfully treated on an outpatient basis. Inpatient treatment is generally indicated only when a disorder is so severe that medical complications arise (e.g., electrolyte imbalances). Unlike anorexia nervosa where patients do not perceive that weight loss is a problem, patients with bulimia nervosa are aware that their eating habits and purging are irregular and when treatment is sought it is usually with this realization, increasing the probability of successful treatment. There are several goals of treatment for bulimia nervosa. Important objectives include establishing a regular eating pattern designed to reduce or eliminate binge–purge cycles, changing the maladaptive thinking associated with the binge–purge cycle, remediating the medical complications and coexisting psychiatric disorders, and preventing relapse. Cognitive behavior therapy has been used to address the distorted thoughts about eating, weight, and body shape. Cognitive behavioral therapies usually include a set number of sessions with specific activities and exercises. In addition to cognitive therapy, exposure plus response prevention has been utilized as a technique based on an anxiety-reduction model. In this treatment, the patient is required to eat a normal amount of food but is prevented from engaging in purging behavior. Theoretically, the elicitation of the anxiety associated with a full stomach, and then the prevention of the response to reduce the anxiety, will lead to a reduction in the anxiety. Both of these therapeutic approaches have been shown to be effective. Following treatment, patients not only improved in relation to the actual act of bingeing and purging, but also showed improvement in self-reported symptoms of depression, self-esteem, and eating disordered thinking. In general, both individual and group approaches can be effective in the treatment of bulimia nervosa. In addition, pharmacologic agents, specifically antidepressants, have been shown to be effective as a component in the treatment of bulimia nervosa. Gastric motility agents and antiaxiolytic agents have been helpful in controlling the feelings of bloating following eating and help to control the anxiety that occurs following a large meal.

PROGNOSIS

Outcome studies suggest that up to 70 percent of bulimic patients continue to abstain from binge–purge behavior as long as 7 to 10 years after treatment.

See also: Anorexia Nervosa; Cognitive-Behavior Therapy; Exposure and Response Prevention; Pharmacological Interventions; Vomiting—Psychogenic

Further Reading

American Psychiatric Association (APA). (1994). *Diagnostic and statistical manual of mental disorders* (4th ed.). Washington, DC: Author.

Herzog, D. B., Keller, M. B., Sacks, N. R., Yeh, C. J., & Lavori, P. W. (1992). Psychiatric comorbidity in treatment-seeking anorexics and bulimics. *Journal of the American Academy of Child and Adolescent Psychiatry, 31,* 810–818.

Hsu, L. K. G. (1990). *Eating disorders.* New York: Guilford.

Keel, P. K., Mitchell, J. E., Miller, K. B., Davis, T. L., & Crow, S. J. (1999). Long-term outcome of bulimia nervosa. *Archives of General Psychiatry, 56,* 63–69.

Linscheid, T. R., & Butz, C. (in press). Anorexia nervosa and bulimia nervosa. In M. C. Roberts (Ed.), *Handbook of Pediatric Psychology* (3rd ed.). New York: Guilford.

THOMAS R. LINSCHEID

Bullies

DEFINITION

Bullies are children or adolescents who frequently, persistently, and intentionally use physical, psychological, or verbal means to intimidate, control, or humiliate one or more other youngsters. Many bullies use overt aggression toward their victims, although relational forms of aggression (e.g., social humiliation via ostracism, exclusion, or rumor) are a prominent feature of many bully–victim relationships. Bullies may act alone or in groups in victimizing others. Some definitions of bullying emphasize an ongoing psychological relationship between bullies and victims, whereby aggression and submissive behavior extends far beyond age-appropriate conflict or social dominance behavior. Some definitions also require a power imbalance between bullies and victims, such that victims lack the physical strength, social support, or psychological resources to defend themselves successfully.

INCIDENCE/PREVALENCE

Studies of the prevalence of bullying have been conducted primarily in schools and suggest that bullying is a common experience for students, although rates differ depending on the reporter (e.g., self, teacher, or peer), the time frame used, and the frequency and behaviors used to define bullying. Studies of bullying in U.S. schools have found that one fourth of children and adolescents admit bullying another student at least once during an academic year. Estimates are lower (7–11 percent) for the percentage of youth who bully others on multiple occasions. Similar rates have been found by studies conducted in other countries, primarily in Europe. Some research suggests that bully–victim problems become less frequent in the high school years with a possible peak around junior high. Bullying typically occurs at school, particularly during times of low or no supervision. In general, boys are more often identified as bullies and use more physical aggression than girls, although bullying girls may rely on relational aggression more frequently than do boys. In addition, boys tend to pick on both boys and girls while girls typically pick on other girls.

CORRELATES

Among males, bullying is associated with aggressive, antisocial behavior and other externalizing symptoms and is also predictive of using coercion and aggression in social relationships during the early adult years. Bullies tend to hold more favorable attitudes toward the use of aggression (e.g., aggression is acceptable and effective) than nonbullying peers. Social environmental features thought to contribute to the onset and maintenance of bullying include exposure (either direct or vicarious) to bully–victim relationships at home or school and inattention to or tolerance of aggression toward vulnerable children and adolescents by adults and peers.

ASSESSMENT

Self-report, peer nominations, and teacher nominations have been used to assess bullying in research studies. Measures typically include items to tap the use of overt and relational forms of aggression during a specified time frame (e.g., last 3 months). Aside from standard clinical procedures to assess aggression (e.g., interviews, behavior rating scales), there are no broadly accepted procedures for evaluating bullying in individual children and adolescents in clinical practice.

TREATMENT

Interventions to address bullying have been almost exclusively school-based and typically include intervention and prevention efforts at multiple levels (i.e., individual, classroom, school, and parents/community). The most extensive early test of a school-based program against bullying was begun by Olweus in the 1970s in Scandinavia. This program consisted of interventions at three levels: the school level, the class level, and the individual level. It also served as a model for numerous other intervention and prevention programs. Although earlier intervention efforts focused on increasing supervision and targeting the behavior of children directly involved in bully–victim relationships, interpersonal dynamics and the role that bystanders play in the prolongation versus reduction of bully–victim problems have received greater attention. Results of the Olweus studies and other similar intervention programs have indicated reductions in bully–victim problems and in general antisocial behavior, increases in student satisfaction, and improved academic performance. However, at least one follow-up study found an increase in bully–victim problems 3 years later. It is unclear what role variation in program fidelity and general age trends (i.e., increases in bully–victim problems at some ages) play in these trends.

PROGNOSIS

Male bullies are at risk for later delinquency and criminal offenses, especially violent crimes. Less is known about the long term risks for female bullies. Persistent bullying that co-occurs with multiple signs of disruptive behavior disorder carries substantial risk for poor outcomes.

See also: Aggression; Conduct Disorder; Victims of Bullies

Further Reading

Committee for Children Web site on bullying. Available at http://www.cfchildren.org/bully.html
Juvonen, J. & Graham, S. (2001). *Peer harassment in school: The plight of the vulnerable and victimized.* New York: Guilford.
Olweus, D. (1993). *Bullying at school. What we know and what we can do.* Oxford, UK: Blackwell.
Ross, D. (1996). *Childhood bullying and teasing: What school personnel, other professionals, and parents can do.* Alexandria, VA: American Counseling Association.
Shafii, M., & Shafii, S. L. (2001). *School violence: Assessment, management, prevention.* Washington, DC: American Psychiatric Press.

BRIDGET K. GAMM
ERIC M. VERNBERG

Burns, Pediatric

DEFINITION

Burn injuries are described in terms of total burn surface area (TBSA) and burn type (degree) and categorized as thermal, radiation, chemical, or electrical. TBSA is calculated through the use of standard charts that display dorsal and ventral views of the body, separated into discrete areas of known percentage of TBSA. Heat intensity and duration of contact determine the extent and depth of skin damage. Injury restricted to the epidermis is a first-degree burn. More extensive injuries to the dermis are called second-degree or partial-thickness burns. Full-thickness (third-degree) burns are injuries involving multiple skin layers and may include injury of subcutaneous tissue and peripheral nerve fibers. Burns are classified as minor, moderate, or severe according to criteria published by the American Burn Association.

INCIDENCE

In the United States, approximately 1.5 million individuals sustain burn injuries each year. Burn injuries are the fourth leading cause of accidental death in children with 5,500 deaths annually. Approximately 70,000 individuals are hospitalized for burn injuries and approximately 50 percent of victims are children and adolescents. Thirty-eight percent of patients hospitalized for burn injuries are less than 15 years of age. Children and adolescents are disproportionately affected with two-thirds of all fatalities occurring in those less than 15 years of age and a male to female ratio of 2:1. For youth (to age 19), fire and burn injuries are the third leading cause of death and second only to motor vehicle accidents for children aged 1–4 years. House fires account for the majority of pediatric fire-related deaths, most deaths due to smoke inhalation as opposed to direct burn insult.

Children less than 5 years of age account for more than 50 percent of all pediatric burn injuries. Expectedly, the manner in which children are injured varies according to the child's level of development. For example, scalds from liquid spills and bathing account for 75–80 percent of burn injuries to infants. In the first 2 years of life, 95 percent of burns occur indoors. As motor abilities increase, toddlers are at risk from pull-down liquid and food spills and from hot tap water. Preschool and school-aged children often are injured in experimental play with lighters, matches, and kitchen

devices (microwaves and stoves). Flame burns tend to be infrequent but are often lethal. Such burns account for 30 percent of admissions but account for 80 percent of the deaths, while scalds account for 50 percent of injuries and 20 percent of fatalities. During adolescence, the majority (60 percent) of injuries occur outside the home and 20 percent are due to scalding injuries within the home.

ASSESSMENT AND TREATMENT

Medical

The treatment of burns consists of three overlapping phases: the emergency period, the acute phase, and the rehabilitation phase. At the scene, emergency treatment involves eliminating the source of heat from the injured person. Standard first-aid treatment is conducted to ensure an unobstructed airway and to evaluate pulmonary, hematologic, and shock status. Upon arrival to the emergency room, continued evaluation and stabilization of respiration occurs. An endotracheal tube placement may be required. A central line is used for fluid infusion and a bladder catheter is placed to assess output. Capillary function increases over the first days after injury and a "fluid shift" occurs. Complications including pulmonary edema and congestive heart failure may result. Vital signs, cardiac functions, temperature, and intravenous (IV) fluids are monitored. Gastrointestinal (GI) functions decrease markedly or cease and patients with more than 20 percent TBSA burns may require a nasogastric tube. Once stabilized, patient care moves to the care of the wound(s). The acute phase of treatment is often the most distressing and traumatic (e.g., repeated IV placements, dressing changes, wound cleansing, grafting). A major concern during this phase is that of serious infection. Treatment includes administration of antibiotics, autografting (transplanting skin from undamaged areas of the patient's body to the site of the injury), and nutritional support. Eschar (burned tissue) must be surgically removed. Debridement procedures that entail vigorous removal of devitalized tissue are conducted one to two times daily. Topical medications are applied to manage wound infection. Partial-thickness burns heal in 3–4 weeks and full-thickness burns in 3–5 weeks. Physiological dressings (transplanted skin from cadavers [heterografts] or animals [xenografts], or artificial preparations) may be required. These dressings are temporary and will be biologically rejected. Autografting is used to treat severe burns. This procedure is often conducted in phases according to the rate of wound healing and the availability of donor material. Patients typically wear pressure dressings and garments to minimize scaring.

During the rehabilitation phase, medical, surgical, physical therapy, nutritional, and self-care procedures continue. Reconstructive surgeries often require repeated hospitalizations over a period of several years.

Psychosocial

A number of premorbid (pre-burn) risk factors have been noted for children who have sustained burn injuries. These include the psychological characteristics and stability of the child, those of the family, and demographic, and environmental factors. A detailed assessment of the child's premorbid cognitive, behavioral, developmental, educational, peer, and family functioning status is important as this information will directly inform intervention strategies during inpatient hospitalization as well as provide important information that will guide posthospital discharge psychological follow-up.

Areas of major concern include the child's mental status, nutritional intake, adherence to treatment, intense itching associated with the healing process, management of pain, symptoms related to the trauma of the burn experience, body image concerns, management of behavior that is perceived to be difficult by the burn unit staff, and finally, issues regarding caregiver and family adjustment to the recovery experience.

Management of disorientation typically includes correcting electrolyte imbalances and ongoing orientation procedures that include the use of visual aids (e.g., clocks, calendars) as well as the child being assigned the same staff members over the course of treatment. Intensive care unit (ICU) psychosis may result from sleep and sensory deprivation associated with long stays in the ICU. Behavioral approaches, including contingency management, have been shown to be useful in increasing caloric as well as fluid intake, thereby decreasing the need for tubal and intravenous feedings. Concerning adherence, caregivers and children are taught to identify barriers to their self-care (wound care, wearing of pressure garments), generating alternative solutions, family decision-making, and use of novel solutions. Contingency management approaches have also shown to be effective in promoting adherence. Behavioral approaches including response interruption and distraction have generally proved effective for younger children in attempting to direct their attention from itching to other more developmentally appropriate activities. Posttraumatic stress disorder as well as associated difficulties including

symptoms of depression-anxiety and/or acting-out behavior are commonly encountered. Timely intervention with validated treatments is needed. Social skills training may prove helpful in teaching youth who have sustained disfiguring burn injuries how to cope with the disfigurement, and how to manage peer taunting, as well as other reactions when interacting in public settings. Body image disturbances may be particularly pronounced in injured adolescents and cognitive-behavioral interventions are available for such difficulties. Because of the increasing recognition that the adequate management of pain is a standard of care in both the acute and rehabilitative phases of treatment for all individuals who have sustained burns, there are a number of drug and psychological treatment protocols available for the sensible management of pain. Finally, familial and caregiver support of the child who has been burned is of central importance. It is imperative to address the needs and concerns of all family members including siblings, throughout the course of hospitalization and recovery.

During the posthospitalization period, the child and family may first confront the reality of recovery that is incomplete and begin to face issues related to permanent scarring and compromise for loss of function. Family stress and school reentry problems are often observed and treatments for such are likely to prove helpful.

PROGNOSIS

Burns account for more days of hospitalization than any other type of injury. In the past two decades, significant advances in medical and surgical care have increased the survival rate of burn victims. Victims now routinely survive massive burns (burns involving more than 80 percent TBSA). The survival rate for patients with burns involving more than 70 percent TBSA is approximately 50 percent. Given the devastating nature of burn injuries, it might be assumed that most youth would fare poorly in terms of their intermediate to long-term adjustment. However, reviews of the outcome literature by Tarnowski and colleagues (1994) have revealed that there exists little empirical evidence to suggest that the *majority* of burn victims exhibit poor postburn adjustment. This conclusion is consistent with the results of recent reviews that indicate that while the recovery period is often protracted, most youth are able to successfully accomplish such recovery. Adjustment appears to be due to several interrelated factors including the nature and extent of patient injury, behavioral risk factors, and child and family psychological resources.

Most experts agree that the majority of pediatric burn injuries are preventable and this remains a priority for future work in this area.

See also: Accidental (Unintentional) Injuries; Coping with Illness; Medical Hospitalization; Medical Rehabilitation, Pediatric; Pain Management

Further Reading

American Burn Association. (1984). Guidelines for service standards and severity classifications in the treatment of burn injuries. *Bulletin of the American College of Surgeons, 69*, 24–28.

Blakeney, P. E., & Meyer, W. J. (1996). Psychosocial recovery of burned patients and reintegration into society. In D. N. Herndon (Ed.), *Total burn care* (pp. 176–192). London: Saunders.

Sheridan, R. L., Hinson, M. I., & Liang M. H. (2000). Long-term outcome of children surviving massive burns. *Journal of the American Medical Association, 283*, 69–73.

Stoddard, F. J. (in press). Care of infants, children and adolescents with burn injuries. In Lewis, M. (Ed.), *Child and adolescent psychiatry: A comprehensive textbook* (3rd ed.), Baltimore: Lippincott Williams & Wilkins.

Tarnowski, K. J. (Ed.). (1994). *Behavioral aspects of pediatric burns*. New York: Plenum.

KENNETH J. TARNOWSKI

Cc

Cancers, Childhood

Childhood cancer is a general term (other terms are malignant, oncologic, and neoplastic) for diseases that are characterized by uncontrolled growth of cells, which, when untreated, can spread (metastasize) to other tissues and organs. Cancer can occur anywhere in the body. The most common type of pediatric cancer is acute lymphocytic leukemia, followed by central nervous system (CNS) tumors and the lymphomas. In most disorders, the etiology is unknown or may have multiple possible causes. More recently, genetic factors, for example, chromosomal mutations, have been isolated in some cancers, which have improved the ability to categorize for risk and provide directions for treatment.

Most children and adolescents seen at pediatric cancer centers are entered into treatment protocols derived from, or part of, ongoing clinical trials. (The enrollment of large numbers of children in these clinical trials is largely responsible for the vastly improved survival rate of childhood cancer over the past 30 years.) The protocol may involve randomization in a clinical trial involving comparison of a new drug or set of drugs with standard care, or comparison of different dosages, or treatment modalities. Treatment is often multi-modal, involving surgery to biopsy or to remove a tumor, radiation to shrink the tumor and kill cells not removable by surgery, and systemic chemotherapy to kill cancer cells throughout the body. Treatment may last from months in Wilms' tumor to 2–3 years in pediatric leukemia. Even after treatment ends, yearly follow-up is important, as late effects of treatment may not occur until several years after treatment has ended.

Over the past 20 years, as survival has increased, much has been learned about the sequelae of pediatric cancer and its treatment. In the year 2010, there will be 1/250 adults who are survivors of pediatric cancer, with many continuing to need medical and psychological care for conditions created by their cancer treatment.

Foremost among the psychological issues for children and families is the fact that, while the prognosis for pediatric cancers has improved significantly over the past 20 years (to about 60–70 percent overall), it is still a potentially fatal disease. Thus, death and survival are major issues when a child is diagnosed with cancer and the possibility lingers through and after treatment. In cases where a genetic etiology or environmental cause is a possibility, parental guilt or blame may be a factor. Children may also search for a cause and attribute blame to their behavior. There are many psychological issues related to the diagnosis and treatment of pediatric cancer. Early coping issues include dealing with fear and anxiety connected with the potentially fatal diagnosis and making decisions about treatment at a time of extreme distress. The importance of a multidisciplinary pediatric oncology team cannot be overestimated. Medical and nursing staff should present the medical information and treatment options, giving the patient and family time to process and discuss at length. A psychosocial team comprised of psychologists, social workers, child life, chaplaincy, school liaison staff, oncology nurses, and oncologists is essential to help the child/adolescent and family to deal with the impact and outcome of pediatric cancer.

Medical/physical effects can vary from temporary effects, for example, hair loss, nausea and vomiting, fatigue, weight gain or loss and procedural pain/distress to permanent sequelae, for example, physical disfigurement, neurological or neurocognitive deficits. Common issues in pediatric cancer include fear and anxiety about the prognosis, treatment, and procedures; pain and discomfort; interruption of normal developmental tasks; changes in appearance and in functioning; separation from family and friends; absences from school and other family and social activities; changes in family functioning, in self-image and interpersonal relationships, and in life goals.

In helping children and families to cope with childhood cancer, adaptation is related to the patient's developmental and cognitive level, personality, previous functioning, coping styles and strategies, and family factors. In fact, parental coping has frequently been found to be one of the most important predictors of the child's effective coping with pediatric cancer, underscoring the need for family-centered approaches. In addition to early child and family assessment and psychosocial intervention, anxiety-reduction techniques, for example, distraction, breathing, relaxation, hypnosis, and imagery, should be taught prior to surgery if possible (with the type of preferred and effective techniques to be tailored to the individual). A multidisciplinary pain team should be involved early to assess and treat surgical pain and, later, phantom pain if it occurs. Side effects of chemotherapy, such as nausea and vomiting, can often be decreased with newer effective antiemetic medications, but behavioral interventions can complement these as well. Although intensive psychological intervention is not necessary for all children and families, it may be necessary at critical times of increased stress: diagnosis and early treatment, reentry into school, development of later school problems, changes in family functioning and resources, development of serious complications from treatment, changes in prognosis and treatment (for example, necessity for bone marrow transplant or other intensive treatment, ending treatment) recurrence or relapse, and probability of the child's death.

Effects from the cancer treatment itself can occur later, sometimes several years after treatment ends: organ dysfunction, infertility, growth problems, and second malignancies. Most pediatric cancer centers have begun multidisciplinary long-term follow-up clinics that include child, adolescent, and young adult survivors of pediatric cancer. It is important for these patients to continue to be followed, not only for late medical effects of treatment, but also for psychological, social, and vocational functioning. When prognosis is poor, the palliative care team should be involved early in treatment to provide continuity of care. In most cases, depending upon the needs and wishes of the family, the oncology team, including the psychosocial team,

continues to be involved with the child's family during and after the child's death to provide support.

See also: Bereavement; Coping with Illness; Ewins Sarcoma; Leukemia; Lymphomas; Neuroblastoma; Osteoblastoma; Parenting the Chronically Ill Child; Retinoblastoma; Wilm's Tumor

Further Reading

Bearison, D., & Mulhern, R. K. (Eds.). *Pediatric Psycho-oncology*. New York: Oxford University Press.
Noll, R. B., & Kazak, A. E. (1997). Psychosocial care. In A. R. Ablin (Ed.), *Supportive care of children with cancer* (pp. 263–273). Baltimore: Johns Hopkins University Press.

MARY JO KUPST
KELLY MALONEY
ANNE B. WARWICK

Cardiovascular Disease

DEFINITION

Cardiovascular disease in children refers to congenital heart disease (CHD), acquired heart disease, and arrhythmias, as well as systemic hypertension (high blood pressure). In addition, considerable research has established that risk factors for adult-onset cardiovascular disease (e.g., hypertension, high cholesterol, coronary artery disease) are established during childhood; furthermore, some children have hypertension and high cholesterol, however, these issues will not be considered in this entry. CHD, acquired heart disease, and arrhythmias will be described in separate sections.

CONGENITAL HEART DISEASE

CHD refers to a variety of disorders involving structural defects to the heart or the coronary blood vessels, and is grouped into acyanotic and cyanotic subtypes. The majority of cases are diagnosed during infancy, with an incidence of approximately 8 in 1,000 live births. In most cases, the etiology of CHD is not known, but occurs during fetal development and is thought to be due to both genetic and environmental factors.

In *acyanotic CHD*, there are holes in the walls of the heart chambers, resulting in blood being shunted away from the body and to the lungs. These are the most common CHD disorders, and include ventricular septal defects (about 28 percent of CHD cases), atrial septal/AV canal defects (about 10 percent of CHD), patent ductus arteriosus (persistence of an arterial communication between the aorta and pulmonary artery, comprising about 10 percent of CHD), and coarctation (constriction) of the aorta (about 5 percent of CHD). Valvular lesions (which obstruct blood flow at the valves) may result in either pulmonic stenosis (thickening of the heart valve between the right ventricle and pulmonary artery; about 10 percent of CHD) or aortic stenosis (thickening of the heart valve between the left ventricle and aorta; about 7 percent of CHD). Cardiomyopathy (disease of the heart muscle) is another type of acyanotic CHD.

In *cyanotic CHD*, there is a communication between the systemic and pulmonary circulations with a shunting of blood away from the lungs, resulting in reduced oxygenation of the blood or cyanosis. These defects include pulmonary atresia (absence of heart valve between the right ventricle and pulmonary artery) and tetralogy of Fallot (a constellation of abnormalities including a ventricular septal defect and abnormality of pulmonary valve), each of which account for about 10 percent of CHD cases, and transposition of the great arteries (TGA), accounting for an additional 5 percent of CHD cases. In TGA, there is a reversal of the aorta and pulmonary arteries, leading to mixing of oxygenated and deoxygenated blood.

Children with CHD may show a variety of symptoms, including fatigue, shortness of breath, growth failure, cough, cyanosis, or chest pain, depending on the type of cardiac defect. Most patients with CHD have mild disease requiring no treatment; however, those with severe disease usually have reduced exercise tolerance and restricted physical activity. Most severe cardiac defects are corrected by surgery during infancy with low mortality rates. However, neurologic complications of cardiac surgery are not uncommon, resulting in increased risk for mental retardation, language and learning disorders, and movement and seizure disorders. Low-flow cardiopulmonary bypass (i.e., an extracorporeal machine that oxygenates and pumps the blood) is increasingly used as a support technique during cardiac surgery rather than hypothermic circulatory arrest (i.e., stopping the heart at a low temperature), as the latter has been associated with greater central nervous system complications postoperatively. Extracorporeal membrane oxygenation (ECMO; prolonged cardiopulmonary bypass) has been successfully used in life-threatening situations after cardiac

surgery. Interventional catheterization has been increasingly used as an alternative to open-heart surgery for repair of certain types of CHD. This involves inserting a catheter to inject dye into the heart circulation to define the anatomy. For example, angioplasty (i.e., balloon catheter dilation of blood vessels) has been successfully used for recurrent coarctation of the aorta, as well as atrial septal defects and patent ductus arteriosus, and valvuloplasty (i.e., balloon catheter dilation of heart valves) has been effectively used for pulmonic and aortic stenosis.

Heart transplantation is now an accepted treatment approach in cases of severe end-stage heart disease where no other treatment options are available. Since 1982, more than 3,500 pediatric heart transplantations have been conducted by various centers throughout the world. One-year survival rates of 75–85 percent and 4-year survival rates of 65 percent have been obtained.

Most children with CHD require medical follow-up at regular intervals. Routine tests for evaluation and monitoring include chest radiographs, electrocardiograms, echocardiography, exercise testing, radionueclide studies, and cardiac catheterization. Because invasive procedures may be stressful for children, routine clinical practice for most patients involves sedation. After surgical repair, some children and parents may fear recurrence of heart-related problems or have unrealistic perceptions concerning restrictions in physical activity. For some children residual problems may exist, requiring further interventions including surgery.

ACQUIRED HEART DISEASE

Acquired heart disease in childhood refers to a variety of disorders that result from bacterial and/or viral infections that damage the heart. These disorders include infective endocarditis (infection of heart valve), rheumatic heart disease, and diseases of the myocardium (heart muscle) and pericardium (tissue around the heart). Normal children may acquire these diseases, but children with CHD are especially vulnerable. Another type of acquired heart disease is coronary artery disease secondary to Kawasaki syndrome, a condition characterized by rash, fever, and enlarged lymph nodes that can result in damage to the coronary arteries. Medical treatment for acquired heart disease generally requires prophylactic drug regimens, and sometimes cardiac surgery is needed to repair structural damage to the heart. When other treatment options are exhausted in severe cases, for example, when myocarditis (infection of the heart muscle) progresses to cardiomyopathy, heart transplantation must be undertaken.

Acquired heart disease is a cause of substantial morbidity and mortality among children. Mortality is low, however, with early diagnosis and treatment. Preventive interventions are, therefore, very important in the medical management of acquired heart disease. A significant problem observed in clinical practice with this patient population is non-adherence with prophylactic drug regimens. Empirical studies of this issue with this population are lacking, however. Because these diseases pose a considerable health risk for children, more research addressing regimen adherence and psychosocial issues of children with acquired heart diseases is needed.

ARRHYTHMIAS

Arrhythmias, or cardiac rhythm disturbances, can result from CHD (both acyanotic and cyanotic subtypes), acquired heart diseases, or acquired systemic disorders. The main risks of an arrhythmia are severe tachycardia (fast heart rate) or bradycardia (slow heart rate), resulting in decreased cardiac output; sudden death may result from a severe untreated arrhythmia. Some rhythm disturbances are fairly common and benign in children, such as premature atrial and ventricular beats. The most common clinically significant arrhythmias are caused by bypass tracts (i.e., atypical conduction patterns) such as Wolff–Parkinson–White syndrome (a type of supraventricular tachyarrhythmia) and congenital heartblock (a type of bradyarrhythmia).

Because of improved diagnostic methods, arrhythmias are now identified more often in children. Children with CHD who have had their defects surgically corrected are at increased risk for arrhythmias. Treatments for arrhythmias include pharmacologic agents, surgery to remove bypass tracts, implanted pacemakers and defibrillators, and heart transplantation in extreme cases that are unresponsive to other interventions. Significant issues in the treatment of pediatric arrhythmias include problems with dosage of medications, variable responses, side effects, and medication adherence. Few studies of psychological and behavioral factors have been conducted with this patient population.

COGNITIVE DEVELOPMENT CORRELATES

Research findings indicate that children with cyanotic CHD may be at risk for some adverse effects on cognitive development, presumably due to inadequate oxygenation of the brain during early development. For example, research by Newburger and colleagues (1984) showed a significant inverse correlation between age at repair (reflecting duration of hypoxia) and IQ for cyanotic children. Another study indicated that children with cyanotic CHD had lower IQ scores than children with acyanotic CHD. There is also evidence that children with CHD who survive cardiac arrest have lower cognitive functioning. Studies have shown that children with CHD, particularly those with cyanotic CHD, are at risk for poor school performance. While findings generally reveal that the IQ of children with CHD is within the normal range, significantly more than expected may have significant verbal-performance IQ discrepancies and require special educational programming. A recent study by Mahle and colleagues (2000) evaluated developmental outcomes of children with hypoplastic left heart syndrome and found that one third had been diagnosed with a learning disability and were receiving special education, with 19 percent having been held back in school.

Cardiac surgical techniques also affect cognitive development. Studies have shown that children who receive low-flow cardiopulmonary bypass as a support technique during cardiac surgery have better developmental outcomes than those who have hypothermic circulatory arrest. Tindall and colleagues (1999) evaluated the neuropsychological functioning of children who had ECMO after cardiac surgery and found significantly more impairment than children receiving cardiac surgery without ECMO or normal children, with lower scores in abstract reasoning and lateralized motor impairment (left hand), as well as lower visual memory and visual-spatial constructive skills. Review of studies of children who received heart transplantation, compared with both cardiac control and normal children, have shown lower scores on developmental, intellectual, and academic functioning. In addition, children receiving transplantation have more difficulties with growth and development, neurologic abnormalites, hearing problems, and speech and language delays.

BEHAVIORAL AND EMOTIONAL FUNCTIONING CORRELATES

A number of studies have investigated the behavioral and emotional functioning of children with CHD. In one study, children with cyanotic CHD (i.e., TGA and TOF) had poorer psychological functioning than a control group of healthy children who had spontaneous recovery of their heart problem, and psychological functioning was predicted by degree of CNS impairment and IQ. A study by Casey and colleagues (1996) examined the behavioral adjustment of children with surgically corrected complex CHD compared to healthy children with innocent heart murmurs. Behavior ratings by teachers revealed that children with CHD were more withdrawn, and more likely to have academic achievement problems. Exercise tolerance and degree of family strain were significant predictors of teacher-rated school functioning. Parent ratings also indicated that children with CHD were more withdrawn, engaged in fewer activities, and had more social problems.

Spurkland and colleagues (1993) examined the behavioral functioning of adolescents with "complex" (i.e., cyanotic) CHD, compared with adolescents who had repaired atrial septal defects and were in good health. Findings revealed that 42 percent of the youths with complex CHD were given *DSM-III* diagnoses versus 27 percent of the acyanotic patients. The most common diagnoses were overanxious disorder and dysthymic disorder. Only one third of youths with complex CHD were functioning normally, with one third having minor to moderate problems, and another third having serious dysfunction. In the acyanotic group, only 4 percent had a major psychiatric disorder, with 54 percent functioning normally and 42 percent considered to have minor to moderate problems. Greater psychopathology was associated with more severe physical impairment. Parent behavior ratings revealed clinically significant problems in 19 percent of the complex group versus only 4 percent in the acyanotic group.

Relatively few studies have considered the longer-term psychological adjustment of children with CHD. Available findings suggest that CHD patients generally report favorable psychosocial adjustment as young adults, with no adverse effects in terms of school and employment. Studies that have examined the psychological adjustment of children following heart transplantation indicate that some patients may be at risk for psychosocial problems following transplantation. In addition, studies suggest that these children may underachieve and have behavior problems at school.

Few studies have examined the psychosocial functioning of children with other types of cardiovascular disorders, although some studies of children with arrhythmias have been reported. For example, in one study children requiring pacemakers did not differ from healthy children on measures of psychosocial adjustment, but they had heightened fears of pacemaker failure and social rejection. DeMaso and colleagues (1990, 2000) examined psychological functioning in 38 children and adolescents before and 3 months after undergoing radio

frequency catheter ablation to correct their arrhythmias. Before ablation, normal psychological functioning was observed. After ablation, patients reported reductions in cardiac-related anxiety and increased enjoyment, with better functioning reported by patients who had curative ablation, suggesting improved quality of life following ablation.

ASSESSMENT

Because of the research findings indicating children with more severe types of CHD are at risk for cognitive and academic problems, as well as psychosocial adjustment difficulties, psychological assessment of these young patients should consider all these aspects of functioning. Social anxiety and social skills may be important to evaluate, particularly for those children who appear different than their peers due to their treatments. Medical regimens may be stressful, not only for the patients but for family members as well. This is particularly true for the post-transplantation regimen, which includes daily doses of immunosuppressive medications that may have considerable side effects, as well as extensive medical follow-up including endomyocardial biopsy. Assessment of adherence problems is an important issue, with studies indicating that up to 30 percent of pediatric patients have significant adherence problems, increasing their chances of graft rejection.

PSYCHOSOCIAL INTERVENTION

Very little psychosocial intervention research has been reported for this patient population. Descriptive studies have documented the high rates of distress commonly seen among young patients during invasive diagnostic procedures, but few intervention studies have been conducted with children who have cardiovascular disease. Available studies suggest that relaxation and imagery techniques without sedation are helpful for pediatric heart transplant patients during endomyocardial biopsy. Campbell and colleagues found that family-based cognitive-behavioral treatment including relaxation and problem-solving resulted in better adjustment in the hospital, as well as at home and school, after discharge from the hospital for cardiac surgery. If, as the available findings suggest, older children with more severe disease experience feelings of vulnerability and fears of social rejection, they may benefit from interventions to increase their social competence and decrease their fears.

See also: Anxiety Disorders; Coping with Illness; Heart Transplantation, Medical hospitalization; Pediatric; Preparation for Medical Procedures; Treatment Adherence: Medical

Further Reading

Alpern, D., Uzark, K., & Dick, M., II (1989). Psychosocial responses of children to cardiac pacemakers. *Journal of Pediatrics, 114,* 494–501.

Campbell, L. A., Kirkpatrick, S. E., Berry, C. C., & Lamberti, J. J. (1995). Preparing children with congential heart disease for cardiac surgery. *Journal of Pediatric Psychology, 20,* 313–328.

Casey, R. A., Sykes, D. H., Craig, B., Power, R., & Mulholland, H. C. (1996). Behavioral adjustment of children with surgically palliated complex congenital heart disease. *Journal of Pediatric Psychology, 21,* 335–352.

DeMaso, D. R., Beardslee, W. R., Silbert, A. R., & Fyler, D. C. (1990). Psychological functioning in children with cyanotic heart defects. *Developmental and Behavioral Pediatrics, 11,* 289–293.

DeMaso, D. R., Spratt, E. G., Vaughan, B. L., D'Angelo, E. J., Van der Feen, J. R., & Walsh, E. (2000). Psychological functioning in children and adolescents undergoing radiofrequency catheter ablation. *Psychosomatics, 41,* 134–139.

Fleisher, B. E., Baum, D., Brudos, G., Burge, M., Carson, E., Constantinou, J., Duckworth, J., Gamberg, P., Klein, P., Luikart, H., Miller, J., Stach, B., & Bernstein, D. (2002). Infant heart transplantation at Stanford: Growth and neurodevelopmental outcome. *Pediatrics, 109,* 1–7.

Fyler, D. C. (Ed.) (1992). *Nadas' Pediatric Cardiology.* Philadelphia: Hanley & Belfus.

Mahle, W. T., Clancy, R. R., Moss, E. M., Gerdes, M., Jobes, D. R., & Wernovsky, G. (2000). Neurodevelopmental outcome and lifestyle assessment in school-aged and adolescent children with hypolastic left heart syndrome. *Pediatrics, 105,* 1082–1089.

Newburger, J. W., Silbert, A. R., Buckley, L. P., & Fyler, D. C. (1984). Cognitive function and age at repair of transportation of the great arteries in children. *New England Journal of Medicine, 310,* 1495–1499.

O'Dougherty, M., Wright, F. S., Loewenson, R. B., & Torres, F. (1985) Cerebral dysfunction after chronic hypoxia in children. *Neurology, 35,* 42–46.

Spurkland, I., Bjornstad, P. G., Lindberg, H., & Seem, E. (1993). Mental health and psychosocial functioning in adolescents with congenital heart disease. A comparison between adolescents born with severe heart defect and atrial septal defect. *Acta Paediatrica, 82,* 71–76.

Tindall, S., Rothermel, R., Delamater, A. M., Pinsky, W., & Klein, M. (1999). Neuropsychological abilities of children with cardiac disease treated with extracorporeal membrane oxygenation. *Developmental Neuropsychology, 16,* 101–115.

Todaro, J. F., Fennell, E. B., Sears, S. F., Rodrigue, J. R., & Roche, A. K. (2000). Cognitive and psychological outcomes in pediatric heart transplantation. *Journal of Pediatric Psychology, 25,* 567–576.

ALAN M. DELAMATER

Celiac Disease

DEFINITION/INCIDENCE/ETIOLOGY

Celiac disease (gluten-sensitive enteropathy) is an immunological disorder that damages the lining of the small intestine in reaction to gluten, a protein found in wheat, rye, and barley. Classic childhood symptoms include some combination of diarrhea, vomiting, abdominal distension, irritability, abdominal pain, anorexia nervosa, and weight loss or failure to gain weight. Less common features include short stature, anemia, seizures, arthralgias, infertility, and hair loss, demonstrating the heterogeneity of this disease. Celiac disease is a lifelong disorder that can present at any age. Approximately 1 in 200 people in North America are affected, however, many cases of celiac disease are undiagnosed. The etiology of celiac disease is unknown, but a genetic predisposition has been confirmed.

ASSESSMENT/TREATMENT/PROGNOSIS

Screening blood tests identify antibodies that develop in untreated celiac disease. Endoscopy with small bowel biopsy is used to confirm the diagnosis. Treatment consists of removing all gluten from the diet, which can be a complex and difficult task. Gluten is present in foods containing wheat, rye, and barley, and it can be hidden in foods and non-food products such as medications. A knowledgeable nutritionist is invaluable in the management of celiac disease. Removal of gluten from the diet results in full clinical remission and restoration of the damage to the small intestine.

PSYCHOSOCIAL CORRELATES

Excluding gluten from the diet results in many daily challenges. Adults with celiac disease and parents of children with celiac disease have reported that their most frequent concern is determining if foods are gluten-free, and they have reported significant difficulty eating in restaurants and at social events. Children and adolescents with celiac disease have reported that they feel different from their peers and envy their peers' unrestricted diets. Adherence to the gluten-free diet can become problematic, particularly in adolescence, with 27–48 percent of adolescents reporting non-adherence. Among adults, one study investigated health-related quality of life and reported significantly lower levels in individuals with celiac disease compared to the general population. A few studies have investigated emotional symptoms in adults with celiac disease and reported significantly more symptoms of depression and anxiety when compared to healthy adults and surgery patients.

See also: Gastrointestinal Disorders

Further Reading

American Gastroenterological Association. (2001). American gastroenterological association medical position statement: Celiac sprue. *Gastroenterology, 120,* 1522–1525.

Farrell, R. J., & Kelly, C. P. (2002). Celiac sprue. *New England Journal of Medicine, 346,* 180–188.

Celiac disease Web sites: www.celiac.org and http://www.celiac.com

LAURA M. MACKNER
WALLACE V. CRANDALL

Central Auditory Processing Disorders

DEFINITION/ETIOLOGY

The terms "central auditory processing" and "auditory processing" are used interchangeably and refer to our understanding of what we hear. Individuals with central auditory processing disorders (CAPD), typically have normal hearing sensitivity; however, they experience difficulty analyzing or making sense of what they hear. Other terms used to define CAPD include problems with auditory perception, central deafness, word deafness, auditory comprehension deficit, and auditory perceptual processing dysfunction.

The prerequisites for auditory processing include: auditory attention, auditory memory, motivation, maturation and integrity of the auditory pathways, decision processes, and use of linguistic cues such as grammar, meaning in context, and lexical representations. Basically, discriminating differences between sounds, identifying speech sounds, sequencing the sounds, auditory figure ground (listening in background), auditory closure (filling in missing information), and auditory memory are all functional skills that comprise auditory processing. Difficulties in any of these areas are considered to be a CAPD.

Causes of CAPD reported in the literature include loss of function from injury or disease and neural

maturational delays from otitis media or prematurity. There also appears to be a genetic component with family members reporting similar central auditory processing problems.

PREVALENCE

The diverse clinical population in which CAPD is observed (i.e., learning disabilities, attention deficit disorders) has made identification of specific prevalence for children difficult. Based on the prevalence of comorbid conditions and testing referrals it is estimated that the prevalence of CAPD in children is between 2 and 3 percent.

CORRELATES

Central auditory processing is important to learning in the classroom. By the time a child is ready for fourth grade, most auditory discrimination, speech and language development, and memory and processing skills are mature and intact. Children with CAPD may demonstrate difficulties in speech, language, and/or learning, especially in the areas of spelling and reading. Common characteristics include appearing hearing impaired, difficulty with phonics or speech sounds, appearing inattentive, easy distractibility by background noise, difficulty following oral directions, and below average academic performance. Many of these characteristics are also present in language disorders, learning disabilities, cognitive disabilities, attention deficit disorders, and attention deficit with hyperactive disorders. Separating the above groups requires cooperation among professionals in order for the appropriate remedial plans to be devised.

The presence of CAPD in diverse clinical populations brings up questions of whether central auditory processing deficits underlie or reflect language disorders. Performance deficits in understanding verbal directions, auditory memory, as well as in academic underachievement and reading difficulties provide a strong link between auditory processing and global cognitive and linguistic functions. This complex link between language and cognitive functions makes it difficult to differentially diagnosis the presence of a CAPD.

By the time the individual is seen by the audiologist for a diagnosis of central auditory processing disorder, a great deal of stress has emerged in the families. Several professionals have likely been consulted and in some cases the test results show adequate language and good cognitive ability. The individual with CAPD and the family may be extremely frustrated. The most common remark that the audiologist will hear is "if the hearing is normal, then the child must be ignoring me." Comorbidity with other disorders will also hinder treatment success if the processing issues are not addressed.

ASSESSMENT

Given that CAPD coexists with other disorders, particularly learning disorders, a differential diagnosis for CAPD is more often an art than a science. The ultimate function of the assessment process should be to identify the strengths and weaknesses of the individual child in order to develop a plan of intervention. Thus, a collaborative effort is required for the assessment of CAPD. To effectively identify the functional deficits, assessment should include physiological (Auditory Brainstem Response and Middle Latency Response Testing) and behavioral audiological evaluation, speech-language evaluation, psycho-educational evaluation and neuropsychological evaluation. Screening tests for CAPD are available for children as young as 3 years; however, the auditory system matures rapidly between 3 and 5 years of age, making it difficult to diagnose a deficit versus normal developmental change. A child 5 years or older may be administered a full central auditory processing test battery.

Often the speech-language pathologist is the first to assess a child who has difficulty listening and following directions. The speech and language pathologist evaluates the linguistic characteristics of the presenting problem. For example, they would look at speech production, speech sounds discrimination, and how well the child follows increasingly more difficult directions. Receptive language (how the child understands language) and expressive language (how the child uses language) would also be evaluated.

The definition of auditory processing problems assumes normal hearing acuity and should be confirmed using basic audiological testing. It is possible for an individual with a hearing impairment to have a central auditory processing disorder, but the assumption is that not enough information is presented for processing if the hearing is impaired. Middle ear problems are also known to affect central auditory performance and this should be assessed before more sophisticated behavioral auditory tests are done. The purpose of the behavioral central auditory processing evaluation completed by the audiologist is to help define the

specific auditory processing difficulties that a child may be experiencing and to recommend appropriate remediation. Performance on auditory processing tests is measured according to chronological age expectancies. The auditory system continues to mature up to age 12 or 13 making it necessary to obtain normative data for each age. To identify an internal processing problem it is necessary to reduce the amount of external information available for processing. The premise of testing is that degraded speech, or speech in noise, will strain the auditory pathways of the central nervous system more than the recognition of unaltered speech or speech in quiet. An individual with normal central auditory processing abilities can, to some extent, compensate for these degraded signals, whereas an individual with a central auditory processing deficit cannot. The psycho-educational and neuropsychological evaluation will provide information concerning the child's learning style and cognitive ability strengths and weaknesses. The pattern of scores also provides information that is useful in separating a generalized learning disability from central auditory processing disorders. Auditory processing disorders will have a discrepancy between the non-verbal and verbal scoring areas with the nonverbal scores being higher. The neuropsychological evaluation will also provide information concerning problems with attention.

TREATMENT

Treatment options include remediation techniques, compensatory strategies, and environmental controls. Remediation techniques include ear training for phoneme and sound recognition, discrimination, sequencing, blending, and strengthening auditory memory and auditory closure. Noise desensitization is an ear-training program that provides practice for listening to a desired signal in the presence of background noise. Noise interference can be handled using environmental and technology modifications; however, provision of practice in a controlled environment by gradually increasing the noise level will help integrate the individual with CAPD into the regular environment. Teaching lip-reading skills provides visual information for the auditory signal and improves attending skills.

Environmental difficulties are associated with the amount of background noise, distance, and distortion of the signal caused by reverberation that may be present. Enhancement of the auditory environment may include: preferred seating to enable the child to easily see the teacher's face and the blackboard, acoustic room treatment to reduce background noise and the echo or reverberation, and use of FM auditory sound systems. An audiologist should complete fitting of system in order to minimize any adverse effects. The teacher wears a wireless microphone, which transmits her speech signal directly to the child's ear or through a strategically placed speaker or small earphones. Smaller class size or individual instruction may be recommended depending on the impact that the auditory processing disorder has on language development.

Classroom teachers can also use specific strategies to assist the child with central auditory processing disorder. A visual display of auditory information can be useful as well as re-stating or rephrasing directions. Using shorter instructions and allowing processing time are useful strategy for the classroom. Compensation strategies that can be taught to the older individual include repetition of what was heard, watching for visual cues, and using context information to figure out the message.

PROGNOSIS

Intervention is successful in providing the individual with compensation strategies that will be useful in any situation that they may encounter. As an adult, the individual with a CAPD will have more control over the environment and they will have the experience that will help them interpret the message in a communication situation. The variables associated with other disabilities will influence the outcome.

See also: Attention-Deficit/Hyperactivity Disorder; Hearing Impairment; Language Development; Learning Disorders

Further Reading

American Speech–Language–Hearing Association; Task Force on Central Auditory Processing Consensus Development. (1996). *American Journal of Audiology, 5*(2), 41–54.

Bellis, T. J. (1997). *Central auditory processing disorders: In the educational setting.* San Diego: Singular Publishing Group.

Katz, Jack. (1992). Classification of auditory processing disorders. In J. Katz, N. Strecker, & D. Henderson (Eds.), *Central auditory processing: A transdisciplinary view.* St. Louis: Mosby.

CAPD: From the Heart of a Mother, Web: http://www.angelfire.com/fl2/capd/

CAPD Parents' Page Resources for Parents of Children with Central Auditory Processing Disorders, Web: http://pages.cthome.net/cbristol/capd.html

Chermak, Gail D., & Musiek, Frank E. (1997). *Central auditory processing disorders: New perspectives.* San Diego: Singular Publishing Group.

Masters, M. G., Stecker, N. A., & Katz, J. (1998). *Central auditory processing disorders: Mostly management.* Boston: Allyn & Bacon.

EVA SAFFER

Central Deafness

See: Central Auditory Processing Disorders

Central Hearing Loss

See: Hearing Impairment

Central Nervous System Tumors

DESCRIPTION

Tumors of the central nervous system (CNS) involve the brain and spinal cord and represent the second most common pediatric cancer after acute lymphoblastic leukemia (20 percent of childhood cancers). About 2,000 children and adolescents are diagnosed with brain tumors each year. The peak incidence in childhood is during the first decade of life, with the male gender being predominant. From 1 to 2 years of age, cerebral tumors are most common, but in older children, cerebellar tumors predominate.

The following are the most common types of brain tumors in children in decreasing incidence: supratentorial astrocytomas (low grade 15–25 percent; high grade 10–15 percent), and high grade (10–15 percent), medulloblastomas (about 20 percent), cerebellar astrocytomas (10–20 percent), brain stem gliomas (10–20 percent), ependymomas (5–10 percent), craniopharyngiomas (6–9 percent), and pineal tumors (0.5–2 percent).

ETIOLOGY

There is an increased risk of CNS tumors in several inherited syndromes, including neurofibromatosis types 1 and 2, von Hippel–Lindau, tuberous sclerosis, and Li–Fraumeni syndrome. However, less than 10 percent of children with brain tumors will have one of these syndromes. Ionizing radiation exposure is related as well to the development of CNS tumors. There is an increased risk of CNS lymphoma with several immune suppression syndromes (Wiskott–Aldrich, ataxia-telengiectasia, and acquired immunodeficiency syndrome) and after solid-organ transplantation. However, the majority of children with brain tumors have no identifiable cause.

PRESENTATION

Presentation depends on the tumor site, age, and developmental level of the child. CNS tumors frequently present with signs and symptoms of increased intracranial pressure (ICP). ICP is caused by infiltration of the tumor and/or obstruction of cerebrospinal fluid (CSF) and leads to hydrocephalus (increased CSF fluid in the ventricles of the brain). Infants may present with lethargy, failure-to-thrive, and loss of developmental milestones. An older child may show poor school performance, fatigue, irritability, morning headaches (which worsen when lying down and become more severe over time), double vision, and vomiting. Symptoms may be mild and difficult to recognize but will progress and become more localizing with time. Supratentorial (above the tentorium separating the cerebrum from the cerebellum) tumors may present with hemiparesis (paralysis on one side of the body), hyper-reflexia (increased reflexivity), seizures, sensory loss, and visual loss. Infratentorial tumors (cerebellum and brainstem) may present with ataxia (loss of muscle coordination), and cranial nerve dysfunction as well as signs and symptoms of increased ICP.

TREATMENT

Treatment of CNS tumors involves several disciplines and modalities. Magnetic resonance imaging (MRI) is usually done preoperatively to assess the location and extent of the tumor. Surgery, either for a biopsy or attempted resection (removal), is usually the first step in therapy. For most tumors, removal of the tumor, or at least gross total resection is related to a better prognosis (although the more extensive the surgery, the greater chance of morbidity). A subset of patients proceed to receive radiation therapy (ranging from about 35 to 54 Gy), chemotherapy, or a combination of both. A small percentage of patients will receive radiation, chemotherapy, or without a biopsy-proven diagnosis due to location (such as brainstem or optic tract tumors), both. The specific treatment for the more commonly seen CNS tumors follows.

Medulloblastomas and primitive neuroectodermal tumors (PNETs) are treated with surgery, craniospinal radiation therapy, and chemotherapy (agents include cisplatin, vincristine, CCNU, and cytoxan). Low grade astrocytomas are treated with either surgery alone, surgery with localized radiation therapy, or surgery with chemotherapy (most common agents include carboplatin and vincristine). High grade gliomas are treated with surgery, radiation therapy, and chemotherapy (agents include prednisone, CCNU, vincristine, procarbazine, carboplatin). High dose chemotherapy with stem cell rescue is also being used for this group of tumors. Ependymomas are primarily treated with surgical excision and radiation therapy. The chemotherapeutic agent, cisplatin, has some activity in these tumors. Brainstem gliomas are treated with radiation therapy. Multiple chemotherapeutic regimens have been tried but none have improved survival over radiation therapy alone.

PROGNOSIS

Outcome for CNS tumors is variable due to the diffuse tumor types and locations. Overall, approximately 65 percent of patients are long-term survivors of brain tumors. However, survival ranges from patients with brainstem gliomas (median survival is less than 1 year) to patients with low-grade gliomas (5-year survival rate over 70 percent). Brain tumors lead other pediatric malignancies in mortality.

Acute and Long-Term Effects

Given the significant morbidity associated with the tumor and treatment, short- and long-term changes in functioning are common in children with CNS tumors. Acute effects of radiation include anorexia nervosa, fatigue, drowsiness, confusion, which typically recede after treatment. However, more serious late effects, depending upon the child's age (those less than 4 years of age are more vulnerable) and dosage of radiation include cortical atrophy and white matter destruction. Other complications of treatment, which also affect normal brain tissue, include significant visual, auditory, and motor dysfunction, seizures, decreased growth, and secondary CNS tumors.

Psychological Issues

In contrast to other pediatric cancers, for example, leukemia, psychological studies of pediatric CNS tumors have been relatively rare until recently. Recent studies of neuropsychological functioning of children with CNS tumors have found that they are at risk for significant and irreversible neurocognitive problems.

Risk factors include: cranial radiation (especially whole brain or supratentorial), young age (less than 4 years old), increased time from treatment, location of the tumor, and presence of hydrocephalus. In addition to decreased IQ and sensorimotor deficits, common sequelae include significant problems in attention, memory, speed of processing, and mathematical ability; these children are frequently placed in special education programs. Sometimes children become frustrated and depressed trying to accomplish tasks that they had previously mastered. Because of lowered processing speed and ability, children may be less able to understand or respond to social cues, resulting in lowered social interaction. Because of their altered appearance, some of which may be permanent (e.g., baldness from radiation, surgical scars or misshapen head, short stature, reduced emotional expression), children may be seen as different and may have more difficulty in the areas of peer acceptance and socialization. They may also become more isolated, preferring not to risk rejection by peers. In addition to one-to-one cognitive/behavioral therapy and therapy to help families deal with CNS tumor sequelae, social skills interventions may be beneficial, as well as participation in oncology-related groups and camps. Children with CNS tumors should be tested longitudinally for at least 5 years after diagnosis, with appropriate school interventions. Currently, there are several studies that are testing the effectiveness of interventions to help improve attention and memory deficits. In addition, they are a group that is at risk for development of psychosocial problems, and should receive psychological intervention to help them cope with treatment and its short- and long-term effects. It is only recently that there have been sufficient numbers of long-term survivors of CNS tumors for psychological studies. However, little is still known about the long-term effects on the quality of life of adult survivors, for example, vocational, social, marital, and physical long-term impact, and more needs to be done to prepare and follow these patients as well as provide help for deficits created by treatment.

See also: Bereavement; Childhood Cancers; Coping with Illness; Parenting the Chronically Ill Child; Preparation for Medical Procedures

Further Reading

Armstrong, F. D., & Mulhern, R. K. (1999). Acute lymphoblastic leukemia and brain tumors. In R. T. Brown (Ed.), *Cognitive aspects of chronic illness in children* (pp. 47–77). New York: Guilford.
Ris, M. D., & Ris, R. B. (1994). Long term neurobehavioral outcome in pediatric brain tumor patients: Review and methodological critique. *Journal of Clinical and Experimental Neuropsychology, 16,* 21–42.
Strother, D. R., Pollack, I. F., Graham Fisher, P., Hunter, J. V., Woo, S. Y., Pomeroy, S. L., & Rorke, L. B. (2002). Tumors of the central nervous system. In P. A. Pizzo & D. G. Poplack (Eds.), *Principles and practice of pediatric oncology* (4th ed., pp. 751–824) Philadelphia: Lippincott, Williams & Wilkins.

MARY JO KUPST
KELLY MALONEY

Cerebral Concussions

See: Traumatic Brain Injury

Cerebral Palsy

DESCRIPTION OF THE DISORDER

Cerebral palsy has been defined as a generic term referring to a family of impairments of muscle tone, muscle control, or locomotion resulting from permanent and nonprogressive defects or lesions of the brain. Children who have cerebral palsy can be divided into two major categories based upon locus of structural central nervous system change: pyramidal and extrapyramidal tracts (pathways) of the nervous system. In the pyramidal tract of the brain, damage occurs in the motor cortex, resulting in spasticity as the predominant symptom. The pyramidal tract is involved with the voluntary control of muscles in the arms and legs (initiating movement). Damage to the nerve fibers or cells in this area results in spastic paralysis. Symptoms vary based upon the region of the brain affected (e.g., hemiplegia in which one side of the body is affected; quadriplegia in which all four limbs are affected). Extrapyramidal cerebral palsy is associated with difficulty in regulating movement and maintaining posture. The most common form of extrapyramidal cerebral palsy is choreoathetoid, marked by abrupt, involuntary movement of the extremities.

ETIOLOGY

There are three distinct groups that delineate causes of cerebral palsy, each having different associations with respect to prevention of the disorder, and amelioration of contributory factors influencing the condition: prenatal factors (before birth), perinatal factors (during the time of birth), and postnatal factors (period immediately after the birth).

INCIDENCE/PREVALENCE

Approximately 9,000 children or 1.4–2.4 per 1,000 births are diagnosed with cerebral palsy each year in the United States, with a total prevalence of one million affected individuals.

CORRELATES

In addition to the primary motor-locomotion symptoms, children with cerebral palsy typically have secondary disabilities including: sensory disorders, seizures, cognitive impairment, heart defects, asthma, dental abnormalities, and speech and language disabilities. Cognitive functioning for children with cerebral palsy varies from above average to mental retardation (approximately half to three quarters of those evaluated with cerebral palsy had some form of cognitive impairment). Caution must be used to avoid misinterpreting physiological neuromuscular symptoms for cognitive ones. For example, the effects of motor impairment may be misleading (e.g., dysarthria or speech dysfluency is not the same as language impairment). One of the major challenges is to separate cognitive impairments from motor impairments in the infant/toddler with cerebral palsy when the speech mechanism is involved. Repeated evaluations by knowledgeable professionals is mandatory.

ASSESSMENT

Immediate postnatal neurological assessment of cerebral palsy is difficult given the maturational state of the infant's central nervous system. Several behavioral symptoms may indicate the existence of cerebral palsy: excessive sleepiness, irritability upon waking, weak cries and poor sucking reflect, apathy toward environment, and unusual sleep position. Clinicians specializing in pediatrics with a thorough knowledge of cerebral palsy are able to make a clinical diagnosis, but most often the delayed motor development of speech is detected by a concerned parent and brought to the attention of his or her family practitioner. Spastic cerebral palsy may be identifiable in the first few months of

life, but choreoathetoid movements may not be detectable for over 18 months.

TREATMENT

Early detection of cerebral palsy enhances the rehabilitation process. Beginning therapy (physical, early cognitive stimulation) within the first few weeks of life increases the probability that motor and developmental function will develop optimally.

Cerebral palsy may be associated with expressive language difficulty. While manual communication may compensate for this functional limitation, motoric deficits associated with cerebral palsy may limit this compensatory strategy. Augmentative communication devices such as electronic communication boards and computers with synthetic voice capability are very useful in promoting language use and socialization. Voice-activated technology can assist with controlling the environment, such as lights, televisions, curtains, doors, and telephones. Depending upon the clarity of speech, a child may be able to use voice-activated word processing programs.

Initial treatment emphases used to incorporate orthopedic surgery techniques, but these have given way to early diagnosis and intervention, placing more emphasis on global remediation of developmental deficits through a variety of physical therapy, occupational therapy (orthotic devices such as braces), medication (to reduce spasticity), and in some instances surgical interventions (hydrocephalus, vascular abnormalities, cysts, or tumors; procedures to correct residual deformities).

Common surgical intervention for children with cerebral palsy ameliorate strabismus, and cleft lip and palate. Children very likely need orthopedic surgery as they mature. Additionally there are state-of-the-art techniques involving the injection of botulinium toxin, baclofin pumps, and selective neurosurgery of the spinal nerve roots (dorsal rhizotomy). These procedures show promise for reducing spasticity, increasing range of motion, and increasing functional skills. The efficacy of these techniques are not yet established with respect to significant and longer-term increases in functional adaptive skills.

PROGNOSIS

The life span of those with cerebral palsy is somewhat less than that of the "normal population."

Prognosis varies by type of cerebral palsy and severity/extent of physical impairment; for example, an individual with severe spastic quadriplegia may not live past the fifth decade. Earlier death is often related to secondary impact of the physical disability, on general health and vitality, for example, mortality associated with pneumonia. Prognosis is also a function of earlier treatments (physical/psychological) and promoting independence in daily skills and life choices.

See also: Health Care Professionals; Individuals with Disabilities Educational Act (IDEA); Parenting the Handicapped Child; Speech and Language Assessment

Further Reading

Batshaw, M. L. (1997). *Children with disabilities* (4th ed.). Baltimore: Brookes.
Kopriva, P., & Taylor, J. R. (1993). Cerebral palsy. In M. G. Brodwin, F. Tellez, & S. K. Brodwin (Eds.), *Medical, psychosocial and vocational aspects of disability* (pp. 519–536). Athens, GA: Elliott and Fitzpatrick.
Web site: United Cerebral Palsy Associations: http://www.ucpa.org

DENNIS C. HARPER

Child and Adolescent Psychiatry

A Child and Adolescent Psychiatrist is a physician who specializes in the evaluation, diagnosis, and treatment of children and adolescents with psychiatric disorders. Training requirements for a child and adolescent psychiatrist usually include 4 years of medical school, a 3-year residency in general psychiatry, and a 2-year fellowship in child and adolescent psychiatry. After completing training, the Child and Adolescent Psychiatrist is eligible to take an examination to become Board certified in General Psychiatry by the American Board of Psychiatry and Neurology. After successfully completing this examination, the Child and Adolescent Psychiatrist is eligible for an additional examination to become Board certified in Child and Adolescent Psychiatry.

Child and Adolescent Psychiatrists receive training to treat infants, children, adolescents, and adults as individuals, couples, families, and groups. They use a variety of treatment techniques such as psychotherapies, behavior therapies, medications, as well as interventions with the school and family. Because of their expertise with medical treatments, psychiatrists are often consulted about prescribing psychotropic medications to children and adolescents. In addition, psychiatrists are often involved in the hospitalization of children and adolescents for psychiatric reasons, such as suicide risks and psychotic disorders. Child and Adolescent Psychiatrists practice in a variety of settings, including private offices, hospitals, clinics and other medical and mental health settings.

See also: Health Care Professionals; Physicians (General, Speciality)

Further Reading

American Academy of Child and Adolescent Psychiatry. (2002). 3615 Wisconsin Avenue, N.W. Washington, DC 20016, http://www.aacap.org/about/q&a.htm

TERRY STANCIN
SUSAN K. SANTOS

Child Maltreatment

DEFINITION

There are currently four recognized forms of child abuse and neglect. These include physical abuse, sexual abuse, neglect, and psychological maltreatment. The four types are increasingly subsumed under the term child maltreatment. It is important to note that there is not a single set of definitions for the forms of abuse that is utilized by all states, tribes, and the federal government. This lack of standardization creates significant problems in obtaining and documenting the actual incidence and prevalence of child maltreatment.

The following are general definitions for the four forms of abuse and neglect:

Physical abuse is defined as a nonaccidental injury that occurs to a child under the age of 18 by a caretaker; it can include beatings, shaking, burns, human bites, or strangulation that results in injuries such as bruises or welts, fractures, brain damage, retinal hemorrhages, or internal injuries.

Sexual abuse is broadly defined as any sexual activity involving a child or adolescent in which consent is not or cannot be given; it includes fondling;

exhibitionism; voyeurism; prostitution of children or adolescents; and oral, vaginal, or anal penetration.

Neglect is broadly defined as the consistent failure of a parent or caregiver to provide children under age 18 with the basic needs for growth and development such as medical or mental health services, food, shelter, nurturance, education, safety and supervision.

Psychological maltreatment is defined as a consistent pattern or an extreme instance of a parent displaying verbal hostility and aggression or being emotionally unavailable to a child. Six types of psychological maltreatment have been described: spurning, terrorizing, isolating, exploiting/corrupting, denying emotional responsiveness, and withholding medical care, mental health services, or education.

PREVALENCE

The most recent figures from the 1999 National Child Abuse and Neglect Reporting System (NCANDS) report that approximately 828,000 children had substantiated cases of abuse and neglect. This is a rate of 11.8 per 1,000 children, and it was estimated that 1,100 children died as a result of child maltreatment. Some 22 fatalities, or 2.1 percent, died while in foster care.

The majority of the cases were substantiated for neglect (58.4 percent), with about one-fifth (21.3 percent) suffering physical abuse and about one-tenth (11.3 percent) experiencing sexual abuse. The average response time for a child protective services (CPS) worker to respond to a report was 63.8 hr, approximately 2.5 days.

The 1999 figures report similar rates overall for males and females, but females are at higher risk for sexual abuse (1.6 per 1,000 for females compared to 0.4 per 1,000 for males). Young children age 0–3 are at highest risk for abuse and neglect and the rates decline as the child's age increases. The rates for race/ethnic groups vary from a low of 4.4 per 1,000 for Asian/Pacific Islander children to 25.2 per 1,000 for African American children. It is alarming to note that children who were abused or neglected prior to 1999 were almost three times as likely to be reabused during the 6 months following their first victimization than children without a prior history of victimization.

See also: Neglect; Physical Abuse; Psychological Maltreatment

Further Reading

Myers, J. E. B., Berliner, L., Briere, J., Hendrix, C. T., Jenny, C., & Reid, T. A. (2002). *The APSAC handbook on child maltreatment* (2nd ed.). Thousand Oaks, CA: Sage.
U.S. Department of Health and Human Services, Children's Bureau. (1999). *Child Maltreatment 1998: Reports from the States to the National Child Abuse and Neglect Data System (NCANDS).* Washington, DC: U.S. Government Printing Office.

BARBARA L. BONNER

Child Psychotherapy

While the term child psychotherapy has often been associated with specific approaches to treatment, any designation of treatments as examples of child psychotherapy must be viewed as somewhat arbitrary, as no one definition has gained universal acceptance. There are, however, some general characteristics of these approaches. Here, child psychotherapy is usually thought of as an interpersonal process, involving a verbal and/or nonverbal interchange between a child who exhibits psychological problems and a therapist who offers help. Within this context, the therapist attempts to gain an understanding of the child's problems and utilize the nature of the relationship and various therapeutic techniques to facilitate personality and behavior change.

Psychodynamic and nondirective/client-centered therapies that focus on the nature of the therapeutic relationship are most often considered as prototypical examples of child psychotherapy. Interpersonal psychotherapy, which has more recently been used with children and adolescents, would also fall under this heading. While child psychotherapy is usually associated with nonbehavioral treatments, emphasizing talk and/or play, cognitive-behavioral approaches can also be seen as "psychotherapeutic." These approaches are not restricted to more traditional behavioral methods but also focus on issues such as problem solving, irrational beliefs, causal attributions, and other types of maladaptive cognitions that may contribute to emotional distress and maladaptive behavior. The emphasis on cognitive factors as they interrelate with affect and behavior results in an approach that overlaps considerably with traditional approaches to child psychotherapy. Overviews of this and other child psychotherapy approaches can be found by considering topics cross-referenced with this listing.

CLINICAL APPLICATIONS OF CHILD PSYCHOTHERAPY

Children versus Adults in Psychotherapy

A major difference in working with adults and children lies in the need to alter therapy techniques to accommodate the child's level of cognitive and emotional development. Children are conceptually more concrete, linguistically less competent, and less introspective than adults. While therapy with verbal adolescents may share many common elements with adult therapy, treatment may have to be altered significantly for the younger child. Play, with its decreased emphasis on verbal communication, can serve as an effective medium of communication to promote constructive personality and behavior change.

Children are also less likely than adults to see themselves as having difficulties or to see the value in talking about their problems. Thus, children are often less than optimally motivated to participate in ongoing treatment or to share a therapist's views on treatment goals.

Children's dependence on caregivers often requires that the therapist deal with persons other than the patient to a much greater degree than is the case in working with adults. In sum, although many of the basic principles of psychotherapy may be similar for adults and children, the immaturity and dependent status of the child may require significant modifications in the application of these principles.

Elements of Change in Psychotherapy

Therapeutic change in child psychotherapy is thought to relate to certain aspects of the therapeutic relationship (general factors) as well as various therapy techniques that may be employed within the context of this relationship (specific factors). *General factors* include providing the child with an opportunity to talk about his/her problems with a therapist who listens and communicates an attitude of acceptance, reinforces appropriate in-therapy behavior, and creates positive expectancies for change. Therapy is enhanced through a therapist who communicates empathy, genuineness, and warmth. *Specific factors* can involve techniques such as *questions* designed to elicit information or encourage the child to continue talking, *clarifications* or *reflection* of feelings to help the child become more aware of the significance of certain behaviors or feelings, *confrontations* which encourage the child to deal with specific therapy-related issues, and *interpretations* that help the child develop important insights into the causes of his/her behavior.

Stages of Psychotherapy

The *initial stage* of therapy lays the foundation for later stages of treatment. Early sessions usually involve providing the child and the parent with information regarding the nature of therapy, developing tentative goals for treatment, and discussing the role of the therapist, patient, and parents in working towards these goals. Here, it is important to discuss the issue of confidentiality with both parent and child, and inform them not only of the importance of confidentiality, but of limitations on confidentiality in psychotherapy. The initial stage of therapy also involves continuing assessment of the presenting problem as well as the development of the patient/parent–therapist relationship. Indeed, the fostering of a positive therapeutic relationship with both the child and parent is viewed by most therapists as critical in determining the outcome of therapy.

The *middle stage* of therapy focuses on using the assessment information and the evolving patient–therapist relationship to affect patient change through the application of various treatment methods. Therapist behaviors designed to facilitate talking about and dealing with important issues, along with techniques such as reflection of feeling and interpretations, are used to help the child develop insight into the nature of their difficulties and "work through" important issues. The actual treatment methods utilized will vary depending upon the orientation of the therapist and the nature of the child's problems.

Timing is crucial when dealing with the *termination stage* of treatment. Issues of termination must be raised so that the child, his or her parents, and the therapist can discuss it without resulting in feelings of rejection by the child. The topic of termination should be approached when most of the treatment goals have been achieved and when the patient, parent, and therapist together feel the child is somewhat better equipped to handle future problems as they arise. During the period between the time a decision to terminate is made and the end of treatment, the therapist can help prepare the child for termination by dealing with separation issues and making plans for the future. Termination is usually accomplished by making the child and parent aware that the therapist will be available should future problems arise and often by setting a specific time for a follow-up appointment to ensure that things continue to go well.

EFFECTIVENESS OF CHILD PSYCHOTHERAPY

Child psychotherapy outcome research continues to lag behind research related to adult psychotherapy both in terms of the number and the quality of studies published. During the past several decades, a number of authors have provided qualitative reviews and critiques of the child psychotherapy research literature. These reviews suggest that, although some studies provide reason to believe that child psychotherapy can result in positive outcomes, methodological limitations often make it difficult to draw firm conclusions regarding efficacy or effectiveness. Recent years have witnessed an increasing number of quantitative outcome studies involving the use of metaanalysis, a statistical method that makes it possible to simultaneously summarize, integrate, and evaluate treatment effects across studies. Two metaanalytic studies, conducted in the mid to late 1980s, evaluated the overall efficacy of various psychotherapeutic treatments for children/adolescents displaying a range of problems. The results of both analyses suggested support for the overall efficacy of treatment when compared to control groups, with more support being found for behavioral over psychodynamic and client-centered approaches. A limitation of these two metaanalyses, however, was their inclusion of a large number of treatment studies that involved children who displayed conditions that were not particularly reflective of those typically seen in clinical practice. Many children participating in these studies were recruited specifically for treatment studies, rather than being clinically referred because of the severity of their problems. Many displayed isolated problems rather than multiple difficulties, as are often seen in clinic patients. Many were seen by clinicians who had been trained in specific treatment methods for specific research studies. These issues make it unclear as to whether these metaanalytic findings provide information regarding the effectiveness of child psychotherapy as it is routinely practiced in clinical settings.

To address this issue of ecological validity, a subsequent metaanalytic study was conducted in 1989 by Weisz and Weiss to evaluate treatment effectiveness with child/adolescent clinic patients displaying a mix of psychological difficulties. The results of this study provided little support for the effectiveness of child and adolescent psychotherapy as is currently practiced in clinical settings. As clinical experience suggests that children and adolescents do often benefit from treatment, there is a need for more sophisticated clinical investigations of child psychotherapy that can provide an empirical basis for clinical practice. Especially needed are studies that yield information regarding which types of therapies are effective for which types of problems, when offered by which types of therapists, and under what conditions.

See also: Client-Centered Therapy; Cognitive–Behavior Therapy; Interpersonal Psychotherapy for Depressed Adolescents; Play Therapy; Psychodynamic Therapy

Further Reading

Johnson, J. H., Rasbury, W. C., & Siegel, L. J. (1997). *Approaches to child treatment: Introduction to theory, research, and practice* (2nd ed.). Boston: Allyn & Bacon.

Weisz, J. R., & Weiss, B. (1989). Assessing the effects of clinical-based psychotherapy with children and adolescents. *Journal of Consulting and Clinical Psychology, 57,* 741–746.

Weisz, J. R., Weiss, B., Alicke, M. D., & Klotz, M. L. (1987). Effectiveness of psychotherapy with children and adolescents: Meta-analytic findings for clinicians. *Journal of Consulting and Clinical Psychology, 55,* 542–549.

JAMES H. JOHNSON
STEVEN K. READER

Child Self-Reports

DEFINITION

Whereas behavioral observation and behavior rating scales can be very useful when assessing perceptible or observable behavior characteristics, self-report scales can be best used for measuring children's personality traits, emotions, cognitions, and psychopathological symptoms. These scales typically contain a large number of items that have to be answered on a forced choice scale (e.g., "yes" or "no"). Some self-reports are rather simple and can be completed by children at age 7, other questionnaires are more complicated and only suitable for older children.

PERSONALITY QUESTIONNAIRES

A commonly used personality measure is the *Adolescent Version of the Minnesota Multiphasic Personality Inventory* (MMPI-A) (1992), which is a downward extension of the well-known adult measure. Scales assess symptoms of depression, anxiety, obsessiveness, paranoia, schizophrenia, psychopathy, conduct problems, alcohol and drug abuse, low self-esteem, and school and family problems, among others. The MMPI-A also includes validity scales that assess attempts to present oneself in a good or bad light, as well as defensiveness and inconsistent responding. The MMPI-A requires advanced reading skills and with a total of 478 "true-false" items the questionnaire is quite lengthy.

A brief self-report scale for measuring personality is the *Junior Version of the Eysenck Personality Questionnaire* (JEPQ) (1975). This 89-item scale which can be employed in youths aged 11 years and above, taps Eysenck's three basic dimensions of personality: extraversion, neuroticism, and psychoticism. The extraversion dimension pertains to characteristics such as sociability, craving for excitement, liveliness, activeness, and dominance. The neuroticism dimension has to do with the ease and frequency with which an individual becomes upset and distressed, with greater moodiness, anxiety, and depression reflecting higher levels of neuroticism. The psychoticism dimension refers to a predisposition to display hostile, manipulative, impulsive, and adventurous behavior.

A more focused personality questionnaire is Harter's *Self-Perception Profile for Children* (SPPC) (1985). The SPPC is a scale assessing a more specific feature of children's personality, namely self-esteem. The scale consists of 36 items that can be allocated to five specific domains (i.e., scholastic competence, social acceptance, athletic competence, physical appearance, and behavioral conduct), as well as global self-worth. Each SPPC item consists of two opposite descriptions, for example, "Some children often forget what they have learned" but "Other children are able to remember all things easily." Children have to choose the description that best fits them and then indicate whether the description is "somewhat true" or "very true" for them.

PSYCHOPATHOLOGICAL SYMPTOMS

Self-report measures are commonly used for assessing internalizing symptoms, about which children's reports may be particularly informative. An example is Kovacs' *Children's Depression Inventory* (CDI) (1981), which is a 27-item inventory for children and adolescents that assesses symptoms of sadness, self-blame, loss of appetite, insomnia, interpersonal relationships, and school adjustment.

Other commonly used instruments are the *Fear Survey Schedule for Children—Revised* (FSSC-R), the *Revised Children's Manifest Anxiety Scale* (RCMAS), and the *Spielberger State-Trait Anxiety Inventory for Children* (STAIC), which all measure anxiety symptomatology. The FSSC-R focuses primarily on phobic symptoms and taps fear of failure and criticism, fear of the unknown, fear of minor injury and small animals, fear of danger and death, and medical fears. The RCMAS is a questionnaire with three anxiety-related subfactors: physiological manifestations of anxiety, worry and oversensitivity, and problems with fear/concentration. The STAIC consists of a state scale that measures present-state and situation-linked anxiety and a trait scale that addresses temporally stable anxiety across situations.

Achenbach's *Youth Self-Report* (YSR) (1991) is the self-report version of the Child Behavior Checklist. The YSR, which can be used in children aged 11 years and above, addresses two broad domains in which problems may manifest themselves. One is externalizing which reflects behavioral problems and the other is internalizing which refers to emotional problems. Factor-analytic procedures performed on the YSR have yielded eight narrow-band factors: withdrawn, somatic complaints, anxious-depressed, social problems, thought problems, attention problems, delinquent behavior, and aggressive behavior.

CLINICAL APPLICATION AND LIMITATIONS

Self-report scales represent a time-efficient way to capture information about children's personality characteristics or psychopathological symptoms. There is evidence to suggest that children with internalizing psychopathology are better than their parents at reporting symptoms, while for those with externalizing disorders the opposite is true. Thus, in particular, when clinicians are faced with children who suffer from emotional problems such as anxiety disorders or depression, use of self-report scales is appropriate. It should be noted, however, that self-report measures are not without methodological limitations. For instance, children may underreport symptoms in order to present themselves more favorably or to avoid therapy. Furthermore, the child's ability to read and to understand the questionnaire items may directly influence the validity of the responses.

See also: Behavior Rating Scales; Screening Instruments; Validity

Further Reading

Achenbach, T. M. (1991). *Manual for the youth self-report*. Burlington, VT: University of Vermont, Department of Psychiatry.

Butcher, J., Williams, C., Graham, J., Archer, R., Tellegen, A., Ben-Porath, Y., & Kaemmer, B. (1992). *Minnesota Multiphasic Personality Inventory—Adolescent: Manual for administration, scoring, and interpretation*. Minneapolis: University of Minnesota Press.

Eysenck, H. J., & Eysenck, S. B. G. (1975). *Manual of the Eysenck Personality Questionnaire (adult and junior)*. London: Hodder & Stoughton.

Harter, S. (1985). *Manual for the Self-Perception Profile for Children*. Denver: University of Denver.

Kovacs, M. (1981). Rating scales to assess depression in school-aged children. *Acta Paedopsychiatrica, 46*, 305–315.

PETER MURIS

Child Temperament

The term temperament is commonly used to refer to individual differences in behavioral style that can be observed as early as infancy and early childhood. These individual differences, which relate more to the "how" rather than the "what" or "why" of behavior, are usually assumed to be biologically based, to be relatively stable across situations and time, and to be influenced in their expression by environmental factors.

Discussions of human temperament date back to the time of Hippocrates (460 BC), who believed temperament to be determined by the predominance of four bodily humors: yellow bile, blood, black bile, and phlegm. More contemporary views of childhood temperament have derived from the work of child psychiatrists Stella Chess and Alexander Thomas and the New York Longitudinal Study (NYLS).

DIMENSIONS AND PATTERNS OF TEMPERAMENT

Thomas and Chess began their research on temperament in the 1950s in response to the then prevailing social atmosphere that highlighted parents as major contributors to childhood behavioral problems. This longitudinal study has now spanned several decades and has provided a wealth of information regarding the nature of child temperament and the relations between temperament and adjustment over time. In their early work, Thomas and Chess defined dimensions of behavior, observable as early as 2–3 months of age, that were thought to differentiate between "Difficult," "Easy," and "Slow-to-Warm-Up" temperament styles. Difficult children were described as showing irregular patterns of eating, sleeping, and elimination (low rhythmicity), tendencies to withdraw in response to new/novel situations, slowness to adapt to new situations, negative mood, and high-intensity emotional responses. Easy children were described as being more predictable in biological functions, as willing to approach new situations, as being quicker to adapt, as having a positive mood, and as showing lower intensity emotional responses. Slow-to-warm-up children were characterized as having a lower activity level, a tendency to withdraw from new situations, as being slower to adapt and, while sometimes displaying a negative mood, as showing less intense emotional responses. It should be noted that Thomas and Chess also delineated additional temperament dimensions of distractibility, attention span/persistence, and threshold of responsiveness, although these have received less attention than those related to Easy, Slow-to-Warm-Up, and Difficult temperament. Of the 141 children in their original sample, 10 percent were classified as "Difficult," 30 percent as "Easy," and 15 percent as "Slow-to-Warm Up," with the others not being easily classified.

Despite the prominence of Thomas and Chess' contribution in present-day conceptualizations of temperament, a range of other dimensions and constellations of temperament characteristics have also been suggested. In reviewing the extensive research in this area, Bates (1989) highlighted a total of seven that he viewed as having adequate support. These included *Negative emotionality* (distress, fear, and anger), *Difficultness,* which overlaps with negative emotionality and includes several NYLS dimensions (e.g., negative mood, withdrawal, low adaptability, high intensity, and low rhythmicity), *Adaptability* (defined in terms of positive/negative reactions to new stimuli), *Reactivity* (response to varying intensities of stimuli), *Activity* (frequency and intensity of motor activity), *Attention regulation* (which incorporates the concepts of distractibility and task persistence), and *Sociability/Positive-emotionality* (enjoying interpersonal interactions and expressing positive emotions).

BIOLOGICAL ASPECTS OF TEMPERAMENT

It is commonly assumed that temperament is biological in origin, as individual differences in temperament can be observed very early in life before the child is subjected to significant socialization. Indeed, twin, family, and adoption studies suggest some genetic contribution to individual differences in temperament. Recent research in the area of neuroscience suggests links between neural structures and the expression of some temperament characteristics. Specifically, approach and avoidance behaviors appear linked to associations between cortical and limbic/brainstem regions. Despite suggestions of the constitutional origin of temperament, it has also been demonstrated that changes in temperament characteristics over time are related to parental characteristics, suggesting that social experience may likewise influence the way in which various aspects of temperament are expressed.

STABILITY OF TEMPERAMENT

Studies investigating the stability of child temperament over time have generally found correlations ranging from 0.25 to 0.82 which vary as a function of age, sex, the temperament dimensions assessed, how temperament is measured, the length of time between assessments, significant life events occurring between assessments, and sample characteristics. Prior (1992) notes that clusters of temperament (i.e., difficult/easy) are more stable across time than specific dimensions, and that stability increases when temperament ratings are at the extreme rather than in the moderate range.

TEMPERAMENT AND LATER OUTCOMES

Research suggests that children with difficult temperament (defined in different ways) are likely to have poorer outcomes than children with easy temperaments. Early findings by Thomas and Chess suggested that 70 percent of the difficult children in their study developed behavioral problems in childhood and adolescence while only 18 percent of easy children developed such problems. Other studies have shown a link between children with difficult temperament and externalizing behavioral problems such as Attention-Deficit/Hyperactivity Disorder (ADHD) and aggressive/antisocial behavior. The relationship between child temperament and internalizing problems is less clear. Generally, the link between measures of temperament and negative outcomes is not particularly strong in infancy but increases with age. While difficult temperament has been linked with later problems, easy temperament may serve as a protective factor for children with psychosocial risk factors.

GOODNESS-OF-FIT

The notion of goodness-of-fit acknowledges the important interaction between child temperament and the child's environment in determining outcomes. Chess and Thomas have defined goodness-of-fit as resulting when the child's abilities, motivation, and temperament are sufficient to meet the expectations and demands of the environment, and have suggested that a poor fit between a child's temperament and the environment can increase the likelihood of negative outcomes. While the focus is often on the fit between child temperament and parenting style, it should be emphasized that goodness-of-fit also relates to the fit between the child and the larger environment.

Consistent with the concept of goodness-of-fit, there is some support for the notion that various aspects of the parent/caregiver–child relationship seems to mediate the relationship between child temperament and later psychological/behavioral difficulties.

FACTORS INFLUENCING THE EXPRESSION OF TEMPERAMENT

In considering the expression of child temperament it is important to consider factors such as gender, socioeconomic status (SES), and culture/ethnicity. There do not appear to be significant gender differences in temperament in infancy. Early sex differences are seen in toddlers and increase with age, specifically as related to activity level and negative emotionality where boys tend to show higher levels than girls. It can be argued that social influences may also play a role here as these behaviors may be more tolerated for boys than girls.

Studies have also shown that a disproportionate number of children with difficult temperaments are from lower SES families, although the specific reasons for these findings are unclear. The importance of considering cultural factors is also highlighted by research suggesting that individuals from different cultural backgrounds often respond differently to temperament questionnaires, resulting in different profiles of child temperament. Different cultures may place different values on identical temperament styles, as noted by Prior (1992).

CLINICAL INTERVENTIONS

Sanson and Rothbart (1995) stress the need for parents to be sensitive and flexible in their interactions with their children and adapt their parenting styles to their child's temperament. This may be particularly important during infancy when children have limited capabilities to control and adapt their responses. In recent years, parenting training programs have been developed with a focus on helping parents cope with difficult child temperament. Sheeber and McDevitt (1998) provide an excellent overview of these programs, including their historical and conceptual bases, interventions, research findings, limitations, and future directions.

See also: Attention-Deficit/Hyperactivity Disorder; Behavioral Observation; Conduct Disorders; Temperament Assessment

Further Reading

Bates, J. E. (1989). Concepts and measures of temperament. In G. A. Kohnstamm, J. E. Bates, & M. K. Rothbart (Eds.), *Temperament in childhood* (pp. 3–26). Chichester, England: Wiley.

Chess, S., & Thomas, A. (1996). *Temperament theory and practice.* New York: Bruner/Mazel.

Prior, M. (1992). Childhood temperament. *Journal of Child Psychology and Psychiatry, 33,* 249–279.

Sanson, A., & Rothbart, M. K. (1995). Child temperament and parenting. In M. H. Bornstein (Ed.), *Handbook of parenting: Vol. 4. Applied and practical parenting* (pp. 299–321). Mahwah, NJ: Erlbaum.

Sheeber, L. B., & McDevitt, S. C. (1998). Temperament-focused parent training. In J. M. Briesmeister & C. E. Schaefer (Eds.), *Handbook of parent training: Parents as co-therapists for children's behavior problems* (2nd ed). New York: Wiley.

JAMES H. JOHNSON
STEVEN K. READER

Childhood

DEFINITION

The study of childhood may be divided by making reference to particular research subtopics or to particular chronological age ranges. The research subdisciplines that comprise the study of childhood include biological/brain development, motor and physical growth, perceptual development and cognitive functioning, language, and social–emotional development. The chronological approach typically divides the period of childhood into the prenatal period (pregnancy to birth), infancy (birth–2 years), early childhood (approximately 2–6 years) and middle childhood (6–12 years).

The childhood years represent a crucial period of successive changes that lead to adolescence and adulthood. One reason why psychologists study the childhood years is to better understand the impact of early experiences on later development. Indeed, the developmental literature is replete with examples of the relations between early development and later outcome, such as the relation between infant visual attention and cognitive outcome in later childhood and the relation between the quality of early attachments to caregivers and later social competence with peers. Other reasons for studying children include the existence of rapid change during the childhood years, social policy applications to improve children's everyday lives, and gaining insight into complex adult processes.

ISSUES IN CHILD DEVELOPMENT RESEARCH

The Nature–Nurture Debate

One of the fundamental issues in the study of development has been the debate over the relative contributions of biology/genetics versus those of the environment/experience to developmental change. Colloquially, this is referred to as the *nature–nurture debate*. Most modern researchers and theorists align themselves with interactionist perspectives that allow for the contributions of both biology and the environment to the development of the child, although in certain topic areas, this controversy is still active.

Other Issues

Other important issues in the field of child development include *continuity versus discontinuity* (i.e., whether development is best characterized in terms of relatively smooth developmental trajectories versus discrete developmental stages) and whether there are *critical or sensitive periods* during the lifespan. During such periods, particular types of experience may be necessary to trigger proper development in various domains of human behavior, for example, the acquisition of a second language. There is considerable variation, however, in the timing and duration of sensitive periods across skills and abilities.

MILESTONES OF DEVELOPMENT

Biological and Brain Development

Important neurological developments appear to occur in early and middle childhood, and such developments are thought to correspond to specific behavioral changes, such as changes in attention, language, visual-spatial, and social abilities. For example, the formation of connections between nerve cells in the brain (*synaptogenesis*) and improvements in the properties of the transmission of signals between nerve cells (through *myelination*) occur over a wide range of years, from the prenatal period through middle childhood and adolescence. In particular, improvements in receptive language correspond to changes in a brain area known as the angular gyrus, and improvements in higher level cognitive functions correspond to changes during childhood in a brain area known as the prefrontal cortex. In addition, the left hemisphere of the brain experiences a growth spurt between 3 and 6 years and then levels off whereas the right hemisphere of the brain matures more gradually between early and middle childhood. Much remains unknown about brain development in childhood due to various obstacles in conducting neurological studies at young ages.

Physical and Motor Development

Physical and motor development during the childhood years is characterized by slow, gradual increments that lead to improvements in gross motor skills (such as increases in the coordination of running, jumping, and throwing) as well fine motor skills (such as improvements that make it easier for children to tie their shoes, draw pictures with increasing precision, and write more legibly). Recently, however, there has been interesting interdisciplinary work in applied topics and developmental research. For example, research on childhood injuries has revealed relations among child temperament, estimates of physical abilities, and unintentional injuries. Specifically, children who were high on extroversion and low on inhibitory control during the toddler and preschool years tended to overestimate their physical abilities and have more unintentional injuries during childhood.

Perceptual Development and Cognitive Functioning

Much of what has traditionally been considered within the realm of cognitive development has come from the theories of Jean Piaget, which emerged during the first half of the 20th century. For example, Piaget's theory holds that children's thinking between 2 and 7 years of age is characterized by the emergence of symbolic thinking and mental representations and limited by semi-logical, egocentric thought. For instance, during this developmental stage, children are unable to understand the social or physical perspective of another person. Between 7 and 11 years, children are able to think logically about concrete objects and events but are unable to reason about the abstract. However, our understanding of cognitive development has grown immensely in recent decades. Research has demonstrated that the use of memory strategies to organize and remember information, problem solving and reasoning, intelligence, and academic skills during childhood have a significant impact on cognitive development. In addition, using knowledge of basic cognitive processes to better understand applied issues has become more prevalent. For example, basic developments in memory have large implications for children's eyewitness testimonials.

Language Skills

There are several important gains in language skills during childhood, such as increases in vocabulary, the mastery of grammatical rules, and pragmatics (i.e., the use of language in a social context such as humor, sarcasm). Furthermore, children are better able to learn a second language as a "native speaker" (i.e., without an accent) than are adults.

Social–Emotional Development

Key social–emotional milestones during early childhood include the emergence of early social relationships (e.g., attachment to caregivers during infancy), self-conscious emotions (e.g., shame, embarrassment, guilt, and pride), altruism, the conscience and morally relevant behaviors, friendships, and an awareness that gender is constant. During middle childhood, children's social–emotional behaviors becomes increasingly more complex. For example, more sophisticated cognitive abilities lead to a better understanding of moral rules and more strategic emotional regulation. Indeed, aggressive children have less skilled social information processing skills and are more likely to attribute ambiguous interactions with peers in a hostile manner.

IMPLICATIONS FOR CLINICAL RESEARCH AND PRACTICE

The importance of early development and experiences for later outcome has large implications for clinical research; as such, early identification of atypical development and implementing intervention programs will greatly impact developmental outcome. Moreover, developmental researchers are particularly cognizant of the mutual influences of all aspects of development on one another, and this perspective is analogous to clinician's understanding of comorbidity among psychological disorders.

See also: Cognitive Development; Developmental Milestones; Language Development; Motor Development

Further Reading

Colombo, J. (1993). *Infant cognition: Predicting later intellectual functioning.* Thousand Oaks, CA: Sage.

Schwebel, D. C., & Plumert, J. M. (1999). Longitudinal and concurrent relations among temperament, ability estimation, and injury proneness. *Child Development, 70,* 700–712.

Shaffer, David R. (2000). *Social and personality development* (4th ed.). Belmont, CA: Wadsworth.

Siegler, R. S. (1998). *Children's thinking* (3rd ed.). Upper Saddle River, NJ: Prentice-Hall.

Thompson, R. A., & Nelson, C. A. (2001). Developmental science and the media: Early brain development. *American Psychologist, 56,* 5–15.

Vasta, R., Haith, M. M., & Miller, S. A. (1999). *Child psychology: The modern science* (3rd ed.). New York: Wiley.

KATHLEEN N. KANNASS
JOHN COLOMBO

Childhood Disintegrative Disorder

DEFINITION

Childhood Disintegrative Disorder (CDD), also referred to as Heller's syndrome or disintegrative psychosis, is a type of Pervasive Developmental Disorder in which a child exhibits typical development (age-appropriate verbal and nonverbal behaviors, play, relationships with others, and adaptive functioning) until the age of 2 years, and then there is a significant loss of development before age 10. Electroencephalogram (EEG) abnormalities and

seizure disorders have been observed in approximately 50 percent of cases. Although individuals with CDD may exhibit behaviors typical of Autistic Disorder (communicative and social deficits, as well as restricted or stereotyped behaviors, activities, and interests), CDD is more severe and has a distinctive developmental onset. Increased activity levels, irritability and anxiety followed by loss of speech and other skills may signal the onset of CDD. Loss of functioning is usually permanent. Typically, CDD is associated with severe mental retardation. Progressive deterioration across the lifespan is common in individuals who have co-morbid neurological illnesses. Due to the rarity of CDD, there is a scarcity of empirical research and a limitation in the understanding of the disorder.

PREVALENCE AND COURSE OF THE DISORDER

Prevalence is estimated to be 1 in every 100,000 children in the United States. Males outnumber females by a ratio of 4 : 1. Although onset may occur as early as 2 years of age, a rapid decline in skills at around 3 or 4 years of age has frequently been observed. Within several months, intellectual, social, and language functioning may decline significantly, causing persistent delay in these areas. Regression in social and emotional development may contribute to difficulty in interacting appropriately with others. A loss in previously acquired skills in areas of expressive or receptive language, social skills or adaptive behavior, bowel or bladder control, play, or motor skills occurs.

ETIOLOGY

Although CDD likely results from neurological insult, it is not known whether it has a genetic basis or is associated with some other pathological condition.

ASSESSMENT

It is important that this disorder be differentiated from other Pervasive Developmental Disorders, as well as Schizophrenia. A thorough assessment involving laboratory work, as well as genetic, psychological, communication, and educational/achievement testing may be helpful in ruling out other conditions (such as Autistic Disorder,

Rett's Disorder, Asperger's Disorder, or dementia) and establishing an appropriate treatment plan. A detailed history of the pregnancy, developmental milestones, and family medical history should be taken. If possible, a review of video tapes and baby books should be conducted to provide supplementary information. Information on the age of onset is especially important considering the diagnostic criteria for the disorder. Observation of the child at play may provide helpful information regarding social, language, cognitive, and motor abilities, as well as any unusual or maladaptive behaviors.

TREATMENT

Currently, there is no cure for CDD. Most treatment techniques focus on symptom management. Psychotropic medications have resulted in mild improvement at best. Antiepileptic medications are often prescribed. Applied behavior analysis methods and special education are aimed at combating further regression of the individual's behaviors, as well as attempting to advance the individual's current abilities in other areas. Family education, participation in a support group, and supportive psychotherapy may be helpful to parents/caregivers, siblings, and extended family.

See also: Applied Behavior Analysis; Autistic Disorder; Mental Retardation; Pervasive Developmental Disorder; Pharmacological Interventions

Further Reading

American Psychiatric Association. (2000). *Diagnostic and statistical manual of mental disorders: DSM-IV* (4th ed., text revision). Washington, DC: Author.
E-medicine. http://www.emedicine.com/ped/topic2654.htm
Malhotra, S., & Gupta, N. (1999). Childhood disintegrative disorder. *Journal of Autism and Developmental Disorders, 29*, 491–498.

AMANDA M. ROEBEL
WILLIAM E. MACLEAN, JR.

Childhood-Onset Schizophrenia

DEFINITION

Schizophrenia is a severe, recurrent, and debilitating neurodevelopmental disorder that affects brain functioning, leading to impairments in thinking, logic, perception, social and personal care skills, and negative symptoms (e.g., social withdrawal, flattening of emotional expression). Childhood-onset schizophrenia (COS), defined as onset at 12 years or younger, appears to be a more severe form of the disorder. The usual onset of schizophrenia is in late adolescence or early adulthood.

PREVALENCE

COS is rare. Estimates of its prevalence range from 0.002 to 0.04 in 100, as compared to 1 in 100 for adult-onset schizophrenia. It is extremely rare in children under age 7.

ETIOLOGY

There is evidence for a genetic factor in some cases. There is an estimated concordance of 40–50 percent for identical twins, and 10 percent for children of a schizophrenic parent. COS may be associated with a relatively higher genetic contribution.

Current research suggests that schizophrenia results from an interaction of inherited vulnerability and early environmental factors, such as a virus before birth or anoxia at birth, that together affect the development of the nervous system. This leads to deviations from normal brain development that affect behavior eventually. The neurotransmitters dopamine and glutamate may be involved. There is some evidence for a loss of grey matter in certain areas of the brain during adolescence and for the possible association between smaller cerebral volume in COS and negative symptoms. Early language difficulties may be related to problems in temporal and frontal lobe development and early transient motor stereotypies implicate developmental abnormalities in the basal ganglia. Some studies report that there is confusing, unclear communication styles in families of schizophrenics, which are associated with the exacerbation of the disorder, but are not causally related to it.

CHILDHOOD-ONSET VERSUS ADULT-ONSET SCHIZOPHRENIA

In COS, there tends to be a more gradual rate of onset with exacerbation of symptoms at 8 years of age, a predominance of males, and more neurodevelopmental abnormalities. While clinically more severe, COS tends to have less differentiated symptomatology and a poorer outcome, and tends to be more resistant to antipsychotic medications. Schizophrenic children tend to have more "odd" characteristics prior to diagnosis.

PREMORBID CHARACTERISTICS

Prior to the onset of the disorder, schizophrenic children tend to have: (1) a social impairment characterized by social withdrawal, aloofness, and atypical peer relationships; (2) a language impairment characterized by disorder of speech rhythm, articulation, and/or language comprehension, or elective mutism; and (3) a motor function impairment characterized by abnormal repetitive movements (stereotypies), poor coordination, neurointegrative problems, and/or restlessness. They may also present with attentional problems, hyperactivity, aggression, disruptive behaviors, anxiety, mood instability, or academic failure. Many children that later develop COS are first diagnosed as having Attention-Deficit/Hyperactivity Disorder (ADHD), Conduct Disorder, or a developmental disorder. None of these premorbid characteristics are specific to COS and may be present in the histories of children with other serious mental health problems.

SYMPTOMS

The criteria for schizophrenia in the Fourth Edition of the *Diagnostic and Statistical Manual for Mental Disorders* (*DSM-IV*), published by the American Psychiatric Association, are the same for onset during childhood or adulthood. To meet the criteria for schizophrenia, the individual must exhibit continuous signs of schizophrenia for at least 6 months, including at least one month with two or more of the core symptoms, which include "delusions, hallucination, disorganized speech, grossly disorganized or catatonic, and negative symptoms (affective flattening, alogia, or avolition)." The child's speech and behavior must be evaluated, however, within the context of developmental, psychosocial, cognitive, and cultural factors. The "positive" symptoms of schizophrenia, hallucinations (false perceptions) and delusions (false fixed beliefs), are also described as characteristics of psychosis.

The majority of children with schizophrenia have auditory hallucinations, delusions, thought disorder, and blunted, flat, or inappropriate affect. Some also display rage reactions, anxiety, and hypersensitivity. The average IQ is between 80 and 90; however, the IQ is likely adversely influenced by the disorder.

Thought disorder may be categorized into four types: (1) illogical thinking, (2) loose associations (a shift in topic without preparing the listener for the change in topic), (3) incoherence, and (4) poverty of content of speech (overuse of nonsubstantive words). Caplan and colleagues (2000) found that of these types, loose associations seem to be specific to COS and are not found in normal children over the age of 7. Illogical thinking is found in children older than age 7 but is not specific to COS. Younger schizophrenic children use more illogical thinking and loose associations than older children. Incoherence and poverty of content are not often found in children with schizophrenia.

SCHIZOPHRENIA-SPECTRUM DISORDERS

A number of researchers have proposed that schizophrenia is the most severe form in a spectrum of disorders. What has emerged from multidisciplinary programs of research is a clustering of biological characteristics and response styles that seems to be associated with the core symptoms of schizophrenia in both adults and children. Some of the characteristics are also found in other apparently related mental disorders, as well as in a significant number of family members who do not have schizophrenia. For example, Yeo and colleagues (1997) have suggested that children with schizophrenia-spectrum disorders have significant brain abnormalities that are similar to those seen in adult schizophrenics.

Multidimensionally Impaired Disorder (MDID) is one such syndrome that may lie on the schizophrenia spectrum. Kumra and colleagues (1998) found that children in this group are significantly impaired, but are less severe than schizophrenic children. MDID children tend to have impaired language or learning disorder, significant attentional deficits, mood outbursts, periodic aggression, and transient hallucinations or delusions under stress. Only a small percentage display thought disorder or flattened affect. They are socially deficient, but more eager to seek social interaction than schizophrenic children. Children with MDID tend to have perceptual disturbances at an earlier age, and are referred for language and behavioral problems more frequently and at an earlier age than schizophrenic children. Overall, a greater percentage of MDID children receive a comorbid diagnosis of ADHD, but they have fewer social problems and show a better outcome than COS. Other researchers have suggested that schizotypal personality disorder is a less severe manifestation in a schizophrenia spectrum.

DIFFERENTIAL DIAGNOSIS

Diagnosis usually includes an extensive evaluation, which may take place over a significant period of time. Distinguishing schizophrenia from other diagnoses is more complex in children because of the typically less differentiated pattern of symptoms and developmental, cognitive, and cultural factors that may account for a child's behavior. For example, a child with a speech and language disorder, mental retardation, developmental delays, bilinguality, or hearing difficulty may mistakenly appear to have problems in thought and communication related to schizophrenia. While a significant number of children with schizophrenia have pervasive developmental delays, few children with developmental delays are schizophrenic.

Since schizophrenia includes a disturbance of attention, a child with schizophrenia may initially be diagnosed with ADHD. There are also other disorders besides schizophrenia that may include symptoms of psychosis. These include Posttraumatic Sress Disorder (PTSD) and dissociative disorders, both of which are mental disorders associated with significant traumatic experiences, as well as mood disorders, such as bipolar disorder and depressive disorder with psychotic features. Since COS may include a history of disturbance in mood, distinguishing bipolar disorder from schizophrenia in a child may be difficult. It is also possible to meet diagnostic criteria for both schizophrenia and a mood disorder.

Features of Obsessive-Compulsive Disorder (OCD), as well as schizotypal and borderline personality disorder may also resemble schizophrenia. Ruling out drug intoxication, withdrawal, or residual states of drug use, particularly involving PCP, other hallucinogens, or stimulants is important. Neurological disorders, including seizures, head trauma, poisoning, tumors, infections, and metabolic disorders may resemble symptoms of schizophrenia. It is not uncommon for a schizophrenic child to receive more than one diagnosis or to have an additional medical condition.

TREATMENT

Treatment is usually multimodal, including antipsychotic medications as well as individual and family therapy. Special education, group therapy, therapeutic recreation, and occupational therapy are often also an integral part of the child's individualized treatment plan. Stabilization of the child's symptoms may need to take place in an inpatient setting if close observation is needed or there is a concern that the child might be dangerous toward himself or others. Case management services and parent support groups are also helpful. Interventions are aimed at reducing the child's psychotic symptoms, treating any co-morbid disorders, promoting the development of age-appropriate skills, and creating a supportive social and emotional environment at home and at school.

The child with disruptive behaviors will usually be better managed if caregivers are aware when the child feels confused, paranoid, or overwhelmed, or is acting on hallucinations or delusions. At such times, adults might help the child feel safe in a quiet place and provide reality-testing (i.e., help the child distinguish between reality and imagination). Behavioral and cognitive–behavioral interventions should be individualized to meet the interests and cognitive and emotional capabilities of the child. These therapies are also likely to be more successful once the child's psychotic symptoms are stabilized. Psychoeducation and structured group experiential exercises on social skills, anger management, communication, problem-solving, leisure skills, and safe and appropriate behavior are beneficial. Individual therapies might also address hygiene, self-care, mood regulation, self-esteem, sexual issues, identity, awareness of personal boundaries, and medication compliance in addition to specific family, peer, or educational issues. Some children may be vulnerable to depression after the onset of the disorder and to thoughts of self-harm. Overall, schizophrenic children will cope better when their environments are reasonably structured and predictable and communications are clear and uncritical. Environments that are noisy, confusing, pressured, or highly emotional may be overwhelming and increase the risk for relapse. In school, children may need encouragement, frequent breaks, and help in negotiating problematic social situations. Families usually need help in understanding the symptoms of schizophrenia, and in adjusting their expectations, home environment, communication, and parenting styles to best support their child's recovery.

See also: Attention-Deficit/Hyperactivity Disorder; Bipolar Disorder; Pervasive Developmental Disorders; Pharmacological Interventions; Social-Skills Training

Further Reading

American Psychiatric Association. (1994). *Diagnostic and statistical manual of mental disorders (DSM-IV), 4th ed.* Washington, DC: Author.

Caplan, R., Guthrie, D., Tang, B., Komo, S., & Asarnow, R. F. (2000). Thought disorder in childhood schizophrenia: Replication and update of concept. *Journal of the American Academy of Child & Adolescent Psychiatry, 39*(6), 771–778.

Kumra, S., Jacobsen, L. K., Lenane, M., Zahn, T. P., Wiggs, E., Alaghband-Rad, J., Castellanos, F. X., Frazier, J. A., McKenna, K., Gordon, C. T., Smith, A., Hamburger, S., & Rapoport, J. L. (1998). Multidimensionally impaired disorder: Is it a variant of very early-onset schizophrenia? *Journal of the American Academy of Child & Adolescent Psychiatry, 37*(1), 91–99.

McClellan, J., Werry, J., Bernet, W., Arnold, V., Beitchman, J., Benson, S., Bukstein, O., Kinlan, J., Rue, D., & Shaw, J. (2001). Practice parameter for the assessment and treatment of children and adolescents with schizophrenia. *Journal of the American Academy of Child & Adolescent Psychiatry, 40*(Suppl. 7), 4S–23S.

Remschmidt, H. (Ed.) (2001). *Schizophrenia in children and adolescents.* New York: Cambridge University Press.

Yeo, R. A., Hodde-Vargas, J., Hendren, R. L., Vargas, L. A., Brooks, W. M., Ford, C. C., Gangestad, S. W., & Hart, B. L. (1997). Brain abnormalities in schizophrenia-spectrum children: Implications for a neurodevelopmental perspective. *Psychiatry Research, 76,* 1–13.

http://www.nimh.nih.gov/events/prschiz.htm
http://www.nimh.nih.gov/publicat/schizoph.htm

LUIS A. VARGAS
MARY C. KAVEN

Children with Parents or Siblings with HIV Infection

Human Immunodeficiency Virus-1 (HIV) is an infectious agent (a retrovirus) that infects and destroys specific blood cells (i.e., CD4 "T-cells") in the human immune system, causing a breakdown of an individual's ability to defend against other infections. When the virus replicates unchecked and compromises the individual's cellular immunologic response system, the likelihood of opportunistic infection increases. Acquired Immune Deficiency Syndrome (AIDS) is diagnosed when the individual's CD4 count drops to below 200 cells per cubic millimeter, and the individual develops a number of opportunistic infections. As no cure for HIV-infection has yet been developed, the ultimate consequence of infection is death—though treatment has significantly improved both the quality and duration of life following infection.

Beyond the devastating impact of the illness on individuals, HIV also has an impact on the families of those who are infected. Among the most vulnerable "silent victims" of the HIV-epidemic are children *affected* by HIV—children with parents or siblings with HIV-infection.

INCIDENCE AND PREVALENCE

Throughout the first two decades of the HIV epidemic, women of color represented the demographic group with the largest increases in incidence rates (i.e., number of new cases per year). In 1992, women accounted for 14 percent of adults or adolescents living with AIDS—by 1999, the proportion had grown to 20 percent. In fact, when the incidence of new cases of HIV was declining in other demographic groups, there was a striking increase in the incidence of HIV attributed to heterosexual contact, especially in women. As a result, both the number of children with HIV and the number of children affected by HIV increased dramatically during those years.

Due to recent improvements in the prenatal care of pregnant women with HIV, the number of new pediatric HIV cases has declined. However, the number of new cases of HIV among women has remained largely stable since the mid-1990s. Thus, while the number of new cases of pediatric AIDS has decreased, the number of children *affected* by a family member's illness continues to grow. Some estimates suggest that the number of AIDS orphans in the United States will reach 125,000 by the year 2010.

CONSEQUENCES OF PARENTAL HIV INFECTION

Parenting Issues

In a recent investigation of parenting behaviors among women, HIV-infected mothers reported poorer mother–child relationship quality and less monitoring of their children's activities than did noninfected mothers, perhaps suggesting that maternal HIV infection may disrupt effective parenting. One reason for the disrupted parenting behaviors may be the physical limitations brought on by a serious chronic illness. Not surprisingly, as individuals progress from "asymptomatic HIV infection" to "symptomatic HIV infection," and finally to a diagnosis of AIDS, the quality of their physical health diminishes. Poorer physical health has been identified as a risk factor for compromised parenting strategies in numerous populations.

Another potential explanation for the relationship between HIV infection and diminished parenting skills is the presence of maternal depressive symptoms. Elevated symptoms of depression have been documented among adults with HIV. Parents with symptoms of depression often experience difficulty facing the challenges of child rearing. This may be particularly true among parents with HIV, who are overrepresented by demographic groups with lower incomes and increased environmental stress.

Perhaps contributing to the constellation of stresses encountered by families affected by HIV is a lack of adequate social support. This may also impact relationships within the family, as parents with inadequate social support are at increased risk for diminished parenting skills. In fact, research suggests that women with HIV and their children reported receiving lower levels of social support than noninfected women and their children. Perceived parental social support has been positively associated with better psychosocial outcomes among several samples of children of HIV-infected mothers and fathers.

Child Behavior Problems

For a number of reasons, noninfected children of parents with HIV are at increased risk for behavior and adjustment problems. Children of mothers with HIV have demonstrated increased risk for depressive symptoms, externalizing problems, and academic difficulties, while children of men with hemophilia and/or HIV infection were at increased risk for poor parent–child relationships. These adjustment problems may be the result of compromised parenting behaviors, diminished social support, or uncertainty regarding the health status of the parent. In one investigation, child medical uncertainty about the parent's illness was more strongly related to child adjustment problems than objective indicators of the parent's illness.

Child behavior problems may also be caused by disruptions in the available coping resources due to parental illness. For example, in a study of families affected by paternal HIV infection and/or hemophilia, illness severity predicted increases in disruptions of the parent–child relationships. Parent–child relationship problems predicted increased use of avoidant coping strategies by the child, which was associated with increased child internalizing problems. Further, the use of avoidant coping strategies by HIV-infected parents and their spouses has been associated with increased behavior problems among their children.

CHILD BEREAVEMENT

Although adults and children with HIV are living longer and healthier lives due to advances in medical management of the illness, there is currently no cure for

AIDS. Thus, children of parents with HIV, and siblings of children with HIV will likely lose a loved one far sooner than what is considered "normal."

Although child bereavement is rarely an uncomplicated process, children who lose loved ones to HIV/AIDS may encounter particular difficulties due to the nature of the illness. For example, in families that have not disclosed the nature of the illness, children must wrestle with what to tell support people regarding the cause of their loved one's death. Currently, the stigma associated with HIV may disrupt the degree of sympathy and support that surviving family members may offer. Further, children may be reluctant to disclose their parent's death because of concern that others will assume that the survivor(s) are HIV infected as well. Finally, in families were the parent or sibling's HIV status has not been disclosed to other family members, the survivors may learn of the loved one's HIV status while they are grieving the loss of the loved one. Any of these complications may impact the child's postgrieving adjustment, and represent issues to be addressed within supportive and/or therapeutic relationships.

EMERGING ISSUES

Permanency Planning

Several issues that directly impact children of parents with HIV recently have been examined in the research literature. For example, given the projections of the number of "AIDS orphans" in the near future, questions regarding custody arrangements for children after the death or incapacitation of their parents must be addressed. Both in the United States and abroad, discussions of "permanency planning" often do not occur among parents with HIV. As a result, children who are orphaned may experience unnecessary transitions in the period immediately following the parent's death. Several programs have been developed to help families make arrangements for children's present and future care. Of particular importance is a coherent and viable plan for the child's custody and welfare in the case of a parent's incapacitation or death. Whether the child is included in these discussions depends primarily on the child him- or herself (e.g., developmental level, disclosure status, preference).

Disclosure

A related issue is the disclosure of HIV status to immediate family members. In several large investigations of mothers with HIV, the majority of children (ages 5–15) were reportedly unaware of their mother's HIV status. When children were told of their parent's illness, the parent was usually the one who disclosed the information. Not surprisingly, no *consistent* findings regarding the benefits or risks associated with disclosure to the child have been reported. Rather, the decision of what and when to tell family members appears to be a highly personal one. Factors that should be considered include (1) the patient's attitude about the illness (e.g., acceptance vs. shame), (2) the child's developmental level, (3) the child's capacity to differentiate public versus private information, and (4) the child's available coping strategies and social support. Disclosure of a child's illness to his or her siblings includes the above considerations, as well as the HIV-infected child's right to privacy.

Need for Psychosocial Services

Given the issues faced by families living with HIV infection, it stands to reason that psychosocial services should be available. Whether the majority of children and families affected by HIV have such services at their disposal remains unclear. The demographic characteristics of children whose parent(s) are HIV-infected suggest that for many, proactive mental health services are not within their reach. However, recent needs assessment surveys suggest that many parents report seeing a need for such services to reinforce their parenting skills, to address their children's concerns regarding illness, and to provide direction through the disclosure process.

See also: Bereavement; Foster Care; Parental Psychopathology; Pediatric Human Immunodeficiency Virus-1 (HIV); Psychological Impact of Parent's Chronic Illness

Further Reading

Armistead, L., & Forehand, R. (1995). For whom the bell tolls: Parenting decisions and challenges faced by mothers who are HIV seropositive. *Clinical Psychology: Science and Practice, 2*, 239–250.

Draimin, B. H., Gamble, I., Shire, A., & Hudis, J. (1998). Improving permanency planning in families with HIV disease. *Child Welfare, 77*, 180–194.

Geballe, S., & Gruendel, J. (1998). The crisis within the crisis: The growing epidemic of AIDS orphans. In S. Books (Ed.), *Invisible children in the society and its schools: Sociocultural, political, and historical studies in education* (pp. 47–65). Mahwah, NJ: Erlbaum.

Roth, J., Siegel, R., & Black, S. (1994). Identifying the mental health needs of children living in families with AIDS or HIV infection. *Community Mental Health Journal, 30*, 581–593.

RIC G. STEELE

Chlamydia

See: Sexually Transmitted Diseases in Adolescents

Chorea: Sydenham's and Huntington's

DEFINITION

The term "chorea" refers to the incessant occurrence of rapid, jerky, involuntary movements. There are two primary types: Sydenham's and Huntington's chorea. Sydenham's chorea is most closely linked with rheumatic fever in childhood, and is characterized by acute involuntary movements that gradually become severe, affecting all motor activities. Choreiform movements typically occur 1–6 months following the initial illness (onset of rheumatic fever). Sydenham's chorea is self-limited and may also be associated with arthritis, skin rash, cardiac difficulties, and behavioral disturbances. Huntington's chorea is a rare hereditary disease usually first evidenced in adulthood, and is characterized by chronic chorea as well as mental deterioration.

Given that Sydenham's chorea primarily affects children (and Huntington's chorea is usually first evidenced in mid-adulthood), Sydenham's chorea is the focus of this entry. Brief information pertaining to Huntington's chorea is also included.

INCIDENCE/PSYCHOLOGICAL CORRELATES

Sydenham's chorea occurs in 10–20 percent of children who have had an acute rheumatic fever attack. Although few children will experience Sydenham's chorea from their first encounter with rheumatic fever, the probability of experiencing it progressively increases to up to 50 percent of affected children with repeated occurrences of rheumatic fever. Females are almost twice as likely to experience Sydenham's chorea than males. Age of onset is typically between 5 and 15 years, with incidence peaking at 8 years of age.

While the involuntary movements associated with chorea may not appear for up to 6 months following the initial illness, psychological symptoms frequently precede the choreiform movements and can present as early as 2 weeks following an initial sore throat associated with rheumatic fever. Mild behavioral symptoms that commonly occur include irritability, emotional instability, crying spells, nightmares, and separation anxiety. It has been suggested that more severe psychiatric symptoms, such as obsessive-compulsive behaviors (contamination fears, fear of harm occurring to a loved one, excessive washing and checking), occur in over 70 percent of children with Sydenham's chorea. Other potential psychiatric responses to chorea include Attention-Deficit/Hyperactivity Disorder (ADHD), tic disorders, and mood disorders. Sydenham's chorea also has been associated with a worsening of ADHD symptoms—in addition to their precipitation—in cases where ADHD symptoms were already present prior to rheumatic fever onset. Less common responses to Sydenham's chorea include delirium and nonaffective psychosis.

The incidence of Huntington's chorea ranges from 4 to 10 individuals per 100,000. Symptoms usually first appear in adulthood (ages 30–45). In addition to the involuntary movements, Huntington's chorea is associated with speech disturbance, cognitive deterioration, and psychiatric symptoms.

ETIOLOGY

Sydenham's chorea is thought to result from an autoimmune inflammatory response involving certain regions of the basal ganglia in the brain. The chorea is a delayed reaction in response to a streptococcal bacterial infection.

Unlike Sydenham's, Huntington's chorea is genetic, caused by an autosomal dominant trait. Mental deterioration is due to degenerative brain changes in the cerebral cortex and basal ganglia.

ASSESSMENT

Sydenham's chorea is generally diagnosed after a thorough medical evaluation including assessment of a prior streptococcal infection and an observation of characteristic symptoms. In addition, a complete neurological evaluation, including magnetic resonance imaging (MRI) and electroencephalogram (EEG), may be performed. Sydenham's chorea must be differentiated from seizures, exposure to toxins, and Huntington's chorea.

The onset of Huntington's chorea is assessed by a comprehensive clinical evaluation, neurological

evaluation, observation of characteristic symptoms, and a complete family history. Genetic testing also has become available recently. A computerized tomography (CT) scan may differentiate a diagnosis of Huntington's disease from other neurodegenerative disorders.

TREATMENT

Few treatments are helpful in decreasing the severity of symptoms associated with Sydenham's chorea. Generally, children with Sydenham's chorea have been diagnosed previously with acute rheumatic fever, and will therefore have been prescribed penicillin or another antibiotic. Current pharmacologic treatment for the symptoms of Sydenham's chorea includes anticonvulsants such as Valproate and Carbamazepine. Only after these treatments have proven ineffective are alternatives such as neuroleptics and steroids considered. Although the psychological symptoms of Sydenham's chorea typically decrease as children physically recover, short-term psychological treatment may be warranted. For example, for children with exacerbation of ADHD symptoms, parents may benefit from supplemental behavior management training. Similarly, cognitive-behavioral therapy may be beneficial for children with the onset of a mood disorder. At a minimum, educating families about Sydenham's chorea could provide reassurance and help those affected to understand and cope with the milder psychological symptoms that frequently occur (e.g., increased irritability or emotional instability).

Currently, there are no treatments that slow, alter, or reverse the progression of Huntington's chorea. Instead, a multidisciplinary team approach is often used to manage the symptoms of Huntington's chorea including psychosocial encouragement, physical therapy, speech therapy, occupational therapy, genetic counseling, and medical assistance.

PROGNOSIS

Sydenham's chorea may subside within a few weeks in some children and most children recover after 3 months. The average duration of illness is 4–6 months, with symptoms ranging anywhere from 1 week to 2 years. Recovery typically includes a return to baseline functioning without lasting impact of physical or behavioral disturbances; death from Sydenham's chorea is extremely rare. Relapses of Sydenham's chorea are not uncommon, particularly within the first two years after initial onset, and some children may therefore be prescribed prophylactic therapy.

Huntington's chorea is a degenerative disease that results in death within approximately 15 years following onset of symptoms.

See also: Acquired Heart Disease; Attention-Deficit/ Hyperactivity Disorders; Neurological Disorders; Obsessive-Compulsive Disorder; Tic Disorders: Tourette's Disorder, Chronic Tic Disorder, and Transient Tic Disorder

Further Reading

Mercandante, M. T., Busatto, G. F., Lombroso, P. J., Prado, L., Rosario-Campos, M. C., do Valle, R., Marques-Dias, M. J., Kiss, M. H., Leckman, J. F., & Miguel, E. C. (2000). The psychiatric symptoms of rheumatic fever. *American Journal of Psychiatry, 157,* 2036–2038.

Moore, D. P. (1996). Neuropsychiatric aspects of Sydenham's Chorea: A comprehensive review. *Journal of Clinical Psychiatry, 57,* 407–414.

Swedo, S. E., Leonard, H. L., Schapiro, M. B., Casey, B. J., Mannheim, G. B., Lenane, M. C., & Rettew, D. C. (1993). Sydenham's Chorea: Physical and psychological symptoms of St. Vitus dance. *Pediatrics, 91,* 706–713.

Swedo, S. E. (1994). Sydenham's chorea: A model for childhood autoimmune neuropsychiatric disorders. *Journal of the American Medical Association, 14,* 1788–1791.

Worldwide Education & Awareness for Movement Disorders (WE MOVE). (2002). Huntington's Disease and Sydenham's Chorea. Retrieved March 12, 2002, from http://www.wemove.org/hd.htm

RANDI STREISAND
LEIGH TAYLOR
MEGAN MURPHY
CLARISSA S. HOLMES

Chronic Tic Disorder

See: Tic Disorder

Cigarette Smoking

DEFINITION

Cigarette smoking continues to be the number one preventable cause of death in the United States, contributing to more than 420,000 deaths each year. Chronic cigarette smoking is associated with a number of serious medical illnesses including cancer, coronary heart disease, and stroke. Although historically conceptualized as an adult health problem, it is becoming clear that cigarette smoking is a pediatric problem.

Evidence for smoking as a pediatric problem is twofold. First, most smokers begin in early adolescence, typically by age 16. Few smokers smoke their first cigarette after high school graduation. Second, exposure to environmental tobacco smoke (ETS) is associated with increased risk for a variety of pediatric illnesses including asthma and sudden infant death syndrome (SIDS). Thus, an understanding of cigarette smoking as a pediatric problem requires knowledge about issues of secondhand smoke exposure *and* known methods to reduce smoking among adolescents.

INCIDENCE

The *Monitoring the Future Study* (2002) has been tracking drug use among high school seniors since 1975. Recent surveys have included data from 8th and 10th graders and allow for comparisons during adolescence. With respect to cigarette smoking, adolescents continue to show a decline in rates as of 2001. Daily smoking among 8th graders is currently about half of that observed in the peak year of 1996. Lifetime prevalence rates in 2001 for 8th, 10th, and 12th graders are 36.6, 52.8, and 61.0, respectively; daily use prevalence rates are 5.5, 12.2, and 19.0, respectively.

Health problems associated with ETS are well documented. Each year, ETS exposure is estimated to be responsible for up to two million ear infections, more than 500,000 doctor visits for asthma, over 400,000 episodes of bronchitis, and almost 200,000 cases of pneumonia in children under 5 years of age. It has been estimated that 38 percent of all children age 2 months to 5 years are exposed to cigarette smoke in the home.

CORRELATES

Smoke exposure has been shown to increase risk for SIDS, particularly prenatal exposure. Studies of postnatal exposure and SIDS is confounded by the overlap between women who smoke during and after pregnancy and it may be impossible to determine the independent relationship between ETS exposure and SIDS. Several studies have reported dose–response relationships between amount of smoking in the home and SIDS, but few studies have adequately measured possible confounding factors such as the infants' sleeping position. One well-controlled study by Klonoff-Cohen and colleagues (1995) reported that children who were exposed to ETS were 3.5 times more likely to be diagnosed with SIDS. Extrapolating this risk to SIDS deaths, the study suggests that as many as 2,000–3,000 deaths in 1993 could be attributed to ETS.

Two major reviews have concluded that ETS exposure is significantly related to the number of asthma episodes and the severity of asthma in children with this disease. Research looking at experimental exposure of children to ETS suggests that while in general ETS exposure increases asthmatic symptoms, there is a "subpopulation of asthmatics who are especially susceptible to ETS exposure" (National Cancer Institute, 1999, p. 203). For these children, protection from ETS exposure is critical.

ETS exposure in children is estimated to increase the risk of lower respiratory infections by 1.5- to 2-fold. While the evidence is not as strong, the relationship between ETS exposure and presence of middle ear effusion is "good," and there is some evidence of an association between ETS exposure and otitis media.

Finally, several studies have consistently linked ETS exposure to more general health effects that can be grouped together as "sensory irritants" such as subjective eye irritation, nasal irritation, odor acuity, and odor "annoyance."

TREATMENT

Several clinical trials have shown that behavioral interventions can reduce children's exposure to ETS. Hovell and colleagues (2000) found that seven counseling sessions with mothers conducted over a 3-month period significantly reduced ETS exposure at a 12-month follow-up. These results were corroborated by measures of cotinine in the children's urine. Thus, it appears that counseling mothers about ETS exposure in children can reduce risk.

Treatment efforts with respect to child and adolescent smoking have primarily focused on prevention of use. Prevention of tobacco use among children has become one of the "cornerstones" of tobacco control programs. School-based programs are needed, and these programs should use evidence-based curricula, ensure tobacco-free policies at the school, and provide teacher training, parental involvement, and cessation services in order to be effective. In addition, counter-marketing efforts are needed to combat media appeal that smoking is a glamorous activity that serves as a "rite of passage" to adulthood. Curricular materials have been developed and are being implemented in several states. It is

recommended that educational efforts begin in elementary schools, and continue through middle school and high school. Details on these programs can be found in the CDC publication *Best Practices for Comprehensive Tobacco Control Programs* (1999), which provides detailed summaries and reference material to developing effective programs.

Two effective methods for smoking prevention are enforcement of laws that prohibit sales to minors and ensuring clean air through nonsmoking schools and public buildings. It has been recommended that all states adopt a policy that identifies retailers who sell tobacco products to minors through the use of frequent checks. Retailers who are not in compliance need civil penalties that should include revocation of licenses for repeated offenders. The removal of vending machines and other self-service displays also should help reduce sales to minors.

SUMMARY AND PROGNOSIS

Efforts to reduce cigarette smoking among children and adolescents appear promising and need to be part of all school programs. While there are only a few controlled studies reported, brief intervention strategies appear promising for reducing child exposure to ETS. However, perhaps the best evidence for aggressive programs to reduce smoking in children is the fact that few adult smokers begin smoking after age 18. Prevention and treatment of childhood smoking may play a pivotal role in addressing this devastating health problem.

See also: Asthma; Otitis Media; Substance Abuse during Pregnancy: Nicotine, Prenatal Exposure; Sudden Infant Death Syndrome

Further Reading

American Cancer Society. (1997) *Cancer facts and figures—1997.* Atlanta, GA: Author.

Centers for Disease Control and Prevention. (1999). *Best practices for comprehensive tobacco control programs—August 1999.* Atlanta, GA: US Department of Health and Human Services.

Hovell, M. F., Zakarian, J. M., Matt, G. E., Hofstetter, C. R., Bernert, J. T., & Perkle, J. (2000). Effect of counseling mothers on their children's exposure to environmental tobacco smoke: Randomized controlled trial. *British Medical Journal, 321,* 337–342.

Johnson, L. D., O'Malley, P. M., & Bachman, J. G. (2002). *Monitoring the Future national results on adolescent drug use: Overview of key findings, 2001* (NIH Publication No. 02-5105). Bethesda, MD: National Institute on Drug Abuse.

Klonoff-Cohen, H. S., Edelstein, S. L., Lefkowitz, E. S., Srinivasan, I. P., Kaegi, D., Chang, J. C., & Wiley, K. J. (1995). The effect of passive smoking and tobacco exposure through breast milk on sudden infant death syndrome. *Journal of the American Medical Association, 273,* 795–798.

National Cancer Institute. (1999). *Health effects of exposure to environmental tobacco smoke: The report of the California Environmental Protection Agency. Smoking and Tobacco Control Monograph No. 10.* (NIH Pub. No. 99-4645). Bethesda, MD: US Department of Health and Human Services.

FRANK L. COLLINS
THAD R. LEFFINGWELL
ERNESTINE GREEN-TURNER
MARY ANNE MCCAFFREE

Classification and Diagnosis

A sound classification system is a prerequisite for both scientific and clinical work. With regard to psychiatric disorders in children and adolescents, Rutter (1997) has suggested that a robust classification system should (1) be reliable and valid; (2) have comprehensive coverage of various disorders; (3) be sensitive to developmental issues; (4) be based on principles and rules which are clearly defined; and (5) contain clinically relevant information. Classification systems that meet these requirements: (i) provide researchers with a common framework for theory formation about the nature of psychiatric disorders; (ii) enable clinicians to communicate effectively with one another about the child's symptoms, prognosis, and treatment selection; and (iii) provide administrators with a rationale for planning and resource allocation.

Diagnosis refers to formal assignment of "cases" to specific categories from current classification systems (e.g., the *Diagnostic and Statistical Manual of Mental Disorders* [*DSM-IV*] [1994] put forth by the American Psychiatric Association or the *International Statistical Classification of Diseases and Related Health Problems* [ICD] [1991] issued by the World Health Organization). Alternatively, diagnoses can emanate from empirically derived taxometric categories, prototypes, or typologies by using a multivariate approach such as the Child Behavior Checklist (CBCL) developed by Achenbach. A diagnosis implies a coherent subset of symptoms, and carries implications about the nature of the disorder, possible etiology, natural history and treatment response.

The two most common approaches to the classification and diagnosis of child psychopathology are the categorical and dimensional approaches. In the categorical approach, psychiatric disorders are divided into categories that represent relatively discrete entities. The *DSM* and ICD represent a categorical system in which the children either meet or do not meet certain criteria for specific disorders. However, knowing that the children have a disorder may not necessarily tell us all about these children and their problems. Although assigning a disorder to a given child facilitates communication among clinicians and other health professionals, concerns have been raised about the negative effects of assigning a label to children, including how others perceive and react to them, and how it might influence children's perception of themselves. Both the *DSM* and ICD assume childhood disorders exist or reside in the child, rather than in the reciprocal interaction between the child and his or her environmental situation.

The dimensional approach in contrast, typically uses standardized tests and statistical techniques (e.g., factor or cluster analysis) to identify sets of items that are interrelated, with each cluster of behaviors constituting a syndrome, as noted by Essau and colleagues (1997). One of the most widely used standardized tests has been the CBCL developed by Achenbach. Although the dimensional approach may be more objective and potentially more reliable than clinically derived classification systems, there are numerous problems associated with its use as well. Among these limitations are the dependency of the derived dimensions on the particular samples studied, the method by which the information was obtained, the characteristics of the informants, and the type of statistical procedures used to determine the dimensions obtained. Furthermore, dimensional approaches may not be sensitive enough to contextual factors that influence the child's psychopathology.

There is much debate about which childhood disorders are best conceptualized as categories and which as dimensions. The extent to which a particular condition should be viewed as a distinct category, or as a continuous dimension, or as both, depends on the validity of the diagnosis under consdieration.

See also: *Diagnostic and Statistical Manual of Mental Disorders*; *International Classification of Diseases and Related Health Problems*; Reliability; Validity

Further Reading

Achenbach, T. M. (1991). *Manual for the Child Behavior Checklist/4-18 and 1991 profile.* Burlington: University of Vermont, Department of Psychiatry.
American Psychiatric Association. (1994). *Diagnostic and statistical manual of mental disorders* (4th ed.). Washington, DC: Author.
Essau, C. A., Feehan, M., & Üstun, B. (1997). Classification and assessment strategies. In C. A. Essau & F. Petermann (Eds.),

Developmental psychopathology: Epidemiology, diagnostics, and treatment (pp. 19–62). London: Harwood Academic Publishers.

Rutter, M. (1977). Classification. In M. Rutter & L. Hersov (Eds.), *Child psychiatry: Modern approaches* (pp. 359–384). Oxford: Blackwell.

World Health Organization. (1993). *The ICD-10 classification of mental and behavioral disorders.* Geneva: Author.

CECILIA A. ESSAU

Clefts of the Lip and Palate

DEFINITION

Cleft lip (CL), cleft palate (CP), and cleft lip and palate (CLP) are the result of a failure of embryological tissue to fuse during the first trimester of fetal development, leaving an opening or fissure in the lip or palate. Clefts can be unilateral, appearing on only one side of the facial midline, or bilateral, involving structures on both sides of midline. In addition, clefts can be either complete or incomplete. Complete CL extends from the lip into the nose and complete CP extends along the entire roof of the mouth. Incomplete presentations involve less extensive areas of the lip or palate. Because the fissures may affect significant sections of the midface and oral cavity, individuals born with orofacial clefts are at increased risk for problems related to feeding and nutrition, speech, hearing, dental development, and physical appearance.

ETIOLOGY

Clefts can be caused by either genetic or environmental factors, with the majority of clefts appearing without a family history of the problem. Such factors as maternal nutritional deficiencies, drug use, and exposure to various toxins have been proposed as possible links to the development of nonhereditary clefts, but conclusive evidence regarding specific environmental risk factors has not been presented.

INCIDENCE

Isolated clefts of the lip or palate are among the most commonly occurring congenital anomalies, appearing in 1 out of every 750 births. Clefts may be associated also with clusters of other birth defects as part of identifiable genetic syndromes. There are over 300 recognized syndromes that include CL, CP, or CLP.

PSYCHOLOGICAL CORRELATES

Families with children born with a cleft lip or palate face numerous challenges from birth through adolescence. During the first few months of life, feeding presents a difficulty for these children due to an inability to form adequate oral suction. Special nipples and bottles are necessary to aid in assuring good nutrition. Most mothers of infants with clefts have significant difficulty breastfeeding and may experience a profound sense of loss because of this. Research regarding early feeding interactions within the mother–child dyad suggests that many mothers of infants with CLP show decreased responsiveness and sensitivity and that the infants may communicate less effectively during feeding than in noncleft comparison dyads. Such problems in early parent–child interactions, combined with the disruptive requirements of medical and surgical care during infancy, have led to concern about the attachment between parent and child. Studies of attachment behavior of children with clefts have yielded inconsistent results. Some studies report decreased responsiveness, playfulness, and imitation of children with clefts within parent–child dyads, but other studies suggest no differences in attachment behaviors of children with clefts and children without.

As children with clefts enter the preschool and school-aged years, concern about social interactions and self-esteem increases. Most research has suggested that children with clefts show a higher level of internalizing behavior problems (e.g., withdrawal, shyness) than comparison children. These internalizing reactions may be related to poorly developed social skills, anxiety regarding facial differences, embarrassment due to unresolved speech or hearing impairments, or a combination of such factors. There is relatively little data on the precise nature of interaction difficulties of children with clefts, although recent information has suggested that children with clefts may be more tentative and less effective in their social interactions. Additionally, they tend to initiate and receive fewer social contacts. Increased internalizing behavior and decreased social contact has often raised questions regarding the self-esteem of children with clefts. It appears, however, that although children's self-concept for appearance is consistently lower than their noncleft peers, global self-concept remains unaffected by having a cleft.

Another concern that arises when children with clefts enter the school environment is that of intellectual and academic ability. Studies of the intellectual abilities of children with clefts consistently place these children in the average range of intellectual functioning; however, when compared to noncleft peers, they tend to score lower on verbal aspects of intelligence. This difficulty in language functioning is also reflected in the higher rates of learning disabilities among children with clefts than is found in the general population. Estimates of the rates of learning disabilities in this group of children range as high as 40 percent, with children with CP having a greater risk for learning disabilities than children with CLP. It appears that in some children with clefts, oral speech mechanisms may be responsible for lower verbal functioning; however, in others, there appears to be a central language processing deficiency evidenced by poor performance on tasks requiring verbal mediation.

ASSESSMENT

Psychological assessment of children with clefts and their families depends on the child's age and the specific reason for consultation. In infancy and toddlerhood it is important that developmental assessments be performed to assure that cognitive and adaptive skills are emerging appropriately. Receptive and expressive verbal abilities should be monitored carefully due to the high risk of linguistic difficulties in young children with clefts. A speech/language pathologist experienced in working with cleft-affected children should be involved early in the child's care. Due to surgical repairs and frequent medical problems (e.g., ear infections, failure-to-thrive) during the child's early years, it is important to monitor the family's coping strategies to assure good adjustment.

During the school-aged and adolescent years, the focus of assessment should be on behavioral and emotional adjustment, social adaptation, and academic achievement. Numerous teacher, parent, and self-report measures of internalizing and externalizing behavior, social skill, and self-concept are available to assist in pinpointing areas of strengths and weaknesses in behavioral and social domains. Psychoeducational evaluation for learning disabilities is imperative for any child with a cleft if academic difficulties at school arise.

TREATMENT

Most children with clefts are treated by a multidisciplinary cleft palate or craniofacial team. The team consists of physicians, surgeons, nurses, dentists, speech pathologists, audiologists, psychologists, social workers and other health care professionals who communicate with each other and the family in developing and coordinating a comprehensive treatment plan. Surgery to close a cleft lip occurs typically at 3 months of age, and the palate is closed at approximately 9 months with additional surgical repairs occurring throughout childhood and adolescence. Speech, dental, and medical interventions also begin in infancy and may continue until adulthood. Psychological treatment can be needed at any time in the individual's lifespan.

Early psychological intervention involves supportive counseling for parents, education regarding normal child development, and helping the family cope with medical and surgical procedures. If families have difficulty accepting their child with a cleft, family support groups or family therapy may be indicated. Developmental stimulation programs may be necessary if normal developmental trajectories are not observed.

As the children become older, social-skills training may be required to assist with initiating and maintaining friendships. Learning strategies for coping with teasing may be especially important in the elementary school years. Issues of social acceptance may also emerge in adolescence and require individual or group therapy to assist with optimal adjustment.

Because children with clefts are at a higher risk for learning disabilities, psychological interventions may involve consultation with schools to assure appropriate school placement. Serving as a liaison between the family and school when disagreements or misunderstandings emerge regarding educational planning can serve a valuable function in the care of the child.

PROGNOSIS

Most children with CL, CP, and CLP develop normally and lead productive lives. However, there is a higher incidence of behavioral and cognitive difficulties in children and adolescents with clefts. In adulthood, few stigmatizing features will remain from the condition if the child receives appropriate and timely treatment from a multidisciplinary team.

See also: Craniofacial Anomalies; Social Development in Childhood; Social-Skills Training; Speech and Language Assessment

Further Reading

Endriga, M. C., & Kapp-Simon, K. A. (1999). Psychological issues in craniofacial care: State of the art. *Cleft Palate—Craniofacial Journal, 36,* 3–11.

Kapp-Simon, K. A., & McGuire, D. E. (1997). Observed social interaction patterns in adolescents with and without craniofacial conditions. *Cleft Palate—Craniofacial Journal, 34,* 380–384.
Kummer, A. W. (2001). *Cleft palate and craniofacial anomalies.*
San Diego: Singular.

STEPHEN R. BOGGS
PHILIP EISENBERG

Client-Centered Therapy

Client-centered therapy focuses on the relationship between the therapist and the child and the process of therapy. If the important conditions of therapy are in place, then the child will develop and use the process of self-actualization. Client-centered therapy is a nondirective approach that follows the lead of the child in the therapy proper. Gaylin (1999) provides a complete discussion of the development and current state of client-centered therapy.

Client-centered or person-centered therapy began with the seminal work of Carl Rogers in the 1940s, 1950s, and 1960s. Self-actualization was central to his theory. As Gaylin described it, self-actualization refers to the tendency of each individual, children and adults, to act in ways that promote the realization of one's potential. The therapist works to facilitate the self-actualization process.

INGREDIENTS OF CLIENT-CENTERED THERAPY

Essential conditions of therapy must be present for change to occur. In 1957, Rogers outlined the importance of the therapist experiencing unconditional positive regard for the client. The therapist is nonjudgmental and accepting of the child. He also stressed the importance of empathy. Listening and empathic understanding is another essential ingredient. Gaylin (1999) describes how the therapist's empathic reflection of the child's reality and frame of reference enables the child to reexperience and reintegrate old experiences and be open to new experiences. Finally, Rogers stressed the importance of the therapist being congruent and integrated in the relationship. The therapist must be aware of his or her own experience and be authentic in the expression of that experience.

Empathic reflection of feeling is the major therapeutic technique. Although this sounds simple, learning to understand, listen, and reflect, requires training and experience. As in other forms of therapy, play is important in client-centered therapy with children. Axline (1947), in her nondirective approach, had the therapist focus on play as a major form of communication for and with the child. The therapist strives to understand and empathize with the child's issues. The therapist trusts the child's developmental process and striving for self-actualization. Crucial ingredients in the therapy for Axline are a warm relationship with the child, acceptance of the child, permissiveness in the relationship so the child can express feelings, reflection of the feelings, respect for the child's ability to solve his/her problems, and a nondirective approach. She stressed the importance of not hurrying the child and establishing limitations only when necessary to anchor the therapy to the world of reality. A wonderful introduction to the use of play in nondirective therapy is provided in Axline's seminal book written in 1964, *Dibbs in Search of Self.*

Moustakas was another leading client-centered theorist who stressed the importance of expression of feelings in play and the importance of the relationship between the child and the therapist. Moustakas discussed the importance of the child and therapist experiencing each other. Genuineness in the relationship is an important aspect of the therapy.

Client-centered family therapy is also being used. Gaylin described the important conditions for client-centered family therapy. The therapist responds to family members as individuals in ways that are consistent with client-centered principles. Empathy and validation of the individual remains a key to therapy, but within the context of the family.

RESEARCH WITH CLIENT-CENTERED THERAPY

Ellinwood and Raskin (1993) pointed out that there is a long tradition of empirical investigation for client-centered therapy. However, there is more research with adult therapy than with child therapy. There are some studies that have found client-centered therapy to be effective. Studies that meet the criteria for empirically validated treatment need to be carried out, however. Research that investigates process variables in the therapy and therapy outcome is especially relevant to the client-centered approach.

The principles of client-centered therapy have influenced many other therapeutic approaches with children. The importance of respecting the child, communicating acceptance, and listening and understanding are important ingredients in many forms of treatment. The client-centered approach holds that these conditions are sufficient for change to occur and that we should trust the child and the therapeutic process to enable this process to occur.

See also: Child Psychotherapy; Cognitive–Behavior Therapy; Family Therapy

Further Reading

Axline, V. M. (1947). *Play therapy.* Boston: Houghton Mifflin.

Ellinwood, C., & Raskin, N. (1993). Client-Centered/ humanistic psychotherapy. In T. Kratochwill & R. Morris (Eds.), *Handbook of psychotherapy with children and adolescents* (pp. 258–277). Needham Heights, MA: Allyn & Bacon.

Gaylin, N. (1999). Client-Centered child and family therapy. In S. Russ & Ollendick (Eds.), *Handbook of psychotherapies with children and families* (pp. 107–120). New York: Kluwer Academic/ Plenum Publishers.

SANDRA W. RUSS

Clinical Child and Adolescent Psychology

In 1995, the American Psychological Association (APA) established the Commission for the Recognition of Specialties and Proficiencies in Professional Psychology (the acronym is CRSPPP, pronounced "crisp"). This Commission provided official recognition for the existing specialties and recognized some new ones. In each case, the APA Council acted on its recommendations, and an archival document was created describing the specialty. The specialty of Clinical Child and Adolescent Psychology in one sense could be considered to have existed since Lightner Witmer founded his first psychology clinic at the University of Pennsylvania in 1896. Witmer's clientele was mostly children. However, since World War II and the emergence of modern Clinical Psychology (with a focus more on adults), the clinical child area was almost overshadowed. It is only rather recently, in 1998, that "Clinical Child Psychology" was recognized as a specialty in its own right by the action of CRSPPP. (The additional term "Adolescent" in the name of the specialty has been added by a consensus of those in the field since 1998 but has not yet made it into the official CRSPPP document.) To state what this specialty involves, one can therefore do no better than quote the corresponding archival document

(obtainable on the APA Website, http://www.apa.org). This is done below together with some elaboration. According to the archival document:

> Clinical Child [and Adolescent] Psychology is a specialty of professional psychology which integrates basic tenets of clinical psychology, developmental psychopathology, and principles of child and family development. Clinical child [and adolescent] psychologists conduct scientific research and provide psychological services to infants, toddlers, children, and adolescents. The research and services in Clinical Child [and Adolescent] Psychology are focused on understanding, preventing, diagnosing and treating psychological, cognitive, emotional, developmental, behavioral, and family problems of children [and adolescents]. Of particular importance to clinical child [and adolescent] psychologists is an understanding of the basic psychological needs of children and the social contexts which influence child development and adjustment.

Like Clinical Psychology, Clinical Child and Adolescent Psychology is a "health service provider" specialty. As the archival definition makes clear, the central topic in Clinical Child and Adolescent Psychology is psychopathology in young persons. It shares this interest with nonpsychological fields such as Psychiatry, Social Work, and Psychiatric Nursing. Although the founder of clinical child and adolescent psychology, Witmer, was an interventionist, much of the clinical work of the pre-World War II generation in the field focused exclusively on psychological assessment of children's cognitive status (typically using the Stanford-Binet test) and personality. Exceptions to this were the famous 1924 studies of Mary Cover Jones desensitizing children's fears and the 1938 development of bell and pad behavioral treatment for bedwetting by the Mowrers. After the war, work with youngsters, like that with adults, broadened out to include psychotherapy and later behavior therapy.

The archival document goes on to describe the training needed to be a Clinical Child [and Adolescent] Psychologist, which may be obtained at either the doctoral or postdoctoral level:

> The preparation of clinical child [and adolescent] psychologists is characterized by: knowledge of normal developmental processes as a prerequisite for distinguishing between normal and abnormal behavior and development, and for understanding developmental factors as they relate to assessment and intervention; normal family processes as they relate to children's development, including the impact of family dynamics, normal family functioning, and child rearing practices on normal child development and on the development of children's problems; child and adolescent psychopathology including epidemiology of children's problems, assessment and classification of problems across the age span, etiological models of child and

adolescent psychopathology, research findings related to etiology, treatment options and treatment efficacy related to specific problems at different ages and knowledge of family and other problems requiring treatment; ... knowledge of the methods of assessment of development, intellect, cognition, personality, mood and affect, and achievement; theories and research evidence for treatments of childhood mental disorders, adjustment reactions of childhood, family problems, and adaptation to stressful conditions or to chronic illness; special ethical and legal issues in research and practice with children; [and] an appropriate appreciation for and understanding of principles of diversity and cultural context as they relate to professional behavior and clinical practice.

In the United States, training in Clinical Child and Adolescent Psychology is usually pursued within an APA-approved PhD or PsyD program, and includes at least a 1-year full-time internship in a health care setting. An alternative is a postdoctoral program with a child and adolescent focus following generic training in such a clinical psychology doctoral program.

According to the archival document, Clinical Child [and Adolescent] Psychologists deal with the following range of problems:

> [P]hysical and/or psychosocial challenges resulting from pre-term birth, serious physical illness, prenatal substance abuse/addiction; severe developmental problems such as pervasive developmental disorders, autism, retardation; mental and emotional disorders such as schizophrenia, attention deficit/hyperactivity disorder, conduct disorder, anxiety, depression; social problems such as delinquency, substance abuse/ dependency, inappropriate sexual conduct; coping difficulties associated with stressors such as parental divorce, remarriage, step parenting, natural disaster or trauma; developmental milestone concerns and difficult temperament characteristics related to such problems as toilet training, tantrums, feeding and sleeping difficulties; cognitive deficits or dysfunction in communication or academic performance; [and] psychological aspects of physical illnesses.

The procedures and techniques used by Clinical Child and Adolescent Psychologists, as listed by the archival document, include the following:

> [I]nterviews, observations, age-normed psychological tests, personality and family assessment measures; behavioral and cognitive-behavioral approaches, play therapy, individual psychotherapy, family therapy and counseling; parent education and training; collaboration with pediatricians to monitor effectiveness of psychoactive medication, deal with medication compliance, or help with issues such as pain management; prevention programs aimed at ... problems and disorders such as social deviance and delinquency; health promotion programs and prevention of abuse and other problems of childhood; multimethod and comprehensive interventions that target children and families across contexts; [and] interdisciplinary consultation.

The boundaries between Clinical Child and Adolescent Psychology and adjacent specialties, both within psychology and outside it are often imprecise. Psychologists should therefore above all adhere to the ethical precept to practice only in those particular domains where they have the competence to do so. The field has the continuing ethical obligation to monitor the efficacy and effectiveness of its interventions through appropriate, controlled research.

See also: Clinical Psychology; Counseling Psychology; Pediatric Psychology; School Psychology; Training Issues

DONALD K. ROUTH

Clinical Child Psychology Organizations

See: Professional Societies in Clinical Child and Pediatric Psychology

Clinical Interviews

See: Interviewing

Clinical Psychology

In 1995, the American Psychological Association (APA) established the Commission for the Recognition of Specialties and Proficiencies in Professional Psychology (the acronym is CRSPPP, pronounced "crisp"). This Commission provided official recognition for existing specialties and recognized some new ones. In each case, its recommendations were acted on by the APA Council, and an archival document was created describing the specialty. The specialty of Clinical Psychology, which had existed for over a century since its founding by Lightner Witmer in 1896, was one of the first such specialties reaffirmed by CRSPPP in 1998. To state what this specialty involves, one can therefore do no better than quote the corresponding archival document (obtainable on the APA Web site, http://www.apa.org). This is done below, together with some elaboration and the addition of historical context to clarify how this specialty came to be what it now is. According to the archival document:

> Clinical Psychology is a general practice and health service provider specialty in professional psychology. Clinical psychologists assess, diagnose, predict, prevent, and treat psychopathology, mental disorders and other individual or group problems to improve behavioral adjustment, adaptation, personal effectiveness and satisfaction. What distinguishes Clinical Psychology as a general practice specialty is the breadth of problems addressed and of populations served. Clinical Psychology, in research, education, training and practice, focuses on individual differences, abnormal behavior, and mental disorders and their prevention, and lifestyle enhancement.

The term "general practice" specialty distinguished Clinical Psychology from more specialized areas such as Neuropsychology that grew out of it. The words "health service provider" apply to Clinical, Counseling, and School Psychology to distinguish them from areas such as Industrial and Organizational Psychology, whose clients tend to be businesses rather than individuals. As the archival definition makes clear, the central topic in Clinical Psychology is human psychopathology. It shares this interest with nonpsychological fields such as Psychiatry, Social Work, and Psychiatric Nursing. Although the founder of Clinical Psychology, Witmer, was an interventionist, most of the pre-World War II generation in the field focused exclusively on psychological assessment of cognitive status and personality. After the war, the field broadened out to include psychotherapy and, later, behavior therapy. At present, practitioners in certain jurisdictions with special additional training are broadening their scope of practice to include the prescription of psychotropic medications as well.

The archival document goes on to describe the training needed to be a Clinical Psychologist:

> Preparation for entry into the specialty begins at the doctoral level and serves as a basis for advanced post-doctoral training in Clinical Psychology or in one or another of the advanced specialties that build on its knowledge and application bases. The substantive areas of basic psychology in which clinical psychologists must have theoretical and scientific knowledge include the biological, social and cognitive/affective bases of behavior and individual differences. In addition, Clinical Psychology has a special focus on the areas of personality and its development and course, and psychopathology and its prevention and remediation.

In the United States, training in Clinical Psychology is usually pursued within an APA-approved PhD or PsyD program in a university and includes at least a 1-year full-time internship in a health care setting. Approved postdoctoral programs are rapidly developing both in Clinical Psychology itself and in its more specialized descendents.

The archival definition next describes assessment in Clinical Psychology:

> Psychological assessment requires knowledge of the developmental and sociocultural normative expectations for the individual(s) assessed. The assessment of attitudinal, cognitive, psychophysiological, affective, and/or behavioral functions of individuals and groups is used to identify and measure unique characteristics which may require modification or amelioration to facilitate performance and social competence.

Clinical assessment traditionally involved cognitive tests, projective measures, and self-report personality questionnaires. Subsequently, it came to include direct behavioral observation and psychophysiological procedures, among others. Most recently, in collaboration with psychiatry, clinical psychology has begun to develop and standardize structured interviews for the formal diagnosis of different types of psychopathology.

Next, the archival document describes intervention:

> The knowledge base of intervention requires mastery of theories of psychotherapy and psychotherapeutic methods and awareness of current literature on effectiveness and emerging interventions. In addition, Clinical Psychology is built on knowledge of principles of behavioral change, clinical decision-making, and the professional and ethical concerns surrounding clinical practice.

Traditional interventions favored by Clinical Psychologists have included psychoeducational and psychosocial approaches such as diagnostic teaching, psychoanalysis, and behavior analysis and therapy. These psychologists have pioneered in formal research on the processes and outcomes of such interventions and have become the de facto experts in this area. The field increasingly favors empirically supported interventions, including those with written treatment manuals.

What populations are the focus of Clinical Psychology? According to the archival document:

> Clinical Psychology services involve the application of psychological principles to the assessment and alleviation of human problems in individuals, families, groups, and communities. Clinical psychologists focus on services to individuals of all ages and may work with a single individual or with groups or families from a variety of ethnic, cultural, and socioeconomic backgrounds who are maladjusted or suffer from mental disorders. Populations include those with medical problems and physical disabilities as well as healthy persons who seek to prevent disorder and/or to improve their adaptation, adjustment, personal development and satisfaction.

As these words may suggest, the boundaries between the specialty of Clinical Psychology and other specialties such as Family Psychology, Health Psychology, and Rehabilitation Psychology are sometimes unclear. Above all, the ethical principle applies that psychologists should only practice in those areas in which they have been trained and are competent; otherwise, they refer patients to others.

Here is what the archival document says about the problems and issues addressed by Clinical Psychology:

> As a general practice specialty, Clinical Psychology focuses on the understanding, assessment, prediction, prevention, and alleviation of problems related to intellectual function; emotional, biological, psychological, and social and behavioral maladjustment, disability, distress, and mental disorder and, therefore, of necessity, enhancement of psychological functioning and prevention of dysfunction.

None of this is to say that Clinical Psychologists are always able to change intractable human problems. Serious problems such as mental retardation, bipolar disorder, and schizophrenia have so far proved to be often resistant to interventions from professionals with many types of backgrounds. It is best to be modest in view of the limitations of what is known and what can presently be accomplished.

Finally, the archival document includes more detail about specific procedures used by Clinical Psychologists in the areas of assessment, intervention, consultation, and supervision. It concludes with the following statement about the importance of research:

> Research is a core activity of Clinical Psychology and includes the development and validation of assessments and interventions related to intellectual, cognitive, emotional, physiological, behavioral, interpersonal, and group functioning; basic research in personality, psychopathology prevention, and behavior change and enhancement; program evaluation; and the review, evaluation, critique, and synthesis of research.

In fact, one of the strengths of clinical psychology has always been its thorough training in research methods and findings in the behavioral sciences. No other mental health discipline even comes close to it in this area.

In summary, clinical psychology focuses mainly on psychopathology, its diagnosis, treatment, prevention, and investigation.

See also: Counseling Psychology; Clinical Child and Adolescent Psychology; Pediatric Psychology; School Psychology

DONALD K. ROUTH

Clinical Utility

Clinical utility refers to a type of validity in which information from an assessment procedure is shown to either directly or indirectly improve clinical practice. Unfortunately, as noted recently by Frick (2000), the development of many assessment instruments have not emphasized this aspect of validity, leading to little overlap between assessment instruments used in research and those used for applied purposes. For example, much of the validity information collected on assessment techniques is correlational or involves documenting mean differences between groups of children on scores from the test. Such group data provide only limited information for interpreting scores for an individual child. Furthermore, and more importantly, Kampaus and Frick (2000) have noted that many assessment techniques have not been validated using clinically important criteria (e.g., predicting response to treatment). In the rare cases when such criteria have been used, the validity of scores across groups of individuals of different sex, developmental levels, cultural groups, or other important characteristics has not been extensively studied.

Vasey and Lonigan (2000) note that clinical utility can be either direct or indirect. Evidence for indirect utility, or conceptual utility, is found when scores from an assessment instrument in some way enhance the understanding of the person being assessed, such as in documenting the severity of impairment associated with an emotional disorder or in documenting the presence of a certain subtype of the disorder. It is hoped that such an enhanced understanding of the subject will also enhance the services provided to the person. However, such treatment benefit is not directly established. In contrast, evidence for direct clinical utility is found when the direct benefit of the scores for making important clinical decisions for individuals assessed by the test can be documented clearly.

There are many forms of direct clinical utility. According to Hayes, Nelson, and Jarett (1987), one of the most important forms of direct clinical utility is treatment utility. Treatment utility refers to the process of documenting that scores from a test enhance treatment outcome for the individual, such as by aiding decisions as to the most appropriate form of treatment that the person should receive. Importantly, to establish such utility, research must not only document that the assessment instrument enhances diagnostic precision (i.e., diagnostic utility). Research must further document that this increase in diagnostic precision enhances treatment outcome. For example, simply showing that a score from a behavior rating scale enhances the accuracy of a diagnosis of Conduct Disorder is not sufficient for establishing direct clinical utility. Research must also document that this increase in diagnostic accuracy actually leads to improved treatment outcome for children with this diagnosis.

Although treatment utility is clearly a very important type of direct clinical utility, there are other types that are also important. Prevention utility is concerned with a test's ability to document children at risk for a certain problematic outcome and, thereby, identify candidates for prevention programs. Treatment-monitoring utility focuses on the usefulness of a test in measuring the effects of treatment. An example of this type of utility is provided by Kamphaus and Frick (2002) with the Conner's Global Index, a 10-item subscale of the Conners Rating Scales-Revised that has been shown to be sensitive to the effects of stimulant medication in the treatment of children with an attention deficit disorder.

One final important concept for understanding clinical utility is the concept of incremental utility. This refers to the usefulness of the scores from a test for enhancing the clinical services provided to an individual over and above the information that is provided by other tests. Specifically, scores on a test may be related to clinically important criteria, like predicting treatment outcome or monitoring response to treatment. However, it is also important to demonstrate that the scores add to the prediction validity of these criteria when used in a battery with other tests. This is a very important aspect of clinical utility, since test scores are rarely used in isolation. Instead, test scores are typically integrated with other assessment information when making important clinical decisions. As a result, it is important to document the usefulness of test scores within a comprehensive battery of tests.

See also: Evidence-Based Treatments; Psychometric Properties of Tests; Risk Assessment and Risk Management; Validity Treatment Outcome Measures

Further Reading

Frick, P. J. (2000). Laboratory and performance-based measures of childhood disorders: Introduction to the special section. *Journal of Clinical Child Psychology, 29,* 475–478.

Hayes, S., Nelson, R., & Jarrett, R. (1987). The treatment utility of assessment: A functional approach to evaluating assessment quality. *American Psychologist, 42,* 963–974.

Kampaus, R. W., & Frick, P. J. (2002). *Clinical assessment of child and adolescent personality and behavior* (2nd ed.). Boston: Allyn & Bacon.

Vasey, M., & Lonigan, C. (2000). Considering the clinical utility of performance-based measures of childhood anxiety. *Journal of Clinical Child Psychology, 29,* 493–508.

JAMIE FARRELL
PAUL J. FRICK

Cocaine, Prenatal Exposure

DEFINITION OF THE PROBLEM

Cocaine is a highly addictive stimulant drug derived from coca leaves that are processed into a variety of forms, which are administered orally, intranasally, intravenously, and through inhalation. Effects can begin in 5 sec up to 5 min, based on the method of ingestion. It produces a "high" by blocking the reabsorption of dopamine, which leads to an abnormally high level of dopamine in the synapses in the brain. This high level of dopamine is responsible for the pleasurable effects associated with cocaine. The effects last approximately 2 hr and cocaine can be detected in the urine up to 4 days after ingestion. Use of cocaine is associated with addiction, irritability and mood disturbances, restlessness, paranoia, auditory hallucinations, nausea, abdominal pain, stroke, cardiac arrest, seizures, respiratory arrest, and death in users. Slang terms for this drug include blow, coke, white, flake, rock, powder, and dime. The use of cocaine has remained fairly stable since 1985 when the current sampling techniques were adopted. Rates of cocaine use are similar across the country and its use occurs equally in both rural and urban areas. The unemployed and those who did not graduate from high school are more likely to use cocaine. In addition, women who use cocaine frequently use other substances that are known to affect fetal development, the most common of which are alcohol, tobacco, and marijuana. Women who use cocaine are also more likely to be victims of domestic violence.

PREVALENCE

Exact figures on the number of women who use cocaine while pregnant are difficult to obtain due to problems of underreporting. However, the National Institute on Drug Abuse estimates that in 1996, 1.1 percent of pregnant women used cocaine. It is estimated that approximately 375,000 children are prenatally exposed to cocaine each year. Identification is dependent on the self-report of the mother and/or toxicology analysis of urine, meconium, or hair. However, testing of infant meconium and maternal hair is the most useful way of screening not only for exposure but also dosage. Unfortunately, drug screening occurs inconsistently and is governed by local policies and procedures.

EFFECTS

Cocaine crosses the placenta and enters the bloodstream of the developing fetus: use early in pregnancy is associated with miscarriage, while use in the later stages of pregnancy is associated with preterm labor and low birth weight. There is not a fetal cocaine withdrawal syndrome as seen in neonatal abstinence syndrome associated with opiates. Furthermore, research has not found evidence for a predictable pattern of dysmorphic features as is seen with Fetal Alcohol Syndrome (FAS).

Studies examining the impact of prenatal exposure to cocaine have been inconsistent in their findings. The primary reason for contradictory findings may be due to the multiple negative environmental factors that may be correlated with study results (e.g., low socioeconomic status (SES), poor prenatal care, nutritional deficits, understimulating home environment, varying levels of cocaine exposure, and use of other drugs associated with problems in child development such as alcohol, tobacco, and marijuana). Cognitive deficits have been found in children with cocaine exposure through 2 years of age, with one study finding 14 percent of the large sample showing scores in the range for mental retardation and 38 percent of the sample showing mild delays. Continued deficits have been reported as the child reaches school age; however, the problems appear to be subtle in nature (e.g., memory and selective attention).

Unfortunately, well-controlled studies investigating speech, language, motor, and social–emotional function are absent in the literature. New research is beginning to target reported behavioral difficulties in children with prenatal exposure to cocaine.

TREATMENT/PROGNOSIS

If cocaine use is identified during pregnancy, drug treatment and prenatal care can help both infant and mother reach their full potential. Reviews of the literature have shown that heavy cocaine users who receive quality prenatal care, independent of drug treatment, show significant improvements in the health and development of their infants. The punitive and criminal atmosphere toward mothers who use cocaine prevents many from seeking prenatal care and/or drug treatment. Comprehensive treatment programs that address both drug (legal and nonlegal) use and other associated factors (such as childcare, healthcare, nutrition, comorbid psychological disorders, domestic violence, socioeconomic status, employment, and education) are recommended. After birth, continued drug treatment and parenting classes become important.

Children with substance exposure should be followed closely with periodic development assessments that examine physical, cognitive, speech–language, motor, and social–emotional development. Due to the current state of the research in this area, there is no conclusive evidence of the exact effects of prenatal cocaine exposure. While such assessments cannot determine a particular cause for any developmental delays, they can identify such delays. Once identified, services can be provided to increase development in this area. Children who were prenatally exposed to cocaine should not be unduly stigmatized or labeled. They should be instead treated with compassion and with rational, research-supported therapies when necessary. Furthermore, as cocaine use is highly associated with factors that put infants and children at risk, it should remain a mental health and public heath concern independent of its unique effects on those children prenatally exposed.

See also: Assessment; Assessment of Global Functioning; Behavior Rating Scales; Effects of Parental Substance Abuse on Children; Family Intervention; Fatal alcohal syndrome; Prenatal Exposure to Methamphetamines; Substance Abuse; Screening Instruments

Further Reading

Curet, L. B., & Hsi, A. C. (2002). Drug abuse during pregnancy. *Clinical Obstetrics and Gynecology, 45*(1), 73–88.

Frank, D. A., Augustyn, M., Knight, W. G., Pell, T., & Zuckerman, B. (2001). Growth, development, and behavior in early childhood following prenatal cocaine exposure: A systematic review. *Journal of the American Medical Association, 285*(12), 1613–1625.

Jacobson, S. W., & Jacobson, J. L. (2001). Alcohol and drug-related effects on development: A new emphasis on contextual factors. *Infant Mental Health Journal, 22,* 416–430.

Singer, L. T., Arendt, R., Minnes, S., Farkes, K., Salvator, A., Kirchner, H. L., & Kliegman, R. (2002). Cognitive and motor outcomes of cocaine exposed infants. *Journal of the American Medical Association, 287,* 1952–1960.

Stanwood, G. D., Levitt, P., Singer, L. T., Arendt, R. E., Delaney-Black, V., Covington, C. Y., Nordstrom-Klee, B., Sokol, R. J., Frank, D. A., Augustyn, M., Knight, W. G., Pell, T., & Zuckerman, B. (2001). Prenatal cocaine exposure as a risk factor for later developmental outcomes. [Special issue]. *Journal of the American Medical Association, 286*(1), 42–47.

LESLIE BUCK
ROBIN H. GURWITCH

Cognitive Development

DEFINITION AND SCOPE OF THE FIELD

The word root *cognit*, which appears in psychological terms such as "cognition" or "cognitive psychology," is derived from the Latin verb *cogitare*, which means "to think." Thus, broadly defined, "cognitive development" is the study of children's thinking, but the field itself actually includes the investigation and exploration of the development of a number of fundamental psychological phenomena. These phenomena include sensory development, perceptual development, the development of attention, age-related changes in learning and memory, language development, and the development of reasoning/problem solving. In addition, topics such as the development of intelligence (i.e., individual differences in cognitive development), social cognition (i.e., the use of cognition in social contexts) and the relationship of cognitive development to educational skills and school achievement are also often considered to be part of this field.

STUDY OF CHILDREN'S THINKING: PAST, PRESENT, AND FUTURE DIRECTIONS

The origin of the field might reasonably be traced to William James' musings about the "blooming, buzzing confusion" that must face an infant or child who is first confronted with a world of stimulation and experience. However, the systematic study of cognitive development in Western civilization is probably more appropriately attributed to the Swiss psychologist Jean Piaget. He published a number of books during the first half of the 20th century on the development of children's reasoning from infancy to adolescence, and developed the first comprehensive theory of cognitive development. This theory was summarized in a classic 1963 volume by John Flavell. Indeed, during the 1950s

through 1970s, a course in cognitive development might have been devoted almost exclusively to Piagetian studies and theory.

However, by the 1980s, the field of cognitive development had changed greatly, being prompted by the emergence of cognitive science and models of information processing. This influence expanded the field beyond the more holistic approaches to higher-order cognitive functions that Piaget emphasized, and prompted consideration of sensory and perceptual function, as well as experimental studies of learning, memory, and language. The 1990s saw two significant advances for the field. First, the contribution of the social environment to cognitive development was recognized and explored. This compelled the inclusion of social cognition within the field, and also prompted a reconsideration of the writings of Lev Vygotsky from the 1920s–1930s as a theoretical influence. Second, the growth of the influence of cognitive neuroscience also prompted further considerations of how age-related cognitive changes were traceable to predictable and systematic changes in the developmental processes within the central nervous system (CNS) including the effects of the early environment on the long-term structure and function of the brain, and the direct measurement of brain functions through imaging and electrophysiological techniques. At the start of the new millennium, linkages between cognitive development and educational concepts are being further explored, leading to the hope, if not expectation, that instructional methods and evaluations may be further influenced by what is known about the basic science of children's thinking, and that the study of cognitive development may become more influenced by functional considerations.

The current state of the field is capably represented by a number of recent textbooks, such as those authored by Bjorklund (1999), Siegler (1998), and Flavell, Miller, and Miller (2002).

CLINICAL RELEVANCE

The field and measurement of development in the cognitive realm constitutes a core set of constructs for the diagnosis and identification of mental retardation. Many emotional disturbances and clinical syndromes can also be identified through measures of cognitive function in children. Some recent research suggests that individual differences in cognitive function in early life may be related to later cognitive ability, thus allowing further progress in the early identification of children at risk for cognitive delays or deficits later in life.

See also: Childhood; Infancy; Language Development; Sensory and Perceptual Development

Further Reading

Bjorklund, D. (1999). *Children's thinking*. Belmont, CA: Wadsworth.
Flavell, J. H. (1963). *The developmental psychology of Jean Piaget*. Princeton, NJ: Van Nostrand.
Flavell, J. H., Miller, P. H., & Miller, S. A. (2002). *Cognitive development*. Englewood, NJ: Prentice-Hall.
Phillips, J. (1981). *Piaget's theory: A primer*. San Francisco, CA: Freeman.
Siegler, R. (1998). *Children's thinking*. Englewood Cliffs, NJ: Prentice-Hall.

JOHN COLOMBO

Cognitive–Behavior Therapy for Children

Cognitive–Behavior Therapy (CBT) for emotional and behavioral disorders of childhood evolved from treatments for adults with these same disorders. CBT approaches with children incorporate the demonstrated positive elements of behavior therapy while considering the cognitive activities of the child in an effort to produce behavioral, cognitive, and affective change. Family and social factors are also considered important.

PREVALENCE OF TARGET CHILDHOOD DISORDERS

Recent epidemiological data suggest that 1 in 10 children have mental health problems severe enough to warrant treatment. Yet, of those children in need of treatment, less than 20 percent receive appropriate services. Indeed, the consequences of untreated childhood disorders are a major problem confronting today's society. CBT is an orientation that guides therapeutic interventions that have been shown to be effective in the treatment of childhood emotional and behavioral disorders.

GUIDING THEORY

CBT represents a perspective that integrates different points of view and considers the child's internal and external environments, including the child's thoughts, feelings, and behavior, as well as important social and interpersonal factors (e.g., peer, family, and school contexts). The CBT model assumes that thoughts, feelings, and behaviors are inextricably linked; therefore, altering one system can lead to changes in the others. An emphasis is also placed on the process of learning, and the CBT model posits that learning is mediated by thought. In other words, not only a situation, but also what the child thinks about that situation, is important to how the child will respond. Accordingly, CBT strategies with children use enactive, performance-based procedures as well as cognitive interventions to produce changes in the child's thinking and behavior. As such, potential historical causes of current childhood disorders are not the focus in CBT. Similarly, pointing fingers of causal blame is not a part of this treatment. Rather, CBT considers the child's current status (e.g., symptoms and level of distress) and works forward to accomplish improvement.

CBT STRATEGIES/TECHNIQUES

CBT uses several strategies to help clients identify maladaptive thoughts and behavior and to foster change. CBT encompasses both cognitive interventions, such as coping self-talk, cognitive restructuring, and problem-solving, and behavioral techniques, including relaxation training, pleasant events scheduling, and self and social reinforcement. These strategies occur in session, as well as through homework, in which the child experiments with and rehearses the material discussed in session. Some examples of homework assignments include maintaining a journal of thoughts, feelings, and behavior, testing hypotheses, and/or practice of behavioral skills. The components of CBT described below are typically implemented in varying amounts and in different ways within particular therapeutic programs.

Several cognitive techniques are characteristic of CBT. Cognitive restructuring refers to the process by which the therapist helps the child to accurately appraise social information by altering aspects of his/her perceptions or beliefs. The first step in cognitive restructuring is to help the child identify his/her maladaptive thoughts or assumptions. Once the child can identify such thoughts, the therapist guides the child to modify them and observe and record the results of these new ways of thinking. Another technique, coping self-talk, shows the child new ways to think about stressful circumstances and encourages the generation and evaluation of alternatives. Problem solving is a related process by which the child and therapist formulate the problem and the major goals for the solution. The child generates alternative solutions and considers each alternative in terms of how well it will help the child to achieve his/her goals. Then, the child selects a solution with which to experiment and, as a last step, evaluates the success of the chosen solution.

Given the inclusion of intervention strategies that are primarily cognitive in nature, it is probable that the effectiveness of CBT is influenced by the child's level of cognitive development. Therefore, it is important for therapists to be aware of their child clients' level of cognitive development and tailor the treatment to their existing and emerging cognitive capacities.

CBT also includes a variety of behavioral procedures. Contingent reinforcement, for example, is the cornerstone of behavior therapy. Contingent reinforcement allows the therapist to change the client's behavior through successive shaping of behavior that approximates the goal. The therapist rewards the child at each step with tangible or social rewards for the performance of a target behavior or for abstention from an undesirable behavior. Another behavioral technique is modeling: the child witnesses another individual, such as someone participating in difficult situations, trying alternative ideas, and experiencing the emotional and behavioral outcomes of such situations and ideas. In symbolic modeling, the child watches videotapes or listens to audiotapes. In live modeling, the therapist actively demonstrates coping responses for the child and then asks the child to participate. When using modeling, it is generally best for the therapist to use a coping model, in which the therapist demonstrates the skills for managing (coping with) frustrations and obstacles that inevitably occur. Role-play practice and exposure to problem situations allows the child opportunities for guided practice of new coping skills. Such role-play or exposure tasks are usually implemented in a gradual manner: the child is initially presented with a mildly difficult situation, followed by increasingly challenging situations.

CBT VERSUS OTHER THERAPEUTIC INTERVENTIONS FOR CHILDREN

CBT differs from other child psychotherapies in several ways. First, a cognitive behavioral therapist is more actively involved in the therapeutic process than a clinician using psychodynamic or play therapy techniques, for example. Also, unlike many other psychotherapies, CBT is manual-based. The treatment manual defines the goals of each session and describes how these goals can be accomplished. The treatment manual provides guidance for the therapist, and the resulting consistency across therapists and settings that result from the use of manual-based treatment allows for empirical evaluation of the treatment. Additionally, CBT differs from others in that it is time-limited (CBT rarely exceeds 15–20 sessions spread out over 7–8 months).

It is also worth noting how CBT differs from both behavior therapy and cognitive therapy. CBT uses various behavioral techniques, but places more importance on the role of the child's social information processing than does traditional behavior therapy. For example, a cognitive behavioral therapist may discuss the client's thoughts before, during, and after an experience and discuss effective strategies to deal with difficult situations. Unlike cognitive treatment, behavioral practice, modeling, and rewards are active ingredients in CBT.

EMPIRICAL SUPPORT FOR CBT

Empirical studies have provided support for the use of CBT for emotional and behavioral disorders of childhood. For instance, as noted by Birmaher and colleagues (1996), several studies have documented the efficacy of CBT for depressed school-age children and adolescents. In addition, CBT has demonstrated efficacy in the treatment of several of the anxiety disorders in children. Controlled clinical trials conducted with children by Kendall and colleagues (1997) have found that, compared to wait-list control, CBT can be effective in reducing self-reported and parent-reported anxiety and diagnoses of an anxiety disorder. Furthermore, treatment gains of CBT for childhood anxiety disorders have been shown to last up to 3.5 years following treatment as demonstrated by Kendall and Southam-Gerow (1996). As reviewed by Lochman (1990), CBT outcome studies have also been conducted with aggressive, conduct-disordered youth. In several studies, children receiving CBT showed greater decreases in aggressive behavior and greater increases in prosocial behavior and adjustment, than children receiving a nondirective therapy or a control condition. Although the efficacy of CBT with aggressive children appears to be promising, results are not entirely supportive. Some data suggest that decreases in aggressive or delinquent behavior may not be maintained over time or may not generalize across situations.

See also: Anxiety Disorders; Conduct Disorder; Child Psychotherapy; Positive Reinforcement

Further Reading

Birmaher, B., Ryan, N. D., Williamson, D. E., & Brent, D. A. (1996). Childhood and adolescent depression: A review of the past 10 years, Part II. *Journal of the American Academy of Child and Adolescent Psychiatry, 35*, 1575–1583.

Kendall, P. C. (1994). Treating anxiety disorders in children: Results of a randomized clinical trial. *Journal of Consulting and Clinical Psychology, 62*, 100–110.

Kendall, P. C., Flannery-Schroeder, E., Panicelli-Mindel, S. M., Southam-Gerow, M. A., Henin, A., & Warman, M. (1997). Therapy for youths with anxiety disorders: A second randomized clinical trial. *Journal of Consulting and Clinical Psychology, 65*, 366–380.

Kendall, P. C., & Southam-Gerow, M. A. (1996). Long-term follow-up of a cognitive behavioral therapy for anxiety disordered youth. *Journal of Consulting and Clinical Psychology, 64*, 724–730.

Lochman, J. E. (1990). Modification of childhood aggression. In M. Hersen & R. M. Eisler (Eds.), *Progress in behavior modification, Volume 25* (pp. 3–22). New York: Guilford.

KRISTINA A. HEDTKE
PHILIP C. KENDALL
SASHA G. ASCHENBRAND
ANTHONY C. PULIAFICO
ALICIA A. HUGHES

Cognitive–Behavioral Play Therapy

DEFINITION

Cognitive–Behavioral Play Therapy (CBPT) is a unique adaptation of cognitive-behavioral therapy for very young children (2 1/2–6 years old). As such, it incorporates traditional cognitive and behavioral interventions within a developmentally appropriate play therapy paradigm. Through use of play, cognitive change is communicated indirectly, often using puppets, stuffed animals, and books to model strategies. Like all play therapies, CBPT is grounded in a positive therapeutic relationship, the use of play as a means of communication, and the notion that the play therapy setting is a safe place for the child to communicate his/her concerns. In contrast with more traditional play therapies, CBPT emphasizes collaboration between the therapist and child in the setting of goals and the selection of play materials and activities. Also, the play is psycho-educational in nature, with an emphasis on the transmission of adaptive coping skills.

METHOD

Of necessity, CBPT emphasizes experiential, rather than verbal, approaches to interacting with the child. One extremely useful mechanism for the transmission of interventions is modeling through play. The therapist uses play materials to identify maladaptive beliefs, counter those beliefs, and provide positive coping statements and skills for the child.

CBPT is usually conducted weekly in individual sessions with the child. Parents are frequently involved in working with the therapist around child management issues, but do not typically participate in therapy sessions, per se.

CBPT can be conceptualized has having four stages. In the Introductory/Orientation stage, the child is prepared for therapy and the therapist often guides the parents in helping to prepare the child for treatment. This may involve teaching the parents how to tell their child about therapy in a developmentally appropriate way, and often includes the parents reading a book about play therapy to the child. Early sessions with the child also serve as an introduction to treatment.

In the Assessment stage, the therapist formulates a sense of the child's perceptions of his/her situation. This is done through the use of unstructured observations, structured play scenarios, and/or structured assessment tools (e.g., the Puppet Sentence Completion Task), in combination with information gathered from the parents.

During the Treatment stage, therapy focuses on teaching more adaptive responses to deal with specific situations faced by the child. Several cognitive and behavioral interventions are utilized during this phase of CBPT, such as contingency management, systematic desensitization, and cognitive change strategies. Reinforcing the gains and successes achieved by the child is vital to their sustainability over time, as well as to the child's achievement of additional successes.

Also during the Treatment stage, generalization and relapse prevention are integrated into the therapy. Generalization of adaptive behaviors to the natural environment is an important component of CBPT; the therapist must build in specific training that helps the child make connections to other settings and individuals. In particular, interventions that address self-control and teach new behaviors are critical. As a rule, all interventions should incorporate the issue of generalization by modeling real life situations as much as possible. In general, reinforcement of skills should come from the natural environment. Adaptive behaviors should be reinforced and emphasized beyond their initial acquisition in order to strengthen and support their continuation. In addition, relapse prevention is a critical focus of this stage of CBPT. That is, the therapist prepares the child for setbacks by working on ways to handle future stressors and life situations. High risk situations are identified, and the child is taught ways of handling such situations, should they arise. As these skills are brought into CBPT, work is also being done with the parents around the same issues.

Finally, the Termination phase of CBPT takes place over several sessions. Preparation for the end of therapy deals with the concrete reality, as well as feelings that the child may have about the end of treatment. Some children benefit from very concrete representation of the ending of treatment (e.g., through calendars or construction chains representing each session).

CLINICAL APPLICATIONS

CBPT has been used with a wide range of populations, with published reports of its use with children with selective mutism, encopresis, fears and phobias, and separation anxiety. It has also been used to treat children who have experienced traumatic life events, such as sexual abuse and divorce. In general, CBPT is an appropriate approach for preschool and early school-age children, as children in these age groups are learning about cause–effect relationships but still lack the language skills for more verbally oriented therapies. Virtually any presenting problem requiring the young child to learn more adaptive coping skills could be treated through CBPT.

EFFECTIVENESS

CBPT is a model of psychotherapy that builds on the principles of cognitive behavior therapy, a well-established, respected therapeutic modality. It is a developmentally sensitive, integrated model of psychotherapy that uses proven techniques and incorporates empirically supported interventions, such as systematic desensitization. Although there has been much interest in play therapy research, CBPT has not been subjected to rigorous empirical study, thus the efficacy of CBPT itself has yet to be determined.

See also: Cognitive–Behavior Therapy; Developmental Issues in Treatment; Developmentally Based Psychotherapy; Play Therapy

Further Reading

Knell, S. M. (1993). *Cognitive–behavioral play therapy*. Northvale, NJ: Jason Aronson. (Soft cover edition published—1995.)
Knell, S. M. (1999). Cognitive behavioral play therapy. In S. W. Russ & T. Ollendick (Eds.), *Handbook of psychotherapies with children and families* (pp. 385–404). New York: Plenum.
Knell, S. M. (2000). Cognitive-behavioral play therapy with children with fears and phobias. In H. G. Kaduson & C. E. Schaefer (Eds.), *Short-term therapies with children* (p. 3027). New York: Guilford.

SUSAN M. KNELL

Colic

DEFINITION

Colic typically appears in infants before 3–4 months of age. It expresses itself as a generalized state of distress in the infant with what appears to be intermittent abdominal pain. The infant appears to be cramping and often will draw the legs up toward the chest, while engaging in inconsolable crying for periods as long as 2–3 hr. Colicky periods typically occur in the afternoon or early evening and seem to resolve spontaneously despite efforts of parents. Colic is only one of many potential reasons for infant crying.

INCIDENCE/PREVALENCE

Colic is a somewhat common phenomenon in infants occurring in approximately 12 percent of all infants.

ETIOLOGY

Interestingly, although colic is one of the world's oldest known forms of distress in infancy, the cause is not known. Theories of etiology include pain, allergies, gastrointestinal disorders, and psychological and neurodevelopmental explanations. There is little evidence for excessive pain or gas as the cause of the colicky behavior noted in infants. Theories of psychological factors as they relate to parental bonding issues were popular some time ago, but have been generally abandoned based on research. Neurodevelopmental explanations postulate that the child is neurologically immature and the distress is a result of the infant's inability to integrate sensory and motor input. No theory has significant research support and the cause of colic remains unspecified.

TREATMENT

Although the cause of colic is unknown and there does not appear to be a relationship between early colic and later feeding problems, it is important for young parents to feel that they are capable of responding and lessening their infant's distress. Parents can be reassured by a pediatrician's testimony that the infant will grow out of the disorder. This is a well-established fact, with disappearance of the symptoms at about 3–4 months of age. Many solutions for addressing colic are on the market and are widely publicized in parent magazines and on the Internet. These solutions include food additives, soothing musical tapes, and prescriptions for swaddling and handling the infant in a certain manner. One interesting treatment device was developed by a parent when he noticed that his infant with colic would calm while riding in the car going about 55 miles per hr. The device attaches to the infants crib and recreates the vibrations and sounds of a car traveling 55 miles per hr. Though this technique does not work for all infants, it has been fairly successful in most instances and the cost is not prohibitive. This may be an appropriate intervention to recommend to parents who are distressed by their inability to comfort their own young infant.

See also: Health Education/Health Promotion; Infancy

Further Reading

Linscheid, T. R., & Rasnake, L. Kaye (2001). Eating problems in children. In C. E. Walker & M. C. Roberts (Eds.), *Handbook of clinical child psychology* (3rd ed., pp. 523–541). New York: Wiley.

Loadman, W., Arnold, K., Bolmer, R., Petrella, R., & Cooper, L. (1987). Reducing the symptoms of infant colic by introduction of vibration/sound based intervention. *Pediatric Research, 21,* 182A.

Barr, R. G., James-Roberts, I., & Keefe, M. R. (2001). *New evidence on unexplained early infant crying: Its origins, nature and management.* St. Louis, MO: Johnson & Johnson Pediatric Institute.

THOMAS R. LINSCHEID

Community Interventions

DEFINITION

Community interventions encompass a variety of programs where professionals meet with youth (identified client) and their families in the natural environment. Typically these settings include the youth's home, school, or other community-based sites, as well as an array of services spanning individual and family therapy, respite care, crisis intervention, psychiatric hospital diversion, case management and advocacy, community outreach and service integration, and parent education and training.

The Child and Adolescent Service System Program (CASSP) initiative in 1986 was an important impetus for this approach to treatment provisions for youth and families. Recognizing that the mental health system was often failing to meet the needs of children with serious emotional disturbances (SED), community-based systems of care for youth and families were created to provide individualized services that are child-centered, family-focused, community-based, least restrictive and culturally competent. This new model of service delivery challenges systems to be flexible and comprehensive enough to meet each child and family's needs so that if treatment is unsuccessful, services are modified rather than withdrawn. As a result, communities have created networks of coordinated local systems of care that wrap services around the youth and family in an effort to maintain the youth in the community. Typically referred to as "wraparound" services, they encompass multiple systems that serve youth and families through the mental health, juvenile justice, educational, and child welfare systems. In addition to serving youth with SED, these services have increasingly been utilized with "at-risk" children as young as preschool age.

DESCRIPTION OF TREATMENT

Due to the individualized nature of these services and variability in community resources, much of the treatment to date has been heterogeneous. Services are often delivered for specific periods of time (i.e., 1–6 months), although some are long-term. Most community interventions are intensive (up to 20 hr a week of direct face-to-face contact), and can often be accessed 24 hr a day, 7 days a week. Community interventions typically include movement of services out of traditional treatment settings into the home or other natural community surroundings to provide support in the least restrictive environment, build parent-professional partnerships, enhance interagency collaboration, and deliver strength-based, culturally competent services. Flexibility in service provision and funding is required to provide individualized wrap around services. Commonly used models include wraparound services, home-based services, and family preservation services.

CLINICAL APPLICATIONS

Intended outcomes for community interventions include maintaining youth in their home (i.e., decreases in psychiatric hospitalization, incarcerations, foster care placements), decreases in problem behaviors, abuse and neglect, and psychiatric symptomatology. Outcomes also include increases in prosocial behaviors, educational attainment, and safety.

EFFECTIVENESS

Effectiveness for community interventions has generally been found to be positive. However, a caveat to this conclusion is that the complexity and variability in the type and quality of community intervention models makes controlled research difficult.

Some short-term intensive programs that utilized strict treatment fidelity and replicable controlled studies have demonstrated strong evidence of effectiveness (i.e., Multisystemic Therapy and Functional Family Therapy). Comparatively high rates of treatment success of these programs have been demonstrated with populations of juvenile delinquents and substance abusers, including decreases in behavioral problems, aggression, incarceration, drug use, and out-of-home placements. In addition, evidence suggestive of decreased risk for child maltreatment has also been established. Research of these short-term community interventions have also demonstrated improvement in family relationships, communication, and school attendance.

Outcome studies for community interventions that involve longer-term service provision are somewhat limited due to the innovative nature of this concept. Available research has demonstrated that community interventions involving wraparound services have led to less restrictive and more stable environments for youth, a significant decrease in overall problem behaviors, fewer abuse-related behaviors, and significant improvements in internalizing and externalizing disorders. Other studies have demonstrated success in safely reuniting abused and neglected children with their families through intensive family based services, and high rates of in-home maintenance for one year after initiation of treatment for youth who were at imminent risk of out-of-home placement. Despite these

improvements in functioning, these interventions are not a catchall, in that serious school and community-related behaviors still occur in youth receiving these services. The cost-effectiveness of community interventions is still unclear, as this variable has only been addressed in a few studies; however, in the short-term these programs appear to be an economical alternative to traditional out-of-home placements.

In summary, community interventions have altered the landscape of traditional mental health services for children and families with SED over the past 15 years. While the most successful community interventions are those that are part of systems of care that have a significant amount of resources available, careful attention should be directed toward understanding how these resources can be examined in light of traditional empirically supported treatments.

See also: Community Mental Health Centers; Family Intervention; Multisystemic Therapy; School-Based Treatments

Further Reading

Burns, B. J., Schoenwald, S. K., Burchard, J. D., Faw, L., & Santos, A. B. (2000). Comprehensive community-based interventions for youth with severe emotional disorders: Multisystemic therapy and the wraparound process. *Journal of Child and Family Studies, 9,* 282–314.
Ghuman, H. S., & Sarles, R. M. (Eds.). (1998). *Handbook of child and adolescent outpatient, day treatment and community psychiatry.* Castelton, NY: Hamilton Printing.
Marsh, D. T., & Fristad, M. A. (Eds.). (2002). *Handbook of serious emotional disturbance in children and adolescents.* New York: Wiley.
Research and Training Center for Children's Mental Health Web site. Available at http://www.fmhi.usf.edu

TAMMY A. LAZICKI-PUDDY
RICHARD W. PUDDY
ERIC M. VERNBERG

Community Mental Health Centers

HISTORY

Mental health interventions in the United States have had an extraordinary history, beginning in colonial times when the mentally ill were isolated in their homes and treated mostly by family members. With industrialization, institutions named asylums were constructed to house those with mental illness in order to "rehabilitate" them so that they could successfully rejoin society, with some early success but then further disappointing results. With the advent of psychiatry, mental hospitals took over the care of the mentally ill, again with the idea that they were to be housed separately for individual care. Unfortunately, for the most part, these institutions did not meet their original goals and often became depositories for the poor, immigrant, and/or insane.

The effects of war on soldiers in World War II set the stage for assessment and early intervention for mental illness. In addition, psychotropic medication made it possible for a larger number of patients to leave mental hospitals and live on their own or with supports from the community. In the 1960s, legislation with federal funding enabled mental health services to be provided in the community. The Federal Acts covered several areas of need in order to provide a continuity of care for a broad spectrum of the populace within their own communities. The services provided ranged from prevention, assessment, and outpatient as well as inpatient treatment, to transitional care and rehabilitation. Five primary areas included outpatient, inpatient, day treatment, emergency, and consulting and educational services. Other areas that Community Mental Health Centers (CMHCs) were encouraged to pursue included diagnostic and rehabilitation services, aftercare services, training, research, and evaluation. Over the next decade, CMHCs developed across the states, working to provide a broad range of services for individuals with differing needs and attempting to integrate mental health with other services.

In the late 1970s and into the 1980s federal dollars for CMHCs were cut back at the same time that the number of state hospital beds were reduced and then many state hospitals were ultimately closed. Because of an influx of chronically ill and tighter financial constraints, services became more linked to clients from specific targeted populations, namely, those with severe and persistent mental health problems as well as the poor. Unfortunately, these factors as well as privatization and managed care have made it more difficult for CMHCs to serve a broad range of community needs. Presently, CMHCs struggle with the issue of how to use public dollars that seem to be targeted for a few with severe mental health disabilities but also serve a broad sector of the community. In the area of public health, the Surgeon General has called for lessening the stigma related to mental illness and its treatment, and making empirically validated protocols available to a wider range of people.

STRENGTHS AND CHALLENGES

In order to fulfill the goals set forth in the legislation of the 1960s, many types of services have been "piloted" in mental health centers. A small sample of these services include partial hospitalization to maintain clients with severe mental illness in their community and build appropriate life skills, emergency screening in conjunction with law enforcement and hospital emergency rooms, and evaluation of the effectiveness of programs. CMHCs have also been crucial in establishing services for children, including early work with child disabilities in the school system, early intervention for children, and case management services for children with severe mental health disabilities. Often, mental health services have differed across CMHCs based on the needs of their particular communities.

CMHCs traditionally work from an ecological model of treatment, concentrating on the individual in the environment and intervening at a systems level. Many of the professionals who have been trained and work in this setting come from a social work background that stresses working with clients from a strength-based perspective and in the client's own environment. This tradition is associated with a current initiative of the American Psychological Association (APA) termed positive psychology, particularly with very difficult clients who have not dealt with traditional services. These programs have particularly focused on foster care children, chronically mentally ill adults, juvenile offenders, and the homeless.

Community mental health has always struggled with funding issues since there is no one centralized health agency to coordinate the necessary range of services for clients. The U.S. mental health service system connects many different sectors and may seem splintered into juvenile justice authority, special education within the school system, social welfare, and others. Because of this, interventions and funding may also be fragmented and create barriers to effective service.

Although the CMHCs have always been called upon to evaluate the clinical services they provide, there has been a tension between academic and applied work. Until recently, most academic institutions have not been interested in doing outcome evaluation projects with CMHCs. However, this kind of partnership could be very powerful in bringing empirically validated programs to a real-life setting with clients who show much diagnostic comorbidity. Currently, the APA has shown a greater emphasis on disseminating empirically validated treatment programs in applied settings.

CMHCs would seem to be a perfect match for this type of agenda and, indeed some communities have forged a successful link between the CMHC and the university setting.

FUTURE PROGRESS

One of the greatest challenges for CMHCs in the future will be realizing the goals set out for them in the 1960s with the cost containment that has come about at the beginning of this new century. Unfortunately, there is a great possibility that CMHCs will suffer the same fate as their predecessors, the asylums and mental hospitals, and become satellites of the welfare system. This would be an unfortunate outcome because it would be a very limited view of what treatment could be accomplished at the community level. Community leaders and citizens should feel empowered to join in discussions concerning the functioning of the mental health center, the functions it serves, and the areas in need of improvement. One area that has been very successful for CMHCs has been using community partnerships with the school, hospitals, social welfare and justice systems, public housing, and other treatment clinics, and providing services more and more in the community. Continuing these services would help to meet the Surgeon General's call for making mental health assessment and treatment more normalized and a part of day-to-day functioning. In addition, the connection between CMHCs and academic institutions would be particularly important to continue the tradition of training practitioners in a community setting and also of combining clinical work with program evaluation. Also, CMHCs should continue to be the leaders in educating the public about disorders and effective treatments and encouraging the community to seek treatment as necessary.

See also: Adjustment Disorders; Community Interventions; Disruptive Behavior Disorders; Health Care Professionals (General), General; Safety and Prevention

Further Reading

Grob, G. N. (1991). *From asylum to community: Mental health policy in modern America.* Princeton, NJ: Princeton University Press.

Isaac, R. J., & Armat, V. C. (1990). *Madness in the streets: How psychiatry and the law abandoned the mentally ill.* New York: Free Press.

Levine, M. (1981). *The history and politics of community mental health.* New York: Oxford University Press.

Mechanic, D. (1998). Emerging trends in mental health policy and practice. *Health Affairs, 17,* 82–98.

U.S. Department of Health and Human Services. (1999). *Mental health: A report of the Surgeon General-Executive Summary.* Rockville, MD: U.S. Author, Substance Abuse and Mental Health Services Administration, Center for Mental Health Services, National Institutes of Health, National Institute of Mental Health.

Julianne M. Smith
Sandra Shaw
S. Douglas Witt

Comorbidity

DEFINITION

Comorbidity has been defined by Wittchen and Essau (1993) as the presence of more than one specific disorder in a person at a specific point in time. This approach makes it possible to determine the occurrence and clustering of disorders over the lifespan of a child. Both the patterns of comorbidity and the temporal sequencing of comorbid disorders can be very different in children.

Although the concept of comorbidity has been described as far back as Hippocrates, Klerman (1990) notes that heightened interest in comorbidity was associated with the shift towards the "neo-Kraepelinian" paradigm during the 1970s, and with the advent of the third edition of the *Diagnostic and Statistical Manual of Mental Disorders* (*DSM-III*, American Psychiatric Association, 1987). The *DSM-III* and the subsequent *DSM* versions provide (i) explicit and operationalized diagnoses; (ii) the reduction of diagnostic hierarchies; (iii) a stronger emphasis on lifetime phenomena; and (iv) an increase in the number of specific diagnostic categories in contrast to the broad and loosely defined generic classes of diagnoses such as neurosis used in earlier versions. The changes inherent in these principles have an impact on clinical and research strategies and findings. That is, due to the higher number of specific diagnoses, use of the lifetime perspective, and the lack of diagnostic hierarchies, children are frequently assigned to more than one diagnostic category.

COMORBID PATTERNS

One of the most consistent findings in childhood psychopathology is the high rate of co-occurrence of disorders; moreover, the degree of comorbidity in children and adolescents is even more common than in adults. As reported by Anderson and colleagues (1987), about 60 percent of children with a diagnosable condition have two or more additional disorders. Furthermore, after reviewing six community studies, Angold and Costello concluded that the presence of one disorder (i.e., depression) in children and adolescents increased the probability for another disorder by at least 20-fold. Among the most common comorbid disorders in children and adolescents are anxiety and depressive disorders, conduct disorder and Attention-Deficit/Hyperactivity Disorder (ADHD), autistic disorder and mental retardation, and Tourette's syndrome and ADHD. Another common comorbid disorder is that of conduct disorder and depression. In fact in the days when masked depression was a popular concept, symptoms of conduct disorder were considered as one of the most frequent "maskers" of depression.

Some studies have also examined the temporal sequence of disorders. For example, among children with both anxiety and depressive disorders, Essau and colleagues (2000) note that anxiety generally precedes rather than follows the depression. Among children with conduct disorder and ADHD, ADHD generally precedes the development of conduct disorder. In fact, impulsivity or hyperactivity components of the ADHD are often considered to be the precursors, responsible for the development of early onset conduct disorder, especially in boys.

POSSIBLE EXPLANATION OF COMORBIDITY

Despite the high comorbidity rates amongst the psychiatric disorders, its meaning for etiological and classification issues remains unclear. There has been much debate as to whether comorbidity is "real" or an artifact. Artifactual explanations include methodological and assessment bias.

Methodological biases include treatment or sampling bias in which children with two or more disorders have a greater chance to be hospitalized or treated. It is argued that the chances of being referred to mental health services is higher for children with a comorbid disorder than for those with only one disorder. Comorbidity found in clinical setting could reflect severe psychopathology and psychosocial impairment; thus, children with comorbid disorders are more likely to be referred than those with non-comorbid disorders.

Assessment bias refers to the lack of discrete diagnostic definitions which may lead to a degree of overlap in the symptom presented (e.g., depressed mood, poor appetite, and sleep disturbance may be present in several other disorders) between different diagnostic categories. Assessment bias also includes the application of diagnostic decision-making hierarchies that may mask the "real" association between disorders.

However, there are also some indicators to support the presence of "true" comorbidity. Rutter (1994), for example, has argued that the core of every disorder is a struggle for adaptation, but the way in which the specific phenotype is expressed depends on environmental conditions and person–environment interactions. Others have argued that the co-occurrence of disorders could be due to etiologic pathways, in which one disorder leads to or causes the second disorder (i.e., causal association), or that the two disorders are manifestations of the same underlying etiologic factors (i.e., common etiology), or that it may reflect different stages of the same disease.

IMPACT OF COMORBIDITY

The presence of comorbid disorders is often associated with impairment in various life domains, the use of mental health services, more police or juvenile court contacts, as well as a negative course and outcome (e.g., chronicity of disorders, elevated rate of suicide attempts).

The frequent co-occurrence of disorders in children illustrates the importance of conducting a comprehensive assessment, not only for the disorder for which the child has been referred, but also other disorders. Second, the high degree of comorbidity also suggests the need to use intervention to deal with multiple disorders.

See also: Anxiety Disorders; Attention-Deficit/Hyperactivity Disorder; Conduct Disorder; Depressive Disorder, Major; *Diagnostic and Statistical Manual of Mental Disorders*

Further Reading

American Psychiatric Association. (1987). *Diagnostic and statistical manual of mental disorders* (3rd Rev. ed.). Washington, DC: Author.

Anderson, J. C., Williams, S., McGee, R., & Silva, P. A. (1987). *DSM-III* disorders in preadolescent children: Prevalence in a large sample from the general population. *Archives of General Psychiatry, 44,* 69–76.

Essau, C. A., Conradt, J., & Petermann, F. (2000). Frequency, comorbidity, and psychosocial impairment of anxiety disorders in adolescents. *Journal of Anxiety Disorders, 14,* 263–279.

Klerman, G. L. (1990). Approaches to the phenomena of comorbidity. In J. D. Maser & C. R. Cloniger (Eds.), *Comorbidity of mood and anxiety disorders* (pp. 13–40). Washington, DC: American Psychiatric Press.

Rutter, M. (1994). Comorbidity: Meanings and mechanisms. *Clinical Psychology: Science and Practice, 1,* 100–103.

Wittchen, H.-U., & Essau, C. A. (1993). Epidemiology of anxiety disorders. In P. J. Wilner (Eds.), *Psychiatry* (pp. 1–25). Philadelphia: Lippincott.

CECILIA A. ESSAU

Conduct Disorder

DEFINITION/CLINICAL PRESENTATION

Conduct Disorder (CD), whether as a diagnostic category or behavioral description, refers to behaviors that represent serious social rule violations, including physical aggression, theft, truancy, or property destruction. Numerous subtypes of Conduct Disorder have been described, focusing on differences such as whether the behaviors are overt (e.g., aggression) or covert (e.g., theft), or whether the behaviors occur primarily when the child is alone or in groups. Perhaps the most common form of subtyping, and the one used in the current *Diagnostic and Statistical Manual of Mental Disorders*, focuses on whether the conduct problems began before or after age 11 (childhood vs. adolescent onset). Children with onset of Conduct Disorder early in life typically have more severe conduct problems, more intellectual and attentional difficulties, and are more likely to come from families that are disrupted. Those children with adolescent onset, on the other hand, typically have less severe problems that remit with time. However, this distinction does not always hold, and in particular, may not be entirely appropriate for describing Conduct Disorder in girls.

PREVALENCE

Conduct Disorder is estimated to occur in 2–9 percent of children. Although the disorder is more common among boys (ratios of approximately 3 or 4 boys to 1 girl), it remains a relatively common mental health concern among girls as well. Conduct Disorder is more prevalent among children of lower socioeconomic status (SES), particularly those living in poor, inner-city neighborhoods. There is little consistent change in the prevalence of the disorder across age. Some symptoms, such as overt aggression, decrease as children age, but other symptoms, such as theft, are more common among older children or adolescents. There is, however, some evidence that rates of the disorder may be increasing over time.

CORRELATES

Conduct Disorder is strongly associated with coercive parenting practices such as a lack of monitoring of the child's behavior, overly or lax harsh punishment, and a lack of warmth. Parents of children with Conduct Disorder also are more likely than other parents to suffer from marital discord, antisocial behavior, depression, and substance abuse themselves. As noted above, Conduct Disorder also is associated with family and neighborhood social disadvantage. Children with the disorder consistently experience difficulties with peers and are likely to associate with other deviant children. These relationships with deviant peers pose a particular risk for the continuation of conduct problems in adolescence. Children with conduct problems frequently have co-occurring problems with Attention-Deficit/Hyperactivity Disorder (ADHD), anxiety and mood disorders, and substance abuse, although the rates and severity of these other disorders may vary between boys and girls. At least for boys with Conduct Disorder, there also is an associated risk of academic and intellectual deficits. For girls, early sexual maturation, coupled with the presence of early behavior problems, increases the risk for Conduct Disorder, and conduct disorder is associated with the probability of teen pregnancy.

ASSESSMENT

Children with conduct problems may minimize and underreport their deviant activities. As a result, heavy emphasis is placed on parent and teacher reports of the child's behavior in assessment. However, during adolescence, the youth's own self-report is an essential component of the assessment adding crucial information regarding covert activities such as substance abuse or delinquent acts. Structured diagnostic interviews, completed by both youth and parent, as well as standardized ratings scales completed by youth, parents, and teachers, such as the Child Behavior Checklist (CBCL) and Youth and Teacher Report Forms developed by Achenbach, are recommended assessment tools. Reports of peer relationships are another important dimension in the assessment of Conduct Disorder, whether gathered via youth self-report, parent/teacher report, or perhaps even peer assessments. Given the associations between conduct problems and academic functioning, evaluation of school behavior and performance is a critical component in the evaluation of Conduct Disorder. Finally, beyond characteristics of the child, assessment also must incorporate evaluation of parenting skills, parent psychological functioning, and marital and family functioning.

TREATMENT

In treating Conduct Disorder, particularly as the severity of the disorder increases, early and/or brief interventions are not typically successful. Instead, multiple services offered over longer periods of time are most often recommended. Treatments that have been identified as effective in reducing child conduct problems include social skills or problem-solving skills training for the child, which focus on teaching the child strategies such as anger control, assertiveness, and interpersonal problem-solving. For parents, behavioral parent management training is highly recommended and teaches skills such as rule-setting and effective use of rewards and consequences. Functional family therapy, focused on intrafamily relationships, and multisystemic therapy, focused on the child and family as well as the surrounding social context including schools and peers, have also been successful in reducing conduct problems. Other approaches such as play therapy or unstructured group therapy are not helpful and may even exacerbate the disorder.

PROGNOSIS

Conduct Disorder unfortunately is quite stable across childhood and adolescence, with approximately 50 percent of children continuing to meet the diagnostic criteria in follow-ups up to 4 years after diagnosis. This stability appears equal for both boys and girls. Conduct Disorder also confers risk for a variety of negative outcomes, ranging from school failure to poor health and being a victim of violence. Children who display frequent and varied conduct problems with an early onset are at the greatest risk for continuation of these problems into adolescence and adulthood. Other child risk factors for continued problems include lower verbal intelligence and the presence of attention-deficit/hyperactivity disorder. Family factors that are

predictive of continued problems include low maternal education or teen parenthood, as well as other indicators of social disadvantage. In contrast, good schools, relationships with nondelinquent peers, and a good relationship with at least one parent stand as protective factors in the outcome of children with conduct disorders.

See also: Aggression; Antisocial Behavior; Attention-Deficit/Hyperactivity Disorder; Delinquent Behavior; Oppositional Defiant Disorder

Futher Reading

American Psychiatric Association. (1994). *Diagnostic and statistical manual of mental disorders* (4th ed.). Washington, DC: Author.

Brestan, E. V., & Eyberg, S. M. (1998). Effective psychosocial treatment of conduct-disordered children and adolescents: 20 years, 82 studies, and 5,272 kids. *Journal of Clinical Child Psychology, 27,* 180–189.

Hill, J., & Maughan, B. (Eds.). (2001). *Conduct disorders in childhood and adolescence.* New York: Cambridge University Press.

Keenan, K., Loeber, R., & Green, S. (1999). Conduct disorder in girls: A review of the literature. *Clinical Child and Family Psychology Review, 2,* 3–20.

Loeber, R., Burke, J. D., Lahey, B. B., Winters, A., & Zera, M. (2000). Oppositional defiant and conduct disorder: A review of the past 10 years, Part I. *Journal of the Academy of Child and Adolescent Psychiatry, 39,* 1468–1484.

CHARLOTTE JOHNSTON
PAUL HOMMERSEN

Conductive Hearing Loss

See: Hearing Impairment

Confidentiality and Privilege

Confidentiality and privilege are distinct concepts. Institutions and professional organizations usually establish practices associated with confidentiality. For example, the American Psychological Association has promulgated ethical principles related to confidentiality in its most recent *Ethical Principles of Psychologists and Code of Conduct* (1992). In contrast, the concept of privilege is defined legally and concerns when it is permissible to divulge confidential information. In most states or provinces, psychologists do not have confidentiality for themselves, but they may raise the privilege of confidentiality on behalf of their patients. At the beginning of the professional relationship, the clinical child or pediatric psychologist should discuss how confidential information will be used and the limits of confidentiality during the informed consent process. In addition, the psychologist should inform the patient if confidential information will be electronically stored or transmitted.

Confidentiality is the centerpiece of any helping relationship in clinical child or pediatric psychology. Protecting confidentiality is a primary obligation for clinical child and pediatric psychologists; it is the bond of trust between the helping professional and the patient. Without the promise of confidentiality, children and families may choose not to divulge private information to the psychologist. Inaccurate or distorted information might lead to inappropriate assessments or interventions because they would be based on false assumptions.

The expectations of confidentiality are different for adults and children. Most young children do not expect confidentiality since parents already know most confidential details about them anyway. In contrast to minors, adults expect that confidential information obtained from a psychologist will not be divulged except when the adult gives written consent to have confidential information released. Adolescents, on the other hand, need more assurances of confidentiality because they often do not want their parents to know the private details of their lives. This situation is often exacerbated by the fact that most adolescents do not volunteer to be seen by a psychologist. Most clinical child and pediatric psychologists who treat adolescents request from parents that confidentially be maintained even though adolescents have no right to confidentiality from a legal perspective.

Clinical child and pediatric psychologists must explain the limits of confidentiality to the children and families before beginning assessment or treatment. When working with children and families, conflicting expectations can exist about how confidential information should be handled. The psychologist should attempt to clarify confidentiality issues for all stakeholders involved. The psychologist must explain confidentiality issues in a way that children or parents with diminished capacity can understand. At the same time, children and their families may have certain expectations of the limits of privacy that may not be appropriate. For example, parents may expect that all information from a psychotherapy session with an 11-year-old child should be revealed to them, but the child may wish to have some information remain private. When working with an entire family, the psychologist must be sure that all family members understand the limits to confidentiality. The expectations for confidentiality may also change during the course of assessment or treatment; the psychologist must clarify the limits to confidentiality continuously during the course of assessment or intervention. For example, if the mother of a 5-year-old patient files for divorce during treatment, the limits of confidentiality should be clarified to both parents especially regarding the release of confidential information. In institutional settings (e.g., hospitals), psychologists must be sensitive to the different expectations children, families, and other health care personnel might have regarding confidentiality. Often in medical settings physicians expect to be informed of all information about their patients, including sensitive personal and confidential information. The child and the parents ultimately have to decide what information is shared with family members or other professionals.

Most states and provinces legally mandate breaking confidentiality in several specific situations. First, clinical child and pediatric psychologists must divulge confidential information if ordered by a court. Second, in all states and provinces helping professionals must inform state or provincial officials of the suspicion of physical, emotional, or sexual abuse. Third, clinical child and pediatric psychologists should always break confidentiality to report imminent danger to the patient or to others. The psychologist must evaluate the potential of danger and disclose that information only to appropriate professional workers, public authorities, the potential victim, and/or the parents as required by state or provincial law. Clinical child and pediatric psychologists must evaluate the risk potential of child and adolescent behaviors (e.g., drug use, alcohol use, sexual behavior) and using their own values, decide if the intensity, frequency, or duration of these behaviors warrants breaking confidentiality. Finally, in many states (e.g., Texas) psychologists are required by law to report any sexual contact between a previous therapist and a patient.

In several instances confidential information can be disclosed without the written consent of the patient or the family. First, information can be disclosed in the course of providing therapeutic services. For example, receptionists and record clerks are exposed to confidential information incidental to their duties. Second, clinical child and pediatric psychologists can obtain appropriate professional consultation in order to promote appropriate care. At the same time, during the consultation, the psychologist only reveals that information relevant to the consultation. Finally, the clinical child or pediatric psychologist can reveal minimal information to insurance companies to facilitate payment of services.

See also: History-Taking; Legal Issues in Clinical Child and Pediatric; Mental Health Records; Psychology; Professional Societies in Clinical Child and Pediatric Psychology

Further Reading

American Psychological Association. (1992). Ethical principles of psychologists and code of conduct. *American Psychologist, 47,* 1597–1611.

Melton, G. B., Ehrenreich, N. S., & Lyons, P. M., Jr. (2001). Ethical and legal issues in mental health services for children. In C. E. Walker & M. C. Roberts (Eds.), *Handbook of clinical child psychology* (3rd ed., pp. 1074–1093). New York: Wiley.

Rae, W. A., Worchel, F. F., & Brunnquell, D. (1995). Ethical and legal issues in pediatric psychology. In M. C. Roberts (Ed.), *Handbook of pediatric psychology* (2nd ed., pp. 19–36). New York: Guilford.

WILLIAM A. RAE

Congenital Adrenal Hyperplasia

DESCRIPTION AND INCIDENCE

The adrenal cortex is a gland responsible for the production of hormones including *glucocorticoids, mineralocorticoids,* and *androgens* (a class of sex hormones). Congenital Adrenal Hyperplasia (CAH) is a genetically inherited disorder that is associated with errors in the synthesis of these hormones, resulting from a deficiency in any one of several enzymes. About 95 percent of all cases are characterized by a deficiency in the enzyme *21-hydroxylase* (or 21-OH). Females with CAH may exhibit ambiguous genitalia (i.e., *intersexuality*) at birth with labial fusion and clitoral enlargement, and may be mistakenly announced as male at birth. CAH in male newborns is not easily identifiable and may be overlooked. In both sexes, late diagnosis or inadequate hormone replacement can result in accelerated growth during childhood and precocious puberty, but eventual short stature during adulthood because of the premature closure of the skeletal growth plates (i.e., *epiphyses*).

There are two major subgroups of 21-hydroxylase CAH: *salt-wasting,* where affected individuals experience varying degrees of salt loss secondary to a deficiency in the production of the hormone aldosterone, and *simple-virilizing* CAH, in which excess androgen production is not accompanied by salt loss. Salt-wasting CAH, experienced by the majority (75 percent) of those affected, is potentially life threatening, particularly during the first few weeks of life prior to diagnosis and treatment. Because of the serious implications of late diagnosis, several states have established a newborn screening test. In the United States, CAH affects approximately 1/11,000 live births but there is considerable variation among ethnic/racial populations.

ETIOLOGY

Transmitted via an autosomal recessive trait, the 21-hydroxylase enzyme deficiency that characterizes the most common form of CAH results in an impaired ability of the adrenal cortex to produce cortisol. Consequently, adrenocorticotropic hormone (ACTH) secretion from the pituitary gland is stimulated, leading to enlargement, or *hyperplasia,* of the adrenal cortex. The enlarged adrenal cortex, along with the blocked metabolic pathway, results in the increased production of androgens. This increase in androgens is responsible for the masculinized (or *virilized*) appearance of the genitalia seen in females. If left untreated, or if metabolic control is not achieved, precocious pubertal development can be observed in both males and females.

ASSESSMENT

In those states in which it is available, newborn screening is the most common way to establish a diagnosis of CAH. This process involves taking a sample of blood placed on filter paper, and testing for the hormone 17-alpha-hydroxyprogesterone (17-OHP), which is elevated in the child with 21-hydroxylase CAH.

Because males with CAH feature a normal genital appearance at birth, newborn screening allows for early detection, diagnosis, and treatment that will avert salt-wasting crises. Although the screening test can yield a false positive result necessitating further testing, the test has proven its utility by significantly reducing the incidence of salt-loss related deaths in states where it is utilized.

ASSOCIATED PSYCHOLOGICAL FEATURES

Although cognitive impairment is not characteristic of CAH, affected children may demonstrate decreased global IQ scores and/or specific cognitive deficits likely resulting from salt-wasting crises during infancy. Also warranting consideration are the more general influences of having a chronic illness and the potential for precocious puberty with associated tall stature in childhood and short stature in adolescence and adulthood. Finally, individuals with CAH may experience psychosocial consequences related to excess prenatal androgen exposure. Extensive animal research conducted since the late 1950s has demonstrated that the brains and behavior of males and females are sexually dimorphic (different), and that these differences result from exposure, at sensitive periods of brain development, to testicular hormones of fetal origin, rather than directly from the genetic sex of the animal. Because of the abnormally high levels of prenatal androgens present in girls with CAH, researchers have examined the behavioral development of these individuals.

A common research strategy used to assess these effects is to focus attention on those behaviors that show significant gender-related variation under normal circumstances, and study these behaviors under conditions where early hormone exposure has been altered due to an endocrine disorder (such as CAH). The behaviors most frequently studied include the pattern of childhood play and propensity toward physical aggression. Cognitive profile, gender identity, and sexual orientation are also domains of interest. Because excess androgen exposure occurs primarily for girls, behavioral research has focused predominantly on females.

Androgen-Related Effects in Girls

Although *gender identity* (i.e., identification of self as either girl/woman or boy/man) is (with few exceptions) unequivocally female in girls and women with CAH, these individuals exhibit a masculine shift in the pattern of gender-typical behaviors. For instance, girls with CAH are more likely to engage in rough-and-tumble play than are unaffected girls. Interestingly, it is girls with the salt-wasting form of CAH that show the most marked gender behavior effects, possibly reflecting the greater severity of this form compared to simple virilizing CAH.

In addition to the behavioral sequelae in childhood, there are also data to suggest that sexual behavior of adolescents and adults with CAH differs significantly from comparison groups. For instance, during adolescence, girls with CAH tend to achieve psychosexual milestones (e.g., dating, kissing, etc.) later than unaffected control subjects. Further, as adults, women with CAH report less heterosexual activity than unaffected comparison subjects. These women are more likely to develop a bisexual or homosexual orientation, as indicated by sexual imagery (erotic/romantic fantasies and dreams) and sexual attractions, and to a lesser extent, overt homosexual activity. However, because the majority of women with CAH are heterosexual, it is thought that factors other than (or in addition to) prenatal androgen exposure are responsible for effects on sexual orientation in women with CAH. As with all of the psychosocial features discussed, sexual orientation is thought to stem from a complex interaction of biological and environmental factors, of which androgen exposure is only one.

Androgen-Related Effects in Boys

Because of the association between androgens and physically aggressive behavior, researchers have examined this domain in boys with CAH. This research, however, does not indicate a significant difference between boys with CAH and unaffected control subjects in terms of this behavior.

TREATMENT

Prenatal Diagnosis and Treatment

CAH can be diagnosed through the use of chorionic villi sampling (CVS) early in pregnancy, though typically, this type of screening is only employed when there has been a history of CAH in the family. Early *in utero* treatment with dexamethasone may help normalize formation of the genitalia in girls and possibly spare affected girls corrective surgery.

Hormone Replacement Therapy

The primary aim of the treatment of CAH is to replace deficient hormones, suppress excess androgen formation, and promote normal growth and development. Glucocorticoid therapy is the basis of treatment for this disorder. By replacing the deficient cortisol and suppressing ACTH production, over-stimulation of the adrenal cortex ceases. This results in the suppression of excessive adrenal androgen production, prevention of further virilization in girls, normalization of accelerated growth, and the normal onset of puberty. After the period of infancy is complete and the condition has been stabilized, glucocorticoid replacement (Cortef®) (administered orally) is the most common treatment. As excessive amounts of cortisol may produce side effects, including growth retardation, dosage must be carefully monitored.

Mineralocorticoid replacement treatment is essential to maintain salt and water homeostasis for patients with the salt-wasting forms of CAH. This is accomplished with the oral administration of fludrocortisone acetate (Florinef®) and the possible addition of dietary salt. Because excessive amounts of mineralocorticoid and salt can result in severe hypertension, blood pressure must be carefully monitored. It is not uncommon for youngsters to "outgrow" the need for daily mineralocorticoid treatment and some may cease to require treatment except on very hot days, or when they are extremely active.

In rare cases where a CAH diagnosis is overlooked and a salt-wasting crisis occurs, emergency care is required. Infants must be treated immediately with intravenous hydration with saline, correction of electrolyte abnormalities, and supplementation with intravenous hydrocortisone.

Psychological Treatment

It is critical that parents and children are educated concerning both the medical and psychological aspects of this condition in a clear and understandable manner. Subsequent family and individual counseling may be necessary to assist with issues that may surface as the patient gets older. For boys and girls, these issues may relate to the experience of precocious puberty and coping with learning disabilities. For girls, concerns may additionally include the genitalia that have an atypical appearance, the discomfort associated with repeated genital examinations, and the possibility of reconstructive genital surgery in early life and again in young adulthood. Because of the likely influence in girls of prenatal androgen exposure on aspects of gender-related behavioral development, families may have questions regarding the relationship between CAH and psychosexual development. It is recommended that counseling of parents (and later, children) begin as soon as the diagnosis is made in an effort to prevent the occurrence of later problems. Such psychoeducational counseling should occur at intervals coinciding with major developmental milestones.

Surgical Management (Females)

For those girls born with masculinized genitalia, surgical management is an additional aspect of treatment. This typically occurs within the first year of life. Because infants do not have the ability to give informed consent, and surgery may damage the sensitivity of genital tissue, the issues surrounding genital reconstruction are entangled and controversial. There are several patient advocacy groups, representing adults with CAH or other medical conditions associated with ambiguous genitalia, which are vehemently opposed to genital surgery at an age when the child is not capable of providing informed consent.

PROGNOSIS

With appropriate medical and psychological intervention, boys and girls with CAH can effectively cope with their condition and go on to maintain healthy and satisfying relationships.

Support Groups

MAGIC Foundation—http://www.magicfoundation.org/, 1327 N. Harlem Avenue, Oak Park, IL 60303; CARES Foundation, Inc.—http://www.caresfoundation.org, P.O. Box 264, Short Hills, NJ 07078.

See also: Coping with Illness; Parenting the Chronically Ill Child; Puberty, Precocious; Sexual Differentiation: Disorders and Clinical Management; Treatment Adherence: Medical

Further Reading

Grumbach, M., & Conte, F. A. (1998). Disorders of sex differentiation. In J. D. Wilson & D. Foster (Eds.), *Williams textbook of endocrinology* (9th ed., pp. 1303–1425). Philadelphia: W.B. Saunders.

Meyer-Bahlburg, H. F. L. (2001). Gender and sexuality in classic congenital adrenal hyperplasia. *Endocrinology and Metabolism Clinics of North America, 30*, 155–168.

Slijper, F. M. E., Drop, S. L. S., Molenaar, J. C., & de Muinck Keizer-Schrama, M. P. F. (1998). Long-term psychological evaluation of intersex children. *Archives of Sexual Behavior, 27*, 125–144.

Zucker, K. J., Bradley, S. J., Oliver, G., Blake, J., Fleming S., & Hood, J. (1996). Psychosexual development of women with congenital adrenal hyperplasia. *Hormones and Behavior, 30*, 300–318.

LAUREN ZURENDA
DAVID E. SANDBERG

Congenital Heart Disease

See: Cardiovascular Disease

Constipation

See: Encopresis

Consumer Satisfaction

DESCRIPTION

Within child mental health services, several facets of consumer satisfaction have been identified and occasionally measured. Satisfaction is generally thought to include how well families' expectations are met, perceptions of treatment effectiveness, family involvement, access to or convenience of services, relationships between professionals and family members, family and parent services (e.g., connections to support groups), and empowerment of families. All aspects of the clients experience are considered, from parking and physical access to warmth of reception and perceptions of staff, to the actual intervention and follow-up. Measurement of consumer satisfaction provides opportunities for identifying areas for service improvement and, on a larger scale, may be used to guide the decisions of policymakers.

Despite increased recognition of the importance of family involvement and satisfaction with services, until recently there had been relatively little systematic research completed on consumer satisfaction with children's mental health services.

Up until the last decade, much of the literature on satisfaction has focused on the adult population. It is only recently that advances have been made in the field of children's mental health. For example, consumer satisfaction ratings collected by pediatric psychologists directed clinicians' attention to improving services, developing new programs, and changing aspects that received less positive ratings from clients. Additionally, consumers' satisfaction ratings have been used to increase understanding of both specific services and entire systems of care.

IMPORTANCE OF CONSUMER SATISFACTION

Parents, children, and professionals all may provide contributions to existing knowledge about the importance of measuring satisfaction with children's

services. Several reasons for the assessment of parental satisfaction have been proposed, including the parents' or primary caregivers' responsibility for their children's welfare and the potential for primary caregivers to be more involved in services with which they are satisfied. Indeed, parents have been the focus of the majority of research examining satisfaction with children's mental health services.

In addition to parental satisfaction, children's satisfaction with services should also be considered, as parents and children may have different experiences of treatment. The perceptions of satisfaction by children and adolescents appear to correlate with different aspects of treatments than does the satisfaction of parents. For example, children have based their ratings of satisfaction on the quality of the child–therapist relationship and changes in symptoms more so than have parents.

Many people other than parents and children themselves are impacted by children's mental health services. Thus, measuring the reports of satisfaction of teachers, physicians, judges, case managers, policymakers, referral sources, and other involved clinicians all are of importance; however, research examining the satisfaction of such individuals has been relatively rare.

MEASUREMENT ISSUES

There is a decided lack of standardized measures of consumer satisfaction with children's mental health services. Initially, information about client satisfaction was collected informally, without concern for psychometric qualities; more recently, measures of satisfaction were created for isolated use with specific programs. Because consumer satisfaction is difficult to accurately assess, many aspects of existing measurements of satisfaction have received criticism.

One such criticism involves the validity of satisfaction measures. Consumers generally report high levels of satisfaction, which may or may not be an accurate representation of their true satisfaction. Clients may not have received an accurate explanation of the purpose of satisfaction measures, which may affect how they respond. They may feel pressured by forces of social desirability to report higher levels of satisfaction than they actually feel or they may even fear that providing negative feedback may jeopardize their access to treatment. In addition, a selection bias often exists, in that it is often only those clients who complete the course of treatment who receive questionnaires about their satisfaction. Dissatisfied clients are more likely to have dropped out of treatment early and may be less likely to be contacted or may fail to respond to mailed questionnaires.

A second criticism of satisfaction research involves the association of satisfaction with treatment effectiveness. Historically, client satisfaction has been confused with quality of care and treatment effectiveness. Some researchers have assumed that consumer satisfaction and treatment effectiveness are implicitly equivalent, while others have hypothesized that consumer satisfaction and treatment effectiveness are entirely different constructs. In general, mixed evidence exists for the relationship between satisfaction and effectiveness. Some studies have found a lack of association between satisfaction and treatment outcomes, or at best, an ambiguous relationship, while satisfaction has been associated with outcome improvements in other studies. Managed care organizations have also created further confusion of the relation between satisfaction and treatment effectiveness by often using satisfaction as a primary outcome variable by which treatments are judged.

In conclusion, consumer satisfaction with children's mental health services is an important pathway to improved services. Efforts should be made to collect information about satisfaction with services from multiples sources and the validity of measurement procedures should be carefully considered.

See also: Evidence-Based Treatments; Global Functioning; Measurement of Behavior Change; Quality of Life; Treatment Goals

Further Reading

Anderson, J. A., Rivera, V. R., & Kutash, K. (1998). Measuring consumer satisfaction with children's mental health services. In M. H. Epstein, K. Kutash, & A. Duchnowski (Eds.), *Outcomes for children and youth with emotional and behavioral disorders and their families: Programs and evaluation best practices* (pp. 455–481). Austin, TX: PRO-ED.

McNaughton, D. (1994). Measuring parent satisfaction with early childhood intervention programs: Current practice, problems, and future perspectives. *Topics in Early Childhood Special Education, 14,* 26–48.

Roberts, M. C., Brown, K. J., & Puddy, R. W. (2002). Service delivery issues and program evaluation in pediatric psychology. *Journal of Clinical Psychology in Medical Settings, 9,* 3–13.

TAMMY A. LAZICKI-PUDDY
CHRISTY A. KLEINSORGE
RICHARD E. BOLES
MICHAEL C. ROBERTS

Conversion Reaction

See: Psychosomatic Disorders

Coping with Illness

DEFINITION

Illness and medical treatments present significant sources of stress to children and adolescents. The ways that children and adolescents respond to and cope with illness- and treatment-related stress are important correlates and possible determinants of emotional adjustment to illness, and potentially with physical health outcomes as well. Research on coping in pediatric populations has included children with cancer, sickle cell disease, chronic and recurrent pain syndromes, diabetes mellitus, and asthma, among other conditions.

Coping refers to conscious volitional efforts to regulate emotion, cognition, behavior, physiology, and the environment in response to stressful events or circumstances. Coping responses have been further distinguished along a variety of dimensions and classified into a number of categories, however, two distinctions have been most widely used. The first distinguishes between problem-focused and emotion-focused coping. Problem-focused coping responses are defined as efforts to change the source of stress and include responses such as information seeking and problem-solving. Emotion-focused coping includes efforts to alter or manage one's emotional reactions to the stressor and has included emotion expression, avoidance, and wishful thinking. An alternative perspective on coping distinguishes responses along a dimension of engagement and disengagement. Engagement responses involve coping efforts that are directed toward either the source of stress or one's emotional response to the stress. Engagement responses have been further distinguished as involving efforts to achieve primary control over the stressor or secondary control responses that reflect efforts to adapt to the stressor. Disengagement responses are efforts to avoid or orient away from the source of stress and one's emotional response.

METHODS

Coping with illness and medical treatment is most often assessed using questionnaires completed either by children/adolescents or by parents reporting on their children's coping. A second method involves the direct observation of coping responses, but this methodology has been used in a limited manner in hospital settings and has been used primarily in research on children coping with medical procedures or procedural pain. Questionnaire measures for the assessment of coping with pain are among the most advanced of pediatric coping scales. For example, the Pain Responses Inventory developed by Walker and colleagues (1991) has well-established reliability and validity for the assessment of coping with Recurrent Abdominal Pain (RAP). A version of the Responses to Stress Questionnaire (RSQ), developed by Compas and associates (2001), has also been adapted for use with RAP. These authors have developed both adolescent self-report and parent-report versions of the RSQ and have shown good correspondence in parent and adolescent reports.

Observation methods have been used primarily to assess procedural pain, and have included reports of the ways that children cope with pain. from parents, professionals, and trained observers. Studies have used observational measures to assess children's coping with venipuncture, immunizations, and coping in anticipation of a surgical procedure. Observational methods have not been extended, however, to studies of the stress associated with chronic or acute illness.

EFFECTIVENESS

Although findings have been mixed, several consistent patterns have emerged. First, engagement responses have been found to be more adaptive than disengagement responses. For example, in a study of children and adolescents coping with RAP, Walker and colleagues (1997) found that passive coping (e.g., self-isolation, behavioral disengagement) correlated positively with pain, somatization symptoms, disability, and depressive symptoms. Active coping (e.g., problem-solving, seeking social support, rest) generally correlated positively with psychological and somatic symptoms, whereas accommodative coping (e.g., acceptance, minimizing pain, self-encouragement, distraction/ignoring) showed mixed results in correlations with outcome variables.

Thomsen and colleagues (2002) also examined coping with pain in a sample of children and adolescents who met criteria for pediatric RAP. These researchers measured three coping factors (primary control engagement coping, secondary control engagement coping, and disengagement coping) that are conceptually similar to the factors of active, accommodative, and passive coping respectively studied by Walker and colleagues (1997). Results demonstrated that both primary control engagement coping (problem-solving, emotional modulation, emotional expression) and secondary control engagement coping (acceptance, distraction, positive thinking, cognitive restructuring) were related to fewer somatic complaints, pain, and symptoms of anxiety and depression. These findings demonstrate that children and adolescents with RAP who deliberately use certain volitional coping strategies when they have stomach pain, such as distracting themselves or talking with someone about the pain, concurrently show lower levels of psychological and somatic symptoms. Disengagement coping (denial, avoidance, and wishful thinking) was generally not related to pain or symptoms of distress.

Several carefully developed, manualized interventions to enhance effective coping with illness and medical procedures have been reported in the literature. This includes interventions to enhance the use of distraction to cope with procedural pain, and the use of active coping strategies to manage chronic conditions such as headache pain. However, no research has been done to determine if teaching coping skills is a critical or active ingredient in interventions for children with chronic illness, and this remains a high priority for future research.

See also: Medical Procedures; Medical Hospitalization; Pain Assessment; Pain Management; Preparation for Medical Procedures, Quality of Life, Recurrent Abdominal Pain

Further Reading

Compas, B. E., Connor-Smith, J. K., Saltzman, H., Thomsen, A. H., & Wadsworth, M. (2001). Coping with stress during childhood and adolescence: Progress, problems, and potential. *Psychological Bulletin, 127*, 87–127.

Rudolph, K. D., Dennig, M. D., & Weisz, J. R. (1995). Determinants and consequences of children's coping in the medical setting: Conceptualization, review, and critique. *Psychological Bulletin, 118*, 328–357.

Thomsen, A. H., Compas, B. E., Colletti, R. B., Stanger, C., Boyer, M., & Konik, B. (2002). Parent reports of coping and stress responses in children with recurrent abdominal pain. *Journal of Pediatric Psychology, 27*, 215–226.

Walker, L. S., Smith, C. A., Garber, J., & Van Slyke, D. A. (1997). Development and validation of the Pain Response Inventory for children. *Psychological Assessment, 9*, 392–405.

BRUCE E. COMPAS

Counseling Psychology

In 1995, the American Psychological Association (APA) established the Commission for the Recognition of Specialties and Proficiencies in Professional Psychology (the acronym is CRSPPP, pronounced "crisp"). This Commission provided official recognition for existing specialties and recognized some new ones. In each case, its recommendations were acted on by the APA Council, and an archival document was created describing the specialty. The specialty of Counseling Psychology, which dates its origins from the writings of Frank Parsons on vocational choice in 1909, was reaffirmed as a specialty by CRSPPP 90 years later, in 1999. To state what this specialty involves, one can therefore do no better than quote the corresponding archival document (obtainable on the APA Web site, http://www.apa.org). This is done selectively below, together with some elaboration and the addition of historical context to clarify how this specialty came to be what it now is. According to the archival document:

> Counseling psychology is a general practice and health service provider specialty in professional psychology. It focuses on personal and interpersonal functioning across the life span and on emotional, social, vocational, educational, health-related, developmental, and organizational concerns. Counseling psychology centers on typical or normal development issues as well as atypical or disordered development as it applies to human experience from individual, family, group, systems, and organizational perspectives. Counseling psychologists help people with physical, emotional, and mental disorders improve well-being, alleviate distress and maladjustment, and resolve crises. In addition, practitioners in this professional specialty provide assessment, diagnosis, and treatment of psychopathology.

The term "general practice specialty" distinguishes Counseling Psychology from more specialized areas such as marital and family counseling. The words "health service provider" apply to Counseling, Clinical, and School Psychology to set them apart from areas such as Organizational and Industrial Psychology whose clients tend to be businesses rather than individuals.

As the archival definition makes clear, the central topic in Counseling Psychology is facilitating optimal development. It shares this interest with narrower or more specialized fields such as vocational counseling, rehabilitation counseling, and mental health counseling. Practitioners in these areas are often trained at the Master's level, whereas Counseling Psychology is a doctoral specialty, usually requiring a PhD or PsyD from an

APA-approved program in a university or free-standing educational institution. Although Counseling Psychology does trace some of its origins to work facilitating vocational choice, it received a great impetus from financial support by the federal government intended to assist World War II veterans readjust to civilian life. The Veterans Administration defined a position of "counseling psychologist" in 1952. The National Defense Education Act in 1958, supporting the training and employment of school guidance counselors, was also important. For historical reasons, training programs in Counseling Psychology are more often located in Schools of Education rather than in Departments of Psychology in Colleges of Arts and Sciences. One distinctive setting in which many Counseling Psychologists work is the University Counseling Center, of which many were founded in the period following World War II. These centers usually provide services to students without additional charge beyond their tuition and fees. In addition, individuals trained as Counseling Psychologists often go into independent practice as psychotherapists, so the present-day overlap of Counseling and Clinical Psychology is substantial, not to mention the fact that much of this same territory is shared with psychiatry and social work.

What is the knowledge base of Counseling Psychology? The archival document approved by CRSPPP continues:

> Building upon a core knowledge base of general psychology (i.e., the biological, cognitive/affective, social and individual bases of behavior, history and systems of psychology) common to the other applied specialties within professional psychology, the competent and skillful practice of Counseling Psychology requires knowledge of career development and vocational behavior, individual differences (including racial, cultural, gender, lifestyle, and economic diversity), psychological measurement and principles of psychological/diagnostic and environment assessment, social and organizational psychology, human life span development, consultation and supervision, psychopathology, learning (cognitive, behavioral), personality, methods of research and evaluation, and individual and group interventions (counseling/ psychotherapy).

Certainly, of all psychological specialties, Counseling Psychology is the most expert in the field of vocational behavior and its measurement, using classic assessment procedures including interest tests developed by such pioneers as Strong, Kuder, and Campbell. Its practical focus on psychotherapy also rivals that of its sibling specialty, Clinical Psychology.

What populations do Counseling Psychologists work with? The archival document describes these broadly:

> Client populations served by Counseling Psychologists can be organized along three dimensions: individuals,

groups (including couples and families), and organizations. Counseling Psychologists work with individual clients of all ages such as children who have behavior problems, late adolescents with educational and career concerns or substance abuse problems; adults facing marital or family difficulties, career shifts, or overcoming disabilities; older adults facing retirement.

The specific problems addressed by Counseling Psychology are many. The archival document provides the following list:

1. Educational and vocational career/work adjustment concerns.
2. Vocational choice, and school/work/retirement transitions.
3. Relationship difficulties, including marital and family [problems].
4. Learning and skill deficits.
5. Stress management and coping.
6. Organizational problems.
7. Adaptation to physical disabilities, disease, or injury.
8. Personal/social adjustment.
9. Personality dysfunction.
10. Mental disorders.

Of these, numbers 1, 2, and 7 seem to be particularly distinctive for Counseling Psychology, but there is considerable overlap with other specialties. A full range of assessment and intervention procedures is used, including psychological testing and interviewing, counseling, psychotherapy, behavior analysis and therapy, and consultation. Counseling Psychologists also perform research to evaluate these kinds of assessment and intervention procedures. They are particularly noted for their research on the supervision process.

In summary, Counseling Psychology is a general practice, health service provider specialty focused on the positive, helping people build on their strengths and overcome limitations.

See also: Clinical Psychology; Clinical Child Psychology Organizations; Pediatric Psychology; School Psychology

DONALD K. ROUTH

Craniofacial Anomalies

DEFINITION

A craniofacial anomaly (CFA) is a condition that affects the structural integrity of the cranium or face. The most common CFA is a cleft of the lip with or without cleft of the palate (see Clefts of the Lip and Palate). Other craniofacial conditions involve different abnormalities of development, such as premature hardening of one or more cranial sutures (craniosynostosis) or asymmetrical growth and development of the skull (e.g., hemifacial mircosomia). CFAs can occur in isolation, or as part of a group of multiple physical malformations that may involve other skeletal structures and organ systems. For example, velocardiofacial syndrome typically involves cleft palate, speech difficulties due to structural abnormalities, heart defects, and differences in facial morphology. Jones provides comprehensive, concise summaries of the characteristics of most identified craniofacial conditions.

ETIOLOGY

CFAs are the result of multiple genetic and environmental factors. A geneticist should evaluate the risk of recurrence for hereditary CFAs. Environmental factors that have been indicated as causal of CFAs include mechanical obstruction *in utero*, maternal heath and nutrition, maternal drug use, and fetal exposure to toxins.

INCIDENCE

Congenital anomalies occur in 3–5 percent of all live births, with CFAs accounting for a significant number of these occurrences. There are many recognized CFAs and associated syndromes. Incidence rates vary with each type of CFA. Table 1 provides a listing of some of the most commonly encountered conditions involving CFAs, characteristic physical features, typical developmental course, and estimated incidence rates.

PSYCHOLOGICAL CORRELATES

Children with CFAs and their families face a wide range of stresses related to the condition and its treatment. After the birth of a child with a CFA, parents must cope with their reactions to the infant with physical disfigurement, unexpected caregiving demands, multiple diagnostic procedures, and the reaction of friends and family to their child's appearance and medical condition. As the child becomes older, both the parent and child must face challenges related to physical, cognitive, and social development. Children with CFAs are at

Table 1. Features of Common Craniofacial Conditions

Craniofacial condition	Physical features	Developmental course	Estimated incidence
Apert Syndrome	Acrocephaly, craniosynostosis (mainly coronal), fusion of the fingers and toes, dental anomalies, widely spaced eyes, concave facial profile (midface hypoplasia), protruding eyes, potential hearing loss secondary to otitis media.	Significant developmental delay, with over 50% of children with Apert syndrome having IQ's < 70.	1:65,000–1:80,500
Craniosynostosis	Abnormally shaped skull resulting from premature fusion of the cranial sutures (metopic, sagittal, coronal, or lambdoid). May be associated with other symptoms if part of a syndrome.	Normal cognitive function in nonsyndromic cases after repair; however, metopic craniosynostosis may result in abnormalities of the forbrain.	1:1,000 (for isolated craniosynostosis)
Crouzon Syndrome	Protruding and wide set eyes, craniosynostosis, conductive hearing loss, poor visual acuity, strabismus or nystagmus, midface hypoplasia.	Normal intelligence to mild mental retardation.	1:60,600
Ectrodactyly Ectodermal Dysplasia-Clefting (EEDC) Syndrome	Small ocular openings, partial absence or malformation of the teeth, cleft lip, abnormalities of midportion of hands (including fused or absent fingers), underdevelopment of cheekbones and jaw, light colored and thin hair, genitourinary abnormalities.	Predominantly normal intellectual functioning.	Rare (exact incidence undetermined)
Frontonasal Dysplasia Sequence	Widely spaced eyes, "widow's peak" hair pattern, broad nasal root, lack of properly formed nasal tip (variability from broad tip to separated nostrils and central cleft lip).	Most are of normal intelligence, with estimates of 8–12% with cognitive impairment.	Rare (exact incidence undetermined)
Hemifacial Microsomia/ Goldenhar Syndrome	All abnormalities tend to be asymmetric and unilateral: Underdevelopment of the cheekbone or jaw (upper or lower), wide mouth, underdevelopment of the facial muscles, small and malformed outer ears. *Note*: When hemifacial microsomia is accompanied by cysts on the eye and vertebral abnormalities it is designated Goldenhar Syndrome.	Most are of normal intelligence, with IQs lower than 85 in 13%.	1:26,500–1:50,000
Moebius Sequence	Facial paralysis, drooping eyelids, potentially crossed eyes, lack of eye movement.	About 15% have cognitive deficits; lack of facial expressions can cause difficulties in social interaction.	Rare (exact incidence undetermined)
Pfeiffer Syndrome	Type 1: Relatively short skull with craniosynostosis, widely spaced eyes, narrow jaw, broad first and last fingers or toes, partial fusion of the central digits. Type 2 and 3: same as above with the addition of clover-leaf skull, bulging eyes, elbow joint immobility.	Type 1 have normal to near normal intellectual ability. Children with Type 2 and Type 3 have increased CNS involvement and often have poor outcomes, including early death.	Rare (exact incidence undetermined)
Pierre Robin Sequence	Underdevelopment of the lower jaw.	Typical development, but must be monitored for breathing difficulties during first month of life.	1:2,000–1:8,500
Stickler Syndrome	Flat faces, prominent eyes, epicanthal folds, underdeveloped midface or jaw, dental anomalies, malformed (large) or poorly functioning joints.	Vision difficulties are common and may lead to blindness.	1:4,000–1:10,000
Treacher Collins Syndrome	Underdevelopment of the cheek bones and lower jaw, partial absence of the lower eyelid and eyelashes, malformation of the outer ear.	Typically of normal intelligence, impaired hearing in 40% of children.	1:10,000
Velocardiofacial Syndrome (Shprintzen Syndrome)	Prominent nose with squared root, narrow eye openings, long face, minor ear anomalies, cardiac defects.	Learning disabilities are common, intelligence is typically in the borderline to average range.	1:8,750–1:14,000

higher risk for problems with behavioral and emotional adjustment, learning disorders, and social competence.

ASSESSMENT

Because a higher risk of developmental delay and learning disabilities exists for children with CFAs, it is important that assessment for such problems begin in infancy and continue periodically through the elementary school years. Assessment of cognitive, motoric, and adaptive progress conducted during the first 3 years may result in early identification of problem areas and provide the opportunity for more effective developmental interventions. When the child reaches school age, periodic psychoeducational assessments are recommended to detect the presence of specific learning disabilities and to assist the school with providing appropriate individual educational plans.

In addition to formal developmental and cognitive assessments, the psychologist working with children with CFAs should provide ongoing screening for behavioral, emotional, and social problems. The diagnostic interview along with broadband child, teacher, and parent report assessment measures are helpful in providing information for decision-making regarding a child's overall psychosocial adjustment.

TREATMENT

An interdisciplinary team approach is accepted nationally as the standard of care for children with CFAs. The complexity of treatment requires input from multiple health care providers and careful coordination of services. Craniofacial teams consist of physicians, surgeons, dentists, geneticists, nurses, speech pathologists, audiologists, social workers, and psychologists. The psychologist's role on the team involves providing assessment and treatment for the diverse problems that may arise in developmental, behavioral, emotional, and social domains. Treatment strategies that may be employed range from assisting the child and family to cope with frequent hospitalizations and medical procedures to individual or group therapy for clinically significant behavioral or emotional problems.

PROGNOSIS

Long-term outcomes for individuals with CFAs vary widely according to diagnostic group. Most individuals with CFAs will have no lasting physical or mental health problems related to their conditions. Others may experience lifelong delays or health problems. See Jones (1997) for prognostic information of specific CFAs.

See also: Clefts of the Lip and Palate; Developmental Issues in Assessment for Treatment; Intellectual Assessment; Social Development in Adolescence; Social Development in Childhood

Further Reading

Endriga, M. C., & Kapp-Simon, K. A. (1999). Psychological issues in craniofacial care: State of the art. *Cleft Palate—Craniofacial Journal, 36*, 3–11.
Jones, K. (1997). *Smith's recognizable patterns of human malformation* (5th ed.). Philadelphia: W.B. Saunders.
Nackashi, J. A., Dedlow, E. R., & Dixon-Wood, V. L. (1997). The craniofacial team: Health supervision and coordination. In K. R. Bzoch (Ed.), *Communicative disorders related to cleft lip and palate* (4th ed., pp. 169–190). Austin, TX: PRO-ED.
Saal, H. M. (2001). The genetics evaluation and common craniofacial syndromes. In A. C. Kummer (Ed.), *Cleft palate and craniofacial anomalies* (pp. 73–100). San Diego: Singular.

STEPHEN R. BOGGS
PHILIP EISENBERG

Crohn's Disease

See: Inflammatory Bowel Disease

Cultural Influences on Assessment

According to Sattler (2001), psychological assessment is the practice of collecting information from a variety of sources regarding an individual's functioning across a variety of contexts. Subsequent to the collection of the assessment information, a professional interprets the information and the results are used to meet a variety of needs (e.g., identification of psychological disorders, enhancement of treatment effects, determination of academic functioning, and qualification for special services).

However, information crucial to the assessment process may be withheld by a test-taker or missed by an assessor when cultural differences exist between the assessor and the person being tested. Disparities in cultural perspectives can and do play a significant role in altering both the process and the outcome of the psychological assessment process. When the assessor is unacquainted with the influence of culture on assessment, the likelihood that the results will be invalid is greatly increased, as noted by Atkinson and Lowe. For example, showing signs of severe physical distress, with few other symptoms, is common way to express psychological distress in certain cultures. If the assessor is unaware of the possible cultural component to this kind of physical complaint, the result could be an incorrect somatic disorder diagnosis or a referral to a medical doctor. More careful investigation of the events surrounding the initiation of the physical symptoms can often lead to a better understanding of the source of the distress and remediation of symptoms.

Several areas in the testing process appear to be especially sensitive to an individual's culture and are especially vulnerable when the culture of the assessor and the test-taker are dissimilar. Influences of culture on assessment primarily revolve around the manner in which the tests are administered and the nature of the assessment tools.

When the content of the items reflect values and beliefs of a culture inconsistent with the person being tested, biased interpretation of the response to those items is likely to occur. Individual performance will likely be misleading or even misrepresent the behavior of the individual being tested.

In addition, for most tests, scores are based on comparison to a standardization sample. That is, the person's responses are compared to a larger sample to determine if the responses are deviant from the general population. However, when the standardization sample is comprised primarily of people who share the same cultural beliefs and are in the majority, when someone from a minority culture takes the test, the likelihood of their score appearing deviant is much higher. That is, when culture is not considered, individuals whose differences appear statistically significant are often perceived to be ill when they may not be. Cultural groups differ as to which behaviors are considered pathological. What is perceived as deviance in one culture may not be viewed as deviance in another culture.

One of the clearest examples of cultural influence on the assessment process is demonstrated when English is not the primary or first language of the assessor and the test-taker. Most often this takes the form of English as a second language for the test-taker. Even when the test-taker (or the assessor) is fluent in English, the possibility for misunderstanding directions or other information crucial to the assessment process allows for bias to enter into the testing experience. When assessors or test-takers assume the meaning of psychological terms, often words not easily translated into other languages, the result is a high probability of invalid assessment results.

Culture may also influence an individual's behavior during the assessment process. Some experts have suggested that lack of exposure and experience with test-taking procedures and materials may contribute to lower test scores for children in some cultures. For example, Atkinson and Lowe (1995) have argued that a child who is unfamiliar with test-taking strategies may be less likely to guess at a test item rather than someone who makes an attempt to solve the same item with problem-solving techniques.

As it applies to psychological testing, the influence of culture has to be recognized and appreciated for its potential to bias assessment results. The commonly used measures are often not culture-free and this should be considered when comparing the responses of individuals who do not share the same cultural values and norms for behavior on which the assessment measures were created. Assessment measures are meant to provide guidelines from which professionals operate. Dana (1993) suggests that professionals should always gather as many sources of information as possible before coming to any conclusions regarding an individual's functioning.

See also: Norms and Normative Data; Test Bias; Psychological Testing; Validity

Further Reading

Armour-Thomas, E. A. (1992). Intellectual assessment of children from culturally diverse backgrounds. *School Psychology Review, 21*, 552–565.

Atkinson, D. R., & Lowe, S. M. (1995). The role of ethnicity, cultural knowledge, and conventional techniques in counseling and psychotherapy. In J. G. Ponterotto, J. M. Casas, L. A. Suzuki, & C. M. Alexander (Eds.), *Handbook of multicultural counseling* (pp. 387–414). Thousand Oaks, CA: Sage.

Dana, R. H. (1993). *Multicultural assessment perspectives for professional psychology* (pp. 91–110). Boston: Allyn & Bacon.

Sattler, J. M. (2001). *Assessment of children* (pp. 1–40). San Diego: Sattler.

YO JACKSON

Culture and Psychopathology

The cultural identification of an individual has a significant relation to the kinds of behavior that individual is likely to display. Culture is a socially constructed experience that includes shared and learned ways of life passed from previous generations to current ones that dictate the values and standards for a group of people. As noted by Gopaul-McNicol and Armour-Thomas (2002), included in the description of culture are a set of rules for acceptable behavior for the members of that culture.

Although rules of culture are rarely if ever formalized, for the mental health community culture, the official rules of unacceptable or psychopathological behavior are summarized in the *Diagnostic and Statistical Manual of Mental Disorders, Fourth Edition (DSM-IV)*, of the American Psychiatric Association. Previous editions of the *DSM* did not comment upon or fully appreciate the influence of culture in the presentation of pathological behaviors; however, the latest edition is different. For various disorders, culture is considered and counsel is provided regarding how a certain diagnosis might be applied to specific cultural groups.

Although it might seem obvious, it is important to consider the nature of the definitions comprising disorders so as to be as free of cultural biases as possible. A lofty goal for sure, as decisions are made, what is chosen as pathological and what is not is influenced by the culture of those creating the definitions. More importantly, when cultural influences are not considered in the application of the diagnostic categories, misdiagnosis is the probable result. When misdiagnosis does occur for people of color and other minorities, it is usually in the more severe direction.

For example, currently there are a disproportionate number of people of color diagnosed with various forms of psychopathology. People of color are seen in disproportionate numbers at mental health clinics, and if misdiagnosed, they are likely to subsequently receive incorrect treatment, thus potentially leading to a worsening of their initial symptoms.

The influence of culture aside, sometimes by virtue of being a member of a specific cultural group, an individual may be at greater risk for psychopathology. For example, according to the 2000 U.S. Census report, African Americans accounted for approximately 12 percent of the U.S. population, but consisted of more than 30 percent of the children living in poverty. Children of color were also overrepresented in classrooms for children with special needs (e.g., learning disabilities, behavior disordered). Clearly, environmental factors affect all individuals, and Caucasian children are also negatively affected by adverse conditions. An impoverished environment creates its own culture so it is important to remember that other environmental variables, such as socioeconomic status (SES), must be considered for their influence on the presenting behavior before a given behavior is diagnosed as pathological.

Although the mental health community has not gone so far as to assert that any one specific culture's way of life is pathological, some behaviors practiced by some groups have not been met with universal approval. For example, physical discipline is not generally encouraged within the field of clinical child and adolescent psychology given the multitude of alternative prosocial approaches to child behavior management. However, in some cultures, the physical disciplining of children for misbehavior is a key part of teaching the child about survival and in fact appears to strengthen the bond between parent and child, as noted by Deater-Deckard, Dodge, Bates, and Pettit (1996). If the parent is from a culture that favors physical discipline, without a consideration of the family's culture, the mental health professional may view the parent's behavior as abusive.

The mental health field has made adjustments through the years as it has grown to appreciate culture-specific behaviors. For example, in some Asian and Native American cultures, seeing visions of people who have died or getting answers to problems via the spirit world are typical and accepted behavior. It was once the case that any demonstration of seeing things that were not physically present was one of the symptoms for the syndrome of psychotic disorders. However, now clinicians have to be careful not to ascribe pathology to this behavior when it is not warranted, as current diagnostic systems appreciate the cultural aspect of this behavior for some individuals.

It is important to note that not all individuals who are a member of a cultural group are necessarily active or traditionally bound to the values and practices of that group. That is, each person is different and may be more or less connected to the traditional beliefs, values, and behaviors of a particular culture. Just like there are degrees and level of severity of pathological behavior, so are there levels of commitment to cultural practices. When members of a cultural group do not strongly identify with that culture, it is not likely that they will accept the group's standard about the kinds of behavior that are unacceptable. Because of vast differences between within each culture, pathological behavior should always be evaluated on a person-by-person basis.

See also: Cultural Influences on Assessment; Gender and Psychopathology; Norms and Normative Data; Psychological Testing

Further Reading

American Psychiatric Association. (1994). *Diagnostic and statistical manual of mental disorders* (4th ed.). Washington, DC: Author.
Dana, R. H. (1993). *Multicultural assessment perspectives for professional psychology* (pp. 79–90). Boston: Allyn & Bacon.

Deater-Deckard, K., Dodge, K. A., Bates, J. E., & Pettit, G. S. (1996). Physical discipline among African American and European American mothers: Links to children's externalizing behavior. *Developmental Psychology, 32,* 1065–1072.

Gopaul-McNicol, S., & Armour-Thomas, E. (2002). *Assessment and culture* (pp. 5–15). Academic Press: San Diego.

United States Census Bureau. (2000, March). *Characteristics of poor children in America.* Washington, DC: Author.

YO JACKSON

Cushing's Disease

DEFINITION

Cushing's disease is an endocrine disorder in which the pituitary gland produces abnormally large quantities of adrenocorticotropic hormone (ACTH). Excess ACTH in the bloodstream stimulates the production and release of cortisol (i.e., hypercortisolism) and other steroid hormones by the adrenal glands. Although similar in symptom presentation, *Cushing's disease* can be differentiated from *Cushing's syndrome* by examining the origin of the disorder. *Cushing's syndrome,* which is also characterized by the overproduction of ACTH, has a nonpituitary origin such as an adrenal gland tumor. Despite its different etiology, the syndrome has similar symptoms, course, and prognosis as Cushing's disease, both of which abate once cortisol hypersecretion ceases. This entry will focus on Cushing's disease.

INCIDENCE

Cushing's syndrome has been estimated to occur in about 13 cases per million people per year. Approximately 70 percent are due to Cushing's disease and 25 percent of cases occur in children. Cushing's disease is four times more common in females than in males.

ETIOLOGY

The most common cause of Cushing's disease is a noncancerous tumor in the pituitary gland, called a pituitary adenoma. Among children and adolescents, 80–85 percent of those with Cushing's disease have a surgically identifiable small tumor (microadenoma) in the pituitary gland, which causes the overproduction of ACTH. Some patients do not have an identifiable pituitary tumor, and it appears that this small group may have a primary hypothalamic disorder.

CORRELATES

The two most reliable indicators of hypercortisolism in children are weight gain and growth retardation. Any child who is overweight disease and not growing should be evaluated for Cushing's syndrome. Unlike adult patients who typically have centralized weight gain in the face ("moon face") and upper back at the base of the neck ("buffalo hump"), children typically present with more generalized weight gain. In addition, children may experience changes in facial appearance such as a florid complexion due to excessive blood (plethora), acne, or excessive hair growth (hirsutism). Frequent viral and bacterial infections, as well as substantial bone loss and undermineralization, are also more common in children with this disease. Pubertal delay or arrest may occur in children with Cushing's disease, with some evidence suggesting that height is most severely compromised in children who have the disease during puberty. Hypertension, osteopenia (decrease in bone volume), diabetes mellitus, and impaired immune function may also occur.

Psychological symptoms typically associated with Cushing's disease are depression with or without agitation, irritability, moodiness, anxiety, insomnia, and personality changes. In addition, patients may experience visual field deficits resulting from a pituitary tumor impinging on the optic nerve. In general, these psychological disturbances are found in adults with Cushing's disease and are less well-described in children.

ASSESSMENT

Diagnosis of Cushing's disease involves demonstrating cortisol excess, as well as distinguishing between a pituitary adenoma and other possible sources of excess ACTH release. Coritsol production and levels vary widely across individuals and time, therefore measuring the quantity of cortisol circulating in the bloodstream is not adequate for diagnosis. Instead, a dexamethasone suppression test is required in which a patient is administered an oral steroid (dexamethasone) in an attempt to decrease the adrenal production of cortisol. Typically, the adrenal glands respond to an increase in cortisol in the bloodstream with a decrease in cortisol production. With Cushing's disease, cortisol production does not diminish in response to the suppression test.

Excess cortisol in the bloodstream is processed by the kidneys and removed as urine waste. Therefore, measuring urine levels of cortisol over a 24-hr period is an additional screening method for Cushing's disease. The Free Cortisol Test requires urine collection for a 24-hr period in a single container to assess cortisol quantities.

After cortisol excess is confirmed through the dexamethasone suppression test and/or the Free Urine Test, the source of the excess is sought. Typically, corticotropin-releasing hormone (CRH) is given in a CRH stimulation test, and blood is drawn to measure ACTH and cortisol. High levels of both hormones generally are indicative of a pituitary adenoma. Additionally, ACTH levels in blood drawn from the small veins that drain the pituitary (petrosal sinuses) can be compared to ACTH blood levels from other venous sources, usually the arm. When ACTH levels are higher in the petrosal sinuses than elsewhere, the source of elevation is likely a pituitary adenoma.

Computerized tomography (CT) and magnetic resonance imaging (MRI) are used in preparation for surgery to evaluate the pituitary and adrenal glands after a diagnosis of Cushing's disease is confirmed. However, a CT or MRI is not diagnostic of Cushing's disease because many healthy people have pituitary or adrenal tumors and are asymptomatic. Further, the presence of a tumor does not ensure that it is the source of increased ACTH production.

The diagnosis of Cushing's disease is often more difficult in children, because they may not respond to diagnostic tests as adults do. For instance, increased concentrations of ACTH and cortisol may be absent. Instead, the first reliable laboratory finding may be a loss of diurnal ACTH rhythm, as evidenced by its continued secretion throughout the afternoon, evening, and nighttime. In addition, children with Cushing's disease may exhibit only partial cortisol suppression in response to low doses of dexamethasone, thereby producing false-negative test results.

The presence of depression is a complicating factor in the assessment and diagnosis of Cushing's disease for all individuals, including children and adolescents. Like individuals with Cushing's disease, patients with endogenous depression that is not associated with the onset of Cushing's disease exhibit abnormally high levels of cortisol secretion, making a differential diagnosis between endogenous depression and Cushing's disease difficult. Blood tests that examine changes in plasma cortisol levels during the evening and after insulin-induced hypoglycemia are two methods available to aid in differentially diagnosing Cushing's disease. Furthermore, patients with endogenous depression do not typically develop the physical symptoms characteristic of Cushing's disease (i.e., moon faces and adipose tissue in the upper back).

TREATMENT

When Cushing's disease is caused by a pituitary adenoma, it can be treated and cured by transphenoidal surgery (TPS; via the nasal passages) to remove the tumor (adenomectomy). Treatment success is immediately apparent in 90 percent of cases following surgery. Some patients may have an immediate postoperative glucocorticoid deficiency in which ACTH-producing cells are suppressed and may take months to recover. Postoperative monitoring is advised as the recurrence rate of Cushing's disease is between 8–14 percent within 2–3 years.

Alternative therapies include bilateral adrenalectomy, primary radiotherapy, hypophysectomy, and medication. Bilateral adrenalectomy, the surgical removal of the adrenal glands, is done only if the pituitary adenoma cannot be removed safely or the source of the excess ACTH production cannot be localized. This procedure is the preferred approach in children after TPS has failed. Primary radiotherapy is indicated only in persons with contraindications to surgery or those who refuse surgery and is effective in 50–83 percent of all cases. This alternative is not ideal for children as large doses of radiation place children at increased risk for cerebral arteritis, leukoencephalopathy, leukemia, bone tumors involving the skull, and congenital defects in subsequent offspring. Hypophysectomy, surgical removal of the pituitary gland, also has significant disadvantages for children in that it eliminates all pituitary hormones including growth hormone, thyroid stimulating hormone (TSH), and gonadotrophins, which can cause growth failure, hypothyroidism, and pubertal failure. Lifetime hormonal replacement is required. Medical management with cyropheptadine, a centrally active serotonin-antagonist, works in less than 50 percent of all patients and has virtually no success in children with Cushing's disease. Additional treatment for psychological symptoms associated with Cushing's disease is not indicated because these symptoms typically remit with medical treatment.

PROGNOSIS

Following appropriate treatment, individuals show significant improvement. With pituitary adenomas, approximately 80 percent of patients are cured with surgery. In addition, psychological sequelae associated with elevated cortisol levels rapidly resolve with lower cortisol levels. When treatment is delayed, patients are at an increased risk for developing diabetes, osteoporosis, and atherosclerosis. Without treatment, Cushing's disease can be fatal.

See also: Depressive Disorder, Major; Growth Hormone Deficiency; Obesity; Puberty, Delayed

Further Reading

Carson-Dewitt, R. (1999). Cushing's syndrome. In D. Olendorf, C. Jeryan, & K. Boyden (Eds.), *Gale encyclopedia of medicine* (pp. 866–869). Detroit, MI: Gale Research.
Devoe, D. J., Miller, W. L., Conte, F. A., Kaplan, S. L., Grumbach, M. M., Rosenthal, S. M., et al. (1997). Long-term outcome in children and adolescents after transsphenoidal surgery for Cushing's disease. *Journal of Clinical Endocrinology and Metabolism, 82* (10), 3196–3202.
Miller, W. L. (2001). The adrenal cortex and its disorders. In C. G. D. Brook, & P. C. Hindmarsh (Eds.), *Clinical pediatric endocrinology* (pp. 356–359). Oxford: Blackwell Science.
Orth, D. N. (1995). Cushing's syndrome. *New England Journal of Medicine, 332*(12), 791–803.
Stevens, A., & Pleet, A. B. (1996). Neuroendocrine disorders. In T. Brandt, L. R. Caplan, J. Dichgans, H. C. Diener, C. Kennard (Eds.), *Neurological disorders: Course and treatment* (pp. 1019–1021). San Diego: Academic Press.

PATRICIA A. LYNCH
ALYSSA M. HERSHBERGER
KATHYRN M. DALFERES
CLARISSA S. HOLMES

Custody Evaluations

DEFINITION

At the time of the legal dissolution of a marriage in which there are minor children, it is necessary for there to be a determination of the legal rights and responsibilities of the divorcing parents. Several different custodial arrangements are possible, and there is an important distinction between legal and physical custody. The parent who has sole legal custody has the right to make major decisions regarding the child, for example, where the child will attend school, and what medical and psychological treatment the child will receive. The primary right of the noncustodial parent is contact with the child. In joint legal custodial arrangements, the parents have

equal rights with respect to the children, and typically are required to consult with each other to arrive at mutually agreeable decisions. Although the courts rarely award split or divided custody of the children, being loath to separate siblings, an arrangement of this nature means that each parent will have sole legal custody of at least one of the children.

Regardless of the assignment of legal custody, there are multiple possible arrangements of physical custody, or the amount of time the child spends in each parent's home. Even though one parent has sole legal custody, the child may spend approximately equal time with each parent. In some joint legal custody arrangements, the child is with one parent the majority of time.

Subsequent to an initial legal determination of custody, parents may decide that the arrangements are not satisfactory. A noncustodial parent may petition the court to change custody to him or her. Petitions are sometimes filed with the court to dissolve joint legal custody and award sole custody to one parent. In some instances, motions may be filed to change visitation, or the amount of time the child spends with the noncustodial parent. The motion may come from the custodial parent who is seeking to limit visitation, or from the noncustodial parent who wishes to have more time with the child.

The legal standard in all states for the initial determination of custody at the time of the divorce is the best interests of the child. States vary in the degree to which the factors that the court is to take into account are specified. Commonly considered factors are the wishes of the parents, the wishes of the child, the nature of the parent–child relationships, the stability of the environment each parent can provide, and the care that has been provided by each of the parents. In recognition of the importance of the child's relationship with both parents, courts are more recently taking into account the degree to which a parent supports the child's relationship with the other parent. In addition, some states have established a rebuttable presumption (i.e., a legal assumption which must be disproved) against awarding custody to a parent who has perpetrated domestic violence.

The courts have long recognized the importance of stability in children's lives. The parent who is petitioning the court to change custody, therefore, has the burden of convincing the court that there have been significant changes since the original decree such that it would be in the child's best interests for custody to be changed.

The majority of custody disputes are resolved without the involvement of mental health professionals.

In some contested cases, psychologists or other mental health professionals may be asked by the parties or appointed by the court to do a custody evaluation. Even in the best of circumstances, custody evaluations are professionally demanding endeavors, fraught with procedural, ethical, and legal complexities. There is a specialized body of knowledge and skills that psychologists must possess in order to practice competently in this area. Performing child custody evaluations has long been the professional service most likely to generate an ethics complaint against a psychologist.

In recognition of the complexity of the field and the vulnerability of psychologists who perform child custody evaluations, a set of aspirational guidelines has been promulgated by the American Psychological Association. Although the *Guidelines for Child Custody Evaluations in Divorce Proceedings* (APA, 1994) do not offer specific directives for conducting custody evaluations, they do provide an invaluable orienting framework for competent, ethical functioning.

For evaluations done at the time the marriage is being dissolved, the most global kind of referral question is likely to revolve around the psychological functioning and needs of the child, the parenting abilities of the mother and father, and the relative "goodness-of-fit" between the former and the latter. In some cases, psychopathology in one or both parents may be raised as a specific issue, but the important focus is always on the ability of a parent to meet the developmental and other important needs specific to the individual child. At times, there may be a circumscribed referral question, such as the psychological competence of an adolescent to state a meaningful preference for his or her custody.

Evaluations done in the context of a motion to modify custody may be similar to those done at the time of the divorce, but the court may also be interested in information concerning what changes might have occurred psychologically in the child since the original custody determination, and what the emotional impact might be of changing the child's current arrangements. Since the laws governing custody vary from state to state, it is imperative that the psychologist be knowledgeable about the laws in the jurisdiction in which he or she is practicing. Knowing what factors the court will consider will help the psychologist determine the appropriate scope and focus of the evaluation. In addition, knowledge of the relevant professional literature regarding children's development and functioning after divorce and the variables that influence it should influence the scope and focus of the evaluation. For example, several states favor as custodian the parent most

likely to foster the child's relationship with the other parent, and the social science literature suggests a better outcome for children who are able to maintain good relationships with both parents; therefore, an important focus of the evaluation would be an assessment of the degree and manner in which each parent supports (or undermines) the child's relationship with the other.

METHODS

It is essential that the evaluator carefully define the referral question(s), who the clients are, fees and payment policies, the procedures to be used and for what purpose, to whom and in what form the results will be presented, and the limits on confidentiality. Not only must these issues be clear in the psychologist's mind but they must also be clarified with the adult parties by obtaining informed consent. Informed assent should also be gotten from children old enough to understand at least some of the pertinent issues.

There is no standard format or set of procedures that has been accepted within the profession as representing the standard of care. Although interviews with the parents and with the child appear to be the most commonly used tool for gathering information, other techniques vary from evaluator to evaluator. There are several important issues regarding the selection of procedures, most of which are addressed in the *Guidelines* published by the APA. Obviously, the procedures should be selected with the referral question(s) in mind. Since the scope of inquiry in custody cases is generally multifaceted, multiple sources and methods of data collection are necessary. A major problem in custody, as well as other forensic evaluations, has been the use of psychological tests to address questions they were not designed to answer. Self-report personality inventories such as the Minnesota Multiphasic Personality Inventory (MMPI) have been used, for example, to draw conclusions about which parent is better able to meet the child's needs without establishing a clear connection between clinical functioning and actual parenting.

Other sources of information are necessary, in addition to direct contact with the parties and child through interviews and the administration of tests and instruments. It is customary for psychologists to review documents such as legal pleadings, school records, medical records, prior evaluation data, and records of past or current psychological treatment. Such records are less vulnerable to distortion, either conscious or unconscious, by parents (and sometimes children) who have a vested interest in the legal outcome. Another frequently used procedure is interviewing collateral contacts as sources of information about the parties and the child. Obviously, if the interest is at least partially successful in minimizing the distortions in the information provided by the parties, professionals (e.g., teachers, pediatricians, treating psychologists) are more helpful as collateral contacts than are relatives, friends, and neighbors.

Subsequent to the performance of the evaluation, the psychologist usually prepares a written report. Opinions vary among psychologists as to the appropriate length of the report. Some argue that attorneys and judges will not read long reports, or will find them burdensome. Others believe that a lengthy report in a custody case may result in settlement since the bulk of the psychologist's findings and opinions that would form the basis for testimony is apparent. However, there is little disagreement that avoiding protracted, hostile litigation is in the child's best interests.

If the psychologist is called to testify, the proper stance is one of impartiality. There is not yet consensus regarding whether psychologists should make recommendations about the legal disposition of the case (e.g., which parent should have custody), but the bulk of scholarly opinion is opposed to so-called ultimate issue testimony.

RELIABILITY AND VALIDITY

It is virtually impossible to assess the psychometric properties of the custody evaluation as a whole, consisting as it does of a plethora of methods and data sources. A crucially important question is whether the instruments are valid for the specific purpose for which they are being used. Psychological tests that comprise part of a standard battery for clinical diagnostic use generally have well-established validity and reliability for assessing psychological characteristics if the normative data are appropriate for the individual tested. There have been efforts to develop techniques for assessing parenting per se, but all of the extant instruments have problems with normative data, validity and/or reliability. It is important that psychologists be circumspect in their selection of procedures and in the inferences and conclusions they draw from them.

See also: Developmental Issues in Assessment for Treatment; Divorce; Expert Testimony; Family Assessment; Psychometric Properties of Tests

Further Reading

American Psychological Association Committee on Professional Practice and Standards. (1994). Guidelines for child custody evaluations in divorce proceedings. *American Psychologist, 49,* 677–680.

Gould, J. W. (1998). *Conducting scientifically crafted child custody evaluations.* Thousand Oaks, CA: Sage.

Gould, J. W., & Stahl, P. M. (2000). The art and science of child custody evaluations: Integrating clinical and forensic mental health models. *Family and Conciliation Courts Review, 38,* 392–414.

Melton, G. B., Petrila, J., Poythress, N. G., & Slobogin, C. (1997). *Psychological evaluations for the courts: A handbook for mental health professionals and lawyers* (2nd ed.). New York: Guilford.

Schaefer, A. B. (2001). Forensic evaluations of children and expert witness testimony. In C. E. Walker & M. C. Roberts (Eds.), *Handbook of clinical child psychology* (3rd ed., pp. 1094–1119). New York: Wiley.

ARLENE B. SCHAEFER

Cystic Fibrosis

DEFINITION

Cystic fibrosis (CF) is the most common terminal genetic disease of Caucasian populations, affecting approximately 1 in 3,400 live births. CF is an autosomal recessive disease that results from a defect in the gene that regulates the transport of sodium and chloride across cell membranes. Consequently, the disease affects several major organ systems including the respiratory, digestive, pancreas, kidney, liver, and reproductive. Although multiple systems are affected, over 90 percent of the morbidity and mortality in patients with CF is a result of chronic respiratory disease.

INCIDENCE

A diagnosis of CF is typically made within the first year of life, with over 80 percent of patients being diagnosed by 4 years of age. It is estimated that in the United States there are currently 30,000 individuals living with CF and, approximately 850 new diagnoses will be made each year. Approximately 1 in every 28 Caucasian Americans are carriers of the defective gene. Although CF affects all races and ethnic groups, it is less common among non-Caucasian populations. For example, CF affects only 1 in 11,500 Hispanics, 1 in 17,000 African Americans, and 1 in 90,000 Asians. Prevalence rates among males and females, and across all socioeconomic levels, have been found to be equivalent.

PSYCHOLOGICAL CORRELATES

Given the extraordinary physical and psychological demands imposed by a chronic illness, it is reasonable to assume that children and adolescents with CF experience increased levels of stress. Sources of stress include altered physical appearance, lack of social relationships, and conflicts with parents and siblings. Furthermore, extensive treatment demands and frequent hospitalizations can affect aspects of daily life including recreation time, family interactions, and peer relationships. In spite of facing a number of disease-specific stressors, children and adolescents with CF adapt to their illness and exhibit rates of psychopathology that are similar to healthy children. In an effort to capture the impact of this chronic illness on daily functioning, disease-specific measures of health-related quality of life have recently been developed.

ETIOLOGY

CF is a genetic autosomal recessive disorder, in which a child must inherit a copy of the recessive gene from both parents. Delta F508 has been identified as the most common defective gene associated with CF and has been documented in 70 percent of individuals diagnosed with CF. However, several hundred different mutations of the gene have now been identified.

ASSESSMENT

The sweat test has been the "gold standard" for diagnosing CF for over 40 years. It is a painless, inexpensive test that provides results within a few hours. The test is used to determine the amount of chloride in an individual's sweat. Levels of chloride above 60 milliequivalents per liter (mEq/l) indicate a positive diagnosis of CF.

Pulmonary function tests (PFTs) assess individuals' lung functioning. Spirometry, the simplest PFT, is typically conducted during routine clinic visits. Although several measurements of lung functioning are calculated based on these tests, the most commonly used measure is forced expired volume in 1 s (FEV_1). It is defined as the volume of air expelled in the first second of a forced expiration, and is typically expressed as a

percentage (FEV_1 percent predicted), standardizing for height, weight, and gender. Disease severity is categorized by FEV_1 percent predicted into three levels: mild (>70 percent), moderate (>40 percent), and severe (<40 percent).

TREATMENT

Due to the impact of the disease on multiple organ systems, the treatment regimen for patients with CF is both complex and time-consuming. First, in order to decrease the thick and sticky mucus from the lungs, nebulized medications are used to open the airways; then, airway clearance techniques (e.g., chest physical therapy, Acapella, The Vest™ Airway Clearance System) are performed to remove the mucus at least twice each day. Finally, patients who are diagnosed as pancreatic insufficient, are also required to increase their calorie intake (150 percent of the daily recommended values) and take replacement enzymes with every meal and snack.

In addition to the daily treatment regimen, individuals with CF are frequently hospitalized to treat pulmonary exacerbations. Approximately 35 percent of patients with CF will be hospitalized in a given year, typically spending 10–14 days in the hospital for treatment with intravenous (IV) antibiotics.

In the later stages of the disease, patients may be listed for a lung transplant. CF is the second most common indication for pediatric lung transplantation, however due to a shortage of donor organs, a significant percent of patients will die while awaiting a transplant. Current statistics indicate that 70 percent of patients with CF survive 1 year posttransplant and 48 percent survive after 5 years. Living-related donor transplants are becoming more common and provide another option for patients awaiting transplantation.

PROGNOSIS

As a result of earlier diagnosis and more aggressive treatment, life expectancy has increased over the past few decades. Median life expectancy is currently 32 years of age, and the projected survival for children born today is approximately 40 years of age. However, gender differences in morbidity and mortality have been documented, with females under the ages of 20 showing greater risk of mortality than males. By age 20, however, no significant differences in survival rates between males and females are found. Newborn screening and early interventions to treat lung infections and inflammation, as well as new drug treatments such as gene therapy, are likely to increase life expectancy and improve quality of life.

See also: Death; Hospitalization—Medical; Lung Transplantation, Pediatric; Quality of life; Treatment Adherence: Medical

Further Reading

Cystic Fibrosis Foundation. (2002). *Facts about lung transplantation.* Retrieved April 27, 2002, from http://www.cff.org/publications09.htm

Kosorok, M. R., Wei, W. H., & Farrell, P. M. (1996). The incidence of cystic fibrosis. *Statistics in Medicine 15*(5), 449–462.

Orenstein, D. M. (2000). *Cystic fibrosis: Medical care.* Philadelphia, PA: Lippincott-Raven.

Quittner, A. L., Espelage, D. L., Opipari, L. C., Carter, B. D., & Eigen, H. (1998). Role strain in couples with and without a chronically ill child: Associations with marital satisfaction, intimacy, and daily mood. *Health Psychology, 17*, 112–124.

Ramsey, B. W. (1997). Management of pulmonary disease in patients with cystic fibrosis. *New England Journal of Medicine, 335*, 179–188.

ALEXANDRA L. QUITTNER
AVANI C. MODI
MELISSA A. DAVIS

Cytomegalovirus Infection

DEFINITION

Cytomegalovirus (CMV) is a member of the herpes virus group. All individuals will have had a CMV infection by the age of 70. In a healthy individual, the primary (first) CMV infection is usually asymptomatic and poses no health risks. However, when a pregnant woman acquires a primary CMV infection, approximately 40 percent of their infants will become infected *in utero* and are born with a congenital CMV infection. Congenital CMV infection is the leading cause of birth defects due to viral infections and the major known cause of severe birth defects such as mental retardation, deafness, and other neurologic problems. In an immunocompromised individual (e.g., an individual with HIV/AIDS or an individual who has a bone-marrow transplant), either a primary or a secondary CMV infection can be a life-threatening illness and may cause serious and even fatal multisystemic disease (see Pediatric Human Immunodeficiency Virus-1).

INCIDENCE

Congenital CMV infection is present in approximately 40,000 (1 percent) of infants born in the United States annually. About 4,000 of these infants have serious neurological defects at birth (e.g., mental retardation, deafness, vision problems) and about 6,000 experience developmental problems later in childhood (e.g., learning disabilities, seizures). The remaining 30,000 infants have no discernable defects or deficits associated with the congenitally acquired infection. There are no known predictors of neurological complications.

PSYCHOSOCIAL ASPECTS

CMV is transmitted via bodily fluids such as saliva, urine, blood, and semen. Children 3 years of age and younger who are in day care are particularly at higher risk for acquiring a primary CMV infection, presumably through the inadvertent sharing of bodily secretions in the day care setting (e.g., mouthing of toys). Usual parental care may expose mothers (and possibly fathers) with their young child's CMV-laden secretions, and, if the parent has not had a prior CMV infection, he or she may acquire a primary CMV infection. A primary CMV infection during pregnancy poses the risk of congenital CMV infection to the infant. Thus, a mother with a young child in day care is at particular risk for exposure to CMV during a subsequent pregnancy. Prevention of a primary CMV infection during pregnancy has the potential to reduce congenital birth defects.

ASSESSMENT

Although cell cultures have been developed to detect the shedding of CMV in urine, saliva, and blood of an individual with an active CMV infection, the viral test is not readily available for all children. Likewise, a CMV culture is not readily available nor is it recommended for pregnant women. Thus, there is no recommended test for CMV infection related to pregnancy for either a pregnant woman or her child. A conservative approach assumes that any pregnant woman with a young child in day care is at risk for acquiring a primary CMV infection from the child in day care and that behavioral practices that reduce exposure of the mother to CMV secretions of the child will reduce the likelihood of acquiring a CMV infection during pregnancy.

TREATMENT

Potential vaccines for preventing CMV infection are in the beginning stages of development and are unlikely to be available for many years. A behavioral preventive regimen has been investigated that includes (1) washing hands frequently (i.e., after exposure to a child's bodily fluids, diaper changes, handling dirty laundry, touching the child's toys and other objects, and bathing the child); (2) wearing protective gloves (i.e., during diaper changes, handling dirty laundry); and (3) reducing intimate contact with the day-care aged child (i.e., avoiding kissing on the mouth, sleeping together, sharing towels and washcloths, and eating or drinking from the child's utensils or cups). The behavioral preventive regimen has been shown to be effective in reducing primary CMV infections in pregnant women, but further clinical trials are needed to establish public health recommendations related to the prevention of CMV infection in women who wish to become pregnant and have children enrolled in day care.

PROGNOSIS

Given that CMV is the leading known cause of birth defects, preventive efforts provide the best prognosis. Women with children enrolled in day care may wish to follow behavioral preventive recommendations to reduce the likelihood that they acquire a primary CMV infection from their young children. However, further research is needed to document the effectiveness of the specific preventive recommendations in reducing primary CMV infections and thereby prevent many congenital birth defects.

See also: Deafness; Mental Retardation; Pediatric Human Immunodeficiency Virus-1 (HIV); Visual Impairment: Low Vision and Blindness

Further Reading

Adler, S. P., Finney, J. W., Manganello, A. M., & Best, A. M. (1996). Prevention of child-to mother transmission of cytomegalovirus by changing behaviors: A randomized controlled trial. *Pediatric Infectious Diseases Journal, 15*, 240–246.

Dobbins, J. G., Adler, S. P., Pass, R. F., Bale, J. F., Jr., Grillner, L., & Stewart, J. A. (1994). The risks of cytomegalovirus transmission in child day care. *Pediatrics, 94* (Suppl.), 1016–1018.

Finney, J. W., Miller, K. M., & Adler, S. P. (1993). Changing protective and risky behaviors to prevent child-to-parent transmission of cytomegalovirus. *Journal of Applied Behavior Analysis, 26,* 471–472.

JACK W. FINNEY

Dd

Day Hospital

See: Day Treatment

Day Treatment

DEFINITION

Day treatment for children, also known as partial hospitalization, has been available in the United States since the 1940s in the form of therapeutic nursery schools. Later the definition was expanded to include adolescents, and day treatment was recognized as playing a critical role along the continuum of care in mental health services for children and adolescents with serious emotional disorders. That is, day treatment programs are less restrictive than inpatient hospitalization programs and more restrictive than traditional outpatient services. This unique feature allows youth to remain in the community without being institutionalized and experiencing permanent or long-term breaks from their family while also providing a structured transitional return to the community for those in residential treatment. Day treatment services provide youth with a balance of treatment intensity by offering services for several hours during the day while allowing them to return to their homes in the evening. Programs typically comprise at least 5–6 hr of treatment per day and are less disruptive to youth's daily routine than is inpatient hospitalization. Day treatment programs tend to vary in their description of populations served, settings, staffing, theoretical approaches, treatment components, and intensity. As a result, there are no universally accepted criteria for what constitutes day treatment. However, day treatment programs are usually considered to be intensive, time-limited, highly structured, multidisciplinary, multimodal, active treatment programs that offer coordinated clinical services within a stable therapeutic milieu. Day treatment programs typically include some combination of the following components: psychiatric evaluation and medication management; special education services; individual, group, and family therapy; crisis intervention; social skills and problem-solving skills; behavior modification emphasizing positive reinforcement procedures; recreational, art, and music therapy; and vocational skills. Day treatment programs focus on building alliances with families and community providers to enlist their cooperation and build collaboration. A variety of educational options are available in this setting, such as self-contained classrooms, home and hospital instruction, continuation programs, and public school placements.

EFFECTIVENESS

Research on day treatment has faced severe difficulties, including methodological limitations (i.e., lack of experimental designs, lack of heterogeneous samples, lack of control or comparison groups, lack of standardized measures, and variations in duration and type of treatments). Despite the sixty-year history of day treatment, studies on children's day treatment programs have been given less attention compared to adult counterparts. Early examinations of day treatment for children

154

focused on descriptive characterizations of programs. This progressed to the single outcome approach, which examined reintegration into the community or educational placements after discharge. Subsequently, multiple outcome approaches evolved to examine reintegration after discharge, cost-effectiveness, clinical status, level of functioning, utilization of behavioral health services after discharge, and patient/family satisfaction. Likewise, recent studies have begun to incorporate control and comparison groups into the study design, allowing some conclusions to be drawn about the effectiveness of day treatment interventions.

Youth in day treatment programs usually have multiple behavioral, neurotic, and psychotic diagnoses, therefore making it difficult to generalize as to the differential effectiveness of a particular program on separate disorders. However, available research does suggest that day treatment programs are less effective for particular groups of children. For example, treatment gains for children and adolescents with severe behavior disorders (attention deficit, conduct disorder) fared less well than other groups (e.g. those with emotional disorders including anxiety and depression) at 18-month follow-up. Those in the psychotic and behaviorally disturbed groups continued to be actively symptomatic and were more frequently in special education or institutional settings after treatment. Conversely, youth that did well in day treatment programs typically were younger at admission, at a higher developmental level, and had a length of stay for over one year. Similarly, other studies have found that children exhibiting school-behavior problems or peer relationship problems have shown marked improvements as a result of participation in day treatment programs. More recently, results of day treatment programs serving severely psychiatrically disturbed truant adolescents have shown marked improvements in truancy and psychiatric symptoms at 6 months after discharge. Additionally, long-term follow-up at one to five years post discharge has found some positive results.

The following general conclusions can be drawn as to the effectiveness of day treatment programs: (1) they appear to promote the reintegration of a portion of youth into the community, (2) they offer modest improvements in individual and family functioning, (3) families play an important role in outcomes following day treatment, (4) they demonstrate effectiveness for a limited population of children, (5) treatment outcomes cannot be generalized to the overall school domain, but do carry over into the child's natural life, and (6) they offer significant reductions in cost and length of stay as compared to inpatient hospitalizations.

In conclusion, in spite of the shortcomings of past research, day treatment continues to effectively serve as an alternative to both inpatient hospitalization and outpatient therapy in impacting cost, length of stay, and individual and family functioning. Careful consideration should be directed at exploring the effectiveness of day treatment components on specific populations in the future.

See also: Community Interventions; Residential Treatment; School-Based Treatments

Further Reading

Flaherty, L. T., & Glassman, S. B. (1998). Day hospital: Planning, staffing, and administration. In H. S. Ghuman & R. M. Sarles (Eds.), *Handbook of child and adolescent outpatient, day treatment and community psychiatry* (pp. 311–321). Castelton, NY: Hamilton Printing.

Kutash, K., & Rivera, V. R. (1995). Effectiveness of children's mental health services: A review of the literature. *Education and Treatment of Children, 18,* 443–477.

McDermott, B. M., McKelvey, R., Roberts, L., & Davies, L. (2002). Severity of children's psychopathology and impairment and its relationship to treatment setting. *Psychiatric Services, 53,* 57–62.

Pazaratz, D. (2001). Theory and structure of a day treatment program for adolescents. *Residential Treatment for Children and Youth, 19,* 29–43.

RICHARD W. PUDDY
MICHAEL C. ROBERTS

Deafness

DEFINITION/ETIOLOGY

Deafness is defined as a hearing impairment that is so severe that the individual is impaired in processing linguistic information through hearing, with or without amplification. Hearing losses greater than 90 dB HL (loudness or intensity of sound measured in units called decibels, dB) are generally considered deaf. Deafness may be viewed as a condition that prevents an individual from receiving sound in all or most of its forms. In contrast, an individual with a hearing loss can generally respond to auditory stimuli, including speech.

There are two models for the definition of the term deaf: the medical and the cultural models. The medical model is the viewpoint that deafness is a functional disorder with all efforts aimed at fixing the deafness. Deafness is seen as a handicap. People holding this viewpoint consider hearing the optimal model and use the auditory methods to obtain the goals of using residual hearing, speech-reading, and speech. The deaf individual is deemed successful if he/she gains good oral skills. Assistive devices such as hearing aids and cochlear implants are used and considered appropriate. A person who has this viewpoint uses the term "deaf" with a lower case "d."

The cultural model of deafness defines the deaf individual as a linguistic minority with a distinct language, culture, and mores. Deafness is viewed as a difference, but not an inferiority. The deaf individual is visual with the natural language of American Sign Language (ASL) or any other naturally occurring signed language. The deaf individual does not need the hearing to be fixed. A deaf individual is successful if he/she attains fluency in ASL. A person with this viewpoint uses the term "Deaf" with a capital "D."

INCIDENCE

Although statistics are gathered on all hearing impairments, the exact number of individuals identified with deafness significant enough to prevent processing of linguistic information through hearing, with or without amplification is unknown. About 1 in every 1000 babies born in the United States has severe hearing loss in both ears. The causes of deafness are the same as for any hearing impairment, genetic or environmental (medication, trauma, or illness). Deafness may be sensorineural with a permanent change within the inner ear. A mixed deafness may also be present that exhibits problems in the middle ear that may fluctuate (ear infections or perforations of the eardrum) and problems with the inner ear (permanent).

CORRELATES

Expressive and receptive language delays may be present due to the severity of the hearing impairment. Literacy, indexed by performance on reading and writing measures, is an issue closely related to language development. Deaf and hard of hearing children obtain an average reading and writing level of third or fourth grade. Reading problems stem largely from an inadequate language system with deficits in vocabulary and complexity of syntactic (sentence) structures.

Society's negative labeling of deaf individuals may contribute to lower self-esteem that has been identified. Deafness may be isolating due to communication

difficulty with individuals who hear and do not use sign language. Due to the delay in language development, some children with hearing impairment may have fewer opportunities for peer interactions, making it difficult to learn "social rules" which may result in reduced social competence. Residential schools provide a vital link in the transmission of Deaf Culture and Language. Children at residential schools are able to communicate in a language readily understood by each other and, therefore, are able to partake in social clubs, sports, and be around deaf role models. This is not to say that mainstream education is unfair for deaf children, but socialization is essential to a child's growth and without a common language socialization may be limited. Deaf children should be encouraged to further their education and to learn that deafness does not mean you cannot grow up to be successful and happy.

ASSESSMENT

The pediatrician and otolaryngologist (ear, nose, and throat specialist) will evaluate the child to determine the cause of the hearing loss and determine its medical management. The audiologist completes the hearing evaluation (also known as audiological evaluation) to determine the degree and type of hearing loss. The physician will use information from the child's medical history, the physical examination, and the hearing test to provide a diagnosis. The audiologist will provide information concerning rehabilitation techniques and will make referrals for additional services such as to the speech–language pathologist, educational psychologist, or the public school. The speech–language pathologist and audiologist will be the primary case managers for the child with a hearing impairment.

TREATMENT

Communication options for families of deaf children are varied and include speech, sign communication (ASL or manually coded English), or fingerspelling. Even though the Deaf Culture supports the use of ASL as the primary language for the Deaf, many Deaf individuals are successful at learning speech. Speech is needed for interaction with hearing sales people, banking personnel, etc.

Language is central to all individuals because it is the means for communicating with others and for thinking and learning. It can be spoken, signed, and written. The essential link to Deaf Culture among the American Deaf community is ASL. This community shares a common sense of pride in their culture and language. ASL is a visual language composed of gestures called signs in combination with various types of nonmanual grammar (mouth morphemes, appropriate facial expression, body movement, etc.). Some of ASL's grammatical features include directional verbs, classifiers, rhetorical questions, and the temporal aspect. ASL has its own grammar that does not follow the grammar of English. English is linear and requires prepositions to create a mental picture of where things are in a sentence, ASL uses the physical space in front of the signer to create the mental picture. A signer can use more than one sign concurrently. In the early 1960s William Stokoe wrote and published Sign Language Structure that proclaimed that ASL was a true language on a par with any spoken language. However, one drawback to using ASL as a sole communication tool is that it does not have an accepted written form. Although individuals choose to remain a part of Deaf Culture, access to literature from other cultures and times should be available. Without a written code to represent ASL, transcription of the literature of other cultures into ASL can only be accomplished by filming it.

A total communication approach to education of the deaf provides a manual coded English sign system, speech-reading, auditory skills, and tactile stimulation to provide language in all sensory systems so that the individual can select the system that provides the most information for learning. Ideally, teachers use sign, writing, mime, speech, pictures, or any other communication method that works. The method of communication should depend upon the needs of the student and the situation. Children are encouraged to work on speech and listening skills. The emphasis in Total communication programming is mainstream education where the child attends regular classes or a class for the hearing impaired within the local school system and may have an interpreter, notetaker, real-time captioning (technology available where the dialogue is simultaneously projected on a screen for reading), or special assistance as needed.

The Deaf Culture has emphasized a bilingual–bicultural education, with ASL taught to the child first and then English taught as a second language. The benefits of such a program are that deaf children receive a language that is highly accessible to them. In the bilingual–bicultural approach, teachers that are native in the language model ASL for the child. If the child attends a residential school, he also has the opportunity to learn from his peers. Since everyone signs ASL at the residential school, the feeling of isolation often found among signing children placed in the mainstream is ameliorated. Since ASL is strongly connected with Deaf Culture,

children in bilingual–bicultural programs have the opportunity to learn about, and participate in, Deaf Culture. This method is particularly useful for deaf children of parents fluent in ASL since the parents already know the target language and can model it correctly.

Cochlear implants involve a surgical procedure in which electrodes are implanted into the inner ear. Candidates for cochlear implant include those who have profound hearing losses that receive no benefit from amplification. Cochlear implants are a controversial rehabilitation option for the deaf. The Deaf Culture holds that the hearing does not need to be fixed. Many reports are available concerning successful use of the cochlear implant in improving language development, speech production, and overall academic achievement.

Individuals who are deaf have many helpful devices available to them. Text telephones (known as TTs, TTYs, or TDDs) enable persons to type phone messages over the telephone network. The Telecommunications Relay Service (TRS) makes it possible for TT users to communicate with virtually anyone (and vice versa) via telephone. The National Institute on Deafness and Other Communication Disorders Information Clearinghouse (telephone: 1-800-241-1044, voice; 1-800-241-1055, TT) makes available lists of TRS numbers by state. There are devices called a Visual Ring Signaler (VRS), which can be connected to the phone and to a lamp, so that when the phone rings the lamp will blink, alerting the deaf person that the phone is ringing. A similar device is available so that when the bell is rung, it signals a light to flash on and off. A device called a baby cry signaler works the same way. One part is in the parents' room and the other in the baby's room. When the baby cries, the device sends a signal to the lamp in the parents' room, which causes it to flash on and off. There are variations in how the lamps will blink so that the phone and the door will have a different signal.

For additional information contact an audiologist or one of the Deaf organizations listed in the Further Reading section.

PROGNOSIS

Communication may be limited for the deaf individual; however, technology is providing access to every aspect of life for the deaf. Telecommunication devices with the National Relay Services open the door to every business. Computer technology is available for real-time captioning for television or for meetings. Whether they communicate using speech or signs, there is no limit on their achievement. Integration into the hearing world or the Deaf Culture will depend on the desire of the deaf person and his or her family members.

See also: Central Auditory Processing Disorders; Hearing Impairment; Language Development; Speech and Language Assessment; Speech and Language Disorders

Further Reading

Gallaudet University, 800 Florida Avenue, NE, Washington, DC 20002, 202-651-5000 TTY/V, Web: http://www.gallaudet.edu/
National Institute on Deafness and Other Communication Disorders Clearinghouse, 31 Center Drive, MSC 2320, Bethesda, MD 20892-2320, 1-800-241-1044 (Voice); 1-800-241-1055 (TT), Web: www.nidcd.nih.gov/
Rollin, W. J. (1987). *The psychology of communication disorders in individuals and their families.* Englewood Cliffs, NJ: Prentice-Hall.
Scheetz, N. A. (2001). *Orientation to deafness* (2nd ed.). Boston: Allyn and Bacon.
Schirmer, B. R. (2001). *Psychological, social and educational dimensions of deafness.* Boston: Allyn and Bacon.

EVA SAFFER

Death

See: Bereavement

Delinquent Behavior

DEFINITION/CLINICAL PRESENTATION

Part of the confusion in defining delinquent behavior is that it has been referred to in many different ways in the literature. For example, it has been referred to as Conduct Disorder (CD), conduct problems, antisocial behavior, youth violence, behavior problems, and as behavior evidenced by delinquents or juvenile offenders. The newest definition of CD is comprised of many behaviors that constitute delinquent behaviors; the primary difference being that CD describes the clinical presentation of the behaviors and delinquency refers to the legal definition of them. Delinquency has been defined by a range of behaviors, such as youth who engage in illegal activity (statutory and criminal), youth who have contact with law enforcement, and those who are adjudicated through juvenile court for a criminal offense. These behaviors violate the rules of a society and result in contact with the juvenile justice system. Originally, the juvenile justice system was set apart from the adult legal system in order to intervene with youth early enough to be able to "rehabilitate" them. However, several sources would agree that the system has become more punitive over time and, as a result, calls to reform the system have been issued. For example, the United States Surgeon General (2001) has asked that youth involved in delinquent behavior be identified appropriately and that empirically validated treatment programs be used with them and their families.

INCIDENCE

Rates of delinquency are often underrepresentations of actual behavior. Since most statistics rely on official contacts with law enforcement, all other illegal activity that is undetected remains unreported. Because of this challenge in obtaining accurate incidence rates of juvenile offending, self-report data become an increasingly important source of information. Arrest rates for violent crimes, including criminal homicide, robbery, aggravated assault, and forcible rape, increased from 1983 to 1993/1994. Factors that played a large role in this increase were youth involvement in gangs, increased drug use, and access and use of guns. However, there has been a decline in arrests since 1993. The overall arrest rate for all crimes committed by juveniles in the United States was 2.4 million in 1999. During this time period, juveniles were involved in 16 percent of all violent crime and 32 percent of all property crime arrests committed in this country. Another indicator of juvenile violence, self-report of crime, shows that the amount of violent behavior has not decreased between 1993 and 1999. One potential reason for this discrepancy between actual arrest rates and self-report of delinquent behavior may be that there has been a decline in youth's use of firearms and some decline in gang membership that has resulted in less severe problem behavior that may not be noticed by the authorities. Other statistics show that 30–40 percent of males and 16–32 percent of females have committed a serious violent offense by the age of 17. There are differences in arrest rates across gender and race, with significantly more males than females arrested, and significantly more African Americans arrested than whites or other minority groups.

CORRELATES

Research concerning delinquent behavior has demonstrated several correlates of this form of antisocial behavior. Many of these youth are diagnosed with Attention-Deficit/Hyperactivity Disorder (ADHD), Oppositional Defiant Disorder (ODD), and/or CD. Youth who evidence delinquent behavior may also have co-occurring depression and/or anxiety as well as substance abuse. They might also engage in early sexual activity as well as truancy and they may drop out of school early. Family correlates of delinquent behavior include family conflict, marital conflict, and parental inconsistency with rules and consequences.

ASSESSMENT

Assessments of adolescents who display delinquent behavior are often court-ordered and are primarily focused on assessing the youth's potential for future harm. Additionally, the assessment may be oriented toward determining if they are amenable to treatment and to the likelihood of future delinquent acts. These evaluations are used to assist in planning probation requirements for the youth as well as potential placement decisions. An evaluation should assess the risk factors associated with future behavior, including past behavior, substance use, social stressors and support, opportunity to commit problem behavior, and characteristics of the residence where they may be placed. In addition, there are several other key areas that are evaluated, including individual, family, peer, and community factors. Individual factors include the range of antisocial behavior, cognitive skills, and personality functioning of the youth. In addition, vocational skills may also be assessed to see how the youth may be able to adapt to his or her environment. Another important area is family dynamics, including parenting strategies, and family conflict as well as warmth. Peer relationships are also an important area, because the best predictor of delinquent behavior is connections with negative peers who display similar behavior. Finally, community factors are considered, such as support systems for the youth and family, as well as neighborhood cohesion or support of delinquent behaviors.

TREATMENT

During the past decade several programs have been empirically validated for the prevention and treatment of delinquent behavior. In general, studies have shown that programs that target multiple systems, including home, school, peers, and neighborhood systems, are family based, short-term, and intensive, and are more effective in treating difficult behavior.

Particular programs identified to show change in juvenile behavior and are cost-effective include Functional Family Therapy, Multidimensional Treatment Foster Care, Multisystemic Therapy, Prenatal and Infancy Home Visitation by Nurses, and the Seattle Social Development Project. Unfortunately, many communities continue to fund programs that have not been shown to be effective, such as gun buyback programs, boot camps, residential programs, milieu treatment, waivers to adult court, and individual counseling.

PROGNOSIS

Much research has been done on the developmental trajectories and risk factors for delinquent youth. There appears to be a developmental pathway to later violent behavior that may begin with less intense problem behaviors, such as stealing, aggression towards others, and/or truancy. Often, these behaviors may progress to more serious problem behaviors, and children may be labeled with ODD, or CD. In addition, two pathways of problem behavior have been described, distinguished by children who begin evidencing problematic behavior at an early age versus those who develop behavior problems in adolescence. Those developing problem behavior at an earlier age are at a higher risk for persistence of violent behavior through adolescence and into adulthood. Further research will continue to delineate the factors related to persistence of delinquent behavior in order to strengthen our treatment of this population. Risk factors (described in assessment section) have been identified by age and also across individual, family, school, peer group, and community domains. In addition, some protective factors have been identified that may assist youth in having a more positive outcome. Having a risk factor does not guarantee that a youth will develop problematic behavior, but when they evidence a higher number of risk factors, there is a greater likelihood they will develop more severe delinquent behavior.

See also: Aggression; Conduct Disorder; Lying; Multisystemic Therapy

Further Reading

Grisso, T. (1998). *Forensic evaluation of juveniles.* Sarasota, Florida: Professional Resource Press.
Loeber, R., & Farrington, D. P. (2000). Young children who commit crime: Epidemiology, developmental origins, risk factors, early interventions, and policy implications. *Development and Psychopathology, 12*, 737–762.

Patterson, G. R., Forgatch, M. S., Yoerger, K. L., & Stoolmiller, M. (1998). Variables that initiate and maintain an early-onset trajectory for juvenile offending. *Development and Psychopathology, 10*, 531–547.

Rutter, M., Giller, H., & Hagell, A. (1998). *Antisocial behavior by young people.* Cambridge, UK: Cambridge University Press.

U.S. Department of Health and Human Services. (2001). *Youth violence: A report of the surgeon general.* Rockville, MD: U.S. Department of Health and Human Services, Centers for Disease Control and Prevention, National Center for Injury Prevention and Control; Substance Abuse and Mental Health Services Administration, Center for Mental Health Services; and National Institutes of Health, National Institute of Mental Health.

JULIANNE M. SMITH
STEPHEN LASSEN

Depressed Adolescents, Interpersonal Psychotherapy

See: Interpersonal Psychotherapy for Depressed Adolescents

Depressive Disorder, Major

DEFINITION

A major depressive episode (MDE) is characterized as at least a two-week period of (1) either depressed or irritable mood lasting most of the day for most days, or a loss of interest or pleasure in most activities, and (2) at least four of the following symptoms: weight loss, failure to make expected weight gains, or excessive weight gain; insomnia or hypersomnia; psychomotor agitation or retardation; fatigue or loss of energy; feelings of worthlessness or guilt; poor concentration; and suicidal or morbid ideation. The symptoms must interfere with family, school, friends, or work, and are not due to other drugs or illness. To meet criteria for major depressive disorder (MDD), manic symptoms must not have ever been present.

The same criteria are used to diagnose depression in children and adults, however certain features may be more salient in young people. Children and adolescents will often present with an irritable mood rather than a depressed mood, and will display more anxiety, somatic complaints, social withdrawal, behavior problems, and low self-esteem.

EPIDEMIOLOGY

The incidence of depression ranges from 0.4 to 2.5 percent in children, and from 0.4 to 8.3 percent in adolescents. The lifetime prevalence rate of MDD in adolescents is 15–20 percent, which is similar to the rates for adults. In children, the rate of MDD in boys is approximately equal to that of girls. However, gender differences emerge in adolescence, as the rate for females is twice that of males.

ETIOLOGY AND RISK FACTORS

The etiology of depression is currently thought to be a combination of genetic and psychosocial factors. Environmental factors are important because individuals at high genetic risk may be more sensitive to environmental stress.

Risk factors for depressive problems include a family history of mood disorders, a stressful family environment, and a negative cognitive style. Children of depressed parents are three times more likely than children of nondepressed parents to experience a major depressive episode, and are at risk for other internalizing and externalizing problems. The family environment of depressed individuals is characterized by more conflict, more communication problems, less support, and more rejection than the families of nondepressed individuals. Depressed children exhibit cognitive distortions. They are more likely to view situations negatively, feel hopeless about their ability to problem-solve, and feel a lack of control over their situation.

PSYCHOSOCIAL SEQUELAE AND COMORBID DISORDERS

Depression is related to a number of associated problems including disruptions in family life, school achievement, and peer relationships. It is often when these disruptions become significant that a family will seek treatment. The seriousness of these associated problems, and their impact on long-term functioning support the need for early and aggressive diagnosis and treatment of depressive disorders.

The presence of comorbid diagnoses in children should be considered the rule rather than the exception. Forty to seventy percent of youth with depression have at least one comorbid diagnosis, and 20–50 percent have at least two. Common comorbid conditions include anxiety disorders, Attention-Deficit/Hyperactivity

Disorder, Oppositional Defiant Disorder (ODD), Conduct Disorder (CD), substance abuse, eating disorders, and learning disorders.

ASSESSMENT

A direct clinical interview with the child or adolescent is essential to obtain information regarding: onset, severity, duration, and frequency of mood, behavior, anxiety, and other symptoms; peer relationships; school functioning; and family environment. Suicide risk should also be assessed. Similarly, a direct clinical interview with the parents is essential, both to cover symptom onset, offset, and duration of depression as well as comorbid conditions. The child's developmental history, medical history, school adjustment, and treatment history should also be obtained, as well as a family history of psychiatric disorders. A complete interview will allow the clinician to make a differential diagnosis, that is, to determine the child's primary and co-occurring mental disorders, and to document physical disorders. As some physical disorders (e.g., anemia, thyroid disease) and medication side effects (e.g., irritable mood, tearfulness on some stimulants) can mimic depression, this is an important component of assessment. Reports obtained from other informants, such as the child's teacher, can also provide useful information regarding symptomatology and functioning in a variety of settings. These reports can be obtained via self-report questionnaires, or behavior checklists, and are particularly useful if the child and parent give discrepant reports regarding the child's problems.

Self-report questionnaires designed to screen for depressive symptoms in children and adolescents include the Children's Depressive Inventory, the Beck Depression Inventory, the Reynolds Child Depression Scale, the Reynolds Adolescent Depression Scale, and the Children's Depression Scale. While these instruments are useful for screening and follow-up, they should not be used alone to make the diagnosis.

TREATMENT

Treatment for childhood depression can be divided into psychosocial interventions and biological treatments. Evidence-based psychosocial treatments include cognitive–behavioral therapy (CBT), family therapy, psychoeducation, and interpersonal therapy. Cognitive–behavioral interventions include techniques designed to identify depressive or negative patterns of thinking and develop more adaptive cognitions.

Behavioral techniques such as social skills training and increasing pleasurable activities may also be included. Family therapy focuses on modifying the maladaptive verbal and behavioral interactions within the family. One goal is to decrease levels of expressed emotion (critical comments and hostility), which has been found to be higher in families of depressed children. Psychoeducation interventions teach families about symptoms of depression, coping strategies for dealing with these symptoms, and strategies for navigating school and mental health systems. Psychoeducation can be presented to individual families, or in multifamily groups. Interpersonal therapy is designed to decrease interpersonal problems associated with depression. The therapist and client often engage in role-play activities to practice interpersonal skills learned in session.

Biological treatments include pharmacotherapy, phototherapy, and electroconvulsive therapy (ECT). Pharmacologic interventions target neurotransmitter systems indicated in depression. Medication safety has improved over the past 10 years, and the number of available agents is increasing. The selective serotonin reuptake inhibitors (SSRIs) are the class of antidepressant medications most commonly indicated for children with depression, because they have fewer side effects than other antidepressants. Phototherapy may be indicated if the child is diagnosed with Seasonal Affective Disorder (SAD) (i.e., depression with a notable seasonal fluctuation). ECT may alter metabolic activity in some regions of the brain. While effective, it is used as a treatment of last resort, when medications and other interventions have been ineffective.

PROGNOSIS

The average length of an MDE is 7–9 months, with 90 percent of episodes lasting less than 2 years. A single major depressive episode is not associated with additional problems. However, children or adolescents who suffer recurrent episodes appear to be left with a "psychosocial scar" that impairs interepisodic functioning, and sensitizes them to future psychological impairment and subsequent depressive episodes. Within 2 years of remission, 40 percent of youth will have another episode; within 5 years, 70 percent will experience a recurrence. To reduce relapse risk, treatment adherence should be monitored. During the final session of "active" treatment, the therapist should review relapse warning signs and instruct the family to return to active treatment if this occurs. Routine follow-up checks can be used as an additional means to detect early warning signs of a recurrence.

Children and adolescents with MDD are at an increased risk of developing bipolar disorder. About 20–50 percent will "switch" into mania and develop bipolar disorder within five years of depression onset. Risk factors for switching include childhood onset depression, psychomotor retardation, psychosis, a family history of bipolar disorder, a very strong family history of depressive disorder, and pharmacologically induced manic symptoms.

See also: Bipolar Disorder; Cognitive-Behavior Therapy; Dysthymic Disorder; Interpersonal Psychotherapy for Depressed Adolescents; Mania; Suicide

Further Reading

American Psychiatric Association. (2000). *Diagnostic and statistical manual of mental disorders* (4th ed., text revision). Washington, DC: Author.

Birmaher, B., Ryan, N. D., Williamson, D. E., Brent, D. A., Kaufman, J., & Dahl, R. E., et al. (1996). Child and adolescent depression: A review of the past 10 years. Part I. *Journal of the American Academy of Child and Adolescent Psychiatry, 35,* 1427–1439.

Kovacs, M. (1997). Depressive disorders in childhood: An impressionistic landscape. *Journal of Child Psychology and Psychiatry, 38,* 287–298.

McClure, E. B., Kubiszyn, T., & Kaslow, N. J. (2002). Advances in the diagnosis and treatment of childhood mood disorders. *Professional Psychology: Research and Practice, 33,* 125–134.

Rohde, P., Lewinsohn, P. M., & Seeley, J. R. (1994). Are adolescents changed by an episode of major depression? *Journal of the American Academy of Child and Adolescent Psychiatry, 33,* 1289–1298.

Wilens, T. E. (1999). *Straight talk about psychiatric medications for kids.* New York: Guilford.

DORY P. SISSON
MARY A. FRISTAD

Dermatology: Dermatitis and Psoriasis

DEFINITION

Dermatitis and psoriasis are common skin diseases characterized by noncontagious irritation and inflammation, often resulting in itching. Dermatitis, also commonly referred to as eczema, can appear as red and itchy rashes, blisters, thickened skin, and greasy-appearing scaling. While the exact cause of dermatitis is not always known, the more common sources of the disease are environmental irritants, and genetic predisposition combined with environmental triggers.

Psoriasis is a chronic incurable skin disease characterized by abnormal rapid growth of immature skin cells that manifests as thick dry skin patches with underlying inflammation and redness. As with some forms of dermatitis, there appears to be a genetic component of psoriasis.

INCIDENCE

Dermatitis, while diagnosed across the lifespan, is commonly experienced by children. Contact dermatitis and atopic dermatitis account for 20 and 10 percent, respectively, of all children diagnosed with the disease. Contact dermatitis is categorized into two types: irritant contact dermatitis, a nonallergic inflammation due to irritants such as poison ivy, and allergic contact dermatitis due to irritants such as detergents. Infants are less likely to develop allergic contact dermatitis, which has been attributed to their limited exposure to potential irritants. Atopic dermatitis refers to a group of skin inflammations that seem to result from a combination of genetic and environmental factors. One type of atopic dermatitis commonly seen in infants is seborrheic dermatitis or cradle cap, a condition of uncertain origin, which typically develops between the ages of 2 and 6 months. Sixty percent of children who develop dermatitis will do so by two years of age, with 90 percent developing the disease by 5 years of age. If a parent has dermatitis or any other predisposition toward development of hypersensitivity reactions against common environmental allergens, then there is a 50 percent chance that the child will also have the disease; however, as many as 30 percent of affected patients have no family members with the disease.

Psoriasis affects between 0.3 and 3 percent of the world's population and approximately 2.6 percent of the U.S. population. As with dermatitis, psoriasis can be diagnosed in childhood; however, the onset of this disease tends to occur later in life. The appearance of psoriasis usually occurs between 15 and 35 years of age, with the average age of diagnosis being 28 years of age. Psoriasis is rarely found in infants. Between 10 and 15 percent of those affected develop psoriasis before the age of 10 and nearly 40 percent develop the disease before age 20. The majority of those who develop psoriasis are Caucasian, and slightly more females than males are affected. Some studies have found that the disease develops earlier and more frequently in colder climates. Approximately 35 percent of persons diagnosed have one or more family members with psoriasis. Estimates of developing psoriasis in one's lifetime is 4 percent in someone with no affected family members, 28 percent in someone with one parent affected, and 68 percent in someone with both parents affected.

PSYCHOLOGICAL CORRELATES

Both psoriasis and dermatitis can have a considerable psychological and social impact on an affected person's life, especially when onset occurs at an early age. Those who experience prominent skin rashes or disease may feel inhibited and embarrassed, making social interactions awkward. Concerns about personal appearance, social rejection, embarrassment for self and family, and guilt may result in depression, anxiety, and social withdrawal. Research indicates that up to 75 percent of individuals with psoriasis may experience reduced self-confidence secondary to the disease, and 8 percent report feeling that their lives are not worth living.

Psychological and emotional stress can trigger onset or worsening of psoriasis and dermatitis flare-ups. Thus, one stressor may easily reinforce the other. With dermatitis, anger, frustration, and embarrassment may cause flushing and itching. Successfully coping with psychologically stressful events and controlling scratching behavior may avoid these stress-triggered flare-ups. Severe cases of psoriasis can be socially disabling and, in rare cases, life-threatening. Psoriasis patients have been found to be at higher risk for substance abuse and are more likely to die from substance abuse than from the disease itself. Some experts believe that heavy drinking and smoking may actually cause biological damage that contributes to the onset of psoriasis.

ETIOLOGY

The cause of dermatitis is not always known. For some forms of the disease, specifically contact dermatitis and neurodermatitis (chronic scaly inflammation of the skin that results in a scratch–itch cycle), the onset is attributed to environmental allergens or irritants such as poison ivy or tightly fitting clothing, whereas stasis dermatitis (itchy rash on lower legs due to poor blood circulation) results from poorly nourished skin secondary to fluid buildup in tissue beneath the skin. The etiology of other forms of dermatitis, such as atopic and seborrheic (resulting in excessive secretion of sebum), remains unclear. Atopic dermatitis is often associated with allergies such as asthma, nasal congestion, and hives, and appears to have a genetic component. Infantile seborrheic dermatitis may be due to gradually diminishing hormones passed from the mother to child prior to birth.

While the exact cause of psoriasis is unknown, environmental triggers of genetic abnormalities in the immune system are generally considered to be the origin of this disease. The immune system is believed to trigger an acceleration of the skin cell cycle. A psoriatic skin cell takes 3–4 days to mature as compared with the standard maturation time of 28–30 days for normal skin cells. The rapid movement of the psoriatic cells to the surface of the skin leads to cell pile up, forming elevated red lesions or plaques.

ASSESSMENT

Diagnosis of dermatitis and psoriasis is usually ascertained by physical examination of the affected area by a physician. Contact dermatitis is characterized by red, dry, and scaly areas with blisters and oozing. In infants, dermatitis is often found on the cheeks and at times on the scalp. As the child ages, the affected areas tend to shift to the arms, legs, chest, back, and in the folds of the arms and legs. Definitive diagnosis of allergic contact dermatitis, one form of contact dermatitis, requires patch testing. Atopic dermatitis is characterized by chronic itching of the affected area but no single symptom definitively distinguishes atopic dermatitis. Therefore, a skin scratch test may be given to rule out other diseases. Seborrheic dermatitis, commonly seen on the scalp and diaper area, is characterized by thick, yellowish scales that occur in patches on the scalp and is accompanied by redness and inflammation in other areas.

Accurate diagnosis of psoriasis can be difficult when symptoms are mild or atypical. Psoriasis most commonly develops as scaly patches or plaques on the scalp, knees, elbows, and torso. Other sites, thought less common, include the nails, palms, soles, genitals, and face. A strong indicator of psoriasis is the presence of small pits in the fingernails. The plaques with underlying inflammation can persist for extended periods of time but periodic flare-ups triggered by cold weather, infection, or stress are more common. In rare cases, a skin biopsy is required to make a definitive diagnosis of psoriasis or dermatitis and to distinguish it from other skin disorders such as fungal infections and drug allergic reactions. Microscopic examination of psoriasis shows excessive dry skin without indication of infection or inflammation.

TREATMENT

Treatment for dermatitis varies according to the etiology of the disease. The main focus of treatment for all forms of dermatitis is avoidance of allergens, specifically chemical irritants, in conjunction with antihistamines. Other lines of treatment for less severe forms include the use of topical emollients, topical antifungals, and topical glucocorticosteroids. Some forms of dermatitis can be treated with ultraviolet (UV) phototherapy.

There are several different types of treatment available for psoriasis, depending on response to treatment and severity of the disease. The first line of treatment is topical medicines, including corticosteroid ointments, vitamin D3 derived medicines, retinoids, and coal tar. Other topical treatments that offer relief but are less effective include bath solutions and moisturizers. The next line of treatment consists of light therapy, which uses different forms of UV light to reduce inflammation and slow skin cell overproduction. Daily, short exposures to natural sunlight may be beneficial to the treatment of psoriasis; however, artificial sunlight (UV phototherapy) is used in a more controlled setting, and can be used for both mild and more severe forms of psoriasis. The last form of medical treatment consists of systemic treatments, which are only used for more severe forms of psoriasis, and include medicines that are taken internally to suppress the immune system. Antibiotics may also be used when infection is indicated as the cause of an outbreak, but are less common.

Clinical studies support the perception that psychological stress can worsen psoriasis. Stress, unexpressed anger, depression, and anxiety are strongly associated with psoriasis flare-ups. Given the relationship between decreased emotional well-being and increased psoriatic symptoms, individuals who have this disease may benefit from psychological counseling. Scratching can also worsen psoriasis and dermatitis/eczema and become a conditioned response. Habit-reversal (i.e., closing hands for 3 min to prevent scratching when feeling itchy), relaxation training, and keeping a diary of stressful situations all have been found helpful in alleviating symptoms and identifying precipitants. For younger children, family/parental intervention to train and reinforce these intervention techniques is important as is monitoring parental responses to reduce secondary gains from differential attention to itching behavior.

PROGNOSIS

The prognosis of dermatitis is determined by the specific form of the disease. Contact dermatitis remediates with the removal or avoidance of the offending irritant or allergen. For children with atopic dermatitis, the prognosis is generally favorable with 90 percent resolution by adulthood. The majority of infants diagnosed with atopic dermatitis have fewer problems with the disease as they grow older. By adolescence, most children have minimal difficulty. A small number of the children will go on to develop a severe form of the disease in adulthood. Many of those affected with atopic dermatitis may have remissions that last for years but the tendency toward dry skin remains.

Psoriasis is an incurable chronic disease that requires continuous treatment. Between 10–30 percent of individuals diagnosed with the disease will also develop psoriatic arthritis, which causes inflammation and stiffness in the soft tissues around the joints. In severe cases, psoriatic arthritis can lead to disabling deterioration of the joints. Each year, approximately 400 people a year are significantly disabled by severe psoriasis and another 400 die from complications. The most serious complications due to the shedding of large areas of the skin include increased susceptibility to secondary infection, and fluid loss resulting in strain on the circulatory system.

See also: Behavior Therapy; Coping with Illness; Developmental Issues in Treatment; Habit Reversal; Psychomatic disorders

Further Reading

American Academy of Dermatology. (2002). Dermatitis, including atopic, contact, seborrheic, and stasis. Retrieved March 19, 2002 from http://www.aad.org/education/dermatitis.htm

Charman, D., & Horne, D. D. (1997). Atopic dermatitis. In A. Baum, S. Newman, J. Weinman, R. West, & C. McManus (Eds.), *Cambridge handbook of psychology, health and medicine* (pp. 372–375). Cambridge, UK: Cambridge University Press.

Larson, D. E. (Rev. ed.). (1996). *Mayo clinic family health book.* New York: William Morrow.

National Psoriasis Foundation. (2002). About psoriasis: Frequently asked questions. Retrieved March 19, 2002 from http://www.psoriasis.org/ b500.htm

DONNA MARSCHALL
SHANNON BECKER
JACFRANZ GUITEAU
MITRA SHAH-HOSSEINI
SMITHA SONNIS
CLARISSA S. HOLMES

Developmental Coordination Disorder

DEFINITION

Developmental Coordination Disorder (DCD) is diagnosed when a child has significant delays in motor coordination skills that interfere with academic achievement and/or activities of daily living and are not due to a diagnosable neurological, sensory, or cognitive deficit (*DSM-IV-TR*, 2000). If mental retardation is present, the motor deficits are greater than those usually associated with retardation alone. Although many different terms have been used to label the diagnosis, including minimal brain dysfunction, developmental dyspraxia, and clumsy child syndrome, as indicated by Dewey and Wilson (2001) DCD is now the recognized term used by most professionals.

Children with DCD can have neurological "soft" signs that may include abnormal reflexes, an awkwardness or poor quality of movement with motor tasks, hypotonia (i.e., low muscle tone), and delayed motor milestones. Learning Disabilities and/or Attention-Deficit/Hyperactivity Disorder are common in children with DCD.

DEVELOPMENTAL COURSE

DCD is not always identified in the first few years of life. Many children with DCD progress through major milestones within the typical timeframe, including learning to sit, walk, and run. Delays in coordination skills may become more apparent as the child approaches 3–4 years of age and should begin to develop more complex motor abilities. The 3–4 year old with DCD may have difficulty learning tasks that require sequencing, such as dressing or activities such as galloping or pedaling a tricycle. Children with DCD often have deficits in motor planning skills that can make it difficult for them to move through a room without bumping into furniture or other people and falling out of or missing a chair when attempting to sit down.

The school-age child with DCD may need more frequent repetition to learn new motor skills, and even after mastering a skill under specific circumstances may not be able to generalize this skill to another situation. For example, the child may learn how to climb on a particular piece of playground equipment at school but is not able to generalize this skill to climb on a different piece of equipment when going to the park with family. Children may also have difficulty with fine motor skills, such as cutting, coloring, handwriting, building with blocks, or managing tools such as getting a pencil out of their pencil box. Due to these difficulties, the child may have difficulty keeping up in the classroom. Children and adolescents with DCD may also find it difficult to keep up with peers in active play or sports activities, and their coordination disorder may have social consequences.

ASSESSMENT

Children with suspected DCD are typically referred to a pediatric occupational therapist or physical therapist. A pediatric occupational therapist has expertise in fine motor development, including using the hands to play with toys, manage tools such as scissors and pencils, and in self-help skills such as eating, dressing, and bathing. Occupational therapists also have expertise in visual–motor development and visual–perceptual development.

A pediatric physical therapist has expertise in gross motor development, including skills that require coordination, strength, and balance. Such activities often include walking, riding a bicycle, climbing on playground equipment, or ball skills.

The assessment should begin with an interview of the parent, and child if appropriate, to identify specific areas of concern. If the child is of school age, the teacher and other educational staff who are familiar with the child should also provide information about the child's current functional abilities and concerns about the child's performance in the educational setting. Based on information gathered from the parent, caregivers, teachers, and child, the therapist can make decisions about how to proceed with the evaluation. If possible, the child should be observed in the natural environment participating in typical daily activities. This may include observation of the child playing at home, playing at the park, in the classroom, in physical education class, or at recess playing with peers. If the therapist is unable to observe the child in these environments, it may be helpful to have the parent videotape the child at home and/or at school. In these settings, the therapist will observe what activities the child is able to do, the quality of movement when performing specific motor skills, and the activities the child has difficulty performing or appears to avoid.

In addition to observation, standardized tests are often used to assist in diagnosing DCD. The Bruininks–Oseretsky Test of Motor Proficiency (BOTMP) and Movement Assessment Battery for Children (M-ABC) are two of the more commonly used tools for assessing motor skills in children (Table 1).

The therapist also assesses muscle strength and flexibility, balance, and quality of movement to determine the extent of the child's motor deficits and to qualify how these deficits may be affecting functional motor skills.

In addition to an occupational therapy and/or physical therapy evaluation, an evaluation by a neurologist, speech–language pathologist, or psychologist may also be needed.

Table 1. Tests Commonly Used to Assist in Identification of Developmental Coordination Disorder

Name of test	Type	Age range	Description
Bruininks–Oseretsky Test of Motor Proficiency	Standardized	4.5–14.5 years	Contains 46 items including gross motor and fine motor composite
Movement Assessment Battery for Children	Standardized	4–12 years	Contains 8 tasks for each of 4 different age groups

TREATMENT

The first step in intervention is identification of the child's functional limitations and identification of the outcomes for the therapy intervention. The family, child, and teacher for the school-age child should all be included in development of the specific outcomes. A variety of treatment approaches have been used when working with children with DCD to improve their motor skills. As noted by Mandich and colleagues (2001), some of the more common approaches include sensory integration therapy, process-oriented treatment, perceptual motor training, and a combination of these approaches. More recent approaches to treatment for children with DCD include task-oriented approaches and cognitive approaches.

In addition to working with the child to improve her or his motor skills, therapy should also include providing information about the child's motor delays and helping parents and teachers understand how these delays may affect the child's daily life. Longitudinal studies conducted by Losse and colleagues (1991) have shown that motor coordination problems continue to be present in adolescence, even for children who received intervention as a young child. Therefore, it is important to also work with the family and teachers to modify activities as needed to help the child or adolescent become more independent and to help the child find areas of strength and activities in which he or she can feel a sense of mastery or success.

See also: Attention-Deficit/Hyperactivity Disorder; Language Disorders; Learning Disorders; Motor Development; Visual–Motor Assessment

Further Reading

American Psychiatric Association. (2000). *Diagnostic and statistical manual of mental Disorders—DSM-IV-TR.* Washington, DC: Author.

Dewey, D., & Wilson, B. N. (2001). Developmental coordination disorder: What is it? *Physical and Occupational Therapy for Children, 20*(2–3), 5–27.

Losse, A., Henderson, S. E., Ellimna, D., Hall, D., Knight, E., & Jongmans, M. (1991). Clumsiness in children—do they grow out of it? A 10-year follow up study. *Developmental Medicine and Child Neurology, 33*, 55–68.

Mandich, A. D., Polatajko, H. J., Macnab, J. J., & Miller, L. T. (2001). Treatment of children with developmental coordination disorder: What is the evidence? *Physical and Occupational Therapy for Children, 20*(2–3), 51–68.

Missiuna, C. (2001). *Children with developmental coordination disorder: Strategies for success.* New York: Haworth Press.

RENE MARIE DAMAN

Developmental Issues in Assessment for Treatment

Developmental issues are an essential consideration in the assessment of child psychopathology. Identifying child psychopathology depends largely on comparisons of child symptoms and behaviors with the behaviors of children at the same mental and chronological age. Children's physical, cognitive, social, and emotional development change so rapidly that behaviors that are normal and expected at one age can be abnormal and symptomatic at the next. For example, a child who is not potty-trained at age 2 would not raise concern, whereas at age 5, it would be a significant problem. Thus, age appropriateness is a primary developmental consideration in the assessment of children, and problem behaviors, by definition, depend on the age of the child.

The assessment of child psychopathology also requires consideration of the age of onset and the chronicity of symptoms. The significance of a symptom may be markedly different if it occurs as an acute reaction to a recent event as opposed to a longstanding behavioral characteristic. Symptoms with early onset and long duration may be particularly resistant to treatment and may require longer treatment and follow-up. Thus, assessment of the severity of psychopathology requires careful consideration of the problem behaviors in relation to the child's age and developmental history.

Because historical information, typically obtained by clinical interview, is necessarily imprecise, information about current symptoms and behaviors is weighed more heavily in assessment decision-making to identify child psychopathology for treatment planning. Current information is relied on exclusively in assessment and decision-making about symptom and behavior changes that result from treatment. Children are evaluated in comparison to children of the same age to provide an estimate of their deviation from the typical or normal developmental path for the constellation of behaviors that are being measured. The traditional methods of measuring children's behavior include parent and teacher rating scales, child self-report measures, and behavioral observations.

Among these methods, parent and teacher rating scales are the most common. Rating scales provide the most easily accessible data for behaviors that may be infrequent or not readily observable, such as lying. They can also provide a more accurate (i.e., valid) picture than self-report measures of disruptive behaviors in young children because young children's behavior is frequently highly salient to the informant. Developmental changes in children's behavior, however, complicate selection of measures. For example, if a rating scale contains age-specific items, or if its standardization resulted in the use of different items at different ages, the scale might function essentially as a different test at each age level in which item content or meaning differs. This situation poses significant problems for therapists intending to evaluate the child's progress over time if the test used at the beginning of treatment is not standardized for children at the time of the later assessment.

Self-report measures are important for assessing the unobservable thoughts and feelings of children. Although it was once believed that preschoolers were not able to recognize or report their emotions reliably due to limited cognitive abilities, researchers have begun to develop age-sensitive measures that result in reliable scores. An example is the "feeling thermometer," a picture depicting different levels of an emotion such as "afraid," which allows young children to point to the level that they feel. Child assessment researchers have also explored the best informant for rating children's problems across the developmental spectrum. Considering age alone, the best informant for a preschooler is typically the primary caregiver. For the school-age child, the best informants may be the parent, teacher, or child, and for a teenager, the best informant is the parent or teenager.

Behavioral observation is the most objective assessment method, with the ability to measure qualities of social interactions that are not validly captured by either rating scales or self-report measures. Comprehensive observational systems, such as the Dyadic Parent–Child Interaction Coding System II, have been developed and standardized for use in both research and clinical practice settings. Observational assessment methods have minimal bias because they do not rely on retrospective recall of children's (or parents') behaviors or the perceptions of informants who may be affected by the problems of the child. They are not easily standardized across ages, however, due to rapid changes in the form and content of children's problem behaviors. Noncompliance, for example, might be measured by coding a young child's response to toy clean-up directions, but like age-inappropriate rating scale items, this situation would not provide a valid test of noncompliance for teenagers.

In summary, developmental considerations are paramount throughout the process of assessment for treatment planning. Measurement methods and instruments must be selected with careful attention to the psychometric properties that support their use for quantifying the current degree of deviation from the normal developmental course and for anticipating future assessment needs. Just as the therapist must consider the child's developmental history when formulating the assessment questions, he or she must also consider whether the current assessment measures need to serve as baseline measures for evaluating future change and, if so, whether the measures have the relevant standardization sample norms for use at the time (age) when the comparisons will need to be made.

See also: Behavior Rating Scales; Behavioral Observation; Child Self-Reports; Developmental Issues in Treatment

Further Reading

Campbell, S. B. (1998). Developmental perspectives. In T. H. Ollendick & M. Hersen (Eds.), *Handbook of child psychopathology* (3rd ed., pp. 3–35). New York: Plenum.

Eyberg, S. M., Schuhmann, E., & Rey, J. (1988). Child and adolescent psychotherapy research: Developmental issues. *Journal of Abnormal Child Psychology, 26,* 71–82.

Eyberg, S. M. (1992). Assessing therapy outcome with preschool children: Progress and problems. *Journal of Clinical Child Psychology, 21,* 306–311.

DANIEL M. BAGNER
SHEILA M. EYBERG

Developmental Issues in Treatment

Consideration of developmental issues is essential for providing optimal treatment to children. Historically, psychological treatments for children have involved downward extensions of interventions used with adults. This practice has resulted in interventions that became successively less appropriate for use with younger children. An increased focus on developmental factors that influence treatment outcome should lead to interventions that are more effective with children. Although age is the most commonly used measure of development, the child's cognitive, emotional, and social development all need to be taken into consideration when selecting an optimal treatment. Developmental factors influence both the procedures used in treatment and the specified goals of intervention.

Preschool-age children are limited in their abilities to understand and verbalize their thoughts and feelings. For this reason, treatment commonly involves either play therapy or parent training to alter parenting style and discipline methods. Effective treatments for young children are increasingly combining these approaches, teaching play therapy skills to parents as one component of treatment to enhance the parent–child relationship and to produce more lasting behavior change. Young children typically express internal distress through their overt behavior, and interventions that seek to change behavior directly are most effective with this age group. By reducing the frequency of symptomatic behaviors in young children to within normal limits, the course of psychopathology is altered, and the child's later functioning in all domains of development is affected.

School-age children have typically developed the necessary cognitive ability and verbal skills to talk about their problems, and they can provide increasingly introspective accounts of their thoughts and feelings within psychotherapy. Further, as they develop insight into their thoughts and feelings, change in their cognitions becomes an appropriate treatment goal in itself. Children often have difficulty determining the motivation for their behavior, however, and until later childhood or adolescence, a continued focus on the direct consequences of their behavior, as opposed to the reasons for their behavior, may be most effective. In addition, parent training continues to be useful with older children, not only to teach behavior management skills but also to address parent–child relationship

issues and teach communication skills. With their increasing ability to understand the perspective of others and the longer-term consequences of their behavior, school-age children are able to use problem-solving methods successfully during cognitive–behavioral therapies.

Children's social development is not only a goal of many treatments, but it also must be considered in selecting the treatment approach and in designing the child's treatment. Children's social development determines the relative influence that different individuals have on them. As preschoolers, children's primary caregivers have the predominant influence on their thoughts, emotions, and behavior and are, therefore, the most effective agents of change. As children enter school, teachers become an additional source of influence and may play a significant role in implementing treatments both in preschool and elementary school settings. Throughout a child's social development, their peers are increasingly influential, and treatments that incorporate a positive peer group may be of particular value during adolescence.

In all treatment approaches with children, the specific techniques that are used must be tailored to the cognitive, emotional, and social development of the child. All treatments involve verbal communication with the child, either directly by the therapist or indirectly by teaching another change agent to communicate in specific ways with the child. Age-appropriate communication is fundamental, and begins with the specific vocabulary and sentence structure that are used in treatment. They must be adjusted to fit the child's receptive language ability to ensure that the child can comprehend the intervention. Children will not usually tell the therapist if they cannot understand the message, and misunderstandings can arise from many sources. Words above a sixth grade reading level, psychological jargon, and words describing emotions other than "mad," "sad," "scared," and "happy" should be used with care. If these words are important to treatment, the clinician must specifically assess the child's understanding and teach the meaning of unfamiliar words. The clinician must also be familiar with the "jargon" of children, including the current media heroes and popular collectibles, at different stages of development.

In the same way that the language of therapy is guided by knowledge of the child's developmental level, the specific techniques used in various treatments must also be tailored directly to the child's developmental level. For example, in behavioral treatments, young children are more responsive to immediate consequences for their behavior whereas older children have the cognitive capacity to respond to delayed consequences. Older children are also able to play a more direct role in the delivery of consequences through the use of self-monitoring and self-reinforcement practices.

In summary, children's cognitive, emotional, and social development influence every treatment decision that must be made. Children's progress is uneven across the dimensions of development, and a thorough understanding of normal child development in each dimension is essential for clinicians working with children. Knowledge of child development guides the determination of appropriate treatment goals and the design of effective interventions. It guides the selection of change agents, the specific techniques and their application, and the targets selected for change. Examination of the developmental issues in treatment provides the framework for effective interventions for children.

See also: Cognitive Development; Developmental Issues in Assessment for Treatment; Developmentally Based Psychotherapy; Emotional Development; Evidence-Based Treatments; Social Development in Adolescence; Social Development in Childhood

Further Reading

Campbell, S. B. (1998). Developmental perspectives. In T. H. Ollendick & M. Hersen (Eds.), *Handbook of child psychopathology* (3rd ed., pp. 3–35). New York: Plenum.

Eyberg, S. M., Schuhmann, E. M., & Rey, J. (1998). Child and adolescent psychotherapy research: Developmental issues. *Journal of Abnormal Child Psychology, 26*(1), 71–82.

Harter, S. (1983). Cognitive-developmental considerations in the conduct of play therapy. In C. E. Schaefer & K. J. O'Connor (Eds.), *Handbook of play therapy* (pp. 95–127). New York: Wiley.

Querido, J. G., Eyberg, S. M., Kanfer, R., & Krahn, G. (2001). The process of the clinical child assessment interview. In C. E. Walker & M. C. Roberts (Eds.), *Handbook of clinical child psychology* (3rd ed.). New York: Wiley.

MICHELLE D. HARWOOD
SHEILA M. EYBERG

Developmental Milestones

Developmental milestones refer to the normative ages at which infants and children attain or acquire certain skills and abilities. The use of milestones in development derives from the "normative approach" in developmental psychology that was championed early on by Arnold Gesell in his longitudinal studies of child development. Reasoning in this approach assumes that development occurs in regular and predictable sequences, with relative invariance in ages of attainment. As such, it should be possible to assess the relative normality of an individual child's development by noting with care if the child attained skills and abilities on the proper developmental schedule. In many cases, these milestones were used as a means to compute the "age-equivalent" status of the individual child, much as the computation of mental age gave rise to the intelligent quotient (IQ).

QUANTIFICATION OF MILESTONES

Most commonly, the average age is usually used as the norm for developmental milestones, although it is important to note that what is considered "normal" for any particular ability always falls within a range of ages. For example, the average age for walking is 12 months, but the normal age range for the onset of walking is anytime between 9 and 17 months. Likewise, there are also intra-individual differences in attaining certain skills and abilities, so that a child could be above the norm in one area (e.g., language) and delayed in another area (e.g., motor development).

Norms are important as they provide a reference point by which to assess individual development, and so early measures of development (such as the Bayley Scales of Infant Development and the Denver Developmental Screening Test) have used developmental milestones to assess the developmental status of infants and toddlers. These assessments are often used by researchers and clinicians to quantify an individual's development, in order to identify those children that may have or be at risk for a developmental delay and benefit from early intervention.

CLINICAL RELEVANCE

Extreme delays in or a complete lack of attaining a particular milestone, or the disappearance of a previously acquired ability (e.g., talking) is often the first indicator a researcher or clinician has that an infant or child may have a developmental problem or disorder. The most commonly used milestones for diagnosing various childhood clinical disorders tend to be those associated with motor, language, and social development (see Table 1). Several childhood disorders listed in the *Diagnostic and Statistical Manual of Mental Disorders* of the American Psychiatric Association list severe delays in attaining milestones as potential criteria for diagnosing a

Table 1. Common Motor, Language, and Social Developmental Milestones

Age (in months)	Motor	Language/Communication	Social
Birth	Reflexive grasp	Cries	Reacts to other people
1	Lifts chin while lying on stomach	Coos (vowel sounds)	
2	Holds head erect when held upright; rolls from side to back		Smiles in response to others
3	Lifts head and chest while lying on stomach; reaches with two hands		Smiles spontaneously
4	Sits with support		"Social" smile
5	Rolls from back to side	Unstructured babbling ("variegated" e.g., goo-da-ga-ba-ma)	
6	Pulls self to sitting position; reaches with one hand		
7	Rolls from back to stomach; sits without support	Structured babbling ("canonical" e.g., babababa)	Plays peek-a-boo
8	Stands with help; creeps (arms pulling body and legs)		
9	Stands holding onto furniture	Imitates speech inflections (prosody)	Begins to fear strangers; takes initiative in contact with others
10	Pulls self up to standing position; crawls (arms and legs alternate)	Uses gestures to make wants known; responds to simple commands	
11	Walks with help; stands alone	Imitation of word sounds (no meaning)	
12	Walks a few steps alone; lowers self from standing to sitting; crawls up and down stairs	Acquisition of first word; one word is used to convey a sentence ("holophrasic" e.g., "ball" = "I want the ball")	Use information about others' emotional expressions to regulate own behavior ("social referencing"); plays pat-a-cake
15	Walks well alone		
18	Runs awkwardly	Vocabulary increases rapidly; easily imitates words heard	Able to recognize self in mirror
19		Begins to combine 2–3 words ("telegraphic" e.g., "Mama up" = "Mama, pick me up")	
23		Uses pronouns (e.g., "mine")	
24	Runs well; walks up and down stairs alone	Uses 4–5 word sentences	Aggression begins to appear; plays alongside other children
36	Can walk on tiptoe, hop on both feet	Uses rule-based/grammar	Interacts with other children during play

particular disorder including autism, developmental coordination disorder, and various communication disorders.

See also: Cognitive Development; Emotional Development; Identity Development; Infancy; Language Development; Memory Development; Moral Development; Motor Development; Perceptual Development

Further Reading

Berns, R. M. (1994). *Topical child development.* Albany, NY: Delmar.

Shaffer, D. R. (2002). *Developmental psychology: Childhood and adolescence* (6th ed.). Belmont, CA: Wadsworth.

Vasta, R., Haith, M. M., & Miller, S. A. (1998). *Child psychology: The modern science* (3rd ed.). New York: Wiley.

D. Jill Shaddy
John Colombo

Developmental Screening

See: Screening Instruments: Behavioral and Developmental

Developmentally Based Psychotherapy

DEFINITION

Although consideration of developmental factors in child and adolescent treatment has a long history (e.g., see the work of Anna Freud [1965]), the emergence of developmental psychopathology as a discipline has underscored the importance of developmental processes for both the development and treatment of child and adolescent psychopathology. As noted by Shirk (1988), a basic assumption of this general approach is that therapeutic change is embedded in a broader class of change processes termed developmental. Interventions aimed at changing thoughts, emotions, or behaviors in children and adolescents occur in a developmental context. Thus, the impact of specific interventions may be constrained or facilitated by developmental processes. Developmentally based psychotherapy, then, does not correspond to a particular type of treatment such as cognitive–behavioral or client-centered therapy, but rather to an orientation that takes developmental processes into consideration in the design and delivery of treatment interventions.

DEVELOPMENTAL FACTORS IN TREATMENT

Three broad types of developmental factors have been considered in relation to child and adolescent treatment: cognitive processes, motivational processes, and family processes. Many child and adolescent interventions involve cognitively based treatment tasks. For example, a central task in cognitive–behavioral therapy (CBT) involves the identification of thoughts that co-occur with feelings. The capacity for self-monitoring and reflecting on cognitions varies across the course of development. Consequently, younger children may lack the conceptual platform for engaging in this task, whereas cognitive growth in late childhood facilitates

self-monitoring. With regard to motivation, children and adolescents rarely refer themselves for treatment. Thus, in contrast to adult treatment, motivation for therapy may be compromised. From a developmental perspective, this means that therapists must attend to processes, for example, the identification of the child's own goals for therapy, that facilitate engagement. These processes themselves may vary with development, for example, a small reward system can be very useful in promoting engagement with younger children, whereas contracts may be more effective with adolescents. Finally, the role of the family in treatment varies with development. For example, with younger children, behavior management training aimed principally at changing parent behavior can be very effective, however given the press toward autonomy and reciprocity in adolescence, interventions that promote communication and negotiation skills for parents and adolescents together may be a better developmental fit. As these examples indicate, treatment interventions are selected and implemented based on developmental factors.

Weisz and Hawley (2002) proposed that developmental research can be used to inform therapists in three ways: *alerting* therapists to issues for which they should be vigilant, *weighing and prioritizing* intervention targets, and *selecting candidate interventions*. With regard to alerting, knowledge of developmental trends heightens awareness of both opportunities and potential perils faced by children of different ages, for example, the emergence of heightened self-consciousness in early adolescence. Awareness of developmental trends can also help therapists to evaluate, weigh, and prioritize particular presenting problems. For example, which among a set of problems is likely to resolve over time because of its normative nature (increase parent–teen bickering), and which represent real developmental hazards (association with older peers). Finally, consistent with previous examples, developmental level intersects with specific treatment tasks such that some tasks may exceed children's capacities.

EVIDENCE FOR DEVELOPMENTAL MODERATORS OF OUTCOME

There is growing evidence that the effectiveness of broad types of treatment is moderated by developmental level, though virtually all of the existing reviews have relied on chronological age as a proxy for development. The most recent analysis of child and adolescent treatment revealed a somewhat larger effect, across all treatments, for adolescents than children.

In particular, samples with more adolescent females showed better outcomes than other groups. Reviews that have examined age-related differences for specific types of treatment have found that older children tend to benefit more from cognitive–behavioral therapy than younger children, as noted by Durlak and colleagues but that younger children benefited more from behavior management therapy than older children. Although these results are consistent with the expectation that the cognitive demands of cognitive–behavioral therapy may exceed the capacities of younger children, studies that directly assess developmental moderators (other than age), are currently rare in the literature.

See also: Child Psychotherapy; Cognitive–Behavior Therapy; Evidence-Based Treatments; Group Psychotherapy

Further Reading

Durlak, J., Fuhrman, T., & Lampman, C. (1991). Effectiveness of cognitive–behavioral therapy for maladapting youth: A meta-analysis. *Psychological Bulletin, 110*, 204–214.

Freud, A. (1965). *Normality and pathology in development*. New York: International Universities Press.

Shirk, S. (1988). *Cognitive development and child psychotherapy*. New York: Plenum.

Weisz, J., & Hawley, K. (2002). Developmental factors in the treatment of adolescents. *Journal of Consulting and Clinical Psychology, 70*, 21–43.

STEPHEN R. SHIRK

Diabetes Mellitus, Type 1

DESCRIPTION AND INCIDENCE

Insulin-dependent (or Type 1) diabetes mellitus (IDDM) is a chronic disease in which the pancreas produces insufficient quantities of the hormone insulin. Insulin regulates the level of glucose (sugar) in the bloodstream by allowing glucose to pass from the bloodstream into cells where it can be broken down and used for energy. Complete failure of the pancreas is characteristic of type 1 diabetes, therefore requiring daily injections of insulin replacement for survival. IDDM differs from type 2 diabetes (or non-insulin-dependent diabetes mellitus, NIDDM). Although individuals with NIDDM continue to produce insulin, the amount available is inadequate to maintain normal blood glucose levels.

Key to the therapeutic goals for IDDM is regulation of blood glucose levels within the normal range. The ideal range for blood glucose levels is between 80 and 120 mg/dl (mg/dl refers to the milligrams of glucose per 100 milliliters of blood). After eating, blood glucose levels can rise to 180 mg/dl. Glucose levels above 180 mg/dl are considered hyperglycemia whereas insulin levels below 70 mg/dl are considered hypoglycemia. Excessive thirst and/or hunger, frequent urination, unusual weight loss, extreme fatigue, irritability, nausea and sweet smelling breath are symptomatic of a hyperglycemic episode. Pronounced hypoglycemia can be associated with seizures, coma, and even death if left untreated because of inadequate concentration of blood glucose to support brain function.

The worldwide incidence of IDDM ranges from 0.6 to 2.5/1,000 children. Incidence in the United States is approximately 1/600 children. This rate is lower than those of Scandinavian countries, equivalent to those in non-Scandinavian and European countries, and higher than those of Asian countries. IDDM occurs equally in males and females. In the United States, incidence is approximately 1.5 times greater in White males than in non-White males. Peak incidence occurs at puberty.

ETIOLOGY

A general cause of IDDM is not known. However, genetic inheritance constitutes a risk factor for its development. Injury to the pancreas caused by viruses may also contribute to disease onset. Destruction of cells in the pancreas that produce insulin may be the result of an autoimmune process in which the immune system produces antibodies which attacks cells or tissues of the organism producing them.

ASSOCIATED COGNITIVE AND OTHER PSYCHOLOGICAL FEATURES

IDDM, in particular an early onset of the condition, is associated with increased risk for learning disabilities. Lower Performance and Full Scale IQ scores are associated with an age of onset prior to 5 years. Academic achievement is also affected more by earlier onset. Arithmetic is less affected than Spelling or Reading. In contrast, lower Verbal IQ scores are associated with onset of diabetes at an older age. Specific neurocognitive deficits in children with IDDM consist of problems of visuospatial processing, verbal ability, visuomotor skill, memory, and attention. These problems may not be apparent, however, until years after the onset of the condition. Visuospatial impairments (one aspect of performance IQ) are usually associated with early onset (prior to age 5) or repeated instances of hypoglycemic seizures in childhood. Verbal deficits are associated with onset of the disease in later childhood.

Mild anxiety and depression can be observed shortly after diagnosis and fade within a 6-month period. Initial emotional response to the diagnosis can predict psychological adaptation for up to 6 years. In contrast to children, depression appears to be more prevalent in adults with IDDM and is also associated with poor glycemic (i.e., blood sugar) control and more severe physical complications (e.g., deterioration of the retina and vision).

Hypoglycemic episodes, which can involve shaking, sweating, and loss of consciousness, can be potentially embarrassing and may have implications for certain types of employment and other activities (e.g., driving) in adolescence and beyond. Extreme fear of hypoglycemic episodes may lead patients to consciously attempt to remain hyperglycemic, placing themselves at risk for long-term complications.

Because the physical symptoms of intense anxiety (e.g., palpitations and sweating) are sometimes observed during episodes of poor glycemic control, it may at times be difficult to distinguish between the two. The diagnosis of an anxiety disorder usually occurs when emotional and behavioral symptoms (e.g., obsessions, compulsions, persistent fears) dominate over physical symptoms, and occur during periods of adequate glycemic control.

Increased risk for eating disorders (such as anorexia nervosa and bulimia nervosa) during adolescence and adulthood may be associated with IDDM (especially in females). Multiple studies have shown that 30–40 percent of adolescent females with diabetes use insulin manipulation as a means of losing weight. Reducing the dose or skipping insulin injections promotes weight loss. Eating disorders may be hard to distinguish from gastroparesis (dilation of the stomach with gastric retention) when vomiting and weight loss occur. Therefore, such disorders may be difficult to diagnose.

TREATMENT

Two types of insulin (short acting and intermediate acting) are typically used in combination to regulate glucose levels. Injections are administered once or twice daily, usually before breakfast and dinner. Glucose levels can be measured by using computerized glucose meters or reagent strips which change color in response to glucose level. Diet and meal planning are also important in glucose regulation. Meals and snacks must be coordinated with the time and amount of insulin injections. The insulin pump can be used instead of injections to regulate blood glucose levels. The pump delivers small amounts of insulin continuously into the bloodstream to maintain a "basal" level of insulin. When food is consumed, whether it is a meal or a snack, the pump can be programmed to release more insulin (bolus). Basal and bolus rates are established by patients and health care providers in the initial stages of pump treatment and can be adjusted to meet the body's changing needs. This method of treatment allows patients to lead a more relaxed lifestyle without strictly regimented meal planning.

Because physical exercise lowers blood glucose by enhancing the utilization of insulin, it is a particularly important lifestyle component for individuals with IDDM. However, excessive exercise without the consumption of sufficient calories may lead to hypoglycemia. Consumption of carbohydrates prior to exercise helps avoid hypoglycemia.

Psychological stress and physical illness can impede insulin action and lead to hyperglycemia. Relaxation training is a common intervention method used to help patients control psychological stress. It is important to note that the effects of stress vary across individuals. While psychological stress may induce hyperglycemia in one person, another may be unaffected.

Strong adherence to the varied aspects of the diabetes treatment regimen is extremely important in order to minimize the long-term medical complications. However, good adherence does not guarantee adequate glycemic control. Knowledge of the disease, child psychosocial adaptation, and family environment can play an important role in treatment adherence. Adolescents with IDDM are known to be less adherent than younger children with IDDM, even though they have a greater knowledge of the disease. Adolescents may be overwhelmed when tasks of adherence to a diabetes regimen are joined with the normal demands of the adolescents' transition into adulthood (dealing with changing body image, new cognitive abilities, forming new peer and intimate relationships, establishing a sense of independence, etc.). This conflict may be associated with poorer adherence during adolescence.

Although good adherence is important, it can sometimes encumber the individual's quality of life.

Those aspects of the diabetes regimen that have a direct effect on a patient's lifestyle are likely to be those that are most associated with poorer adherence. The general Health Belief Model (HBM), comprising several distinct components, has been employed to account for variability in adherence to therapeutic regimens. First is the concept of susceptibility, or the belief that the individual is vulnerable to a disease and its consequences. Second is seriousness, or how intensely the disease is perceived to negatively impact the individual's life. Third is the belief that a certain treatment regimen will be effective in reducing the severity of the disease. The fourth is the belief that the *costs* (psychological, physical, or economic) associated with the treatment will be outweighed by the benefits. The fifth is self-efficacy, or the belief that the individual is capable of carrying out the treatment regimen without difficulty. Self-efficacy and the belief that the treatment will reduce severity of the disease show the strongest association with adherence in adolescents with IDDM. If an adolescent with IDDM believes that he/she can actually carry out the tasks associated with treatment, and that completing these tasks will help avoid complications, then they are more likely to adhere to the treatment.

Psychosocial interventions, alone or in combination with psychotropic medication, can be employed to treat depression in individuals with IDDM. However, special caution needs to be exercised in prescribing psychotropic medication that stimulates appetite and may contribute to hyperglycemia. Also, certain serotonin-reuptake inhibitors can potentiate insulin action and suppress appetite leading to hypoglycemic episodes. Other interventions, such as psychotherapy groups, self-help consumer support groups, and "diabetes camps" can serve to facilitate the adaptive coping of children (and their families) faced with the developmental challenges associated with diabetes. These interventions are often aimed at enhancing social skills, in particular, assertive behavior, which can be used as effective coping techniques in interpersonal situations related to diabetes.

PROGNOSIS

Long-term complications of diabetes can include eye problems (such as cataracts and blindness), kidney disease, heart attack, stroke, numbness, and/or pain in legs, and increased infections (especially of skin, upper and lower extremities, legs, and feet). These poor outcomes are associated with prolonged poor glycemic control. Increased depression in adults occurs with onset of long-term complications. Regulation of blood sugar through insulin injections, diet, and exercise can allow IDDM patients to live a relatively normal life.

SUPPORT/CONSUMER GROUPS

American Diabetes Association, 1660 Duke Street, Alexandria, VA 22314, (800) 232-3472, www.diabetes.org; Juvenile Diabetes Research Foundation International, 120 Wall Street, New York, NY 10005-4001, (800) 533-2873, www.jdfcure.org

See also: Coping with Illness; Diabetes Mellitus, Type 2; Hypoglycemia; Parenting the Chronically Ill Child; Treatment Adherence: Medical

Further Reading

Bond, G., Aiken, L., & Somerville, S. (1992). The Health Belief Model and adolescents with insulin-dependent diabetes mellitus. *Health Psychology, 11*, 190–198.

Jacobson, A. (1996). The psychological care of patients with insulin-dependent diabetes mellitus. *The New England Journal of Medicine, 334*, 1249–1253.

Johnson, S. (1995). Insulin-dependent diabetes mellitus in childhood. In M. C. Roberts (Ed.), *Handbook of pediatric psychology* (pp. 263–285). New York: Guilford.

Rovet, J., Ehrlich, R., Czuchta, D., & Akler, M. (1993). Psychoeducational characteristics of children and adolescents with insulin-dependent diabetes mellitus. *Journal of Learning Disabilities, 26*, 7–22.

Rubin, R., & Peyrot, M. (1992). Psychosocial problems and interventions in diabetes. *Diabetes Care, 15*, 1640–1657.

TERESA WIECH
DAVID E. SANDBERG

Diabetes Mellitus, Type 2

DEFINITION

Type 2 diabetes mellitus is one of several types of disorders characterized by high blood glucose, including type 1 diabetes, gestational diabetes mellitus, and diabetes secondary to other conditions. In type 2 diabetes, high blood glucose is the result of the pancreas producing insufficient quantities of the hormone insulin, as well as insulin resistance. In contrast, in type 1 diabetes there is an eventual absolute deficiency of insulin production, due to an autoimmune process resulting in destruction of the insulin-producing beta cells. Insulin regulates the level of glucose in the blood by allowing glucose to pass from the blood into cells where it can be broken down and used for energy. The symptoms of type 2 diabetes include high blood glucose, and associated excessive thirst, urination, and hunger.

ETIOLOGY

Type 2 diabetes, formerly referred to as non-insulin-dependent diabetes mellitus or adult-onset diabetes, is thought to result from a combination of insulin resistance and beta-cell dysfunction. Peripheral insulin resistance, in which cells resist the action of insulin at the receptor level, occurs early in the disease course. This is initially compensated for by increased production of insulin, or hyperinsulinemia. Over time, insulin secretion declines, and hyperglycemia results (high blood glucose). There is no single cause of type 2 diabetes, although it is generally believed to be the result of genetic, physiologic, and lifestyle factors, including obesity and physical inactivity.

INCIDENCE/PREVALENCE

A dramatic increase in the incidence of type 2 diabetes has been documented in recent years, even among children. Previously, only 1–2 percent of children with diabetes were classified as having type 2 diabetes; however, according to the American Diabetes Association, this incidence has more recently increased to 8–45 percent. In one study conducted in Ohio, the number of patients in the age range of 10–19-years old who were diagnosed with type 2 diabetes increased tenfold between 1982 and 1995, and accounted for 33 percent of all newly diagnosed cases. In addition to studies reporting increases in Ohio and California, the ADA reported increases in the incidence of pediatric type 2 diabetes among children in Pennsylvania, Chicago, Tokyo, Bangladesh, Libya, and specifically, among aboriginal populations in Australia and Canada, as well as among the Pima Indians, where the prevalence is highest. Epidemiologic studies reviewed by Fagot-Campagna and colleagues (2000) suggest that type 2 diabetes in children has an incidence of 1–50/1,000, depending upon the ethnic group surveyed. For example, among 15–19-year- old North American Indians, the prevalence per 1000 has been estimated as 51 for Pima Indians, 4.5 for all U.S.

American Indians, and 2.3 for First Nation peoples (Canadian Indians). From 1967–1976 to 1987–1996, the prevalence of type 2 diabetes has increased sixfold for Pima Indian adolescents. The mean age at diagnosis for new pediatric cases of type 2 diabetes is 13 years.

RISK FACTORS

Research indicates that genetic, behavioral, and environmental factors may increase risk for type 2 diabetes. The increase in incidence of type 2 diabetes in children has been paralleled by an increase in the incidence of pediatric obesity across all ethnic, age, and gender groups. It is currently estimated that 25 percent of children are overweight, with higher incidences reported in minority children. Although genetic factors play an important role in the increased incidence of type 2 diabetes, the fact that the prevalence of childhood obesity has increased over the last two decades suggests a greater impact of environmental factors. Childhood obesity may be the mediating factor between a predisposition for type 2 diabetes and development of the disease. Studies have shown that obesity and a positive family history of type 2 diabetes are nearly always present in children and adolescents with type 2 diabetes, with 85 percent of children with type 2 diabetes being either overweight or obese at diagnosis. A study that compared characteristics of type 1 diabetes to type 2 diabetes found 96 percent of children with type 2 diabetes were overweight or obese as opposed to only 24 percent of children with type 1 diabetes. Research indicates that body mass index (BMI) (weight in kilograms divided by the square of height in meters) is a significant predictor of fasting glucose and insulin in children of all ages and genders. Recent findings also show that obese children are at high risk for having impaired glucose tolerance, a metabolic precursor to type 2 diabetes. Impaired glucose tolerance is diagnosed on the basis of a standardized oral glucose tolerance test, and defined as fasting glucose less than 126 mg/dl, and a 2-hr value of 140–199 mg/dl. In a study of 167 obese children and adolescents referred for obesity, Sinha and colleagues (2002) administered oral glucose tolerance tests and found that 25 percent of obese children and 21 percent of obese adolescents had impaired glucose tolerance, with an additional 4 percent having type 2 diabetes.

Studies have also demonstrated that minority groups may be at the greatest risk for developing type 2 diabetes. Pinhas-Hamiel and colleagues (1992) documented that 69 percent of youth with type 2 diabetes in Cincinnati, Ohio, were African American. Scott and colleagues (1997), in a study in Arkansas investigating differences in children with type 1 versus type 2 diabetes, found that 74 percent of children with type 2 diabetes were African American, as opposed to only 18 percent of children with type 1. Racial differences in correlates of type 2 diabetes have also been demonstrated in nondiabetic children, with African-American children demonstrating lower insulin sensitivity and higher insulin secretion, after controlling for BMI and/or visceral fat accumulation.

Hispanic children are another minority group at increased risk for developing type 2 diabetes, as indicated by a recent study by Neufeld and colleagues (1998) that found 31 percent of newly diagnosed Mexican American diabetic children had type 2 diabetes. This increased risk in Mexican-American children may be related to behavioral factors as well. Recent research findings indicate that Mexican American children consume a higher percentage of calories from fat and saturated fat, have lower consumption of fruits and vegetables, increased body fat, lower physical fitness, and a sedentary lifestyle. Another study demonstrated increased BMI, insulin, glucose, triglycerides, and systolic blood pressure, as well as lower HDL cholesterol, all consistent with early appearance of the insulin resistance syndrome in Mexican-American children. In a study of young Hispanic children (including mostly those of Cuban, Nicaraguan, and Mexican-American backgrounds), Delamater and colleagues (2001) found an interaction of obesity and family history of type 2 diabetes, with the greatest insulin resistance observed in obese children with a positive family history of type 2 diabetes.

TREATMENT

Little is known about how to effectively intervene with youth who have type 2 diabetes, but clearly weight control must be an integral part of treatment. The goal of medical intervention is normalization of blood glucose in order to prevent acute and long-term health complications. The ADA has recommended that all children with type 2 diabetes should receive comprehensive self-management education, including self-monitoring of blood glucose and behavior modification for changing lifestyle habits to improve dietary intake and increase physical activity. For most children, pharmacological treatment is also necessary, not only to improve glycemia, but also to potentially reduce insulin resistance and preserve beta-cell function. Medications such as Metformin are typically used clinically in the

treatment of type 2 diabetes in youth, but few controlled studies evaluating its efficacy are available. In addition, little is known about behavioral and psychosocial issues affecting treatment for type 2 diabetes in children and adolescents.

Interventions with youth who have type 2 diabetes must also involve the entire family, as family influences are significant in this patient population. Although effective family-based, behavioral interventions exist for the treatment of obesity in children, these interventions have not yet been conducted with youth who have type 2 diabetes. Because weight reduction is an essential aspect of treatment for type 2 diabetes, future studies should evaluate the effects of these interventions for type 2 diabetes in youth, as well as behavioral interventions to enhance adherence to other aspects of the medical regimen.

PROGNOSIS

Type 2 diabetes affects an estimated 15 million adults in the United States and is a cause of significant morbidity and excess mortality. The health complications associated with poorly controlled diabetes include cardiovascular disease, renal disease, blindness, and limb amputations. Given the significant health risks associated with diabetes, programs should be developed to screen at-risk groups, for example, those children who are obese, of ethnic minority status, and/or who have a positive family history for type 2 diabetes. Secondary prevention efforts should be put in place, so that these high-risk children can receive weight control and/or other interventions that may reduce their risks of developing type 2 diabetes. More research addressing the prevention of type 2 diabetes as well as intervention for those with type 2 diabetes is needed.

See also: Diabetes Mellitus, Type 1; Family Assessment; Family Intervention; Obesity; Treatment Adherence—Behavioral and Medical

Further Reading

American Diabetes Association. (2000). Type 2 diabetes in children and adolescents. *Diabetes Care, 23*, 381–389.

Delamater, A., Brito, A., Applegate, B., Casteleiro, V., Patino, A., Sabogal, C., & Goldberg, R. (2001). Obesity and family history increase metabolic risk in Hispanic children. *Annals of Behavioral Medicine, 23* (Suppl.), S130.

Fagot-Campagna, A., Pettitt, D. J., Engelgau, M., Burrows, N. R., Geiss, L., Valdez, R., Beckles, G. L., Saaddine, J., Gregg, E., Williamson, D., & Venkat Narayan, K. M. (2000). Type 2 diabetes among North American children and adolescents: An epidemiologic review and a public health perspective. *Journal of Pediatrics, 136*, 664–672.

Neufeld, N. D., Raffel, L. J., Landon, C., Chen, Y. D. I., & Vadheim, C. M. (1998). Early presentation of type 2 diabetes in Mexican-American youth. *Diabetes Care, 21*, 80–86.

Pinhas-Hamiel, O., Dolan, L. M., Daniels, S. R., Standiford, D., Khoury, P. R., & Zeitler, P. (1996). Increased incidence of non-insulin-dependent diabetes mellitus among adolescents. *The Journal of Pediatrics, 128*, 608–615.

Scott, C. R., Smith, J. M., Michaeleen, C., & Pihoker, C. (1997). Characteristics of youth-onset noninsulin-diabetes mellitus and insulin-dependent diabetes mellitus at diagnosis. *Pediatrics, 100*, 84–91.

Sinha, R., Fisch, G., Teague, B., Tamborlane, W., Banyas, B., Allen, K., Savoye, M., Rieger, V., Taksali, S., Barbetta, G., Sherwin, R., & Caprio, S. (2002). Prevalence of impaired glucose tolerance among children and adolescents with marked obesity. *New England Journal of Medicine, 346*, 802–810.

ALAN M. DELAMATER
ANNA MARIA PATINO

Diagnostic and Statistical Manual for Primary Care (*DSM-PC*), Child and Adolescent Version

PURPOSE AND CLINICAL UTILITY

The *Diagnostic and Statistical Manual for Primary Care (DSM-PC)*, Child and Adolescent Version is a manual for coding of behavioral and developmental problems that present in primary care settings. The manual was intended to help primary care practitioners, including pediatricians, identify behavioral and developmental problems and relevant stressful environmental situations so that they can either provide intervention or refer children for more intensive mental health services.

The *DSM-PC* fills the need for a coding system that facilitates pediatricians' abilities to describe and diagnose the wide range of problems that are seen in primary care practice. Currently, the most frequently used diagnostic system for the classification of behavioral problems is the American Psychiatric Association's *Diagnostic and Statistical Manual of Mental Disorders, Fourth Edition (DSM-IV)*. This system includes mental disorders that are more serious and much less prevalent than the broad spectrum of behavioral and developmental problems that are commonly encountered in pediatric primary care.

The *DSM-PC* has several potential uses for pediatric psychologists, especially for those who work with pediatric colleagues in primary care. For example, use of the *DSM-PC* may increase pediatricians' abilities to make appropriate referrals and communicate effectively with psychologists concerning the management of behavioral and developmental problems. Psychologists can also use the *DSM-PC* to teach their pediatric colleagues about the spectrum of behavioral and developmental problems that present in primary care settings. Finally, psychologists and pediatricians can use the *DSM-PC* to conduct research on the incidence, prevalence, stability, and management of behavioral and developmental problems that are encountered in primary care settings.

ORGANIZATION AND CONTENT OF THE *DSM-PC*

The *DSM-PC* includes a Table of Contents, Introduction, and the two core content areas: (1) Situations, and (2) Child Manifestations. The appendices include a list of presenting complaints and page numbers, a section on diagnostic vignettes, which provide case material useful to practice coding in order to become familiar with the *DSM-PC* system, and a section that summarizes selected diagnostic criteria of the *DSM-IV* that are most likely to be used by pediatricians (e.g., Attention-Deficit/Hyperactivity Disorder [ADHD]).

Situations

The Situations section was designed to help practitioners to describe and evaluate the impact of stressful situations (e.g., divorce, changes in family situation) that can affect children's mental health, to assess the potential consequences of such adverse situations on children and families, and to identify factors that may make a child more vulnerable to the development of behavioral disorders and/or influence the management of behavioral disorders. The major categories of situations are the following: Challenges to primary support group, (e.g., marital discord/divorce), Changes in caregiving (e.g., physical illness of parent), Functional changes in family (e.g., addition of a sibling), Community of social challenges (e.g., acculturation), Educational challenges (e.g., parental illiteracy), Parent or adolescent occupational challenges, Unemployment housing challenges (e.g., homelessness), Economic challenge (e.g., poverty/inadequate financial status), Inadequate access to health and/or mental health services, Legal system or crime problem (e.g., parent or juvenile crime), Other environmental situations (e.g., natural disaster), and Health-related situations (e.g., chronic or acute health conditions).

Child Manifestations

The second major content area of the *DSM-PC*, Child Manifestations, describes behavioral symptoms. This section is organized into twelve specific sections or behavioral clusters, each of which begins with examples of symptoms that describe concerns typically described by parents (e.g., "My child is not talking"). The behavioral clusters include the following: Developmental competency (e.g., learning and developmental problems), Impulsivity, hyperactivity, or inattention, Negative antisocial behaviors, Substance use/abuse, Emotions and mood (e.g., sadness and anxiety), Somatic and sleep behaviors, Feeding, eating, and elimination, Illness-related behaviors (e.g., noncompliance with treatment), Sexual behavior, and Atypical behaviors (e.g., ritualistic behavior).

Each cluster description has a similar format that includes the cluster title, presenting complaints, definitions and symptoms, as well as information about epidemiology and etiology. This format was developed to help primary care clinicians consider the following issues for each cluster: (1) the spectrum of severity of each child's presenting problems; (2) common presentations of behavioral problems during various periods of development (e.g., infancy, early and middle childhood, and adolescence); and (3) differential diagnosis.

Spectrum of Problem Severity

One of the unique features of the *DSM-PC* is the concept that children demonstrate symptoms that vary along a continuum from normal variations to severe disorders that are divided into clinically relevant levels. For example, behavioral and developmental problems are divided into three categories: (1) *developmental variations*, defined as behaviors that parents may raise as a concern with their child's primary care provider, but are within the range of what is expected for the child's age; (2) *problems* that reflect behaviors serious enough to disrupt the child's functioning with peers, in school, and/or in the family, but do not involve a sufficient level of symptom severity to warrant the diagnosis of a mental disorder based on the *DSM-IV*; and (3) *disorders* as they are defined in the *DSM-IV*, which include conditions such as ADHD that are commonly treated in primary care settings.

Future directions for potential applications of the *DSM-PC* include the following: using the *DSM-PC* to help psychologists categorize the problems they see in primary care settings, incorporating the *DSM-PC* in training of psychologists and pediatricians, conducting research on the incidence and prevalence of a broad range of developmental and behavioral problems seen in primary care, including the patterns of stability and change in these problems, and describing the incidence and prevalence of various environmental stressors experienced by children who present in primary care.

See also: Adolescence; Childhood; *Diagnostic and Statistical Manual of Mental Disorders*; Infancy; Parenting Practices

Further Reading

American Psychiatric Association. (1994). *Diagnostic and statistical manual of mental disorders, DSM-IV* (4th ed.). Washington, DC: Author.

Drotar, D. (1999). The diagnostic and statistical manual for primary care (DSM-PC), child and adolescent version: What pediatric psychologists need to know. *Journal of Pediatric Psychology, 24,* 369–380.

Wolraich, M. L., Felice, M. E., & Drotar, D. (Eds.). (1996). *The classification of child and adolescent mental diagnosis in primary care: Diagnosis and statistical manual for primary care (DSM-PC), child and adolescent version.* Elk Grove, IL: American Academy of Pediatrics.

DENNIS DROTAR

Diagnostic and Statistical Manual of Mental Disorders

The *Diagnostic and Statistical Manual of Mental Disorders (DSM)* developed in the United States is a widely used classification system around the world. In the first version of the *DSM*, two categories of childhood disorders (adjustment reaction and childhood schizophrenia) were included, and in the subsequent *DSM-II*, the category "Behavioral Disorder of Childhood and Adolescence" was added. The later versions of the *DSM* (*DSM-III, DSM-III-R, DSM-IV*) have included an expanded number of diagnostic categories specific to children and adolescents. Since the introduction of *DSM-III*, the criteria for making the diagnosis of psychiatric disorders in terms of their symptoms, duration, and associated features have been explicitly and more clearly described.

The most recent edition, *DSM-IV*, categorizes psychiatric disorders into 16 major diagnostic classes, with the first section being devoted to "Disorders Usually First Diagnosed in Infancy, Childhood, or Adolescence." *DSM-IV* continues to apply the multiaxial system introduced in *DSM-III*, with minor modifications. The use of a multiaxial system allows assessment of several domains of information about the children, including the presence of certain types of disorders, aspects of the environment (i.e., stressors), and areas of functioning that may be overlooked if the focus is based on a single presenting problem. The multiaxial system in *DSM-IV* includes 5 axes, which each patient can be evaluated on:

Axis I	Clinical disorders
	Other conditions that may be a focus of clinical attention
Axis II	Personality disorders
	Mental retardation
Axis III	General medical conditions
Axis IV	Psychosocial and environmental problems
Axis V	Global assessment of functioning

Axis I contains various types of clinical disorders, with the exception of mental retardation and personality disorders. Included in this axis are diagnostic categories labelled "Disorders Usually First Diagnosed in Infancy, Childhood, or Adolescence." The disorders which fall under these categories include: mental retardation, learning disorders, motor skills disorders, communication disorders, pervasive developmental disorders, attention-deficit/disruptive behavior disorder, feeding and eating disorders of infancy or early childhood, tic disorders, elimination disorders, and other disorders of infancy, childhood, or adolescence (e.g., separation anxiety disorders, selective mutism). In addition to these disorders, there are a series of other diagnoses that are not specific to children; however, with minor modifications, they are for the most part applicable for children and adolescents (e.g., anxiety, depressive disorders, eating disorders, somatoform disorders, substance use disorders). Each child can receive more than one disorder listed in Axis I. In such instances, comorbidity is said to occur.

Axis II includes personality disorders and mental retardation. These two disorders are listed on a separate axis to ensure that consideration be given to them in the presence of more acute Axis I disorders. It also contains prominent maladaptive personality features that fail to meet the threshold for a personality disorder.

Axis III is used to report general medical conditions that may be relevant for the understanding and management of the child's psychiatric problems. In some children, medical condition may have a direct influence in the development of psychiatric disorders (e.g., difficulty with sleeping may lead to depression), whereas, in other children, psychiatric disorders may be a reaction to certain medical condition (e.g., depression as a reaction to having a diagnosis of cancer). Although some medical conditions have no direct relationship to the psychiatric disorders, they may have important prognostic or treatment implication.

Axis IV assesses psychosocial and environmental factors that may be important in the initiation or exacerbation of the disorder. Some examples of psychosocial and environmental problems include negative life events, lack of support or personal resources, family or other interpersonal stress.

Axis V is used to report the clinician's ratings of the child's overall level of impairment. For this purpose, the Global Assessment of Functioning Scale is used. The Global Assessment of Functioning Scale ranges from 1 to 100, with a low score being indicative of greater impairment, and a high score being indicative of mild, transient, or absence of significant impairment.

Each disorder in *DSM-IV* is described along the following headings: Diagnostic features; Subtypes and/or specifiers; Recording procedures; Associated features and disorders; Specific culture, age, and gender features; Prevalence; Course; Familial pattern; and Differential diagnosis.

DSM-IV also employs the concept of diagnostic hierarchies in that children who meet the criteria for the diagnoses lower in the hierarchy are generally not given that lower diagnosis. Hierarchies are used in three instances: first, the presence of a psychiatric disorder due to a general medical condition or a substance-induced disorder preempts other diagnoses with the same symptoms. Second, the application of hierarchies requires that more pervasive disorders (e.g., schizophrenia) preempt less pervasive disorders (e.g., dysthymic disorder). Third, they are useful when differential diagnostic decisions are not straightforward to make, and when there is a need to have an immediate clinical plan.

Although much improvement has been made in the latest version of *DSM*, it has been criticized on several grounds by Essau and colleagues (1997). For some disorders (e.g., anxiety and depressive disorders), the same adult criteria have been applied to children and adolescents. Little is known about the validity or the reliability of these criteria when applied to children. Moreover, the *DSM* system is not sensitive enough to developmental issues, which makes it difficult to decide whether symptoms occur frequently enough to be clinically significant since certain problematic behaviors may be developmentally appropriate. Another criticism is related to the notion of unidimensionality and symptom equivalency. That is, generally, once one or two cardinal symptoms are evident (e.g., depressed mood for major depressive episode), all subsequent symptoms (e.g., loss of appetite, suicidal ideation) are given equal weight in making the diagnosis. Achenbach (1995) has indicated that the thresholds of symptomatology in the *DSM-IV* used to determine presence of a disorder have historically been arbitrarily determined, as reflected by changes in the number of symptoms that have to be met in the different versions of the *DSM*. *DSM-IV* has also been criticized for focusing little attention on the complex transactions and setting influences that are important in understanding and treating various child behavior disorders, as noted by Jensen and Hoagwood (1997).

See also: Classification and Diagnosis; Global Functioning; International Classification of Diseases and Related Health Problems; Quality of Life

Further Reading

Achenbach, T. M. (1995). Developmental issues in assessment, taxonomy, and diagnosis of child and adolescent psychopathology. In D. Cicchetti & D. J. Cohen (Eds.), *Developmental psychopathology. Volume 1: Theory and methods* (pp. 57–80). New York: Wiley.

American Psychiatric Association. (1994). *Diagnostic and statistical manual of mental disorders* (4th ed.). Washington, DC: Author.

Essau, C. A., Feehan, M., & Üstun, B. (1997). Classification and assessment strategies. In C. A. Essau & F. Petermann (Eds.), *Developmental psychopathology: Epidemiology, diagnostics, and treatment* (pp. 19–62). London: Harwood Academic.

Jensen, P. S., & Hoagwood, K. (1997). The book of names: DSM-IV in context. *Development and Psychopathology, 9,* 231–249.

CECILIA A. ESSAU

Diagnostic Interview

See: Interviewing

Dialysis

BRIEF DESCRIPTION AND INDICATIONS

The accumulation of harmful waste products, hypertension, excess fluid, and underproduction of red blood

cells often occur when kidneys fail to function normally. Dialysis is a process in which blood is removed from the body, cleaned and filtered, and then returned to the body. Typically used with patients who have lost at least 80 percent of kidney function, dialysis essentially performs the normal functions of a healthy kidney. Approximately 60 percent of children with end-stage renal disease receive dialysis treatments.

There are two types of dialysis: hemodialysis and peritoneal dialysis. Hemodialysis (Figure 1) involves the use of a dialyzer, which essentially removes and filters blood to eliminate excess water, salt, and harmful wastes, and to restore proper balance of potassium, sodium, calcium, and bicarbonate. Prior to initiating hemodialysis treatment, access to a high flow bloodstream is surgically created via an arteriovenous fistula or graft. A fistula is created surgically in the wrist or upper forearm and involves connecting an artery to a vein to permit arterial blood to flow directly into the vein. If a fistula cannot be constructed due to small blood vessels, a graft is used to join an artery and a vein in the patient's upper arm, lower arm, or thigh. The graft can come either from the patient (e.g., a vein in the thigh) or artificially constructed using polytetrafluoroethylene. While home-based treatments are possible, hemodialysis is usually done in a dialysis center three times a week and each treatment typically lasts 3–5 hr. Common complications include vascular access problems, infection, clotting, poor blood flow, muscle cramps, and hypotension.

In contrast to hemodialysis, peritoneal dialysis (Figure 2) is usually done at home. Using the peritoneal membrane (the transparent serous membrane lining the abdominal cavity) as a natural filter, a dialysis solution (mixture of minerals and dextrose) travels through

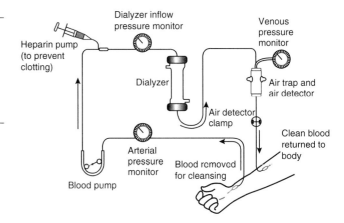

Figure 1. Hemodialysis (from http://www.niddk.nih.gov/health/kidney/).

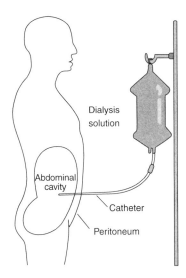

Figure 2. Peritoneal dialysis (from http://www.niddk.nih.gov/health/kidney/).

a surgically implanted abdominal catheter and draws excess water, salt, and harmful wastes from the blood vessels in the peritoneal membrane. The "used" dialysis solution is then drained from the peritoneal membrane and exchanged for fresh dialysis solution. With continuous ambulatory peritoneal dialysis, the dialysis solution remains in the peritoneum for 4–6 hr before being drained and exchanged for fresh dialysis solution. No equipment is necessary since the patient manages the entire exchange. With continuous cycler-assisted peritoneal dialysis, a machine is used to conduct three to five exchanges during the night while the patient sleeps. In some instances, both types of peritoneal dialysis methods are used. Abdominal infection (i.e., peritonitis) is the most common complication associated with peritoneal dialysis. Other complications include hypovolemia (low blood volume), hypervolemia (abnormal increase in blood volume), and dialysate retention and leakage.

OUTCOMES

It is important to emphasize that dialysis is not a cure for renal failure. For most children with renal failure, the eventual treatment goal is kidney transplantation, which offers a better chance for longer survival and improved quality of life. Approximately 70 percent of children whose onset of end-stage renal disease occurred between birth and age 4 will survive at least 5 years of dialysis treatment, compared to 82 percent of children whose end-stage renal disease was diagnosed after age 4. The most common causes of death for children receiving dialysis include infection, cardiac arrest, and cerebrovascular disease. Females are at higher mortality risk than males.

Children with nutritional and growth problems prior to dialysis initiation tend to have more complications during dialysis treatment and are at higher risk of death when compared to children with normal height. While the precise relationship between dialysis dose and growth and development is not clear, it is commonly believed that underdialysis affects the cognitive and physical development of children. Consequently, these outcomes should be formally assessed and monitored on a regular basis.

The psychological ramifications of dialysis have not been systematically examined. Nevertheless, there are a variety of potential psychological issues that warrant careful attention and evaluation. These include the impact of frequent school absences due to hemodialysis and hospitalizations on academic achievement and the development of healthy peer relationships, limitations on physical activities, resources for coping with declining health status, short stature, disfiguring surgical scars, and family stress.

See also: Cardiovascular Disease; Coping with Illness; Kidney Transplantation, Pediatric; Parenting the Chronically Ill Child; Quality of Life

Further Reading

Furth, S. L., Stablein, D., Fine, R. N., Powe, N. R., & Fivush, B. A. (2002). Adverse clinical outcomes associated with short stature at dialysis initiation: A report of the North American Pediatric Renal Transplant Cooperative Study. *Pediatrics, 109,* 909–913.
Schweitzer, J. B., & Hobbs, S. A. (1995). Renal and liver disease: End-stage and transplantation issue. In M. C. Roberts (Ed.), *Handbook of pediatric psychology* (2nd ed., pp. 425–445). New York: Guilford.

JAMES R. RODRIGUE
WILLEM J. VAN DER WERF
STEPHANIE TOY

Diarrhea

DEFINITION

Diarrhea is a common problem for young children, and complications can include dehydration, malnutrition, and in some cases even death. Diarrhea is classified as acute (less than 2–3 weeks), of which infectious diarrhea is the most common, and chronic (more than 2–3 weeks), which may be due to a variety of underlying disorders such as cystic fibrosis, celiac disease, inflammatory bowel disease, or overconsumption of nonabsorbable sugars. This entry will focus on chronic nonspecific diarrhea. For information on acute/infectious diarrhea, see Gastrointestinal Disorders.

CHRONIC NONSPECIFIC DIARRHEA

Definition/Incidence/Etiology

Chronic nonspecific diarrhea refers to an often distressing, but medically insignificant condition in young children. Chronic nonspecific diarrhea is defined by recurrent, painless passage of three or more large, unformed stools, for four or more weeks, without evidence of organic cause. Onset occurs between 6 and 36 months of age. Chronic nonspecific diarrhea is reported to be a frequent complaint, but specific incidence rates are unavailable. The etiology of chronic nonspecific diarrhea is unknown.

Psychosocial Correlates

Clinical experience suggests that children with chronic nonspecific diarrhea do not have more psychosocial difficulties than healthy children. However, some research suggests that children with chronic nonspecific diarrhea have a significantly higher frequency of sleeping problems, crying, irritability, digestive problems other than diarrhea, overactivity, discipline problems, and higher levels of environmental and family stress than healthy children. These studies are limited by small sample sizes, lack of standardized measures, and limited information regarding recruitment and inclusion criteria, so caution is warranted in drawing conclusions about the psychosocial functioning of children with chronic nonspecific diarrhea.

Assessment/Treatment/Prognosis

Diagnosis is made after organic causes such as enteric infections, ingestion of laxatives, urinary tract infection, and antibiotic use are ruled out. Dietary intake is also assessed to exclude diarrhea due to excessive fruit juice or sorbitol consumption, excessive carbohydrate ingestion with low fat intake, and food allergies. Children can recover spontaneously, but may benefit from treatment focusing on parent behavior management skills. In one small study, parents who learned behavioral strategies such as positive reinforcement and time-out procedures reported significant improvements in diarrhea and behavior problems after treatment and at a 6-month follow-up. In a biofeedback study, a small group of adolescents and adults were taught to control intestinal movement via audible feedback of bowel sounds. All five patients demonstrated improved bowel function.

See also: Biofeedback; Gastrointestinal Disorders; Parent Training

Further Reading

Rasquin-Weber, A., Hyman, P. E., Cucchiara, S., Fleisher, D. R., Hyams, J. S., Milla, P. J., & Staiano, A. (1999). Childhood functional gastrointestinal disorders. *Gut, 45*(Suppl. II), II60–II68.
Winnail, S. D., Artz, L. M., Geiger, B. F., Petri, C. J., Bailey, R., & Mason, J. W. (2001). Diarrhea management training in early childhood settings. *Early Childhood Education Journal, 28*, 231–236.

Laura M. Makhner
Kellee N. Sims-Clark
Wallace V. Crandall

Differential Social Reinforcement/ Positive Attention

DESCRIPTION OF TREATMENT

Differential social reinforcement is a procedure used to decrease maladaptive behavior and increase appropriate behavior. This procedure involves attending to and reinforcing appropriate behavior, and not attending to (i.e., ignoring) or reinforcing inappropriate behavior. When this is done, the attention-based behaviors that were given positive attention will increase, and the behaviors that were ignored, eventually, will decrease. Although ignored behaviors will eventually decrease, it is important to note that the immediate effect of ignoring is an increase or worsening of maladaptive behaviors called an extinction burst. After the initial increase, attention-seeking behaviors that continue to receive no attention will decrease over time.

The use of differential social reinforcement involves four steps. First, the maladaptive behavior must be identified. During this process, a functional analysis should be conducted to determine the conditions under which (i.e., "why") the behavior is being exhibited. If the behavior is maintained by receiving attention, then differential social reinforcement is an appropriate procedure to use to decrease the behavior. For example, conducting a functional analysis may indicate that a 5-year-old boy steals cookies whenever his mother leaves the room because the taste of cookies is reinforcing for him, whereas a 6-year-old girl whines whenever her mother leaves the room because her mother reenters the room and provides her with attention (e.g., "What's wrong honey? Don't whine. Mommy's here."). Differential social reinforcement would be an appropriate technique to use to decrease the girl's whining behavior, which functions to obtain attention. However, this technique (which would involve ignoring the theft of the cookies) is likely to be ineffective for cookie stealing because the purpose of the stealing was to obtain the cookie, not to obtain attention.

The second step when using differential social reinforcement is to identify alternative, appropriate behaviors. These behaviors should be incompatible with the maladaptive behavior. For example, "using your big girl voice" (alternative behavior) is incompatible with whining (maladaptive behavior), and talking softly (alternative behavior) is incompatible with yelling (maladaptive behavior).

The third step is to reinforce alternative, appropriate behaviors by providing positive attention. An effective and appropriate type of positive attention is called "labeled praise." A labeled praise informs individuals of what, specifically, about their behavior is praiseworthy (e.g., "I like the way that you are using your inside voice." "Great job keeping your hands to yourself."). Labeled praise increases the probability that the behavior being praised will increase in the future. Thus, labeled praises frequently are used to reinforce behaviors that are incompatible with the problem behavior (e.g., playing gently, using kind words). For individuals who are less verbal, positive and incompatible behaviors are reinforced with eye contact, touches, smiles, and enthusiastic voice intonations.

The final step in the process is to remove attention for inappropriate behaviors (i.e., remove reinforcers). When ignoring inappropriate behavior, it is important to ignore it entirely and consistently. In other words, the entire inappropriate behavior must be ignored (e.g., complete 30 seconds of whining), and every instance of

the inappropriate behavior must be ignored. Using active ignoring techniques will make it more evident to the individual that attention is being removed. Active ignoring consists of removing all of one's attention with such techniques as avoiding eye contact, turning head, turning entire body, and leaving the room.

The following is an example of using differential social reinforcement with an adolescent, Franklin, with mental retardation who squeals loudly whenever the staff at his day treatment program are interacting with other individuals. The identified problem behavior that the staff wanted to decrease was loud squealing. Conducting a functional analysis indicated that Franklin squealed loudly only when staff began a task with other individuals, and ceased only when that staff person provided attention to Franklin (e.g., provided eye contact, criticized, frowned). Thus, Franklin's squealing behavior was being reinforced and maintained by the staff's attention. Therefore, an incompatible behavior, vocalizing softly, was chosen to reinforce. Whenever Franklin exhibited any soft vocalization (e.g., moans, words, grunts), the staff provided him with an enthusiastic labeled praise for that behavior (e.g., "I really like how you are talking softly!") including eye contact and smiling. In addition, whenever Franklin squealed loudly, the staff turned their back to him and removed all of their attention (e.g., ignored). At first, Franklin squealed louder when he was ignored, but eventually, this behavior decreased, and Franklin began vocalizing softly more often.

CLINICAL APPLICATIONS

Differential social reinforcement can be used to decrease any type of maladaptive behaviors and increase any appropriate behaviors that are maintained by attention. Additionally, this procedure can be used in various settings with any population. For example, differential social reinforcement would be appropriate in a school setting for a disruptive child that hits other children for negative attention, or in a nursing home setting for a resident that uses inappropriate language to receive a reaction from other residents.

EFFECTIVENESS

Differential social reinforcement has proven to be effective in several settings such as schools, nursing homes, dentist's offices, daycare centers, homes, and at the work place. Also, this procedure is effective with different types of populations (e.g., children, adolescents, individuals with mental retardation, college students, individuals with psychological problems, adults, older adults).

See also: Behavior and Functional Analysis; Parent Training; Parent–Child Interaction Therapy; Positive Reinforcement

Further Reading

Hembree-Kigin, T. L., & McNeil, C. B. (1995). *Parent–child interaction therapy.* New York: Plenum Press.

Martin, G., & Pear, J. (1996). *Behavior modification: What it is and how to do it* (5th ed.). Upper Saddle River, NJ: Prentice Hall.

Miltenberger, R. G. (2001). *Behavior modification: Principles and procedures* (2nd ed.). Pacific Grove, CA: Brooks/Cole.

Zeiler, M. D. (1976). Positive reinforcement and the elimination of reinforced responses. *Journal of the Experimental Analysis of Behavior, 26,* 37–44.

CHERYL B. MCNEIL
HOLLY A. FILCHECK

Diffuse Axonal Injuries

See: Traumatic Brain Injury

Disruptive Behavior Disorders

DESCRIPTION

The *Diagnostic and Statistical Manual of Mental Disorders, Fourth Edition* (*DSM-IV*) is the most commonly used classification scheme for mental disorders in North America and much of the world. The *DSM-IV* groups disorders into major categories, one of which is Disorders usually first diagnosed in infancy, childhood, or adolescence. Within this categorization, there are 10 sections, including a section for Attention-deficit and disruptive behavior disorders. This section includes the diagnoses of Attention-Deficit/Hyperactivity Disorder (ADHD), Oppositional Defiant Disorder (ODD), and Conduct Disorder (CD). ADHD describes excessive levels of inattention and/or impulsivity and hyperactivity. ODD refers to a pattern of behavior that is negative, hostile, and defiant toward authority. Finally, CD is characterized by behaviors that violate the basic rights of others

and/or are contrary to major social norms and rules. Many feel that ODD is better seen as a developmental precursor to CD, rather than as a distinct disorder.

All of these disorders are more common among boys than girls and show evidence of a moderate degree of stability over time (even into adulthood). In general, the disruptive disorders are associated with increased likelihood of child academic and cognitive problems, poor peer relationships, and parenting and family difficulties. Children who have both ADHD and ODD/CD diagnoses experience more serious and persistent problems than children who have only ADHD or only ODD or CD. Assessment of these disorders must include information from several sources and should focus not only on the child's behavior, but also on the family and school context. Effective treatments include medication (for ADHD), child skills training, and parent and family interventions.

See also: Attention-Deficit/Hyperactivity Disorder; Conduct Disorder; Oppositional Defiant Disorder; Parent Training

Further Reading

American Psychiatric Association. (1994). *Diagnostic and statistical manual of mental disorders* (4th ed.). Washington, DC: Author.

Quay, H. C., & Hogan, A. E. (1999). *Handbook of disruptive behavior disorders.* New York: Kluwer Academic/Plenum.

CHARLOTTE JOHNSTON

Divorce

In 1950, the number of children involved in divorces stood at 6.3 per 1,000 children under 18 years of age. By 1980, that rate rose to 17.3 per 1,000 children, reflecting a 175 percent increase. With divorce named as the fastest growing marital status category, the United States Census Bureau reported in 1998 that almost 10 million children 18 years and younger were living in one-parent households as a result of divorce (7 million children) or parental separation (3 million children).

FACTORS INFLUENCING CHILDREN'S ADJUSTMENT TO DIVORCE

Although the divorce process involves substantial life changes for children, including new living arrangements, parental separation, and economic changes, not every child exhibits negative reactions to divorce, and the magnitude of the reaction is not consistent across children. In fact, a majority of children of divorce fall within the average range of emotional adjustment on standardized measures. However, specific characteristics of the parental relationship, the child, and the time since divorce, play a significant role in determining how children adjust to the experience of their parents' divorce.

SHORT-TERM EFFECTS OF DIVORCE

The time surrounding the initial separation and divorce is when most children and parents are attempting to cope with changes in their environment (school, workplace, and community), family structure and routine, and socioeconomic status (SES). Children observed during this time frequently react with considerable anger toward one or both parents, pervasive sadness, feelings of loss, and disruptions in concentration and academic functioning.

LONG-TERM EFFECTS OF DIVORCE

The long-term impact of divorce tends to reflect the family's ability to adapt to the changes necessitated by the divorce. Most children show improved functioning after two years, as family members learn to cope with the change and with the new family arrangements. This adaptation by the family is associated with a lessening in intensity of the stressors surrounding the dissolution of the marriage. Child maladjustment may persist, however, if parental conflict persists over time.

EFFECTS OF CHILD AGE AND SEX ON CHILDREN'S ADJUSTMENT TO DIVORCE

Early theories of child adjustment to divorce suggested that children coped with parental separation differently depending on their stage of cognitive and emotional development. For example, some theorists believed that preschoolers had more difficulty coping than older children because they were cognitively unable to appreciate the complexity of their parents' feelings and often felt as if they were to blame for their parents' troubles. Others believed that adolescents were more affected by divorce because of their longer exposure to parental conflict and more pronounced feelings of responsibility for parent separation. Sex differences

were also reported in the early literature, with boys found to experience more deleterious effects from the divorce itself, and girls found to be more affected by remarriage.

Despite the many theories, the empirical literature examining children's adjustment at various ages is sparse, and has been relatively inconclusive. The inconsistent findings may have been due to flaws in methodology. Similarly, current research examining sex differences in children's adjustment to divorce has called into question many of the earlier findings. Specifically, the newer studies have not found differences in boys' and girls' academic achievement, conduct, or psychological adjustment, with the exception that boys from divorced families exhibit more difficulty than girls in social adjustment. The disappearance of child sex effects in divorce research has been attributed to a recent increase in the involvement of fathers with their children following divorce. In turn, the increased paternal involvement has been attributed to rises in rates of joint custody and in the number of father-headed households, as well as to societal changes in perception of the fathers' parental role.

EFFECTS OF PARENT CONFLICT ON CHILDREN'S ADJUSTMENT TO DIVORCE

Conflict between parents has been consistently identified as a major source of child maladjustment in separating and divorced families. Children who experience higher levels of postdivorce conflict between their parents tend to have more difficulty than children whose parents show little conflict. A large body of research actually suggests that it is not the divorce or separation per se that affects child adjustment, but rather the parental conflict and hostility that accompany the divorce process. Specifically, frequent and intense marital conflict is a more powerful predictor of children's postdivorce adjustment than other divorce-related variables such as the loss of a parent or the economic changes that occur as a result of the divorce.

Conflict between divorced parents normally declines in the long run, with about one quarter of divorced parents being able to maintain a cooperative, mutually supportive relationship with one another. The majority of parents, however, develop parallel, disengaged parenting patterns with little communication or cooperation but also little active undermining of the other parent. Between 8 and 12 percent of divorced parents continue to have high-conflict relationships as long as 3 years after their divorce.

ASSESSMENT

Children having difficulty coping with their parents' divorce typically present to a clinic with problems such as anxiety, depression, disruptive behavior, peer relationship problems, and academic difficulties. Ideally, assessment would include all parties involved in the child's caregiving. Realistically, the assessment may need to be conducted in stages, as some parents may not agree to be seen at the same time. A sound evaluation should include a clinical interview with the child and all caregivers, psychological tests that assess child *and* parent functioning in a variety of domains (i.e., cognitive, behavioral, and emotional functioning), and behavioral observations of parent–child interactions. Information should also be gathered from teachers or day care providers to determine the extent of the child's problems.

TREATMENT

Under ideal circumstances, custodial and non-custodial parents work together to form a functional and conflict-free coparenting relationship. A positive coparenting relationship is one in which both parents are invested in the child, value the other parent's involvement with the child, respect the judgments of the other parent, and desire to communicate with the other parent. Parents who can maintain a positive coparenting relationship help to ease the transitions resulting from the dissolution of the marriage by providing some level of consistency and stability in the children's lives. Research confirms that cooperation in the parenting role is more predictive of child adjustment than conflict in other areas of the marriage.

Because the coparenting relationship plays such an important role in children's adjustment to divorce, it is frequently the focus of parent-oriented treatments during the divorce process. In fact, many states have developed court-mandated courses for parents who file for divorce that focus on developing a strong coparenting relationship. Key components of these programs include education about the effects of the parents' relationship quality on child adjustment as well as training in communication and problem-solving, conflict resolution, parenting skills and discipline techniques, and stress management.

A fundamental strategy in helping children adjust during the divorce process is to have the parents talk together with the child about the divorce on a developmentally appropriate level. Specifically, the parents should tell the child what parts of the child's life will change (e.g., mother and father will no longer live together) and what parts will stay the same (e.g., child will go to the same school). Parents should reassure the child that although they no longer live with one another, they both still love the child very much. Parents should also tell the child the agreed-upon plans for where the child will live and when the child will see the other parent.

Clinic-based interventions can range from individual play therapy to group intervention programs. These interventions typically focus on providing a supportive environment to help children identify and express feelings related to the divorce, educating children about the divorce process to clarify any misconceptions, and teaching the children appropriate coping skills. Bibliotherapy is another widely used intervention strategy for children, and many children's books are available that help children understand and cope with the divorce process.

See also: Adolescent Parenting; Domestic Violence; Family Therapy

Further Reading

Bearss, K., & Eyberg, S. M. (2002). *The parenting alliance in divorce: Its relation to child adjustment.* Manuscript submitted for publication.

Emery, R. E. (1999). *Marriage, divorce, and children's adjustment* (2nd ed.). Thousand Oaks, CA: Sage.

Hetherington, E. M. (1999). *Coping with divorce, single parenting, and remarriage: A risk and resiliency perspective.* Mahwah, NJ: Erlbaum.

Wallerstein, J. S., Lewis, J., & Blakeslee, S. (2000). *The unexpected legacy of divorce: A 25 year landmark study.* New York: Hyperion.

KAREN BEARSS
SHEILA M. EYBERG

Domestic Violence

DEFINITION

Domestic violence is defined as significant conflict between adult intimate partners, including those that are married or cohabiting. The range of behavior that constitutes domestic violence involves a pattern of assaultive or threatening physical, sexual, or psychological attacks.

INCIDENCE

The incidence rates of domestic violence are difficult to calculate. National surveys and federal reports estimate that between one and four million women are the victims of domestic violence annually, with one in four women experiencing domestic violence in their adult lifetime. Using data from surveys of family violence and extrapolating the number of expected children in those homes, it is estimated that more than three million children are exposed to domestic violence annually. An additional concern is the high rate of co-occurrence of domestic violence and child abuse. The Department of Justice estimates that in homes where domestic violence occurs, children are 1,500 times more likely to be abused.

RISK FACTORS

Domestic violence occurs across all race, gender, and socioeconomic classes. Risk for domestic violence may be higher when women are pregnant or in families who are isolated, have problems with substance abuse, are impoverished, unemployed, or where either parents has a childhood history of exposure to domestic violence or child abuse. Children in families of domestic violence are more at risk when their parents have psychiatric problems, substance abuse issues, or intellectual deficits.

EFFECTS OF EXPOSURE TO DOMESTIC VIOLENCE

For children and adolescents, exposure to domestic violence can include directly witnessing, overhearing, or observing the aftermath of the violence (e.g., broken objects, physical injuries, tension between parents). Estimates indicate that between 40 and 80 percent of children are present during domestic violence episodes. Furthermore, children in homes with domestic violence are at a greater risk of also being physically abused. Domestic violence is further detrimental for children because it interferes with both parents' ability to parent effectively. The presence of domestic violence has been linked to parental depression, irritability, and stress, which are also known to negatively impact parenting. Thus, children exposed to domestic violence can be harmed in three distinct ways: witnessing the violence, increased risk of direct abuse, and impairments in parenting associated with the violence.

Children of all ages, from infancy to adolescence, can be negatively impacted by exposure to domestic violence and may display symptomatology similar to that seen in abused children. Infants and toddlers may show disturbances in eating and sleeping patterns, frequent irritability and fussiness, increased clinging behaviors, disturbances in attachment, or failure to thrive. School-age children are more likely to have academic difficulties, elevated rates of aggression and bullying, depression, anxiety, and disturbances in social functioning. They are also at risk for the development of posttraumatic stress symptoms, including hyperarousal, sleep disturbances, regressive behaviors, avoidance, numbing, and reexperiencing the violence (often seen in play reenactment in younger children). Adolescents exposed to domestic violence show higher rates of internalizing problems, delinquent behaviors, and posttraumatic stress symptoms, including depression, withdrawal, suicidal ideation, substance abuse, criminal behaviors, and sexual promiscuity. In comparison to adolescents from nonviolent homes, they are more aggressive with friends, dating partners, and disliked peers.

While exposure to domestic violence is clearly associated with child maladjustment, several factors are associated with increased risk of negative outcomes for children. Domestic violence that involves frequent and intense conflict, conflict that is specifically about the child, and the child experiencing self-blame, leads to more distress for children. For children who are also physically abused, the negative effects are compounded. The majority of research and clinical practice focuses on the maladjustment in children exposed to domestic violence; however, it is equally important to consider the 50–60 percent of children and adolescents from these adverse situations who do *not* exhibit clinical symptomatology. Adult social support, peer support, and a positive maternal relationship have been shown to buffer the negative effects of domestic violence on children and adolescents.

ASSESSMENT OF CHILDREN

A multimodal, multimeasure method of assessment is recommended to gain an overall understanding of children's responses to domestic violence exposure. This should include reports from the child, caregivers, and others who have contact with the child (i.e., teachers). Three areas to be assessed with children exposed to domestic violence include: risk and safety, history of exposure to violence, and well-being. It is critical to determine the level of current violence in the home, potential harm to the child, and children's perception of safety. Based on this initial assessment, a comprehensive safety plan should be developed with children to help them in future incidents of violence.

Assessment of the child's exposure to violence can be helpful in better understanding of their experiences. The partner violence version of the Conflict Tactics Scales has been adapted to measure children's witnessing of violence and is the most commonly used measure in this field. Other measures of family conflict include the Family Environment Scale and the Children's Perception of Interparental Conflict Scale. An interview protocol may also be utilized to gather information about the child's exposure to violence. A variety of standardized instruments are available to assess children's social, emotional, and behavioral functioning (i.e., depression, anxiety, trauma symptoms), and may be utilized with children exposed to domestic violence to assess their well-being.

TREATMENT OF CHILDREN

There is limited empirical research on the efficacy of treatment interventions for children exposed to domestic violence. Clinical interventions should consider a child's developmental level, history of exposure to violence and other forms of abuse, and current level of impairment in functioning. Structured group treatment lasting 6–10 sessions is often utilized with children exposed to domestic violence. Key components of treatment include education about family violence and correcting attributions of self-blame; improving emotional security and self-competence; social skills training; teaching constructive coping skills for anger management and conflict resolution; reducing anxiety; helping the child to adopt healthy beliefs about interpersonal relationships and the use of aggression; and safety planning. Group interventions are thought to be best for children experiencing mild to moderate disturbances in functioning. However, for children with severe symptomatology or for those who have been chronically exposed to severe levels of violence, more in-depth, long-term therapy may be necessary.

PROGNOSIS

Poor prognosis is expected for children exposed to chronic and severe domestic violence, those who have also experienced abuse, and those with limited social support, particularly those with poor maternal relationship.

See also: Child Maltreatment; Exposure to Violence; Parenting Practices; Posttraumatic Stress Disorder in Children; Risk and Protective Factors; Violence

Further Reading

American Psychological Association. (1996). *Violence and the family: Report of the American Psychological Association Presidential Task Force on violence and the family.* Washington, DC: Author.

Edelson, J. L. (1999). Children's witnessing of adult domestic violence. *Journal of Interpersonal Violence, 14*(8), 839–870.

Holden, G. W., Geffner, R., & Jouriles, E. N. (1998). *Children exposed to marital violence: Theory, research, and applied issues.* Washington, DC: American Psychological Association.

Kilpatrick, K. L., Litt, M., & Williams, L. M. (1997). Post-traumatic stress disorder in child witnesses to domestic violence. *American Journal of Orthopsychiatry, 67*(4), 639–644.

Kolbo, J. R., Blakely, E. H., & Engleman, D. (1996). Children who witness domestic violence: A review of empirical literature. *Journal of Interpersonal Violence, 11*(2), 281–293.

Margolin, G. (1998). Effects of domestic violence on children. In P. K. Trickett & C. J. Shellenbach (Eds.), *Violence against children in the family and the community.* Washington, DC: American Psychological Association.

Minnesota Center Against Violence and Abuse. http://www.mincava.umn.edu

The National Center for Children Exposed to Violence. http://www.nccev.org

MICHELLE KEES
BARBARA L. BONNER

Down Syndrome

DEFINITION

Down syndrome is a chromosomal disorder associated with mental retardation. Children with Down syndrome have a typical physical appearance that can include a small head circumference, flattened face with a recessed bridge of the nose, upward slanting eyes, small ears and mouth, protruding tongue, short, broad hands and feet, stubby fingers, broad neck, and stocky appearance. Down syndrome has several associated medical conditions including congenital gastrointestinal and cardiac abnormalities, obesity, diabetes, hypothyroidism, eye problems such as myopia, strabismus, nystagmus, and cataracts, mild to moderate conductive hearing loss secondary to chronic middle ear infections, sleep apnea, hair loss, and low muscle tone. Infants and young children with Down syndrome are also at increased risk for acute leukemia as compared to the general population. Neuroanatomic studies of people with Down syndrome show a markedly reduced cortex and cerebellum relative to matched controls. Moreover, there is an immaturity of brain development evident in both neurons and their synaptic connections. Most people with Down syndrome function within the mild to moderate range of mental retardation on standardized intelligence tests. Some function in the borderline or low average ranges and only a few have severe mental retardation. Within the intellectual realm, there are greater deficits in verbal-linguistic skills relative to visual-spatial skills. Delayed language acquisition appears to play a primary role in deceleration of overall intellectual development in longitudinal studies of infants and young children with Down syndrome. Performance on adaptive behavior measures is generally commensurate with intellectual test results. Although children with Down syndrome are at lower risk for serious psychopathology, conduct problems, such as oppositional and defiant behavior, are common.

PREVALENCE AND COURSE

Down syndrome occurs in 1:700 to 1:1000 live births. Boys outnumber girls 1.3 to 1.0 and the disorder occurs in all racial and ethnic groups. It can be detected prenatally through chromosomal analysis. If prenatal diagnosis is not conducted, Down syndrome is generally diagnosed soon after birth because health professionals are very familiar with its physical characteristics. Children with Down syndrome attain early developmental milestones at much later ages than typically developing children. Delays in gross motor and expressive language development are quite prominent. For example, in children with Down syndrome, independent sitting is usually attained at 1 year of age while independent walking is not achieved until an average age of 2 years. Given early identification of Down syndrome, children typically participate in early intervention programs and receive comprehensive special education services upon attaining school age. It is generally believed that such involvement maximizes developmental potential and may have long-term implications for independence, community functioning, and quality of life.

ETIOLOGY

Ninety-five percent of Down syndrome cases are due to trisomy of chromosome 21. Trisomy occurs when

a child inherits three copies of a particular chromosome from his parents instead of two copies. It results from nondisjunction during meiosis prior to ovulation. In nearly all cases the nondisjunction is maternal in origin and is significantly related to maternal age. Women older than 35 at the time of conception are at significantly greater risk for having a child with a chromosomal disorder such as Down syndrome. The remaining 5 percent of Down syndrome births result from translocation in which a portion of chromosome 21 attaches to another chromosome or from mosaicism due to an error in cell division soon after conception. Mosaicism occurs when not every cell contains the trisomy condition. Children with mosaicism typically have less obvious physical features and less severe cognitive, language, and adaptive behavior impairments. For example, children with mosaicism typically have higher IQ scores, by 12–15 points on average, than children with trisomy 21.

ASSESSMENT

Down syndrome can be readily detected through chromosomal analysis prenatally or postnatally. Given that Down syndrome typically arises from meiotic nondisjunction, there is no carrier status that can be detected through genetic counseling. Although maternal age is a significant risk factor for chromosomal disorders including Down syndrome, the majority of children with Down syndrome are born to younger mothers. Children with Down syndrome should receive comprehensive developmental evaluations throughout early childhood to monitor progress and assess the need for ancillary services.

TREATMENT

Although there is no cure for Down syndrome, various treatment methods may enhance functioning. Infants and young children with Down syndrome are often involved in early intervention programs designed to maximize their developmental potential. Children and adolescents of school-age with Down syndrome benefit from academic curricula that embed reading, writing, and arithmetic skills with teaching of daily living and personal–social skills. The ability to care for oneself, maintain good interpersonal relationships, and exhibit appropriate work habits and behaviors is crucial to successful transition from school to work and from home to community living. Behavioral parent training may be effective in managing oppositional and defiant

Dual Diagnosis **190**

behaviors. Parent groups and family education programs may provide support to parents, siblings, and extended family.

See also: Fragile X Syndrome; Group Psychotherapy; Mental Retardation; Parent Training; Psychological Testing

Further Reading

Dykens, E. M., Hodapp, R. M., & Finucane, B. M. (2000). *Genetics and mental retardation syndromes: A new look at behavior and interventions*. Baltimore: Paul H. Brookes.
National Down Syndrome Congress. http://www.ndsccenter.org
National Down Syndrome Society. http://www.ndss.org
Pueschel, S. M., & Pueschel, J. K. (Eds.). (1992). *Biomedical concerns in persons with Down syndrome*. Baltimore: Paul H. Brookes.

WILLIAM E. MACLEAN, JR.

Drug Use

See: Substance Abuse

Dual Diagnosis: Mental Retardation and Psychiatric Disorders

Children with mental retardation are at greater risk than their normally developing peers for psychiatric disorders and behavior problems. Prevalence studies suggest rates 4 to 5 times greater than that of children with typical intellectual and adaptive functioning. Frequent diagnoses include, Oppositional-Defiant Disorder (ODD), Conduct Disorder (CD), mood disorders, anxiety disorders, Attention-Deficit/Hyperactivity Disorder (ADHD), stereotyped movement disorder (with self-injury), and adjustment disorders. Increased risk of psychopathology has been linked to communication difficulties, inadequate social skills development, and immature emotion regulation. Certain diagnoses show substantial co-occurrence with mental retardation such as Autistic disorder and other Pervasive Developmental Disorders (PDD).

Although the American Psychiatric Association's *Diagnostic and Statistical Manual of Mental Disorders (DSM)* does a fair job of providing a psychiatric nomenclature for most children and adolescents, there is concern about its validity for children and adolescents with

mental retardation. Moreover, studies suggest that existing *DSM* disorder categories may be more adequate for children with mild mental retardation than for children with severe or profound mental retardation. Therefore, the field has established an additional clinical focus on behavior disorders that occur with increased frequency in children with mental retardation such as aggressive behavior, property destruction, and socially offensive behaviors, among others. The common element among these topographies is that the behavior is worthy of assessment and treatment but does not meet criteria for a *DSM* diagnosis. In many instances, behavior disorders are unintentionally maintained by social responses from parents or teachers. For example, some behaviors are maintained by positive reinforcement such as social attention while others are reinforced through negative reinforcement such as avoidance or escape. In short, mental and behavioral disorders exhibited by children with mental retardation are a significant clinical issue. These conditions are associated with frequent referrals for educational assistance, more restrictive placements in educational and residential settings, and limited child participation in community activities.

Research on behavioral aspects of particular etiologies has yielded some useful information on psychiatric disorders among people with mental retardation. Table 1 presents an overview of typical intellectual functioning level and associated mental disorders for several etiologies.

ASSESSMENT OF PSYCHOPATHOLOGY

The assessment of psychological/behavioral difficulties in children with mental retardation requires a sound understanding of psychopathology, child development, and mental retardation. Thus, parents and service providers are strongly encouraged to seek out professionals with specialized training or expertise in the field of mental retardation when making referrals for assessments and interventions. In addition, comprehensive, multimodal assessments are highly recommended for the evaluation of psychopathology in children with mental retardation. Three major modes of assessment are described below.

Clinical Interviews

A thorough assessment of psychopathology in children with mental retardation involves informal clinical interviews with the child (when applicable), parents, direct care providers, teachers, and other informants who

Table 1. Etiologies Associated with Mental Retardation and their Behavioral Features

Etiology	Typical IQ range	Behavioral features
Down syndrome	50–60	Conduct disorder, oppositional behaviors, temper tantrums, and depression.
Fragile X syndrome	24–40 (males) 60–85 (females)	Males: ADHD, PDD, self-injurious behaviors, and autistic-like behaviors. Females: anxiety, depression, schizoid personality, and attention problems.
Fetal alcohol syndrome	50–85	ADHD, oppositional and defiant behaviors.
Prader–Willi syndrome	60	Compulsive behavior such as hoarding and storing food, and skin picking, whining, and complaining.
Rett's syndrome	<40	Repetitive hand-washing movements, autistic-like behaviors, seizures, dementia, neurological and developmental declines in infancy and early childhood.
Smith–Magenis syndrome	50–70	Stereotyped movement disorder (with self-injury), oppositional and defiant behaviors, hyperactivity.
Williams syndrome	50–60	Excessive anxiety and ADHD.

are familiar with the child. The information gathered from such interviews is often helpful in determining the frequency, settings, situations, reinforcing qualities, and possible functions of undesired behavior. Standardized clinical interviews may also assist the assessment process by focusing on specific symptoms for diagnostic clarity. However, many structured clinical interviews lack normative data for people with mental retardation.

Rating Scales

Several brief screening measures have been developed to assess psychopathology in children with mental retardation. Rating scales may be used to measure broad categories of behavior or a specific form of psychopathology. Several rating scales have been designed with both parent and teacher versions of the measure to assess behavior in multiple settings. At the present time, rating scales for children with mental retardation should be used with caution and only in conjunction with clinical interviews as the utility of such measures are much less broad and promising than similar instruments designed for normally developing children.

Behavior Observations

Direct behavior observations play a vital role in the assessment of psychopathology in children with mental retardation. An advantage of observation systems lies in the flexibility in which they can be administered. A trained observer can code a wide variety of behaviors or a single behavior in a continuous or time limited manner. In addition, a child's behavior can be easily observed in an unobtrusive manner in multiple settings. For more infrequent behavior problems, primary caregivers may be instructed to videotape episodes of

the undesired behavior for later analysis. Finally, behavior observations can be conducted in a systematic manner to test specific hypotheses about causal and maintaining factors of undesired behavior.

TREATMENT

Several treatment approaches have been shown to effectively reduce behavior problems in people with mental retardation. For people with mild intellectual impairments, traditional psychotherapy may produce beneficial results. Other forms of intervention include special education programs, physical therapy, occupational therapy, speech–language therapy, skills training, and psychoeducational programs.

Behavior therapy is perhaps the most widely used and researched form of treatment for people with mental retardation and severe behavior problems. Often, behavior problems are related to communication deficits. Interventions such as Functional Communication Training are very helpful in increasing communication abilities and reducing problem behaviors among children with severe mental retardation. Additionally, pharmacotherapy, when administered by a medical professional with specialized training with people with mental retardation, may be a useful addition to a behavior management plan.

See also: Behavior and Functional Analysis; Behavior Therapy; Mental Retardation; Pharmacological Interventions

Further Reading

Dykens, E. M., Hodapp, R. M., & Finucane, B. M. (2000). *Genetics and mental retardation: A new look at behavior and interventions.* Baltimore, MD: Paul H. Brookes.

Griffiths, D. M., Gardner, W. I., & Nugent, J. A. (Eds.). (1999). *Behavioral supports: Individual centered interventions. A multimodal functional approach.* Kingston, NY: NADD Press.

Reiss, S., & Aman, M. G. (Eds.). (1998). *Psychotropic medications and developmental disabilities: The international consensus handbook.* Baltimore, MD: Paul H. Brookes.

Rojahn, J., & Schroeder, S. R. (1991). Behavioral assessment. In J. L. Matson & J. A. Mulick (Eds.), *Handbook of mental retardation* (2nd ed., pp. 240–259). Elmsford, NY: Pergamon Press.

Rojahn, J., & Tassé, M. J. (1996). Psychopathology in mental retardation. In J. W. Jacobson & J. A. Mulick (Eds.), *Manual of diagnosis and professional practice in mental retardation* (pp. 147–156). Washington, DC: American Psychological Association.

MICHAEL L. MILLER
WILLIAM E. MACLEAN, JR.

Dysthymic Disorder

DEFINITION

Dysthymic Disorder (DD) in children is characterized by depressed or irritable mood that lasts most of the day and occurs more days than not for at least one year. During periods of depressed mood or irritability, children with DD experience at least two of the following symptoms: changes in appetite, sleep difficulty (e.g., sleeping too much, being unable to fall asleep), low energy or fatigue, low self-esteem, poor concentration or difficulty making decisions, and/or feelings of hopelessness. To diagnose a child with DD, these symptoms must be severe enough to cause significant distress or interference in the child's social, academic, or family functioning. In addition, there cannot be a period of more than 2 months without symptoms. If the child meets criteria for a Major Depressive Episode (MDE), this supercedes the diagnosis of DD. Other symptoms reported in children with early-onset DD include feelings of being unloved, anger, physical complaints, anxiety, and disobedience.

In children, it is often difficult to differentiate between DD and the more episodic mood disturbances of Major Depressive Disorder (MDD), which can have prodrome (i.e., premonitory symptoms) and residual (i.e., long lasting) phases. To make this distinction, it is necessary to take a careful longitudinal history of symptom onset, offset, and duration. It is not uncommon for children to be diagnosed with "Double Depression" in which a major depressive episode is superimposed on preexisting DD.

INCIDENCE/COMORBIDITY

The incidence rate of DD has been estimated as 0.6–1.7 percent of children and 1.6–8.0 percent of adolescents. Typically, DD presents at an earlier age than MDD. In the Pittsburgh Longitudinal Study, the earliest age of onset for clinic-based children with DD was 5 years, with a mean age of 8.7 years. In comparison, children whose first depressive episode was an MDD had a mean age of 10.9 years. Despite differences in age of onset, as many as 70 percent of early-onset DD patients will develop a superimposed episode of MDD. Children with DD are also at high risk for other psychiatric disorders. Anxiety disorders, Conduct Disorder (CD), and Attention-Deficit/Hyperactivity Disorder (ADHD) are the most common comorbid conditions. In addition, it is estimated that 13 percent of children with DD will develop bipolar disorder within five years of their first depressive episode.

COURSE

The average duration of DD is 4 years. Put in perspective, this amount of time for a child or adolescent includes the majority of the elementary school years or all of the high school years. As a result, individuals with early-onset DD spend large portions of their childhood having significant impairment in school, social, or familial areas of their life. These difficulties interfere with normal child development. Due to the extremely high risk for future anxiety and depressive disorders, the long-term outcome of children with DD is mixed. Research suggests children with DD have greater levels of impairment and a higher rate of relapse when compared to children with MDD.

There is also a strong association between depressive disorders and suicide. The majority of suicide attempts occur in the context of psychiatric disorders with depressive features. Moreover, it is estimated that one third of children with MDD or DD will attempt suicide by the time they reach 17 years of age.

ASSESSMENT

Early diagnosis and treatment of DD is critical to reduce the occurrence and severity of future episodes. To diagnose DD, it is important to complete a comprehensive interview in which information about the child's developmental history, medical history, family history of psychiatric disorders, school adjustment, history of behavioral, anxiety, mood, and other symptom onset, offset, and duration, and treatment history are ascertained. This allows for the completion of the child's differential diagnosis. That is, their primary diagnosis, co-occurring diagnoses, and any physical diagnoses or treatment side effects can be determined. As some physical disorders (e.g., anemia, thyroid disease) and medication side effects can mimic depression, this is an important component of assessment.

To ensure accurate diagnosis, information should be gathered using a variety of methods and informants. In addition to collecting information about symptoms, it is also important to evaluate children's cognitive and interpersonal functioning. Teacher self-report forms (e.g., the Teacher Report Form [TRF], the Conner's Teacher Rating Scale, and the Home and Community Social and Behavioral Scales [HCSBS]) are often used to assess a child's school functioning. In addition to being useful diagnostically, understanding a child's cognitive and interpersonal functioning is important for determining the type and course of treatment.

TREATMENT

Very few treatments have been designed specifically for DD. One study suggests treatment with antidepressants may be effective for treating chronic depression. However, more research is needed to determine the efficacy of pharmacologic treatments for DD.

No specific psychosocial interventions exist for treating DD in children. Research on adults with DD has suggested that treatments designed for MDD can be modified to treat the chronic symptoms of DD. For example, several cognitive approaches have been found to reduce depressive symptoms in adult patients with DD. Research is needed on the efficacy of such treatments for children with DD.

Due to the long course of DD and its high level of impairment and comorbidity, psychoeducation may be a useful treatment strategy for parents of and children with DD. The goal of such treatment would be to improve both symptom management and family functioning so that the child could recover from the DD in a healthier environment. Investigation of such programs is another important area for future research in pediatric depressive disorders.

See also: Bipolar Disorder; Cognitive–Behavior Therapy; Cognitive–Behavioral Play Therapy; Major Depressive Disorder; Suicide

Further Reading

American Psychiatric Association. (2000). *Diagnostic and statistical manual of mental disorders* (text revision). Washington, DC: Author.

Birmaher, B., Ryan, N. D., Williamson, D. E., Brent, D. A., Kaufman, J., Dahl, R. E., Perel, J., & Nelson, B. (1996). Childhood and adolescent depression: A review of the past 10 years. Part I. *Journal of the American Academy of Child and Adolescent Psychiatry, 35,* 1427–1439.

Birmaher, B., Ryan, N. D., Williamson, D. E., & Brent, D. A. (1996). Childhood and adolescent depression: A review of the past 10 years. Part II. *Journal of the American Academy of Child and Adolescent Psychiatry, 35,* 1575–1583.

Kovacs, M. (1997). Depressive disorders in childhood: An impressionistic landscape. *Journal of Child Psychology and Psychiatry, 38,* 287–298.

Kovacs, M., Feinberg, T. L., Crouse-Novak, M. A., Paulauskas, S. L., & Finkelstein, R. (1984). Depressive disorders in childhood: A longitudinal prospective study of characteristics and recovery. *Archives of General Psychiatry, 41,* 229–237.

KRISTEN E. HOLDERLE
MARY A. FRISTAD

Ee

Ear Infections

See: Otitis Media

Early Childhood Caries

DEFINITION

Early Childhood Caries (ECC) is an infectious disease characterized by dental decay of the primary dentition in children 5 years of age and younger (Figure 1). ECC presents a pattern consistent with anterior to

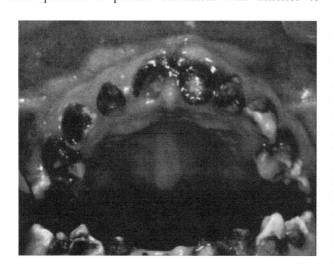

Figure 1. A 4-year-old child with severe ECC.

posterior embryological development and tooth eruption. Specifically, it initially, and most severely, affects the upper front teeth (maxillary incisors), followed by the primary molars. Except in severe disease, the lower front teeth generally are less involved, due to protection from the tongue. Multiple descriptive terms (e.g., nursing caries, nursing bottle caries, and baby-bottle tooth decay) have been coined to describe this process and its presumed causation. However, only in the 1990s did a consensus definition begin to evolve, benefiting and standardizing the empirical study of ECC, its causes, and contributing cultural, environmental, family system, behavioral, and psychological factors.

INCIDENCE/PREVALENCE

ECC is the most common chronic disease of childhood. The 1998 National Health and Nutrition Examination Survey (NHANES III) calculated overall prevalence rates ranging from 8.4 percent in 2-year-old children to 40.4 percent in 5-year-olds, with significantly higher rates reported among low socioeconomic and minority groups, including African Americans and Hispanic Americans. For reasons that are as yet poorly defined (e.g., limited access to care, individual genetic and psychosocial vulnerabilities, mediation by factors that also increase their risk for prematurity), low-income children experience 2–5 times more caries than higher income groups. In aboriginal groups prevalence rates range from 65 to 70 percent. Statistics notwithstanding, the Surgeon General's Report considers ECC a "silent epidemic," affecting the most vulnerable populations.

194

ETIOLOGY

ECC is a multifactorial disease with *Streptococcus mutans* as the primary bacterial pathogen. A chronic infectious process, it begins with the transmission of bacteria to the child during the course of primary tooth eruption. These bacteria convert foods, especially sugar and starch, into acid. Based on the persistent nature of bacterial-produced acid exposure, the impact of this process can vary from minimal enamel demineralization to severe and rampant decay resulting in a cavity (hole in the tooth). Depending on other host factors (e.g., saliva physiology, immunological host response, and inappropriate tooth formation), rapid deterioration of tooth structure may occur. If left untreated, bacteria are able to infiltrate the nerve, leading to a tooth abscess and death of the nerve and blood vessels that under healthy conditions give the tooth vitality. This process can result in premature loss of primary teeth that are important for function, dental development, and aesthetics.

Developmental tooth defects also have been positively correlated to ECC, likely due to subsequently increased bacterial retention and colonization of *S. mutans*. Interestingly, greater prevalence of enamel tooth defects is found among preterm, low birth-weight children, a group that has demonstrated higher prevalence of ECC. In addition, emerging associations among maternal periodontal disease, restricted fetal growth, and infant prematurity support an underlying "maternal oral to systemic disease connection."

Psychosocial and behavioral factors are also important in the development of this disease. Inadequate oral hygiene behaviors, as well as frequent or prolonged exposure to cariogenic foods (those high in sugar and starch), increase the risk of dental decay. Inappropriate feeding practices, including bedtime or naptime use of the bottle or sippy cup and prolonged nocturnal breast-feeding, are risk factors. Moreover, the quality of parenting and "goodness-of-fit" between child and caregiver can also contribute to ECC. For example, parenting stress and depression can be posited to interfere with a caregiver's provision of the oral health care necessary for the prevention of ECC. Similarly, parental report of a child's shy or "difficult" temperament profile correlates with increased caries risk, perhaps mediated by difficulties in dietary and oral health care.

CORRELATES

ECC can be devastating to the child and family. Adverse health consequences range from initially unrecognized physical changes and only mild discomfort, to heightened sensitivity and severe pain from carious teeth. The latter consequences of ECC may result in decreased caloric intake and "failure to thrive"; a syndrome that can affect brain growth, cognitive development, and future learning potential. Importantly, ECC increases the physical risk that a child will experience future dental caries. In addition, early caregiver-mediated oral hygiene and/or cariogenic diet choices may fail to establish healthy behavioral routines, contributing to subsequent internalization of poor oral health practices by the autonomous child, adolescent, and adult.

Oral rehabilitation is not without risk, especially for children who require conscious sedation or general anesthesia. In addition to the psychological impact of premature primary tooth loss, emotional distress experienced during restoration can result in the development of fearfulness, anxiety, and phobias. Additional family burdens of ECC include the parents' time away from work, travel requirements for those who live in communities more distant from treatment centers, plus the fiscal and emotional cost of restorative dental surgery.

DENTAL AND PSYCHOLOGICAL INTERVENTIONS

Generally, destroyed tooth structure does not regenerate. Dental treatment preserves children's teeth. Early recognition of dental disease and prompt treatment is less painful and less expensive than restoration following extensive decay. Once a cavitated lesion has formed, drilling out and removing the damaged tissue serve to halt the decay. The compromised tooth structure is then replaced by a restorative material such as silver alloy or composite resin. Crowns may be used if decay is extensive and/or there is limited tooth structure with which to work. A root canal may be required if the nerve in a tooth dies from decay or from a traumatic blow.

Psychological interventions may utilize peer modeling and guided doll play for educational and emotional preparation for dental procedures. Play therapy may ameliorate a child's perceptions of painful examination and treatment experiences, helping them master their anxious apprehensions regarding procedures and fearfulness of dental staff. Parenting skills training and child cognitive behavioral therapies may help enhance adherence to prescribed oral hygiene practices.

PREVENTION

ECC is a preventable disease. However, once initiated, the disease is neither self-limiting nor responsive to short-term pharmacological management, and requires invasive oral rehabilitation. Thus, "producing health," rather than "restoring health," is the focus of the following standard recommendations to help prevent ECC:

1. Promote pre- and postnatal maternal nutrition and oral health. This can help reduce formation of children's tooth defects while teeth are forming, as well as limit the transmission of *S. mutans* from mother to child in the early years of life.
2. Encourage initiation of appropriate behavioral routines for sleep and feeding by the time of first tooth eruption (~6 months of age). Avoid bedtime bottle or nocturnal breast-feeding, as well as practices that accomplish soothing the baby or toddler primarily via feeding. From a dental standpoint, transitioning to a "sippy cup" at 12 months is recommended. Encourage water between meals and discourage frequent consumption (i.e., snacking) of cariogenic foods. "Grazing" or frequent snacking increases the duration that acids are in contact with the tooth surface. The type of cariogenic food, and the timing and frequency of ingestion are more important than the amount. Sticky foods (e.g., candy, raisins) are more harmful because they remain on the surface of the teeth for prolonged periods of time.
3. Begin oral hygiene practices as soon as the first tooth erupts using an infant (Stage 1) toothbrush. Toothpaste designed specifically for infants can be used. Shifting to fluoridated toothpaste, as a source of topical fluoride in preschool aged children, should occur once the child is able to spit. Introduction of fluoride toothpaste can occur earlier if the child is at high risk for dental disease, albeit with caution regarding the possibility of swallowing too much fluoride. Floss as soon as teeth are touching or in contact. As the child matures, a matter-of-fact routine of proper brushing at least twice a day and flossing at least daily should be established, with the child gradually assuming responsibility for oral health behaviors as his or her effective skills develop and the caregiver's motivation and routines are internalized.
4. Recommend the initial dental visit to take place by the first birthday. This is consistent with the American Academy of Pediatrics Bright Futures Dental Guidelines.
5. Assess systemic fluoride level of water supplies and need for supplementation. Fluoride is a mineral that acts like a vitamin to strengthen the teeth. Appropriate levels are important, as too much fluoride may increase the risk of tooth weakness and staining, while too little fluoride increases the risk for caries development.
6. Apply dental sealant to correct developmental imperfections of tooth enamel when indicated. This material creates a smooth and easy to clean surface that decreases the penetration and accumulation of food and bacteria. Sealants fail at an annual rate of 5–10 percent but, overall, reduce the probability of developing a carious lesion on pit and fissure surfaces of teeth.

CONCLUSION

ECC is an important public health concern associated with a number of negative and debilitating sequelae. While ECC is associated largely with lower socioeconomic status (SES) and ethnic minority groups, evidence suggests that these factors do not cause ECC, but rather, mirror increased representation of environmental, behavioral, medical, and/or genetic differences that affect the greater ECC prevalence. The creation of a heuristic model to help guide our understanding of the natural history of caries within a developmental context will serve to direct effective and efficient preventive and intervention strategies, as well as aid in guiding future research.

See also: Behavioral Dentistry; Health Education/Health Promotion; Parenting Practices; Risk and Protective Factors; Treatment Adherence—Behavioral

Further Reading

Drury, T. F., Horowitz, A. M., Ismail, A. I., Maertens, M. P., Rozier, R. G., & Selwitz, R. H. (1999). Diagnosing and reporting early childhood caries for research purposes. A report of a workshop sponsored by NIDCR, HRSA and HCFA. *Journal of Public Health Dentistry, 59,* 192–197.

Mouradian, W. E., Wehr, E., & Crall, J. J. (2000). Disparities in children's oral health and access to dental care. *Journal of American Medical Association, 284,* 2625–2631.

Quiñonez, R., Keels, M. A., Vann, W., Jr., McIver, T., Heller, K., & Whitt, K. (2001). Early childhood caries: Psychosocial and biological risk factors in a high-risk population. *Caries Research, 35*(5), 376–383.

Quiñonez, R., Santos, R., Wilson, S., & Cross, H. (2001). Temperament and early childhood caries. *Pediatric Dentistry, 23*(1), 5–10.

U.S. Department of Health and Human Services. (2000). Oral Health in America. A report of the Surgeon General. Rockville, MD: USDHHS, National Institute of Dental and Craniofacial Research, National Institute of Health.

Vargas, C. M., Crall, J. J., & Schneider, D. A. (1998). Sociodemographic distribution of pediatric dental caries: NHANES III 1988–1994. *Journal of American Dental Association, 129*, 1229–1238.

ROCIO BEATRIZ QUIÑONEZ
J. KENNETH WHITT

Early Intervention

DESCRIPTION OF TREATMENT

Early intervention is typically thought of as a particular type of prevention strategy. Specifically, there are three levels of prevention: primary (also referred to as universal) prevention attempts to avoid the appearance of the disorder altogether; secondary (also referred to as selective) prevention strives for early diagnosis and treatment to shorten the duration of or reduce the ill effects of the problem; and tertiary (i.e., targeted) prevention aims to reduce limitations caused by the disorder and helps to speed the recovery process after the problem has occurred. Early intervention falls under the secondary prevention category.

Certain legal guidelines have recognized the need for early intervention strategies for all individuals. In 1975, Public Law No. 94-142 (Education for All Handicapped Children Act) ensured education for children with special needs. Public Law No. 99-457 extended these services to infants and toddlers aged 0–3 years. Then, in 1987, the United States Department of Education developed the Individuals with Disabilities Education Act (IDEA; Public Law No. 101-476), which was created to assist states in offering early intervention strategies to eligible children. Eligible infants and toddlers include children with developmental delays, those with a diagnosed physical or mental condition that may cause a developmental delay, and those deemed at-risk by the state. Although IDEA does not mandate that states create early intervention programs, funding is provided for states that choose to provide such programs. Currently all 50 states in the United States provide some type of early intervention services.

Because of federal regulations, early intervention for children aged 0–3 years has been implemented for a variety of issues encountered early in life. These services have varied from interventions for child-specific problems such as autism to more general social concerns such as poverty. The overall goal of early intervention is to foster positive environments for infants and toddlers as well as thwart developmental delays. The following section provides a sampling of the many early intervention programs available to date.

CLINICAL APPLICATIONS

Early and continuous intervention is highly recommended for children diagnosed with autism and other pervasive developmental disorders (PDDs). Although several early intervention programs are available, behavioral treatment approaches, such as Lovaas' discrete trial training, have received the most support. Behavioral programs for autism typically begin when the child is 2 years old and include highly structured instruction for the child about how to attend to and respond to social cues in the environment as well as appropriate academic material. Initial treatment involves rapport building and teaching the children how to pay appropriate attention (e.g., sitting in their chair, attending to materials). Children are then presented developmentally appropriate academic material in a highly structured manner involving prompting, shaping, and imitation until the desired skill is learned. This method is also used to teach appropriate social behavior (e.g., making eye contact, spontaneous communication). After the skills are learned in teacher-directed therapy sessions, the skills are generalized to the natural environment.

Programs have also been designed for children at-risk for other disabilities or delays. Some interventions, for example, the individual caregiver–child therapy model, focus on improving the child's communication abilities. Consistent with this model, professionals work directly with the child and provide a model for the parent of the correct interaction style to improve child's communication skills. Other approaches have concentrated on the child's emotional development. Greenspan, for example, developed a technique called "floor time" that involves teaching parents how to engage their child in developmentally appropriate play designed to improve socioemotional processes. These types of early intervention programs help to foster appropriate development in infants and toddlers who are at-risk for or display early signs of delays or disabilities.

Because the parent–child interaction is of great importance to proper emotional and social development of the infant, some interventions focus directly on altering and enhancing the interactions between parents and their infant or toddler. This may be achieved through watching videotapes of and modeling appropriate interactions for the parent. Other techniques, such as triadic strategies, strive to change the parent–child interaction through play. The therapist, parent, and child all work together to build on the parent's strengths through contextual and interpersonal support. The therapist helps establish a supportive atmosphere in the context of play. Through modeling and direct instruction, the therapist helps the parent to recognize behaviors that can facilitate development and to focus on the strengths of the interaction. The therapist instills parental confidence by helping the parent to acknowledge his or her own accomplishments. Similar techniques have also been used to prevent young children's behavior problems from worsening. For example, Parent–Child Interaction Therapy (PCIT) combines play therapy and behavior therapy to strengthen the parent–child bond while increasing parenting skills (e.g., maintaining appropriate expectations of the child, discipline consistency) and subsequently reducing child noncompliance and other behavior problems. Parents learn how to enjoy interactions with their children, foster development, and gain confidence in their parenting abilities.

Early intervention programs have also focused on averting future academic difficulties often encountered by children in high-risk families (e.g., families living in poverty). For example, programs such as the Abecedarian Project have been developed to reduce the risk of developmental delays and future academic failure for at-risk children. The Abecedarian Project targeted healthy infants who were born into impoverished families with high numbers of the following risk factors: low parental education levels, low familial income, single parent households, poor maternal social support, siblings experiencing academic difficulties, receipt of welfare, low parental IQ, parents working at unskilled jobs, and need for counseling or other community services. Infants enrolled in the project were divided into four groups. First, half of the children in this program received an early childhood education program beginning at 6 weeks of age and ending once the children entered kindergarten. The other half served as a control group. Both the intervention and control groups were then divided further into two additional groups, those who received 3 years of school-age intervention and those who did not. Results indicated that the early education program (i.e., from 6 weeks to 5 years) demonstrated the most lasting positive effects

on academic achievement when compared to similar children who had not received this part of the intervention.

Early Head Start is another program designed to address the developmental and intellectual needs of children from birth to 3 years. This program is essentially a downward extension of the Head Start program and provides early education for infants and toddlers, parent education, physical and mental health services, nutritional education, and family support for low-income families. Families can obtain services in their home, at a center, or both. Initial results have been positive. Children, 2 years of age, enrolled in Early Head Start have demonstrated higher cognitive development and larger vocabularies than control children. Additionally, their home environments have been more supportive of intellectual development and their mothers have had better parenting skills and were more likely to use play to help stimulate and support their children's development.

Although thwarting future developmental problems is important, it is equally important to ensure that the basic needs of the infant or toddler are met. The Special Supplemental Nutritional Program for Women, Infants, and Children (WIC) provides food, nutritional education, and referrals to health care and social services for low-income mothers and their children up to 5 years of age. The idea behind this program is to circumvent health problems that stem from poor nutrition. This program has been effective at meeting this goal, especially for mothers and infants.

Finally, early interventions have been created for infants and toddlers who are at risk for being abused. These programs do not focus on the child per se, but rather focus on fostering a safe environment for the child in order to thwart future developmental, physical, and emotional problems. Many states offer early intervention programs for families at high risk for abuse or neglect. One type of early intervention, parent aide programs, offers support for and appropriate role models of good parenting for parents at risk of becoming abusive. For example, the Vermont Parent/Child Centers provide childcare, play groups, parent education, support, and drop-in or home-based services for families identified as high risk for abuse. A newer concept in abuse prevention is wraparound service. Wrap-around service includes an interdisciplinary team made up of the parent, child, service coordinator, child/parent advocate, and other professionals deemed to be necessary. Services are individualized to the needs of the family and change as the needs of the family change.

EFFECTIVENESS

Early intervention programs have proven effective in reducing the negative effects of several problems encountered early in life, including developmental disorders, dysfunctional parent–child interactional style, familial low income, nutritional deficits, and risk for abuse or neglect. Thus, early intervention programs have been successful in reducing developmental delays and cognitive impairments as well as improving the environment of the child to foster future appropriate development.

See also: Head Start; Mental Retardation; Parent–Child Interaction Therapy; Parent Training; Pervasive Developmental Disorders—Not Otherwise Specified

Further Reading

Crane, J. (Ed.). (1998). *Social programs that work.* New York: Russell Sage Foundation.

Raikes, H. H., & Love, J. M. (2002). Early Head Start: A dynamic new program for infants and toddlers and their families. *Infant Mental Health Journal, 23*(1–2), 1–13.

Singer, G. H., Powers, L. E., & Olson, A. L. (Eds.). (1996). *Redefining family support: Innovations in public–private partnerships.* Baltimore, MD: Paul H. Brookes.

Zeanah, C. H. (Ed.). (2000). *Handbook of infant mental health* (2nd ed.). New York: Guilford.

CHERYL B. MCNEIL
REBECCA S. BERNARD

Eating Disorders

See: Anorexia Nervosa; Bulimia Nervosa; Obesity

Effects of Parental Substance Abuse on Children

DEFINITION OF THE PROBLEM

Substance abuse is a growing problem in the United States. This includes both legal (e.g., cigarettes, alcohol, prescription medications) and illegal (e.g., cocaine, methamphetamines, opiates) substances. It is estimated that 11–13 percent of pregnant women use drugs or drink alcohol during their pregnancies. The percentage of pregnant women who smoke cigarettes is close to 20 percent. Substance use during pregnancy can have long-lasting developmental and behavioral consequences for children. For example, alcohol use during pregnancy is the leading known cause of mental retardation in children in the United States. In addition to the prenatal effects, environmental factors must also be considered. It is estimated that 10 million children live in homes where substance abuse is present. Of these, close to 400,000 children are maltreated each year. This may be an underestimate, given the numbers of cases that go unreported or unfounded. The United States reports anywhere from 20 to 90 percent of all child maltreatment cases involve substance abuse. Furthermore, substance abuse is also strongly correlated with domestic violence. The overall result is an increasing number of children placed in foster care each year due to substance abuse by caregivers. For example, two thirds of the children in foster care in California and Illinois have at least one parent with a substance abuse problem. Unfortunately, while the number of children entering the foster care system continues to climb, the number of available homes for these children is on the decline. Costs for care of children with prenatal exposure as well as other children impacted by substance abuse are staggering. For example, the financial cost related to substance abuse during pregnancy is estimated at between $22.3 million and $125 million annually. The National Center on Addiction and Substance Abuse (1999) estimates that the Child Protective Services system spends approximately $10 billion per year due to substance abuse problems; this figure does not take into account medical and legal costs related to the children.

PROGNOSIS

In general, some of the risk factors for child maltreatment include low socioeconomic status (SES) caregiver stress, history of child maltreatment, and poor parenting skills. However, there are other risk factors that are unique to children living in homes where substance abuse is present. Allocation of resources such as time and money for food/clothing may be focused on securing the next "high" or "fix" rather than spending these resources on the children. Due to drug-seeking behaviors, caregivers are more likely to be involved in illegal activities such as theft, burglary, and prostitution than are caregivers not involved in substance abuse. As a result, troubles with the law and time in jail are common in this population. Caregivers who abuse substances are also at increased risk for comorbid mental health diagnoses (e.g., depression, anxiety disorders, bipolar, personality disorders). Furthermore, they are at increased risk for physical health problems such as hepatitis, HIV/AIDS, and sexually transmitted diseases. When mental and/or physical health concerns are present, the ability to effectively provide for the needs of children may be compromised. Finally, as parents use substances, children attend to these behaviors, increasing their risk for substance abuse.

Health risks also exist for children living in homes where substance abuse is present. Accidental ingestion of substances left within easy reach can occur or adults who abuse substances in the home may proffer substances. Unfortunately, this may result in hospitalization or even death. Fumes common during manufacture of drugs may also cause health risks to children as well as risk of physical harm due to burns or explosions. Children of substance abusers are at increased risk for attachment problems. Parenting is often inconsistent, resulting in harsh punishments that are generally unpredictable in nature. Furthermore, due to separation that may occur shortly after birth because of involvement of Child Protective Services and/or extended hospital stays, babies with prenatal substance exposure may have inconsistent caregivers. With the increase in methamphetamine production in the United States, more law enforcement raids on these labs are being conducted. Children found in the home during these raids are generally placed in shelters following a check of medical status and potential decontamination procedures. The result of these unpredictable and frightening experiences has been a reported increase in posttraumatic stress reactions in children from these homes. Posttraumatic Stress Disorder (PTSD) has also been reported in children who have been physically or sexually abused; again, this risk is increased in substance abusing environments.

Behaviors of neonates prenatally exposed to substances are often difficult for their caregivers. Caregivers of these children generally report less satisfaction with parenting, more negative perceptions of their children, and greater levels of stress than do caregivers of children without exposure. Problems with feeding, sleep, state regulation, and consolability are challenging in and of themselves. Parents who are actively using substances may not have the patience required to care for the infants, thus increasing the risk for abuse and/or neglect.

The dynamics of families who are impacted by substance abuse are often dysfunctional. Children may assume many parental responsibilities such as caring for younger siblings, housekeeping, and cooking. They may also feel responsible for meeting the needs of the caregiver. When domestic violence is present, these children may try to take the role of family peacemaker.

Other children may take the role of family scapegoat. In other words, they may bear the brunt of caregiver anger, frustration, and demands. Self-esteem in children reared in substance abusing families is often low. Peer relationships may also be affected, as children are unlikely to bring friends home to an unpredictable or negative environment, resulting in feelings of isolation. Although many children reared in difficult family situations are resilient, the risk for problems (academic, social, emotional, and behavioral) in this population is high.

INTERVENTIONS

Substance abuse treatment programs involving the courts are expanding across the United States. When substance abuse is a problem in a family, two issues are paramount: child safety and intervention. The safety issues are often addressed by removing the children from the care of the parents until progress is made in substance abuse treatment. For children that remain with the parents, monitoring of treatment plans and home environment is important. Many different models of substance abuse treatment exist ranging from self-help (e.g., Alcoholics Anonymous) to short-term programs to long-term residential programs. Some programs allow children to accompany parents into treatment while others do not. For substance abuse treatment to be most effective, gender-specific services are strongly recommended. Treatment should also be multimodal in nature, going beyond treating only the substance abuse problem. Issues of parenting, physical and mental health, pediatric care, education/job training should also be incorporated into treatment plans. Long-term follow-up services are strongly recommended. Treatment intervention services for children are also important. Services focused on issues ranging from parent–child interactions to effective coping strategies, anger management, and substance abuse education may be incorporated into these services. By addressing the entire family system that has been adversely impacted by substance abuse, both the caregiver(s) and the child may be helped to reach their full potential.

See also: Child Maltreatment; Family Assessment; Family Intervention; Fetal Alcohol Syndrome; Prenatal Exposure to Methamphetamines

Further Reading

Ammerman, R., Kolko, D., Kirisci, L., Backson, T., & Dawes, M. (1999). Child abuse potential in parents with histories of substance use disorder. *Child Abuse and Neglect, 23*, 1225–1238.

Bays, J. (1990). Substance abuse and child abuse: The impact of addiction on the child. *Pediatric Clinics of North America, 37,* 881–904.

Johnson, J., & Leff, M. (1999). Children of substance abusers: Overview of research findings. *Pediatrics, 103*(5), 1085–1099.

National Center on Addiction and Substance Abuse (1999). *No safe haven: Children of substance abusing parents.* New York: Author, Columbia University.

ROBIN H. GURWITCH

Emotional Abuse

See: Psychological Maltreatment

Emotional Development

DEFINITION

Emotional states are complex reactions that are accompanied by affective states (i.e., feelings). The development of these emotional states begins with the expression of primary emotions at birth and continues to the expression of more complex emotions with age. The development of emotions seems to be related to the maturation of the brain, but can be altered by environmental influences. Each emotion is expressed in a certain way (e.g., crying, smiling, frowning) and is accompanied by certain neurochemical processes in the body. Individuals differ in the ways in which emotions are elicited and how they are expressed. In addition, each society has rules that govern how and when certain emotions are to be expressed.

INFANT EMOTIONAL DEVELOPMENT

The primary emotions that infants display at birth are interest, distress, disgust, and contentment. These emotions are displayed through facial expressions, which become more distinct with age, and can be measured using a scale such as Izard's Facial Expression Scoring Manual. Between 2 and 7 months of age, other basic emotions emerge (anger, sadness, joy, surprise, and fear). The emergence of these emotions may depend upon the opportunity to experience them.

The expression of these primary emotions in infants takes on three distinct forms: crying, smiling,

and laughing. The expression of emotions is important in infancy because it is an infant's means of communication. When the infant's emotional expressions gain a response, the infant acquires a sense of control over its environment. Crying is the way in which infants express their vital needs. At first their cries signify physical discomfort, and later cries signify psychological discomfort as well. If the infant's cries are reinforced by caregivers, the infant will gain confidence that their actions will bring results, and by the end of the first year, infants whose cries have been reinforced will cry less and use other communicative acts in place of crying to communicate their needs. Smiling is another way that infants communicate with caregivers. The first smile that appears soon after birth occurs as a result of central nervous system activity and is independent of sensory stimulation. However, smiles soon begin to occur during the second week in response to care giving activities (feeding, caregiver's sounds, etc.). By one month of age the infant's smiles are increasing in frequency and are socially directed, and by the second month of age, infants begin to selectively smile more at familiar people. Laughing also develops early in infancy (by about 4 months of age) and is related to sensations and events that the infant enjoys as well as occurrences that may frighten the infant. Laughing increases with age and cognitive development, and is generally seen in response to inconsistencies in the environment.

CHILDHOOD EMOTIONAL DEVELOPMENT

Complex Emotions

During the second year, children begin to express more complex emotions (embarrassment, shame, guilt, envy, and pride). Emotions such as embarrassment are considered "self-conscious" emotions and do not appear until the child has achieved self-recognition and an understanding that they are separate from other people and objects. Emotions such as shame, guilt, and pride are considered "self-evaluative" emotions and the attainment of these emotions generally requires that both self-recognition and an understanding of rules are acquired. The development of more complex emotions reflects the ability of children to consider their actions and measure them against societal rules, which marks the beginning of moral understanding.

Fears

Fears may stem from a number of sources including frightening images on television, conditioning, and underlying anxieties. Temporary fears are very common in young children. In midchildhood (around 6 years of age), children are likely to be afraid of things like the dark, monsters, and thunderstorms mainly because of their inability to separate make-believe from reality. As children age, they are more likely to be afraid of bodily injury and physical danger because of their understanding of cause and effect relationships and because they have a greater number of previous experiences from which to acquire fears.

Altruism

Altruism develops as the child is able to understand how another person might feel, and as the child gains a sense of responsibility for others' feelings. This may begin as early as 2 years of age. However, spontaneous self-sacrifice is uncommon in toddlers and preschoolers, but becomes more common during elementary years.

SOCIETAL DISPLAY RULES

All societies have rules on how and when certain emotions are to be displayed. Children learn and acquire these rules with age, and the acquisition of these rules plays an important role in the child's social development. Children are taught display rules very early in life. For example, mothers of infants in the United States become increasingly responsive to positive emotional displays (smiling, laughing), and become less responsive to negative emotional displays (crying, screaming). Therefore, the infant learns to suppress their expression of negative emotions.

From infancy through childhood, children are learning how to suppress certain emotional displays in accordance with societal standards. As children mature, they are able to use various behaviors to replace socially inappropriate emotional displays. For example, a child 2 years of age may bite his/her lips to suppress anger, and a preschooler may convey his/her feelings in an appropriate manner using their language abilities. The suppression of emotions is often very difficult for young children but with age children become better at being emotionally deceptive. Abiding societal display rules may also entail intensifying the expression of some emotions (e.g., feeling of guilt when you cause anguish, excitement at receiving a birthday present, or pride in an achievement). By encouraging children to intensify certain emotional displays, the children will learn about display rules and about how they should feel in certain situations.

UNDERSTANDING OTHERS' EMOTIONS

Emotional development also entails learning how to recognize and interpret the emotional displays of others. The ability to interpret and understand others' emotions is central to the development of social cognition. Although there is some debate about when infants are able to differentiate emotional expressions, it has been shown that 3-month-olds have a preference for happy faces over sad or neutral faces. Between 8 and 10 months of age, infants develop the ability to use social referencing to interpret and use the emotions of caregivers to regulate their own actions, and with age, social referencing extends to the emotional expression of persons other than caregivers. By 4–5 years of age, children are able to explain why others are expressing certain emotions but focus on external events as causes; however, by 8 years of age, children are able to focus on internal events as causes of emotional expressions. By 7–9 years of age, children are able to understand that people can experience more than one emotion at a time. In addition, older children are able to interpret contradicting emotional cues and infer the proper emotion. The development of emotional interpretation and understanding often parallels the child's cognitive development.

CLINICAL IMPLICATIONS

Acute fears, anxieties, acting-out behaviors, and sad moods are very common during childhood; however, for some children these emotions and behavioral expressions can become extreme or chronic, requiring professional intervention. Just as children learn to label emotions, to talk about emotions, and to use language about emotions to guide behavior, so must they learn to regulate emotions and behaviors. Emotional regulation refers to the ability to initiate, maintain and modulate the occurrence, intensity or internal feeling states and emotion-related physiological processes; behavior regulation refers to the ability to control emotionally driven behavior (facial or bodily reactions, aggression, etc.). Children face many challenges in learning to regulate their emotions and behavior including: (1) tolerating frustration; (2) coping with fear and anxiety; (3) defending themselves and their property; (4) tolerating being alone; and (5) negotiating friendships. Learning to regulate one's emotions is learned through experiences in interacting with others, modeling others' behavior, and environmental circumstances such as the death of a loved one or child abuse. Inborn temperamental characteristics also play a role in how one reacts to a variety of stimuli or situations. In addition, cognitive and language skills play a critical role in the ability to self-regulate and help the child gain the ability to intentionally apply strategies for regulation.

The inability to regulate one's emotions is associated with behavior problems: externalizing problems (e.g., oppositional-defiant behavior, conduct problems) for children who are underregulated, and internalizing problems (e.g., depression, anxiety) for those who are overregulated. For example, Caspi and colleagues (1996) found that children who were underregulated (irritable, impulsive, lacking in persistence, had trouble sitting, and had rough and uncontrolled behavior) at 3 years of age were more likely to fit a diagnosis for antisocial personality disorder and to be involved in criminal activity at 21 years of age. In contrast, overregulated 3-year-olds were more likely to meet diagnostic criteria for depression at age 21 years. Thus, a child's emotional development plays a major role in a child's ability to adjust or cope with life circumstances, and the focus of psychological intervention is often on helping children learn to regulate their emotions and behavior.

See also: Attachment; Identity Development; Moral Development

Further Reading

Caspi, A., Moffitt, T. E., Newman, K. L., & Silva, P. A. (1996). Behavioral observations at age 3 predict adult psychiatric disorders: Longitudinal evidence from a birth cohort. *Archives of General Psychiatry, 53,* 1033–1039.

Gowen, J. W., & Nebrig, J. B. (2002). Enhancing early emotional development: Guiding parents of young children. Baltimore, MD: Paul H. Brookes.

Papalia, D. E., & Olds, S. W. (Eds.). (1995). *Human development* (6th ed.). New York: McGraw-Hill.

Salisch, M. V. (2001). Children's emotional development: Challenges in their relationships to parents, peers, and friends. *International Journal of Behavioral Development, 25,* 310–319.

Shaffer, D. R. (Ed.). (1998). *Developmental psychology: Childhood and adolescence* (5th ed.). Pacific Grove CA: Brooks/Cole.

CHRISTA J. ANDERSON
JOHN COLOMBO

Empirically Supported Treatments

See: Evidence-Based Treatments

Encopresis*

DEFINITION/PREVALENCE

The essential feature of encopresis is that the child repeatedly passes feces in inappropriate places such as in clothing or on the floor. The passage of feces can be involuntary or intentional. The *Diagnostic and Statistical Manual of Mental Disorders, Fourth Edition* of the American Psychiatric Association (*DSM-IV*) requires a chronological or developmental age of at least 4 years and inappropriate passage of feces at least once a month for a minimum of 3 months for a diagnosis of encopresis. Since this is, by definition, a functional disorder, *DSM-IV* specifies that the condition not be due to a physiological or general medical problem. *DSM-IV* further stipulates that the presence or absence of constipation and the resultant overflow incontinence be indicated as present or absent. Approximately 5–7 percent of children experience difficulty with encopresis. The incidence is four or five times more common in boys than in girls.

Three subtypes or categories of encopresis have been identified. The first category of encopresis is the most common. This is retentive encopresis or encopresis based on chronic constipation. While this seems paradoxical (that constipation causes soiling), it is the most common cause (80–90 percent of cases). Second, there are cases of soiling that appear to be due to stress-induced diarrhea and loose bowels. Third, there are children who can be described as manipulative soilers. These children soil when there is a secondary benefit such as passively expressing anger toward their parents, avoiding a test at school, or some similar social stimulus. The soiling appears to be at least partially deliberate and under voluntary control. It is relatively rare in occurrence.

ETIOLOGY

There are three general approaches to understanding the etiology of encopresis: biological, emotional, and learning. Although encopresis is, by definition, a functional disorder and therefore not the result of a basic organic dysfunction, some notions regarding the etiology of encopresis involve a biological or physiological underlay.

*The views expressed in this article are those of the author(s) and do not necessarily reflect the official policy or position of the Department of the Navy, Department of Defense, or the U.S. Government.

Hereditary factors and developmental delay have been proposed as possible bases for encopresis; however, it is unlikely that such factors play a significant role in most cases of encopresis. One biological factor that definitely requires medical evaluation prior to treatment for encopresis is Hirschsprung's disease or aganglionic megacolon. This is a condition in which the colon lacks sufficient nerve supply to function normally. It is present at birth and is quickly diagnosed in severe cases but can go undetected until later in life in mild cases. Treatment involves surgical removal of the section of the colon that is defective.

Early mental health literature on encopresis often assumed a psychodynamic etiology to the problem. Thus, this symptom was sometimes thought of as a sign of unconscious conflict. Studies have generally failed to support psychodynamic hypotheses, and psychotherapy has a very modest success rate (if it helps at all) with children who have encopresis. Thus, while emotional factors may be involved in some children who are encopretic, this notion does not satisfactorily account for the etiology of the problem.

Consideration of the three subcategories of encopresis within a learning theory framework suggests several possible explanations for the behavior. First, manipulative soiling appears to follow a reinforcement model. Use of soiling to successfully manipulate the environment serves to reinforce the child's soiling behavior. Chronic diarrhea and irritable bowel syndrome can be understood as symptoms of children in which stress and anxiety lead to impaired bowel control and loss of successful performance of previously learned toileting behaviors. Associated with this might well be an inherited predisposition to react with intestinal distress in difficult situations along with a failure to learn effective coping behaviors to reduce stress.

Finally, as noted, the most common form of encopresis is based on constipation. Poor dietary choices and failure to establish good toilet habits, both of which are learned, play a role in development of this disorder. In addition, children may learn to voluntarily withhold stools for various reasons. This withholding can readily precipitate constipation. Children, for example, may withhold stools while playing outside because they do not wish to take time to return to the house to go to the bathroom. When a child becomes chronically constipated, the stools create an impaction in the colon. When food leaves the stomach to enter the intestine, it is a liquid. Ordinarily, the fluid is extracted as it makes its way through the intestinal tract and solid waste is expelled at the end. However, when impaction is present, a liquid mass forms a pool at the point of impaction and leaks around it, resulting in soiling of the underclothing without any sensation of a bowel movement because the seepage is a passive process. At times, large masses of solid fecal material

loosen and are expelled. Thus, constipation is the root cause of soiling.

ASSESSMENT

Assessment of the child with encopresis should begin with a medical examination to rule out organic disease that could be causing the condition. If no such disease is present, a psychological evaluation should be performed to determine the etiology of the problem and to rule out serious psychopathology. This can generally be accomplished by interview, though psychological testing is sometimes needed. If serious psychopathology is present, it may be wise to treat this first and to attempt treatment of the encopresis later. The interview should establish the etiology of the problem and obtain information necessary to implement a behavior modification program for treatment.

TREATMENT

Consideration of the three categories of encopresis described suggests that different treatments are advisable for the different etiologies. With respect to manipulative soiling, a combination of behavioral and family therapy is indicated. Efforts should be made to teach the child more effective ways of coping with the environment, and the parents should be taught ways to communicate with and respond appropriately to their child. Sources of reinforcement supporting the soiling behavior should be removed and more appropriate behavior rewarded. Behavioral treatment programs have been described by Walker and his colleagues (1981).

Chronic diarrhea or irritable bowel syndrome is best addressed through stress reduction and the acquisition of effective coping skills. A variety of approaches such as relaxation training, stress inoculation training, assertiveness training, and general stress management procedures may be effective in managing diarrhea in these patients. In addition, supportive psychotherapy as well as certain medications are sometimes useful. Antidiarrhea medications as well as antianxiety and antidepressant medications are often used by physicians.

Since 80–90 percent of children diagnosed as encopretic fall in the category of retentive or constipation-based encopresis, a number of treatments have been developed for dealing with these cases. The standard medical treatment for constipation-based encopresis involves thorough evacuation of the bowel through laxatives and/or enemas followed by oral administration of 1–3 teaspoons of mineral oil 2–3 times a day for a period of 3 months to a year. A very thorough position statement on the medical treatment of this disorder has been prepared by the North American Society for Pediatric Gastroenterology and Nutrition.

The most effective behavioral treatments combine medical procedures with behavioral conditioning procedures such as positive reinforcement, punishment, cleanliness training, and periodic toileting. Treatment programs involving enemas and suppositories along with positive reinforcement for bowel movements, mild aversive consequences for soiled under clothing, and diet manipulation (a high fiber diet with restrictions on milk and cheese) reported virtually 100 percent effectiveness. Useful clinical protocols for the application of these procedures may be found in the writings of Howe and Walker (1992).

PROGNOSIS

The prognosis for all forms of encopresis is very good. Proper treatment based on the etiology of the problem is highly successful. The problem becomes infrequent in adolescence and rare in adults.

See also: Developmental Issues in Assessment for Treatment; Developmental Issues in Treatment; Gastrointestinal Disorders; Irritable Bowel Syndrome

Further Reading

American Psychiatric Association. (1994). *Diagnostic and statistical manual of mental disorders* (4th ed., Rev.). Washington, DC: Author.

Angelides, A., & Fitzgerald, J. F. (1981). Pharmacologic advances in the treatment of gastrointestinal diseases. *Pediatric Clinics of North America, 28,* 95–112.

Baker, S. S., Liptak, G. S., Colletti, R. B., Croffie, J. M., DiLorenzo, C., Ector, W., & Nurko, S. (1999). Constipation in infants and children: Evaluation and treatment. *Journal of Pediatric Gastroenterology and Nutrition, 29,* 612–626.

Howe, A. C., & Walker, C. E. (1992). Behavioral management of toilet training, enuresis, and encopresis. *Pediatric Clinics of North America, 39*(3), 413–432.

Walker, C. E., Hedberg, A. G., Clement, P. W., & Wright, L. (1981). *Clinical procedures for behavior therapy.* Englewood Cliffs, NJ: Prentice-Hall.

C. EUGENE WALKER
DREW C. MESSER†

†I am a military service member. This work was prepared as part of my official duties. Title 17 U.S.C. 105 provides that "Copyright protection under this title is not available for any work of the United States Government." Title 17 U.S.C. 101 defines a United States Government work as a work prepared by a military service member or employee of the United States Government as part of that person's official duties.

Endocrine Disorders

See: Congenital Adrena Hyperplasia; Diabetes Mellitus, Type 1; Diabetes Mellitus, Type 2; Clinical Gigantism and Acromegaly: Growth Hormone Deficiency; Gynecomastia; Hyperthryroidism, Acquired: Hypothyroidism, Acquired; Hypothyroidism, Congenital; Klincfelter Syndrome; Nonnan Syndrome; Prader Willi Syndrome; Puberty, Delayed; Puberty, Normal: Puberty, Precocious; Sexual Differentiation: Disorders and Clinical Management; Short Stature: Psychological Aspects

Enuresis*

DEFINITION/PREVALENCE

The essential feature of enuresis is that the child repeatedly voids urine in inappropriate places such as wetting the clothes during the day or wetting the bed at night. The *Diagnostic and Statistical Manual* of the American Psychiatric Association (*DSM-IV*) criteria include (1) may be involuntary or intentional; (2) the child must have reached a chronological or developmental equivalent age of 5 years; (3) the problem must have clinical significance due to either a frequency of twice a week for at least three consecutive months or associated with distress/impairment in social, academic (occupational), or other important areas; and (4) be functional in etiology. Whether the wetting is diurnal (daytime), nocturnal (nighttime), or both should be specified. Though not included in essential *DSM-IV* criteria, differentiating whether it is primary/continuous, which refers to wetting existing from birth, or secondary, which is usually defined as enuresis following a period of urinary continence lasting at least 6 months, is often of interest. Approximately 7 percent of males and 3 percent of females at age 5 have enuresis; by age 10 it is 3 percent and 2 percent, respectively; by age 18 it is one percent for males and less than one percent for females. There is a 15 percent spontaneous remission rate per year for untreated enuresis.

*The views expressed in this article are those of the author(s) and do not necessarily reflect the official policy or position of the Department of the Navy, Department of Defense, or the U.S. Government.

ETIOLOGY

There are three general approaches to understanding the etiology of enuresis: biological, emotional, and learning. Although enuresis is, by definition, a functional disorder and therefore not the result of a basic organic dysfunction, numerous ideas regarding the etiology of enuresis presuppose some biological or physiological underlay creating the problem. The two main biological theories that have received a reasonable amount of support from the research literature are that the disorder may be inherited genetically and that it might involve developmental delay of the nervous system. Another theory with some support is that decreased production of antidiuretic hormone (ADH) by some children may result in overproduction of urine at night and consequently wetting of the bed.

At one time, mental health workers generally assumed that enuresis was primarily a symptom of emotional disorder. Enuresis was conceptualized as an expression of neurotic or emotional conflict. The idea that there was an intrinsic relationship between enuresis and various types of neurotic or emotional conflict probably resulted from a bias in referral patterns to mental health professionals and is not given much credence today.

The third, and probably most widely accepted view regarding the etiology of enuresis, assumes a problem in learning to be the major cause. At birth, the process of urination is governed by reflex action. After long experience, adults learn to delay the reflexive behavior of urination for relatively long periods of time. During their developmental years, children are attempting to master the learning task of controlling a reflexive behavior. Children with enuresis may be viewed as children who are experiencing difficulty in learning this control mechanism.

ASSESSMENT

Assessment of the child with enuresis should begin with a medical examination to rule out any organic diseases that could be causing the condition. If no such disease is present, a psychological evaluation should be performed to determine the etiology of the problem and to rule out serious pathology. This generally can be accomplished by interview, though psychological testing is sometimes needed. If serious psychopathology is present, it may be wise to treat this first and to attempt treatment of the enuresis later. The interview should establish the etiology of the problem and obtain information necessary to implement a behavior modification program for treatment.

TREATMENT

In considering possible treatments for enuresis, one would be well advised to consider the discomfort of the problem versus the danger and possible consequences of the attempted cure. Since there is a steady progression in "spontaneous" remission each year, and the incidence of enuresis persisting into adulthood is very low, there is some question as to whether or not enuresis should be treated at all and if so at what age. Reasons for treatment include sanitation concerns, the degree of family conflict and parent–child antagonism, and embarrassment, teasing, and ostracism of the child by other children which may have significant effects on the child's emotional well-being and self-esteem.

Over a period of five decades there have been dozens of demonstrations of the effectiveness of alarm system training. This system involves a sensor that sounds a bell or alarm when the child urinates. The child is thus awakened and goes to the bathroom. Application of such systems for a period of 8–12 weeks can be expected to result in between a 75 and 90 percent success rate in initial arrest of bed-wetting. Reliable and reasonably inexpensive equipment can be obtained from numerous places (see http://bedwettingstore.com). A recent development in this area is the invention of a miniature ultrasonic sensor that is worn on a belt around the abdomen. This sensor determines urine volume in the bladder and sounds an alarm at a predetermined point.

Two popular books are available on the market to assist parents in using behavioral treatment programs for dealing with bedwetting. These are *Toilet Training in Less Than a Day* (Azrin & Foxx, 1989) and *Bedwetting: A Guide for Parents and Children* (Houts & Liebert, 1984). Use of the programs described in these books is highly successful, especially if pursued under professional supervision, and should be the first attempt at treatment for most children. Other approaches may be attempted if the behavioral approach is unsuccessful.

There are three medications that are currently prescribed with some frequency for enuresis. The most commonly prescribed medication is imipramine (Tofranil). Research has indicated that this medication has some usefulness and success in the treatment of enuresis. Unfortunately, less than 50 percent of children treated with this become completely dry. The remainder shows only a reduction in frequency or no effect. When the medication is terminated, most children who have been treated with imipramine relapse. Other medications increasing in popularity are desmopressin acetate (DDAVP) and oxybutynin chloride (Ditropan). DDAVP is a synthetic form of vasopressin, a hormone that stimulates the kidneys to concentrate urine. Concentration of urine reduces the volume of urine produced during the night and enables some children to sleep through the night without wetting. Ditropan reduces spasms of the bladder and thus increases the capacity of the bladder.

PROGNOSIS

The prognosis for enuresis is very good. Proper treatment based on the etiology of the problem is highly successful. Enuresis persisting into adulthood is rare.

See also: Developmental Issues in Assessment for Treatment; Developmental Issues in Treatment; Encopresis

Further Reading

American Psychiatric Association. (1994). *Diagnostic and statistical manual of mental disorders* (4th ed., Rev.). Washington, DC: Author.

Azrin, N. H., & Foxx, R. M. (1989). *Toilet training in less than a day.* New York: Pocket Books.

Petrician, P., & Sawan, M. A. (1998). Design of a miniaturized ultrasonic bladder volume monitor and subsequent preliminary evaluation on 41 enuretic patients. *Transactions on Rehabilitation Engineering, 6*(1), 66–74.

Houts, A. C., & Liebert, R. M. (1984). *Bedwetting: a guide for parents and children.* Springfield, IL: Charles C. Thomas.

DREW C. MESSER†
C. EUGENE WALKER

†I am a military service member. This work was prepared as part of my official duties. Title 17 U.S.C. 105 provides that "Copyright protection under this title is not available for any work of the United States Government." Title 17 U.S.C. 101 defines a United States Government work as a work prepared by a military service member or employee of the United States Government as part of that person's official duties.

Environmental Tobacco Smoke

See: Cigarette Smoking

Environmental Toxins

Environmental toxins are agents in the air, water, and earth's crust that may have an adverse effect on health, learning, and behavior. Toxins may attack the body at the molar level of behavior, at the level of the organ system, the organelle, the cellular, and the molecular levels. Many naturally occurring chemicals in the environment are toxic above some threshold level. There are even more man-made chemicals produced in huge quantities each year, which may have the potential for developmental toxicity. For instance, in 1997, there were about 4 billion pounds of conventional pesticides used in the United States, 1.2 billion of which were used for agricultural purposes or in homes, and whose toxicity for children was very poorly understood. Only a handful of environmental toxins have been extensively researched for their neurotoxicity in children. These are heavy metals, that is, lead, methyl mercury, cadmium, manganese; polychlorinated biphenyls (PCBs); organic solvents; pesticides and herbicides, that is, organophosphates like chlordane and malathion; environmental tobacco smoke; radiation; and endotoxins. In 1998, there were 2,863 such high-production chemicals produced in the United States at a rate of more than 1 million pounds per year. Yet, only 7 percent have a full set of basic toxicity test data on them. Environmental toxins loom on the horizon as a major threat to children's health and development.

See also: Cigarette Smoking; Effects of Parental Substance Abuse on Children; Lead Poisoning

Further Reading

Klaassen, C. D. (1996). *Casarett & Doul's toxicology: The basic science of poisons* (5th ed.). New York: McGraw-Hill.

Spencer, P. S., & Schaumburg, H. H. (2000). *Experimental and clinical neurotoxicology* (2nd ed.). New York: Oxford University Press.

STEPHEN R. SCHROEDER

Epidural Hematomas

See: Traumatic Brain Injury

Epilepsy

DEFINITION

Epilepsy is a medical condition in which the affected individual experiences recurrent seizures. A seizure is an abnormal electrical discharge in the brain that can cause a sudden and involuntary change in behavior due to this abnormal firing of collections of brain cells (neurons). The term seizure disorder is often used to describe both the recurrence of these involuntary electrical discharges and the different types of behavioral changes that occur as a result of the abnormal brain activity.

PREVALENCE

Epilepsy and seizures have been described as one of the most common neurological disorders and can affect people of all ages from infancy to old age. Approximately 11 percent of the general population may experience a single seizure over the span of their lifetime whereas a smaller number will suffer from repeated seizures. It is estimated that somewhere between 125,000 and 300,000 children suffer from some form of epilepsy. The ratio of males to females varies somewhat according to the age of onset and the type of the seizure disorder. The specific percentages for each type of epileptic seizure in childhood are not firmly established; however, generalized seizures are more common than partial seizures.

CLASSIFICATION OF THE EPILEPSIES

Epilepsy is sometimes classified according to etiology into two broad categories: (1) symptomatic and (2) idiopathic epilepsy. *Symptomatic* epilepsy refers to that group of epileptic conditions for which the cause of the seizures is known. Metabolic disorders, brain tumors, malformations of the blood vessels of the brain and traumatic brain injury are examples of medical conditions that can cause epilepsy. The term *idiopathic* (or cryptogenic) epilepsy is used to describe those epilepsies for which a clear etiology is not ascertained. As advances have been made in structural and metabolic brain imaging, it is now easier to identify microscopic structural abnormalities that can give rise to a variety of epilepsy syndromes in children.

Since 1981, an international system has been used that classifies seizures according to the characteristic brain localization features of the seizures. In this system, there are two broad categories of seizures: partial and generalized. In 1989, this system of classification was revised to include descriptions of specific epilepsy syndromes. An epilepsy syndrome is a collection of behavioral and laboratory signs that characterize a particular type of epilepsy. Behavioral signs are any changes in cognitive, sensory, motor, or emotional functioning that

accompany a clinical seizure. These changes may also occur at the onset of a seizure or in the time between seizures. When describing the clinical phases of a seizure, four phases are used: (1) the *aura* which refers to the initial phenomena of a seizure that is sometimes experienced as a "warning" that a seizure will occur; (2) the seizure phase (also called the *ictal phase*); (3) the time following a seizure in which the patient is slowly recovering to normal functioning (called the *post-ictal phase*) and; (4) the time period in between seizures (called the *inter-ictal phase*). Information about the different forms of epilepsy is provided in the sections that follow.

PARTIAL SEIZURES

Partial seizures are seizures that originate from a focal change in electrical activity in a portion of one cerebral hemisphere. They are also referred to as focal or local seizures. Partial seizures are further classified as one of three types: a *simple partial seizure*, a *complex partial seizure*, and a *partial seizure with secondary generalization*. Simple and complex partial seizures differ in whether or not consciousness is impaired during the seizure. During simple partial seizures, there is no impairment of consciousness, whereas during complex partial seizures, consciousness is impaired. Consciousness refers to the degree to which the individual having the seizure is aware of and/or responsive to stimuli in his or her environment. Degree of impairment of consciousness can vary from complete loss of awareness to minimal or no impairment of awareness.

Simple Partial Seizures
Clinical Features

Simple partial seizures may present with a variety of clinical manifestations. Although the symptoms or signs of simple partial seizures may vary between individuals, they tend to be consistent from seizure to seizure for an individual child. Based upon the focus of the seizure activity in the brain, the individual may show motor signs such as jerking of a limb, somatosensory symptoms such as sensations of tingling or numbness on a part of the body, autonomic symptoms such as flushing of the skin, or "psychic" symptoms (involving higher brain functions such as emotion).

Simple partial seizures with motor signs are also referred to as focal motor seizures. Motor signs may involve any part of the body, depending upon where on the motor strip the seizure activity originates. In some children, focal motor seizures may spread to adjacent areas of the motor strip in the brain, causing motor symptoms in a sequence of body parts. This is known as an epileptic "march," or Jacksonian seizure. Simple partial seizures may involve somatosensory or special sensory symptoms. These seizures originate in areas of the brain responsible for the sensory functions (sight, hearing, taste, touch, and smell). The most common somatosensory symptoms are a feeling of "pins-and-needles" or numbness. Like the motor signs, somatosensory symptoms may also exhibit marching if the seizure activity spreads to adjacent sensory areas. Depending upon the sensory function involved, symptoms can range from simple (e.g., flashing lights or sounds) to quite complex (e.g., visual or auditory hallucinations). Simple partial seizures with autonomic symptoms can include sweating, vomiting, flushing, piloerection (i.e. sensation of "hairs standing on end"), pallor, and pupil dilation. Finally, simple partial seizures may include "psychic" symptoms, which often involve affective symptoms such as anger, fear, or pleasure; flashbacks or déjà vu (feeling that a new experience has been experienced before); and impaired speech, or dysphasia. The patient may be completely aware of these various symptoms yet experience no control over their onset, type, or duration.

Complex Partial Seizures

Clinical Features

Unlike simple partial seizures, consciousness is impaired in complex partial seizures. These seizures may begin as a simple partial seizure with a subsequent change in consciousness, or consciousness may be impaired from the initial onset of seizure activity. Sometimes, the impairment of consciousness looks like a staring spell and may be mistaken for another form of epilepsy called petit mal. More often, the impairment in consciousness is accompanied by involuntary motor activity called *automatisms*. Automatisms may consist of a continuation of an activity that was occurring when the seizure began, or they may be a new activity that starts with the impairment of consciousness. Examples of automatisms frequently seen in children with complex partial seizures are chewing, lip smacking, grimacing, rocking, fumbling with nearby objects, crying, yelling, and walking or running around. Because automatisms occur during a state of impaired consciousness, the child does not recall the actions after the seizure. Complex partial seizures may be brief, lasting for seconds, or may continue for up to 2 or 3 min. These may or may not be accompanied by loss of bowel or bladder control. The child is typically unaware of the seizure. The post-ictal phase may also be brief or

may last for longer periods of up to several hours. Some children are able to quickly resume ongoing activities while other children may complain of feeling tired and need to nap before returning to their activities.

Assessment

Classifying seizure type can be difficult, particularly in children. However, proper classification of seizure greatly impacts treatment. Assessing epilepsy syndromes requires considering seizure type along with information from physical examinations, family and patient history, and diagnostic testing such as electroencephalograms (EEGs) and magnetic resonance imaging (MRI). Often, a home or hospital videotape of a seizure may help the clinician to classify the type of seizure. In addition, children with partial seizures may need to undergo a comprehensive neuropsychological evaluation to determine whether the seizure disorder or its treatment has resulted in cognitive problems that can adversely affect academic performance and learning.

Generalized Seizures

Definition and Classification

Generalized epileptic seizures are seizures in which the first clinical changes indicate initial, synchronous involvement of both hemispheres. Generalized seizures can be classified as either convulsive or nonconvulsive. Six types of generalized seizures are recognized (see Table 1).

Absence seizures, also called "petit mal seizures," are most common in childhood. They usually begin between the ages of 6 and 12, and rarely begin after the age of 20. This type of seizure involves a sudden, brief lapse of consciousness, eye blinking, staring, and other minor facial movements. Absence seizures last from a few seconds to a minute, during which time the patient will be unresponsive. These seizures may occur many times a day and possibly result in poor school performance. Approximately 40 percent of these

Table 1. Generalized Seizure Classification (Convulsive or Nonconvulsive)

1. Typical absence seizures (petit mal)
   Atypical
2. Myoclonic seizures
3. Clonic seizures
4. Tonic seizures
5. Tonic–clonic seizures (grand mal)
6. Atonic seizures

From the Commission on Classification and Terminology of the International League against Epilepsy, 1981.

patients recover, but others develop additional types of seizures that continue into later life.

Atypical absence seizures involve more pronounced muscle movement, which may include rhythmic convulsions, rigidity, or falling down. This type of seizure may be followed by a period of confusion, and recovery may take longer than the typical absence seizures. However, full recovery is usually achieved after a few-seconds with no persisting confusion. The patient does not have any recollection of the event.

Myoclonic seizures involve quick jerks of muscles that are sudden, brief, shock-like contractions. These contractions can occur in one or several areas of the body, either simultaneously or sequentially. Consciousness is not usually impaired. Myoclonic seizures usually occur in specific epilepsy syndromes although they can occur alone.

Tonic seizures involve the continuous tightening of facial and body muscles, with rigid, violent muscular contractions where the arms bend and the legs extend in a strained position. There is usually a deviation of the eyes and of the head toward one side. Consciousness is impaired. Tonic seizures are most common in children.

Clonic seizures are also common in children, involving the alternating of contractions and relaxation of muscle groups in succession. Consciousness is impaired.

Tonic–clonic seizures (grand mal seizures) begin suddenly. A person experiencing this type of seizure sometimes experiences a vague ill-described warning. The individual typically cries out and falls to the ground. There is a tonic phase characterized by a sudden sharp continuous contraction of muscles, which may last from 15 to 45 s, after which time short periods of relaxation occur. With increased frequency of the relaxation periods, the clonic phase begins, involving alternating contraction and relaxation of muscles. At the end of this stage, deep respiration occurs and is accompanied by a relaxing of all the muscles in the body. Sometimes a loss of urine occurs as the muscles of the bladder relax. Full consciousness may not return for 10–15 min, with confusion and fatigue possibly lasting for hours or even days.

Atonic seizures involve a sudden loss of muscle tone in the back and legs, causing the patient to suddenly drop to the floor (drop attacks). These attacks typically last for only a few seconds and may occur without a loss of consciousness.

Etiology and Assessment

Generalized epileptic seizures, like partial seizures, can arise due to a number of medical conditions such as brain malformations, metabolic disorders, tumors of the central nervous system (CNS), traumatic brain injuries, renal disease as well as a number of developmental disorders associated with genetic/chromosomal abnormalities. In order to diagnose the possible causes of the seizures, children will routinely undergo one or more EEGs, along with blood or urine chemistry analysis and some type of brain-imaging study such as a computerized tomography (CT) scan or MRI scan. In some centers, SPECT scans (measures of brain metabolism) may also be conducted. At this point in time, functional neuroimaging studies are still being investigated for their potential usefulness in characterizing different types of epilepsy.

Generalized Epilepsy Syndromes

In an epilepsy syndrome, a group of signs and symptoms are used to collectively define the seizure disorder. Epilepsy syndromes are characterized by both the clinical features of the seizure phenomena and by the results from diagnostic testing. Typical diagnostic testing will include an EEG, MRI, CT, position imaging tomography (PET), and/or SPECT scans. The generalized epilepsies are most common in children with different syndromes occurring at different ages of onset (newborns, infants, children, and older children and adolescents). Epilepsy syndromes are divided into primary (idiopathic) and secondary (symptomatic) types. Primary types are usually not associated with structural lesions of the brain and are often characterized as a non progressive, genetically determined disturbance that is usually age-related. Examples of primary generalized epilepsies are absence seizures, bilaterally synchronous myoclonic seizures, and/or tonic–clonic seizures. Interictal periods of EEGs are described as normal except for characteristic, bilaterally synchronous epileptiform discharges. This type of generalized seizure is usually responsive to medications and often disappears by adolescence or early adulthood. Secondary seizures are due to diffuse or multifocal lesions of the brain.

Patients with secondary seizures may have mixed types of generalized epileptic seizures, commonly associated with neurological and psychological signs and symptoms of diffuse cerebral lesions. The typical interictal EEG pattern consists of irregular and often asynchronous epileptiform discharges superimposed on diffusely abnormal baseline rhythms. In addition, the seizures respond poorly to treatment and do not resolve with time.

Idiopathic with age-related onset syndromes include benign neonatal familial convulsions (a rare syndrome involving generalized seizures that only occur during the first week of life); childhood absence; and juvenile myoclonic epilepsy (which begins during teenage years and involves myoclonic, absence, and generalized tonic–clonic seizures).

Symptomatic and/or idiopathic epilepsy consists of a mixed set of syndromes sharing similar clinical characteristics. Unlike children diagnosed with idiopathic age-related epilepsy who have intelligence in the normal range, children in this classification are often mentally retarded. A number of different idiopathic epilepsy childhood syndromes have been described.

West's Syndrome, also known as Infantile Spasms, consists of a characteristic triad: infantile spasms, arrest of psychomotor development, and hypsarrhythmia (continuous high amplitude, irregular, and asynchronous sharp and slow waves occurring in a chaotic fashion). Onset peaks between ages 4 and 7 months and is always present before 1 year. The characteristic seizure in this syndrome involves bending of the neck, waist, arms, and legs with the arms either drawn away from or toward the body, lasting only a few seconds. Infants who suffer from this syndrome usually achieve normal development until the spasms begin, resulting in the arrest of psychomotor development in the child. Half of children with infantile spasms develop Lennox–Gastaut Syndrome.

Lennox–Gastaut Syndrome consists of a combination of seizures including: axial tonic attacks, tonic–clonic seizures, atypical absence seizures, and atonic seizures. The onset of this syndrome occurs between 1 and 8 years of age, and often results in developmental delays that may include language delays from which the child may not recover.

Treatment

There are currently over 20 different anticonvulsant drugs available to treat the variety of childhood epilepsies. The principle of anticonvulsant drug therapy is to control the frequency or severity of seizures while minimizing adverse side effects of drug therapy. Side effects of drug therapy can be physical (e.g., rash, appetite suppression), physiologic (e.g., blood chemistry changes, liver dysfunction), cognitive (e.g., poor concentration, confusion), affective (e.g., mood changes, irritability) and/or any combination of these areas of functioning. Most children on any type of anticonvulsant medication will require routine blood level checks to be sure that the medication is in the proper level in the bloodstream and that there are no changes in blood chemistries or other organ systems.

Anticonvulsant medications that are used in the treatment of partial seizures in children include carbamazepine, phenytoin, and, less frequently, primidone or phenobarbital. In addition, valproic acid, clonazepam, and clorazepate may be added to the regimen if the former treatments are not successful. Among the medications utilized in the treatment of generalized seizures or epileptic syndromes are: valproic acid, lamotrigine, topiramate, zonisamide, carbamazepine, gabapentin, and phenobarbital. Infantile spasms are sometimes treated with steroids to reduce the frequency of seizures that can occur over 100 times per day.

In general, anticonvulsant medication typically is successful in reducing or controlling seizures. It is estimated that 60 percent of seizure disorders will be controlled by a single medication. Another 15 percent are controlled by the use of two or more medications.

If anticonvulsant medications are not effective, a ketogenic diet may also be instituted to try to control the seizures. A ketogenic diet is one that is extremely high in the proportion of fats and very low in the proportion of carbohydrates that make up the total diet. This is most often used when the child is unable to tolerate the side effects of anticonvulsant medications. About 1 percent of children will be put on a ketogenic diet to control their seizures. Finally, vagus nerve stimulators have also been utilized to treat some generalized epilepsies. These devices stimulate the vagus nerve which then causes cortical electrical activity to desynchronize and stop the seizure. Currently less than 1 percent of children have been treated with a vagus nerve stimulator to control their seizures.

Surgical treatments of intractable epilepsy are also now utilized in children. Surgery is most often considered when the child has a focal lesion that continues to cause epileptic seizures despite multiple attempts to control the seizures with combinations of anticonvulsants. In this type of surgery, sometimes called a lesionectomy, the seizure focus is surgically removed from the brain. Occasionally, surgery will be offered that disconnects a seizure focus from adjacent brain areas or the opposite hemisphere in order to prevent the spread of the seizure. Surgical treatment for epilepsy is typically considered only after all other types of interventions have been tried and failed. Only about 0.2 percent of patients have surgery for epilepsy.

Because epilepsy and its treatment can often cause cognitive difficulties, it is helpful to obtain a comprehensive neuropsychological evaluation for the child. The purpose of this evaluation is to identify any cognitive difficulties that may contribute to learning problems in school. Similarly, some children with epilepsy experience problems in adjusting to their disorder and may need supportive counseling when problems with anxiety, depression, self-esteem, or compliance become apparent. Adolescents seem to be particularly vulnerable to adjusting to having epilepsy, likely due to the limitations posed by epilepsy at a time in their lives when separation and independence are important tasks in development. Conflicts over disclosing their seizure disorder, driving, and compliance are common in this age group. Family counseling can also be helpful in handling the effects of having a child with epilepsy on both the parents and siblings of the affected child.

Psychological Correlates

Because of the many different types of seizures, the variety of antiepileptic drugs that may be used singly or in combination, and the number of different causes of epilepsy, psychological correlates of this disorder vary widely by age of onset, etiology, medication use, and seizure control obtained. Among the idiopathic seizures, the greatest risk for cognitive, behavioral, and adjustment problems occurs in children whose seizures are poorly controlled or require multiple anticonvulsant medications or who have experienced episodes of status epilepticus.

Poorly controlled seizure disorders almost always affect school progress and may result in developmental delays. Parents of children with poorly controlled seizures are often stressed by the complications of medical management of the disorders, which can affect siblings of the affected child as well. Behavioral disorders reported in children with poorly controlled seizures include: irritability, emotionality, problems in attention and concentration, hyperactivity, sleep disorders, and oppositionality. While many of these same problems are reported among children with symptomatic epilepsies, there is an additional burden of dealing with the neurological, genetic, or medical disorder that has given rise to the child's seizure disorder. Educating the parents about their child's type of epilepsy and helping them to understand the effects of anticonvulsant treatment is critical to successful management of seizure disorders. Parents may also need to work closely with their child's school in order to ensure that appropriate educational interventions are made available to the child. Among the childhood epilepsies, children with well-controlled partial epilepsies and those with uncomplicated generalized epilepsy (such as petit mal epilepsy) are reported to have the fewest problems in psychological adjustment and cognitive outcomes.

Febrile Seizures
Definition and Incidence

Febrile seizures are seizures that occur in association with a febrile illness that is not caused by a central nervous system infection. It is the most common form of childhood seizures and occurs in 2–5 percent of the population. The onset of febrile seizures peaks at between 18 and 22 months of age, although a large number of children may experience febrile seizures as early as age 6 months. Most febrile seizures have their onset before 5 years of age. These seizures can continue to occur up to about age 10 years. Prevalence estimates vary by race and ethnicity, ranging from 3.5 percent of Caucasian children to 4.2 percent of African-American children and up to 9–10 percent of Japanese children.

Risk factors for febrile seizures have been identified in population-based studies. These include: family history of febrile seizures in a first or second degree relative; neonatal nursery stay of greater than 30 days; developmental delay; and day care attendance. If a child has two or more of these risk factors, they have a 30 percent chance of developing febrile seizures.

The explicit causes of febrile seizures are still unknown. Animal studies have demonstrated that the risk of seizures is associated with younger age/maturity and temperature elevation. However, most febrile seizures in children do not occur at the peak temperature level of the fever or during the rise in temperature.

Clinical Features of Febrile Seizures

Febrile seizures may be simple or complex in their phenomenology. Simple febrile seizures are relatively brief (less than 10–15 min) generalized seizures and typically consist of a single seizure episode for that febrile illness. Complex febrile seizures last longer, can recur over the course of the febrile illness and may have partial onset followed by secondary generalization. Sometimes febrile seizures last longer than 30 min with no signs of recovery during this time period. This clinical event is called a "febrile status epilepticus." A prolonged seizure of this type accounts for approximately 5 percent of febrile seizures.

Assessment

Because febrile seizures, by definition, occur in the context of a febrile illness, assessment of the seizure includes ruling out infections of the central nervous system (e.g., meningitis or encephalitis) and metabolic/electrolyte imbalances due to the febrile illness. Accidental poisoning and other causes of acute symptomatic epilepsy are also part of the differential diagnosis. Laboratory studies of blood and urine samples may be ordered by the treating physician. A spinal tap to allow examination of cerebral spinal fluid for signs of infection or bleeding is common. Unlike other seizures, however, an EEG and neuroimaging studies are not routinely ordered for febrile seizures as they are of limited help in the diagnostic process.

Treatment

Typical treatment for a febrile seizure involves ruling out other causes for a seizure, reducing the fever and treating any infection that is identified (e.g., otitis media) or middle prescribe antiepileptic medications because of the potential for adverse side effects for what is believed to be a benign condition. However, if a child suffers from recurrent or prolonged complex febrile seizures, a physician may prescribe the use of rectal diazepam (Valium) as a prophylactic to abort or limit the intensity or recurrence of a seizure.

Pseudoseizures

Definition

Pseudoseizures are behavioral events that mimic some aspects of seizure behavior but are not accompanied by abnormal electrical discharges in the brain. They are sometimes called "nonelectrical seizures." Pseudoseizures are less common in children than in adults. However, as with adult patients with seizure disorders, pseudoseizures can occur even when the patient has a diagnosed seizure disorder. Typically, pseudoseizures begin within the first decade of life and may continue into adulthood.

Characteristics

Most pseudoseizures consist of prolonged episodes of staring during which the child is unresponsive. Other pseudoseizures may consist of shaking and trembling of the body or thrashing of the legs and arms and may include pelvic thrusting. Despite this motor activity, the child is rarely injured during a pseudoseizure. Incontinence of urine can occur but is rare. Because pseudoseizures can sometimes mimic a typical seeizure in an individual with seizure disorder, these are often confused with epilepsy.

Assessment

Diagnosing pseudoseizures requires a careful history since these seizures often occur in individuals with a history of abuse or in response to environmental stressors. In addition, a video-linked EEG will help to determine whether the apparent seizure is accompanied by diagnostic changes in the EEG. Psychological evaluations may also provide information about the factors that may be contributing to the development of pseudoseizures.

Treatment

Pseudoseizures do not respond to antiepileptic medications. Interventions typically include treating the psychological factors that have contributed to the onset or maintenance of pseudoseizures. Behavioral management training for the parents of a child with pseudoseizures can also be helpful. In certain instances, individual psychotherapy may also be implemented and is of particular help in adolescent patients. However, parents may need to be the focus of interventions when the child is developmentally delayed or mentally retarded.

See also: Coping with Illness; Neurological Disorders; Neurologic Examination; Neuropsychological Assessment

Further Reading

Commission on Classification and Terminology of the International League Against Epilepsy. (1981). Proposal for revised clinical and electroencephalographic classification of epileptic seizures. *Epilepsia, 22,* 489–501.
Commission on Classification and Terminology of the International League Against Epilepsy. (1985). Proposal for classification of epilepsies and epileptic syndromes. *Epilepsia, 26*(3), 268–278.
International League against Epilepsy. (1989). Commission on Classification and Terminology of the International League Against Epilepsy. Proposal for revised classification of epilepsies and epileptic syndromes. *Epilepsia, 30,* 389–399.
Leppik, I. E. (2000). *Managing your epilepsy: Advice from a distinguished expert in seizures and epilepsy.* Newtown, PA: Handbooks in Health Care Co.
Sheth, R. D. (Ed.) (2002). Pediatric epilepsy: Current challenges. *Journal of Child Neurology, 17*(Suppl. 2), 2S1–2S42.

EILEEN B. FENNELL
DANIELLE A. BECKER
SUSAN BONGIOLATTI

Ethical Issues

The Ethical Principles of Psychologists and the Code of Conduct of the American Psychological Association

(APA Ethics Code) guide clinical child and pediatric psychologists in their assessment, consultation, intervention, and research with children and families. Because of the special vulnerabilities of children and the complexities involved in coordinating with schools, health care facilities, and families, psychological services for children, adolescents, and families require an exceptionally high standard of ethical behavior. The APA Ethics Code is written broadly to apply to psychologists with varied roles in many different professional contexts. The ethical guidelines are written primarily with adults in mind and, as a result, they may not always apply to the special needs of children. In this regard, "special needs" of children might include not only the child, but also other family members as well during assessment, intervention, or research. Legal standards for minors are very different than those for adults. Because of their diminished cognitive capacity, children cannot be fully informed about an assessment, intervention, or research project when compared to adults. Clinical child and pediatric psychologists have a moral obligation to advocate for children because of their special vulnerabilities. The psychologist must aspire to maintain the highest legal and ethical practices in working with children and families. At the same time, it is also recognized that ethical dilemmas will occur that will challenge the clinical child and pediatric psychologist.

The APA Ethics Code provides a common set of values with which psychologists can develop their scientific and professional behaviors. Six general principles are specified in the APA Ethics Code. Although they are not considered enforceable rules per se, psychologists must consider these principles when considering an ethical course of action.

The first principle specifies that psychologists should strive to maintain high standards of competence in their work. Obviously, clinical child and pediatric psychologists have special training and expertise in working with children and families. At the same time, they should be aware of the limitations of their expertise and not practice outside the boundaries of their competence. The psychologist should determine if he or she has had adequate experience and/or training to perform the service requested. For example, clinical child or pediatric psychologists who are not trained in psychotherapy with young children should not treat young children since they may not have the specific expertise required. Overall, clinical child and pediatric psychologists should protect the welfare of the children and families with whom they work and make appropriate use of relevant professional resources as needed.

The second principle indicates that psychologists should promote accuracy and honesty in all professional endeavors. Above all, psychologists should be fair, honest, and respectful of others. Clinical child and pediatric psychologists should be keenly aware of their own values and belief systems, since their biases could influence the psychological services they provide. When working with children and families, psychologists should attempt to clarify their role with all parties involved and try to avoid potential conflicts. The psychologist should avoid any dual relationship that could compromise integrity of the psychological services and could damage the patient. Dual relationships can occur, particularly when working with families since children, parents, and other family members may have different expectations for the provision of the professional services provided by the psychologist.

The third principle concerns professional and scientific responsibility in their psychological practice by establishing trustful relationships, maintaining awareness of their professional responsibilities, and upholding standards of conduct. Clinical child and pediatric psychologists should develop cooperative alliances with other professionals (e.g., psychiatrists) and institutions (e.g., schools) in order to serve the best interests of their patients. Psychologists should uphold professional standards of conduct that include accepting responsibility for their actions, clarifying their roles, and adapting their methods to fit the needs of different populations. Although the psychologist's standards of moral behavior are regarded as a personal matter, psychologists do not compromise their professional duties because of actions taken based on their own moral standards. This would have the effect of reducing the public trust in the profession of psychology. As part of their ethical responsibilities, psychologists consult with other professionals in order to avoid unethical conduct by themselves or with others.

The fourth principle refers to psychologists treating all people equitably and respecting their fundamental dignity, rights, and worth. Clinical child and pediatric psychologists should respect the rights of confidentiality, self-determination, autonomy, and privacy for their patients. At the same time, psychologists should be aware of the fact that legal mandates might conflict with their patient's rights. For example, according to legal mandates in all states and provinces, confidentiality can be breached without permission if there is a suspicion of child abuse. Obviously, the psychologist must take into account the fact that children cannot have the same kind of autonomy and self-determination as adults; minors have far less autonomy and self-determination as defined by law. Psychologists must also aware of any cultural, role, or individual differences (e.g., ethnicity, age, gender, disability) which could affect the psychological services provided. Psychologists must adjust their interventions to fit the needs of any special population with whom they work. For example, when engaging in psychotherapy with an immigrant child from an Asian culture, the psychologist must engage in culturally competent interventions during the therapy process. Psychologists must not let biases or discrimination affect their provision of psychological services.

The fifth principle indicates that psychologists should always attempt to help their patients while also striving to cause no harm to them. Clinical child and pediatric psychologists continually consider the welfare and rights of those to whom they provide services and must always attempt to contribute to their welfare through their professional activities. Clinical child and pediatric psychologists have a special responsibility to be mindful of the power differential between themselves and the children with whom they provide services. When working with children and families, practitioners must be very careful not to mislead or exploit their patients in any way both during and after their professional interactions.

Finally, the sixth principle concerns the fact that psychologists must be aware of not only their responsibilities to their patients but also their professional responsibilities to the society and the community as a whole. In this regard psychologists contribute to the welfare of society by working to eliminate distress and suffering. Psychologists should contribute to the initiation of public policy matters that can potentially positively affect society and should encourage the development of laws that would serve the best interests of their patients. Clinical child and pediatric psychologists are encouraged to provide a portion of their professional services for minimal or no compensation.

The APA Ethics Code sets forth enforceable rules for work-related conduct for psychologists that are applied by the American Psychological Association, courts, state or provincial psychology boards, and other public bodies. For the most recently published version of the APA Ethics Code (1992), rules are divided into eight categories as follows: (1) General Standards, (2) Evaluation, Assessment, or Intervention, (3) Advertising and Other Public Statements, (4) Therapy, (5) Privacy and Confidentiality, (6) Teaching, Training Supervision, Research, and Publishing, (7) Forensic Activities, and (8) Resolving Ethical Issues. When a clinical child or pediatric psychologist makes a decision regarding professional behavior, the psychologist must take into account applicable laws, state or provincial psychology board rules, and the APA Ethics Code. For the most part, the psychologist should follow the APA Ethics Code unless it is in conflict with existing law. If the Ethics Code conflicts with the law, the psychologist should make known his or her commitment to the Ethics Code and try to responsibly resolve the conflict.

Specific procedures for filing, investigating, and resolving complaints of unethical conduct are described in the 1996 Report of the APA Ethics Committee. The APA can take several actions in response to a violation of the Ethics Code, which include actions such as censure, reprimand, termination of APA membership, and referral to other governmental or professional entities.

See also: Confidentiality and Privilege; Mental Health Records; Training Issues; Written Reports

Further Reading

American Psychological Association. (1992). Ethical principles of psychologists and code of conduct. *American Psychologist, 47,* 1597–1611.

American Psychological Association. (1997). Report of the Ethics Committee, 1996. *American Psychologist, 52,* 897–905.

Koocher, G. P., & Keith-Spiegel, P. (1998). *Ethics in psychology: Professional standards and cases* (2nd ed.). New York: Oxford.

Melton, G. B., Ehrenreich, N. S., & Lyons, P. M., Jr. (2001). Ethical and legal issues in mental health services for children. In C. E. Walker & M. C. Roberts (Eds.), *Handbook of clinical child psychology* (3rd ed., pp. 1074–1093). New York: Wiley.

Rae, W. A., Worchel, F. F., & Brunnquell, D. (1995). Ethical and legal issues in pediatric psychology. In M. C. Roberts (Ed.), *Handbook of pediatric psychology* (2nd ed., pp. 19–36). New York: Guilford.

WILLIAM A. RAE

Evidence-Based Treatments

BACKGROUND

According to a recent review by Kazdin (2000), over 550 psychological treatments for childhood disorders exist. Unfortunately, for a vast majority of these treatments, we know very little about their effectiveness. Furthermore, many therapists continue to judge the utility of therapeutic techniques by relying on their own clinical intuition, subjective reports of outcome by individual clients, and comparisons with their past clinical experiences. This more "intuitive" approach, though important, has limited utility in developing and evaluating treatments that might be more effective and useful in clinical practice.

Contemporary researchers have responded to this problem by generating criteria by which treatments can be evaluated more systematically. One way of evaluating treatments is based on the degree and quality of research evidence found in support for that treatment. The impetus for this type of evaluation comes from at least three sources. First, until recently, results from research and clinical practice have largely failed to inform each other and there has been a wide chasm between research and practice. Research was not considered relevant to the practice of clinicians in applied settings and the complexity of applied clinical practice was seemingly not well-addressed in research studies. There remains an increasing need to advance accountability and exchange between clinicians and researchers. Second, given the increasing demands of managed health care, and health care costs more generally, there remains a need to identify efficient and effective treatment options. Psychologists have a professional and ethical responsibility to identify, promulgate, and use treatments that help ameliorate psychological problems and that, as a result, have considerable evidence for their efficacy. Third, given the large number of available treatment options, there is interest in determining the most appropriate way both to train mental health professionals and to advance the skill level of more seasoned clinicians. It is unlikely that all 550 treatments identified by Kazdin (2000) are equally effective or that any one clinician could possibly learn all of them.

Evidence-Based Treatment (EBT) is a categorization used to describe those treatments that have been empirically evaluated and have withstood a set of criteria used to identify clinically sound methods of helping children and their families with psychological problems. Separate efforts to identify EBTs have been undertaken by different professional organizations, including the Evidence-Based Mental Health Movement and the American Psychological Association's (APA) Society of Clinical Psychology (Division 12) Task Force on Promotion and Dissemination of Psychological Procedures. Although the terminology differs across these independent efforts, their general goals and assumptions are similar. Namely, the movement to identify treatments with empirical evidence is based on the view that scientific evidence should be used in the selection and training of treatment interventions. EBTs are based on a given set of scientific criteria that are used to evaluate the treatment and reflect how the treatment selected fares in light of those specified criteria as compared to other treatments.

APPROACH

EBTs are used to identify the therapeutic ingredients required to obtain a successful therapeutic outcome and the research methods that are applied to arrive at that outcome. Generally, this involves four primary steps. First, it is necessary to determine whether the study that tested the treatment is internally valid. Internal validity addresses whether the findings, indeed, reflect the effects of the treatment itself (rather than some other aspect such as the mere passage of time or some other phenomenon that might be present in the therapeutic situation). The internal validity of a study is increased when study participants are randomly assigned to the treatment and to treatment alternatives (e.g., waiting list, "control" treatment) and when the researchers who evaluate the treatments are not aware of (i.e., "blind") the assignment status of participants. Additionally, clear specification of the treatment (e.g., by following explicit guidelines or a treatment manual) increases the likelihood that differences in participants following treatment reflect differences in the treatments, not extraneous factors.

Second, the outcome of the study must be successful. However, this seemingly straightforward goal is actually quite elusive. The improvement of a child's dysfunction can be evaluated by many methods, including standardized behavior rating scales that are normed for the child's age and gender, direct observation of a child's behavior by clinicians or caregivers, sophisticated psychological tests, and/or self-report measures of mood and cognitions. Changes can occur in many expected (and unexpected) domains. Results of the study depend on the treatment outcomes of interest. For example, a social skills group may intend to enhance a child's social problem solving skills and improve the child's social behavior, but instead produces noticeable effects only on the child's self-report of friendships. Was this treatment ineffective? Surely, self-reports of increased friendships are important; yet, the treatment did not have the intended treatment effects. Similarly, a treatment may result in changes based on parent reports but not on the reports of teachers or the child himself. Is this treatment effective? As is evident, defining successful treatment outcome can be a difficult task.

Third, results of the study should not just be statistically significant; rather, they should also be clinically meaningful. Too frequently, researchers have concluded that treatments are effective when only minimal and trivial, albeit statistically significant, changes have occurred. Statistical significance does not necessarily mean that the changes are meaningful ones. In other words, an EBT should be able to demonstrate that important and noticeable changes did, in fact, occur for a child and his or her family. This can be measured in a standardized way across studies, using a number of possible scientific formulas. For example, EBTs may be evaluated by calculating the "Number Needed to Treat," which is the number of children who received a favorable outcome with a particular treatment when a poor outcome was found for a child in a control or comparison group. Ideally, for every child who does not respond to a given treatment, a large number will. In general, EBTs aspire to a 4:1 ratio, meaning that about 80 percent of the children respond favorably to the given treatment.

Fourth, evaluation of an EBT should include the applicability of the intervention to the individual child and his or her family. This requires a consideration of both the participants in the study and the results obtained in that study. Specifically, participants involved in empirical testing should reflect the population of individuals for whom the treatment is intended to apply. For example, if a parent training program is tested with parents of young children, the results may not be "generalizable" or applicable to parents of older children, let alone adolescents. Also, treatment outcomes may be relevant to specific goals (e.g., decrease symptoms of conduct disorder, reduce level of depression) or more generalized goals (e.g., improve classroom behavior, increase self-concept). These points have important implications for the application of treatments in clinical practice. It is possible that a treatment that works well for one type of problem or child may prove harmful, or at least ineffective, for another.

OVERALL EVALUATION

The list of EBTs is much smaller than the overall collection of documented treatments. However, there are several effective treatments for the more common childhood psychological problems encountered in clinical practice, including anxiety/fear/phobias, depression, Oppositional Defiant Disorder (ODD) and Conduct Disorder (CD), substance use disorder, and attention deficit hyperactivity disorder, as well as a host of common pediatric problems (e.g., recurrent abdominal pain, headache, etc.). The selection of EBTs for these common problems in the clinical setting is a positive way to expand upon a clinician's repertoire of available treatment options while also increasing the likelihood of treatment success. EBTs also offer a more straightforward approach to treatment that incorporates a set of guidelines or a manual to assist the therapy process.

They also recommend reliable and valid assessment tools to evaluate the treatment outcome. Moreover, evolving research suggests that clinicians are beginning to prefer such materials in their therapeutic work in that it provides them structure while also allowing for flexibility in addressing individual child and family needs.

LIMITATIONS AND FUTURE DIRECTIONS

Although EBTs provide an important starting point from which to build a collection of tools used in clinical practice, there remain some criticisms about the ease of applying EBTs outside the research setting. Many controls are set in place to insure that a study is methodologically sound in research settings. However, a stringent set of criteria about treatment participants and treatment delivery may not be appropriate in some clinical settings where a diversity of child needs and treatment limitations may be found. As a result, findings of clinical research may not always transfer to the outcomes of clinical practice. In addition, it is important to note that a lack of empirical evidence in support of a treatment does not necessarily mean that the treatment itself is of poor quality or that it is ineffective. A vast majority of EBTs are derived from behavioral, cognitive–behavioral, and interpersonal principles. However, empirical evaluation simply has not yet occurred for a number of frequently used alternative approaches (e.g., play therapy, psychodynamic psychotherapy). It is imperative that these procedures be evaluated if they are going to be used in clinical practice on an ongoing basis.

Clearly there remains a need to further investigate the criteria used to define an EBT and to consider the implications of identifying treatments as having supporting empirical evidence. Overall, however, the movement to use EBTs is an important advance in the care of children and their families who require psychological treatment. Moreover, this movement has set the foundation for a favorable trend in clinical research and practice and may help bridge the gap between these two professional activities.

See also: Behavior Therapy; Cognitive–Behavior Therapy; Interpersonal Psychotherapy for Depressed Adolescents; Measurement of Behavior Change

Further Reading

Chambless, D. L., & Hollon, S. D. (1998). Defining empirically supported therapies. *Journal of Consulting and Clinical Psychology, 66*, 7–18.

Chorpita, B. F., Yim, L. M., Donkervoet, J. C., Arensdorf, A., Amundsen, M. J., McGee, C., Serrano, A., Yates, A., Burns, J. A., & Morelli, P. (2002). Toward large-scale implementation of empirically supported treatment for children: A review and observations by the Hawaii Empirical Basis to Services Task Force. *Clinical Psychology: Science and Practice, 9,* 165–190.

Hawley, K. M., & Weisz, J. R. (2002). Increasing the relevance of evidence-based treatment review to practitioners and consumers. *Clinical Psychology: Science and Practice, 9,* 225–230.

Kazdin, A. E. (2000). *Psychotherapy for children and adolescents: Directions for research and practice.* New York: Oxford University Press.

Ollendick, T. H., & King, N. J. (2000). Empirically supported treatments for children and adolescents. In P. C. Kendall (Ed.), Child and adolescent therapy: Cognitive behavioral procedures (2nd ed., pp. 386–425). New York: Guilford.

HEATHER K. ALVAREZ
THOMAS H. OLLENDICK

Ewing's Sarcoma

DESCRIPTION

Ewing's sarcoma and peripheral primitive neuroectodermal tumors (also called Ewing's sarcoma family tumors (ESFT) are malignant tumors of the bone and soft tissue and are the second most common primary bone cancer in childhood and adolescence. They are neural (parasympathetic) in origin. The annual incidence in the United States is 2.1 cases per million children. Eighty to ninety percent of patients are less than 20 years of age at diagnosis, with most (about two thirds) between the ages of 10 and 20. Males are diagnosed more often than females.

ETIOLOGY

The etiology is unknown. There is no known association with congenital diseases of childhood or with the familial cancer syndrome. Chromosomal translocations (t11;t22) (q24;q12) are common in greater than 95 percent of patients. The MIC2 gene is strongly associated with ESFT.

PRESENTATION

The most frequent presenting symptoms are: local pain (85–96 percent), local swelling (60–61 percent),

fever (21–30 percent), and pathological fracture (16 percent). Symptoms can be present for several months before diagnosis (3–10 months), with shorter duration for patients with a palpable mass. The most common sites are the extremities, central axis, and pelvis chest wall. Head, neck, or paravertebral areas are less common sites for Ewing's sarcoma.

TREATMENT

Treatment is determined by location of the primary tumor and the presence or absence of metastases, for example, spread of the disease. Twenty to thirty percent of patients will have metastases at diagnosis, and common sites are lung, bone, bone marrow, and pleura. Treatment involves surgery (e.g., amputation versus limb salvage), and/or radiation (to decrease incidence of local recurrences) with multiagent chemotherapy (varying doses and timing of vincristine, doxorubicin, actinomycin-D, cyclophosphamide with addition of other agents). New treatments involve dose intensification and addition of drugs called camptothecans, all of which involve more time spent in the hospital, more clinic visits, and the possibility of more side effects due to the increased intensity of therapy.

Acute complications include mucositis, diarrhea, desquamation, that is, shedding of the skin (from radiation). Late effects, depending on the site of the tumor, type, and intensity of treatment can include cardiac toxicity, arrest of bone growth or irregular growth after radiation, fibrosis, neurologic problems, physical effects due to loss of a limb, and second malignancies. With the exception of radiation-related sequelae, the psychological impact on the child/adolescent is similar to that of osteosarcoma.

PROGNOSIS

Overall 5-year disease-free survival for localized Ewing's sarcoma treated with surgery, radiation, and multiagent chemotherapy is about 55–60 percent. Localized distal tumors have a 5-year survival of 75 percent, while those who have metastases at diagnosis have a 20–30 percent 5-year survival rate. Favorable prognostic factors include no metastases at diagnosis, location in distal bones and ribs, no soft tissue extension, no neural differentiation, tumor size less than 100 cc, low serum LDH levels, female gender, younger age (less than 10 years), and a good initial response to treatment.

Prognosis for recurrent disease is generally poor. Length of survival depends on site and extent of recurrence, aggressiveness of the tumor, previous treatment, and time to failure.

See also: Bone and Soft Tissue Tumors; Childhood Cancers; Osteosarcoma; Coping with Chronic Illness; Parenting the Chronically Ill Child; Treatment Adherence; Treatment Adherence: Medical

Further Reading

Ginsberg, J. P., Woo, S. Y., Johnson, M. E., Hicks, M. J., & Horowitz, M. E. (2002). Ewing's sarcoma family of tumors. In P. A. Pizzo & D. G. Poplack (Eds.), *Principles and practice of pediatric oncology* (4th ed., pp. 973–1016). Philadelphia: Lippincott, Williams & Wilkins.
Helligenstein, E., & Holland, J. C. (1989). Malignant bone tumors. In J. C. Holland & J. Rowland (Eds.). *Handbook of Psycho-oncology* (pp. 250–253). New York: Oxford University Press.
West, D. C. (2000). Ewing sarcoma family of tumors. *Current Opinion in Oncology, 12,* 323–329.

MARY JO KUPST
ANNE B. WARWICK

Excessive Sleepiness

DEFINITION

Excessive sleepiness is a condition in which the child feels very drowsy during the day and has an overwhelming urge to fall asleep, even after getting enough nighttime sleep. Children with excessive sleepiness generally sleep more than 2 hr a night longer than the average for his or her age, or require daily naps beyond the preschool years.

INCIDENCE/ETIOLOGY

Approximately 5–10 percent of individuals who present to sleep disorders clinics report symptoms of daytime sleepiness. Excessive sleepiness can occur in children of any age, but is most common in those between the ages of 6 and 10 years. Genetic influences seem to be involved in a portion of the cases, as 39 percent of people with hypersomnia also have a family history of the disorder. A significant subgroup of individuals diagnosed with hypersomnia were previously exposed to a viral infection such as mononucleosis, hepatitis, and viral pneumonia, which suggests that there may be more than one cause of the disorder.

CORRELATES

Children with excessive sleepiness fall asleep quickly and have good sleep efficiency, but may have difficulty waking up in the morning, often appearing confused, combative, or ataxic. Excessive sleepiness in children has been associated with disturbances in mood and affect; behavioral problems (aggressiveness, hyperactivity, and poor impulse control); neurocognitve deficits (attention, memory, and executive functions); and performance deficits (academic, social). Teachers are usually the first to notice these problems, and a child is often described as performing poorly because of inattention, laziness, or overactivity.

ASSESSMENT

Rating scales can be used as a subjective measure of excessive sleepiness while physiological tests can be used as a more objective measure. The *Multiple Sleep Latency Test* is a well-validated test of the underlying physiologic tendency to fall asleep during usual waking hours. In addition, behavioral and performance measures can be used to assess for excessive daytime sleepiness.

TREATMENT

Since the cause of excessive sleepiness varies from child to child, treatment depends on the cause of the disturbance and the individual needs of the child. The most common treatment for excessive sleepiness is determining the interfering cause (i.e., environmental disturbances, fear, obstructive sleep apnea) and then designing a treatment plan to address it. Some children may only require an intervention that involves decreasing the amount of environmental interference (e.g., structuring daily routines of sleep, eating, exercise and social activities), while others may require medical attention and a more intensive treatment plan in an attempt to treat their disorder. Monitors for sleep apnea, sleep aides, or even surgery to reduce an obstructed airway may be required as part of the treatment for children with severe excessive daytime sleepiness.

PROGNOSIS

Once the cause of excessive sleepiness has been determined, children tend to respond quickly and positively to individualized treatment plans.

See also: Narcolepsy; Obstructive Sleep Apnea; Sleep Patterns, Normal

Further Reading

Anders, T. F., & Eiben, L. A. (1997). Pediatric sleep disorders: A review of the past 10 years. *Journal of the American Academy of Child and Adolescent Psychiatry, 36*, 9–20.

Guilleminault, C., & Pelayo, R. (2000). Idiopathic central nervous system hypersomnia. In M. H. Kryger, T. Roth, & W. C. Dement (Eds.), *Principles and practice of sleep medicine* (3rd ed., pp. 687–692). Philadelphia: W. B. Saunders.

National Sleep Foundation, 1522 K Street, NW, Suite 500, Washington, DC 20005, Phone: (202) 347-3471, Fax: (202) 347-3472, E-mail: nsf@sleepfoundation.org, www.sleepfoundation.org

V. Mark Durand
Kristin V. Christodulu

Expert Testimony

DEFINITION

Testimony is evidence in the form of statements made by witnesses, usually orally, to the trier of fact (the judge or jury), pertinent to the legal matter before the court. Lay witnesses are limited to the presentation of information they have perceived through their senses. A common example of a lay witness is an eyewitness who was present when an incident in question occurred, and testifies about his or her observations.

According to Rule 702 of the Federal Rules of Evidence, adopted by most states in the United States, an expert witness is an individual who, by virtue of specialized education, training, or experience, possesses knowledge or expertise that is not commonly possessed by the average person. Expert witnesses may present testimony in the form of professional opinions. The primary legal restriction on the testimony of experts is that their testimony be relevant to the matter at hand and helpful (rather than prejudicial) to the trier of fact in understanding and deciding the case. Psychologists have a long history of participation in the legal system, but their involvement as expert witnesses has been increasing greatly in recent years.

PROCEDURES

When an expert takes the stand to testify, he or she is required to take an oath to tell the truth, just as all witnesses are. The oath has special meaning for psychologists, however, because ethical standards require that data which form the basis for their testimony be presented in an objective and unbiased manner. Being an advocate for one side in a case suggests that the psychologist is selectively presenting data that support one party's position and withholding unfavorable or disconfirmatory findings. The functional role supported by most psychologist experts is that of educator, rather than advocate, whose testimony would be the same regardless of which side called him or her to testify.

Once the expert has been sworn in, the usual procedure is for the attorney of the party who called the psychologist to present the qualifications of the psychologist. By consulting with the attorney prior to the trial or hearing, the psychologist can insure that case-specific qualifications are emphasized. Naturally, it is the ethical responsibility of the attorney to have ascertained before participating in the case that he or she has the appropriate qualifications, that is, that the psychologist is competent in the area. The other side may stipulate that the psychologist is an expert in the area claimed, or may challenge the credentials of the expert to testify in the case; the latter procedure is known as *voir dire*. If the psychologist is qualified as an expert, the next phase ensues.

Although the testimony of experts has long been subject to challenges as to its admissibility, in recent years such testimony has been subject to even greater scrutiny. Since the decision in 1993 in a federal case referred to as *Daubert*, judges have been given more responsibilities as "gatekeepers" of scientific evidence. As such, they are charged with barring the admission of scientific testimony that does not meet certain standards, such as evidence of professional peer review and psychometric soundness. Psychologists who present themselves as expert witnesses may find the psychological tests or other procedures they have used to establish credibility challenged before the trial and ruled inadmissible. In the least, such scrutiny makes it even more imperative for psychologists to be well informed about the psychometric properties and research basis for their techniques.

If there is no *Daubert* challenge, or if all evidence has been ruled admissible, the next phase of the trial or hearing ensues. First, there is a direct examination by the attorney who called the expert. Careful preparation with the lawyer before the trial or hearing is most likely to result in the psychologist being able to give complete, ethical, and competent testimony. The attorney representing the other party may object to the questions being asked or the answers being given during the direct examination. Court room protocol dictates that the witness refrain from offering further testimony until the judge decides whether or not to uphold the objection.

Once the direct examination is finished, the other attorney will conduct a cross-examination in which the procedures, findings, and/or opinions of the expert may be challenged. After the cross-examination, the first attorney has the opportunity to conduct a redirect examination in an attempt to explain or rehabilitate the testimony given during the cross-examination. There is also allowance for a recross-examination of the expert. The process can be a grueling one, particularly if the cross-examination is extremely aggressive. The adversarial system is founded on the belief that the process by which evidence is presented and challenged will result in the emergence of a true picture. At times, however, an attorney will launch an attack on the psychologist, rather than challenging the testimony. As a result, unfortunately, many qualified psychologists will not participate in the legal system or will refuse to provide services to individuals if there is the specter of possible legal involvement.

PSYCHOLOGISTS' TESTIMONY

A psychologist may be asked to provide expert testimony in a wide variety of cases involving children. A psychologist may appear as a scientific expert who has had no actual contact with the litigant. The psychologist's testimony in these instances typically consists of research findings in a particular area. For example, a psychologist might testify about the research on the suggestibility of children's recall to help the trier of fact decide how much weight to give a child's testimony. As a rebuttal witness, a psychologist might be called upon to critique or dispute the procedures, interpretations, or opinions of another psychologist who testified in a case. In this latter position, for example, a psychologist might be called upon to rebut the testimony of another psychologist that projective test results prove that a child was sexually abused.

Most frequently, psychologists are asked to conduct an evaluation of an individual or individuals and then testify to their findings. The request may come from any of a variety of sources, including a litigant, an attorney, or an agency, or the psychologist may be appointed by the court. Many of the cases involving children, such as child custody, abuse and neglect, and termination and adoption proceedings, are emotionally charged and fraught with competing demands and interests. If possible, psychologists usually prefer being appointed as the court's expert to maintain a formalized, neutral position. Regardless of the nature of their retention in a case, it is incumbent upon the psychologist to clarify who the client is. In addition, the psychologist has the responsibility for understanding the nature of the referral question(s), the relevant psycholegal issue(s), the pertinent research, and the limits on confidentiality. Furthermore, it is the responsibility of the psychologist to clarify with the appropriate parties issues of confidentiality, the nature and scope of the evaluation, the role of the psychologist, fees and payment policies, and who the client is. The psychologist is obligated to obtain informed consent from adult clients and from the parents of minor clients (and assent from minors who are capable of giving it), or from legal representatives as appropriate.

It is apparent that the testimony of psychologists exposes the profession to the public; therefore, it is essential that psychologists who offer themselves as experts in the public arena of the court room understand the special ethical and professional practice issues that are involved in their participation in the legal system. The responsibility is no less weighty when a psychologist reluctantly becomes a witness. For example, a psychologist who has been treating a child of divorced parents may find himself or herself with a subpoena to appear in court, with records in hand, to testify in a hearing in which one of the parents is moving to modify custody. It behooves the psychologist to clarify an appropriate response to the request for records and testimony with an experienced colleague; independent legal counsel may also be prudent. While there are many thorny legal and ethical issues involved in this relatively common scenario, it is fundamentally important for the psychologist to avoid giving opinions about the legal matter at hand. In this situation, the treating psychologist is a fact witness whose appropriate scope of testimony might include the reason the child is receiving treatment, what kind of treatment is being provided, and what the prognosis is. The psychologist, not having done the necessary kind of evaluation, is in no position to offer a professional expert opinion as to which parent should have custody.

Finally, it should be noted that the latter type of opinion, which addresses the legal matter the court is deciding, is called ultimate issue testimony. For numerous reasons, the bulk of scholarly opinion is that psychologists as expert witnesses are not qualified to offer ultimate issue testimony and should therefore refrain from doing so. Examples in addition to telling the court which parent should have custody are testifying that a child was sexually abused or that it is in a child's best interests for a parent's legal rights to be terminated.

It should be obvious that psychologists' participation in the legal system is a complex endeavor involving a specialized body of knowledge and skills. One source of guidance for psychologists who provide expert testimony is the *Specialty Guidelines for Forensic Psychologists* (Committee on Ethical Guidelines for Forensic Psychologists, 1991). As is true of other guidelines for psychologists, they are not mandatory but aspirational in nature. Any psychologist who regularly offers expert testimony, as well as those who find themselves reluctantly making an appearance in court, will find the *Guidelines* indispensible.

See also: Custody Evaluations; Ethical Issues; Legal Issues in Child and Pediatric Psychology; Psychometric Properties of Tests; Termination of Parental Rights

Further Reading

Blau, T. H. (1998). *The psychologist as expert witness* (2nd ed.). New York: Wiley.

Brodsky, S. L. (1999). *The expert witness: More maxims and guidelines for testifying in court.* Washington, DC: American Psychological Association.

Committee on Ethical Guidelines for Forensic Psychologists. (1991). Specialty guidelines for forensic psychologists. *Law and Human Behavior, 15,* 655–665.

Melton, G. B., Petrila, J., Poythress, N. G., & Slobogin, C. (1997). *Psychological evaluations for the courts: A handbook for mental health professionals and lawyers* (2nd ed.). New York: Guilford Press.

Schaefer, A. B. (2001). Forensic evaluations of children and expert witness testimony. In C. E. Walker & M. C. Roberts (Eds.), *Handbook of clinical child psychology* (3rd ed., pp. 1094–1119). New York: Wiley.

ARLENE B. SCHAEFER

Expiratory Apnea

See: Breath-Holding Spells

Exposure and Response Prevention

EXPOSURE

Exposure is a behavior therapy technique used in the treatment of childhood fears and phobias. Exposure is based on the idea that anxiety is maintained by avoidance of the fear-eliciting stimulus. The reduction in anxiety associated with this avoidance serves to both reinforce that behavior and strengthen the underlying fear response. During exposure treatment, the child is asked to deliberately come into contact with anxiety-provoking stimuli and to remain in contact with the stimuli for a given period of time. Over the course of the exposure, the individual comes to realize that the expected feared consequences associated with the stimulus are not going to occur. This cognitive correction, along with a decrease in physiologic arousal due to autonomic habituation, serves to reduce heightened anxiety and over repeated trials can lead to eventual elimination of the fear response.

There are two types of exposure: in vivo and imaginal. In vivo exposure involves exposure to actual stimuli as encountered in one's environment. Interoceptive exposure, a specific form of in vivo exposure, involves exposure to bodily sensations or symptoms and is used for the treatment of panic disorder. In interoceptive exposure, feared bodily sensations (e.g., dizziness, increased heart rate) are induced until the child realizes that the feared consequence (e.g., going crazy, death) will not occur.

Imaginal exposure entails exposure to imagined anxiety-provoking situations or objects in lieu of direct exposure. Imaginal exposure is used when in vivo exposure is not possible. Most often, this is due to stimuli being internally based (e.g., urges, thoughts), not easily accessible or immediately available (e.g., public speaking), or not amenable to re-creation (e.g., fear of stabbing a loved one). Imaginal exposure is also used as an initial step when in vivo exposure is too anxiety-provoking for the patient. Exposure can take many forms in addition to direct or imaginal contact with the feared stimulus, including drawing pictures of, and/or writing, telling, or listening to stories about feared situations or objects, as well as virtual presentation of the stimuli.

METHOD FOR CONDUCTING EXPOSURES

Exposures are typically conducted in graded fashion with milder symptoms exposed first. A fear hierarchy, or list of specific feared situations and/or objects arranged in order from least to most feared, is used to guide graded exposure. Depending on the disorder and stage of treatment, hierarchies may consist of a relatively broad range of disparate symptoms (i.e., touching doorknobs in public places, checking to make sure the stove is off, counting sidewalk cracks for obsessive-compulsive disorder [OCD]) or a series of smaller steps related to one specific symptom (e.g., placing finger on public doorknob, placing palm on doorknob, holding hand on doorknob for 2 min). Child self-reports of anxiety or distress are obtained at frequent intervals throughout the exposure and each specific trial is continued until the child's reported anxiety drops to at least 50 percent below the highest level reported during the exposure. Exposure can be conducted in almost any setting and may occur with the therapist present or assigned as homework. When possible, specific exposure exercises should be modeled by the therapist prior to asking the child to do them.

RESPONSE PREVENTION

For patients with OCD, exposure is typically paired with response prevention. Response prevention involves blocking the performance of rituals or other behaviors (i.e., avoidance) performed to reduce anxiety or other noxious feelings associated with obsessions. As an example, a child with contaminations fears and associated compulsive handwashing might be asked to touch a contaminated surface (exposure) and then refrain from washing (response prevention). By limiting the opportunity to reduce anxiety through ritualizing or avoidance, response prevention allows for greater levels of cognitive correction and autonomic habituation. Once an exposure to a given fear item has begun, the child is instructed to resist urges to ritualize in response to that stimulus both in treatment and nontreatment settings.

CLINICAL APPLICATIONS AND EFFECTIVENESS

The efficacy of exposure and response prevention for childhood anxiety disorders has been demonstrated in multiple rigorously controlled studies. Exposure is the treatment of choice for specific phobias, and when paired with response prevention, for OCD. Exposure is also a key component of cognitive-behavioral treatments for other anxiety disorders such as separation anxiety, social anxiety, and generalized anxiety disorders (GAD). Interoceptive exposure is a primary component in cognitive-behavioral therapy (CBT) used in the treatment of panic disorder.

See also: Anxiety Disorders; Behavior Therapy; Cognitive–Behavior Therapy; Evidence-Based Treatments; Obsessive-Compulsive Disorder

Further Reading

Ollendick, T. H., & King, N. (1998). Empirically supported treatments for children with phobic and anxiety disorders. *Journal of Clinical Child Psychology, 27*, 156–167.

Piacentini, J. (1999). Cognitive behavioral therapy of childhood OCD. *Child and Adolescent Psychiatric Clinics of North America, 3*, 599–616.

JOHN PIACENTINI
TAMI ROBLEK

Exposure to Violence

DEFINITION

Exposure to violence has been categorized along the multiple dimensions that might potentially influence its impact on children and adolescents. Community-based violence, which occurs outside an individual's home and is perpetrated by someone outside of the individual's family, has been distinguished from family-based, domestic violence perpetrated by close relatives or household members. Violence from intentional human actions directed toward harming others has been distinguished from accidents, natural disasters, and self-harm. Intentional violence is often subdivided into three categories: interpersonal, situational, and predatory. Interpersonal violence is characterized by violent acts that occur between individuals who have ongoing relationships with each other. Situational violence involves intentionally harmful acts that are not necessarily directed specifically toward the injured parties, and is often associated with social factors such as poverty, social upheaval, and elevated levels of criminal activity. Predatory violence includes harmful actions occurring as part of a pattern of criminal or antisocial behavior.

The degree of direct exposure to the violence (direct victimization, witnessing, vicarious witnessing) is another potentially important distinction. Direct victimization is perpetrated upon the individual. Witnessing involves any direct observation of a violent act as it is occurring. Vicarious witnessing occurs when an individual has been told or has heard an account of violent event.

INCIDENCE

Children's exposure to violence varies widely. Greatest exposure has been found among minority youth who live in poor inner-city communities. The majority of children in these areas often report having directly witnessed one or more acts of serious violence (e.g., stabbing, shooting) at home or in the community. Youth-on-youth violence is a significant source of exposure.

Recent national surveys in the United States estimate that 1 in 12 high school students is threatened or injured with a weapon each year. Juveniles under the age of 18 years are involved in approximately one quarter of all serious violent victimizations, including 14 percent of sexual assaults, 30 percent of robberies, and 27 percent of aggravated assaults. Juveniles are twice as likely as adults to commit serious violent crimes in groups, enhancing the possibility for more juveniles to witness or perpetrate violence. Domestic abuse is a primary source of direct exposure as a victim or witness for younger children.

Exposure to violence in the media is ubiquitous. By some estimates, the average sixth grader in the United States has seen 8,000 murders and 100,000 acts of violence on television.

CORRELATES

Effects of exposure to violence depend on numerous individual and contextual factors. These include proximity to violent acts; developmental timing of exposure events; the nature, intensity, and duration of exposure, the relationship between the perpetrator and victim; and individual and family coping resources. Many aspects of cognitive, social, emotional, and psychophysiological functioning may be significantly affected by exposure to violence. The most frequently reported internalizing effects include posttraumatic stress symptoms, depression, withdrawal, disregulation, dissociative reactions, and declines in cognitive performance. Other potential effects include increased antisocial behavior, reduced threshold for using violence reactively or instrumentally (i.e., to get what one wants), drug use, and carrying a weapon. Social information processing may also be affected by repeated exposure to violence (e.g., approval of aggression as a social response, problems with the interpretation of social cues, perceived positive outcomes for the use of aggression). Attachment relationships may be adversely affected, especially when domestic violence is involved. Intense and prolonged exposure to violence is believed to influence psychophysiological features such as autonomic reactivity.

ASSESSMENT

Assessment of violence exposure ideally should include information from multiple sources. Several self-report and parent-report measures of exposure have been developed to tap different aspects of exposure. It is often useful to compare objective indicators of exposure (e.g., police or protective service reports)

to self-reports. Children, adolescents, and parents may be extremely reticent to disclose certain forms of exposure (e.g., domestic violence) because of shame or fear of the consequences of disclosure. Gauging the effects of exposure requires comprehensive techniques for measuring both internalizing and externalizing symptoms.

TREATMENT

Numerous model programs have been developed for violence prevention and intervention for violence-exposed children and adolescents. Many of these are part of complex school- and community-based efforts that address multiple risk factors and settings. Clinical treatment protocols for specific forms of violence (e.g., single-incident trauma, sexual abuse) have been developed in recent years, and evidence-based approaches are increasingly becoming available. Developmental considerations influence the selection and delivery of appropriate treatments and preventive interventions.

PROGNOSIS

The potential effects of violence exposure are numerous and complex. Gauging the short- and long-term effects on exposed children and adolescents requires consideration of the extent and context of exposure, individual and family characteristics, and cultural factors influencing the understanding and lessons drawn from violent events.

See also: Aggression; Child Treatment; Community Interventions; Posttraumatic Stress Disorder

Further Reading

Dahlberg, L. L., Toal, S. B., & Behrens, C. B. (1998). *The measurement of violence-related attitudes, beliefs, and behaviors among youths: A compendium of instruments*. Atlanta, GA: Centers for Disease Control and Prevention, National Center for Injury Prevention and Control.

Jacobson, W. B. (2000). *Safe from the start: Taking action on children exposed to violence*. U.S. Department of Justice, Office of Justice Programs, Office of Juvenile Justice and Delinquency Prevention: Washington, DC [Available at http://www.ncjrs.org/pdffiles1/ojjdp/182789.pdf.]

Osofsky, J. D. (1997). *Children in a violent society*. New York. Guilford.

Weist, M. D., & Cooley-Quille, M. (Eds.). (2001). Violence and youth. [Special section]. *Journal of Clinical Child Psychology, 30*, 147–239.

AARON C. STRATMAN
ERIC M. VERNBERG

Extinction

According to the principles of applied behavior analysis, behaviors are maintained through reinforcement. That is, a behavior continues to occur because on all or some occurrences it is followed by some form of reinforcement. Consider, for example, the child who plays nicely and his mother praises him for it. That child is more likely to play nicely in the future. Unfortunately, reinforcement will also maintain behaviors that parents do not like. Consider the child who cries after being put to bed and is then picked up by his parent. The parent's attention reinforces the child's crying and on future occasions when the child is put to bed he is likely to cry again until the parent picks him up. Both of these behaviors will continue to occur as long as the reinforcement is provided when the behavior occurs.

Extinction is a term that is used in two ways. First, it is used to describe the process that occurs when a behavior disappears as a result of the reinforcement being withdrawn. Second, it is used to describe an intervention procedure that is used in an attempt to remove an undesirable behavior. Here the term is used in the latter sense, that is, as a procedure to remove an undesirable behavior.

Extinction as an intervention procedure aims at breaking the connection of behavior and reinforcement. It relies on the fact that never reinforcing a behavior will result in the decreased frequency of the behavior. When extinction is being used, reinforcement of the undesirable behavior must never occur. Even if there is an occasional reinforcement of the behavior, extinction will be less likely to be successful. If the child's behavior is periodically reinforced, it is technically on an intermittent schedule of reinforcement and the behavior will likely continue and persist.

In order for extinction to work effectively, it is essential to identify the reinforcers maintaining the behavior, and then to remove them. Therefore, a key element in the successful use of the extinction procedure is to conduct a detailed assessment of the behavior and its associated reinforcers.

Extinction procedures are frequently used for behaviors that are not serious or dangerous, but rather are ongoing and disruptive, such as nagging, attention seeking, and bedtime crying.

An initial effect of extinction is that the behavior may temporarily increase in intensity. This is known as an extinction burst. Consider the example of the child who cries when put to bed until a parent picks him up. If the parent begins to use extinction (not giving attention for the crying), the child is likely to cry harder and longer in an attempt to gain access to the reinforcement. It is important that during the extinction burst reinforcement is not given at any stage, otherwise the child simply learns to engage in the behavior more intensely and longer in order to obtain the desired reinforcement. Extinction bursts generally do not last more than a few sessions if reinforcement is consistently withheld. In addition, the use of reinforcement for appropriate behavior reduces the likelihood of extinction bursts occurring.

It is important to note that if a behavior is intrinsically reinforced, that is, if the reinforcement is part of the behavior and not separate from it (e.g., for self-stimulatory behaviors), extinction will not be effective as it is not possible to remove the intrinsic reinforcement.

See also: Applied Behavior Analysis; Behavior Modification; Positive Reinforcement

Further Reading

Grant, L., & Evans, A. (1994). *Principles of behavior.* New York: Harper Collins.
Hudson, A. (1998). Applied behavior analysis. In A. Bellack, M. Hersen (Series Eds.), & T. Ollendick (Vol. Ed.), *Comprehensive clinical psychology (Vol. 5). Children and adolescents: Clinical formulation and treatment* (pp. 107–129). New York: Pergamon.
Lerman, D. C., Iwata, B. A., & Wallace, M. D. (1999). Side effects of extinction: Prevalence of bursting and aggression during the treatment of self-injurious behavior. *Journal of Applied Behavior Analysis, 32,* 1–8.

EMMA LITTLE
ALAN HUDSON

Eye-Movement Desensitization and Reprocessing

DEFINITION

Eye-movement desensitization and reprocessing (EMDR) is a therapeutic technique developed by Shapiro (1995) that has been proposed as a treatment for Posttraumatic Stress Disorder (PTSD) and other psychopathological conditions. During EMDR, children imaginally expose themselves to a traumatic or aversive memory, while simultaneously engaging in lateral eye movements that are induced by the therapist. The idea is that through the eye movements, negative memories are emotionally processed and assimilated.

METHOD

EMDR sessions can be conducted by the mental health professional who has received the special training courses that are organized by Shapiro's EMDR Institute. The basic protocol that is followed in each EMDR treatment is straightforward and is probably suitable for children and adolescents, although the procedure may require some simplification when applying it to younger children. The protocol starts with asking children to describe the aversive event and to identify the most disturbing image of this event. Next, children formulate a negative (e.g., "I am worthless") and a positive (e.g., "I am in control") cognition in relation to the aversive experience. Following this, children rate the credibility of the positive cognition (i.e., validity of cognition; VOC) on a 7-point scale (1 = *not at all credible*, 7 = *very credible*). Then, children describe their physical anxiety response during the experience and rate the level of disturbance on a 10-point Subjective Units of Disturbance Scale (SUDS; 1 = *no disturbance at all*, 10 = *highest disturbance possible*). Finally, children are asked to bring up their most disturbing image of the negative experience and to generate the accompanying negative cognition and the physical anxiety response. When children signal that they have been able to do this, the first set of horizontal eye movements (24 saccades) is carried out. Following this, children are instructed to blank out the image and to take a deep breath. After a brief pause, children are asked to describe their images, feelings, and/or thoughts. As long as descriptions have a negative content, new sets of eye movements are initiated. When the reported image, feeling, and/or thought has a neutral content, children are instructed to reimagine the negative experience and to rate the level of disturbance on a SUDS. The eye movement procedure is repeated until children report a SUDS score of 1 (no disturbance at all). At this point, the positive cognition is installed, that is, children reimagine the negative experience and simultaneously generate the positive cognition. While doing so, eye movements are initiated again. After each set, children rate the credibility of the positive cognition (VOC) and this is repeated until a score of 7 (very credible) is reached.

During an EMDR session that usually lasts for 1 hr, the therapist tries to desensitize the aversive experience and install the positive cognition employing the eye-movements technique. For patients who find the eye movements physically uncomfortable, and this is relatively often the case with children, alternative forms of stimulation (hand taps and sounds) can be used. Each EMDR session also includes a "body scan," which actually is a guided relaxation exercise that is used to calm down the patient before he/she leaves the therapist's office.

EMDR is based on the assumption that traumatic or aversive memories play a pivotal role in a broad range of psychopathological conditions. The dysfunctional nature of such memories is most evident in PTSD. In Shapiro's (1995, p. 30) words: "When someone experiences a severe trauma, it appears that an imbalance may occur in the nervous system, caused perhaps by changes in neurotransmitters, adrenaline, and so forth. Due to this imbalance, the system is unable to function and the information acquired at the time of the event, including images, sounds, affect, and physical sensations is maintained neurologically in its disturbing state. Therefore, the original material, which is held in this distressing, excitatory state-dependent form, continues to be triggered by a variety of internal and external stimuli and is expressed in the form of nightmares, flashbacks, and intrusive thoughts, the so-called positive symptoms of PTSD." Shapiro (1995) assumes that the eye movements (or other rhythmic stimulation) rebalance the nervous system, shift information that is dysfunctionally locked in the nervous system, and/or catalyze the appropriate biochemical balance. It should be mentioned that several authors, including Muris and Merckelbach (1999), have been critical of the theoretical foundations underlying the use of EMDR.

CLINICAL APPLICATION AND EMPIRICAL STATUS

Although initially developed as a treatment procedure for PTSD, EMDR has been proposed as an effective intervention for a broad range of mental disorders, including typical childhood problems such as specific phobias, separation anxiety disorder, reactive attachment disorder, and disruptive disorders (DD). So far, however, these claims have not been substantiated. Available therapy outcome research indicates that only in the case of PTSD in adults, EMDR yields positive effects that are comparable with those reached by cognitive-behavior therapy (CBT). For other types of psychopathology, convincing evidence in support of its efficacy is still lacking. Moreover, the empirical status of EMDR is highly questionable since its theoretical basis is speculative and research has shown that the treatment procedure is just as effective without the eye movements.

See also: Attachment Behavior Therapy, Specific Phobia; Cognitive–Behavior Therapy; Posttraumatic Stress Disorder (PTSD)

Further Reading

Davidson, P. R., & Parker, K. C. H. (2001). Eye movement desensitization and reprocessing (EMDR): A meta-analysis. *Journal of Consulting and Clinical Psychology, 69,* 305–316.

Muris, P., & Merckelbach, H. (1999). Traumatic memories, eye movements, phobia, and panic. A critical note on the proliferation of EMDR. *Journal of Anxiety Disorders, 13,* 208–224.

Shapiro, F. (1995). *Eye movement desensitization and reprocessing. Basic principles, protocols, and procedures.* New York: Guilford.

Tinker, R. H., & Wilson, S. A. (1999). *Through the eyes of a child: EMDR with children.* New York: Norton.

PETER MURIS

Ff

Failure-to-Thrive

DEFINITION

Traditionally, failure-to-thrive (FTT) has been a diagnosis of infancy and early childhood and is often characterized into two types, organic and nonorganic. Central to both subtypes is the failure of an infant or young child to make expected weight gains or to actually lose weight during a period of normally active growth. Organic reasons for FTT include gastrointestinal, cardiac, renal, or metabolic disorders. Nonorganic failure-to-thrive (NOFTT) is a common term used to describe those infants or children for whom no medical (organic) reason could be found for the failure to gain at an expected rate. Absence of a medical explanation lead to the assumption that the failure was related to psychosocial factors. The fourth edition of the *Diagnostic and Statistic Manual of Mental Disorders* (*DSM-IV*) (1994) published by the American Psychiatric Association includes a diagnosis of Feeding Disorder of Infancy and Early Childhood (307.59), defined as a feeding disturbance described by a failure to eat adequate amounts to produce normal weight gain, or resulting in significant weight loss that is not associated with a medical condition, or is better explained by another mental disorder or lack of available food. *DSM IV* specifies that the onset of the disorder be before age 6 years.

INCIDENCE/PSYCHOLOGICAL CORRELATES

As many as 1–5 percent of pediatric hospital admissions are for FTT and there have been estimates that 3.5–20 percent of children in rural and urban ambulatory care clinics present with FTT. Children with prematurity and developmental delays are at higher risk for FTT. The condition of FTT poses numerous threats to the child. These range from the medical effects of malnutrition and dehydration to disruptive effects of interruptions in caregiving due to hospitalizations, and other social or psychological interventions. Children with FTT are believed to be at increased risk for behavioral and learning problems, poor ego development, and decreased resiliency. The condition often leads to removal from the mother or original caretaker by a +social service agency, setting the stage for adjustment difficulties. This often occurs following a hospitalization in which it is documented that the infant or child does gain weight when fed by trained caregivers. The disturbed interaction in the feeding situation is likely indicative of compromised parenting skills in other areas, suggesting possible problems in bonding, emotional support, or behavior management.

ASSESSMENT

The assessment of a child with NOFTT involves three areas: developmental assessment, examination of environmental and social variables in the family, and assessment of specific feeding behaviors and behavioral interactions between the primary caregiver (usually the mother) and the child during the feeding process. Developmental assessment should include standardized measures of the child's cognitive and adaptive development. The assessment of family functioning and the child's social environment is usually accomplished by clinical interview and the use of standardized assessment

228

instruments such as the Family Environment Scale and marital adjustment inventories. Behavioral observation of the actual feeding process is necessary to determine ineffective feeding practices and to identify strategies for behavior change. It is important to resist drawing conclusion about the cause of feeding problems from behavioral observations if the child is extremely malnourished, as some behaviors of the child or feeder may be the result of undernutrition or parent frustrations, rather than the cause.

TREATMENT

Interventions for NOFTT can be broad-based, directed at producing changes in the infant's social and physical environment, or more specific to the feeding situation. Broad-based approaches are usually intense, multielement interventions addressing the social and economic needs of families. Included are social welfare interventions, early intervention for developmental issues, and supportive counseling with parents and family. The results of broad-based interventions have not been encouraging to date. However, the need to consider social and emotional support is so intrinsically sensible and this area should not be neglected in treatment planning. The effectiveness of behavioral treatment methods for treating a variety of feeding problems are now well documented. These methods use contingency based procedures to increase acceptance of increased quantity of foods or to change the child's ability or willingness to accept a greater variety and texture of foods by mouth. Parents are taught to be aware of the child's cues during the feeding situation and how to provide positive reinforcement in the form of praise and interaction to the child for compliance with feeding requests. Methods for decreasing noncompliance, behavioral acting out, and stalling are also taught and demonstrated. The goal is not only to increase the child's weight but also to make the feeding situation pleasant and successful for the parent so as to foster a sense of confidence in the parent's ability to care for the child.

PROGNOSIS

The prognosis for NOFTT is generally good if the variety of contributory etiological factors can be addressed. Treatment must be intense and instituted early to avoid the developmental and emotional sequelae the child can accrue from poor nutrition and unsuccessful parent–child interactions around feeding. Social, supportive, economic, and behavioral interventions are all part of a successful treatment program.

See also: Behavioral Observation; Behavior and Functional Analysis; Behavior Modification; Behavior Rating Scales; Differential Social Reinforcement/Positive Attention; Gastrointestinal Disorders; Rumination

Further Reading

American Psychiatric Association (APA). (1994). *Diagnostic and statistical manual of mental disorders* (4th ed.). Washington, DC: Author.

Linscheid, T. R., & Bennett-Murphy, L. (1999). Feeding disorders of infancy and early childhood. In S. D. Netherton, D. Holmes, & C. E. Walker (Eds.), *Child & adolescent psychological disorders* (pp. 139–155). New York: Oxford University Press.

Linscheid, T. R., & Rasnake, L. K. (2001). Eating problems in children. In C. E. Walker & M. C. Roberts (Eds.), *Handbook of clinical child psychology* (3rd ed., pp. 523–544). New York: Wiley.

THOMAS R. LINSCHEID

Families Who Are Homeless

DESCRIPTION OF FAMILIES WHO ARE HOMELESS

Families who are homeless live in places they do not perceive as their own homes. This includes families living in places not designed for human habitation (e.g., cars, on the street, parks, empty buildings), families in temporary housing situations (e.g., shelters, motels), families living with friends or relatives on a temporary basis, and those in situations where they must immediately leave their current living arrangement because of safety, financial, or other reasons. Thus, homeless families are not simply defined as those living in homeless shelters. In fact, more homeless families may live outside of shelters than in them. Homelessness affects families across all ethnic groups; however, minority families are overrepresented among the homeless. Homeless families, compared to homeless individuals, have lower rates of substance abuse and mental health problems. Homeless parents are more likely to be women, and female-headed families are the fastest growing subgroup of the homeless, thought to comprise one third of the 2.5 million homeless people in the United States (U.S. Conference of Mayors, 1987). Often, these mothers are escaping from abusive environments.

What factors contribute to homelessness? Homelessness among families appears to be related to poverty, lack of affordable housing, and lack of social support. These families have more difficulty accessing social services, and they appear to know less about the procedures for getting services. Families who do not know how to access services and who do not speak English are less likely to access services, and are therefore more likely to experience long-term homelessness. A lack of resources among relatives is also related to homelessness.

EFFECTS OF HOMELESSNESS ON THE FAMILY

Homelessness and associated poverty place significant stress on families. Most homeless families are single-parent, female-headed families, usually young female mothers with 2–3 children. Homeless mothers report family stressors specific to homelessness and shelter life, including being unable to fulfill parental roles (e.g., provide food, shelter, effective discipline); public parenting (e.g., other shelter residents or relatives interfering with parenting); and shelter rules (e.g., rigid meal times, lack of access to kitchen, curfews, rules barring male children from shelters, rules requiring parents to be with children at all times). In addition, homeless mothers have higher rates of depression than nonhomeless mothers, and parental depression has been shown to have detrimental effects on children's mental health and behavior.

Child distress has been shown to have negative effects on parent–child relationships, and homeless children have higher rates of distress than children in the general population. Older children may experience more distress than younger children. Their lives may be more disrupted and they may experience feelings of embarrassment. Sometimes the family is broken up with children placed in foster care, or dispersed to stay with relatives. In addition, some shelters do not allow male children, so a male child may be sent to live apart from the family. On a more positive note, many families report that they are closer as a result of living in close quarters and coming together during a crisis.

EFFECTS OF HOMELESSNESS ON CHILDREN

Development and Mental Health

Poverty places children at risk for many psychological and behavioral disorders (e.g., Oppositional Defiant Disorder [ODD], Conduct Disorder [CD], learning disorders, mild mental retardation, Attention-Deficit/Hyperactivity Disorder [ADHD]). Thus, it is difficult to determine what effects homelessness has on children's mental health beyond the effects of poverty. Research comparing homeless children with poorly housed children has found that homeless children have higher rates of internalizing disorders (e.g., depression, anxiety). In general, children living in poverty have higher rates of developmental delays, including delays in cognitive skills, language, and motor skills; most homeless children can be included in this group. Less clear is whether homeless children experience higher rates of abuse than low-income housed children or children in the general population.

The effects of homelessness and poverty on children's development may accumulate over time. For example, initially children may not differ on developmental tests; however, differences begin to emerge as the children get older, with older children who are homeless performing more poorly on measures of development than low-income housed children. This finding suggests that, over time, the negative effects of poverty and homelessness on children's development increase.

Physical Health

Children who are homeless have less access to, and receive fewer, health care services, including well-child care and dental care. Homeless children, along with low-income housed children, have higher levels of respiratory infection, diarrhea and asthma, and lower rates of immunization compared to children in the general population. Homeless children may experience delayed outpatient care, and may use emergency room services at a higher rate than housed children.

Living in close proximity with other families and sharing facilities puts children living in shelters at higher risk for infectious disease, and enteric infections like *Salmonella*. They do not appear to be at greater risk for chronic illness than poor, housed children, unless they have lived in an inappropriate place, such as a garage, park, car, or empty building. Malnutrition and anemia are more common among homeless children, and they are at risk for obesity—they are more likely to eat in fast-food restaurants and to experience longer periods of food deprivation than housed children.

Academic Performance

Homeless children have poorer academic performance than peers in the general population. However, their performance is similar to that of poor, housed peers. Homelessness and poverty place children at greater risk for school absence and transitions from one school to another. Homelessness and shelter life may make it difficult to complete homework or access resources necessary for academic success.

CONCLUSION

Clinical child and pediatric psychology has been involved in the development and provision of mental health services to poor and homeless families, often in public sector clinics and hospitals. School psychologists are also faced with the problems posed by this segment of the school population. Policymakers, governmental agencies, and health care professionals need to understand and be involved in the issues of homelessness and the improvement of children's conditions in this country.

See also: Domestic Violence

Further Reading

Buckner, J. C., Bassuk, E. L., & Weinreb, L. F. (2001). Predictors of academic achievement among homeless and low-income housed children. *Journal of School Psychology, 39,* 45–69.
Buckner, J. C., Bassuk, E. L., Weinreb, L. F., & Brooks, M. G. (1999). Homelessness and its relation to the mental health and behavior of low-income school-age children. *Developmental Psychology, 35,* 246–257.
Coll, C. G., Buckner, J. C., Brooks, M. G., Weinreb, L. F., & Bassuk, E. L. (1998). The developmental status and adaptive behavior of homeless and low-income housed infants and toddlers. *American Journal of Public Health, 88,* 1371–1374.
Dornbusch, S. M. (1994). Additional perspectives on homeless families. *American Behavioral Scientist, 37,* 404–411.

REBECCA J. JOHNSON
MICHAEL C. ROBERTS

Family Assessment

BACKGROUND

In order to understand infants, children, and adolescents, it is essential to understand the family contexts in which they live. Development unfolds not only in the individual child but also throughout the entire family system. Children and parents, for example, have reciprocal relationships, which change over time. Families

are remarkably diverse social settings. There is no one "normal" family but rather a multitude of family structures and patterns of functioning. The term *family assessment* refers broadly to both formal and informal methods of learning about a particular family. While changes in the family in the United States are widely acknowledged (e.g., recognition of divorce, remarriage, grandparent-headed families, single parenting, adoption, and gay and lesbian-headed families), there are some general guidelines which are helpful in assessing families.

Basic, but often overlooked, is the question "Who is in the family?" Family membership should be defined by the family itself (e.g., whom do you consider your family?). There are potentially several different family constellations for each family. For example, biological and legal linkages can define a family, but so can function (Who helps to parent?) and circumstances (Who do you call when you have an emergency? Who joins family celebrations?). Unfortunately, our understanding of families is based primarily on the perspective of mothers. The neglect of fathers in this work results in a biased understanding and one that can be remedied by strategic inclusion of fathers. As complex systems, families are in constant change. Thus, the family structure itself, or its function, may differ based on the age of children across the lifespan, as well as in response to external demands on the family. Families reflect the broader social ecology in which they live. Understanding families with respect to fundamental parameters such as ethnicity is critical. Finally, families interact with other systems and can be appreciated within the networks of family, health, school, and community settings.

GENERAL APPROACHES TO FAMILY ASSESSMENT

There are many ways in which family assessments may be conducted, including unstructured and structured interviews, genograms, self-report questionnaires, and observational methodologies. Illustrations of these approaches show the complexity of families and the many pertinent facets of family structure and function. These approaches can be used individually or can be combined.

In an *unstructured interview*, one may ask about family structure, roles, and functioning as part of the process of understanding the interpersonal dynamics of the family system. Before doing so, it is essential to establish connections with each member of the family, sometimes in family therapy called joining or using Acceptance, Respect, Curiosity, Honesty (ARCH, see Miccucci [1998]). One might ask, for example, how each member of the family is related to each other and elicit the perception of each family member of the problem and possible solutions. In the course of this discussion, important aspects of the family history, themes that characterize the family, and ways in which the family system operates are identified.

Structured interviews provide a series of topics or questions, which are covered, usually in a proscribed order. The interview protocol might include both general and specific questions, such as: How many children are in the family and how many live in the home? Who do you go to for help (what kinds of help)? When did the problem begin? How has it affected parents, siblings, relationships with the school? How is conflict handled at home? What has your family done to cope with their concerns?

The best known approach to understanding a family graphically is the use of *genograms*. The genogram builds on a basic family pedigree (family tree) but provides more detailed information about the structure of the family, including a timeline of events. The genogram shows not only family structure but also a visual portrayal of the closeness and conflict in family relationships. The genogram also shows how family patterns may repeat themselves in different parts of the family, or across generations (e.g., the presence of substance abuse, patterns of deaths or divorces, repeated alienation of sons from fathers, etc.). The genogram can be used with either individuals or families.

Perhaps the most common approach to family assessment is use of *family self-report questionnaires*. There are many questionnaires and the selection of which to use is determined by what aspects of functioning are most critical. (The reader is referred to Toulitatos [2000] and colleagues for a compendium of information about measures). In each instance, key elements of family functioning are measured (e.g., cohesiveness, conflict, values, rules, organization). These questionnaires have the advantage of being psychometrically established and with normative data. Their disadvantage is that they generate relatively broad data and may not be sufficiently specific to the concerns of particular groups of families. Another disadvantage is that these scales are administered to individual family members and therefore reflect the biases of the person completing them.

A related approach to assessing families is to use measures of different aspects of family functioning. In this way, more specific information is obtained about several different relationships in the family. For example, parenting stress, marital satisfaction, social support, parent–child conflict, and sibling relationships may all be measured using standardized self-report questionnaires. Using the data obtained, a richer understanding of family functioning may be obtained than with a general family questionnaire.

Observational approaches to family assessment add an important element, the more objective perspective of those outside the family. Well validated observational measures of family functioning are available. Observers may conduct ratings based on live observation or may analyze videotaped interviews. Although some emphasize clinical functioning of families, these approaches are generally limited to research settings, given the need for trained staff, space, and equipment in order to utilize these approaches.

SPECIALIZED FAMILY ASSESSMENT

Sometimes a more general family assessment approach may not yield sufficient information related to a particular issue (e.g., child abuse, divorce, substance abuse, Attention-Deficit/Hyperactivity Disorder [ADHD], autistic spectrum disorders, chronic and acute child health problems). In order to refine the process and content of family assessment, the specific research and clinical theory and practice literatures related to these areas should be consulted, particularly with regard to issue-specific assessment approaches.

See also: Assessment; Behavior Rating Scales; Child Self-Reports; Family Intervention; History-Taking; Interviewing; Social Support

Further Reading

McGoldrick, M., Gerson, R., & Shellenberger, S. (1999). *Genograms: Assessment and Intervention* (2nd ed.). New York: Norton.
McGoldrick, M., Giordano, J., & Pearce, J. (1996). *Ethnicity and Family Therapy* (2nd ed.). New York: Guilford.
Micucci, J. (1998). *The adolescent in family therapy: Breaking the cycle of conflict and control.* New York: Guilford.
Power, T., DuPaul, G., Shapiro, E., & Kazak, A. (2003). *Promoting children's health: Integrating health, school, family and community systems.* New York: Guilford.
Seagull, E. (2000). Beyond mothers and children: Finding the family in pediatric psychology. *Journal of Pediatric Psychology, 25,* 161–169.
Touliatos, J., Straus, M., & Perlmutter, B. (2000). *Handbook of family measurement techniques.* Thousand Oaks, CA: Sage.
Walsh, F. (2002). *Normal family processes* (3rd ed.). New York: Guilford.

ANNE E. KAZAK

Family Intervention

BACKGROUND

Family interventions have in common a focus on behavior in the context of the family, the inclusion of multiple family members in treatment, and the belief that change in the interpersonal context of the family is essential to fostering lasting improvement in child-related difficulties. There are many different therapeutic approaches that fall under the broad rubric of family intervention. The field of family intervention is multidisciplinary, with many contributions made by psychiatrists, sociologists, social workers, nurses, and other family researchers. Although family therapy and psychoeducational approaches are often considered distinct, we include them together to provide a comprehensive overview of family intervention relevant to children and their families.

FAMILY THERAPY AND PSYCHOEDUCATIONAL APPROACHES

Family therapy, the most intense and well known type of family intervention, is generally directed toward remedying distress of one or more family members. There are many different schools of family therapy, each with a specific theoretical orientation (e.g., behavioral, psychoanalytic, experiential, cognitive-behavioral, structural) and techniques that promote change consistent with the theoretical approach. Information about family therapy approaches can be found in comprehensive textbooks and handbooks such as Nichols (2000). A more recent movement in family therapy is toward integrative models that identify core components of family interventions that supercede particular theories and techniques in order to integrate treatment approaches.

Structural and behavioral family therapy approaches are best known in child and pediatric psychology. Minuchin and colleagues conducted structural family therapy with inner-city children and families and also explored the idea that family functioning might affect the course of treatment for childhood diseases such as asthma, diabetes, and eating disorders. Although little empirical investigation has been devoted to structural family therapy, the legacy of engaging difficult-to-treat families in family therapy, the notions of family hierarchy, leadership, boundaries, and focused intervention techniques provided by this model are enduring.

Behavioral family therapy models have been evaluated more thoroughly, with evidence suggesting that applying a behavioral (and/or cognitive behavioral) approach in work with multiple members of the family is effective, across a range of childhood behavioral and health concerns. These include acting out disorders and pediatric chronic illnesses such as cystic fibrosis, diabetes, and cancer. Research on families of youth with antisocial behavior and substance abuse has also shown the effectiveness of family treatment approaches that treat adolescents in the context of their families and other social systems.

Psychoeducational interventions are effective in changing family systems, but often have a more explicit educational emphasis (e.g., learning how a behavior problem or medical condition impacts families) rather than a targeted approach to decrease symptoms or reduce psychopathological responses. Psychoeducational approaches may be more readily offered (and accepted) by a larger number of families than family therapy.

OTHER APPROACHES TO FAMILY INTERVENTION

There are many other interventions that are utilized with families, including direct services to families, that are provided in many clinic and hospital settings. These may include, for example, family-centered care in pediatric health settings, mental health and social services in community agencies, and school based intervention and prevention programs focused on specific needs of children and their families such as divorce, bereavement, nutrition, disease management, or social skills. Family systems approaches are also integrated into consultation models in health care. The latter model views systemic variables (in this case of the child's healthcare team) as part of the conceptualization of the problem and also as integral to the intervention.

USING FAMILY INTERVENTIONS

Family interventions can and must be used in a flexible manner. For example, a family intervention should include the relevant members of the family system, but this must be viewed flexibly and in accord with the family's definition of the family. Despite the ongoing association of "family" with two parents of one or more children living independently from extended family, this does not reflect the reality of American families today. Families may have one parent, two parents of the same sex, or have another family member functioning in the role of parent. They may be a foster family, an adoptive family, or a family that has had one or more remarriages, with half-siblings and stepsiblings. The socioeconomic, ethnic, and racial background of family members is also critical in formulating intervention approaches and considering how to engage families of diverse structures and background. Yet, all families share common goals regarding the growth and development of their members and a quest for overall well-being and strategies for handling difficulties as they arise. Family interventions are complex and may appear relatively uncontrolled when compared with some traditional research designs. However, given the importance of understanding children in the context of their families, the future is promising for creative, integrative approaches, which address the concerns of families across a broad spectrum of developmental stages and life circumstances.

See also: Family Assessment; Multisystemic Therapy; Parent–Child Interaction Therapy; Parent Training

Further Reading

Barkley, R., Robin, A., & Edwards, G. (1999). *Defiant teens.* New York: Guilford.

Henggeler, S., Schoenwald, S., Rowland, M., Borduin, C., & Cunningham, P. (1998). *Multisystemic treatment of antisocial behavior in children and adolescents.* New York: Guilford.

Kazak, A., Simms, S., & Rourke, M. (2002). Family systems practice in pediatric psychology. *Journal of Pediatric Psychology, 27,* 133–143.

Liddle, H. (2002). *Troubled teens: Multidimensional family therapy.* New York: Norton.

Mikesell, R., Lusterman, D. D., & McDaniel, S. (1995). *Integrating family therapy: Handbook of family psychology and systems theory.* Washington, DC: American Psychological Association.

Nichols, M. (2000). *Family therapy: Concepts and methods* (5th ed.). New York: Allyn & Bacon.

Spirito, A., & Kazak, A. (in press). *Effective interventions in pediatric psychology.* New York: Oxford University Press.

ANNE E. KAZAK

Family Physician

A family physician is a physician, doctor of medicine (MD), or doctor of osteopathy (DO) who specializes in the comprehensive health care for the individual and family. The family physician provides health care to patients of all ages, from infants to the elderly. After completing four years of medical school, the family physician undergoes three years of residency training. During residency, the physician gains clinical experience in a wide variety of medical specialties including pediatrics, adult medicine, obstetrics, gynecology, and general surgery. After completion of residency the physician is qualified to practice as a family physician. Some family physicians may decide to pursue a fellowship in geriatrics, obstetrics, rural medicine, or sports medicine.

All physicians, including resident physicians, require a medical license granted by the state in which they practice. After completion of residency, many family practitioners seek certification from the American Board of Family Practice (ABFP). This requires the family physician to have graduated from an accredited medical school, completed three years of residency training, attained a valid, unrestricted state license to practice medicine, and completed a comprehensive examination covering all aspects of family practice. Many family practitioners are members of the American Academy of Family Physicians (AAFP). The AAFP is a medical organization that was founded in 1947 to promote improved health care in the United States, to advance the specialty of family practice, and to serve the professional needs of its members.

The role of the family physician is to provide continuing and comprehensive medical care, health maintenance, and preventive health care to all members of the family regardless of age, sex, or type of problem. The family physician is responsible for the diagnosis and treatment of acute medical problems such as infections like ear infections or strep throat, heart attacks, and musculoskeletal injuries. The family physician provides care for gynecological problems such as sexually transmitted diseases and some may perform basic surgical procedures like an appendectomy or hernia repair. Chronic medical conditions the family physician may diagnose and treat include asthma, diabetes, high blood pressure, and depression. Some family physicians may provide obstetrical care for pregnant women including prenatal care and uncomplicated vaginal deliveries. The services provided by the family physician during health maintenance and prevention visits include a complete medical history, physical exam, screening tests, and disease prevention. For the child, this may include immunizations and blood work to check for anemia or lead poisoning; for a young woman this may include a routine pelvic exam, PAP smear, and ordering a mammogram; and for a man this may include screening for prostate cancer and high cholesterol. Another crucial part of the health maintenance visit is to focus on any psychosocial concerns that the patient or the family may have. The family physician may have greater insight into these concerns because of the unique opportunity to know and care for the patient and the patient's family. Many family physicians manage psychiatric problems such as Attention-Deficit/ Hyperactivity Disorder (ADHD), depression, and anxiety by prescribing medications and providing counseling both alone and in collaboration with a psychologist or psychiatrist.

The family physician may serve as the coordinator of the health care of patients of all ages. Insurance companies often mandate the family physician, as the primary care provider, to serve as the "gatekeeper" for access to subspecialty services. The family physician is often the first to address medical, behavioral, and psychosocial concerns of the patient and then determines the need for subspecialty care, like pediatrics or pediatric subspecialties. The family physician continues to provide follow-up care of ongoing medical needs in conjunction with other subspecialties, serving as a stable health care provider throughout the life of the patient.

See also: Health Care Professionals (General); Physicians (General, Specialty)

Further Reading

American Academy of Family Physicians. (2002). AAFP official definitions of "family practice" and "family physician." http://www.aafp.org/about/300_c.html

American Board of Family Physicians, Inc. (2002). Definitions and policies. http://www.abfp.org/

Sugar-Webb, J. (2000). *Opportunities in physician careers.* Chicago: IL: VGM Career Horizons, 36–40.

TERRY STANCIN
SUSAN K. SANTOS

Family Therapy

See: Family Intervention

Father's Role in Treatment

Parent involvement in psychological treatments for children is increasing for internalizing (e.g., anxiety, depression) as well as externalizing disorders (e.g., attention deficit hyperactivity disorder, conduct problems). For example, among the treatments for children's conduct problems, all of the evidence-based treatments depend on parent participation to a significant extent. Because fathers are typically not the primary caregivers,

however, interventions involving parents are usually focused on the mother. Fathers are sometimes encouraged to attend treatment as well, on the assumption that their involvement will be beneficial to the child's treatment, and some therapists hold evening or weekend sessions to accommodate fathers who work on weekdays.

The involvement of fathers in parent training interventions is thought to benefit the family's progress in a number of ways. When both parents attend sessions together, they are likely to provide greater consistency for the child at home in the rules for acceptable behavior and in enforcing the rules. The parents are also likely to support one another more effectively in their shared parenting efforts and goals. Furthermore, the father's involvement allows therapists to capitalize on the father's unique position in the family as a male role model for the child.

Involving fathers in parent training, however, presents a number of obstacles for the family and for service delivery. Because fathers are not typically the primary caregiver, their availability to attend treatment sessions during working hours is often more limited. Furthermore, if treatment is scheduled when fathers are not working, the fathers in treatment are not available to care for siblings who may come home from school as well. Finally, clinic staffing for evening or weekend appointments is a costly undertaking, particularly in the absence of strong evidence to suggest that father involvement makes a difference to treatment outcome.

A metaanalysis conducted by Couplin and Houts in 1991 revealed only 13 (37 percent) studies on parent training interventions in a 7-year period (1981–1988) that even mentioned father involvement. Only one of the 13 studies explored the impact of father involvement on treatment outcome. In that study, Webster-Stratton (1985) compared involved-father families with absent-father families who participated in a parent training intervention focused on teaching the parents play skills and operant techniques to help manage their child with conduct problems. Involved-father families were defined as those in which a father or father figure living in the child's home or elsewhere provided some of the child's care and was willing to attend some of the child's treatment, whereas absent-father families were those in which no father or father figure lived in the home or attended treatment. At the end of treatment, results showed no differences in the children's behavior in the two groups. One year later, however, children in the involved-father families were observed to be more compliant with their mothers than children from the absent-father families, and the mothers in involved-father families were also less critical of their children.

Recently, Bagner and Eyberg (2002) examined the effect of father involvement in Parent–Child Interaction Therapy (PCIT) by comparing three groups: (1) involved-father families, (2) uninvolved-father families, and (3) absent-father families. A father or father figure lived in the home with the child in both the involved- and uninvolved-father families, but the father attended at least one treatment session in the involved-father families and none of the sessions in the uninvolved-father families. Absent-father families were those with no father or father figure living in the home or attending any sessions of the child's treatment. The PCIT sessions were offered at times convenient for all family members, which resulted in an unexpectedly low number of uninvolved-father families for study. Over half (54 percent) of involved fathers attended 100 percent of the treatment sessions. Only 5 percent of the fathers attended less than 60 percent of the treatment sessions. The high number of fathers involved in treatment suggests that fathers are interested in participating in their child's treatment if it is scheduled at a time they are available. Because there were so few uninvolved-father families in the study, however, few conclusions could be drawn about the effect of uninvolved fathers on treatment outcome.

Results from both the Webster-Stratton (1985) and the Bagner and Eyberg (2002) studies were consistent in finding little evidence to suggest father involvement in treatment affected treatment progress or immediate treatment outcome. In fact, in the Bagner and Eyberg study, mothers from the absent-father families actually reported greater improvements in child behavior at the end of treatment. Bagner and Eyberg reassessed the families' progress at a 4-month follow-up. At that time, results indicated that although the children from the father-involved families maintained their initial improvements at follow-up, the mothers in absent-father families reported significant declines in the children's behavior after treatment ended.

In summary, although research on father involvement in parent training is very limited, the evidence is consistent in suggesting that fathers play a significant role in the maintenance of treatment gains, at least for young children with conduct problems. Although there are yet no data to support the widely held belief that it is important to involve both parents from two-parent families in treatment, the fact that so many fathers are willing to participate in their child's treatment suggests that they should be included until conclusive data indicate otherwise. Evidence also suggests that for absent-father families, it may be particularly important to schedule regular follow-ups so that booster treatment can be provided if needed. It may also be useful to recommend involvement in a parent support group for mothers who are socially isolated.

See also: Conduct Disorder; Fathers' Roles in Abnormal Child Development; Mothers' and Fathers' Roles in Normal Child Development; Parent–Child Interaction Therapy

Further Reading

Bagner, D. M., & Eyberg, S. M. (2002). *Father involvement in Parent–Child Interaction Therapy.* Manuscript in preparation.

Couplin, J. W., & Houts, A. C. (1991). Father involvement in parent training for oppositional child behavior: Progress or stagnation? *Child & Family Behavior Therapy, 13,* 29–51.

Webster-Stratton, C. (1985). The effects of father involvement in parent training for conduct problem children. *Journal of Clinical Psychology and Psychiatry, 26,* 801–810.

DANIEL M. BAGNER
SHEILA M. EYBERG

Fathers' Roles in Abnormal Child Development

See: Mothers' and Fathers' Roles in Abnormal Child Development

Fathers' Roles in Normal Child Development

See: Mothers' and Fathers' Roles in Normal Child Development

Febrile Seizures

See: Epilepsy

Feeding Disorders

See: Failure-to-Thrive, Food Refusal, Food Selectivity, Rumination, Pica

Fetal Alcohol Syndrome (FAS)

DEFINITION OF THE PROBLEM

Fetal alcohol syndrome (FAS) was first identified in French medical journals in 1968, and then the English-language medical journals five years later. The syndrome is characterized by growth retardation, central nervous system (CNS) dysfunction, and a pattern of specific anomalies, particularly distortions of the form and structure of the face (facial dysmorphology). New findings suggest that FAS has specific structural brain abnormalities detected by magnetic resonance imaging (MRI), affecting preferentially the midline structures, basal ganglia, cerebellar vermis, and corpus callosum. However, diagnosis continues to be made solely on the clinical judgment of a physician. FAS is a clinical condition that occurs as a direct result of the mother's alcohol consumption during pregnancy. The Institute of Medicine suggested that alcohol exceeds all other substances of abuse in its deleterious effects on the fetus. As a result of maternal drinking, children with FAS and alcohol-related neurodevelopmental disorders (ARND), face a host of primary and secondary disabilities. Primary disabilities are those inherent in the diagnosis of FAS/ARND as a result of CNS dysfunction. Secondary disabilities are those that a person is not born with (e.g., school disruption, mental health difficulties, social skills problems, etc.) that could, in principle, be ameliorated through improved understanding and appropriate interventions. Drinking at any point during pregnancy can cause problems in the developing fetus. As a result, the American Medical Association and the American Academy of Pediatrics have stated that abstinence throughout pregnancy is the only safe practice.

PREVALENCE

The prevalence of FAS is uncertain. The March of Dimes estimates that FAS occurs in 1 out of 750 births. Others estimate the average birth prevalence of FAS in the United States to range from 0.33–3.7 per 1,000 live births. In Native Americans, the risk is even greater with Southwestern tribes ranging from 3.9–33.3 per 1,000 women of childbearing age. It has been suggested that the variability and inconsistency across studies are due primarily to difficulties with definitions, diagnostic criteria, and methods of assessment. However counted,

FAS is now the leading known cause of mental retardation in the United States, a staggering rate for a condition that, in theory, is totally preventable. The estimated cost for rearing a child with FAS is close to $600,000. The emotional cost to the child and caregivers and the child's lost potential is immeasurable.

Studies looking only at those children who meet full criteria for FAS will underestimate the number of children who have significant difficulties that can be directly attributed to maternal alcohol use. The terms ARND and Alcohol Related Birth Defects (ARBD) are used to describe children with impairments as a result of alcohol exposure during pregnancy, but without the full spectrum of FAS; these terms replaced the term Fetal Alcohol Effects (FAE). Approximately 50,000 babies are born with ARND each year in the United States.

PSYCHOSOCIAL CORRELATES

Behavioral consequences of FAS/ARND often occur without problems in growth and physical development. It is the brain dysfunction caused by prenatal alcohol exposure, not the facial dysmorphology or physical growth impairment, that has the most serious functional consequences for affected individuals and their families. Brain dysfunction underlies the problem behaviors that lead to trouble in daily life, including learning disabilities, poor school performance, poor social skills and poor understanding of social rules and expectations, poor impulse and behavioral control, hyperactivity, problems with attention and concentration, and poor judgment and adaptive behavior problems. Many children with FAS/ARND are also diagnosed with Attention-Deficit Hyperactive/Disorder (ADHD). CNS dysfunction can also be expressed in speech/language difficulties, particularly language processing, and motor skill deficits.

Problems may be particularly difficult for the children with ARND who have few to no dysmorphic facial features and therefore, appear normal to others. Indeed, only about 25 percent of children with FAS and less than 10 percent of children with ARND readily qualify for special education services if mental retardation is used as a sole criterion. For example, the Intelligent Quotient (IQ) score of a child with FAS averages around 79 and that of a child with ARND around 90 (for the general population scores in the normal range are between 85 and 115). However, the adaptive behavior scores of both diagnostic groups is less than 70 (61 and 67, respectively). Streissguth (1997), a leading expert in the area of FAS, and her colleagues found that of children with FAS/ARND, 90 percent had mental health problems and 60 percent had disruptive school experiences characterized by suspension, expulsion, or dropping out. Other significant problems were noted as the children reached young adulthood (e.g., trouble with the law, substance abuse issues, homelessness, joblessness). Clearly, these problems go beyond what is expected based solely on IQ.

Caregivers' perceptions of children with prenatal exposure to alcohol and other drugs are more negative than those of children without exposure. Furthermore, these caregivers report significantly higher levels of stress. The difficult behaviors often seen in the children, together with the caregivers' perceptions and stress, increase the risk for child abuse/neglect and disruptive foster care placements.

PSYCHOLOGICAL ASSESSMENT AND INTERVENTION

Ongoing comprehensive evaluations are recommended for children with prenatal exposure to alcohol. As the difficulties faced by children with FAS (and alcohol-related disabilities) and their families change with age, assessments can help to identify areas of deficits as well as strengths in these children. Assessments should incorporate not only measures of IQ and executive functioning, but also other areas of development such as language processing, visuospatial and motor abilities, and behavior and social-emotional functioning. Measures of attention and concentration are also recommended. Finally, ongoing evaluations of caregivers' stress and family functioning are important.

Most children with FAS and problems related to alcohol exposure require some special education services through the local school system. As many children also meet criteria for ADHD, medication management is often part of a family's treatment plan. Consultation with a mental health professional with expertise in this area can be extremely helpful to the family in terms of both education related to FAS and behavior management issues.

Finally, as this syndrome and related problems are wholly preventable, special efforts should be taken in educating childbearing women about the dangers of alcohol use during pregnancy. Motivational interviewing techniques have been found to be effective in interventions with individuals abusing alcohol. In general, improving and increasing treatment services for women who abuse alcohol are critical to reducing the number of children and families impacted by FAS and related problems.

PROGNOSIS

The prognosis for children with FAS and alcohol-related disabilities is, unfortunately, not promising. As noted above, children are at increased risk for a variety of problems. They are also at increased risk for specific learning disabilities (e.g., arithmetic), problems with memory, judgment, abstract reasoning, and poor adaptive functioning. Through early assessment of the child and the caregivers, relative strengths can be identified. Targeted services can then address these areas of strength as well as deficits to enhance the ability of helping the child reach his/her full potential.

See also: Attention-Deficit/Hyperactivity Disorder; Behavior Modification; Child Maltreatment; Effects of Parental Substance Abuse on Children; Family Intervention; Substance Abuse

Further Reading

Astley, S., & Clarren, S. (2000). Diagnosing the full spectrum of fetal alcohol-exposed individuals: Introducing the 4-digit diagnostic code. *Alcohol, 35,* 400–410.
Institute of Medicine (IOM), Stratton, K. R., Howe, C. J., & Battaglia, F. C. (Eds.). (1996). *Fetal alcohol syndrome: Diagnosis, epidemiology, prevention, and treatment.* Washington, DC: National Academy Press.
Kleinfield, J. M., & Wescott, S. (Eds.). (1993). *Fantastic Antone Succeeds.* Fairbanks: University of Alaska Press.
Kleinfield, J. M., & Wescott, S. (Eds.). (2000). *Fantastic Antone Grows Up.* Fairbanks: University of Alaska Press.
Streissguth, A. (1997). *Fetal alcohol syndrome: A guide for families and communities.* Baltimore: Paul H. Brookes.
http://www.nofas.org

ROBIN H. GURWITCH
JOHN J. MULVIHILL

Fictitious Disorder

See: Psychosomatic Disorders

Finger Sucking

DEFINITION

Sucking itself is an essential human activity that begins reflexively and continues because of the psychophysiological results it produces (see Etiology below). Nonnutritional sucking (NNS), a virtually universal human activity in early life, occurs when children suck objects that are incapable of providing nutrition such as fingers, toes, portions of the caregivers' body, or objects designed ad hoc, termed pacifiers in American culture and dummies in others. Although pacifier usage is common, finger sucking is the most commonly observed form of NNS by a wide margin. Finger sucking involves one readily observed core behavior (i.e., finger or fingers in mouth) and virtually all formal definitions include the operation of two lips touching or closing over at least one finger. Some add topographical detail describing where the finger is placed (against the roof of the mouth) or the location of adjacent fingers (curled over the bridge of the nose or fisted with the other fingers). Lastly, some definitions include age and location criteria in order to distinguish potentially harmful from harmless finger sucking. For example, finger sucking can be considered chronic when it occurs in two or more social environments (e.g., home and school) after the age of five as suggested by Friman and Schmitt (1989).

INCIDENCE

In neonates, estimated rates of finger sucking reach as high as 95 percent. In fact, finger sucking is so prevalent in newborns that its absence is sometimes interpreted as a risk factor for physical or developmental problems. With its reflexive onset, almost universal early presence, and development benefits, finger sucking is not typically even discussed as a habit until the toddler years. As many as 50 percent of children between the ages of 2 and 3 years exhibit the habit and the average age of stopping is around 4 years. The habit remains common at later ages, however, occurring in up to 25 percent of 5-year-old and 11 percent of 10-year-old children.

CORRELATES

Finger sucking is healthful or at least harmless for very young children but continued practice beyond the age of 4 or 5 years increasingly places the children at risk for a variety of unhealthful physical and psychological outcomes. The most common physical risk involves problematic formation of teeth. Chronic sucking can have an effect on developing dentition (e.g., malocclusion) that is virtually the opposite of the effect produced by dental braces and can require extensive (and expensive) orthodontic intervention for repair. Other physical risks include deformity of the finger, infection in the fingernail, and accidental poisoning. The most common psychological risk involves adverse social

reaction and even rejection. A study of thumb sucking in first-grade children conducted by Friman and colleagues (2001) showed that those who sucked fingers were viewed as less attractive and intelligent and less preferred as seatmates, classmates, neighbors, and friends than nonsucking peers. Other psychological risks include problematic interactions with parents. Finger sucking is also often correlated with other self-soothing behaviors such as object attachment (e.g., Linus in the syndicated cartoon Peanuts) and self-stimulatory behaviors such as hair pulling (i.e., trichotillomania). Concern about finger sucking, persistent from Freud to the present day, involves the belief that its practice reflects underlying psychopathology. A substantial and growing body of research has dismissed this concern, however, for all but a very tiny minority of finger sucking children. Additionally, the extensive number and problematic nature of problems in this minority usually renders sucking a secondary concern.

ETIOLOGY

The primary cause of extended finger sucking has been alluded to above. Specifically, finger sucking produces a psychophysiological effect and reduced arousal (e.g., self-soothing, comforting, etc.) that is habit-forming. A large body of scientific evidence has demonstrated this effect, especially in very young children, but most adults have witnessed the effect by watching crying children seek comfort from their thumb or finger or calm down quickly when given a pacifier. In technical terms, finger sucking is maintained in two ways. One involves positive reinforcement and it results from the pleasure obtained from the act. The other involves negative reinforcement and it involves the relief obtained from the act. Very early in life the procurement of pleasure and relief via sucking is normal and expected but chronic practice beyond the age of 5 years may suggest a deficiency in more mature methods of procuring these psychological commodities.

ASSESSMENT

Assessment of finger sucking itself is straightforward, merely involving direct observation. Special attention should be paid to the age of the child and location and duration of the sucking. Sucking in very young children or in older children that occurs in only one location (e.g., bed) for short durations is harmless. However, extensive sucking occurring in more than one social environment (e.g., home and school) exhibited by children older than 5 years requires additional assessment (and usually treatment). Additional assessments focus on correlated psychological, medical, and dental problems. Psychological assessment is readily conducted via parent and child interviews and parental completion of a standardized behavior problem checklist. Medical and dental assessments are obtained via referral to the children's primary care providers.

TREATMENT

Effective treatment for finger sucking usually requires multiple components. One involves a short moratorium (e.g., at least 2 weeks) on parental attention devoted to the habit and a substantial increase in parental attention to and demonstrable affection for preferred child behavior. Additionally, it is helpful to prescribe a daily allotment (e.g., 5–15 min) of special parental time spent with the child along with a daily increase in physical affection. Another component involves a short problem-solving interview with the child targeting their reasons for sucking and specifying strategies for quitting and benefits for doing so. Effective treatment also usually involves a motivational component. A method for younger children (e.g., 4–7 years) involves a grab bag filled with 25–50 slips of paper upon which small deliverable rewards are described. These should include tangible (e.g., dime, sticker, small toy) and activity-based (e.g., 10 min special time with dad, 15 min of extra bedtime, etc.) items. Each day spent with no adult observations of finger sucking allows the picking of one slip from the bag and delivery of the reward it describes. A method for older children involves a dot-to-dot drawing of an item the child desires and the parents can afford. The number of dots is determined by the cost of the item (e.g., 1 dot for every 50 cents). Each day spent with no adult observations of finger sucking allows the connecting of two dots. Dots thus connected are not to be unconnected under any circumstances. When all the dots are connected, the parents purchase and provide the item to the child. Lastly, some method of modifying the pleasurable basis of the sucking is usually employed (e.g., tape or bitter taste on the finger, mittens). The form of the modification does not seem to matter although the results of study using taste have been impressive. Another type of intervention altogether involves dental appliances but because it is highly invasive, it should be reserved for extreme cases.

PROGNOSIS

By the age of 14 years, most finger sucking children have stopped sucking their fingers or suck their fingers so privately and infrequently that the possibility of harm is nonexistent. Additionally any problems caused by the sucking, even in chronic cases, have also usually been remediated by then.

See also: Behavior Modification; Interviewing; Nail Biting; Positive Reinforcement; Trichotillomania

Further Reading

Friman, P. C., Byrd, M. R., & Oksol, E. M. (2001). Oral digital habits: Demographics, phenomenology, causes, functions, and clinical associations. In D. W. Woods & R. Miltenberger (Eds.), *Tic disorders, trichotillomania, and other repetitive behavior disorders: Behavioral approaches to analysis and treatment* (pp. 197–222). New York: Kluwer Academic/Plenum.

Friman, P. C., & Leibowitz, J. M. (1990). An effective and acceptable treatment alternative for chronic thumb and finger sucking. *The Journal of Pediatric Psychology, 15*, 57–65.

Friman, P. C., & Schmitt, B. D. (1989). Thumb sucking: Guidelines for pediatricians. *Clinical Pediatrics, 28*, 438–440.

PATRICK C. FRIMAN

Firesetting

DEFINITION

Despite the apparent severity of both firesetting and playing with matches, there is no standard definition for either of these two childhood behaviors. Firesetting is commonly used to describe those incidents involving any unsanctioned use of fire that produces at least some damage to property whereas matchplay is usually reserved for those incidents involving some form of fireplay in the absence of any damage, such as lighting matches or playing with fire from the stove. Of course, a child's involvement with fire and the consequences that ensue may vary widely, thus making it difficult to clearly describe these incidents. It is also important to understand that descriptive details regarding an incident are often provided by different informants and methods, including fire departments that generate data the number of fires to which they have responded, government agencies that document arrest records, and survey researchers who examine the characteristics or impact of involvement with fire.

INCIDENCE

Children playing with or setting a fire is a major contributor to fire injuries and death in both children and adolescents. In 1997, as reported by Hall (2001), children playing with fire accounted for 65,000 fires that resulted in 284 civilian deaths and 2,158 civilian injuries. An estimated 9,200 juveniles were arrested for arson in 1999, of whom 89 percent were males and 67 percent were under the age of 15. Juveniles accounted for 54 percent of all arrests for arson that year. This makes arson the only crime for which juveniles make up a majority of all arrests. The overall magnitude of the impact of firesetting and arson attributable to youth in this country is difficult to ascertain, but includes both heightened property damage costs (estimated at $283 million dollars in 1998) and various medical and psychological sequelae following burn trauma (e.g., hospitalization, posttraumatic stress, depression).

ETIOLOGY

Although few studies have systematically examined the causes of children's fires, the various reasons or motives attributed to them have been described, often in the context of general clinical descriptions of different subgroups of firesetters. For example, cases have been described as "curiosity" (i.e., accidental fires due to curiosity or experimentation), "pathological" (i.e., serious firesetting characterized by frequent, intentional, concealed, and destructive incidents, as well as clinical problems), "cry for help" (i.e., fires due to a need for attention or assistance in dealing with a recent stressor or crisis), and "delinquent" (i.e., fires that reflect more generalized involvement in antisocial behavior, especially due to peer pressure and delinquency). Some practitioners also describe a group of severely disturbed firesetters. There is only anecdotal support for these subtypes, however. The findings suggest more overlap than uniqueness in the primary characteristics of most firesetters. Other conceptualizations of firesetting motives have been proposed, but have not been subject to empirical evaluation.

Survey or interview data have described various motives that may underlie the firesetting incidents (i.e., for fun, to see what would happen, boredom, wanting to destroy something). Some evidence has shown that heightened (versus low) curiosity was associated with greater psychopathology (e.g., externalizing and internalizing behavior problems, hostility, inappropriate social behavior), firesetting risk (e.g., curiosity, exposure to materials, community complaints, early experiences), and fire involvement (e.g., fire interest, matchplay, firesetting recidivism). Heightened (versus low) anger was associated with certain firesetting risk measures (e.g., involvement in fire-related acts, knowledge about

combustibles, exposure, complaints, use of mild punishment) and fire involvement (i.e., matchplay).

ASSESSMENT: CHARACTERISTICS AND CORRELATES

Case Screening

Alternative measures have been used to screen and/or triage children and adolescents who may have engaged in firesetting behavior. Early screening instruments were developed for different age groups and sought to classify cases into little, definite, and extreme risk for recidivism, primarily by evaluating the clinical severity of the child and his/her family, and both the details and seriousness of the fire incident. Although these tools are common in fire departments across the country, there is little empirical data to suggest their validity or usefulness. Other instruments as suggested by Wilcox and Kolko (2002) may simplify the screening process.

Firesetting Details and History

Additional measures capture aspects of a child's firesetting incident. These tools document parameters of their children's most serious incidents, such as details of the incident (e.g., how materials were obtained, site of fire, type of property damage), behavioral and emotional antecedents (e.g., aggression/defiance, depression/withdrawal, rule violations), possible motives for the fire, and consequences following the fire. It is also important to conduct a structured approach to collecting information about the nature and extent of a child's firesetting history by asking questions that quantify both the occurrence and frequency of firesetting or matchplay incidents (e.g., does child like fire, did child play with matches, did child burn something or set anything on fire, how many times did this occur, was fire department called?).

Fire Risks and Correlates

Child and family characteristics that relate directly to a child's access to, interest in, and exposure to fire materials have been specified in order to promote an understanding of factors that may increase a child's risk for firesetting. These instruments can be completed by both parents and children. The content of these measures includes certain fire-related factors (e.g., curiosity about fire, exposure to peer/family models, fire skill/competence or knowledge) that have been found to differentiate firesetters from non-firesetters. Other measures address additional variables related to the child's firesetting incident, fire history, motivation, and personality, among other factors.

Clinical Characteristics/Functioning

Given the heterogeneity in the backgrounds and clinical characteristics of firesetting children and youth, it is important to point out that no specific "profile" of the juvenile firesetter has been reported. However, research by the author has shown that firesetters have been found to differ from nonfiresetters in certain child, parent, and family characteristics. Child characteristics of firesetters have included heightened child dysfunction, such as aggression and covert behaviors, and occasionally conduct disorder, hostility, impulsivity, and emotional reactivity. Some evidence has suggested that adolescent firesetters were more likely to have a history of sexual abuse and inhalant abuse, to receive higher scores on the schizophrenia and mania scales of the Minnesota Multiphasic Personality Inventory (MMPI), and to have a childhood history of firesetting.

In terms of the parental correlates of firesetting behavior, high levels of personal or relationship problems have been reported, such as psychiatric distress, marital discord, less child acceptance, and greater difficulties with parenting practices (e.g., less monitoring, discipline, and involvement in prosocial activities) than parents of nonfiresetters. Firesetters have described their parent's child rearing practices as reflecting greater anxiety induction, lax discipline, and nonenforcement of rules or consequences. On family measures, firesetters have been found to experience more stressful life events than nonfiresetters. These findings implicate a broad clinical picture implicating both child and family variables. However, the role of these variables in the origins of a given firesetting incident are virtually unknown at this time.

INTERVENTION

Although there are many specific procedures for working with firesetters, there are two common approaches to intervention which vary by target: (1) the child's fire-specific experiences, interests, or motives, or (2) specific behavioral or environmental characteristics related to the child's and family's clinical functioning. This distinction reflects the usual forms of expertise that are available to serve this population, notably, the fire service (fire education) and mental health practitioners (psychological treatment). Contemporary programs often integrate these two approaches.

Fire Service Approaches and Fire Safety Education

Perhaps the most common intervention used with this population involves fire safety education (FSE) consisting of instruction in safety skills/practices and, more recently, fire science principles. Training often includes exposure to a didactic emphasizing protection (e.g., fire drills) and prevention skills (e.g., using matches safely), such as training in fire science and evacuation and assistance skills. These concepts are often tailored to the developmental status of the child and the nature of the child's firesetting history and motives, among other characteristics of the learning environment.

Psychological Services and Treatment Approaches

Treatment applications designed to alter behavioral dysfunction and environmental conditions have incorporated several cognitive-behavioral treatment (CBT) procedures, occasionally, in combination with fire safety training. Specific procedures for children include graphs that depict the personal context of a fire, contingency management, prosocial, anger-control, problem-solving, and assertive skills training. Procedures for use with parents have been directed towards child management, use of home programs, self-control and stress management, and family skills training in problem-solving and communication. Comprehensive treatments have targeted child self-control, parent management skills, and/or positive family interactions, with some interventions incorporating several procedures (e.g., contingencies and/or behavioral training skills).

PROGNOSIS AND OUTCOME

Much of the evidence for reductions in the frequency and severity of firesetting has been reported by fire departments anecdotally or in case reports or uncontrolled studies in the research literature. In general, most community programs report low recidivism rates. This optimistic impression is consistent with the results of recent controlled studies that have included fire safety and clinical intervention components that have reported significant reductions in the frequency of firesetting after intervention, with modest 1-year recidivism rates.

Kolko (2002) also found evidence for greater improvement in reducing involvement with fire among children who received FSE or CBT relative to those who had a firefighter visit the home. Thus, alternative approaches are available to help the child or adolescent firesetter and his parent. Where applicable, clinical services may complement the administration of fire safety education due to the large population of firesetters who may set multiple fires and exhibit psychosocial maladjustment, who are referred to fire service and mental health systems for intervention, and who exhibit factors in the two primary risk-factor domains.

See also: Aggression; Antisocial Behavior; Cognitive–Behavior Therapy; Conduct Disorder; Disruptive Behavior Disorders

Further Reading

Hall, J. R. (2000). *Children playing with fire.* Quincy, MA: National Fire Protection Agency.
Kolko, D. J. (2002). Research studies on the problem. In D. J. Kolko (Ed.), *Handbook on firesetting in children and youth.* New York: Kluwer Academic/Plenum.
Kolko, D. J. (2001). Efficacy of cognitive-behavioral treatment and fire safety education for firesetting children: Initial and follow-up outcomes. *Journal of Child Psychology and Psychiatry and Allied Disciplines.*
Wilcox, D. K., & Kolko, D. J. (2002). Assessing recent firesetting behavior and taking a firesetting history. In D. J. Kolko (Ed.), *Handbook on firesetting in children and youth* (pp. 47–89). New York: Kluwer Academic/Plenum.

DAVID J. KOLKO

Food Allergy

DEFINITION/INCIDENCE/ETIOLOGY

Food allergy occurs when the body mistakenly believes that a food is harmful and creates antibodies to that food. When the food is eaten, the antibodies trigger the release of histamine and other chemicals, which results in allergic symptoms. Symptoms can include itching, abdominal pain, diarrhea, vomiting, hives, rashes, asthma, and anaphylaxis, which is a severe, immediate immune response that can result in life-threatening respiratory distress, shock, hives, and swelling. The foods that most commonly cause allergic reactions are milk, eggs, peanuts, tree nuts such as walnuts or cashews, fish, shellfish, soy, and wheat. Food allergy is a specific type of food intolerance, which is a general category of adverse reactions to food that can be caused by enzyme deficiencies, pharmacologic effects, and allergies. Food intolerance occurs in 8 percent of children, but food allergy occurs in only 1–2 percent. Studies have consistently demonstrated that people tend to overestimate the prevalence of food allergy and intolerance in themselves and their children. Several studies have reported that 16–28 percent of adults report having food allergies, and that 19 percent of parents reported that their child had food intolerance. In the adult studies, double-blind placebo-controlled food challenges (see below) of those reporting food allergy lent support to much lower actual prevalence rates.

ASSESSMENT/TREATMENT/PROGNOSIS

Diagnosis is made through a thorough history, allergy testing, and an "elimination and challenge" in which the suspected food is eliminated from the diet and then reintroduced. In some people, a double-blind placebo-controlled food challenge may be used. In this type of food challenge, the suspected food is eliminated from the diet. Then that food, as well as neutral foods, are hidden in a capsule for reintroduction, and symptoms are observed after ingestion. If an individual has a history of an anaphylactic reaction, reintroduction of the suspected food does not take place. Skin and blood tests may also be conducted, but both have high false-positive and false-negative rates. Treatment involves eliminating the food from the diet. A dietitian is helpful in identifying hidden sources of the food and suggesting alternative ingredients. Epinephrine is used for anaphylactic reactions. The course of cow milk allergy, the most common childhood allergy, is well studied, and as many as 78–87 percent of children outgrow milk allergies by age 6.

PSYCHOSOCIAL CORRELATES

Two studies examining health-related quality of life (QOL) in children with food allergies have been conducted. One study reported that the QOL of children with confirmed peanut allergy was similar to that of children with rheumatological disease, but no healthy comparison group was employed. The other study reported that levels of QOL for children with food allergies were significantly lower than the published norms for healthy children in the areas of mental health, general health, parental emotional impact, and limitation in family activities. However, this study used a sample of members of the Food Allergy and Anaphylaxis Network, and food allergies were not confirmed. Research in adults has demonstrated that individuals with confirmed food allergies differ from those who feel that they have food allergies that are not confirmed via elimination and challenge. Adults with unconfirmed food allergies report significantly more somatic, anxiety, and depressive symptoms, as well as significantly higher levels of overall emotional distress than those with confirmed food allergies.

See also: Gastrointestinal Disorders

Further Reading

Knibb, R. C., Armstrong, A., Booth, D. A., Platts, R. G., Booth, I. W., & MacDonald, A. (1999). Psychological characteristics of people with perceived food intolerance in a community sample. *Journal of Psychosomatic Research, 47,* 545–554.
Food Allergy and Anaphylaxis Network Web site: http://www.foodallergy.org.

LAURA M. MACKNER
WALLACE V. CRANDALL

Food Refusal

DEFINITION

Some infants and children engage in total oral food refusal. As a subtype of food refusal, some children will consume liquids but refuse all solid or soft textured foods. This problem occurs most frequently in children who, because of medical complications, have been fed by artificial means, such as nasogastric tube, gastrostomy tube, or total parenteral nutrition (TPN; intravenous infusion of nutrients and calories). This phenomenon is differentiated from food selectivity, in which children will consume solid foods by mouth but are overly selective as to texture or taste. It is generally thought that children who have complicated oral motor deficiencies are not categorized as having food refusal. The assumption is that food refusal is a voluntary act and that normal chewing/swallowing mechanisms are intact. Food refusal can sometimes occur in children who have been eating normally and then undergo a medical procedure that necessitates artificial feedings for a short duration. It is not uncommon for some children to refuse oral feedings following this period of artificial feeding.

INCIDENCE/PREVALENCE

It is difficult to get a firm estimate of the number of children with feeding problems who present with total food refusal. Most published estimates report feeding problems across a broad spectrum of difficulties. These estimates, however, range from 2–45 percent of the population, depending on the nature of the problem studied. Medical conditions, such as prematurity, gastroesophageal reflux, and bronchial pulmonary dysplasia (inadequate development of the lungs leading to tracheostomy and difficulty breathing—hence difficulty eating as breathing is interrupted), dramatically increase the risk for food refusal, as these conditions often require artificial supplementation. It is likely that the incidence of childhood food refusal will increase given its association with conditions that are on the increase (e.g., prematurity, low birth weight).

ASSESSMENT

Assessment of a child with total food refusal involves documentation of the number of calories received through feeding tubes, the child's nutritional needs for growth, and the child's current medical status. In addition, direct observation of the child during attempts to feed provides important information about the child's response. This observation lends information as to the child's behavioral response to prompts to eat. The observed response may be phobic in nature if the child shows anxiety and fear with the introduction of food into the oral cavity. The response may appear to be more manipulative in an effort to encourage the feeder to discontinue the feeding situation. It is important to note whether food can actually be introduced into the child's mouth and, if so, if it elicits choking or gagging responses. There are no standardized behavioral instruments designed to assess food refusal per se; history and direct observations are the most important components of the assessment.

TREATMENT

There are two main components to the treatment of children with food refusal. The first is often called appetite manipulation and requires arranging artificial feedings or access to currently accepted foods (usually liquids) so as to induce hunger in the child at the time of the feeding treatment sessions. This is an essential component. Many children who have had artificial feedings have not developed a sense of hunger. Artificial feedings are usually done slowly over long periods of time, so that the child never experiences a normal cyclical hunger/hunger cessation following food intake pattern. Without this history, children do not recognize the feeling of distress induced by hunger. Therefore, an important treatment component is to introduce the cyclical introduction of food after extended periods without calorie supplementation so that the child begins to learn the relationship between hunger and hunger cessation through food intake.

The second major component of treatment involves the utilization of behavioral modification procedures to provide reinforcement for food acceptance and consumption accompanied by procedures designed to discourage negative behaviors at mealtimes. It is often necessary to conduct behavioral feeding treatments on an inpatient medical unit in a hospital. This setting provides close medical monitoring of the patient's hydration and weight status and allows for intense and consistent behavioral intervention treatment sessions. The phobic nature of resistance to food is an important component in designing treatments for these problems. Children who have not experienced food in the oral cavity and normal chewing and swallowing until a time period well past the normal introduction of solids often exhibit a phobic-like response to foods. It is necessary to desensitize this fear by the continual presentation of food into the mouth until the child can acquire the confidence that chewing and swallowing will not result in choking. Food refusal can emerge following an incident of choking or severe sore throat in children who previously consumed solid food normally. Treatment procedures for this phenomenon are the same as those described for infants who have been artificially fed and never experienced oral feeding. Time to recovery for choking-phobia difficulties is significantly faster than for children who have never eaten.

PROGNOSIS

Recent research suggests that the behavioral interventions described above are very effective in treating food refusal in children. Differential reinforcement procedures are particularly effective. Several treatment programs have reported that the treatment of food refusal in children with gastrostomy tubes results in removal of the tube in approximately 90 percent of the children.

See also: Behavior Modification; Differential Social Reinforcement/Positive Attention; Gastroesophageal Reflux Disease; Systematic Desensitization

Further Reading

Kedesdy, J. H., & Budd, K. S., (1998). *Childhood feeding disorders: Biobehavioral assessment and intervention.* Baltimore, MD: Paul H. Brookes.

Linscheid, T. R., & Rasnake, L. K. (2001). *Eating problems in children.* In. E. Walker, & M. C. Roberts (Eds.), *Handbook of Clinical Child Psychology* (3rd ed., pp. 523–541). New York: Guilford.

THOMAS R. LINSCHEID

Food Selectivity

DEFINITION

Food selectivity occurs when an infant or child selectively limits foods to either texture or type. Children who do not follow the normal developmental pattern and progress to solid foods at the appropriate age are said to have a food selectivity problem based on texture regardless of the range of taste that they are willing to consume. On the other hand, many other children are fully capable of chewing and swallowing rather difficult textures but limit their intake to only one or two foods. Restriction in the range of type and texture of food is particularly common in certain conditions such as autism and developmental delay.

INCIDENCE/PREVALENCE

A realistic estimate of the percentage of children who present with food selectivity is not available. Almost all children have some degree of food selectivity. Problems become noteworthy only when there are gross nutritional or social abnormalities or difficulties that accrue as a result of the child's eating habits. Estimates of feeding problems have ranged from 2 percent of the population to as high as 45 percent of the population. It is likely that the severity of food selectivity problems requiring professional intervention is in the range of 2–4 percent of the population of infants and children. High-risk populations such as those children with early medical problems or developmental disabilities may have a higher incidence.

ASSESSMENT

The assessment of food selectivity problems in children requires a multicomponent approach. Nutritional and medical assessments are necessary to determine the degree to which the child's eating habits are affecting normal growth development and to determine the presence of ancillary medical problems. It is also important to assess the child by direct observation of the child in the feeding situation. This yields information about the child's behavior during the meal, techniques that are utilized by the caregiver or parent, the level of emotional distress during the meal, and offer indications as to whether or not there may be oral motor components of the feeding problem. This is particularly relevant in children who fail to progress from soft or pureed textures to normal solid foods. If oral motor problems are suspected a referral to a neurologist or occupational therapist or speech therapist for further assessment is warranted. In assessing the seriousness of the problem, there are feeding interaction scales and questionnaires that allow for comparison of the child's problem with normative samples.

TREATMENT

Behavioral interventions have been shown to be effective in the treatment of chronic food selectivity. Depending on the specific nature of a child's difficulty (e.g., texture vs. variety), behavioral interventions can be developed to systematically reinforce acceptance of textured foods or a greater variety of foods. Refusal to accept certain foods and textures can be discouraged through the use of behavioral procedures such as timeout, extinction, and removal of privileges. In addition to the behavioral procedures, it is necessary to structure the child's intake to ensure they are maximally hungry at the treatment meal occasions. This is usually accomplished by restricting any calorie intake between meals, allowing access to water or other noncaloric liquids only. This ensures that the child stays hydrated during the treatment, but is not able to obtain relief from hunger between treatment meals. For those children who eat a limited variety of foods, reinforcement of the consumption of new foods can be accomplished by the presentation of a favorite food contingent upon acceptance of the new food. For children with texture-related problems, fading of the soft textured food into an intermediate stage of lumpy food, and then eventually to a solid consistency food is a procedure that is frequently utilized.

PROGNOSIS

Prognosis for the remediation of food selectivity problems is excellent. Behavioral research reports

provide ample empirical support for the effectiveness of these treatments.

See also: Behavior Modification; Differential Social Reinforcement/Positive Attention; Food Refusal, Positive Reinforcement; Time Out

Further Reading

Kedesdy, J. H., & Budd, K. S., (1998). *Childhood feeding disorders: Biobehavioral assessment and intervention.* Baltimore, MD: Paul H. Brookes.
Linscheid, T. R., & Rasnake, L. K. (2001). Eating problems in children. In E. Walker & M. C. Roberts (Eds.), *Handbook of clinical child psychology* (3rd. ed., pp. 523–541). New York: Guilford.

THOMAS R. LINSCHEID

Foster Care

Foster care is the general term for out-of-home care for children who cannot be safely cared for by their parents. Although originally conceived to provide abused and neglected children a safe family environment while their parents addressed problems that caused the maltreatment, foster care has increasingly been used for juvenile offenders and status offenders. Foster care is intended to be temporary care. Unfortunately, the burgeoning numbers of maltreated children and other youth needing homes, the increased complexities of the problems facing parents, and the overwhelmed child protection and legal systems have resulted in foster care as the place where many children grow up. The Adoption and Safe Families Act of 1997 represents a federal attempt to address "foster care drift" and require states to move children to permanent living situations in a timely fashion. The verdict is still out as to whether the goals of the Act have been realized.

There are four general categories of foster care: family (non-relative) foster care, kinship care, treatment (or therapeutic) foster care, and residential group care. Please see *Residential Treatment* for group care that has a specific treatment focus.

FAMILY FOSTER CARE

Family foster care has been the most common means of providing out-of-home care for children who cannot remain with their parents. Family foster care involves nonrelative nonprofessionals providing room, board, and supervision to children in their homes. Foster parents are reimbursed for the costs of caring for the children and their homes need to be licensed in order to receive these reimbursements. Licensing standards typically include requirements about the acceptability of the physical home (safety, cleanliness, sufficient space, etc.), criminal checks for the adults in the home, and training for the foster parents. Public or private child protection agencies monitor children's placements in foster homes.

There is limited research about characteristics of foster parents, but some general features of typical foster families are known. The majority of foster homes have two foster parents and their average age is the midforties. Half of the families would be considered middle class and a substantial minority would be considered working class or low income. The majority of the foster parents completed high school, but between 15 and 20 percent did not. Less than 20 percent had completed college. The vast majority of foster parents actively participate in organized religious activities.

There is also limited research on determining the relationship between foster parent characteristics and foster placement success. Foster families from working or low income levels are more successful than those from higher socioeconomic statuses (SES) although it is possible that the "match" between the child's SES and the foster family's SES contributes to this effect, rather than the level of SES itself. High levels of foster parent stress have been associated with foster placement failures and foster parent training has been associated with reducing failures.

Adult outcomes for children who had been in care have been explored, considering a number of placement factors. Children who were in family foster care do better as adults than children who spent all or part of their time in group or residential care. They completed more education, were less likely to be arrested, were less likely to report substance abuse problems, and had stronger social networks. The number of placements that a child experienced also was related to outcomes. The fewer placements a child experienced was associated with more education, lower arrest rate, increased life satisfaction, and other positive outcomes. Surprisingly, longer, as compared to briefer, stays in family foster care were associated with a number of benefits including overall generally improved adult functioning. Not surprisingly, the benefits were greatest for children who had long stays with one stable, healthy foster family. However, the research has not demonstrated that stable family foster care caused the positive outcomes for children. It is equally possible that children who enter the foster care system with more serious problems are more likely to be placed in group or residential care, are more likely to disrupt placements, and are less likely to have a single stable family foster care long-term placement.

KINSHIP CARE

Kinship care refers to foster care by relatives of the child(ren). There has been enormous growth in kinship care over the past decade and in some states there are more children in kinship homes than in nonrelative family foster homes. Many states have policies that support a preference for kinship placement over nonrelative placement. A 1979 Supreme Court decision held that states were required to provide foster care (*Miller v. Yoakum*) reimbursements to relatives who met the same licensing requirements as nonrelatives. The rapid growth in kinship care has been viewed as a result of the huge increase of children needing out-of-home placement, the shortage of nonrelative foster homes to meet the demand, the natural obligation that many relatives feel they have to care for children in their extended families, and the availability of reimbursement to assist low-income kin families in providing care. Further, there have been attitudinal shifts among decision makers about the relative merits and drawbacks of placing children with their extended families rather than with people who are unknown to them.

There is a modest, yet growing, body of research that supports the shift to kinship placement as a preferred placement alternative for children. Children in kinship homes, especially kinship homes that are licensed, seem to be safer from further maltreatment than are children in nonrelative foster homes. It is difficult to determine whether this effect is caused by selection factors (relatives may not volunteer to care for more disturbed children who may have a greater risk to be a victim of further abuse), monitoring factors (nonrelative foster homes may receive more services and consequently be more closely monitored), or whether relatives provide safer homes for children in their own families. In any event, there is no evidence that relative placement presents a safety risk to children.

Children's self reports indicate a general preference for kinship homes. Children are equally likely to report that they feel safe in both kinship and foster family homes. However, they are more likely to report that they are happy and feel loved in kinship homes as compared to foster homes.

Stability of placements and likelihood of reunification with parents have been explored. Kinship placements appear to be more stable than foster family homes with children, in one study, experiencing an average of less than two placement changes in kinship homes and approximately three placement changes in foster family homes. Additionally, placement changes in kinship care typically involved moving from one relative to another, not to a foster family. Children in kinship placement are reunified with their parents at the same rate, but the time to reunification is much longer. When children are not reunified with their parents, children in kinship care are less likely to be adopted than children in foster care. Relatives are apparently reluctant to force termination of the parental rights of their relatives since they are already "family." These relatives often state that they have made a lifelong commitment to the children, despite the lack of legal permanence. Whether these informal permanent arrangements are sufficient to meet the goals of permanency for children is as yet unsettled.

As discussed above, it is not clear if some of the more positive outcomes for kinship care are a result of selection factors in that relatives may be less likely to take the most behaviorally or emotionally disturbed children into their homes. These children generally have the least placement stability and are the least likely to be reunified with their parents. Random assignment to foster family or kinship care would be considered unethical, so the relative effectiveness of the two types of family placements may never be completely known.

TREATMENT FOSTER CARE

Treatment foster care is also referred to as therapeutic foster care, specialized foster care, and family-based foster care treatment. All terms refer to a nonrelative family-based approach to providing treatment to seriously emotionally or behaviorally disturbed children, serious youthful offenders, or children with serious developmental disabilities. Treatment foster care is considered a less restrictive treatment environment for children and youth who would otherwise need to be in group residential care because their problems make them unable to be safely and effectively cared for in a typical family home.

Treatment foster care is distinguished from most group care programs in that there are only one or two children placed in a home; families are recruited, trained, supported and considered professional; and the children are integrated into the public school system.

Additional features of most treatment foster care programs are the inclusion of biological parents in the treatment program and provision of transitional and aftercare services. Treatment foster care programs cost less than one-third of the costs of residential centers or group homes serving the same types of children and problems.

Research on the effectiveness of treatment foster care is impressive. First, it should be noted that children and adolescents in treatment foster care have similar problems to those served in group and residential care. Still, most children and youth improve while they are in the treatment foster care placements and several follow-up studies have demonstrated better adjustment and better discharge stability as compared to youth who were in group or residential settings. Follow-up studies also demonstrate that youth offenders in treatment foster care had lower rates of recidivism and were more likely to return to their families than youth in group or residential care.

GROUP CARE

An alternative to family-based foster care for maltreated children, juvenile offenders, and status offenders is group residential care. States differ in specific numbers of children that are permitted to live in group homes, but the term "group home" typically refers to relatively small residential care facilities. Therapeutic group homes are small group residential programs that have a substantial treatment component. General group homes typically do not have a treatment component and have developed because there have not been sufficient family settings available or willing to provide homes to youth needing foster care placements. Emergency shelter refers to small group facilities designed to provide housing and supervision to children and youth for a brief time while more suitable placements can be found. Unfortunately, placement shortages sometimes result in shelters becoming long-term placements for children and youth.

Family-focused interventions and post-placement planning and services have been identified as critical components to group care effectiveness. Most of the research on group care has been as a comparison to family foster care or kinship care. The evidence suggests that group care is the least optimal placement within the foster care system. Compared to individuals who were in family foster care or kinship care, youth who have spent time in group care facilities have, as adults, lower educational attainment and psychosocial adjustment and higher arrest rates. Children in group care settings were significantly less likely to report that they felt safe, loved, or happy than did children in family foster care or kinship care. As discussed above, it is possible that more troubled youth enter group care rather than the other settings. However, there is some evidence that there are negative effects on high-risk youth when they are grouped together. In any event, a conservative conclusion is that there is no evidence that supports group homes as an optimal placement for children and youth who cannot live with their parents.

See also: Divorce; Group Psychotherapy; Parenting Practices; Residential Treatment

Further Reading

Berrick, J. D. (1998). When children cannot remain home: Foster family care and kinship care. *The Future of Children*, (Spring 1998), 72–87.

Chamberlain, P. (2000). What works in treatment foster care. In M. P. Kluger, G. Alexander, & P. A. Curtis. (Eds.), *What works in child welfare*. Washington, DC: CWLA Press.

Curtis, P. A., Dale Jr., G., & Kendall, J. C. (Eds.). (1999). *The foster care crisis: Translating research into policy and practice*. Lincoln, NE: University of Nebraska Press.

Dishion, T. J., McCord, J., & Poulin, F. (1999). When interventions harm: Peer groups and problem behavior. *American Psychologist 54*, 755–764.

Haugaard, J., & Hazan, C. (2002). Foster parenting. In M. H. Bornstein (Ed.), *Handbook of parenting: Vol. 1. Children and parenting* (2nd ed., pp. 313–328). Mahwah, NJ: Erlbaum.

McDonald, T. P., Allen, R. I., Westerfelt, A., & Piliavin, I. (1996). *Assessing the long-term effects of foster care: A research synthesis*. Washington, DC: CWLA Press.

Miller v. Youakum, 1979, 440 U.S. 125.

Whittaker, J. K. (2000). What works in residential child care and treatment: Partnerships with families. In M. P. Kluger, G. Alexander, & P. A. Curtis. (Eds.), *What works in child welfare*. Washington, DC: CWLA Press.

VICTORIA WEISZ

Fragile X Syndrome

DEFINITION

Fragile X Syndrome, also known as Martin Bell syndrome, is the most common cause of inherited mental retardation. The syndrome involves social, emotional, and communication difficulties and a range of cognitive impairment, from mild learning disabilities to severe mental retardation. Fragile X is frequently associated with autism, self-injurious behavior, Attention-Deficit/Hyperactivity Disorder (ADHD), anxiety, and mood problems. Certain physical characteristics also accompany Fragile X syndrome in males, such as a high arched palate, large and protruding ears, a long face, prominent jaw, flat feet, and large testicles. Mitral valve prolapse may occur in as many as 80 percent of males with Fragile X. In general, females do not manifest an altered physical appearance. Generally, Fragile X results in greater functional impairment for males than for females. For example, most males with the disorder will have severe intellectual disability, while only one third of females will have intellectual test scores in the mentally retarded range. Similarly, females may exhibit an impaired ability to relate to others, while males with this diagnosis may demonstrate impairment in communication and social skills commensurate with an additional diagnosis of autism.

PREVALENCE AND COURSE OF THE DISORDER

Prevalence is estimated to be 1 per 2,000 males and at least 1 per 4,000 females. However, the symptoms that appear in individuals with Fragile X vary widely, contributing to the difficulty of accurate diagnosis. Some suggest that many individuals with Fragile X have yet to be diagnosed, indicating that we may be underestimating the prevalence of this disorder. The majority of children with Fragile X show no readily observable physical characteristics at birth. Diagnosis typically occurs in early childhood given delayed or atypical development is detected and referral for genetic testing is made. Some individuals will exhibit a significant decline in their IQ as the disorder progresses. However, instead of losing skills, there is a slowing in the rate of acquisition of cognitive skills, thus resulting in an eventual decline in IQ scores. A similar trajectory has also been reported for adaptive behavior skills. Typically, males and females with this diagnosis experience characteristics of the disorder for the duration of the lifespan.

ETIOLOGY

Scientists discovered FMR1, the gene that causes Fragile X, in 1991. This gene is located on the X chromosome. The disorder is transmitted through families, being passed by the mother to either male or female children and by the father to only his female children.

One in 259 women may be a Fragile X permutation carrier and therefore is at risk of having children with the syndrome. The prevalence of the mutation among men in the general population is not known. Those carrying the genetic permutation typically have neither physical signs of Fragile X syndrome nor cognitive or behavioral impairments. As the mutation is passed from one generation to the next, it actually expands in size—eventually causing a fragile site to develop on the X-chromosome. In these cases, a full mutation is said to have occurred and, as a result, little if any FMR1 protein is produced by that gene. This protein is believed to be vital for normal brain development. Females are less affected due to the fact that they have two X chromosomes; therefore, one chromosome may have a normal FMR1 gene.

ASSESSMENT

Direct deoxyribonucleic (DNA) testing of the FMR1 gene can identify normal, permutation, and full mutation size gene sequences, allowing family members to learn whether or not they are permutation carriers. Usually, the DNA for Fragile X testing is taken from blood samples, fetal cells in amniotic fluid, or other tissues. Following the birth of a child with Fragile X, it may be recommended that the family obtain genetic counseling to become aware of the possibility of having more children with this disorder. Individuals who have mental retardation or autism with no known etiology should be tested for Fragile X Syndrome. Given the co-occurrence of significant learning and behavioral problems, a comprehensive developmental evaluation is warranted as well as referral for early intervention services.

TREATMENT

Although there is no cure for Fragile X, various treatment methods may enhance functioning. For example, individualized education plans should emphasize cognitive, communication, and social skills. Regarding the classroom setting, an optimal environment would utilize techniques to reduce visual and auditory distracters, emphasize the overall meanings of concepts, have a standard daily routine, and use calming strategies. Stimulants and other medications normally used to treat ADHD have shown positive effects. Additionally, selective serotonin reuptake inhibitors (SSRIs) may be used to address difficulties with shyness, social anxiety, and aggression. Supportive psychotherapy (individual,

group, or family) may benefit higher functioning individuals with Fragile X. Similarly, parent groups and family education programs may provide supports to parents, siblings, and extended family.

See also: Applied Behavior Analysis; Autistic Disorder; Mental Retardation; Group Psychotherapy; Pharmacological Interventions

Further Reading

Center for the study of autism. http://www.autism.org/fragilex.html
Dykens, E. M., Hodap, R. M., & Finucane, B. M. (2000). *Genetics and mental retardation syndromes*. Baltimore, MD: Paul H. Brookes.
Fragile X Association of Washington State. http://www.wafragilex.org/
FRAXA Research Foundation-Fragile X. http://www.fraxa.org/html
Hagerman, R. J. (1999). *Neurodevelopmental disorders: Diagnosis and treatment*. New York: Oxford University Press.

AMANDA M. ROEBEL
WILLIAM E. MACLEAN, JR.

Functional Analysis

See: Behavior and Functional Analysis

Functional Dyspepsia

DEFINITION/INCIDENCE/ETIOLOGY

Functional dyspepsia refers to persistent or recurrent abdominal pain or discomfort in the upper abdomen unrelated to changes in bowel habits, and without evidence of an organic disease. The syndrome is characterized by symptoms lasting at least 12 weeks during the last 12 months. Symptoms include epigastric pain, fullness, early satiety, bloating, belching, nausea, vomiting, and heartburn. The incidence in children is unknown, but between 3 and 23 percent of adults experience functional dyspepsia. There are several possible physiological mechanisms (e.g., gut dysmotility, visceral hypersensitivity), as well as psychological factors (depression, anxiety, poor coping skills) and environmental factors (negative life events, family stress) that may contribute to functional dyspepsia, but the cause remains unknown.

PSYCHOLOGICAL CORRELATES

Psychosocial correlates of functional dyspepsia have not been investigated in children, but have been fairly well-studied in adults. Adults with functional dyspepsia report significantly more anxiety and depressive symptoms, as well as higher levels of overall psychological distress than healthy adults. Psychiatric diagnoses are also more prevalent in adults with functional dyspepsia. One study reported that individuals with functional dyspepsia use less flexible coping strategies and are less likely to use social support, distraction, or relaxation as coping strategies. Among those with functional dyspepsia, individuals with significant symptoms of anxiety and/or depression report more frequent dyspeptic symptoms and are more likely to seek medical care.

ASSESSMENT/TREATMENT

Diagnosis of functional dyspepsia is made after organic causes (esophagitis, gastritis, duodentitis, ulcer) are excluded, often through endoscopy. Dietary, psychological, and social factors that could contribute to symptoms are also assessed. Treatment includes both medical and psychological strategies. Medical treatment includes acid suppressive medicines, prokinetic agents, and low-dose tricyclic antidepressants. In one study, adults with functional dyspepsia who participated in cognitive-behavioral therapy focusing on coping skills and stress management reported significant reductions in dyspeptic symptoms as well as in depression and anxiety when compared to a control group. Treatment gains were maintained at a 1-year follow-up.

See also: Cognitive–Behavioral Play Therapy; Gastrointestinal Disorders; Irritable Bowel Syndrome; Recurrent Abdominal Pain

Further Reading

Olden, K. W. (1998). Are psychosocial factors of aetiological importance in functional dyspepsia? *Bailliere's Clinical Gastroenterology, 12,* 556–571.

Rasquin-Weber, A., Hyman, P. E., Cucchiara, S., Fleisher, D. R., Hyams, J. S., Milla, P. J., & Staiano, A. (1999). Childhood functional gastrointestinal disorders. *Gut, 45* (Suppl. II), II60–II68.

Laura M. Mackner
Kellee N. Sims-Clark
Wallace V. Crandall

Gg

Gastroesophageal Reflux Disease

DEFINITION/INCIDENCE/ETIOLOGY

Gastroesophageal reflux (GER) is a normal, common event involving the return of the stomach's contents into the esophagus when the sphincter between the stomach and esophagus temporarily relaxes. In infants, GER often results in spitting up or vomiting. In older children, symptoms of GER are typically regurgitation, heartburn, and intermittent vomiting. GER is very common in infancy, with two thirds of infants exhibiting the sole symptom of vomiting. Most of these infants have no other complications, and the vomiting spontaneously resolves by 9–12 months of age. A small proportion of infants and children develop gastroesophageal reflux disease (GERD), which is characterized by complications such as inflammation of the esophagus (esophagitis), poor weight gain, and perhaps reactive airway disease, recurrent pneumonia, laryngitis, and/or obstructive apnea. Symptoms of GERD in infants include recurrent vomiting, irritability, loss of appetite, difficulty swallowing, back-arching, and vomiting of blood. Symptoms of GERD in children include intermittent vomiting, regurgitation, heartburn, difficulty swallowing, chest pain, and vomiting of blood.

ASSESSMENT/TREATMENT

There are numerous diagnostic tests for assessing GERD. A thorough history and physical examination typically determines which diagnostic tests are used. The tests might include esophageal pH monitoring, esophagoscopy, and/or upper gastrointestinal (GI) contrast study, and swallowing studies. Uncomplicated infant reflux does not require treatment. If treatment is indicated, acid-suppressive and prokinetic medications are often used. Surgery is rarely needed. Thickening infant formula with rice cereal may decrease the frequency of vomiting, but does not change the amount of reflux. It is recommended that children and adolescents elevate the head of their bed during sleep and maintain an upright position after meals. Limiting trigger foods plus caffeine, alcohol, and tobacco smoke exposure may also be useful.

PSYCHOSOCIAL CORRELATES

The psychosocial correlates of GERD have not been studied in children. Results from adult studies investigating emotional functioning have been mixed, with some studies reporting higher levels of anxiety and depressive symptoms in adults with GERD versus healthy adults. A study comparing people with GERD who sought medical treatment to a community sample of those with GERD (who had not sought treatment) and a healthy comparison sample reported that when symptom severity was equal in the GERD groups, those who sought treatment had significantly higher levels of anxiety and less adequate social support. Given this finding, differences in sampling (differences in severity, community vs. referred samples) may contribute to the mixed results.

It has also been suggested that stress may play a role in GERD. The role of acute stress was investigated in a well-designed experiment in which adults with

GERD consumed a meal and then participated in stressful and nonstressful situations. Acid in the esophagus was measured via esophageal pH monitoring, and subjects also provided subjective reflux symptom ratings. During the stressful situations, pulse rates and blood pressure levels significantly increased, but the acid activity in the esophagus did not. However, a subset of subjects reported significant increases in subjective symptom ratings during the stressful situations despite no change in esophageal pH. Taken together with the results on emotional functioning, it may be the case that only a subset of adults with GERD have greater psychological difficulty and perceive reflux symptoms during stress, whereas most of those with GERD do not have increased emotional difficulty. This subset of individuals with GERD may be experiencing functional dyspepsia, which may be exacerbated during stress and may account for the increased symptoms reported during stressful situations.

See also: Functional Dyspepsia; Gastrointestinal Disorders

Further Reading

Bradley, L. A., Richter, J. E., Pulliam, T. J., Haile, J. M., Scarinci, I. C., Schan, C. A., Dalton, C. B., & Salley, A. N. (1993). The relationship between stress and symptoms of gastroesophageal reflux: The influence of psychosocial factors. *American Journal of Gastroenterology, 88,* 11–19.

Rudolph, C. D., Mazur, L. J., Liptak, G. S., Baker, R. D., Boyle, J. T., Colletti, R. B., Gerson, W. T., & Werlin, S. L. (2001). Guidelines for evaluation and treatment of gastroesophageal reflux in infants and children: Recommendations of the North American Society for Pediatric Gastroenterology and Nutrition. *Journal of Pediatric Gastroenterology and Nutrition, 32,* S1–S29.

LAURA M. MACKNER
WALLACE V. CRANDALL

Gastrointestinal Disorders

Gastrointestinal disorders encompass a wide range of conditions that highlight the complex interactions of biological and psychosocial factors. The brain and the gut are intimately linked, and emotional distress can result in abdominal discomfort and changes in bowel function even in healthy individuals. The interactions of biological and psychosocial factors may be most evident in the "functional" gastrointestinal disorders, disorders that are not associated with any known structural or biochemical abnormalities. However, both biological and psychosocial factors play a large role in the "organic" disorders as well. For example, emotional distress can result in a worsening of symptoms and increased health care usage, and living with a gastrointestinal disorder can result in increased emotional distress. Additionally, some individuals may experience both organic and functional symptoms, underscoring the intricate links between biological and psychosocial factors. Despite the potential for interesting research examining these factors, with the exception of recurrent abdominal pain, psychosocial issues in children with gastrointestinal disorders have not been well studied. Table 1 describes several

Table 1. Gastrointestinal Disorders

Disease	Symptoms	Incidence/ Prevalence	Management/ Treatment	Prognosis
Celiac disease	Diarrhea, vomiting, abdominal distension, irritability, abdominal pain, anorexia nervosa, weight loss, anemia and many others	1 in 200	Elimination of gluten from diet, including wheat, rye, and barley	Removal of gluten results in full remission and restoration of small intestine to normal
Chronic intestinal pseudo-obstruction	Constipation, urinary retention, abdominal distension, vomiting, failure to pass meconium	100 births per year	Treat disorders causing or exacerbating symptoms, prokinetic medications, anti-biotics, nutritional support	Depending on severity, mortality may reach 33% within the first year
Diarrhea Acute/Infectious	Watery or loose stool, increased stool output, sometimes bloody stool	In children under 5 years, 1–2 episodes per year	Oral rehydration solutions, rapid reintroduction of normal feeding, probiotics, occasionally antibiotics	Brief, self-limited course

(Continued)

Table 1. (*Continued*)

Disease	Incidence/ Symptoms	Management/ Prevalence	Treatment	Prognosis
Chronic/Nonspecific	3 or more large unformed stools for 4 or more weeks with no organic cause	Reportedly common	Dietary education, parent behavior management training	Generally self-limited course
Food allergy	Itching, abdominal pain, diarrhea, vomiting, hives, rash, asthma, anaphylaxis	1–2%	Elimination of suspected food from diet	Elimination of specific food results in remission of symptoms. 78–87% of children outgrow food allergies by age 6
Functional dyspepsia	At least 12 weeks of epigastric pain, bloating, belching, nausea with no organic cause	3–23% in adults	Acid suppressive medications, prokinetic agents, tricyclic antidepressants, psychotherapy	Not reported
Gallstone disease	Abdominal pain, nausea, vomiting	0.15–0.22%	Removal of gallbladder, analgesic medications, dissolving agents	No symptoms after surgery
Gastroesophageal reflux disease	Recurrent episodes of stomach contents returning to esophagus. In infants, vomiting, spitting up, weight loss. In older children, heartburn.	Reflux occurs in 67% of infants, but complications occur in 8%	Smaller, more frequent feedings, thicken food, remain upright after meals, acid-suppressive & prokinetic medications, occasionally surgery	Reflux spontaneously resolves in most infants
Hirschsprung's disease	Absence or delay in passage of meconium, constipation, vomiting, abdominal distension, growth delay, enterocolitis	1 in 5,000 births	Surgery	With no enterocolitis, mortality rate 4%. With enterocolitis, mortality rate 33%. Fecal incontinence, constipation, diarrhea, & abdominal distension can persist after surgery.
Inflammatory bowel disease	Abdominal pain, diarrhea, rectal bleeding, weight loss	6 in 100,000	Aminosalicylates, corticosteroids Immunosuppressive medications, antibiotics, biologic agents, surgery	Variable
Irritable bowel syndrome	At least 12 weeks of abdominal pain, change in frequency of stool, change in appearance of stool with no organic cause	6–14%	Tricyclic antidepressants, anticholinergic medications, fiber, psychotherapy	Symptoms worsen or remain stable in 24–57% of untreated adults. Up to 94% improve with psychotherapy
Liver disease Hepatitis (A, B, C)	Can be asymptomatic, fatigue, fever, nausea, abdominal pain, weight loss, rash, jaundice	1–6%	Immune globulin if exposed, interferon, antiviral agents, immune modulatory therapies	Hepatitis A: Symptoms resolve 2–3 weeks after onset. Hepatitis B, C: Variable course, becomes chronic in 10–50%, cirrhosis, cancer, and liver failure rare
Gilbert's Syndrome	Elevated serum bilirubin, usually no symptoms, mild jaundice	5%	None needed	No negative implications for health
Steatosis	Excess fat in liver due to obesity, diabetes, metabolic disorders. Usually asymptomatic, mild jaundice	47–85% in obese adults	Treat primary disease (e.g., obesity)	May progress to steatohepatitis (inflamed fatty liver) or cirrhosis

(*Continued*)

Table 1. (*Continued*)

Disease	Incidence/ Symptoms	Management/ Prevalence	Treatment	Prognosis
Pancreatitis	Abdominal pain, anorexia nervosa, nausea, vomiting	Unknown	Analgesia, removal of gastric secretions via nasogastric suction, fasting, surgery	Variable course, mortality rate 9% in adults
Peptic ulcer disease	Episodic epigastric pain, may be associated with vomiting and nocturnal awakening in children	5–10% in adults, rare in children	Eliminating *H. pylori* infection via antibiotics and acid-suppressive medication	Successful treatment of *H. pylori* results in complete recovery
Recurrent abdominal pain	3 or more episodes of abdominal pain over a 3-month period that is severe enough to interfere with routine functioning with no organic cause	10–20%	Fiber, cognitive– behavioral therapy	87% improve with psychotherapy
Short bowel syndrome	After surgical resection of the small intestine, diarrhea, malabsorption of nutrients, growth delay	Unknown	Total parenteral nutrition, tube feeding; if oral feeding, frequent, small meals; antidiarrheals, acid suppressive medications, pancreatic enzymes, antibiotics	Influenced by age, length and location of bowel resected

gastrointestinal disorders, and additional chapters are provided for the disorders in which psychosocial issues have been addressed.

See also: Celiac Disease; Diarrhea; Functional Dyspepsia; Inflammatory Bowel Disease; Irritable Bowel Syndrome; Peptic Ulcer Disease

LAURA M. MACKNER
KELLEE N. SIMS CLARK
WALLACE V. CRANDALL

Gay and Lesbian Partners

See: Sexual Orientation: Homosexuality

Gay and Lesbian Youth

See: Sexual Orientation: Homosexuality

Gender and Psychopathology

Frick and Silverthorn (2001) have shown that between 9 and 22 percent of preschoolers, children, and adolescents have significant behavioral and emotional problems at any given time. However, these overall rates of psychopathology conceal important gender differences in prevalence that vary across developmental stages. In general, prior to adolescence, more boys than girls are diagnosed as having a psychopathological condition. In contrast, during adolescence, prevalence rates shift, with some studies finding that girls and boys are diagnosed at equal rates and others finding that girls are diagnosed more often than boys.

INTERNALIZING DISORDERS

Differences in the prevalence of disorders not only vary by age and gender, but also by type of diagnosis. In general, internalizing disorders (e.g., depressive disorders and anxiety disorders) are typically thought of as "female" disorders. However, this is not always the case across development. For example, prior to puberty, boys are more often diagnosed with Major Depressive Disorder than are girls, typically by a 2:1 ratio. However, this ratio switches in adolescence, becoming 2 : 1 in favor of girls, a trend that continues into adulthood. This shift in gender prevalence is due to an increase of depression in girls during midpuberty accompanied by a decrease of depression in boys. Angold and colleagues (1998) have identified several reasons for this shift in gender prevalence in depression including the role of pubertal hormones, the role of stress experiences and stress responsivity, the influence of adherence to feminine stereotypes, and the role of specific cognitive response styles that may place girls at greater risk for depression after puberty and protect older boys.

Results are less consistent for gender differences in the prevalence of anxiety disorders in youth and may vary depending on the type of anxiety disorder. For example, during childhood, more boys than girls are diagnosed with Generalized Anxiety Disorder (GAD), whereas after approximately age 9 more girls than boys are diagnosed with GAD. In contrast, during both childhood and adolescence, more girls than boys are diagnosed with Separation Anxiety Disorder, Simple Phobia, and Social Phobia.

EXTERNALIZING DISORDERS

There are also gender differences in the prevalence of externalizing disorders, although these are quite different from the gender differences found for anxiety and depression. For example, more boys than girls are diagnosed with Attention-Deficit/Hyperactivity Disorder (ADHD), with ratios varying from 4 : 1 in community samples to 9 : 1 in clinical samples. This male predominance seems to be somewhat consistent across development. However, these overall rates of ADHD obscure important gender differences in the prevalence of ADHD subtypes. Specifically, more girls are diagnosed with the Predominantly Inattentive Type of ADHD than with the Combined type or the Primarily Hyperactive-Impulsive type, as recently reported by Biederman and associates (2002). Despite the differences in prevalence rates, when girls do show ADHD, the symptom presentation appears to be quite similar to the symptom presentation found in boys. One important gender difference in the expression of ADHD appears to be in the age-of-onset of the disorder and the age at which children with ADHD are referred for treatment. Specifically, girls with the Predominantly Inattentive type of ADHD appear to have a later age of onset than boys, despite being referred for treatment at a similar age than boys. In contrast, Silverthorn, Frick, and colleagues (1996) have noted that when girls have ADHD-C, they appear to be referred at an earlier age than boys, despite showing a similar age of onset.

Gender differences in the diagnosis of Oppositional Defiant Disorder (ODD) and Conduct Disorder (CD) are more complex and show greater variation across development. In general, boys and girls tend to show similar levels of conduct problems prior to age 5. In contrast, more boys than girls manifest conduct problems during childhood and adolescence, although the male predominance decreases somewhat in adolescence from about 4 : 1 in childhood to about 2 : 1 in adolescence. There is some controversy as to whether the differences in prevalence rates in childhood and adolescence are real differences in the rates of conduct problems for boys and girls or whether they are an artifact of diagnostic definitions that are not sensitive to sex differences in how conduct problems are expressed. For example, it has been argued that girls are less often diagnosed with severe conduct problems because they manifest more indirect or relational aggression rather than overt, physical aggression. Others have argued that girls manifest similar types of behaviors, but that they should be diagnosed using a more lenient criterion that compares girls to other girls rather than to mixed samples of girls and boys. Still others, such as Moffit and Caspi (2001) and Silverthorn and Frick (1999) have argued that girls manifest similar antisocial behaviors as boys, but that girls are less likely to experience the necessary precursors (both familial and genetic) that lead to the development of antisocial behavior.

One additional source of controversy is whether developmental models to explain the onset and causes of severe conduct problems are equally valid for girls and boys. Specifically, it is generally accepted that girls are less likely to show a childhood-onset to their severe conduct problems, accounting for the changes in the gender ratio found between childhood and adolescence. However, it is not clear whether or not when girls do develop severe antisocial behavior in adolescence that it is a sign of a less severe and less chronic disturbance, as it is in boys. There is some evidence that, despite the adolescent-onset, many antisocial girls show the familial, individual, and interpersonal deficits and the negative outcome in late adolescence and adulthood that make them more similar to boys who show a childhood-onset to their conduct problems. Regardless, it appears that when girls manifest severe conduct problems, they are more likely than boys to experience comorbid conditions, particularly internalizing disorders.

See also: Adolescence; Attention-Deficit/Hyperactivity Disorder; Conduct Disorder; Delinquent Behavior; Depressive Disorder; Social Development in Adolescence; Social Development in Childhood

Further Reading

Angold, A., Costello, E. J., & Worthman, C. M. (1998). Puberty and depression: The roles of age, pubertal status and pubertal timing. *Psychological Medicine, 28,* 51–61.

Biederman, J., Mick, E., Faraone, S. V., Braaten, E., Doyle, A., Spencer, T., et al. (2002). Influence of gender on attention deficit hyperactivity disorder in children referred to a psychiatric clinic. *The American Journal of Psychiatry, 159,* 36–42.

Frick, P. J., & Silverthorn, P. (2001). Psychopathology in children. In H. E. Adams & P. Sutker (Eds.), *Comprehensive handbook of psychopathology* (3rd ed., pp. 879–919). New York: Kluwer Academic/Plenum.

Moffitt, T. E., & Caspi, A. (2001). Childhood predictors differentiate life-course persistent and adolescent-limited antisocial pathways, among males and females. *Development and Psychopathology, 13,* 355–375.

Silverthorn, P., & Frick, P. J. (1999). Developmental pathways to antisocial behavior: The delayed-onset pathway in girls. *Development and Psychopathology, 11,* 101–126.

Silverthorn, P., Frick, P. J., Kuper, K., & Ott, J. (1996). Attention Deficit Hyperactivity Disorder and sex: A test of two etiological models to explain the male predominance. *Journal of Clinical Child Psychology, 25,* 52–59.

PERSEPHANIE SILVERTHORN
PAUL J. FRICK

Gender Identity Disorder

DEFINITION

The American Psychiatric Association's *Diagnostic and Statistical Manual of Mental Disorders, Fourth Edition* (*DSM-IV*) criteria for Gender Identity Disorder (GID) include two central features: (1) strong and persistent cross-gender identification as manifested in a desire to be or belief that one is the opposite sex, and preferences for stereotypical cross-gender clothing, activities, or playmates and roles in fantasy or make-believe play; and (2) persistent discomfort with one's own sex as manifested in aversion to one's own genitalia, or sex-typed behavior, activities or clothing. Symptoms of GID typically begin to appear between 2 and 4 years of age and include: (1) identity statements indicating that one is or wishes to be a member of the opposite sex; (2) cross-dressing which may occur in public and can have an obsessive or driven quality resulting in tantrums when prohibited; (3) cross-sex toy and role play;

(4) preference for opposite sex peers and avoidance of same-sex peers; (5) cross-sex mannerisms and voice quality; (6) anatomic dysphoria, wherein the child expresses dislike of or tries to hide his or her genitalia; and (7) preference for (among girls) or avoidance of (among boys) rough and tumble play. Many of these symptoms appear to be age-dependent, at least for boys. Cross-gender behavior and explicit statements about wishing to be the opposite sex decrease with age among boys, probably because of the social stigma associated with these behaviors. GID in both boys and girls often co-occurs with other forms of psychopathology, particularly internalizing disorders. Older children and adolescents with GID have higher rates of comorbid psychopathology than do younger children, which may reflect the cumulative effects of peer rejection and social isolation that almost inevitably accompany GID.

EPIDEMIOLOGY

GID is a relatively rare disorder. Although instances of cross-gender behavior among preschool children are quite common, it is not known how many of these children would actually fulfill all the criteria for a *DSM-IV* diagnosis of GID. In a nonclinical sample of 4- to 5-year-olds, 6 percent of boys and 11.8 percent of girls were reported by their mothers to sometimes or frequently behave like the opposite sex. Further, 1.3 percent of boys and 5.0 percent of girls were reported to sometimes or frequently express a wish to be the opposite sex. Higher rates of cross-sex-typed behaviors are typically found in clinical samples, although less so for girls than boys.

Referral rates are much higher for boys than girls (6–7:1), raising the question of whether the prevalence of GID is actually higher for boys than for girls. It may be that boys are more vulnerable to GID because masculine development is dependent on prenatal androgen secretion whereas feminine development occurs in the absence of prenatal androgens. Alternatively, the higher referral rates for boys may be due to the fact that society has less tolerance for cross-gender behavior in boys than girls. Referral rates for adolescent boys and girls with gender disturbance are much more similar (1.4:1).

ETIOLOGY

Biological factors, particularly prenatal hormone secretion, may predispose children to problems with gender identity. Variations in prenatal hormone exposure (i.e., increases or decreases in androgens) have been shown to influence later behavior (without altering external genital structures) of both animals and humans. Female fetuses exposed to androgens prenatally exhibit behaviors more typical of males after birth, whereas male fetuses that are not exposed to sufficient levels of androgens exhibit more typically feminine behaviors. The causes of variations in hormone secretion during pregnancy are not yet well understood. In rats, prenatal maternal stress has been linked with decreased androgen secretion and later demasculinized behavior in the male offspring. To date, however, this phenomenon has not been observed in humans.

Further evidence for a biological contribution to GID is found in studies that indicate that boys with GID are more likely to be later born and have more brothers than sisters when compared to boys without GID. It is hypothesized (but not proven) that antibodies to one or more of the hormones needed for sexual differentiation (including testosterone) produced by the mother of a male fetus may reduce the biological activity of these hormones and that this effect might increase over several pregnancies involving a male fetus.

Evidence for the role of the social environment in GID is found in studies that show successful formation of gender identity in children born with ambiguous genitalia and assigned to one sex or another shortly after birth. Other research demonstrates higher rates of parental and family dysfunction for children with GID than for controls. Moreover, clinical experience indicates that parents of children with GID often respond neutrally or positively to their children's early cross-gender behavior, thus potentially increasing this behavior through differential reinforcement.

Taken together, research on etiology of GID suggests that this disorder probably results from an interaction between biological and environmental factors. Fetal sex hormones influence brain development which subsequently mediates behavior. This process creates a predisposition to behave as a male or female. The social environment then functions to reinforce or discourage cross- or same-gender behavior and identification.

TREATMENT

Treatment of GID has generated some controversy. One argument is that treatment reinforces a sexist view of child rearing. Others have questioned the ethics of treating GID in an ettempt to prevent homosexuality (although it is not clear that treatment is effective in this regard). Another view proposes that early treatment of GID may at least alleviate the peer relationship and self-esteem problems that accompany the disorder. This approach advocates intervention to eliminate cross-gender behaviors and to replace them with behaviors that are consistent with the child's physical sex. Alternatively, intervention might acknowledge and affirm the child's cross-gender preference and then help the child learn how to express this preference in a manner that allows for both good peer relations and a positive self-image.

When treatment is offered, a behavioral approach is most common. This approach assumes that cross-gender behavior is learned and, therefore, can be changed by manipulating the consequences for cross- and same-gender behavior. Behavioral treatment provides opportunities and positive reinforcement for engaging in gender-appropriate behavior and choosing gender-appropriate games and toys. Verbal feedback is given about appropriate and inappropriate gender behavior, and cross-gender behavior is extinguished by ignoring. Self-esteem enhancement focused on gender-related issues is also an important component of treatment in most cases of GID. Parental involvement is essential to the success of treatment; parents can contribute by ensuring that the program is implemented consistently across settings and people. Treatment of any accompanying parental or family psychopathology is essential to maximize the effectiveness of the treatment program.

LONG-TERM PROGNOSIS

Homosexuality

There is a strong relationship between early cross-gender behavior and later homosexuality. A majority (60–80 percent) of boys with GID have a homosexual or bisexual orientation as adults. It is important to note that the association between cross-gender behavior in childhood and later homosexuality is not absolute; a substantial minority of homosexual adults do not recall engaging in cross-gender behavior during childhood and some children with gender disturbance do not adopt a homosexual orientation as adults. Deviant gender identity for most boys with GID normalizes with development and most adult homosexuals do not demonstrate gender identity or gender role problems as adults. The reason why gender identity appears to normalize with development is not yet clear. It may be, however, that gender identity problems are resolved through the process of determining one's sexual orientation.

Transsexualism

GID and transsexualism (adults who have persistent gender identity problems and wish to undergo sex reassignment) are also associated. Although few children with GID become transsexuals as adults, almost all adult transsexuals (both male and female) recall cross-gender behavior as children. Zucker and Bradley (1995) suggest that the transition from childhood to adolescence may be a critical time for the development of transsexualism. They note that children who maintain a consistent cross-gender identification as they move through adolescence are most at risk for transsexualism.

Transvestitism

Transvestitism (male heterosexuals who cross-dress for purposes of sexual arousal) is not related to GID and, in fact, the clinical picture for this disorder is quite different than that of GID. Transvestites typically do not have gender problems as children and are usually quite securely masculine as adults. Moreover, they clearly demonstrate masculine gender roles. The function of cross-dressing appears to distinguish potential transvestitism from GID. Cross-dressing among gender-disturbed boys is done for the purpose of enhancing identification with the opposite sex (typically employing outer clothing) as opposed to a soothing or erotic function (typically involving female underwear) for transvestites.

See also: Adolescence; Emotional Development; Identity Development; Self-Concept/Self-Image; Sexual Development; Sexual Orientation: Homosexuality

Further Reading

American Psychiatric Association. (1994). *Diagnostic and statistical manual of mental disorders* (4th ed.). Washington, DC: Author.

Bradley, S. J., & Zucker, K. J., (1997). Gender identity disorder: A review of the past 10 years. *Journal of the American Academy of Child and Adolescent Psychiatry, 36*, 872–880.

Rekers, G. A., & Kilgus, M. D. (1995). Differential diagnosis and rationale for treatment of gender identity disorders and transvestitism. In G. A. Rekers (Ed.), *Handbook of child and adolescent sexual problems* (pp. 225–289). New York: Lexington Books.

Zucker, K. J., & Bradley, S. J. (1995). *Gender identity disorder and psychosexual problems in children and adolescents.* New York: Guilford.

BETTY N. GORDON

Generalized Anxiety Disorder

DESCRIPTION/CLINICAL PRESENTATION

Generalized Anxiety Disorder (GAD) was recently included in the fourth edition of the *Diagnostic and* *Statistical Manual of Mental Disorders* (*DSM-IV*) as a disorder appropriate for diagnosis in childhood and adolescence. The core features of GAD include excessive and preoccupying worry that is difficult to control. The worry is not focused on a specific situation or object and is not related to a recent stressor. In addition to worry, the child must experience at least one physical symptom/complaint including stomachaches, muscle aches, sleep disturbance, fatigue, concentration difficulties, and/or irritability. Because all children worry or have short periods when they may worry excessively, *DSM-IV* requires that the physical symptom(s) and excessive uncontrollable worry be present for at least 6 months before assigning a diagnosis of GAD.

PREVALENCE AND CORRELATES

Most of the information on the prevalence and correlates of GAD in youth is derived from studies using the *DSM-III* and *DSM-III-R* overanxious disorder (OAD) diagnostic category, which is now subsumed under GAD in *DSM-IV*. The prevalence of OAD in child and adolescent samples was found to range from 3 to 12 percent in community samples and 6 to 12 percent in clinical samples. Children with OAD tend to be older than children with other anxiety disorders such as separation anxiety disorder, specific phobias, and social phobia.

Most of the information on the correlates of GAD is from studies using heterogeneous samples of children with anxiety disorders, including GAD. As noted by Messer and Beidel (1994), these studies generally have found that children with anxiety disorders have high trait anxiety, temperaments that are less flexible and more rigid, and have less physical and cognitive self-confidence than children without any disorder. Also, the family environments of children with anxiety disorders tend to promote less independence for the child.

ASSESSMENT

A variety of semi-structured (e.g., Anxiety Disorders Interview Schedule for *DSM-IV*: Child and Parent Versions) and structured (e.g., Diagnostic Interview Schedule for Children) diagnostic interviews are available for assessing GAD in children and adolescents. In addition, there are measures that assess symptoms of general anxiety, such as the Revised Children's Manifest Anxiety Scale and the State-Trait Anxiety Inventory for Children. Self-rating scales that contain subscales to assess *DSM-IV* GAD symptoms are the

Multidimensional Anxiety Scale for Children and the Screen for Anxiety and Related Emotional Disorders. Both of these scales also discriminate children with GAD from children with other types of phobic and anxiety disorders. These assessment tools are frequently used in the initial assessment of GAD as well as in the continued monitoring of treatment response. When assessing GAD, it is important to thoroughly assess for the presence of comorbid psychiatric disorders including other anxiety, mood, and externalizing disorders.

TREATMENT

Silverman and Berman (2001) reported that considerable evidence has been accumulated demonstrating the efficacy of exposure-based cognitive-behavior therapy (CBT) for reducing childhood anxiety disorders in general, and *DSM-III-R* OAD and *DSM-IV* GAD in particular. CBT has been found to be efficacious in treating anxiety disorders in children, including GAD, whether delivered using an individual child format, a format that involves increased parental involvement, and a format that involves increased peer involvement. Overall, results from these studies indicate positive treatment gains for up to 1-year posttreatment. In addition, a follow-up study conducted by Barrett and colleagues showed positive treatment gains were maintained for up to 7 years post-treatment. There also is preliminary evidence that treatment for GAD may be improved if treatment is matched or prescribed in accordance with the specific needs or circumstances of the child (e.g., emphasize cognitive therapy for children who worry excessively; emphasize relaxation training for children who display excessive physiological symptoms).

The pharmacological literature on the treatment of childhood anxiety disorders, including GAD, is in its infancy when compared to the literature on exposure-based CBT, as noted by Stock and associates (2001). Birmaher and colleagues examined the efficacy of the anti-depressant Fluoxetine (i.e., Prozac) in 21 children with separation anxiety disorder, social phobia, as well as overanxious disorder; 81 percent of the children displayed moderate to marked improvement of their anxiety symptoms and no side effects were reported by any of the children. Because research is so sparse, pharmacological interventions have been recommended with only the more difficult or "resistant" cases, rather than the front-line approach to be used with all cases.

See also: Behavioral Diaries; Cognitive–Behavioral Play Therapy; Headache; Parent Training; Problem-Solving Training

Further Reading

Messer, S. C., & Beidel, D. C. (1994). Psychosocial correlates of childhood anxiety disorders. *Journal of the American Academy of Child and Adolescent Psychiatry, 33*, 975–983.

Silverman, W. K., & Berman, S. L. (2001). Psychosocial interventions for anxiety disorders in children: Status and future directions. In W. K Silverman & P. D. A Treffers (Eds.), *Anxiety disorders in children and adolescents: Research, assessment and intervention* (pp. 313–334). Cambridge, UK: Cambridge University Press.

Stock, S. L., Werry, J. S., & McClellan, J. M. (2001). Pharmacological treatment of paediatric anxiety. In W. K Silverman & P. D. A. Treffers (eds.), *Anxiety disorders in children and adolescents: Research, assessment and intervention* (pp. 335–367). Cambridge, UK: Cambridge University Press.

LISSETTE M. SAAVEDRA
BARBARA LOPEZ
WENDY K. SILVERMAN

Genetic Counseling

Genetic counseling is a process intended to help individuals and families understand the ramifications associated with the present occurrence (and risk of recurrence) of any condition in which a genetic etiology is known or suspected. Genetic counselors often work in tandem with clinical geneticists (M.D.s) who diagnose and treat genetic conditions. Genetic counseling typically involves (1) provision of information about diagnosis and prognosis, (2) assistance in understanding the role of heredity to the disorder and the risk of recurrence in the family, (3) assistance in understanding the options for dealing with risk, including prenatal diagnosis, (4) non-directive assistance in selecting courses of action that are consistent with family goals and values, and (5) supportive counseling to help individuals and families cope with the psychological burden imposed by discovery of a genetic disorder and the emotional complexity that results from genetic and reproductive risks. Genetic counseling may also involve referral to relevant community support groups and to financial, social, and educational services necessary for optimal care as well as for emotional and psychological adjustment. Common indications for genetic counseling include the presence of birth defects, developmental delay, short stature, metabolic disorders, dysmorphic features, significant behavioral disorder, infertility, neuromuscular disorders, and pregnancy after the age of 35. Genetic counselors are typically Masters-level professionals who are board certified by the American

Board of Genetic Counseling to provide services in the medical genetics specialty of genetic counseling.

See also: Behavioral Genetics; Health Education/Health Promotion; Risk and Protective Factors

Further Reading

Cassidy, S. B., & Allanson, J. E. (2001). *Management of genetic syndromes*. New York: Wiley.
Robinson, A., & Linden, M. G. (1993), *Clinical genetics handbook*. Boston: Blackwell Scientific.

KEITH D. ALLEN

Genital Herpes

See: Sexually Transmitted Diseases in Adolescents

Genital Warts

See: Sexually Transmitted Diseases in Adolescents

Genogram

See: Family Assessment

Genotype

See: Behavioral Genetics

Gestational Age

See: Prematurity: Birth Weight and Gestational Age

Gigantism and Acromegaly

DESCRIPTION AND INCIDENCE

Gigantism is a disease caused by overproduction of growth hormone (GH) before the fusion of the epiphyses.* Overproduction of GH in adults (after the epiphyses are fused) is referred to as *acromegaly*. Children with gigantism experience rapid linear growth and can reach a stature of eight feet tall or more by adulthood. Other clinical manifestations of the disease include coarsening of facial features including broadening of the nose, enlargement of the tongue and mandible and separation of the teeth. Enlarged hands and feet, thickened fingers and toes, and thickened skin with increased oiliness and sweating are also symptomatic of the disease.

Gigantism/acromegaly is a very rare disease with an annual incidence of 3–4/1,000,000 cases. There is no bias towards race. In adults, GH excess occurs in men and women equally.

ETIOLOGY

Overproduction of GH is most commonly caused by a tumor made up of somatotrophs (GH-secreting cells) or mammosomatotrophs (GH and prolactin-secreting cells). Another possible cause of gigantism and acromegaly is an oversecretion of GH releasing hormone (GHRH). This may result from tumors of the hypothalamus or pancreas.

ASSOCIATED PSYCHOLOGICAL FEATURES

Due to the rarity of the disease, there is little research on the psychological adaptation of individuals with gigantism or acromegaly. Patients with pituitary tumors may experience impairment of memory. Irritability and depression are symptomatic features of acromegaly. However, it remains uncertain whether these problems are due to hormonal imbalance or a psychological response to the disfigurement caused by the disease. Sleep apnea is also common in acromegaly and can lead to emotional distress and lifestyle changes. Loss of initiative and decreased libido are also common in acromegaly. There is no research that relates GH excess to any impairment in intellect. Assessments of neuropsychological functioning, psychopathology, or quality of life have not appeared in the medical or psychological literature on gigantism or acromegaly.

---

*Epiphyses are the ends of long bones that are separated from the rest of the bone with cartilage. As growth occurs, the ends become attached or fused to the rest of the bone.

TREATMENT

The goal of treatment for gigantism and acromegaly is to normalize GH levels (3–5 ng/ml). Transsphenoidal surgery (through or across the sphenoid bone, a large bone at the base of the skull), in which the entire tumor is removed, may be curative. Radiation therapy has also been successful. More recently, pharmacological therapy has been successful in normalizing GH levels. Drug categories used in treatment include somatostatin analogues, such as Octreotide, dopamine analogues, such as Bromocriptine (Parlodel) and Cabergoline (Dostinex), and GH-receptor antagonists, such as Pegvisomant (Somavert).

PROGNOSIS

Patients with GH excess are at higher risk for developing diabetes mellitus, hypertension, and cardiovascular disease. Without treatment, complications of the lungs, heart, and brain can cause death. However, patients can live a normal life span with treatment.

RESOURCES AND SUPPORT GROUPS

The Pituitary Foundation, P.O. Box 1944, Bristol BS99 2UB, United Kingdom, Web site: http://www.pituitary.org.uk/, E-mail: helpline@pituitary.org.uk; The Pituitary Tumor Network Association, P.O. Box 1958, Thousand Oaks, CA 91358, Web site: http://www.pituitary.com/

See also: Coping with Illness; Parenting the Chronically Ill Child

Further Reading

Furman, K., & Ezzat, S. (1998). Psychological features of acromegaly. *Psychotherapy and Psychosomatics, 67*, 147–153.

Cohen, P. (2000). Hyperpituitarism, tall stature, and overgrowth syndromes. In R. E. Behrman, R. Kliegman, & H. B. Jenson (Eds.), *Nelson textbook of pediatrics* (pp. 1685–1687). Philadelphia, PA: W.B. Saunders.

Teresa Wiech
David E. Sandberg

Global Functioning

Global functioning typically refers to a clinician's judgment of a youth's overall level of functioning in performing various roles and day-to-day activities, as would be observed in school, at home, and in interactions with others in general. Assessment of global functioning is considered so important that it was incorporated in the multiaxial system of the American Psychiatric Association's *Diagnostic and Statistical Manual of Mental Disorders, Fourth Edition* (*DSM-IV*) as Axis V, or more specifically, as Global Assessment of Functioning (GAF). The GAF was derived from the Global Assessment Scale (GAS), authored by Jean Endicott and colleagues in 1976, which was in turn derived from the Health-Sickness Rating Scale developed by Lester Luborsky in 1962. The clinician is instructed to consider psychological, social, and occupational functioning on a hypothetical continuum of mental health-illness in assigning the youth a score from 1 to 100, using 10 anchor descriptions. A higher score indicates better functioning. The clinician rates the youth's lowest level of functioning during a time period that is specified by the clinician (e.g., last month, last year). The 10 anchor descriptions consist primarily of symptom descriptions with some examples of impaired functioning. For the most part, functioning is measured by the lack of impairment (e.g., the anchor for a score 90 begins with "absence of minimal symptoms"). David Shaffer and colleagues modified the anchor descriptions in 1983 to reflect examples pertinent to children, with this adaptation referred to as the Children's Global Assessment Scale (CGAS). There is no training for scoring the CGAS or GAF. It is assumed they can be readily used by professionals who have had formal educational and clinical experience in working with a variety of childhood psychiatric disorders.

In the narrative introduction to *DSM-IV*, impairment in functioning is stipulated as a criterion for receiving a diagnosis. In order to meet the criteria for a disorder, the individual must have impairment in one or more important areas of functioning or experience significant distress. In general, impairment is not defined in the diagnostic criteria, although for some diagnoses, a vague statement is included about the disturbance causing clinically significant impairment in social, academic, or occupational functioning.

A diagnosis consists of a constellation of symptoms, whereas impairment reflects the consequences or effects of symptoms on day-to-day functioning. Level of functioning is regarded as a more rigorous criterion for need for treatment than presence of a set of symptoms. Epidemiological research, in which community rather than clinical samples are studied, has confirmed the need to incorporate the requirement of impairment when trying to identify youths in need of services. Without this requirement, the proportion of youths meeting criteria for diagnosis has consistently been inordinately high. Epidemiological studies have also demonstrated that even when youths did not meet diagnostic criteria for any common diagnosis, youths with functional impairment were as likely to receive specialty mental health services as were youths that had both a diagnosis and impairment.

In fact, when the Center for Mental Health Services (CMHS) of the Substance Abuse and Mental Health Services Administration operationalized the definition of Serious Emotional Disturbance (SED), they required the presence of diagnosis and functional impairment which substantially interferes with or limits the child's role or functioning in family, school, or community activities. In applying for federal block grant funds from CMHS, each state must demonstrate that they are meeting the needs of youths with SED. In addition, this operationalized definition of SED is used to determine prevalence rates for the purpose of identifying the mental health needs of children at a national and state level.

Various measures, which yield a global score or a total score reflecting on functioning, have been widely used and include the CGAS, Columbia Impairment Scale (CIS) developed by Bird and colleagues (1996) and the Child and Adolescent Functional Assessment Scale (CAFAS) authored by Hodges (2000). The CGAS yields one numeric value; the CIS generates a total score from 13 items; and the CAFAS generates a total sum based on scores for eight subscales assessing various domains of functioning. The CGAS has typically been used in research published in the psychiatric literature, such as medication studies. The CIS was developed for epidemiological studies in the hope that parents and youths could complete the measure. However, parents tend to score their children as healthier than they are, as judged by nonclinician raters who scored the CGAS after detailed interviews with the child and parent. As a result, the nonclinician CGAS has been recommended over the CIS as a measure of impairment in epidemiological studies. The version for the youth is not recommended because of consistently poor psychometric properties (i.e., its reliability and validity). The CAFAS is widely used to evaluate outcome in applied clinical settings and in clinical research. The CAFAS consists of a set of behavioral descriptions (e.g., expelled from school, bullies peers) which are grouped into levels of impairment (e.g., severe, moderate, etc.) for each domain (e.g., school, home, etc.). According to an annual survey on how the states are evaluating their children's services, conducted by the Georgetown University National Technical Assistance Center for Children's Mental Health, the CAFAS is used by approximately 25 states. In addition, the 67 System of Care Initiative sites

awarded grants by the CMHS use the CAFAS as an outcome measure. There is considerable evidence of criterion-related and predictive validity of the CAFAS.

In addition to the role of identifying need for treatment, measures of global level of functioning, according to *DSM-IV*, are useful in measuring the impact of treatment, in predicting the outcome of treatment, and in planning treatment. While no rationale or justification is given for these assertions in *DSM-IV*, the empirical literature does support them. Numerous studies have used the CGAS and the CAFAS to demonstrate the impact of intervention on improvement in functioning. Global measures of functioning are commonly used as quality assurance or performance indicators to monitor quality of care and to ensure accountability of providers. In fact, functioning has come to be viewed as an important criterion for assessing treatment outcome because it ensures that clinically meaningful and significant change has taken place. Showing change in symptom counts is not considered sufficient for demonstrating efficacy for an evidence-based treatment. To be considered efficacious, the treatment should demonstrate an impact on the child's everyday functioning in the real world. There is evidence to suggest that impacting functioning is more difficult to accomplish than reducing symptoms, based on the findings of a community sample study, which examined the relationship between service dose and outcome.

The assertion that the level of functioning at the onset of treatment is a prognostic indicator of eventual outcome also has empirical support. A higher level of impairment is associated with poorer response to psychotherapy. In addition, in a community study in which youths were evaluated 5–7 years after their initial assessment, the findings indicated that the likelihood of having a diagnosis and functional impairment in adolescents was much higher for those with a diagnosis and impairment as a child, compared to healthy children.

It makes intuitive sense that global functioning would be useful in treatment planning because the score would have implications for level of care decisions and for documenting the need for more intensive or costly treatments. In fact, studies using the CAFAS have shown that a higher degree of impairment at intake means that the individual is much more likely to need a stronger intervention. Higher measures of impairment on the CAFAS have been shown to correspond to a more intensive level of care, more restrictive or therapeutic placement, and more serious psychiatric disorders. Also, prediction studies have shown that higher measures of impairment on the CAFAS at intake were significantly related to more restrictive care, higher cost, more bed days, and more days of services at 6 and 12 months postintake, more restrictive living arrangement and higher number of days in out-of-family care at 6 months, significantly greater likelihood of contact with the law and poor school attendance at 6 months postintake, and significantly greater likelihood of recidivism during the year after discharge from a juvenile justice residential placement facility. The assertions that global functioning is important in identifying need for service, in treatment planning, in assessing the impact of treatment, and in predicting the response to treatment are thus supported by the literature.

See also: Behavior Rating Scales; Classification and Diagnosis; Clinical Utility; Risk Assessment and Risk Management

Further Reading

Bird, H. R, Andrews, H., Schwab-Stone, M., Goodman, S., Dulcan, M., Richters, J., Rubio-Stipec, M., Moore, R. E, Chiang, P., Hoven, C., Canino, G., Fisher, P., & Gould, M. S. (1996). Global measures of impairment for epidemiologic and clinical use with children and adolescents. *International Journal of Methods in Psychiatric Research, 6*, 295–307.

Hodges, K., & Kim, C. S. (2000). Psychometric study of the Child and Adolescent Functional Assessment Scale: Prediction of contact with the law and poor school attendance. *Journal of Abnormal Child Psychology, 28*(3), 287–297.

Manteuffel, B., & Stephens, R. L. (2002). Overview of the national evaluation of the comprehensive community mental health services for children and their families program and summary of current findings. *Children's Services: Social Policy, Research, and Practice, 5*(1), 3–20.

KAY HODGES

Glycogen Storage Disease

DEFINITION

Glycogen storage disease is an autosomal recessive disorder that results in the absence or deficiency of glucose-6-phosphatase that affects the function of the kidney, liver, and lining of the intestine. There are several types of glycogen storage disease (Ia, Ib), each with variations in clinical symptoms.

INCIDENCE

Glycogen storage disease is rare, occurring in 1 of 20,000 live births.

DIAGNOSIS

The diagnosis of glycogen storage disease involves laboratory findings of abnormal lactate and lipid values, a clinical presentation of enlarged liver and/or seizures, and often physical features of puffy cheeks, thin extremities, short stature, and bulging abdomen. A definitive diagnosis requires a liver biopsy. The diagnosis is sometimes made in newborns based on findings of hypoglycemia and lactic acidosis, but most often occurs at 3–4 months of age when the enlarged spleen and seizures are noticed.

CLINICAL SYMPTOMS

In addition to enlarged liver (hepatomegaly) and seizures, clinical symptoms include hypoglycemia and lactic acidosis after fasting, elevated urea and lipid levels, intermittent diarrhea, and easy bruising and prolonged bleeding. Type Ib additionally produces low white blood cell counts (neutropenia) and an increase in the risk for bacterial infections. Puberty is often delayed, but long-term fertility is usually unaffected. As children age into adolescence and young adulthood, gout may present as a symptom, and tumors (benign or malignant) of the liver may develop. Later, pulmonary hypertension and osteoporosis can occur.

TREATMENT

Treatment focuses on maintaining normal blood glucose levels, and primarily involves modification of diet (adding corn starch, limiting fructose and galactose). Dietary supplements of multivitamins and calcium are needed. Allopurinol is given to reduce the levels of uric acid in the system, and granulocyte-macrophage colony stimulating factors (GMCSF) are given to correct low white blood cell counts and reduce the severity of bacterial infections. Because of the risk of prolonged bleeding, good metabolic control should be established and bleeding status evaluated prior to any surgery.

The primary behavioral intervention needed for children with glycogen storage disease is support for parents and children in maintaining the dietary regimen. Attention to changes in adherence with the dietary requirements is important at each developmental transition point.

PROGNOSIS

Prior to early diagnosis and dietary treatment, most children with glycogen storage disease died, and those who survived had many of the clinical symptoms described above. Early treatment appears to have improved the immediate outcome, but long-term outcomes are unknown.

See also: Bleeding Disorders; Bone Marrow Failure and Primary Immunodeficiency; Failure-to-Thrive; Medical Adherence; Short Stature: Psychological Aspects; Storage Diseases; Treatment Adherence

Further Reading

Chen, Y. T. (2000). Defects in metabolism of carbohydrates. In R. E. Behrman, R. M. Kleigman, & H. B. Jenson (Eds.), *Nelson textbook of pediatrics* (16th ed., pp. 406–413). Philadelphia: W.B. Saunders.

F. DANIEL ARMSTRONG

Gonorrhea

See: Sexually Transmitted Diseases in Adolescents

Grief

See: Bereavement

Group Homes

See: Residential Treatment

Group Psychotherapy

Although child treatment often focuses on the individual child, many clinicians have highlighted the distinct advantages of treating children in groups. One obvious advantage of this approach is that it may be more efficient, as several children can be seen in the same amount of time that would usually be spent treating a single child. Additionally, it has been argued that group therapy is the most effective form of treatment for some children such as those with relationship problems, those who are shy, withdrawn and deficient in social skills, or those who are overly aggressive. Here, the socially withdrawn child may learn that it is safe to be more outgoing, and thus develop skills necessary to behave in this manner, while the socializing influence of the group may result in the aggressive child adopting more desirable ways of interacting. As the social interactions within group therapy more closely approximate the child's real world, one might also expect greater generalization of changes to the natural environment than with individual therapy.

Group therapy often provides children with a better understanding of how their behavior is seen by others. And it often helps them learn first hand that their problems are not unique and that effective ways of dealing with problems can often be found by learning how others have dealt with them. These potential advantages suggest that group treatments can have much to offer, especially in cases where problems in the area of peer relationships are of concern.

GROUP COMPOSITION

The nature of therapy groups for children/adolescents varies widely. Most group models recommend 4–8 children per group, with groups for younger children being smaller. Children in groups are usually of similar age in order to maximize similarity of interests and capabilities. Groups can differ in gender but a balance of males and females appears to be important. Usually, groups meet weekly for one-hour-long sessions, although playgroups with young children may be shorter than this and activity group sessions may last up to 2 hr in length. Length of treatment can range from 10 sessions with play therapy groups to 2 years with activity group therapies. Contraindications for group therapy include psychosis, mental retardation, sexually acting-out behaviors, extreme aggression, and sociopathic tendencies.

GROUP THERAPY METHODS

Activity Group Therapy (AGT)

AGT, like the approach to follow, originated in the early 1930s and 1940s with the work of S. R. Slavson, a psychiatrist who worked at the Madelyn Borg Child Guidance Institute in New York. AGT can be viewed as a non-directive, psychoanalytically oriented treatment approach for children ages 8–12 with mildly disordered behavior (i.e., withdrawal, social anxiety) and who have the capacity for relating to peers. The context for therapy consists of children engaging in a range of activities instead of simply talking or playing. This focus on activities is thought to provide an initial avenue for the expression of conflict and a basic framework for the interaction among group members. As therapy progresses, it is assumed that involvement with activities becomes secondary to the interaction among group members and that therapeutic change occurs primarily through such interactions. In AGT, the therapist makes few interpretations and takes a permissive and neutral stance towards children's behavior during sessions. This is intended to create a milieu where working through of important conflicts can be accomplished.

Activity-Interview Group Psychotherapy (A-IGP)

Although this approach is similar to AGT in involving children in a range of therapeutic activities, it was developed for older children displaying more serious problems. Here, the therapist's use of limit setting and guidance makes A-IGP more structured than AGT, and hence more suitable for children and adolescents who are more seriously disturbed. Consistent with the psychoanalytic base of A-IGP, the therapist interprets significant individual and group conflicts during both group activities and group discussions. These interpretations are intended to help the child/adolescent gain insight into the nature of his/her difficulties and resolve internal emotional conflicts.

Group Play Therapy

This psychoanalytically based approach is often utilized for younger children and emphasizes play as the medium of communication. The playgroup, with its symbolic use of play materials and activities, can provide the child with a protective buffer during exploration of emotionally laden thoughts and feelings and a safe environment within which to express and deal with a wide range of problems. This approach is seen as especially useful for children who may have suffered trauma or emotional distress (i.e., physical/sexual abuse, neglect), and who are unable or unwilling to process their experience solely through verbal means.

Behavioral Group Therapy

As the name suggests, this approach focuses on using behavioral principles to modify child and adolescent behavior. A wide range of problematic behaviors can be addressed, including those of an interpersonal (i.e., poor social skills, aggressive behavior, withdrawal) and more intrapersonal (anxiety, stress) nature. Groups are usually composed of 4–8 children of mixed gender who are relatively similar in age. Therapy approaches such as cognitive restructuring and problem solving can also be taught and incorporated into group discussions, making such groups more cognitive-behavioral in nature and applicable to a wider range of problems.

Specialized Groups

These groups often focus on specific issues experienced by children and adolescents. Specialized groups have been used with children displaying a range of chronic illnesses such as diabetes, cystic fibrosis, and cancer. Here, common issues often include children's feelings about their illness, treatment-related concerns, and social adaptation. Other special groups for whom group therapy is often provided include children of divorce, children who have lost a parent through death, children who have experienced trauma from physical or sexual abuse and children of alcoholic parents.

Adolescent Groups

As their participants are older, adolescent groups are typically more verbal in nature than are child groups. Common topics often focus on peer interactions, sexuality, substance use, autonomy, and dealing with authority as well as other issues raised by group members. Inpatient groups frequently deal with issues related to substance abuse (as opposed to substance use), more serious sexually related issues such as rape and sexual abuse, as well as social skills and other interpersonal issues common to adolescents. Inpatient groups also commonly utilize various activities such as recreation, dance, music, and art along with regular group meetings. Educational groups focusing on sexuality, drug education, and suicide prevention, as well as various self-help groups, are also commonly provided for adolescents as well.

EFFECTIVENESS

Despite a therapy outcome literature fraught with methodological problems, one can draw some limited conclusions regarding the issue of effectiveness. For example, a 1976 review found approximately equal numbers of studies yielding positive and null effects, with behavioral groups showing the most evidence of effectiveness.

A more recent metaanalysis of 56 outcome studies published between 1974 and 1997 (Hoag and Burlingame (1997)) has suggested that child/adolescent group therapy is comparable in effectiveness to individual therapy. Here, patients who received group therapy had better outcomes than 73 percent of patients who did not receive group treatment, although psychoanalytic and nondirective group therapy approaches did not seem to be as effective as other approaches.

While there is some support for the effectiveness of certain group therapy approaches there is a need for additional studies comparing group treatments with relevant control groups, studies with larger sample sizes, studies that focus on a wider range of presenting problems, including more severe psychopathology, and studies that focus on specific treatment variables that may be associated with differential outcomes.

See also: Behavior Modification; Client-Centered Therapy; Cognitive–Behavior Therapy; Evidence-Based Treatments; Play Therapy; Psychodynamic Therapy

Further Reading

Dagley, J. C., Gazda, G. M., Eppinger, S. J., & Stewart, E. A. (1994). Group psychotherapy research with children, preadolescents, and adolescents. In A. Fuhriman & G. M. Burlingame (Eds.), *Handbook of group psychotherapy* (pp. 340–369). New York: Wiley.
Hoag, M. J., & Burlingame, G. M. (1997). Evaluating the effectiveness of child and adolescent group treatment: A meta-analytic review. *Journal of Clinical Child Psychology, 26,* 234–246.
Lomonaco, S., Scheidlinger, S., & Aronson, S. (2000). Five decades of children's group treatment: An overview. *Journal of Child and Adolescent Group Therapy, 10,* 77–97.

JAMES H. JOHNSON
STEVEN K. READER

Growth Disorders

See: Congenital Adrenal Hyperplasia; Endocrine Disorders; Feeding Disorders; Gigantism and Acromegaly; Growth Hormone Deficiency; Gynedomastia; Hypothyroidism, Acquired; Hypothyroidism, Congenital; Noonan Syndrome; Prader-Willi Syndrome; Puberty, Delayed; Puberty, Normal; Puberty, Precocious; Short Stature, Psychological Aspects

Growth Hormone Deficiency

DESCRIPTION AND PREVALENCE

The pituitary gland, which is divided into two lobes (the anterior and posterior pituitary), rests in a depression in the base of the skull and secretes hormones influencing body growth, metabolism, and the activity of other endocrine glands. It is sometimes referred to as the "master gland," a reference to its regulatory role in regard to several other endocrine glands. Growth Hormone (GH) is an anterior pituitary hormone and is best recognized for its growth-promoting actions in children and adolescents. GH is also understood to exert important metabolic and body composition benefits in adulthood. Pituitary GH secretion is stimulated by GH-releasing hormone from the hypothalamus, a region of the brain controlling the anterior pituitary gland. The prevalence of GH deficiency (GHD) in children in the United States has been estimated at approximately 1 in 3,500 and is twice as common in boys than in girls.

ETIOLOGY

GHD may result from disruption of the GH axis in the higher brain, hypothalamus, or pituitary. The pituitary gland may be congenitally small, deformed, or absent. It may be damaged by trauma or tumors of the central nervous system. Therapeutic radiation of tumors of the brain is an additional cause. Disease factors in the etiology of GHD may also be responsible for deficits of other pituitary hormones. An additional cause of GHD is physical or psychological abuse and/or neglect. While most instances of isolated GHD are idiopathic (of unknown cause), specific disease states are typically responsible when GHD is associated with multiple pituitary hormone deficiencies (MPHD). It is thus understandable that psychological adaptation, including intellectual functioning, will vary according to the etiology of the pituitary insufficiency (hypopituitarism).

ASSESSMENT

In a child with short stature and slow growth whose medical history and pattern of growth over time suggest GHD, testing requires the measurement of IGF-I (insulin-like growth factor 1) / IGFBP-3 (IGF-binding protein) levels in blood and GH stimulation tests. In suspected

GHD, two pharmacological GH stimulation tests are required. These tests are performed either on an inpatient or outpatient basis. Because these tests are far from perfect in differentiating between a normal and abnormal functioning GH axis, it is important that the clinician integrates all available data (clinical, growth history, radiological, and biochemical) when making a diagnosis.

ASSOCIATED PSYCHOLOGICAL FEATURES

The psychosocial and educational adaptation of individuals with GHD has been the focus of many studies. The majority of the difficulties experienced by these individuals in their daily functioning has been (mis)attributed to short stature, the most visibly salient characteristic in childhood of untreated GHD. (The social consequences of short stature are reviewed elsewhere [see *Short Stature: Psychological Aspects*]).

There is, however, increasing evidence that the psychosocial or psychiatric problems sometimes reported in GHD are due to factors other than short stature. For example, it was recently demonstrated in a relatively large study of adults previously treated for GHD that the subgroup with MPHD was experiencing a poorer quality of life than those with isolated GHD, in spite of comparable heights. Those with isolated GHD were indistinguishable in their daily functioning from healthy siblings. This same study failed to demonstrate an association between the relative amounts of growth achieved during GH therapy and psychological outcome variables assessed in adulthood. Nor was adult height predictive of quality of life or psychological distress. In a different study comparing adults with hypopituitarism, largely with MPHD, and equally short but untreated healthy volunteers, individuals with hypopituitarism exhibited impaired cardiovascular reactivity to a social-stress test. Those with MPHD also showed lower assertiveness but greater "neuroticism" than comparison subjects.

Higher than expected rates of grade retention or academic underachievement are commonly reported among those with GHD. Studies of isolated GHD, however, have revealed intellectual functioning that falls in the average range. There remains a question of whether GHD may be associated with specific cognitive deficits. In contrast, those with MPHD are more likely to exhibit lower IQ and experience school problems. In a recent study of children and adolescents receiving GH therapy, between 18 and 29 percent of youths were performing poorly in at least one of four key academic domains, and 26 percent had been classified as educationally "handicapped." Those with pathological growth failure, for example, MPHD, septo-optic dysplasia or intrauterine growth retardation, exhibited greater academic failure than those with isolated GHD or idiopathic (healthy) short stature. Most importantly, neither the severity of short stature, nor the growth-responsiveness to treatment was significantly related to academic functioning. Such differences in academic performance between subgroups of patients with short stature once again strongly suggest that factors other than stressful psychosocial experiences related to height are responsible for the observed deficits.

TREATMENT

GHD is treated with daily subcutaneous injections of GH. In the case of children and adolescents, the first year of treatment is associated with the largest increase in growth velocity (catch-up growth). This faster-than-normal growth rate slowly declines over time, but it continues to be greater than would occur without treatment. Treatment is often associated with an increase in the child's appetite and loss of body fat. GH therapy continues over several years and typically ends when maximum growth potential has been achieved. Individuals receiving GH therapy should not expect to achieve an adult height in excess of what would be expected based upon family genetic potential. The risk of unfulfilled expectations is real and can be countered with adequate counseling prior to and during the course of treatment. The prescribing of GH to individuals with childhood-onset GHD should be restricted to pediatric endocrinologists.

Not all children with GHD will remain deficient in adulthood. For this reason, it is important that as each GH deficient teen reaches adulthood, studies should be performed to determine need for continuing therapy. The justification for lifelong GH replacement stems from its beneficial effects on body composition, bone density, lipid metabolism, cardiovascular function, and physical performance.

PROGNOSIS

With timely diagnosis and treatment, children with GHD can achieve their full growth potential. Derived gains beyond improved growth velocity and taller relative height stature should not be expected. However, individual children and adolescents for whom short stature represents a challenge to their positive self-image may experience a sense of relief with the onset of treatment.

See also: Coping with Illness; Short Stature: Psychological Aspects

Further Reading

Sandberg, D. E., MacGillivray, M. H., Clopper, R. R., Fung, C., LeRoux, L., & Alliger, D. E. (1998). Quality of life (QOL) among formerly treated child-onset growth hormone-deficient (GHD) adults: A comparison with unaffected siblings. *Journal of Clinical Endocrinology & Metabolism, 83,* 1134–1142.

Sandberg, D. E., Ognibene, T. C., Brook, A. E., Barrick, C., Shine, B., & Grundner, W. (1998). Academic adjustment among children and adolescents receiving growth hormone therapy. *Children's Health Care, 27,* 265–282.

Sandberg, D. E., & Voss, L. (in press). The psychosocial consequences of short stature: A review of the evidence. *Baillière's Best Practice & Research. Clinical Endocrinology and Metabolism.*

DAVID E. SANDBERG

Gynecomastia

DESCRIPTION AND INCIDENCE

Gynecomastia is the development of unilateral or bilateral palpable breast tissue in males. It usually begins with a small lump beneath the nipple that may be tender. Enlargement of breasts is usually uneven. Gynecomastia can occur in newborns (which is associated with galactorrhea or milk flow), adolescents, and the elderly.

Gynecomastia is common, especially in adolescence. Approximately 60 percent of boys develop some sort of subareolar growth in the breast during adolescence, which spontaneously regresses (transient gynecomastia). The median age of onset is 14 years.

ETIOLOGY

In newborns, gynecomastia can result from the presence of maternal or placental estrogens. In adolescents, during the normal course of puberty, breast tissue develops when estradiol reaches adult levels prior to testosterone. Exposure to drugs that contain or act as estrogens (such as dermal ointments, cosmetic creams, oral contraceptives, estrogen-injected animal meat, etc.) can result in the development of gynecomastia. Drugs that inhibit the synthesis of testosterone (ketocanazole, metronidazole) or restrain the action of testosterone by blocking testosterone receptors (spironolactone and antiandrogens such as cyproterone, flutamide, zanoterone and bicalutamide) can also produce gynecomastia.

Careful investigation of a patient's drug history (including indirect exposure to estrogens) and a limited endocrine work-up (in which elevated levels of plasma estradiol or urinary 17-ketosteriods may be present) can help determine the cause of the gynecomastia. In adults, gynecomastia can result from chronic liver disease due to increased concentrations of plasma estrogens. In rare cases, the secretion of estrogen by tumors can result in gynecomastia. Gynecomastia can also appear as a feature of clinical syndromes such as Klinefelter syndrome, Reifenstein's syndrome, primary hypogonadism, and untreated hyperthyroidism.

DIAGNOSIS

Gynecomastia may be difficult to distinguish from lipomastia, which is breast enlargement due to adipose tissue (fatty tissue). However, a definitive diagnosis can be made through the use of mammography or ultrasonography.

ASSOCIATED PSYCHOLOGICAL FEATURES

The development of breast tissue in an adolescent boy can be emotionally distressing. Based on clinical experience, embarrassment can cause the affected individual to avoid social activities in which the chest is exposed or otherwise noticeable (swimming and other sports). In extreme cases this situation is associated with a depressed mood and/or anxious state. The influence of gynecomastia on psychosocial adaptation has been associated with the age of onset of the disorder; young adolescent boys (9–12 years) show little effect, whereas older boys are sensitized to the social significance of having breasts and may feel insecure about their masculinity. Systematic research on the psychological features associated with gynecomastia is scarce.

TREATMENT

If the amount of breast tissue is less than 3–4 centimeters in diameter, gynecomastia usually regresses spontaneously within approximately three months. When treating boys with gynecomastia, it is important to reassure them, and their families, of the temporary nature of the disorder. If the condition persists, treatment with the androgen dihydrotestosterone can improve symptoms. If the amount of breast tissue is more than 3–4 centimeters in diameter, it is less likely to regress spontaneously. If the condition does not subside over time or with medical treatment, surgery can be considered to address psychological or cosmetic concerns.

PROGNOSIS

Gynecomastia is typically a short-lived condition. In newborns, breast development is usually reversed within a few weeks. In most adolescents, gynecomastia resolves once the estrogen/testosterone ratio achieves a normative balance. In most cases, the condition does not persist for more than 1–3 years. Gynecomastia does not place boys at an increased risk for developing breast cancer except when it is associated with Klinefelter syndrome.

See also: Adolescence; Klinefelter Syndrome; Sexual Development

Further Reading

Jenkins, M. (1985). Adolescent gynecomastia. In F. Lifshitz (Ed.), *Pediatric endocrinology: A clinical guide* (pp. 171–178). New York: Marcel Dekker.

Frantz, A., & Wilson, J. (1998). Endocrine disorders of the breast. In J. Wilson, D. Foster, H. Kronenberg, & P. Larsen (Eds.), *Williams textbook of endocrinology* 9th ed. (pp. 877–900). Philadelphia, PA: W.B. Saunders.

TERESA WIECH
TOM MAZUR
DAVID E. SANDBERG

Hh

Habit Reversal

DEFINITION

Habit reversal is a multicomponent treatment procedure for repetitive behavior problems. The child is taught the procedure in session and asked to implement it outside of session. Habit reversal as originally developed by Azrin and Nunn (1973) consisted of 13 treatment components separated into four phases: (1) awareness training, (2) competing response training, (3) motivation procedures, and (4) generalization training. Extensive research since then has yielded a much simplified version consisting of only four components divided into just three phases (awareness training, competing response training, and social support training). Simplified habit reversal (SHR) has been found to be as effective as the more complex prototype and it will be described here.

METHOD

The entire SHR procedure can be taught to children in one session and this teaching is reinforced in subsequent booster sessions as needed. The teaching begins with awareness training. It has two components: response description and response detection. Response description involves requiring children to thoroughly describe their target repetitive behaviors and all preceding behaviors or "warning signs," both public and private (collectively referred to as target behaviors hereafter). Response detection initially involves therapist

simulation of the target behaviors and child detection of the simulations. When children can readily detect the clinician's simulations, they are asked to begin detecting in-session occurrences of their own target behaviors. If the target behaviors do not occur in session, the children are asked to simulate them and practice detecting their simulations. After the therapist determines that the children can adequately detect their target behaviors, competing response training begins.

Competing response training involves teaching children to engage in behaviors that are incompatible with the target behaviors for at least 1 min contingent on the emission of (or urge to emit) those behaviors (see Table 1 for a sample of competing responses). Initially, the therapist models the proper use of competing responses contingent on the emission of simulated target behaviors. Then children practice exhibiting competing responses contingent upon emission of actual target behaviors. As in awareness training, if the target behaviors do not naturally occur in session, children

Table 1. Examples of Competing Responses

Repetitive behavior	Competing response
Vocal tics	Diaphragmatic breathing
Motor tics	
Shoulder jerking	Depress shoulders
Arm flapping	Press arms against sides
Head jerking/shaking	Tense neck
Jaw stretching	Press lips together
Hard eye blinking	Tense eyes open
Nail biting	Make fists with hands
Thumb/finger sucking	Make fists with hands
Hair pulling	Make fists with hands
Skin picking	Make fists with hands

practice on simulated occurrences. Lastly, children are instructed to continue to use the competing response outside whenever the emission of, or urge to emit, target behaviors occurs. Then social support training begins.

Social support training involves teaching important persons in the children's life (e.g., parents or teachers) to assist the children with correct implementation of the competing response outside of treatment sessions. Specifically, the social support person is taught to: (1) prompt children's use of competing responses when they exhibit the target behaviors and (2) praise (reinforce) correct use of the competing responses.

Although the three phases of habit reversal can be taught in one session, booster sessions are usually needed to strengthen the teaching and maintain practice of treatment components. During booster sessions children are asked to demonstrate the proper use of the SHR procedure. If any components are forgotten or not demonstrated correctly, they are reviewed according to the procedure used in the initial session. The booster sessions are also used to address any concerns or problems experienced by the client.

CLINICAL APPLICATIONS

SHR has been found to be an effective treatment for many repetitive behaviors including: motor and vocal tics, nail biting, thumb/finger sucking, hair pulling, skin picking, and cheek biting. Modified versions of the procedure have been used to treat stuttering and aggressive behaviors. The procedure has been found effective for treating repetitive behaviors in children, adolescents, and adults of different genders and ethnicities. Despite the simplification of SHR compared to the complex prototype, it may be difficult for preschool-age children to learn and practice and there is little research on its use with them.

EFFECTIVENESS

Habit reversal is currently listed as a "probably efficacious" treatment for habit behaviors on the American Psychological Association's list of empirically validated treatments. The initial evaluation by Azrin and Nunn (1973) convincingly demonstrated the effectiveness of the full habit reversal treatment. This investigation included 12 participants (age range 5–64) with a variety of repetitive behaviors including motor and vocal tics, hair pulling, thumb/finger sucking, and nail biting. Results

showed virtual elimination of the repetitive behaviors as a result of treatment, with results being maintained for 11 of the 12 participants at a 5-month follow-up. Subsequent research has shown that the simplified version (SHR) is as effective as the original procedure. Research also shows that the competing response is probably the most important component of the treatment and may be necessary for SHR to be effective. Additional research indicates that practice of the competing response should occur for one minute or longer.

See also: Nail Biting; Stereotypic Movement Disorder; Tic Disorders: Tourette's Disorder, Chronic Tic Disorder, and Transient Tic Disorder; Trichotillomania

Further Reading

Azrin, N. H., & Nunn, R. G. (1973). Habit reversal: A method of eliminating nervous habits and tics. *Behaviour Research and Therapy, 11*, 619–628.

Miltenberger, R. G., Fuqua, R. W., & Woods, D. W. (1996). Applying behavior analysis to clinical problems: Review and analysis of habit reversal. *Journal of Applied Behavior Analysis, 31*, 447–469.

Woods, D. W., & Twohig, M. P. (2001). Habit reversal manual for oral-digital habits. In D. W. Woods & R. G. Miltenberger (Eds.), *Tic disorders, trichotillomania, and other repetitive behavior disorders: Behavioral approaches to analysis and treatment* (241–268). Norwell, MA: Kluwer Academic.

MICHAEL TWOHIG
PATRICK C. FRIMAN

Hair-Pulling

See: Trichotillomania

Hashimoto's Encephalopathy

DEFINITION AND SYMPTOMS

Hashimoto's encephalopathy (HE) is a disorder characterized by persistent or relapsing neurologic and/or neuropsychiatric deficits that are associated with elevated blood concentrations of antithyroid antibodies, reflecting the body's autoimmune "attack" on the thyroid. The clinical presentation varies and may include seizures, altered consciousness, involuntary movements, psychotic episodes, and hallucinations. Confusion, memory impairments, and apathy may also be evident. In adults, HE usually begins with an acute stroke-like event, or as an insidious decline in cognitive functioning. The clinical picture in adolescents with HE is often an abrupt, sometimes subclinical, onset of seizures and encephalopathy that is characterized by confusion, as well as other mental status changes such as hallucinations. A pattern of progressive cognitive deterioration manifested only as a drop in school performance may be present.

INCIDENCE

Relatively few pediatric cases are described in the clinical literature, making it difficult to estimate prevalence or incidence. Based upon available data, the average age at presentation is around 14 years in females. HE in males is so rarely reported that abstracted incidence or age of onset statistics may be even less reliable.

ETIOLOGY

In the absence of definitive neuropathologic findings, the mechanism of effects causing HE remains poorly defined. An immune-mediated pathophysiology, such as an autoimmune cerebral vasculitis or an anti-neuronal antibody-mediated reaction is strongly suspected, with a few authors proposing a toxic effect of thyroid-releasing hormone on the central nervous system. Canton and colleagues (2000) have proposed the term "encephalopathy associated to autoimmune thyroid disease" as a more descriptive nomenclature.

MEDICAL ASSESSMENT

HE is variously diagnosed by antithyroid antibody levels, elevated cerebral spinal fluid (CSF) protein, focal neurologic findings, electroencephalogram (EEG) tracings, and/or neuropsychological test results. However, the primary diagnostic test is evaluation for thyroid autoantibodies, which may remain elevated despite clinical improvement. (Indeed, thyroid autoantibody titers should be considered even when thyroid function tests are normal since patients often develop this syndrome when in an euthyroid, or only mildly hypothyroid, state.)

Diffuse background slowing is the most common EEG abnormality in adolescents with HE, with the temporal lobe sometimes being specifically affected. In young patients with HE, neuroimaging studies are neither sensitive nor specific. Computerized axial tomography (CAT) is usually normal, although it may reveal cerebral atrophy or ventricular dilation. Cranial magnetic resonance imaging (MRI) is more sensitive, but not more specific in detection. Cranial magnetic resonance angiography (MRA) may be helpful during an acute episode. Neuropsychological testing can define performance deficits, and/or uncover significant scatter among cognitive abilities that may be inconsistent with past academic history.

DIFFERENTIAL DIAGNOSIS

Due to its diffuse neurological and psychiatric symptomatology, HE may be underdiagnosed, especially at initial presentation. Diagnosis is complicated by the multiple possible etiologies of acute mental status changes in children and adolescents, including trauma, vascular lesions, developing structural abnormalities, and seizures, as well as a variety of infectious and toxic-metabolic encephalopathies. Accurate psychiatric/psychological diagnosis often benefits from the inclusion of organic brain syndrome (OBS), including HE, in the differential diagnosis whenever otherwise unexplained confusion and hallucinations occur, even in the apparent absence of associated seizure activity or focal neurological signs. A case example demonstrates the difficulties in the diagnosis of HE.

The authors consulted on a 14-year-old patient who, after several inconclusive efforts at diagnosis, was found to have HE. By history, the patient had had two seizure-like episodes. Each was atypical, characterized by altered consciousness and followed by an extended period of confusion. Neurological and physical exams were unremarkable. Video EEG conducted during a hospital admission was normal. Consulting pediatric psychologists were asked to consider the possibilities of pseudoseizures, depression, and anorexia nervosa in this thin young woman. No diagnosis ensued during an otherwise unremarkable hospital stay. The patient returned 12 h following discharge with another seizure-like episode, a stuporous state lasting about 14 h, episodic confusion, and autonomic dysregulation. Over the next two days, her mental status was characterized by auditory, visual, and olfactory hallucinations. These symptoms were judged to evidence an OBS; however, no hypothesized etiologic process fit the picture and no toxin was identified. Repeated EEG and neuroimaging studies were negative and could not confirm epileptic activity. The nature of her affect and content of her verbalizations were sufficiently specific to raise the possibility of Posttraumatic

Stress Disorder (PTSD) with psychotic features. This triggered an investigation for possible chronic sexual abuse. During a subsequent admission to an adolescent inpatient psychiatry unit for continued diagnosis and management of her psychotic symptoms, both PTSD and Munchausen's by Proxy Syndrome (MbPS) were considered briefly as she again became symptomatic immediately following a parental visit. However, she progressed to status epilepticus, with accompanying development of tachycardia, hypertension, mydriasis, and delirium, followed by agitation and social disinhibition. A concurrent EEG found diffuse slowing, as well as generalized and periodic lateralized epileptiform discharges over the left hemisphere. Otherwise, besides a positive test for antithyroid antibodies, only a fortuitous MRA that revealed irregular areas of mild narrowing of both middle cerebral arteries, consistent with a CNS vasculopathy, was positive. Indeed, even the repeat MRA one week later appeared normal. This patient responded well to steroid treatment. Follow-up at 6 and 12 months demonstrated continued recovery, with a lessening of the 40 point split between her Verbal and Performance IQ found on a WISC-III administered just prior to initial discharge, however, not before her cognitive functioning had dropped further in the aftermath of the final episode.

In the absence of either physical findings on initial exam or confirmatory neuroimaging results, a high index of suspicion is necessary to differentiate between rare metabolic disorders and toxic encephalopathy. In adolescent girls who present with recurrent or progressive encephalopathy, thyroid autoantibodies should be considered, since early intervention can rapidly reverse clinical symptoms and may prevent additional morbidity that may result from undiagnosed HE.

MEDICAL TREATMENT

Clinical improvement is evident in patients treated with steroids. However, reoccurrence of symptoms when the corticosteroids are withdrawn, or even while taking them, has been reported.

PSYCHOLOGICAL ASSESSMENT AND INTERVENTIONS

Progress toward normalization of EEG patterns and reduction of neuropsychological deficits are accepted benchmarks for monitoring response to and duration of steroid medication therapy. Adolescents with HE may be left with mild cognitive sequellae even when early

recognition and prompt treatment are instituted. Thus, repeated psychoeducational or neuropsychological testing is required to both assess for signs of relapse and assure that appropriate environmental supports are in place for immediate coping, as well as for longer-term psychosocial and academic adaptation. Psychological interventions may help the adolescent and her family adapt to their experiences with HE. Mental health professionals can also monitor success of social reentry, assure that effective environmental accommodations are implemented, facilitate a return to more normal family routines, and encourage, within the bounds of appropriate expectations, increasingly more autonomous functioning.

See also: Bone Marrow Failure and Primary Immunodeficiency; Coping with Illness; Epilepsy; Neurological Disorders; Neuropsychological Assessment

Further Reading

Canton, A., de Fabregas, O., Tintor, M., Mesa, J., Codina, A., & Simo, R. (2000). Encephalopathy associated to autoimmune thyroid disease: A more appropriate term for an underestimated condition? *Journal of Neurologic Science, 176,* 65–69.

Isik, U., Tennison, M., & D'Cruz, O. (2001). Recurrent encephalopathy and seizures in an adolescent girl. *Clinical Pediatrics, 40,* 273–275.

Shaws, P. J., Walls, T. J., & Newman, P. K. (1991). Hashimoto's encephalopathy: A steroid responsive disorder associated with high antithyroid antibody titers—report of 5 cases. *Neurology, 41,* 228–233.

Vasconcellos, E., Pina-Garza, J. E., Fakhoury, T., & Finichel, G. M. (1999). Pediatric manifestations of Hashimoto's encephalopathy. *Pediatric Neurology, 20,* 394–398.

J. KENNETH WHITT
ELENA LEA

Head Start

HISTORY AND DEFINITION

Head Start is a program that was created in 1965 to ensure that economically disadvantaged 3–5-year-old children would begin school at the same readiness level as more privileged children. As part of President Johnson's "War on Poverty," Head Start was created through the Office of Economic Opportunity. To this day, the mission of Head Start is not only to provide an academic advantage to these children, but also to provide them with social, emotional, and health advantages that they might not otherwise receive. Furthermore, children in Head Start are given mental health services, nutritional education, and hot meals. Even though all Head Start schools follow this general mission, each community adapts its program to meet local needs and uses local resources to meet these goals. It is common for children in Head Start to attend preschool at a local center for several hours each day, as part of a more comprehensive program. Yet, individualized, home-based options are also available. Specific services typically include health and developmental screenings (e.g., dental, vision, speech, hearing), parent education, home visits, and family support.

HEAD START PROGRAMS

Since Head Start's inception, several programs have been implemented in an attempt to better serve the Head Start population. For example, the Education for Parenthood program was developed to teach parenting and child abuse prevention skills to adolescents. Also, Parent and Child Development Centers were created and used to evaluate parents' roles in infant development. A support program for children up to age 8, the Child and Family Resource Program, was created to provide additional services (e.g., child care, health services) to parents. Furthermore, Head Start created programs to provide school-aged children with services. These programs—Project Follow Through, Project Developmental Continuity, and the Head Start Transition Project—attempted to continue the benefits of Head Start through elementary school. To address the competency of child care staff in Head Start, The Child Development Associate program was created to provide training to these individuals.

The most recent Head Start program is Early Head Start, which began in 1995 and services children under the age of 3 years. Early Head Start's mission is to provide economically disadvantaged infants and toddlers with increased social, emotional, health, and academic opportunities. Specifically, Early Head Start provides services such as child care, home visits, case management, and parent education beginning before birth. Just as with Head Start, this program follows specific principles (e.g., parent involvement, prevention, comprehensiveness), but each program differs, taking into account individual community needs (e.g., home-based services).

Preliminary research on this program suggests that it has some positive effects. Specifically, children in the Early Head Start program have higher cognitive

development scores as assessed at age 2 than children not in the program. Also, parents reported that these children have larger vocabularies and use more complex sentences than control children. Additionally, the parents of Early Head Start children have been found to be more supportive, sensitive, and stimulating of their children's cognitive development (e.g., language, reading, parent-child play), than families of children not in an early intervention program. Although the effects of these programs are modest, overall research concerning Early Head Start suggests that this is a promising program for economically disadvantaged infants and toddlers.

PARENTAL INVOLVEMENT

Because Head Start was started as a community-based program, parental involvement has been a key component. For example, parents volunteer to aid in the classroom, attend meetings and workshops addressing parenting skills, and allow Head Start staff to visit their homes. Parent involvement in Head Start has had a positive effect on parent functioning in addition to providing services to Head Start schools. Specifically, parent volunteers have increased career development opportunities compared to parents that do not volunteer in the Head Start classroom.

RESEARCH/EFFECTIVENESS

A great deal of research has been conducted concerning the effects of Head Start on the children's social, emotional, health, and academic development. Compared to children not in preschool, children in Head Start have increased receptive vocabulary, IQ scores, sociocognitive skills, and motor inhibition skills at the end of the year. Additionally, children in Head Start have demonstrated gains in social competency. Furthermore, these children receive more health care and better nutrition than economically disadvantaged children not in Head Start. Concerning long-term effects, Head Start children missed fewer days of school once in elementary school. Because much research has replicated these findings, some consider Head Start to be the most effective program developed during the "War on Poverty."

In contrast to these positive findings, some research suggests that there are limitations to the success of Head Start. For example, some studies have found that children who complete Head Start are not at the same level as children who complete some other preschool programs (e.g., private preschools) when they enter elementary school. Also, the gains that are achieved while in Head Start (e.g., cognitive, social) have not been shown to maintain over time. Advocates of Head Start suggest, however, that one year of Head Start should not be expected to be sufficient to provide children with an even start throughout high school, considering all of the stressors associated with being economically disadvantaged (e.g., less opportunities). Efforts to expand services through the development of Early Head Start and other programs are expected to enhance its effectiveness and address some of the current concerns. Yet, future investigations are needed to determine Head Start's overall impact on the lives of economically disadvantaged children.

See also: Early Intervention; Intellectual Assessment; Parent Training

Further Reading

Head Start research and evaluation Web site (n.d.). Retrieved May 10, 2002, from http://www.acf.dhhs.gov/programs/hsre
Raikes, H. H., & Love, J. L. (2002). Early Head Start: A dynamic new program for infants and toddlers and their families. *Infant Mental Health Journal, 23,* 1–13.
Zigler, E., F., & Muenchow, S. (1992). *Head Start: The inside story of America's most successful educational experiment.* New York: Basic Books.
Zigler, E. F., & Styfco, S. (1994). Head Start: Criticisms in a constructive context. *American Psychologist, 49,* 127–132.

HOLLY A. FILCHECK
CHERYL B. MCNEIL

Headache

DEFINITION

Loosely defined by the International Headache Society as "pain located above the orbitomeatal line," headaches (HA) are a common complaint among children and can present with a variety of associated symptoms, which include nausea, photosensitivity, ringing in ears, and double vision. HA, especially if recurrent, can cause considerable distress to the child, and lead to difficulties in school and at home.

EPIDEMIOLOGY

HA is the single most common reason for referral to a pediatric neurologist. As children age, the prevalence of HA increases dramatically. It has been reported that by age 3, 3–8 percent have had HA; by age 5, 19.5 percent have had HA; by age 7, 37–51.5 percent have had HA; and by age 15, 57–82 percent have had HA. Gender does not appear to affect the occurrence of HA until puberty, when girls tend to have more HA than boys. The role of ethnic and socioeconomic factors in pediatric HA has received little attention thus far.

CLASSIFICATION OF HEADACHE

Currently, HA can be classified into one of five categories based on the temporal pattern of their symptoms and severity:

1. acute, which is a single event with no prior HA events;
2. acute recurrent, which involves the repetition of HA events of similar severity;
3. chronic progressive, which worsen in frequency and severity across time;
4. chronic nonprogressive, which maintain their level of frequency and severity across time; and
5. mixed, which is a combination of acute and chronic conditions.

CAUSES

The majority of HA are referred to as "primary HA," in that they are the primary presenting problem, and no underlying significant pathology is suspected. While the mechanisms of HA involve the rapid expansion and contraction of vasculature (blood vessels) precipitating excitatory potentials in pain receptors in the vasculature, many physiological and emotional factors have been shown to serve as trigger mechanisms. These HA may be due to exacerbations of existing medical conditions (e.g., allergies, low blood sugar, high blood pressure, dental disease), exposure to certain foods or medications, normal developmental changes (e.g., puberty), or seemingly nonsignificant events (e.g., bump on the head). Emotional distress (e.g., trouble at school or home) may also manifest as or exacerbate HA. Although the majority of HA are not due to serious neurological disease, HA are associated with brain tumors, vascular disruption, and increased intracranial pressure, so a thorough medical examination is warranted.

ASSESSMENT

When evaluating a child with HA, a thorough history of the events will examine whether the child has one or more types, of HA, when or how they began, if the course is stable or progressive, how long they last, where the pain is, what the pain is like, what the associate symptoms are, what triggers them, and what makes them feel better or worse. Information should be gathered from both the child and parents. A thorough evaluation of the child and family's reaction to the HA is essential, and should include evaluating reinforcement contingencies, avoidance behaviors, stress, and depression or anxiety as contributing factors. A medical and family history is also useful, as are recent physical and neurological examinations. Several clinical assessment scales have been developed that are appropriate for children as young as 3–5 years old. Similarly, a child's drawings can provide insight into the type of pain he/she experiences.

TREATMENT

Although there are a number of pharmacological and medical interventions for HA, many parents prefer psychological and nonpharmacological treatments. Initial reassurance can allay fears from the parent and child that the HA is not a sign of a serious neurological disease. Education in the proper use of analgesic medications (i.e., useful at the first sign of an HA, but not as a daily preventive tool) can minimize HA events. Changes in lifestyle (e.g., regular sleep patterns, avoiding chaotic and overtaxing schedules, avoiding foods that trigger HA) have been shown to decrease HA frequency and severity. Stress management and various relaxation techniques (e.g., progressive muscle relaxation, guided imagery, self-hypnosis) have also been useful. Cognitive restructuring may allow the child to identify and challenge negative thoughts surrounding his/her HA (e.g., "my headache will never go away"). In thermal biofeedback, the child learns to affect skin temperature as a way of exerting control over his/her own body and HA. Lastly, individual or family therapy may be beneficial in addressing causes for emotional distress within the child, which may manifest as or exacerbate HA. Effective management of HA often requires a multimodal approach in which several of the above methods are incorporated into an individual treatment plan.

See also: Cognitive–Behavior Therapy; Migraines; Pain Assessment; Pain Management; Stress Management

Further Reading

McGrath, P. A., & Hillier, L. M. (2001). *The child with headache: Diagnosis and treatment.* Seattle: IASP Press.

Winner, P., & Rothner, A. D. (2001). *Headache in children and adolescents.* Lewiston, NY: B.C. Decker.

KEVIN DUFF
JAMES SCOTT

Health Care Professionals (General)

Modern pediatric health care depends upon the skills and services of a variety of professionals who care for children and adolescents. Interdisciplinary collaboration and coordination of care between medical, mental health, and other providers now represents the state of the art in health care.

Medical care providers include *physicians (MD or DO)*. They are medical doctors who prevent, diagnose, and treat diseases and problematic health conditions. Primary care physicians (general *pediatricians and family medicine physicians*) treat general medical problems and usually assume primary responsibility for overseeing the comprehensive health care of and services for children and adolescents. Other physicians focus on one area of medicine such as surgery, radiology, ophthalmology, otolaryngology, dermatology, orthopedics, and a number of other specialty medical fields.

Physicians rely on the assistance of other medical professionals. *Nurses* are medical providers who care for sick and injured children and assist with prevention of illness and health promotion. A *registered nurse* (RN) may assist physicians during treatments and examinations, monitor a child's condition, give medications and vaccinations, and keep patient medical records up-to-date. A *licensed practical nurse* (LPN) assists registered nurses by providing routine patient care. Advanced practice nurses, such as nurse practitioners and certified nurse midwives, are registered nurses who have completed specialized training. *Pediatric nurse practitioners* (PNP) perform many important functions that were once done only by physicians, including giving physical examinations, diagnosing and treating minor illnesses, and sometimes prescribing medications. Nurse practitioners also provide health education and advice to families. Like nurse practitioners, a *physician assistant* (PA) provides some aspects of basic medical care under the supervision of a physician. They take medical histories, perform physical examinations, order tests and procedures, and make preliminary diagnoses; and some prescribe medication.

There are other medical professionals involved in pediatric care. *Chiropractors* (DC) manipulate or adjust the spine and other parts of the body to treat some conditions such as back pain. *Dentists* (DDS or DDM) prevent, diagnose, and treat problems of the teeth, jaws, and gums. *Optometrists* (OD) diagnose vision problems and prescribe and fit corrective eyeglasses and contact lenses. *Podiatrists* (DPM) diagnose, treat, and prevent diseases and conditions of the foot and lower leg.

Mental health providers are playing an increasingly important role in health care of children. *Pediatric and child clinical psychologists* (PhD or PsyD) are doctors involved in prevention, diagnosis, and treatment of child and adolescent mental disorders. In addition, psychologists are often integral to the treatment of children with medical conditions by facilitating adjustment (e.g., by teaching effective coping techniques) or by identifying and treating stress-related medical problems (e.g., headaches). *Child and adolescent psychiatrists* are physicians who specialize in diagnosing and treating mental disorders. Because of their expertise with medical treatments, psychiatrists are often consulted about prescribing psychotropic medications to children and adolescents.

Medical social workers (MSW or LISW) help children and their families cope with the social and emotional aspects of illness. Social workers provide counseling and support and help patients arrange for care after leaving the hospital. In emergency room and clinic settings, social workers are often called in to provide family social support and to link families to needed outpatient community services.

There are several kinds of therapists and other professionals who provide specialized treatments or services that are an important part of many child treatment plans. *Physical therapists* (PT) use physical means such as exercise to improve a child's ability to move or function normally. *Occupational therapists* (OT) help children with illnesses or disabilities develop, recover, or maintain skills necessary for work or daily living. *Speech–language therapists/pathologists* (SLP) work with children with speech and language problems, such as delayed speech onset, articulation problems, and aphasia. Physical, occupational, and speech therapists play a particularly vital role in the ongoing care of children with developmental disabilities. *Audiologists* (MA, FAAA) detect and diagnose hearing problems, and may fit children with hearing aids. *Recreational therapists* guide patients in games, dance, arts and crafts, or other enjoyable activities to maintain physical and emotional well-being. Likewise, *child life workers* facilitate a child's adjustment to hospitalization or medical procedures through play, distraction techniques, and facilitating social activities between patients. *Respiratory therapists* (CRT or RRT) provide evaluations and treatments for children who have respiratory problems from disorders such as cystic fibrosis, asthma, and bronchiopulmonary dysplasia (BPD). *Dietitians* (RD), also called nutritionists, evaluate and plan balanced diets for children and adolescents and assist in evaluating and treating feeding problems. *Pharmacists* (PharmBS or PharmD) fill prescriptions for medications written by physicians and other health practitioners. They also provide patients with instructions on how to take the medication and inform them of possible side effects. *Genetic counselors* work with individuals and families to understand the ramifications of a current genetic condition or the risk of occurrence/recurrence of a genetic condition.

Some medical services require high levels of a special technical skill. *Medical technologists* perform laboratory tests. *Radiology technologists* prepare children for imaging procedures such as X-rays, ultrasound, computed tomography (CT), and magnetic resonance imaging (MRI). *Emergency medical technicians* (EMTs) and/or paramedics arrive by helicopter or ambulance to the scenes of emergencies, administer urgent medical care to critically ill or injured people, and then transport them to medical facilities.

Many children with chronic illnesses receive care from a team of health professionals. For example, many children with cancer receive treatment from several cancer physician specialists including a pediatric oncologist (who prescribes cancer drugs), radiation oncologists (who use radiation to shrink tumors), and surgeons. Moreover, cancer care teams may also include pediatric psychologists, social workers, child life workers, and specially trained nurses.

See also: Child and Adolescent Psychiatrist; Clinical Child and Adolescent Psychology; Family Physician; Genetic Counseling; Nursing; Pediatrician; Pediatric Psychology; Physician (General, Specialty); Physician Assistant

Further Reading

Garnick, M. B. (2002, March 6). *Medicine*, World Book Online Americas Edition, http://www.aolsvc.worldbook.aol.com/wbol/wbPage/na/ar/co/353160

Snock, I. D., & D'Orazio, L. (1998). *Opportunities in Health and Medical Careers* (pp. 26–27). Chicago, IL: VGM Career Horizons.

Swanson, B. M. (2000). *Careers in health care* (pp. 205–210). Chicago, IL: VGM Career Horizons.

TERRY STANCIN
SUSAN K. SANTOS

Health Care Use

DEFINITION

Health care use (also called health care utilization) refers to patterns of medical and mental health care use. Families vary widely in their use of pediatric health care services: Some families are low users of pediatric services whereas other families are high users. Patterns of use often vary across types of medical services; some families rely on primary care services, while others may depend on emergency departments or specialty care clinics. Health services research has shown that approximately one in eight children can be considered high users; this group accounts for a disproportionate share of all ambulatory health care use in pediatric settings. A similar number of children can be considered low users, and these children may not receive optimal health care services to protect health and promote child development.

CORRELATES

Variations in health care use have been related to many factors.

Child Factors

- Younger children have higher use than older children
- White children have higher use than African American and Hispanic children
- More (and varied) health problems are associated with higher use
- Child psychiatric/psychological distress is associated with higher use
- Past high use is associated with future high use

Parent Factors

- Mother's higher use is associated with higher use for child
- Father's higher use is associated with higher use for child
- Mother's lower social support is associated with higher use for child
- Mother's psychological distress is associated with higher use for child
- Mother's employment outside the home is associated with lower use for child

Family Factors

- Smaller family size is associated with higher use for child
- Having health insurance is associated with higher use for child
- Lower family income is associated with lower use of primary care, but higher use of emergency department services
- Easier access is associated with higher use for child
- Higher family conflict is associated with higher use for child

CONSEQUENCES OF LOWER AND HIGHER HEALTH CARE USE

Lower pediatric health care use may be associated with reduced receipt of preventive care, lack of early treatment for acute illnesses which leads to long-term health problems, incomplete immunizations, and unmet and undetected health and mental health needs. Higher health care use (in the absence of a diagnosed chronic or severe illness) may be associated with increased receipt of unnecessary medical tests and treatments, increased propensity to use care excessively across later childhood and into adulthood, and excessive vigilance for minor and common signs and symptoms. Patterns of high use also place a strain on the health care system that is already burdened by high costs and restricted access for many individuals.

IMPLICATIONS

The United States Department of Health and Human Services' goals for *Healthy People 2010* include appropriate access to, and use of, pediatric health care to promote child health and development. Changes in the nation's health care system are needed to ensure equal access to health care and optimal use of available health care services. Families with lower use of pediatric services may need increased access (e.g., a regular source of primary care, affordable health insurance) and encouragement or interventions to seek appropriate levels of health care (e.g., home visits to promote health care use, reminders for immunizations and health supervision appointments). Families with higher use of pediatric services may benefit from referral to specialty services to address complex health and mental health problems in the child, parent, or family that are not easily addressed in primary care. As managed care services become even more common in the United States, we should expect better distribution of the use of pediatric health care services by reducing unnecessarily high use and increasing unusually low use. By providing more optimal levels of health care use for greater numbers of children, we will be better able to document the effects of health care use on children's health outcomes.

See also: Health Care Professionals; Measurement of Behavior Change; Psychological Consultation with Physicians

Further Reading

Janicke, D. M., & Finney, J. W. (2001). Children's primary health care services: A social-cognitive model of sustained high use. *Clinical Psychology: Science and Practice, 8*, 228–241.

Janicke, D. M., Finney, J. W., & Riley, A. W. (2001). Children's health care use: A prospective investigation of factors related to care-seeking. *Medical Care, 39*, 990–1001.

Szilagyi, P. G. (1998). Managed care for children: Effect on access to care and utilization of health services. *The Future of Children, 8,* 39–59.

U. S. Department of Health and Human Services. (2000). *Healthy People 2010* (2nd ed., Vols. 1 and 2). Washington, DC: U.S. Government Printing Office.

JACK W. FINNEY
DAVID M. JANICKE

Health Education/Health Promotion

DEFINITION

Health education (health promotion) entails providing information and learning experiences that promote healthy lifestyles and discourage health-risk behaviors, thereby preventing disease and injury, and enhancing individual health and development. Pediatric health education focuses on the role of parents in promoting child health, especially for infants and young children. For older children and adolescents, parental health education is supplemented with individually oriented behavioral health promotion. The U.S. Department of Health and Human Services' *Healthy People 2010* sets specific objectives for child and adolescent health promotion, including enhancing educational and community-based health programs, increasing physical activity and fitness, improving nutrition, reducing the use of tobacco, alcohol, and other drugs, preventing injuries, and decreasing cancer risks. Objectives for prenatal and infant health promotion include increasing breastfeeding and immunizations, improving access to, and use of, prenatal and infant health care services, as well as encouraging health-enhancing behaviors and discouraging health-risk behaviors among pregnant women and new mothers in order to optimize prenatal and early-infancy development.

METHODS

Health education may occur in health care settings, schools, and communities, as well as through mass media (e.g., radio, television, the Internet). During health-care supervision (well-baby/well-child) visits, primary care providers may conduct individual health education interactions with parents and children, addressing a range of age-appropriate matters on child development—nutrition, exercise, sleep, safety/injury prevention, parenting, health risks, and responsible sexual behavior. In schools, health education is common as part of the physical education curriculum, and is often supplemented with special campaigns focused on specific topics (e.g., nutrition, smoking, physical fitness, drug abuse, prevention of sexually transmitted diseases). Community programs have been focused on nutrition, exercise, and obesity prevention, and statewide programs around the country have targeted drunk driving, firearms risks to children, bicycle helmet use, and home fire safety, among other health topics. Many of these larger public health education campaigns have employed multiple components and strategies, supplementing conventional public service announcements and other media information with incentives for healthy behavior (e.g., gun buy-back programs to encourage parents to disarm; distribution of free home smoke alarms for those who cannot afford them). In addition, legislation (e.g., prohibiting smoking in public buildings), community standards (e.g., intensive enforcement of antidrunk driving laws), and municipal planning projects (e.g., construction of walking paths and bicycle lanes) are important aspects of community health promotion initiatives.

CLINICAL APPLICATION

Health education programs provide factual health-related information based on current scientific and medical knowledge. Although the provision of information is a basic component of all health education programs, the goal of most health education programs is to influence immediate or long-term behavior. Health education often entails providing health-related advice aimed at persuading individuals to engage in health-promoting behaviors, or not to engage in health-risk behaviors. Persuasive health education may be targeted at changing current health behaviors (e.g., smoking cessation, increasing physical exercise), or at influencing future health behaviors (e.g., drug resistance education programs for children; infant car-seat education programs for expectant parents).

An extensive body of scientific research has been conducted on factors that influence health-related behaviors; most viable models of health-related behavior change now include numerous considerations beyond the target individual's factual health-related knowledge. Health-related behavior therapies address the mechanisms by which unhealthy behaviors are initiated and maintained, and employ behavioral strategies (e.g., monitoring and recording target behaviors, goal-setting and selective reinforcement, fading, extinction, rearranging environmental contingencies, enlisting social support) to decrease unhealthy behaviors and increase healthy alternatives. Individual beliefs, attitudes, expectations, emotions, motivations, and cognitions may intervene between objective knowledge and behavior; cognitive–behavioral treatments may address these influences on health behavior. Many health education programs have incorporated aspects of clinical behavioral and cognitive therapies in an attempt to increase receptivity to persuasive health messages and provide more effective advice for individuals who attempt the (often difficult) behavior changes recommended by health education messages.

EFFECTIVENESS

Individual, short-term effects of health education programs are limited. Most health-related behaviors are complex, multiply determined, and resistant to change; influencing these behaviors often requires additional intervention beyond the provision of factual information and persuasive appeals. Education alone does not adequately address the clinical needs of many individuals with problematic health-related behaviors. For example, most smokers know that cigarettes pose serious immediate and long-terms risks to their health, and yet they continue to smoke. However, health education programs may be of value, and may confer considerable benefit, even if they cannot be demonstrated to influence the behavior of any given individual. Many health education messages represent newly accepted or developing social standards about health behavior; as

these standards change, the process of their dissemination may be made faster and more thorough by the elaborate provision of consistent health education messages.

Although targets of health education may be resistant to behavior-change messages (e.g., antidrunk-driving campaigns may be least persuasive to the most dangerous offenders), health education messages reach secondary targets—individuals who may not engage in a given risky health behavior themselves, but who may influence the health behavior of those around them (e.g., family members, friends, neighbors, teachers, and employers). Persuasive health appeals may influence broader social perceptions and encourage naturalistic sociocultural influences to exert their powerful effects on individual behavior. The social influence of health education campaigns can be seen in recent reductions in alcohol consumption by pregnant women and in cigarette smoking, as well as in recent increases in seatbelt use. Public perceptions and social acceptance of these health-related behaviors, all of which were targets of extensive public health initiatives, have changed substantially in recent years. Improvements in these behaviors reflect sociocultural and attitudinal changes, and underscore the importance of health education in influencing the health behavior standards of communities and society.

See also: Adolescent Health; Cigarette Smoking; Community Interventions; Injury Prevention; Safety and Prevention

Further Reading

U.S. Department of Health and Human Services. (2000). *Healthy people 2010* (2nd ed., Vols. 1 and 2). Washington, DC: U.S. Government Printing Office.
U.S. Public Health Service. (1998). *The clinician's handbook of preventive services* (2nd ed.). McLean, VA: International Medical.
Wurtele, S. K. (1995). Health promotion. In M. C. Roberts (Ed.), *Handbook of pediatric psychology* (2nd ed., pp. 200–216). New York: Guilford.

Web Sites

http://www.healthbehavior.com/index3.shtml—The Center of Excellence in Education for Health, Inc., web pages provide individual, family, school, community, and worksite health education information.
http://www.mayoclinic.com/—The Mayo Clinic web pages have a wide range of health education information for children and families.
http://www.medem.com/MedLB/bufferpage_aap.cfm—*Medem's Medical Library* includes a range of patient education information from several partner medical societies, including the American Association of Pediatrics.

JACK W. FINNEY
KIRSTEN BRADBURY

Health Psychology

See: Pediatric Psychology

Health-Related Quality of Life

See: Quality of Life

Hearing Development

See: Sensory and Perceptual Development

Hearing Evaluation

See: Hearing Impairment

Hearing Impairment

DEFINITION/ETIOLOGY

Hearing impairment results from a number of causes and is described by the type and degree of hearing loss. Sound is measured by its loudness or intensity (measured in units called decibels, dB) with 0 representing soft sounds and good hearing and 110 representing loud sounds and poor hearing. Sound may be described using frequency or pitch (measured in units called hertz, Hz) with 250 Hz representing lower pitch sounds such as a drum and 8000 Hz representing high-pitch sounds such as bells. Impairments in hearing may exist in only one ear or in both ears. Degree of hearing loss is related to the extent that the disorder is interrupting normal function and is generally described as slight (15–26 dB), mild (26–40 dB), moderate (41–55 dB), severe (71–90 dB), or profound (90 dB or greater), depending upon how well a person can hear the intensities or frequencies associated with speech. Definition of deaf is considered to be hearing losses greater than 90 dB HL or any hearing level where use of hearing for communication is not possible.

The type of hearing loss is related to the location of the disorder within the auditory system and includes conductive, sensorineural, mixed, or central hearing losses. A *conductive hearing loss* is a type of hearing impairment caused by diseases or obstructions in the outer or middle ear. Conductive hearing losses may affect all frequencies of hearing evenly and are generally less than 60 dB. They account for 5–10 percent of all hearing loss. Depending on the cause of the conductive hearing loss, the hearing may fluctuate. A person with a conductive hearing loss usually can be helped medically or surgically. Examples of conductive losses are wax, ear infections (otitis media), rupture of the eardrum, and deformity of the outer or middle ear structure. If the otolaryngologist (ear, nose, and throat specialist [ENT]) determines that the hearing loss is not medically correctable, the individuals with a conductive loss usually do well with amplification.

Sensorineural hearing losses involve damage to the sensory nerves of the inner ear. These losses, which usually cannot be surgically or medically corrected, can range from mild to profound and they often affect the person's ability to hear certain pitch sounds. Sensorineural deafness affects both loudness and fidelity of sound, making the sound distorted. Amplification is the usual rehabilitation technique; however, it will not return the hearing to normal levels. Different causes of sensorineural losses are: heredity, diseases such as bacterial meningitis, injury, and excessive noise.

A mixed hearing loss refers to a combination of conductive and sensorineural loss and means that the problem occurs in both the outer or middle and the inner ear. Mixed losses cause difficulty with both distortion and loudness. As conductive losses tend to fluctuate, depending on the nature of the loss, mixed losses may also fluctuate.

Central hearing loss involves the pathways from the inner ear and the auditory centers in the brain. This kind of loss involves the brain end of the process rather than the hearing end. The ability to detect the sounds is usually good, though the understanding of sounds is extremely poor.

Another consideration in determining the impact of the hearing loss is the time of onset of deafness. A *congenital or prelingual hearing loss* is defined as reduced hearing sensitivity that exists at or dating from birth. *Acquired or postlingual hearing impairment* can be defined as reduced sensitivity that occurs after the child has learned the parents' native spoken language and is the result of injury or disease. The *progressive hearing loss* is one that worsens over time and will require repeated testing to monitor the hearing. The impact of the hearing impairment on communication is greater for the child that does not have an auditory memory of sound (prelingual). A child who has never had the opportunity to learn his parents' language is in a different position than the child who has language well established before losing the hearing (postlingual). However, this is only true for children of hearing parents since children of deaf parents learn American Sign Language (ASL) or whatever sign system their parents use.

PREVALENCE/INCIDENCE

Hearing loss and deafness affect individuals of all ages and may occur across the life span from infancy through old age. The U.S. Department of Education (2000) reports that during the 1998–99 school year, 70,813 students aged 6–21 (or 1.3 percent of all students with disabilities) received special education services under the category of "hearing impairment." The number of children with hearing loss and deafness may be higher, since many of these students may have multiple disabilities and may be served under other categories. About 1 in every 1,000 babies born in the United States has severe hearing loss in both ears. An additional 5 per 1,000 are born with moderate hearing loss. Because of these high rates, since 1994, there has been universal screening of newborns for hearing loss.

CORRELATES

Auditory linked acquisition of language is related to early maturational periods in the infant's life. The longer the auditory language stimulation is delayed, the less efficient the language facility will be. The process for learning language is the same for all humans, regardless of culture, with the parents' modeling their own language. When a child is deaf and the parents are hearing, this process is altered. Even mild early childhood hearing loss affects speech and language development as well as social development. The hearing impairment may cause a receptive or expressive language disorder that will require special services.

Many individuals with hearing impairment do not have a positive perception of themselves because they feel different from those using hearing aids. However, if a parent or caregiver feels competent and adjusts to the unexpected presence of the hearing impairment, children will more likely feel accepted and a positive self-concept will emerge. Due to the delay in language development,

some children with hearing impairment may have fewer opportunities for peer interactions, making it difficult to learn "social rules" which may result in reduced social competence.

Upon receiving a diagnosis of hearing impairment, parents often find themselves having feelings of guilt, anger, or feelings of uncertainty, depending on their knowledge of hearing impairment. They may face a communication dilemma and must relearn how to communicate with the hearing impaired child. Information concerning modes of communication such as oral (speech), sign language, signing exact English, or a combination of all of these will help the parents make decisions concerning the educational needs of the child. The audiologist or speech–language pathologist will help them with this information.

ASSESSMENT

The pediatrician and otolaryngologist will evaluate the child to determine the cause of the hearing loss and determine medical management of the hearing loss. The audiologist completes the hearing evaluation (also known as audiological evaluation) to determine the degree and type of hearing loss. The physician will use information from the child's medical history, the physical examination, and the audiological evaluation to provide a diagnosis. The audiologist will provide information concerning rehabilitation techniques and will make referrals for additional services to the speech–language pathologist, educational psychologist, or the public school. The speech–language pathologist and audiologist will be the primary case managers for the child with a hearing impairment.

A thorough history will be the starting point for the examination. The risk factors for hearing loss include family history of hereditary childhood hearing loss, abnormalities of the head, being born with certain infections that were contracted while in the womb, meningitis, birth weight under about $3\frac{1}{3}$ pounds (1.5 kilograms), need of a ventilator after birth for five days or more, jaundice severe enough to require a blood transfusion, administration of certain medications (e.g., Kanamycin, streptomycin, chloroquine) which are known to have hearing loss as a possible side effect, parent or caregiver's concerns about hearing loss, or any type of development delay including speech and language.

The purpose of the diagnostic hearing tests is to determine the type and degree of hearing impairment and provide information concerning the possible impact on the child's communication and educational skills.

The hearing evaluation will include a combination of behavioral tests (tests that require a response from the child) and physiological tests (tests that do not require a response from the child). An examination of the external ear canal will be completed to see if there is any earwax (also called cerumen), ear drainage, or deformities of the ear canal or external ear. Tympanometry is a physiological test of middle ear function, which provides information concerning mobility of the eardrum, physical ear canal volume, and peak pressure. Middle ear pathologies such as middle ear fluid, perforations, and eustachian tube dysfunction will be identified using tympanometry. The basic pure tone audiometry will result in a chart of the hearing known as an audiogram. The measurement of the different tones (frequencies) important for speech is completed and charted at the quietest level the child would respond 50 percent of the time. Different techniques are available to obtain tone thresholds depending on the age of the child. Speech audiometry assesses the ability to detect and understand speech. The speech recognition threshold identifies the quietest level that the child will respond to two-syllable words (i.e., baseball). Speech recognition tests measure the ability to repeat back words at a comfortable loudness level. These tests are presented in an ideal condition and usually do not represent the child's ability to recognize and understand when in a classroom or home setting.

Physiological measures are available for the very young child, the child who is shy, and the child that is not cooperative. The Otoacoustic Emission (OAE) test is considered a screening tool, which provides information about the inner ear sensory nerve function. It is a very quick test, usually taking no more than two minutes per ear with no discomfort. A small earphone is placed in the ear canal, which will present low level clicking sounds or tones and measure the response to those sounds. When the response is present within normal limits, hearing is estimated to be normal. Absences of a response require additional testing in order to be completed. The primary difficulty with this test is that the child needs in order to be quiet during the testing and responses may be absent if there is a middle ear pathology or excessive earwax.

The most sensitive physiological test is called the Auditory Brain Stem Response (ABR or BAER) test. This is a noninvasive test in which sensors called electrodes (which look like circular bandages with wires coming out) are attached to the head. Sound pulses are given in each ear, and the electrodes will detect brain waves that will be recorded on paper. It takes about an hour to complete and will provide information concerning the whole auditory system response to sound. The child need not do anything but relax and not move around. Many patients drift off into natural sleep. Young children, those who are anxious about the test procedure, and those who experience difficulty sitting still for an extended length of time may require a mild sedative for test results to be reliable. The test is not a hearing test; however, normal response is associated with normal hearing acuity. Measurement of the quietest level that a brain response is present will give an estimate of the hearing levels.

TREATMENT

Most children with a hearing impairment will benefit from some form of amplification. Even a small amount of sound provided to the profound hearing loss will bring about environmental awareness of sound for safety and will improve speech-reading and understanding ability. Hearing aids make sounds louder and are available in several types, including behind-the-ear hearing aids, in-the-ear hearing aids, and in-the-canal hearing aids. The degree of hearing loss and the age of the child will determine the type of hearing aid needed. A behind-the-ear hearing aid may be recommended for the young child because children are growing rapidly until the age of 10 or 11. Other technology available includes the cochlear implant, which is an electronic device with part of the device implanted in the inner ear and part of the device worn outside. The cochlear implant provides sound information to the individual by directly stimulating the auditory nerve fibers in the inner ear, enabling them to perceive sound. Assistive devices may also be used to improve the detrimental effects of distance, background noise, and reverberation. For example, an FM system picks up the sound at the source, amplifies it, and sends it to the child using his personal hearing aid with an FM receiver attached.

Hearing loss or deafness does not affect a person's intellectual capacity or ability to learn. However, children who are either hard of hearing or deaf generally require some form of special education services in order to receive an adequate education. Such services may include speech, language, and auditory training from a specialist; amplification systems; services of an interpreter for those students who use manual communication; preferential seating in the class to facilitate speech-reading; captioned films/videos; assistance of a notetaker, who takes notes for the student with a hearing loss, so that the student can fully attend to the instructions; instruction for the teacher and peers in alternate communication methods, such as sign language; and counseling.

PROGNOSIS

Communication may be limited for the hearing impaired; however, technology is providing access to every aspect of life. Amplification and cochlear implants will allow easy access to sounds in the environment. There should be no limitation on achievement and interaction in society.

For additional information, contact an audiologist or one of the listed hearing impairment organizations.

See also: Central Auditory Processing Disorders; Deafness; Language Development; Speech and Language Assessment

Further Reading

Alexander Graham Bell Association for the Deaf, Inc., 3417 Volta Place, NW, Washington, DC 20007, (202) 337-5220 (Voice/TT), Web site: http://www.agbell.org
American Academy of Audiology, 8300 Greensboro Drive, Suite 750, McLean, VA 22102-3611, Web site: http://www.audiology.com/index.php
American Speech–Language Hearing Association, 10801 Rockville Pike, Rockville, MD 20852, (301) 897-5700 (Voice/TT); 1-800-638-8255 (Helpline), Web site: http://www.asha.org
Luterman, D. M. (1991). *When your child is deaf: A guide for parents.* Parkton, MD: York Press. (Tel.: 1-800-962-2763. Web site: http://www.yorkpress.com/index.html)
Northern, J. L., & Downs, M. P. (1991). *Hearing in children* (4th ed.). Baltimore: Williams and Wilkins.
Stach, B. A. (1998). *Clinical audiology: An introduction.* San Diego: Singular Publishing Group.

EVA SAFFER

Heart Transplantation, Pediatric

BRIEF DESCRIPTION

The heart is the hollow muscular organ that receives blood from the veins and pumps it through the arteries by alternate dilation and contraction. Since 1984, heart transplantation has been a viable therapeutic intervention for children with myopathic (muscular disease) and complex structural heart diseases. By definition, heart transplantation involves the replacement of a severely damaged heart with one from a cadaver organ donor. For some pediatric patients, extensive aortic reconstruction is necessary during transplant surgery. The aorta is the main artery of the body, carrying blood from the left ventricle of the heart to arteries in all organs and body parts. In June 2001, there were 277 children under 18 years of age wait-listed for heart transplantation in the United States. This number represents 6.6 percent of the 4,200 total patients awaiting heart transplantation. Fifteen to twenty percent of children waiting for heart transplantation will die because suitable donor organs are not available.

Since 1990, there have been approximately 2,900 pediatric heart transplants performed in the United States. Today, pediatric heart transplants account for about 13 percent of all heart transplants performed in the United States, with half of these occurring in children less than 5 years of age. Over one third of all pediatric heart transplants have been done during the child's first year of life.

INDICATIONS

In pediatric populations, heart transplantation is usually considered for those who have complex congenital heart disease and end-stage cardiomyopathy. Hypoplastic left heart syndrome (i.e. underdevelopment of the left side of the heart), the fourth most common congenital heart anomaly, is the most frequent indication for heart transplantation in infants.

OUTCOMES

Overall, pediatric patient survival rates are generally as good as those seen in adults—87 percent at 1 year, 73 percent at 3 years, and 67 percent at 5 years. However, while older children and adolescents have survival rates that are nearly identical to those of adults, infants have the lowest survival rates.

Early postoperative complications can include seizures, hyperperfusion syndrome, kidney (renal) failure, and infections. Possible long-term complications can include hypertension, graft vasculopathy (a thickening of the innermost wall of the graft vessel), arrhythmias, renal failure, and neoplastic diseases. Retransplantation may occur in up to 5 percent of cases, most commonly due to coronary artery disease, acute rejection, or chronic rejection.

For many pediatric heart transplant recipients, there is a return to normal growth. Yet, linear growth appears to increase mainly for children less than 5 years of age—the mean height values approach the 40th percentile for age, with a corresponding gain in body weight. In contrast, adolescent heart transplant recipients, while benefiting from weight gain following surgery, generally do not demonstrate any significant increase in height.

PSYCHOLOGICAL CONSIDERATIONS

Pediatric psychologists are generally involved in the psychological evaluation of children and families at the time they are being considered for heart transplantation. The nature and extent of these evaluations varies by transplant program, but generally includes an assessment of child development, adherence history, quality of life, psychological adaptation and coping, and family resources. In addition to assessment-based services, psychological interventions are developed and implemented as needed to enhance both pre- and post-transplant health outcomes.

Approximately 20 percent of children with heart disease requiring transplantation may experience impairment in cognitive development and functioning secondary to low cardiac output, cardiac arrhythmias, and acute anoxic effects. While improved quality of life has been reported following pediatric heart transplantation, there are few published studies substantiating such outcomes.

See also: Cardiovascular Disease; Parenting the Chronically Ill Child; Quality of Life

Further Reading

Boucek, M. M., Faro, A., Novick, R. J., Bennett, L. E., Keck, B. M., & Hosenpud, J. D. (2001). The Registry of the International Society for Heart and Lung Transplantation: Fourth official pediatric report—2000. *Journal of Heart and Lung Transplantation, 20,* 39–52.

Fortuna, R. S., Chinnock, R. E., & Bailey, L. L. (1999). Heart transplantation among 233 infants during the first six months of life: The Loma Linda experience. Loma Linda Pediatric Heart Transplant Group. *Clinical Transplantation, 13,* 263–272.

Fricker, F. J., Addonizio, L., Bernstein, D., Boucek, M., Boucek, R., Canter, C., Chinnock, R., Chin, C., Kichuk, M., Lamour, J., Pietra, B., Morrow, R., Rotundo, K., Shaddy, R., Schuette, E. P., Schowengerdt, K. O., Sondheimer, H., & Webber, S. (1999). Heart transplantation in children: Indications. Report of the Ad Hoc Subcommittee of the Pediatric Committee of the American Society of Transplantation (AST). *Pediatric Transplantation, 3,* 333–342.

Scientific Registry of Transplant Recipients Home Page. http://www.ustransplant.org (Accessed May 2002).

Todaro, J. F., Fennell, E. B., Sears, S. F., Rodrigue, J. R., & Roche, A. K. (2000). A review of cognitive and psychological outcomes in pediatric heart transplant recipients. *Journal of Pediatric Psychology, 25,* 567–576.

United Network for Organ Sharing Home Page. http://www.unos.org (Accessed May 2002).

JAMES R. RODRIGUE
F. JAY FRICKER

Helicobacter pylori

See: Peptic Ulcer Disease

Hematomas

See: Traumatic Brain Injury

Hemophilia

See: Hereditary Coagulation Disorders

Hereditary Coagulation Disorders

DEFINITION

The three most common hereditary bleeding disorders are hemophilia A (Factor VIII deficiency), hemophilia B (Factor IX deficiency), and von Willebrand's disease (vWf protein deficiency). Hemophilia A and B are both X chromosome-linked recessive disorders, with the gene carried by females but the disease experienced almost exclusively in males, although some females who are carriers may develop hemophilic symptoms. von Willebrand's disease is an autosomal disorder that is equally distributed among males and females, and typically involves a very mild set of symptoms.

In humans, blood clotting requires adequate numbers of the blood cells that perform this function (the platelets), and the presence of a series of proteins (clotting factors) that permit the platelets to function. There are a number of these proteins, or factors, that are activated as part of a chain of events that lead to clotting. If one of the major factors is missing or does not function properly, the clotting sequence is altered, and clotting does not occur. In hemophilia, the bone marrow usually produces enough platelets, but specific genetic mutations occur that produce deficiencies in two of the factors in the chain, Factors VIII and IX. Deficiencies in either or both of these factors (or any of the other clotting proteins) disrupts the sequence of events that lead to clotting, and thus produce the characteristic symptom of prolonged bleeding. Deficiencies may occur for any of the proteins in the clotting sequence, but the severity of clinical outcome depends on which factors are deficient. The most severe bleeding problems are in hemophilia and are associated with Factor VIII (Hemophilia A) or Factor IX (Hemophilia B). The clinical symptoms of both types of hemophilia are different, but treatment requires replacement of the specific factor that is deficient, leading to the distinction between the two types. When a factor deficiency occurs, bleeding occurs that damages tissue and, in some cases, can be fatal. The concentration of factor determines the severity of each type of hemophilia: severe, moderate, or mild. In von Willebrand's disease, the deficiency is in the vWf protein. When the vWF protein is present, platelets adhere to it, triggering activation of a sequence that "recruits" other platelets and permits clotting. When the vWf protein is deficient, this platelet "recruiting" process does not occur, and bleeding results.

INCIDENCE

Hemophilia occurs in approximately one in 5,000 males (1 percent of the population) with the majority (85 percent) having hemophilia A. von Willebrand's Disease occurs in about 1 percent of the population, although the symptoms are often so mild that this incidence may be an underestimate.

DIAGNOSIS

The diagnosis of hemophilia and von Willebrand's disease can be made on the basis of known genetics (a family history if the mother is a known carrier), but more frequently the diagnosis is made following the onset of clinical symptoms. The most common times for a diagnosis are when a young boy is circumcised, or when he begins to walk and experiences an ankle bleed. Tests of bleeding time and genetic studies are used to confirm the diagnosis.

CLINICAL SYMPTOMS

For most individuals with hemophilia, the most frequent site of bleeding is in the deep joints and muscles, and most develop what is called a "target joint," where repeated bleeds occur, although bleeding is not limited to this target joint. These bleeds are usually first noticed when the child begins to walk. Bleeding into these joints results in swelling, pain, and ultimately arthritis and restricted use of the joint. In severe cases, contractures (extreme limitation of joint movement) can occur.

Traumatic injury in children with hemophilia may lead to serious symptoms not associated with joint bleeds. Trauma to the head or abdomen may result in bleeding that results in vital organ injury, and this can lead to death if not treated.

Von Willebrand's disease is associated with mild bleeding, usually in connection with surgery, menstrual periods, nosebleeds, or bleeding from the gums. In the most severe forms, gastrointestinal bleeding may occur, and in extreme cases this can result in shock.

TREATMENT

Treatment of hemophilia and more serious cases of von Willebrand's disease involves intravenous infusion of concentrated factor replacement. Some of these factor replacements are derived directly from human or animal (pig) blood plasma, while recent genetic advances have led to the production of recombinant factors (factors that are produced by genetically splicing a human factor gene onto a nonhuman cell that can be grown in the laboratory). Recombinant factors are not derived from blood products, so they do not carry the risk of disease transmission (e.g., HIV or hepatitis), but may be contaminated by the traces of nonhuman proteins produced by the host cell. Since some individuals with hemophilia develop inhibitory antibodies to the factor replacement, treatment may vary across individuals with the same type of hemophilia. As repeated bleeds occur, the likelihood of joint injury occurs. These will often require orthopedic treatment, physical therapy, and sometimes surgery. For von Willebrand's disease, treatment usually involves intravenous treatment with desmopressin (DDAVP).

Care of the child with hemophilia should occur in a comprehensive hemophilia center with a team of professionals that include a physician (hematologist), nurse, orthopedic surgeon, social worker, psychologist, physical therapist, dentist, financial counselor, and possibly an infectious disease specialist. In the 1980s, many children treated for hemophilia were exposed to HIV contaminated factor, and required treatment for both HIV and hemophilia. Since careful screening of the blood supply was put into place, the incidence of HIV in children with hemophilia has all but disappeared.

Behavioral support for children with hemophilia and their families primarily focuses on coping with the diagnosis, assisting in the development of parenting strategies that minimize the risk of bleeds, supporting children who are unable to engage in high-risk physical activities, and assisting with adherence to prophylactic factor regimens to prevent bleeds.

PROGNOSIS

Aggressive management of bleeds and use of prophylactic factor treatment has resulted in a dramatic change in the outlook for children with hemophilia. Most severe consequences of hemophilia can now be prevented, allowing children to live normal, active lives with minimal restrictions. Serious consequences are now limited to severe abdominal or head bleeds, with some children occasionally experiencing long-term orthopedic complications.

See also: Bleeding Disorders; Bone Marrow Failure and Primary Immunodeficiency; Kidney Transplantation, Pediatric; Leukemia; Liver Transplantation; Orthopedic Disabilities; Pediatric Human Immunodeficiency Virus-1 (HIV); Platlet Abnormalities—Thrombocytopenia; Self-Management

Further Reading

Kelly, L. A. (1996). *My blood doesn't have muscles: How children understand hemophilia from preschool to adolescence.* King of Prussia, PA: Centeon, L.L.C.

Kelly, L. A. (1999). *Raising a child with hemophilia: A practical guide for parents.* King of Prussia, PA: Centeon L.L.C.

Montgomery, R. R., Gill, J. C., & Scott, J. P. (1998). Hemophilia and von Willebrand's Disease. In D. G. Nathan & S. H. Orkin (Eds.), *Nathan and Oski's hematology of infancy and childhood* (5th ed., pp. 1631–1659). Philadelphia: W.B. Saunders.

Paper, R., & Kelly, L. A. (2002). *A guide to living with von Willebrand's disease.* King of Prussia, PA: Aventis Behring L.L.C.

F. DANIEL ARMSTRONG

Herpes labialis

See: Sexually Transmitted Diseases in Adolescents

High Blood Pressure

DEFINITION

Blood pressure increases when there is an increase in blood output from the heart, or when there is increased resistance to blood flow in the blood vessels. Elevated blood pressure (hypertension) may be either primary (no identifiable cause) or secondary (related to a disease process). In infants and young children, secondary hypertension is most common, and the underlying cause differs with age.

INCIDENCE

Hypertension occurs in approximately 1–2 percent of school-age children. The most common reason for hypertension in children is a problem with the renal system (80–85 percent), and a urinary tract infection leading to obstruction is present in 25–50 percent of children with secondary hypertension. Other causes include abnormalities in the thyroid, parathyroid, and adrenal glands, neurologic conditions (e.g., Guillain-Barré syndrome), and other brain tumors. Environmental toxins and drugs (e.g., cocaine, tobacco) may also produce hypertension.

Primary hypertension is more common in adolescents than younger children, and is usually related to a strong family history of essential hypertension (e.g., father, mother, or grandparents had high blood pressure or other forms of cardiovascular disease).

DIAGNOSIS

The diagnosis of hypertension is made by repeated measurement of systolic and diastolic blood pressure using age-appropriate norms. Considerations of ethnicity should also be included when assessing high blood pressure, as racial differences have been found in adults.

CLINICAL SYMPTOMS

The symptoms of hypertension are not usually specific, and may include failure-to-thrive, low-grade fever, and excessive crying in children under 3 years of age. In older children, headaches, nausea, and rapid heart beat may occur. In severe cases, seizures, cardiac failure, blindness, or renal failure may occur.

TREATMENT

Emergency treatment of severe hypertension usually requires hospitalization. For moderate to severe chronic hypertension, oral medications may be used. For mild to moderate hypertension, dietary changes (reduced salt, low fat diet, high calcium, high potassium), weight reduction, and exercise are the most common types of treatment. Family support for lifestyle changes is essential.

PROGNOSIS

When carefully managed, the prognosis for high blood pressure is good, but some children may require lifetime medication. If untreated, serious long-term complications may include stroke, heart failure, renal failure, and damage to the retinas of the eye.

See also: Cardiovascular Disease; Endocrine Disorders; Feeding Disorders; Growth Disorders; Neurofibromatosis; Obesity; Visual Impairment: Low Vision and Blindness

Further Reading

Bernstein, D. (2000). Systemic hypertension. In R. E. Behrman, R. M. Kleigman, & H. B. Jenson (Eds.), *Nelson textbook of pediatrics* (16th ed., pp. 1450–1455). Philadelphia: W.B. Saunders.
Pediatric On Call. (2002). Parent corner: Hypertension (high blood pressure) in children. http://www.pediatriconcall.com/forpatients/CommonChild/hypertension1.asp

F. DANIEL ARMSTRONG

Hirschsprung's Disease

DEFINITION/INCIDENCE/ETIOLOGY

Hirschsprung's disease is a congenital disease that is caused by an absence of the nerve cells that enable intestinal muscles to move stool through the intestines. The internal anal sphincter is affected as well and does not function normally. Stool cannot pass through the affected areas, so obstruction may result. One of the earliest symptoms of Hirschsprung's disease is failure or difficulty passing meconium, an infant's first bowel movement, within the first 48 hr of life. Abdominal distension and vomiting are also common symptoms in these infants. Some children have a more insidious course, with symptoms of constipation, diarrhea, vomiting, abdominal distension, and growth delay. Enterocolitis, severe inflammation of the bowel wall, is a potentially life-threatening complication. Around 80 percent of infants with Hirschsprung's disease are diagnosed in the first year, but 8 percent may not be recognized until childhood. Hirschsprung's disease occurs in about 1 in 5,000 births. It is more common in males and in first-degree relatives.

ASSESSMENT/TREATMENT/PROGNOSIS

Hirschsprung's disease is diagnosed via barium enema, anal manometry, and/or rectal biopsy. Treatment consists of surgery to remove the affected area of the intestine and to rejoin unaffected areas. Some children continue to experience fecal incontinence, constipation, diarrhea, and abdominal distension after surgery, although reported incidence rates of these problems vary widely (e.g., 0–80 percent for incontinence) and may be related to the abnormally functioning internal anal sphincter, the surgical procedure, and/or the section and amount of bowel removed. Children may also lack a normal urge sensation, which contributes to the risk of constipation and incontinence.

PSYCHOSOCIAL CORRELATES AND TREATMENT

Little research has examined psychosocial functioning in children with Hirschsprung's disease. One study reported no significant differences in the behavioral/emotional functioning of children with Hirschsprung's disease compared to healthy children. However, in this study, fecal incontinence was significantly associated with worse psychosocial functioning. Another study reported that 19.5 percent of children with Hirschsprung's disease had significant behavioral/emotional problems, but no comparison group was employed. Additionally, these authors found no relationship between fecal incontinence and psychosocial functioning.

One study reported on a behavioral intervention aimed at teaching toileting behaviors and defecation skills in children with Hirschsprung's disease. The intervention consisted of education, relaxation strategies, extinction of any fear related to toileting, incorporation of a regular schedule of toileting, and shaping toileting skills so that the child learned to evacuate feces voluntarily and independently. If necessary, children were also taught correct straining techniques, in which biofeedback was occasionally used. At the end of treatment, 88 percent of children had good defecation behavior and good continence, and 75 percent were free of constipation.

See also: Behavior Therapy; Biofeedback, Relaxation Training; Encopresis; Gastrointestinal Disorders

Further Reading

Diseth, T. H., Bjornland, K., Novik, T. S., & Emblem, R. (1997). Bowel function, mental health, and psychosocial function in adolescents with Hirschsprung's disease. *Archives of Disease in Childhood*, 76, 100–106.

van Kuyk, E. M., Brugman-Boezeman, A. T. M., Wissink-Essink, M., Severijnen, R. S. V. M., Festen, C., & Bleijenberg, G. (2000). Defecation problems in children with Hirschsprung's disease: A biopsychosocial approach. *Pediatric Surgery International*, 16, 312–316.

Laura M. Mackner
Wallace V. Crandall

History-Taking

History-taking is a form of interview through which a clinician obtains background information about a client's personal history and current life circumstances in order to better understand the nature and causes of his/her psychological difficulties. However, history-taking is not only a fact-gathering exercise, it also provides a relatively nonthreatening introduction to assessment and therapy, creating the context in which the therapist and client may start to develop a constructive working relationship. Thus, the skills of taking a good personal history are related to the style of interviewing, in addition to the content and structure of the interview.

The information obtained during history-taking assists the therapist to identify a range of factors that will help in designing an appropriate therapy program. The history-taking interview focuses primarily on life history issues, rather than an in-depth analysis of the presenting problem. The main aim is to obtain information about the client's life history and personal circumstances that may have played a part in the development of the current difficulties. These factors include those that placed the individual at increased risk of or increased vulnerability for developing the problem of concern. These factors may be related to the client's previous family environment, life experiences, or early temperament. The therapist is also interested is knowing about previous factors or events that may have protected the client against developing further difficulties. In addition to identifying possible causal factors, the interviewer may wish to know about any factors within the client's life that might be currently influencing the presenting problem. Similarly, it is important to collect information about variables that might affect the outcome of treatment. There is now a good deal of research that demonstrates ways in which individual client characteristics influence treatment outcome and guides the therapist to select the type of treatment approach that is most likely to be effective.

BASIC SKILLS OF HISTORY-TAKING

It is important that the interviewer gains the client's trust early on in the interview process, making him/her feel welcome and comfortable and ensuring privacy. The client needs to be reassured about issues of confidentiality and yet be made aware of any reporting requirements that the therapist may have. Skills that are important in the development of positive therapist–client relationships come into play right from the start of the history-taking interview, including listening skills, empathy, warmth, and positive regard. The interviewer needs to use a balance of open-ended and closed questions in order to obtain the material in an efficient manner, while allowing the client to provide more detailed information of significance and to guide the interview to key issues in the personal history.

The interviewer is likely to have limited time available for history-taking and many clients have experienced long and complex lives. It is important, therefore, to obtain a quick biosketch of the client's life and return later to key life points that require further exploration. History-taking is only one element of the assessment process and is generally followed by a more detailed assessment of the client's presenting problems. These methods may include a detailed cognitive–behavioral and/or diagnostic interview, psychological questionnaires, or observation techniques.

Table 1. Checklist for History-Taking

Personal Details • Name • Age • Date of birth • Gender • Ethnic origins • Reason for referral • Referral source		
Personal history	Historical	Current
• Birth history (gestation, delivery) and developmental milestones		
• Family structure (parents, siblings, children, adoption)		
• Family relationships (quality)		
• Friendship patterns and social supports		
• Recreational activities and interests		
• Schooling and education		
• Employment: occupations, duration of positions		
• Living environment		
• Close relationships: courtships, engagements, defactos, marriages, separations, divorces		
• Financial circumstances, income, debts		
• Trauma events		
• Bereavements		
• Major life changes/events and stressors		
• General health, illness, injuries, operations, hospitalizations, accidents		
• Substance use (tobacco, alcohol, prescription/nonprescription drugs)		
• Lifestyle, exercise, and diet		
• Sexual development, relationships, preferences, puberty/menarche, abuse		
• Family psychiatric history		
• Personal psychiatric history, diagnoses, treatments		
• Temperament and personality		
• Religious beliefs and activities		
• Legal issues: convictions, arrests, incarcerations, lawsuits		
• The presenting problem (nature, dates of onset, duration, course treatment, and outcomes)		

THE CONTENT OF HISTORY-TAKING

Table 1 presents a checklist that can be used to prompt coverage of key issues in a client's personal history. In addition to the historical perspective, the interviewer is interested in the client's current personal circumstances that may impact upon their psychological health. Clearly, some of the content areas are inappropriate for some clients. For example, sexual relationship history is not generally appropriate for children, and indeed may not be relevant to some presenting problems among adults. Thus, the topics included in history-taking should be selected according to the relevance to a particular client. Furthermore, the interviewer may choose to take a developmental approach, covering a breadth of topics relevant to various stages of the client's life, or a categorical approach, whereby each area of the personal background is investigated separately.

See also: Classification and Diagnosis; Interviewing; Mental Status Examination; Psychological Testing

SUSAN HILARY SPENCE

HIV

See: Pediatric Human Immunodeficiency Virus-1 (HIV)

Home-Based Report Cards

See: Token Economies

Homelessness

See: Families Who Are Homeless; Running Away

Homosexuality

See: Sexual Orientation: Homosexuality

Hospitalization—Medical

See: Medical Hospitalization

Hospitalization—Psychiatric

See: Residential Treatment

Human Papilloma Virus

See: Sexually Transmitted Diseases in Adolescents

Human-Made Disasters

DEFINITION

Human-made disasters include overwhelming events that cause serious injury, loss of life, and property destruction as a result of the failure or faulty use technology. Human error or negligence is often involved, but intentionally harmful acts of violence are specifically excluded from these types of disasters. Some definitions focus only on events that affect large numbers of people in a single venue and episode, such as toxic waste spills, dam breaks, nuclear accidents, and mass transportation accidents. Other definitions include extreme events that affect only a few individuals at a time, yet, cumulatively represent a large source of trauma exposure (e.g., residential fires, motor vehicle crashes).

INCIDENCE

Human-made disasters affect millions of children and adolescents worldwide each year. Incidence of specific types of human-made disasters varies widely. Industrialized nations have more rigorously enforced safety standards compared to less developed countries, yet, also have highly mobile populations and large numbers of transportation-related trauma exposure. For example, over 400,000 children and adolescents 15 or younger in the United States are injured in motor vehicle accidents annually. Efforts at industrialization and growing populations in less developed countries increase the risk of human-made disasters such as toxic waste spills and mass transportation disasters.

CORRELATES

Human-made disasters are not always marked by a readily identifiable acute traumatic event. For example, toxic waste spills and nuclear accidents may not be immediately recognized as disasters or even as events requiring quick intervention due to lack of knowledge, concealment, or misinformation. The effects of such phenomena may be insidious and their pernicious effects may, in part, be magnified by chaotic and disorganized reactions from the community fueled by fear, misinformation, and residential evacuations. In these circumstances physical effects of exposure may be ambiguous and the psychological and behavioral reactions of parents are often strong predictors of their children's adjustment.

In the case of mass transportation disasters, residential fires, and motor vehicle accidents, trauma exposure is often sudden and dramatic. Exposure to grotesque scenes, loss of life, and imminent, overwhelming threat pose risks for acute stress reactions and long-term psychological effects, including posttraumatic stress disorder. Mass transportation disasters often occur away from survivors' home communities and the experience is often shared with strangers. This poses a challenge in terms of having later opportunities to talk with others who have been through the same experience.

ASSESSMENT

Evaluation of the nature of trauma exposure is a key aspect of assessment. This includes systematic inquiry regarding primary elements of trauma exposure (e.g., perceived life threat, exposure to grotesque scenes, personal injury, harm to others) and the individual's understanding of what happened and why. Important features of the postdisaster recovery environment to be assessed include ongoing disruptions and adversity since exposure (including economic hardships and physical impairments), access to supportive social relationships, and functioning of primary caregivers. Exposure-related posttraumatic stress symptoms (reexperiencing phenomena, psychic numbing or avoidance, hyperarousal) and associated features require careful assessment, including direct questioning of children rather than relying solely on adult informants. Depression, separation anxiety, and disaster-related fears or phobias are relatively common sequelae of extreme exposure involving loss of life or serious injury and should be carefully assessed.

TREATMENT

Treatment strategies vary by the point at which mental health contact is made, the severity and duration of traumatic exposure, and the extent of emotional distress shown or reported by the child or caregivers. Emergency services provided shortly after disasters focus on psychological first aid (e.g., support activation, debriefing or crisis-reduction counseling), information-giving, and support for adaptive functioning of the child and family. As the immediate crisis recedes, interventions for persistent trauma-related symptoms using time-limited, disaster-focused protocols are often helpful.

PROGNOSIS

Exposure-related symptoms typically diminish with time, although focused, evidence-based interventions appear to reduce the duration and intensity of psychological effects. Individual differences in reactions are well-documented, as are effects for features of the recovery environment.

See also: Natural Disasters; Terrorism Disasters; Posttraumatic Stress Disorder; Stress Management

Further Reading

Hickman, A. J., & Blanchard, E. B. (Eds.). (1999). *The international handbook of road accidents and psychological trauma: Current understanding, treatment, and law*. Amsterdam: Elsevier.
Hobfall, S. E., & de Vries, M. W. (Eds.). (1995). *Extreme stress and communities: Impact and intervention*. Dordrecht, the Netherlands: Kluwer Academic.
La Greca, A. M., Silverman, W. K., Vernberg, E. M., & Roberts, M. C. (Eds.). (2002). *Helping children cope with disasters and terrorism*. Washington, DC: American Psychological Association.

ERIC M. VERNBERG
R. ENRIQUE VARELA

Huntington's Chorea

See: Chorea: Sydenham's and Huntington's

Hydrocephalus

DEFINITION

Hydrocephalus is a complex and serious brain disorder that is related to abnormal flow patterns of the cerebral spinal fluid between the ventricles of the brain. If there is a blockage in the passages between the ventricles or infection causing inflammation and swelling, pressure can build up in the brain and affect adjacent areas of the brain, causing damage, and death if untreated. It is often associated with the occurrence of myelomeningocele, especially spina bifida, where it occurs in 65–90 percent of the cases, depending on the location of the lesion. Its causes, however, are many and varied.

ETIOLOGY

There are at least five classes of causes for hydrocephalus, some of which are congenital and some of which are acquired: (1) brain malformations such as Chiari malformation in which the brainstem and part of the cerebellum are displaced downward toward the neck rather than in the skull, causing complications in breathing, swallowing, and motor development; (2) genetic processes such as X-linked or autosomal recessive disorders; (3) inflammation of the meninges or the ventricles; (4) chemical irritants such as subarachnoid or ventricular blood; and (5) tumors and hemorrhages. Problems may occur due to blockage or failure to reabsorb the cerebral spinal fluid.

ASSESSMENT

Hydrocephalus can be diagnosed by ultrasonography during the prenatal period and by computed tomography (CT) or magnetic resonance imagery (MRI) in later childhood. Clinical signs and symptoms of conditions associated with hydrocephalus are (1) enlarged ventricles with symptoms including vomiting, headaches, irritability, lethargy, poor feeding, paralysis of upward gaze, seizures, and changes in muscle tone. In infants, additional signs are bulging fontanelle, enlarging head, splitting of the sutures, and strabismus; (2) progressive change in head size or ventricle size even without other signs of intracranial pressure; (3) enlarged ventricles in a child with a large head for age. Children often have learning difficulties, especially executive functions, in school, but they may vary greatly depending on the nature of the pathophysiology.

TREATMENT

Hydrocephalus is treated with a shunting procedure. The most common shunt is a tube with a valve implanted into the enlarged ventricle and running under the skin, emptying into the abdominal cavity. Shunts often become blocked and have to be repaired or replaced. Recognition of shunt failure and prompt referral to a neurosurgeon for treatment is very important. This can be a significant patient management issue. Families must be aware of the seriousness of shunt infections and how to evaluate the clinical signs. Shunt failure can be a life-threatening event.

PROGNOSIS

In the United States, virtually all infants and children with hydrocephalus receive shunt systems. Before shunts, children had less than a 20 percent chance of reaching adulthood, with most deaths occurring before two years of age. Now treated children can have normal intellectual development, although many have a variety of neuropsychological disorders. The most important factors affecting prognosis are: (1) cause of the hydrocephalus; (2) duration of the condition prior to shunting, and (3) associated brain abnormalities. Shunt failure is also a risk factor. It occurs most frequently in the first months after placement, but it can also fail after years or decades. Hydrocephalus is one of the most complex and difficult pediatric disorders to manage, but proper management makes a tremendous difference in improving children's outcomes.

See also: Spina Bifida

Further Reading

Batshaw, M. L. (1997). *Children with disabilities* (4th ed.). Baltimore, MD: Paul H. Brookes.

Fletcher, J. M., Bohan, T. P., Brandt, M. E., Brookshire, B. L., Beaver, S. R., Francis, D. J., Davidson, K. C., Thompson, N. M., & Minor, M. E. (1992). Cerebral white matter and cognition in hydrocephalic children. *Archives of Neurology, 49*, 818–824.

Kinsman, S. L. (1996). Childhood-acquired hydrocephalus. In A. J. Capute & P. J. Accardo (Eds.), *Developmental disabilities in infancy and childhood* (2nd ed., Vol. II, pp. 179–188) Baltimore, MD: Paul H. Brookes.

Vernet, O., & Rilliet, B.(2001). Late complications of ventriculoatrial or ventriculoperitoneal shunts. *Lancet, 358*(9293), 1569–1570.

STEPHEN R. SCHROEDER

Hypertension

See: High Blood Pressure

Hyperthyroidism, Acquired

DESCRIPTION AND INCIDENCE

Acquired hyperthyroidism is a condition characterized by the excessive production of thyroid hormone (thyroxine) in a person who was born with a normally functioning thyroid gland. Because this overproduction causes an acceleration of bodily functions, mental and physical energy reserves can become exhausted; as a result, affected children are likely to experience behavioral and emotional changes. Other physical symptoms may include an enlarged thyroid gland, a sudden growth spurt, heat intolerance, rapid fingernail growth, and protruding (exophthalmos) and irritated eyes. Affecting around 1/500–1000 children, onset can occur any time after birth, but in more than two thirds of childhood cases, symptoms begin to show between 10 and 15 years.

ETIOLOGY

Although there are several reasons why acquired hyperthyroidism might arise, in at least 95 percent of cases seen in childhood, the overproduction of thyroid hormone is caused by an autoimmune condition known as Graves' disease. Autoimmunity refers to a process in which the immune system produces antibodies that attack cells or tissues of the organism producing them. In approximately 60 percent of patients with hyperthyroidism, there is a family history of autoimmune thyroid disease present.

ASSESSMENT

The preliminary steps of the diagnostic procedure for hyperthyroidism are the same as those employed for other thyroid disorders: A comprehensive physical evaluation and family history is obtained, along with blood tests to check for the level of thyroid hormone and its stimulating factor. Low levels of thyroid stimulating hormone (TSH) in conjunction with elevated thyroid hormone confirm the diagnosis of hyperthyroidism. Additional studies are then ordered to determine the specific cause of the disorder and to plan for recommended treatment.

ASSOCIATED PSYCHOLOGICAL FEATURES

Children with acquired hyperthyroidism may demonstrate a number of behavioral and emotional changes as a result of their condition. Most affected children will experience a change in sleeping patterns. While the body normally slows down during sleep in unaffected individuals, the body continues to speed in a person with hyperthyroidism. This heightened metabolic state, associated with sleeplessness and insomnia, can result in extreme mental and physical exhaustion, and accompanying mood changes. Children with hyperthyroidism may seem irritable or exhibiting a difficult temperament.

TREATMENT

Acquired hyperthyroidism can be treated effectively with antithyroid medication, and the excessive production of thyroid hormone is usually brought to normal levels within weeks (though it may take longer). Unfortunately, the bodies of some children are not able to tolerate antithyroid medication and may exhibit allergic reactions including fever, hives, or a rash. Additionally, 1/300 children on antithyroid medication will experience agranulocytosis, a condition in which white blood cell count drops markedly, thereby affecting the immune system's ability to resist infection. Symptoms of agranulocytosis include fever, sore throat, and mouth sores. If any of these symptoms are observed, parents should terminate treatment and contact the child's physician immediately.

In cases in which the use of antithyroid medication is contraindicated, or where patients are not good surgical candidates, radioactive iodine treatment is recommended. This treatment typically results in hypothyroidism and is subsequently treated with thyroxine (levothyroxine, taken orally). Although there has been some suggestion that radioiodine may cause leukemia or other cancers, there is currently no evidence to support this claim.

PROGNOSIS

With appropriate treatment, acquired hyperthyroidism can be successfully controlled. Symptoms are generally reversible following treatment, and the long-term prognosis for children with acquired hyperthyroidism is excellent.

See also: Hypothyroidism, Acquired; Hypothyroidism, Congenital; Treatment Adherence: Medical

Further Reading

Cooper, D. S. (2001). *Medical management of thyroid disease.* New York: Marcel Dekker.
Dallas, J. S., & Foley, T. P. (1996). Hyperthyroidism. In F. Lifshitz (Ed.), *Pediatric endocrinology: A clinical guide* (pp. 401–414). New York: Marcel Dekker.
Hauser, P., & Rovet, J. (1999). *Thyroid diseases of infancy and childhood: Effects on behavior and intellectual development.* Washington, DC: American Psychiatric Press.

LAUREN ZURENDA
DAVID E. SANDBERG

Hypnosis

See: Pediatric Hypnosis

Hypoglycemia

DEFINITION

The literal meaning of hypoglycemia is "low blood sugar." Hypoglycemia occurs when blood sugar or glucose levels (BGLs) are inadequate to meet the body's need for energy. Some debate exists over the precise definition of hypoglycemia because symptoms can occur at different BGLs in different individuals according to age, weight, gender, concurrent disease(s), emotion, physical activity, and dietary history. However, the general consensus is that preterm infants experience hypoglycemia at or below a BGL of 20 milligrams of glucose per deciliter of blood (mg/dl); older infants at or below 40 mg/dl; and children at or below 50 mg/dl. Symptoms are often elicited at higher BGLs in children (i.e., 65 mg/dl) and it has been suggested that this more liberal cutoff be utilized, because of the undesirable health consequences related to untreated severe hypoglycemia, which can include loss of consciousness. Isolated or idiopathic hypoglycemia, with no underlying medical cause, is very rare in children.

INCIDENCE

Because many diverse medical conditions can produce hypoglycemia, incidence rates vary based on etiology. In relatively infrequent disorders such as infants small for gestational age (SGA), hypoglycemia occurs in 13 to 44 percent of cases; the incidence rate for children with pituitary hormone deficiency varies from 11 to 27 percent. When the total prevalence of affected children is considered, hypoglyccmia is most often secondary to insulin-dependent diabetes mellitus (IDDM), with an incidence of 6–20 percent of those receiving conventional insulin treatment. Children with diabetes who receive intensified insulin treatment, often administered via an insulin pump, may experience a threefold increase in hypoglycemia compared with conventionally treated children.

ETIOLOGY

Hypoglycemia results when blood glucose levels are inadequate to meet bodily demands; either through reduced blood glucose supplies or through increased glucose use. Hypoglycemia is most common during extended periods of fasting or during illness; and rarely occurs in healthy individuals. Medical conditions that have been related to a reduction of glucose supply primarily include: disorders of growth (SGA infants, intrauterine growth retardation, prematurity, hypopituitarism, growth hormone deficiency, congenital hypothyroidism), and insulin-dependent diabetes mellitus (IDDM). Some metabolic disorders, such as glycogen storage disorders and galactosemia, can also result in hypoglycemia via glucose reduction. In contrast, disorders that produce hypoglycemia via increased glucose utilization are relatively rare, and most are not covered here. The more common perinatal conditions related to increased glucose utilization, and subsequent hypoglycemia, are: infants born to mothers who have diabetes, transient neonatal hyperinsulinism, perinatal asphyxiation, or large for gestational age babies.

PSYCHOLOGICAL CORRELATES

The psychological correlates of hypoglycemia are usually short-term, but can impact social functioning and school performance. Hypoglycemia can result in argumentative or irritable behavior as well as dizziness, confusion, and clumsiness. During a hypoglycemic episode, a child may be misunderstood by peers or feel embarrassed because of these atypical behaviors. Hypoglycemia also can produce a temporary decline in mental efficiency, flexibility, and reaction time, resulting in diminished attention and slower responses that may negatively affect learning or testing in school. After treatment, and a return to normal blood glucose levels (80–120 mg/dl), behavioral and cognitive functioning usually is normalized, often after a period of cognitive adaptation (i.e., approximately 30–45 min).

ASSESSMENT

Blood glucose levels can be measured from a variety of sources (arterial, venous, capillary, or whole blood serum). Most over-the-counter blood glucose monitors use capillary blood obtained from a finger prick. A thorough physical examination with medical history, and urinalysis, is necessary to determine the cause of hypoglycemia. Diagnosis is often difficult because of the transient nature of hypoglycemia and the subjective nature of the physical symptoms. Neuroglycopenic symptoms, which result from low blood glucose in the brain, include headache, dizziness, confusion, drowsiness, odd behavior, irritability, or slurred speech. During moderate to severe hypoglycemia (BGLs $\leq$ 40 mg/dl), more severe neurologic symptoms may occur and include amnesia, seizures, unconsciousness, and coma. Adrenergic symptoms, which result from the autonomic system, also occur during hypoglycemia and may include irregular heart beat (palpitations), tremor, weakness, or sweating. Some children experience mild hypoglycemia without any physical symptoms, making its detection very difficult until severe hypoglycemia results with its symptoms of seizures or unconsciousness. In older youth, particularly adolescents, the symptoms of hypoglycemia may be mistaken for intoxication.

TREATMENT

In diabetes and most other conditions that produce hypoglycemia, frequent snacks or meals can minimize its occurrence. Once hypoglycemia occurs, immediate treatment consists of having a child eat or drink a readily absorbed glucose source (usually high in fructose or sugar, i.e., candy or fruit juice) to normalize BGLs

Table 1. Common Etiologies and Treatments of
Hypoglycemia in Children

Etiology	Treatment
Hypopituitarism, growth hormone deficiency	Growth hormone replacement, cortisol, as needed
Congenital hypothyroidism	Thyroid replacement hormone
Small for gestational age infants	Frequent feedings
IDDM	Ingestion of 15 mg fast-acting carbohydrates (fruit, juice, sugar packets, candy, commercially prepared items), glucose (naturally occurring sugar) or glucagon (a protein hormone promoting sugar content of blood) administration
Hyperinsulinism	Glucose administration, Diazoxide, Somatostatin, pancreatectomy
Glycogen storage disorders Type 1	Glucose infusion, uncooked cornstarch, multivitamins and calcium, restrict fructose and galactose intake
Galactosemia	Galactose-restricted diet

rapidly. In the advent of severe hypoglycemia and its symptoms of nausea or unconsciousness, intravenous glucose or glucose suppositories may be required. Additional treatment should be tailored to the etiology of hypoglycemia (see Table 1).

PROGNOSIS

In infants, transient hypoglycemia often resolves within 1–2 days. If hypoglycemia continually occurs after eating in a child who has not had gastrointestinal surgery, it may be an early indicator of Type II (non-insulin-dependent) diabetes. Although discrete episodes of mild hypoglycemia may remit rather quickly with prompt administration of glucose (typically lasting only 10–30 min), hypoglycemia is likely to reoccur until the underlying medical condition is stabilized and/or treated.

Because the brain is critically dependent upon the body's immediately available BGLs, compromised cognitive functioning is the main risk of hypoglycemia. Infants and young children appear to be at particularly increased risk, because they are unable to communicate their symptoms to caregiving adults. In newborns, hypoglycemia may result in damage to several areas in the brain including the cerebral cortex, hippocampus, and caudate nucleus. Mild cognitive difficulties,

particularly in attention, processing speed, verbal memory, and visual-spatial skills, have been reported in children with diabetes who experience repeated severe hypoglycemic episodes, which results in seizures or unconsciousness, in the first 4–6 years of life. Slower learning and/or memory problems may also occur, although mental retardation is uncommon. Although cognitive difficulties have been reported in older children with diabetes, controversy exists over whether these problems are related solely to hypoglycemia, chronic hyperglycemia, early onset of the disease, or some combination of these factors.

In general, the prognosis for children experiencing hypoglycemia is favorable when mild episodes are treated quickly. However, untreated hypoglycemia has a poor prognosis, as it can result in permanent brain/neuronal damage secondary to seizures, coma, or accidents. Death also may result from severe hypoglycemia if left untreated.

See also: Diabetes Mellitus, Type 1; Diabetes Mellitus, Type 2; Glycogen Storage Disease; Hypothyroidism, Congenital; Metabolic Disorder; Prematurity: Birth Weight and Gestational Age; Prematurity Outcomes; Short Stature: Psychological Aspects; Storage Diseases

Further Reading

Becker, D. J., & Ryan, C. M. (2000). Hypoglycemia: A complication of diabetes therapy in children. *Trends in Endocrinology and Metabolism, 11*(5), 198–202.

Chavez, H., Ozolins, D., & Lozek, J. D. (1999). Hypoglycemia and propanolol in pediatric behavioral disorders. *Pediatrics, 103,* 1290–1299.

Kaplan, D., & Birrer, R. (1999). Assessing and treating hypoglycemic events. *Patient Care, 33,* 22–36.

Lteif, A. N., & Schwenk, W. F. (1999). Hypoglycemia in infants and children. *Endocrinology and Metabolism Clinics of North America, 28*(3), 619–646.

McAulay, V., Deary, I. J., & Frier, B. M., (2001). Symptoms of hypoglycemia in people with diabetes. *Diabetic Medicine, 18,* 690–705.

Raine, J. E., Donaldson, M., Gregory, J. W., & Savage, M. O. (2001). *Practical Endocrinology and Diabetes in Children.* London, U.K: Blackwell Science.

Ryan C. M., and Becker, D. J. (1999). Hypoglycemia in children with type 1 diabetes mellitus. *Endocrinology and Metabolism Clinics of North America, 28*(4), 883–900.

World Health Organization. (1997). *Hypoglycemia of the Newborn,* 1–66.

KELLY B. VAN SCHAICK
SARI A. SOUTOR
LAUREN ZIMMERMAN
CLARISSA S. HOLMES

Hypoparathyroidism

DESCRIPTION AND INCIDENCE

Hypoparathyroidism (HP) refers to a band of disorders characterized by a deficiency in *parathyroid hormone* (PTH). As PTH serves to regulate the amount of calcium and phosphorus in bone and blood, a deficiency in this hormone results in the abnormal metabolism of these minerals. Consequently, individuals with HP exhibit deficient blood levels of calcium and elevated levels of phosphorus. Abnormal levels of these minerals may result in a tingling sensation of the lips, fingers, and toes, muscle cramps, or muscle spasms that can cause pain of varying degrees. Spasms of the larynx can cause children with HP to have difficulty breathing. Rarely, affected individuals experience convulsions or seizures. Other associated features of HP include abdominal pain, dry hair and skin, brittle nails, tooth malformation, and cataracts. Postponement in treatment of this disorder can lead to growth retardation, developmental delays, learning disabilities, or death; fortunately, early intervention can prevent these effects.

HP affects 4 in 100,000 people and can occur at any age. Risk factors include family history of parathyroid disorder, history of certain autoimmune endocrine diseases, or recent thyroid or neck surgery.

ETIOLOGY

There are multiple causes of HP. The condition may result from a deficiency in PTH secretion, the inability to produce an active form of PTH, or the inability of the kidneys and bones to respond to PTH. Those with *congenital HP* are born without parathyroid glands; this defect is characteristic of a childhood disorder known as *DiGeorge syndrome*. Although individuals with congenital HP lack parathyroid glands at birth, symptoms may not present until later in life, typically within the first 24 months. In a minority of cases, symptoms do not emerge until several years later. A transient form of HP can occur as a result of overactive maternal parathyroid glands. The excess calcium enters the fetus and suppresses parathyroid function, thereby resulting in low calcium levels.

Acquired HP is an autoimmune disorder, resulting from the immune system's development of antibodies that attack parathyroid tissues in an attempt to reject what is perceived as foreign tissue. Children may also develop hypothyroidism due to accidental injury to the parathyroid glands during head or neck surgery.

Patients with HP typically have no family history of the disease; however, there are congenital cases that seem to be familial in origin. Autosomal dominant, autosomal recessive, and X-linked inheritance have been reported.

ASSESSMENT

Children who show signs of HP should be referred to a pediatric endocrinologist for a comprehensive evaluation. This evaluation features a family history, a physical examination, and several laboratory tests. Tests showing low PTH levels, low calcium levels, high phosphorus levels, or sometimes, low magnesium levels indicate a diagnosis of HP. High-resolution chromosome analysis may also be used to detect gene mutations in cases where the affected individual presents with cardiac anomalies and dysmorphic features.

ASSOCIATED PSYCHOLOGICAL FEATURES

Although children with HP are at a greater risk than unaffected children for the development of cognitive deficits and problems with psychological adaptation, these features are not an inherent part of the condition. Lower performance IQ scores and learning disabilities, however, are common among children with HP, and developmental milestones are typically achieved later than the expected age for healthy children. Language acquisition is delayed in many children with HP, and it is also common for these children to show difficulties with nonverbal learning, abstract reasoning, and mathematics. Children with HP are at risk for mental retardation as well. Although the reason for the association between mental retardation and HP has not yet been established, it has been suggested that *hypoxia* (inadequate oxygen tension at the cellular level) stemming from *hypocalcemic* (low calcium) seizures may be a contributing factor.

Children with HP are also thought to be at greater risk for psychiatric symptoms than are healthy children, though data concerning this issue are inconsistent. Perhaps more common than psychiatric symptoms, are difficulties with psychosocial adjustment that may affect any child with a chronic illness. Additionally, children with HP may experience difficulties related to delayed growth (see *Short Stature: Psychological Aspects* for further details).

TREATMENT

The goal of treatment for HP is to restore mineral balance within the body. Life-long treatment with oral calcium carbonate and Vitamin D supplements is typically necessary. Because overtreatment can result in *hypercalcemia*, or high blood calcium, and impaired kidney function, it is critical that blood levels are monitored consistently to ensure proper dosage. A diet that is high in calcium and low in phosphorus is recommended in addition to therapy.

If it happens that an affected child experiences an acute, life-threatening seizure or prolonged muscle contractions (*tetany*), intravenous infusion of calcium must be administered. In such cases, precautions must be taken in an effort to prevent laryngeal spasms that could lead to breathing difficulties, and heart monitoring for abnormal rhythms should be continued until the person is stabilized. Once the episode has passed, treatment continues with oral supplements.

In addition to medical management, it is necessary for parents and children to receive psychoeducational counseling where they are given the opportunity to ask any questions that they may have. Children with HP may also benefit from psychological intervention where they can learn to cope with problems related to their condition. For the child who experiences developmental delays or learning disabilities, it is essential that remedial educational services be provided.

PROGNOSIS

When treatment begins early, growth retardation and developmental delays can be prevented and prognosis is good, though there are some symptoms that are irreversible. These include dental changes, cataracts, and brain calcifications.

See also: Coping with Illness; Learning Disorders; Mental Retardation; Short Stature: Psychological Aspects

Further Reading

Perheentupa, J. (1996). Hypoparathyroidism and mineral homeostasis. In F. Lifshitz (Ed.), *Pediatric endocrinology* (3rd ed., pp. 433–471). New York: Marcel Dekker

LAUREN ZURENDA
DAVID E. SANDBERG

Hypothyroidism, Acquired

DESCRIPTION AND INCIDENCE

Acquired Hypothyroidism is a condition characterized by a deficiency in thyroid hormone (*thyroxine*). Although the clinical presentation varies among individuals, most affected children feature a *goiter*, or enlarged thyroid gland. Additional, nonspecific symptoms include physical weakness, lethargy, decreased appetite (but with mild obesity), cold intolerance, constipation, and dry skin. Most affected children demonstrate growth deceleration with delayed skeletal maturation and puberty (rarely precocious puberty), and girls may feature *galactorrhea* (i.e., flow of milk at times other than nursing).

Though difficult to ascertain with accuracy, the incidence of acquired hypothyroidism is estimated at 1/500 to 1,000 school age children. Observed more often in girls than boys, onset typically occurs during childhood or adolescence.

ETIOLOGY

The most common cause of acquired hypothyroidism in children and teenagers is *Hashimoto's thyroiditis* (autoimmune chronic lymphocytic thyroiditis), an autoimmune condition resulting from the immune system's production of antibodies that attack thyroid tissue and impair glandular function. Acquired hypothyroidism occurs with increased frequency in other autoimmune-mediated diseases as well, especially insulin-dependent diabetes mellitus and Down, Klinefelter, and Turner syndromes. While acquired hypothyroidism appears to run in families, a specific mode of inheritance has yet to be identified.

ASSESSMENT

The diagnostic procedure for suspected thyroid disorders includes a comprehensive physical evaluation and detailed family history, along with tests for thyroid function. Specifically, these tests include the measurement of thyroid stimulating hormone (TSH), thyroxine (T$_4$), and thyroid antibodies. Because individuals with acquired hypothyroidism may not experience clinical symptoms, it is common for the diagnostic procedure to begin when a patient presents with an enlarged thyroid gland during a routine check-up examination.

ASSOCIATED PSYCHOLOGICAL FEATURES

Although acquired hypothyroidism shares some common features with *congenital hypothyroidism*, it is important to distinguish between the two. Perhaps the most important distinction concerns the potential for impaired intellectual functioning stemming from damage to the central nervous system. Where as newborns with congenital hypothyroidism will experience central nervous system damage if the condition is left untreated, children with acquired hypothyroidism under the age of 3 years will not, so long as the child receives prompt and adequate treatment. When onset occurs later in childhood or during adolescence, affected children are not at risk for related central nervous system damage.

However, because a deficiency in thyroid hormone does adversely affect energy levels, most children with hypothyroidism will demonstrate deterioration in academic performance. With appropriate medical intervention, performance in school improves in response to the increase in energy levels.

TREATMENT

As with congenital hypothyroidism, acquired hypothyroidism is treated with daily doses of thyroid hormone (*levothyroxine*) taken orally. As mentioned previously, when symptoms emerge prior to age 3, prompt treatment is essential to prevent damage to the central nervous system. For all affected children, regardless of age of onset, treatment should begin as early as possible to allow for the achievement of full genetic growth potential. Undesirable side effects, such as irritability, restlessness, decreased attention span, a restless sleep or insomnia are often observed in cases where a return to normal thyroid hormone levels is achieved too rapidly; for this reason, dosing must be carefully monitored.

PROGNOSIS

When prompt and appropriate treatment is administered early in the development of the disorder, prognosis is excellent and almost all features are reversible. One feature that may not be reversible is final height.

While prepubertal children with severe hypothyroidism and short stature typically experience a period of "catch-up growth" following treatment, some have incomplete catch-up and never achieve their full genetic growth potential.

See also: Down Syndrome; Hypothyroidism, Congenital; Hyperthyroidism, Acquired; Klinefelter Syndrome; Turner Syndrome; Treatment Adherence: Medical

Further Reading

Cooper, D. S. (2001). *Medical management of thyroid disease.* New York: Marcel Dekker.

Dallas, J. S., & Foley, T. P. (1996). Hypothyroidism. In F. Lifshitz (Ed.) *Pediatric endocrinology: A clinical guide* (pp. 391–399). New York: Marcel Dekker.

Hauser, P., & Rovet, J. (1999). *Thyroid diseases in infancy and childhood: Effects on behavior and intellectual development.* Washington, DC: American Psychiatric Press.

LAUREN ZURENDA
DAVID E. SANDBERG

Hypothyroidism, Congenital

DESCRIPTION AND INCIDENCE

Early in fetal development, the thyroid gland "descends" from the base of the tongue to its final destination just below the thyroid cartilage (i.e., Adam's apple) in the front of the neck. By the end of the first trimester, the thyroid gland is not only located in its normal location in the neck, but it is also capable of collecting iodine and other raw materials from the fetal circulation for the production of thyroid hormone, *thyroxine.*

Abnormalities along the hypothalamic–pituitary–thyroid neuroendocrine axis during fetal life can result in harmful effects manifest in certain organ systems, including the central nervous system and skeleton. If left untreated, congenital hypothyroidism (CH) can lead to impaired bodily growth, as well as a marked reduction in brain size. This latter condition is termed *cretinism* and is accompanied by severe mental retardation. Fortunately, the introduction of newborn screening for all children born after 1974 has made early diagnosis and treatment possible; as a result, severe mental retardation as a consequence of CH has essentially been eliminated. Most infants with CH appear indistinguishable at birth. However, the continuous maintenance of proper thyroid hormone levels from the newborn period through childhood is absolutely essential for normal postnatal physical growth and brain development.

CH affects 1 in 4,000 births, occurring equally among males and females.

ETIOLOGY

CH is caused by a deficiency in thyroxine (T_4), a hormone responsible for the regulation of metabolic processes. The deficiency can result from an abnormality anywhere along the hypothalamic–pituitary–thyroid axis. When the site of defect is the thyroid gland itself (i.e., primary hypothyroidism), there are several forms the condition can take: the gland may be entirely absent (*athyreosis*); it may function inadequately (*dyshormonogenesis*); or it may be abnormally positioned (*ectopic*). There is thought to be an association between etiological factors and the severity of clinical features; as might be expected, individuals who lack a thyroid gland (athyreosis) tend to exhibit the most severe symptoms.

ASSESSMENT

In addition to severe mental retardation, untreated CH may result in feeding problems, failure-to-thrive, constipation, hypotonia (poor muscle tone), excessive sleeping, protruding tongue, and hoarse voice. However, since nearly all affected infants have the advantages of early intervention, the problem is corrected before these symptoms can emerge. The primary screening test for CH is the measurement of thyroxine and thyroid-stimulating hormone (TSH) from blood collected by heelstick the day after birth and adsorbed onto filter paper. Because false positives are common, an infant who tests positive on the initial test will be given the test again to confirm the diagnosis. The screening test programs for CH are very effective, and serve to identify virtually all children with CH.

ASSOCIATED PSYCHOLOGICAL FEATURES

Findings from the most encouraging longitudinal studies have demonstrated that global intelligence, as well as the relationship between intelligence and school achievement scores, is virtually identical in children with CH diagnosed at birth and unaffected children. Unfortunately, these optimistic findings are tempered by data indicating a deterioration during adolescence of adherence to the hormone replacement regimen (with associated thyroid hormone insufficiency). Insofar as improvement in treatment adherence brings about an enhancement in cognitive functioning, the importance of maintaining adequate thyroid hormone replacement clearly extends beyond childhood.

Although the finding that CH children function intellectually in the average range has been replicated in multiple studies, it has also been reported that a subgroup—those with athyreosis—perform poorly compared to unaffected children. This relative deficiency in intellectual potential is thought to reflect impairment caused by prenatal hypothyroidism that is not completely countered by early postnatal treatment. In these children, early development is characterized by delays in locomotor skill and speech acquisition, followed by deficits in language and auditory perception, visual-spatial organization, and numeracy.

In addition to the possibility of slightly inferior global intelligence, some studies have suggested the presence of selective neurocognitive deficits in children with CH. Unfortunately, little consensus exists concerning the particular type or extent of impairment. The problems identified include speech and language delays, poorer motor function (especially balance), and weaker perceptual-motor abilities. It has been suggested that children with this form of CH exhibit a cognitive profile resembling that of children with nonverbal learning disabilities. There is also an association between CH and hearing loss, which must be considered as a factor whenever language delays are observed.

TREATMENT

When newborn screening indicates a diagnosis of CH, infants are treated with thyroxine replacement (levothyroxine, taken orally) within the first few weeks after birth. Although treatment is required throughout their lifetime, parents should be aware of the critical nature of the first 3–4 weeks, as strong adherence to medical recommendations is essential. Some researchers have observed cognitive deficits and lethargy in children treated with thyroxine and have attributed these deficits to inadequate dosing. Thus, they recommend that higher dosages be prescribed in the early stages of childhood, when the brain is experiencing major growth and development. The potential long-term benefits of treatment with higher dosages of thyroxine must, however, be balanced against the drawbacks of behavioral difficulties observed in children with relatively elevated blood levels of thyroxine (e.g., restlessness and distractibility). Given the potential risks of inadequate or excessive dosing, thyroxine replacement therapy must be monitored closely.

Although there are data to suggest that the athyreotic subgroup of CH children may remain at risk for the development of cognitive and learning deficits, it is not known whether these deficits exhibit recovery over time. Inasmuch as the athyreotic subgroup of children with CH appears to be at greater risk for learning problems, they are good candidates for early educational assessment and targeted remediation to forestall the development of academic delay.

PROGNOSIS

Prompt normalization and maintenance of thyroid hormone levels makes normal development of the central nervous system likely in most cases of CH.

Although some affected individuals may remain at risk for cognitive and learning deficits due to a deficiency in prenatal thyroid hormone, the development of newborn screening procedures has allowed for the early diagnosis and treatment of the condition. Early treatment is accompanied by an excellent prognosis for an otherwise debilitating condition.

See also: Hyperthyroidism, Acquired; Hypothyroidism, Acquired; Learning Disorders; Treatment Adherence: Medical

Further Reading

Cooper, D. (2001). *Medical management of thyroid disease.* New York: Marcel Dekker.

Dallas, J. S., & Foley, T. P. (1996). Hypothyroidism. In F. Lifshitz (Ed.), *Pediatric endocrinology: A clinical guide* (pp. 391–399). New York: Marcel Dekker.

Hauser, P., & Rovet, J. (1999). *Thyroid diseases of infancy and childhood: Effects on behavior and intellectual development.* Washington, DC: American Psychiatric Press.

LAUREN ZURENDA
DAVID E. SANDBERG

Ii

Identity Development

DEFINITION

Identity development refers to the ways in which individuals view themselves in relation to the world around them. Identity encompasses one's self-concept, self-knowledge, self-worth, and self-esteem. The development of identity begins early in infancy with self-awareness and self-recognition, and continues into adolescence and young adulthood with the forging of an identity.

INFANCY

Identity development begins when infants first recognize that they are separate from other people and things. The first step toward acquiring this separation from other things comes from the knowledge of personal agency, which is the infant's understanding that they are the cause of certain events. This understanding is usually seen around 2 months of age and is generally developed through interactions with responsive caregivers. Once infants have the knowledge that they can manipulate their environment, they can begin to understand their separation from other people and things. This understanding comes through the development of self-awareness, which is seen in infants between 4 and 10 months of age. At this stage in development, infants' level of self-awareness is egocentric in that they tend to understand other things only in relation to themselves and do not use other cues in their environment.

By 18 months of age, infants show signs of self-recognition, which is typically measured by recording the infants' reactions to their mirror reflections. This test of self-recognition is used to determine whether the infants' reactions indicate that they are looking at the reflection more because they can manipulate it or because they recognize it as themselves. The development of self-recognition seems to be independent of culture because infants from cultures who have never been exposed to mirrors display self-recognition at the same time as infants who have been exposed to mirrors. The infants' ability to recognize themselves seems to be closely related to their level of cognitive development and social experiences. The development of self-recognition is important not only to the development of identity but also to the development of social, emotional, and cognitive abilities.

EARLY CHILDHOOD

Once the child has achieved self-recognition, they begin to notice the ways that they are similar and different from others. Through this recognition children begin to form both a categorical self and a gender identity. The categorical self is formed through the categorization of the self by dimensions that are noticed in others. During this stage in development, children use dimensions such as gender, age, and some evaluative dimensions to categorize themselves and they incorporate these categories into their self-concept.

Early childhood is also the time when children begin to adopt others' behaviors, attitudes, and beliefs.

In addition, children are beginning to form their gender identity by identifying with a caregiver who is generally of the same sex. Beginning at age 2 years, children will observe and model the same sex caregiver and by 3 years of age they will have a good idea to which sex they belong. However, it is not until about 4 years of age that children achieve gender constancy, which is the understanding that their sex will remain the same.

During this period, children are also beginning to develop "theory of mind," which is the ability to distinguish the public from the private self. By 3 years of age, children are able to understand that others cannot observe their thoughts, but do not yet understand that thoughts differ between people and that their thoughts are not always correct. However, by 5 years of age, children are able to understand that their thoughts may be inaccurate and that others may not share their thoughts. The development of "theory of mind" is important because children learn to distinguish between their private selves and their public selves, which is important for social development as well as the development of identity.

MIDDLE CHILDHOOD

During middle childhood, there is a developmental shift in how children describe themselves. During early childhood, children focus on their external qualities to describe and categorize themselves, but during middle childhood, they begin to focus on their inner qualities and incorporate these into descriptions of themselves. However, they view these psychological labels (inner qualities) as stable and unchanging (i.e., they believe they possess the same psychological characteristics in all situations), and it is not until adolescence (about 15 years of age) that children begin to understand that their psychological characteristics are not the same in all situations.

With the shift in self-concept to the incorporation of psychological labels comes the development of self-esteem. Self-concept refers to one's view of oneself while self-esteem is defined as how one evaluates oneself, that is, the discrepancy between one's actual self-concept and the ideal standard that they have set for themselves. Children begin to judge themselves based on how well their real selves correspond to their ideal standards. Consistent with cognitive development, preschool children tend to view themselves in terms of concrete attributes such as physical characteristics and possessions. Preschoolers also tend to think of themselves in either-or terms, for example, as "nice"

or "mean," "good" or "bad." At this time, self-concept and self-esteem are largely tied to feedback from parents and other significant others. During the middle childhood years, however, children begin to think of themselves in more abstract terms and their sense of self becomes increasingly dependent on how they think others, especially peers, perceive them. Self-esteem is also developed when children begin to learn that they have certain proficiencies that others may not possess. Children learn about their abilities by comparing themselves with their peers and thus a sense of competence is developed. This competence and hence self-esteem is further enhanced through social support by caregivers, teachers, and peers for their goals and achievements.

ADOLESCENCE

During adolescence, the goal of identity development is to become a unique adult with a purpose or specific role in life. To achieve this goal, adolescents are faced with what Erikson termed an "identity crisis." During the identity crisis, adolescents may fall into one or more of James Marcia's four categories of identity status: identity diffusion, foreclosure, moratorium, or identity achievement. Identity diffusion is a stage in which the adolescents have not yet begun to think about their identity or future. This is often seen in young adolescents, but may be seen in older adolescents and adults as well. Identity foreclosure is a stage in which the adolescent has achieved an identity without going through the process of evaluating other identities. This stage is often seen in adolescents who have a close bond with their parents and have accepted the identity that their parents have given them. The moratorium stage is the phase in which adolescents go through the traditional identity crisis. During this stage, adolescents are actively exploring who and what they want to become without making any definite identity commitments. Finally, identity achievement is the stage in which adolescents have resolved their identity crisis by making a commitment to an identity.

Most adolescents 12–18 years of age have neither entered their identity crisis (identity diffusion) nor have accepted the identity that was chosen for them (foreclosure). It is generally not until adolescents are 21 years of age or older that they enter their identity crisis (moratorium) or have achieved a stable identity (identity achievement). However, the formation of an identity is not fixed. Adults often reevaluate their identities, commonly after major life changes (e.g., divorce, death of a spouse, going back to school, or an employment change). In addition, adolescents may commit to an identity in one domain (i.e., occupation, political beliefs, and religious beliefs) and may not have made a commitment to an identity in other domains.

CLINICAL CONSIDERATIONS

The formation of a positive self-concept, self-esteem, and the establishment of an identity is healthy and adaptive, and the failure to form an identity or positive self-image may result in unhealthy behaviors and attitudes. Low self-esteem is associated with a number of psychiatric diagnoses (e.g., depression) and also with poor academic achievement and peer relationship problems. High self-esteem, on the other hand, has been shown to buffer the effects of stress. Conversely, successful coping with stressful events can foster a sense of mastery and thus enhances self-esteem. Adults have many opportunities to bolster children's self-esteem. They can reward, punish, or ignore their children's successful experiences; they can expose their children to mildly stressful experiences and help them cope; or they can shield them from every adversity, denying them the experience of mastery and consequent self-confidence. The failure to form an identity during adolescence may result in depression and low self-confidence or may result in the formation of a negative identity. The negative identity may involve delinquency and is often viewed by the individual as a means to obtain self-worth.

See also: Adolescence; Attachment; Emotional Development; Parenting Practices; Risk and Protective Factors; Social Development in Childhood; Social Development in Adolescence

Further Reading

Meeus, W. (1996). Studies of identity development in adolescence: An overview of research and some new data. *Journal of Youth and Adolescence, 25*, 569–598.

Meeus, W., Iedema, J., Helsen, M., & Vollebergh, W. (1999). Patterns of adolescent identity development: Review of literature and longitudinal analysis. *Developmental Review, 19*, 419–461.

Papalia, D. E., & Olds, S. W. (Eds.). (1995). *Human development* (6th ed.). New York: McGraw-Hill.

CHRISTA J. ANDERSON
JOHN COLOMBO

Idiopathic Thrombocytopenic Purpura

See: Platelet Abnormalities

Immunodeficiency

See: Bone Marrow Failure and Primary Immunodeficiency

Individuals with Disabilities Education Act (IDEA)

HISTORY

An outcome of civil rights movements for free and appropriate education for all children was a law enacted to provide federally mandated services for children with conditions that inhibit learning. First established in 1975 as the Education for All Handicapped Children Act of 1975 (PL 94-1420), the law covered children who were of school age, although some states choose to broaden the age range. Throughout the years, the law has been changed to provide services for children of ages 3 through 21 years, although some states may provide services for more extended age ranges. The law has also been changed to add categories for eligibility, as well as to incorporate person-first language so that children are identified first, with the disability named second, through the Individuals with Disabilities Education Act, 1990 (IDEA, 1990). Currently, children are served under IDEA 1997, and with reauthorization of this law enacted in the year 2002. There are several key concepts that are incorporated in IDEA 1997.

KEY CONCEPTS

Free and Appropriate Public Education (FAPE) means that every child identified with a disability is entitled to public education that is appropriate for that child and is at no additional cost to his or her parents.

Local Education Agency (LEA) is the school district in which the child who is eligible for services resides. The LEA is responsible for implementing state and federal regulations, and providing placement and services.

Least Restrictive Environment (LRE) means that children with IDEA eligibilities are served in the classroom along with their peers whenever possible. This process has been called mainstreaming, inclusion, and integration. There is typically a range of placements, from total inclusion in the regular education classroom to residency in state schools. This placement is determined by the Individualized Educational Plan (IEP) team.

The IEP team is a group of people who determine eligibility, placement, and the individualized educational plan for the student. The IEP team is composed of multidisciplinary members that must by law include the parents, the student (as appropriate), regular education and special education teachers, and LEA representatives for provision of services (typically an administrator) and interpretation of assessment findings (typically someone who specializes in assessment). Other members may be included such as related services personnel (e.g., speech therapist, occupational therapist, physical therapist, mobility specialist). The team is also responsible for taking into account other factors that may affect educational needs such as behavior, language proficiency, and vision and hearing impairments. The name of this team varies from state to state, but all teams must address both federal and legal mandates.

The IEP is created by the team members and includes eight components. There must be a statement of the student's present level of educational performance that includes how the disability affects educational performance and participation in educational activities. There must be measurable annual goals that include short-term objectives that monitor progress. A statement indicating special education services, as well as supplementary aids, services, program modifications, and support that assist the child in advancing toward annual goals, participating in general curriculum as well as extracurricular activities, and learning and participating with peers in all activities, must be included. The degree of LRE must be explained if the child is not in the regular education classroom full time. Children must participate in state- or districtwide assessments, and if modifications are needed to do so, they must be indicated. The commencement, frequency, location, and duration of services and modifications must be stated. Transition needs and services must be stated as the student prepares to move from the schools into society. This typically starts at age 14. How the student progresses toward meeting annual goals is measured and how this is reported to the parent must be indicated.

Eligibility for special education services is based on having one or more disabilities that interfere with learning, as well as a need for special education and related services related to their disability. The eligibilities include mental retardation; hearing impairments, including deafness, speech, or language impairments; vision impairments, including blindness; serious emotional disturbance; orthopedic impairments; autism; traumatic brain injury; and other health impairments which can

also include Attention-Deficit/Hyperactivity Disorder (ADHD), and specific learning disability. Specific learning disability refers to a disorder in one or more of the processes involved in understanding or using spoken or written language that may manifest itself in poor ability to listen, think, speak, read, write, spell, or do mathematical calculations.

Procedural safeguards include several provisions such as independent educational evaluations, prior written notice of any meetings about their children, parental consent, access to educational records, opportunity to present complaints, continued placement of student during due process hearings, placement of student in interim alternative educational settings for disciplinary reasons, mediation, due process hearings, state-level appeals, civil actions, and attorneys' fees. Implications for parents: IDEA 1997 provides for rights and protections as well as due process. While parents are integral to the processes, parents alone cannot determine the placement and services. Rather, these must come from the committee. Parents must sign release of information forms to have school records released to outside agencies, including their own mental health provider.

IMPLICATIONS FOR CLINICIANS

Clinicians outside the school settings may have their reports released by the parents to the schools, and may obtain school reports only if parents sign to release this information. Outside clinician reports can be considered but need not be used by the IEP team. Clinicians outside the school setting may be utilized for independent educational evaluations. Clinicians in this situation must be aware that they cannot dictate placement, and that their recommendations can only be considered or may or may not be implemented. Since educational eligibility is determined by federal and state law, DSM diagnoses may be considered, but will not be the sole determinant of eligibility; rather, eligibility is determined by the committee.

See also: Autistic Disorder; Language Development; Language Disorders, Learning Disorders; Underachievement

Resources

http://www.NICHY.org, http://www.ed.gov/offices/OSERS/OSEP, Pub.L.No.94-142, 89 Stat. 975, Pub.L.No.101-479, 104 Stat. 1103, Pub.L.No.105-17, 111 Stat. 82

CONSTANCE J. FOURNIER

Infancy

DEFINITIONS

The period of infancy has traditionally been defined in terms of specific ages, such as birth to 3 years of age. Perhaps more accurately, the period of infancy (the label deriving from the Greek *infans*, meaning "without reason or language") may be defined as the period of life that predates the development of complex communicative abilities. If considered this way, infancy may be generally thought to span the period between birth and 18–24 months of age. It is worth noting that this definition of infancy also implies the inclusion of prenatal behavioral development as a proper topic. Despite the characterization of the newborn infant as a *tabula rasa* ("blank slate"), it has long been known that the newborn infant enters the world with a considerable history of prenatal experience, preferences, and responses.

THEORY AND RESEARCH

The study of infancy was largely ignored as a topic of empirical study in developmental psychology until the 1950s. However, over the last 50 years, scientific work on infant development has been generally incorporated into the realm of developmental science, and as a result, a number of journals devoted to empirical work in this area have emerged. These more specialized journals include *Infancy, Infant Behavior and Development,* and *Infant and Child Development.* In addition, a number of summary texts are available on the topic of infancy, most notably those by Fogel (2001), Bornstein and Lamb (1992), and Snow (1998).

STAGES OF DEVELOPMENT WITHIN INFANCY

Investigators have identified several different periods during infancy in which behavioral reorganizations take place. For example, the neonatal period (i.e., birth to 6–8 weeks postnatal) is dominated by major changes in behavioral states such as sleeping, waking, crying/fussiness, and various types of alertness. The period of 2–6 months of age may be characterized as a time during which visual attention predominates. The infant becomes increasingly active, cognitively sophisticated,

and social during the period from 6 to 12 months of age. At or around 12 months of age, when the infant begins using words or meaningful sounds, the primary focus of infant development changes to language, which combines the products of the cognitive system within the social context. At the same time, during the second year, the infant becomes increasingly able to drive his/her own interactions with the environment, rather than being driven by stimuli or events in the environment.

TOPIC AREAS WITHIN INFANCY

In addition to characterizing infancy in terms of time periods or behavioral domains, the study of infancy may also be defined by particular topics. For example, coverage of infancy in college classes or in terms of research subdisciplines may be divided into areas that include basic brain/central nervous system (CNS) development, motor development, sensory development, perceptual/attentional development, development of higher order cognitive functions (memory, categorization, problem solving, representation), language development, and social development.

RELEVANCE TO CLINICAL RESEARCH AND PRACTICE

Decades of research have shown that the central nervous system is not fully mature at birth, and that both the structure and function of the brain may be strongly affected by rearing conditions that are encountered during the early part of the lifespan. As such, the period of infancy has generally been regarded as a type of "critical period" during which the individual child can be greatly affected by his/her environment. For example, it is commonly considered that the child may be considered to be highly vulnerable to stimulus deprivation and abnormal environmental conditions during infancy, but also that the development of the child can be appreciably enhanced by exposure to a variety of stimulation and optimal input. As such, clinical interests in infancy will logically involve the efficacy, efficiency, and necessity of early intervention in infants at risk for developmental delay or disorder. An important corollary to this focus is on the early identification of individuals at risk for such developmental delay or disorder so that early intervention may be implemented.

See also: Attachment; Cognitive Development; Developmental Milestones; Early Intervention; Emotional Development; Language Development; Memory Development; Prematurity

Outcomes; Prenatal Development; Sudden Infant Death Syndrome

Further Reading

Bornstein, M. H., & Lamb, M. (1992). *Development in infancy* (3rd ed.). Columbus, OH: McGraw-Hill.
Colombo, J. (2001). The development of visual attention in infancy. *Annual Review of Psychology, 52*, 337–367.
Fogel, A. (2001). *Infancy: Infant, family and society.* St. Paul, MN: West.
Snow, C. W. (1998). *Infant development* (2nd ed.). Upper Saddle River, NJ: Prentice-Hall.

JOHN COLOMBO

Infant Assessment

The developmental assessment of children in the first 3 years of life has received new attention from psychology, special education, and related fields in the last several decades (Smith, Pretzel, & Landry, 2001), as well as from the society at large. The 1986 passage of Public Law 99-457, with funding for services to children ages 0–3, and the improved survival of very premature infants were two factors that accelerated the emphasis on infants and toddlers. The most important factor, though, has been the rapid expansion of the field of early intervention. Intensive, family-friendly, and developmentally appropriate intervention for infants and toddlers has been shown to make a real difference in outcome both for the child and the family (Bagnato & Neisworth, 1991; Meisels & Fenichel, 1996). For such services to be effective, assessments are needed to identify the children who need and can benefit from services, provide guidance in developing appropriate individualized programs, track progress, and inform parents about their children's strengths and challenges. Infant and toddler assessments are also needed to assess the effectiveness of innovative medical and developmental treatment approaches for infants.

METHODS

There are many ways to classify assessment approaches for infants and toddlers. Some of these include whether the instrument is designed for screening or in-depth assessment; the amount of structure used; the domains covered; the use of normative versus criterion or curriculum-based reference; and the emphasis on observation versus elicited behavior. However, infant assessments generally share some common characteristics that distinguish them from assessments designed for older children.

First, they generally involve much more parental participation. Most infant assessments are developed with the assumption that a parent will be present and involved in the assessment process. Information provided by the parent is a key part of the data gathered and the parent is seen as a central member of the assessment team.

Second, the infant is not expected to cooperate with adult demands in the same way as the older child is. Rather, the examiner is expected to keep the child interested, intrigued, and motivated to respond to the test items, which are designed to be appealing. Most infant assessments allow the examiner flexibility in the order in which items are presented so as to keep the infant's attention and participation at an optimal level. The actual process of most infant assessments appears to be a playful and enjoyable interaction between the examiner and the child, using a variety of materials, with varying degrees of involvement and assistance by the parent. Even in the more structured infant assessments, time spent observing the infant in free play and in interaction with the parent is crucial to understanding the child's overall function and to interpreting the more formalized assessment results. Even more than with older children, the examiner must accommodate to the child's need to be rested, fed, and physically well. Positioning the infant to facilitate his or her ability to interact with the examiner and the assessment materials is always crucial, and may require special equipment or other modifications when infants have motor delays or disabilities. The examiner must also be especially sensitive to the possibility that the infant may have undiagnosed sensory disabilities, such as hearing or visual impairments.

Third, professionals evaluating infants face a special challenge in sorting out the contribution of motor, cognitive, language, and social–emotional development on the performance of each child. While different assessment instruments approach this task differently, it requires careful observation to tease out cognition and problem-solving skills independent of motor and social competence in infants and toddlers, and due caution in drawing conclusions and making predictions. Similarly, in the second and third years of life, language maturation may have a significant impact on the accuracy of the assessment of the child's cognitive skills. The examiner must be very aware of the child's relative strengths in each of these areas of development, and must be sensitive to the interplay among them in order to obtain a meaningful, holistic assessment. For example, if a child does not succeed at an item requiring him to stack blocks, the reason may lie in a problem with any of the following: the fine motor skill of grasping and placing the block, the gross motor capacity to sit and use the arms freely, the ability to inhibit the impulse to drop or throw toys, attention to or comprehension of verbal instructions or visual demonstration, confidence in trying a new task, or the cognitive understanding of the concept of stacking. Each one of these possibilities indicates an important finding that should be part of the total assessment result, and is far more important than the mere observation of "failure to stack blocks." While some instruments that focus specifically on a particular domain such as language or motor skills are available, most infant assessments are comprehensive and attempt to provide information on the range of areas important to each child's development.

Fourth, infant assessment activities tend to be the most transdisciplinary of any age group. Psychologists, developmental pediatricians and nurse practitioners, physical therapists, occupational therapists,

speech–language pathologists, special educators, and child development specialists may each function in the role of assessing multiple aspects of the development of an individual infant, although ideally each examiner has access to colleagues in other disciplines for consultation and assistance.

In light of all of these issues, some authors such as Meisels and Fenicel have argued for a decreased role for norm-referenced and standardized assessments in infancy, in favor of naturalistic, observational, and play-based assessments (Meisels & Fenichel, 1996). These approaches have been quite useful in settings with the appropriate resources to accomplish them properly.

Table 1 provides a summary of some of the commonly used approaches to infant assessment. It includes screening tests, which are designed to briefly look at the developmental progress of large numbers of children to select the children that need more in-depth attention, as well as tests that evaluate individual children in-depth for the purposes of classification and of designing interventions. The table includes a representative selection of the dozens of instruments available, emphasizing those that cover multiple developmental domains.

Table 1. Infant Assessment Approaches (Partial List)

Name and author	Publisher and year	Purpose	Age range	Areas assessed	Special features
Ages and Stages Questionnaire, Bricker, D., Squires, J., and Mounts, L.	Brookes, 1999	Developmental screening, surveillance	0–48 month(s)	Communication gross/fine motor, problem solving, personal–social	Completed by parent or parent/ professional together; English and Spanish versions
Brigance Screens, Brigance, A. N. and Billerica, M. A.	Curriculum Associates, Inc., 1978	Developmental screening	21–90 months	Speech–Language, motor, readiness, general knowledge	Combines observation, elicitation
Parents' Evaluation of Developmental Status (PEDS), Glaseoe, F. P.	Ellsworth and Vandemeer Press, Ltd., 1997	Developmental screening	0–8 years	Language, motor, behavioral, social; 1–2 questions each	English and Spanish versions, elicits parent's concerns
Denver Developmental Screening Test—II, Frankenburg, W. K. and Dodds, J. B.	Denver Developmental Materials, 1990	Developmental screening	0–6 years	Cognitive, motor, adaptive, language	Revision of one of the first screening tests published
Bayley Infant Neurodevelopmental Screener (BINS), Aylward, G. S.	Psychological Corporation, 1995	Screen infants at risk for developmental delay or neurological impairment	3–24 months	Neurological functions/ intactness, receptive functions, expressive functions, cognitive processes	Yields high, moderate, low risk score
Bayley Scales of Infant Development— II, Bayley, N.	Psychological Corporation, 1993	Norm-referenced evaluation	1–42 months	Mental, motor, behavioral scales	Extensive national norms. All elicited items

(Continued)

Table 1. (*Continued*)

Name and author	Publisher and year	Purpose	Age range	Areas assessed	Special features
Mullen Scales of Early Learning, Mullen, E. M.	American Guidance Service, 1995	Norm-referenced evaluation	0–7 years	Visual receptor, fine motor, receptive language, expressive language, gross motor	Offers separate scale scores and early learning composite. All elicited items
Transdisciplinary Play-Based Assessment, Lindner, T. W.	Brookes, 1990	Individualized, developmental functional assessment	6 months– 6 years	Cognitive, social–emotional, communications, sensorimotor	Structured play observation; yields detailed summary rather than score
Fagan Test of Infant Intelligence, Fagan, J. and Shepherd, P. A.	Infatest Corp, 1985	Assessment of information-processing ability as a measure of intelligence independent of motor skills	5, 7, 9, and 12 months	Information-processing assessed through novelty preference	Paradigm is quite different from traditional tests
Battelle Developmental Inventory, Newborg, J. et al.	Riverside Publishing, 1984	Developmental screening and diagnostic evaluation	0–8 years	Personal–social, adaptive, motor, communication, cognitive	Linked to curriculum guides
Brigance Inventory of Early Development—Revised, Brigance, A. N.	Curriculum Associates, 1998	Diagnostic evaluation for intervention	0–7 years	Varies depending on age—covers range of areas	Criterion-referenced, offers curriculum guide
Assessment, Evaluation, and Programming System (AEPS) for Infants and Children, Bricker, D.	Brookes, 1993	Assessment/evaluation for intervention	0–3 years (version for older children available)	Fine and gross motor, adaptive, cognitive, social	Curriculum-based; corresponding intervention plan available
The Carolina Curriculum for Infants and Toddlers with Special Needs, Johnson-Martin, N. M. et al.	Brookes, 1991	Assessment/ intervention for children with mild to severe special needs	0–2 years (version for older children available)	Cognition, communication, social adaptation, fine and gross motor	Assessment leads directly to curriculum with specific teaching guidelines
Hawaii Early Learning Profile (HELP®), Parks, S. et al.	Vort, 1997	Assessment/ Intervention	0–3 years (version for older children available)	Cognitive, language, gross and fine motor, social, self-help	Array of curriculum and family education items available

RELIABILITY AND VALIDITY ISSUES

Infant assessment presents some complex psychometric issues. These issues are different for screening versus diagnostic tests. Screening tests are useful to the extent that they accurately predict which children do and do not prove to have developmental delays when given full evaluations. Information about these characteristics is generally published for each screening test, and is described as the test's sensitivity and specificity. This information should be used to judge the appropriateness of the screening test selected for a particular purpose. Such tests may be used in pediatric offices during routine health surveillance or as part of community-wide "child-find" efforts. They should never be used to diagnose or label individual children.

The purpose of most infant assessment is to identify children who can benefit from intervention and to guide that intervention, rather than to predict later IQ. This issue, and the rapid change that is the hallmark of infancy, make the standards of test–retest reliability and predictive validity that are applied to assessments of older individuals less appropriate for infants. In addition, different kinds of skills must be assessed at different ages. For example, on the Bayley-II Mental Development Index, items that require sensorimotor manipulation make up much of the test during the first year, while language items become dominant in the second year. In general, as children become older, the test-retest reliability and predictive validity of assessment instruments improve, and they are clearly higher for children who fall at the more extreme ends of the developmental spectrum. In addition, repeated assessments over time provide much more reliable information about the long-term potential of the individual child, and more accurate guidance about his order current and long-term needs, than do single assessments. For this reason, most psychologists and other developmental specialists try to follow at-risk infants and toddlers longitudinally. Definitive diagnoses of developmental disabilities are often deferred until the child is at least 2 or 3 years old, has received intervention services, and has been assessed over time along multiple dimensions.

See also: Developmental Issues in Assessment for Treatment; Developmental Milestones; Individuals with Disabilities Education Act (IDEA); Infancy; Neonatal Assessment; Prematurity Outcomes; Psychometric Properties of Tests; Screening Instruments: Behavioral and Developmental

Further Reading

Bagnato, S. J., & Neisworth, J. T. (1991). *Assessment for early intervention: Best practices for professionals*. New York: Guilford.

Culbertson, J. L., & Willis, D. J. (Eds.). (1993). *Testing young children: A reference guide for developmental, psychoeducational, and psychosocial assessments*. Austin, TX: Pro-ed.

Meisels, S. J., & Fenichel, E. (Eds.). (1996). *New visions for the developmental assessment of infants and young children*. Washington, DC: Zero to Three.

Singer, L. T., & Zeskind, P. S. (2001). *Biobehavioral assessment of the infant*. New York: Guilford.

Smith, T., Pretzel, R., & Landry, K. (2001). Infant assessment. In R. J. Simeonsson & S. L. Rosenthal (Eds.), *Psychological and developmental assessment: Children with disabilities and chronic conditions*. New York: Guilford.

Wyly, M. V. (1997). *Infant assessment*. Boulder, CO: Westview Press.

MELISSA R. JOHNSON

Infantile Amnesia

See: Memory Development

Infectious Diseases

See: Pediatric Infectious Diseases

Inflammatory Bowel Disease

DEFINITION/INCIDENCE/ETIOLOGY

Inflammatory bowel disease (IBD), which includes Crohn's disease and ulcerative colitis, is caused by uncontrolled inflammation in the gastrointestinal (GI) tract. It is a chronic disease with a variable relapsing and remitting course. The most common symptoms include abdominal pain, diarrhea, rectal bleeding, and weight loss, and associated symptoms can include fever, arthritis, and perianal disease. IBD occurs in 6 of every 100,000 children, with approximately one-fourth of all cases occurring in people under the age of 20. The etiology of IBD is unknown, although genetic and microbial factors are both known to be involved.

PSYCHOLOGICAL CORRELATES

Children with IBD have reported concerns about missing school, taking medicine, experiencing flare-ups, missing out on sport and social activities, and lacking energy. However, much of the research on psychosocial issues in pediatric IBD is limited by methodological problems and mixed results. Some studies have reported significantly more behavioral/emotional and social problems in children with IBD than healthy comparison children, whereas other studies have reported functioning within normal ranges. When children with IBD do display emotional problems, they seem to be more prone to internalizing problems such as depression and anxiety rather than externalizing problems. Additionally, the relationship between psychosocial difficulties and health status is unclear. Some studies report increased difficulties with more severe disease, whereas others have not found this relationship.

ASSESSMENT/TREATMENT

Diagnosis is based on history, physical exam, laboratory evaluation, radiographic studies, and endoscopy/colonoscopy. There is no cure for IBD, so the focus of treatment involves controlling the inflammation. Medications include aminosalicylates, corticosteroids, immunosuppressive medications, antibiotics, and biologic agents. Patients often take many medications several times a day, and adherence can become a concern. Surgery also may be required.

The effects of psychotherapy have not been studied in children, but in adults, there is some support for cognitive–behavioral techniques. Two adult studies found that cognitive–behavioral strategies aimed at stress management and pain management resulted in decreases in IBD symptoms compared to control groups. Another study investigating cognitive–behavioral therapy reported that subjects in the treatment group reported less stress, depression, and anxiety than the control group, which consisted of symptom monitoring. However, IBD symptoms decreased in both groups, so no group differences were found in disease outcomes. A study examining psychodynamic therapy found no significant differences in disease outcome or psychosocial variables.

See also: Cognitive–Behavioral Play Therapy; Gastrointestinal Disorders

Further Reading

Crohn's and Colitis Foundation of America (CCFA) Web site: http://www.ccfa.org

Drossman, D. A. (2000). Psychosocial factors in ulcerative colitis and Crohn's disease. In J. B. Kirsner (Ed.), *Inflammatory bowel disease* (5th ed., pp. 342–357). Philadelphia: W.B. Saunders.

Rice, H. E., & Chuang, E. (1999). Current management of pediatric inflammatory bowel disease. *Seminars in Pediatric Surgery, 8,* 221–228.

Shanahan, F. (2001). Inflammatory bowel disease: Immunodiagnostics, immunotherapeutics, and ecotherapeutics. *Gastroenterology, 120,* 622–635.

LAURA M. MACKNER
WALLACE V. CRANDALL

Informed Consent

The clinical child and pediatric psychologist must obtain informed consent prior to assessment or intervention by fully explaining the potential risks and benefits. Four essential elements are involved in informed consent with children and their parents or guardians. First and foremost, informed consent requires competence to understand the risks and benefits of the assessment or intervention. Since children cannot always understand all the ramifications of making these decisions for themselves, the legally responsible person (e.g., parent) must give permission for participation. Although it is best practice to obtain permission from both parents for services, it is usually not legally required by most states or provinces. Because of their diminished capacity and lack of life experience, minors are not legally allowed to consent to services except in rare circumstances (e.g., suicide assessment). Even though there is no legal necessity to obtain consent from minors, an attempt is made to have children assent to assessment or treatment since a child who agrees to participate is generally more cooperative which in turn may lead to a better outcome. At all times, clinical child and pediatric psychologists should inform children of the proposed interventions in a manner commensurate with their psychological capabilities, seek their assent to those interventions, and consider their preferences and best interests. Obtaining consent from parents or guardians is legally required and once the consent has been given regarding the assessment or intervention, the child's desires become irrelevant from a legal point of view.

The second element requires that the child and parent be provided information about the assessment or intervention that might affect their willingness to participate. The clinical child or pediatric psychologist should provide an explanation that is clear, comprehensive, and unambiguous. The psychologist should make reasonable efforts to answer questions and to avoid any misunderstandings about the nature of the assessment or intervention. The goal of the explanation is to ensure that the child and parents are fully knowledgeable about the services they are about to receive. Within the context of the explanation, the child and parent should be fully informed about any potential risks and benefits inherent in the services. In addition, the explanation should be given in a manner appropriate for the developmental and cognitive understanding of the child and parent.

The third element requires that the child and parent participate in the assessment or intervention voluntarily. Although the child is usually brought in for services by the parent, it is still helpful to get the child's assent to participate. Regardless of whether the child assents or not, the parents retain the legal right of consent. The clinical child or pediatric psychologist must not coerce or inappropriately influence participation in psychological services. In most cases assessment or intervention that is coerced is not effective. The psychologist should also be cognizant of the power differential in their relationship that could influence participation. In medical settings, physicians usually refer patients for psychological services and parents might believe that if they decline psychological services, their future medical care might be affected. In these settings pediatric psychologists should restate the voluntary nature of obtaining psychological services.

The fourth and final element requires that the informed consent should be appropriately documented. Although not required by ethical guidelines, it is the best practice to obtain written consent rather than oral consent. In either case, documentation of the consent is required regardless of whether the consent was obtained orally or in writing.

Clinical child and pediatric psychologists should be especially careful with informed consent with families. Whether with assessment or intervention activities, the psychologist should delineate the nature of the professional relationship with the child and with other family members at the onset of professional contact. If an assessment is conducted, the psychologist should clarify who is being assessed and how information will be used. If an intervention is conducted, the psychologist should inform all parties who will be the focus of treatment and how information will be shared with other family members. If a role conflict becomes apparent, the psychologist should modify or clarify his or her role accordingly and, if no resolution appears evident, should withdraw from providing services.

A number of exceptions exist to informed consent practices for children and adolescents. The legal aspects of providing psychological services and the minimum age of consent vary from state to state. The exceptions to informed consent fall into two distinct areas. In the first area, a minor can legally consent to assessment or intervention for certain kinds of presenting problems. For example, depending upon the state or province in which the individual resides, minors can obtain psychological services independent of parental consent for physical or sexual abuse, pregnancy, sexually transmitted diseases, drug use or addiction, and suicidal or homicidal ideation. In the same way, in most states and provinces, minors can obtain emergency services at their own request if the minor has diminished capacity and/or if the minor is in danger to self or others. In the second area, the legal status of the minor determines how the informed consent is obtained. In most states and provinces, an individual younger than 18 years who is in the military, married, or living independently from parents and financially

self-supporting is regarded as an "emancipated minor." Also, informed consent is not necessary if a minor has been compelled by a court to obtain an assessment or intervention. Like adults, the court can involuntarily hospitalize minors if they are a danger to themselves, a danger to others, or have diminished capacity to care for themselves.

See also: Confidentiality and Privilege; Ethical Issues; Legal Issues in Child and Pediatric Psychology; Mental Health Records; Training Issues

Further Reading

American Psychological Association. (1992). Ethical principles of psychologists and code of conduct. *American Psychologist, 47,* 1597–1611.

Melton, G. B., Ehrenreich, N. S., & Lyons, P. M., Jr. (2001). Ethical and legal issues in mental health services for children. In C. E. Walker & M. C. Roberts (Eds.), *Handbook of clinical child psychology* (3rd ed., pp. 1074–1093). New York: Wiley.

Rae, W. A., Worchel, F. F., & Brunnquell, D. (1995). Ethical and legal issues in pediatric psychology. In M. C. Roberts (Ed.), *Handbook of pediatric psychology* (2nd ed., pp. 19–36). New York: Guilford.

WILLIAM A. RAE

Initiating and Maintaining Sleep

DEFINITION

Insomnia is one of the most common sleep disorders. People are considered to have insomnia if they have trouble falling asleep at night (difficulty initiating sleep), if they wake up frequently or too early and cannot go back to sleep (difficulty maintaining sleep), or even if they sleep a reasonable number of hours but are still not rested the next day (nonrestorative sleep). Bedtime resistance, as well as difficulty in falling or remaining asleep, are among the common sleep problems exhibited by children. Young children frequently cry, have tantrums, or misbehave at bedtime and often do not resettle without significant parental intervention when they wake in the middle of the night.

INCIDENCE/ETIOLOGY

Almost one-third of the general population reports some symptoms of insomnia during any given year, and

17 percent indicate that their problems are severe. Estimates of insomnia among healthy young children range from 25 percent to more than 40 percent. In addition, sleep disturbances do not tend to go away if left untreated. For example, the prevalence rates of sleep disorders in adults are similar to those found in children, suggesting that people experiencing sleep disturbances as children continue to experience them as adults. Growing evidence points to both biological as well as cultural explanations for poor sleep among adolescents. Many children and adolescents who have difficulty initiating and maintaining sleep have a history of "light" or easily disturbed sleep. However, sleep difficulties in children may also arise from an irregular sleep schedule (e.g., inconsistent bedtime and wake-up times), poor sleep habits (e.g., unstructured bedtime routine, caffeine intake too close to bedtime), and parental behavior in response to sleep disturbance (e.g., increased parental attention).

CORRELATES

Chronic insomnia may lead to decreased feelings of well-being during the day, including a deterioration of mood and motivation; decreased attention, energy, and concentration; and an increase in fatigue. Sleep difficulties have also been associated with increased child irritability during the day as well as increased behavior problems (e.g., eating problems, crying, and temper tantrums). In clinical populations, sleep difficulties have been associated with depression, depressive symptoms, and posttraumatic stress. Associations between attention-deficit/hyperactivity disorder (ADHD) and sleep problems have also been reported in clinical populations (although there is limited empirical support for this association). Additionally, parents of children with persistent sleep difficulties report negative effects that extend beyond the immediate hassle of a bedtime or nighttime tantrum (e.g., parental stress, family tension, maternal depression).

ASSESSMENT

A daily sleep diary that includes the time the child was put to bed, the time the child fell asleep, the time and duration of nighttime awakenings, a description of nighttime awakenings, the time the child awoke, and the time and duration of naps is an invaluable tool when assessing for difficulties in initiating and maintaining sleep. In addition, a sleep assessment interview can provide more specific information regarding the type of disturbance, as well as the frequency, duration, and intensity of the disturbance. A sleep problem scale (e.g., Albany Sleep Problem Scale) is a useful tool to obtain information about the type of sleep problem the child is experiencing (e.g., bedtime and night waking, sleep schedules, nightmares, etc.).

TREATMENT

Numerous behavioral interventions have been successful in reducing this sleep difficulty. Behavioral procedures used to treat difficulties in initiating and maintaining sleep include bedtime routines, graduated extinction, scheduled awakenings, bedtime fading, and sleep restriction. *Bedtime routines* include a series of relaxing activities to help children with the transition to sleep, and generally include activities such as taking a bath, changing into pajamas, and reading a story. Extinction procedures involve ignoring the child's cry or other vocalizations/requests. *Graduated extinction* is a variation of ignoring which involves ignoring bedtime (or nighttime) crying for progressively longer periods of time before attending to the child. *Scheduled awakening* involves partially waking the child 15–60 min before a spontaneous awakening and then letting him/her fall back to sleep. Scheduled awakenings are reduced and eventually eliminated when the child no longer experiences spontaneous awakenings. *Bedtime fading* involves selecting a time for bed when the child is likely to fall asleep with little difficulty and within 15 minutes. If the individual falls asleep with little resistance, then the bedtime is faded back in small increments until the desired bedtime is achieved. Sleep restriction involves restricting the amount of time in bed to the total amount of time asleep, thereby reducing the time spent in bed not sleeping. Despite the success of behavioral interventions in the treatment of sleep difficulties, the use of medication is a very common treatment for insomnia in both adults and children. Pharmacological treatments, however, appear to have little long-term benefit on the sleep patterns of children. According to most sleep professionals, medication is usually recommended only as a short-term answer to a sleep problem—usually for no more than a few weeks. One of the concerns about medication is *dependence*—the possibility of becoming addicted to sleep medication. Another problem with some medications is *insomnia rebound*—the sleep problems do not just come back after the person stops taking the medication, they come back worse than before. In addition to fears that people will become addicted to these medications and have a difficult time getting away from their use, there are concerns that the sleep problems will not be "cured" even after a period of time on medication.

PROGNOSIS

Difficulties in initiating and maintaining sleep do not tend to go away if left untreated. Although treatment can be very effective for many children, some children are biologically vulnerable to having disturbed sleep patterns and will continue to remain vulnerable despite successful intervention.

See also: Depressive Disorder, Major; Excessive Sleepiness; Post-Traumatic Stress Disorder; Sleep Patterns, Normal; Sleep–Wake Cycle Problems

Further Reading

Durand, V. M., Mindell, J. A., Maptsone, E., & Gernert-Dott, P. (1995). Treatment of multiple sleep disorders in children. In C. E. Schaefer (Ed.), *Clinical handbook of sleep disorders in children* (pp. 311–333). Northvale, NJ: Jason Aronson.
Schroeder, C. S., & Gordon, B. N. (2002). *Assessment and treatment of childhood problems: A clinician's guide* (Rev. ed.). New York: Guilford.
Stores, C., & Wiggs, L. (1998). Clinical services for sleep disorders. *Archives of Disease in Childhood, 79,* 495–497.

National Sleep Foundation, 1522 K Street, NW, Suite 500, Washington, DC 20005, Phone: (202) 347-3471, Fax: (202) 347-3472, E-mail: nsf@sleepfoundation.org, www.sleepfoundation.org

V. MARK DURAND
KRISTIN V. CHRISTODULU

Injury Prevention

The alarming prevalence of childhood injuries in the United States goes undisputed (see Accidental [Unintentional] Injuries). Both professionals and caretakers agree that a large portion of childhood injuries are preventable. The importance of injury prevention has been noted in the Society of Pediatric Psychology's task force on the Prevention of Unintentional Injuries report that stated "An injury is the outcome of a behavior–environment interaction that leads to death or damage. Perhaps the most effective mode of injury control is prevention. Prevention can be directed

toward changes in behavior or environment, or in the complex interaction of the two" (Finney et al., 1993, p. 500). There are various strategies to the prevention of unintentional injuries in children, also described as injury control.

PASSIVE VERSUS ACTIVE INJURY PREVENTION STRATEGIES

Passive prevention strategies make safety modifications that typically affect a large number of people but do not require a continuous individual effort. Passive interventions, sometimes referred to as structural interventions, are generally the most effective methods to decrease the overall incidence of injury and are often a result of legislative action. The 1970s and 1980s were fruitful in passing legislation to help keep children safe through passive strategies. For example, the Poison Prevention Packaging Act of 1970 required manufacturers of potentially dangerous household substances to use child-proof packaging for their products. There was a significant decrease in deaths due to poisoning in children as a result of this and similar child-safety packaging legislation. In addition, environmental modifications such as flame-retardant sleepwear for children have resulted in fewer burn deaths and an increase in survival rates for fire victims in sleepwear. Asphyxiation deaths due to children getting trapped inside large appliances has decreased significantly since the passage of the Refrigerator Safety Act, which banned the production of appliances with doors that could not be opened from the inside.

In some legislation, however, parents are still left primarily responsible for keeping their child safe. For example, while all 50 states now require that children be properly restrained while in a motor vehicle, parents must be willing to purchase the seat and use it regularly in order to keep the child safe. Similarly, installation and maintenance of smoke detectors for homes requires action by those who would benefit. These are considered active strategies. These types of regulations for safety are only powerful in keeping children safe if proper enforcement is in place.

While passive prevention efforts have been very effective in many instances, it would be impossible and potentially unethical to control a family's environment to the level necessary to reduce all potential hazards. Therefore, active prevention efforts are needed. Active prevention strategies require varying levels of caregiver participation and generally have a much lower overall success rate.

Table 1. Some Exemplary Injury Prevention Programs

Program	Main goals	Components	Primary outcomes
Roberts and colleagues	Community-wide intervention to increase use of child car safety devices in Tuscaloosa, Alabama	Rewards for children when all passengers were wearing appropriate restraint. Community resources (e.g., PTA) mobilized	Increased baseline compliance levels (percentage of cars in which all passengers were properly restrained) by 272%
Jones and colleagues	Teach grade-school children fire safety	Multifaceted behavioral program; simulated fire situations; shaping, modeling, rehearsal, reinforcement	Significant improvements in safety behaviors and self-reports of fire safety skills. Gains maintained 2 weeks after training
Peterson and colleagues	Targeted elementary-school children who are often home alone (i.e., latchkey kids) to increase home safety skills	Parents supervised in the training of their children using protocols in three areas—everyday happenings, emergencies, and strangers. Rehearsal and feedback	Children learned safety skills; 6-month follow-up skills remained with most children
Seattle Children's Helmet Campaign	Community intervention to increase bicycle helmet use	Multimedia exposure, coupons for parents for helmets; school and health care programs	Observations showed that helmet use among 5–12-year-olds increased from 5.5% in 1987 to 40% in 1992
Lutzker's Project 12-ways and Project SafeCare	Targeted parents with history of neglect to teach home safety precautions	Home environment checks, parent training	Substantial decreases in environmental hazards at 1 year follow-up
Children Can't Fly	Community intervention to reduce falls from windows in New York City	Home visitors installed free window guards; community coalition	50% reduction in all falls in target area; 35% reduction in deaths from fall

APPROACHES TO INJURY PREVENTION

Several active strategies for improving safety behaviors have been employed. Educational approaches typically have a lecture component followed by the distribution of safety materials. There is generally little or no follow-up with families that participate in the education. Most of these programs have not been systematically evaluated and evidence supporting their effectiveness in reducing childhood injuries is often lacking. More comprehensive and multifaceted approaches to injury prevention have been researched, and while typically more expensive, many have been effective in reducing injuries.

In general, programs that have been most successful in preventing childhood injury have required more extensive efforts including the provision of incentives and rewards for appropriate preventive behaviors, rehearsal, performance feedback, and booster sessions. These interventions can be delivered to specific individuals or communitywide. Table 1 describes some successful prevention interventions. While this list is not exhaustive, these programs represent areas of success and provide direction for future prevention programs.

See also: Accidental (Unintentional) Injuries; Safety and Prevention

Further Reading

Alexander, K., & Roberts, M. C. (in press). Unintentional injuries in childhood and adolescence: Epidemiology, assessment and management. In L. L. Hayman, M. M. Mahon, & J. R. Turner (Eds.), *Health and behavior in childhood and adolescence: Cross-disciplinary perspectives.* New York: Springer.

Durlak, J. A. (1997). *Successful prevention programs for children and adolescents.* New York: Plenum.

Finney, J. W., Christophersen, E. R., Friman, P. C., Kalnins, I. V., Maddux, J. E., Peterson, L., Roberts, M. C., & Wolraich, M. (1993). Society of Pediatric Psychology Task Force Report: Pediatric psychology and injury control. *Journal of Pediatric Psychology, 18,* 499–526.

Jones, R. T., & Zaharopoulos, V. (1994). Prevention. In K. J. Tarnowski (Ed.), *Behavioral aspects of pediatric burns* (pp. 243–264). New York: Plenum.

Lutzker, J. R., & Bigelow, K. M. (2002). *Reducing child maltreatment: A guidebook for parent services.* New York: Guilford.

Peterson, L., Mori, L., Selby, V., & Rosen, B. N. (1988). Community interventions in children's injury prevention: Differing costs and differing benefits. *Journal of Community Psychology, 16*, 62–73.

Rivara, F. P., Thompson, D. C., Thompson, R. S., Rogers, L. W., Alexander, B., Felix, D., & Bergman, A. B. (1994). The Seattle children's bicycle helmet campaign: Changes in helmet use and head injury admissions. *Pediatrics, 93*, 567–569.

Roberts, M. C., Layfield, D. A., & Fanurik, D. (1992). Motivating children's use of car safety devices. *Advances in Developmental and Behavioral Pediatrics, 10*, 61–88.

Spiegel, C. N., & Lindaman, F. C. (1977). Children Can't Fly: A program to prevent childhood morbidity and mortality from window falls. *American Journal of Public Health, 67*, 1143–1147.

KERI J. BROWN
SUNNYE E. MAYES
MICHAEL C. ROBERTS

Insulin-Dependent Diabetes Mellitus

See: Diabetes Mellitus, Type 1

Intellectual Assessment

DEFINITION

Researchers have been studying the nature of intelligence for well over a century, and yet there is still no consensus regarding the definition of the construct. There seems to be as many definitions or conceptualizations of intelligence as there are theorists in the field. Nevertheless, the dominant approach appears to be that of researchers who propose a hierarchical model of intelligence with *g* (variously called general ability, abstract reasoning ability, mental ability) at the top and other types of intelligence at varying levels below. Broadly speaking, intelligence is a general mental ability reflecting a person's ability to reason, plan, think abstractly, learn from experience, and solve problems quickly. Intelligence, as so defined, can be measured and current intelligence tests measure it quite well.

STANDARDIZATION

In general all tests of intelligence are developed and standardized using a large group of people (usually around 2,000) that reflect the demographic characteristics of the population according to the most recent census data at the time of the test standardization. For most tests, sampling is stratified within each age group by gender (equal number of males and females at each age level tested), geographic region (usually West, South, Northeast, and North Central), race/ethnicity (whites, blacks, Asians, and Hispanics), and level of education of the individual (or parent if a child is being tested). Level of education is commonly used as a measure of socioeconomic status. The major tests of intelligence published within the past 20 years have done an excellent job of selecting a normative sample truly representative of the U.S. population.

INTELLIGENCE QUOTIENT (IQ) SCORES

Intelligence Scores follow a normal distribution that is a bell-shaped curve, with a mean IQ score of 100 and a standard deviation (SD) of 15. For most tests, IQ scores between 90 and 109 are classified as Average. Scores between 110 and 119 are labeled High Average; scores between 120 and 129 are classified as Well Above Average or Superior and scores of 130 or above are classified as Very Superior or Gifted. At the other end of the distribution, scores between 80 and 89 are Low Average; scores between 70 and 79 are classified as Borderline or Well Below Average, and scores below 70 are classified as Intellectually Deficient (Mental Retardation). Approximately 3 percent of the population has scores below 70 or above 130.

RELIABILITY AND VALIDITY

In general, the current measures of intelligence have excellent reliability and validity. The various tests correlate well with each other and with measures of academic achievement. Research shows that IQ scores predict educational and occupational status and job training performance in different occupations quite well.

GROUP DIFFERENCES

Intelligence tests standardized within the past 15–20 years are not biased against any native-born English-speaking ethnic or racial group within the United States. Members of all ethnic groups are found at every IQ level and IQ scores have been found to predict academic and job performance equally well for all ethnic and socioeconomic groups. However, this does not mean that there are not differences in scores among various ethnic groups. Research has shown that the IQ distribution for various ethnic groups has the same shape (normal curve) but with differing means. The curves for some groups (Jews and East Asians) are centered somewhat higher than for whites in general. The normal curves for other groups (blacks and Hispanics) are centered somewhat lower than non-Hispanic whites. Intelligence scores are remarkably stable over time; nevertheless, when educational or other placement decisions are to be made, a current assessment should be completed as changes do occur. Additional information about the points above can be found in major textbooks in assessment and/or psychological testing and professional journals.

ARE WE GETTING SMARTER?

The major IQ tests are updated approximately every 12–15 years. Research has shown that without a re-norming of the test, the average IQ score would increase about 3 points per decade. The cause of the gains is unknown, but it is a worldwide phenomenon. Many reasons for the increase (e.g., better nutrition, more schooling, greater sophistication about test taking, etc.) have been proposed but we really do not know why the rise in test scores occurs. Test publishers deal with this rise by restandardizing the test. Restandardization serves two functions: keeping the mean IQ score anchored at 100 and revising items/subtests that are no longer appropriate for the current culture.

COMMONLY USED INDIVIDUAL INTELLIGENCE TESTS

Because of space limitations, only the two most commonly used individual tests of intelligence will be discussed here. Perhaps the best-known measure of intelligence is the Stanford–Binet Intelligence Scale. Originally developed by Alfred Binet, a French psychologist, the test has undergone a number of revisions since 1916. Three types of standard scores are provided: standard age scores (SAS) for the 15 subtests (e.g., vocabulary, number series, etc.; Mean = 50, SD = 8); four area standard age scores (Verbal Reasoning, Abstract/Visual Reasoning, Quantitative Reasoning, Short-Term Memory; Mean = 100, SD = 16); and a Composite Score. The Composite SAS represents a global measure of the individual's intellectual ability.

By far, the most frequently used measures of intelligence are those developed by David Wechsler: the Wechsler Adult Intelligence Scale (WAIS); the Wechsler

Intelligence Scale for Children (WISC); and the Wechsler Preschool and Primary Scale of Intelligence (WPPSI). All of the Wechsler IQ tests provide one overall score (Full Scale IQ score), reflecting Wechsler's view of intelligence as a global attribute of an individual and a Verbal IQ and a Performance IQ score. The verbal subtests rely heavily on verbal skills such as vocabulary, factual information, social comprehension, and abstract verbal reasoning, whereas the performance scale is less verbally laden and measures such nonverbal reasoning skills as perceptual organization and psychomotor speed. In addition, various other factor scores such as Verbal Comprehension, Perceptual Organization, Processing Speed, Working Memory (WAIS), and Freedom From Distractibility (WISC) can be obtained. These factor scores often provide a more complete picture of an individual's ability profile, particularly when there are substantial differences between the Verbal and Performance IQ scores.

OTHER MEASURES OF INTELLIGENCE

The tests discussed above represent the most commonly used comprehensive individual measures of intelligence. There are many other measures of intelligence but space precludes mentioning them. To find out more about other intelligence tests as well as additional information about the tests discussed or points made in this review, the reader is referred to Sattler (2001).

CLINICAL UTILITY

Intelligence tests are appropriate and useful for a number of different purposes. Most often intelligence tests are given in the context of a more comprehensive evaluation. Scores on IQ tests are only a sample of a person's behavior and are highly dependent upon the person's motivation and cooperation. Test scores do not measure traits directly; instead these scores allow us to make inferences about the traits. These inferences are only as good as the reliability and validity of the test and must take into consideration the individual's cultural background, language, and physical characteristics, for example, vision, hearing, and handicapping conditions. Temporary conditions, such as fatigue, anxiety, illness, and stress, can also influence the scores.

CONCLUSIONS

Intelligence tests yield valuable information about an individual's ability. However, it is important to remember that IQ scores are just that—scores. Hopefully, these scores are related to many measures of daily functioning but this is not always true. In addition to reflecting basic cognitive ability, the scores also reflect the individual's personality, motivation, and test-taking skills. Any assessment must be accompanied by relevant background and history, and interpretation of the scores should consider the cultural background of the individual.

See also: Academic Achievement; Cognitive Development; Mental Retardation; School Age Assessment; Speech and Language Assessment

Further Reading

Sattler, J. M. (2001). *Assessment of children: Cognitive applications* (4th ed.). San Diego: Jerome M. Sattler.
http://www.apa.org/science/testing.html

JEAN SPRUILL
LAURA STOPPELBEIN

International Classification of Diseases and Related Health Problems

The International Classification of Diseases and Related Health Problems (ICD) is a widely used classification system, of which chapter F is devoted solely to psychiatric disorders. The chapter is divided into 10 groups, with each category denoted by the letter F followed by a number for the main group (e.g., F40 Phobic Anxiety Disorders). A fourth character is given (e.g., F40.1 Social Phobia) if a further subdivision is needed.

In the latest version of the ICD (ICD-10) published in 1993, the disorders with an onset in childhood or adolescence have been expanded and classified into three groups: those comprising mental retardation (F70–F79), disorders of psychological development (F80–F89) (e.g., specific developmental disorders of speech and language or of scholastic skills), and those comprising behavioral and emotional disorders with onset usually occurring in childhood and adolescence (F90–F98) (e.g., hyperkinetic disorders, conduct disorders, mixed disorders of conduct and emotions).

ICD-10 is available in several versions in order to serve several purposes, namely: (1) clinical descriptions and diagnostic guidelines; (2) diagnostic criteria for research purposes; (3) primary care version; and (4) multiaspect (axial) systems. The clinical descriptions and diagnostic guidelines contain descriptions of each

disorder, and allow for some clinical judgment in making the diagnosis. The diagnostic criteria for research contain specific criteria that have to be fulfilled before assigning a diagnosis. Thus, the diagnostic criteria are more precise and less flexible than the criteria used for clinical purposes. The primary care version has been adapted for use in primary care settings, which contains a simpler description of each disorder compared to those in the main classification system. The broad categories listed in the primary care version of ICD-10 are: dementia, delirium, eating disorders, acute psychotic disorder, chronic psychotic disorder, depression, and bipolar disorder.

Similar to the fourth edition of the *Diagnostic and Statistical Manual of Mental Disorders (DSM-IV)* published by the American Psychiatric Association, the ICD-10 is a multiaxial system, which allows simultaneous assessment of the various aspects of the child's psychological problems. The multiaxial classifications of child and adolescent psychiatric disorders in ICD-10 contain six axes (compared to only three in adult disorders):

Axis I   Clinical psychiatric syndromes
Axis II   Specific disorders of psychological development
Axis III Intellectual level
Axis IV   Medical conditions
Axis V   Associated abnormal psychological situations
Axis VI   Global assessment of psychosocial functioning

Axis I includes coding for disorders that are generally of little relevance for children, although some of these disorders can apply to childhood and adolescence, such as schizophrenia and schizotypal and delusional disorders (F20–F29). Axis II contains specific delays in disorders of psychological development, independent of their origin, except when delays are solely due to poor schooling. Some examples of disorders listed under Axis II are specific developmental disorders of speech and language of scholastic skills. Axis III is used to describe a child's current level of general intellectual functioning. The child can be described as having "intellectual level within the normal range" to "profound mental retardation." Axis IV provides coding of nonpsychiatric medical conditions. Axis V provides coding of abnormal psychosocial situations (e.g., abnormal intrafamilial relationships, abnormal qualities of upbringing, acute life events, and societal stressors) that may be relevant for the development of psychiatric disorders or for therapeutic planning. Axis VI reflects the child's psychological, social, and occupational functioning at the time of examination. It deals with disability in functioning as a consequence of psychiatric disorders, specific disorders of psychological development, or mental retardation.

Unlike its earlier versions, Essau and colleagues (1997) have noted that ICD-10 is very similar to *DSM-IV* in its categorization approach, although some differences still exist in style. The ICD-10 lists the codes and names of the disorders with a glossary describing each disorder, whereas in *DSM-IV*, each disorder is presented under different categories (e.g., diagnostic features, onset, and course). As a general rule, ICD-10 does not include interference with the performance of social roles as part of the diagnostic criteria, whereas *DSM-IV* does. An exception is made for some of the disorders of childhood and adolescence, in which some form of interference with social behavior and relationships is included among the diagnostic criteria. The complicated and interactive nature of many disorders of childhood and adolescence makes it necessary to include the social criteria. In *DSM-IV*, diagnostic criteria include significant distress and impairment in social, occupational, or other important areas of functioning. In ICD-10, the International Classification of Impairments, Disabilities and Handicaps can be used to assess psychosocial impairment. Another difference is related to the multiaxial system. ICD-10 places all the diagnoses included in the *DSM-IV* Axes I, II, and III on one axis.

Although ICD-10 represents a major advance from previous editions, it has been open to criticism. The same criticisms as those made about the *DSM-IV* can be applied to the ICD-10 as well, including being not sensitive enough to developmental issues, issues related to the notion of unidimensionality, and symptom equivalency, as well as the arbitrariness of symptom thresholds for distinguishing the presence or absence of a disorder.

See also: Classification and Diagnosis; Comorbidity; *Diagnostic and Statistical Manual of Mental Disorders*; Interviewing

Further Reading

American Psychiatric Association. (1994). *Diagnostic and statistical manual of mental disorders* (4th ed.). Washington: Author.

Essau, C. A., Feehan, M., & Üstun, B. (1997). Classification and assessment strategies. In C. A. Essau & F. Petermann (Eds.), *Developmental psychopathology: Epidemiology, diagnostics, and treatment* (pp. 19–62). London: Harwood Academic Publishers.

World Health Organization. (1993). *The ICD-10 classification of mental and behavioral disorders*. Geneva: World Health Organization.

http://www.who.int/msa/mnh/ems/icd10/icd10.htm

CECILIA A. ESSAU

Interpersonal Psychotherapy for Depressed Adolescents

DEFINITION

Interpersonal psychotherapy is a time-limited therapy that is specified in a manual and tested in clinical trials. The goals of treatment are to reduce the adolescent's symptoms and to improve the quality of his/her current interpersonal and social functioning. According to this treatment model, there are many possible causes of depression, but regardless of the cause, depression is associated with how things are going in the patient's personal life and with his or her relationships. Through weekly individual therapy, the therapist helps the adolescent identify specific strategies for managing the interpersonal difficulties related to his or her depression more successfully. Ideally, parents are involved in the treatment periodically to receive psychoeducation about depression and the treatment, to participate in sessions on improving communication, and to review the adolescent's progress in treatment and receive follow-up recommendations.

METHOD

Interpersonal Psychotherapy—Adolescents (IPT-A) is designed as a once weekly, 12-week individual psychotherapy treatment. If there is a crisis, the therapist and patient may meet for an additional session if the crisis is short-term and manageable as an outpatient. IPT-A is an active treatment protocol with a large psychoeducational component aimed at building the adolescent's competencies and skills. It is structured and organized in a way such that the adolescent can take an increasingly more active role in the treatment as it progresses. The focus of the treatment is on chronic relationship problems related to the adolescent's depression. This treatment differs from more psychodynamic approaches to treatment in its focus on current rather than past relationship issues.

The treatment is divided into three phases: (1) the initial phase, (2) the middle phase, and (3) the termination phase. Each phase takes approximately four sessions. The *initial phase* focuses on diagnosing the depression, educating about the illness, exploring the patient's significant relationships, and identifying the problem area that will be the focus of the remainder of treatment. Problem areas are key aspects of one's life circumstances or relationships that appear to be related to one's depression. The identified problem areas of IPT-A include grief reactions, interpersonal conflicts (such as parent–child disputes or peer conflicts), difficulty making transitions between stages in life, single-parent families, and social isolation/communication problems.

During the *middle phase* of treatment, the therapist focuses on identifying specific strategies that help the adolescents negotiate their interpersonal difficulties within one or two problem areas more successfully. More specifically, the therapist teaches the patient to link depressive symptoms to difficulties in one or more of these areas and to link improvement in mood to using effective interpersonal strategies including constructive and direct communication.

For example, adolescents are taught communication skills to express their feelings regarding conflicts or disappointments in their relationships and life circumstances such as an absent father, an inconsistent father, or conflict about dating rules. Techniques include expression of affect, clarification of expectations for relationships, communication analysis, interpersonal problem-solving, and role-playing new methods of interaction.

The goal of the *termination phase* is to clarify warning symptoms of future depressive episodes, identify successful strategies used in the middle phase, foster generalization of skills to future situations, emphasize mastery of new interpersonal skills, and discuss the need for further treatment.

CLINICAL APPLICATIONS

IPT-A was designed to treat adolescents aged 12–18 years with depression. There are many different types of depression. The initial research on this treatment included only adolescents who had Major Depression (MDD). Many of the adolescents also reported comorbid anxiety disorders. Currently, an effectiveness study is being conducted which includes adolescents with other forms of depression (Dysthymia, Depression Not Otherwise Specified, and Adjustment Disorder with Depressed Mood) as well as additional comorbid disorders such as Conduct Disorder, Attention-Deficit/Hyperactivity Disorder, and Eating Disorders. The results from this latter project are not yet available. The adolescents for all of these studies have been primarily from low socioeconomic status (SES), single-parent Latino families in an urban environment.

Based on clinical experience, we have ascertained several patient conditions associated with the optimal likelihood of success of IPT-A. Adolescents whose families are supportive of and willing to participate in treatment are more likely to benefit from IPT-A. This appears to be due to a combination of improved treatment compliance and increased receptivity of the family members to the changes in interpersonal/communication strategies. IPT-A is not recommended for patients who have a long-standing history of severe interpersonal problems; rather, it is most suited to those who have an identifiable interpersonal event that precipitated or exacerbated a depressive episode, who are motivated to be in treatment or to "feel better" and willing to receive time-limited treatment. IPT-A as an outpatient treatment is not appropriate for the treatment of adolescents who are currently actively suicidal, homicidal, psychotic, bipolar, or substance abusing.

EFFECTIVENESS

Mufson and colleagues have been engaged in a programmatic study of IPT-A (including randomized, controlled trials in hospital and community settings) in a sample of minority, underprivileged, urban, depressed adolescents. Additionally, IPT-A has also been studied in a controlled trial in Puerto Rico by Rossello and Bernal (1999).

Mufson and colleagues' first controlled clinical trial of IPT-A was conducted with a sample of 48 clinic-referred adolescents with a diagnosis of MDD. In this study, IPT-A was compared to a clinical management control group (supportive therapy once a month). Results showed that those adolescents who received IPT-A, as compared to clinical management, reported significantly greater reductions in depressive symptomatology and greater improvements in overall social functioning and certain social problem-solving skills. Specifically, they reported greater improvement in functioning with friends and in the ability to generate alternative solutions to problems, as well as solution implementation and verification, measured by the Social Problem Solving Inventory. Additionally, significantly more IPT-A patients as compared to control patients met recovery criteria for depression (75 percent compared to 46 percent, respectively) and completed the 12-week protocol (88 percent compared to 46 percent, respectively).

In a study of 71 adolescents in Puerto Rico, Rossello and Bernal contrasted cognitive-behavior therapy (CBT) to IPT to waitlist with adolescents diagnosed with MDD and/or Dysthymia. Both IPT and CBT significantly reduced depressive symptoms in comparison to waitlist control with IPT showing a little more benefit than CBT for improving general functioning. Depression recovery rates were 82 percent for IPT and 59 percent for CBT.

Despite the limitations, these two studies of IPT-A together suggest that it is an acceptable and efficacious treatment for adolescent depression in a specialty mental health setting. Its effectiveness in a community setting is still under study.

See also: Adolescence; Cognitive-Behavior Therapy; Evidence-Based Treatments; Group Psychotherapy; Major Depressive Disorder

Further Reading

Mufson, L., Moreau, D., Weissman, M. M., & Klerman, G. (1993). *Interpersonal psychotherapy for depressed adolescents.* New York: Guilford.

Mufson, L., Weissman, M. M., Moreau, D., & Garfinkel, R. (1999). Efficacy of interpersonal psychotherapy for depressed adolescents. *Archives of General Psychiatry, 56,* 573–579.

Mufson, L., Moreau, D., Weissman, M. M., Wickramaratne, P., & Samoilov, A. (1994). The modification of interpersonal psychotherapy with depressed adolescents (IPT-A): Phase I and II studies. *Journal of the American Academy of Child and Adolescent Psychiatry, 33*(5), 695–705.

Rossello, J., & Bernal, G. (1999). The efficacy of cognitive-behavioral and interpersonal treatments of depression in Puerto Rican adolescents. *Journal of Consulting and Clinical Psychology, 67*(5), 734–745.

LAURA MUFSON

Interpretive Conference

DEFINITION

An interpretive conference is a session following the psychological evaluation of a child, in which the clinician reports the evaluation findings to the family. In addition to explaining assessment results, the clinician works to clarify the meaning of diagnostic information, answer all of the child's and parents' questions, help the family cope emotionally with the new knowledge, and assist them in making plans to carry out recommendations. The interpretive conference typically lasts between an hour and an hour-and-a-half.

PREPARATION

Writing the evaluation report before the interpretive conference is highly recommended because it helps to ensure that interview and test results have been thoughtfully interpreted and integrated, and any missing pieces can be obtained during the conference itself. It also allows the clinician to obtain in advance all of the information the family will need to follow through with the recommendations that will be made, such as telephone numbers and addresses for the resources located in their community. Before the conference, the clinician should also decide who will actually attend the session. Except when children are very young (below school age), it is important to include them. It is also important to have both parents attend, if possible, and to ask if they would like anyone else to attend, such as other relatives or a teacher. With preadolescent and younger children, it is normally best to present findings first to the parents alone and then to the child in a joint session with the parents present. With older children and adolescents, evaluation feedback is sometimes presented first to the child alone, and in this case, the parents should be invited to join the session at the end to review and clarify the child's understanding of the material that has been presented. Otherwise, material may be presented to both adolescents and parents at the same time. Additionally, the physical location of the interpretive conference should be a quiet, uninterrupted room with comfortable chairs. Tissues should be made available in case of need.

CONTENT

The clinician should begin the interpretive conference by restating the questions and concerns expressed by the child and/or parents in the initial evaluation. The clinician may then describe the standardized tests that were used in the evaluation to address the questions, followed by the specific test results. The clinician should present the results using simple, jargon-free language and frequently check to make sure that all parties understand the information being presented. Reporting test scores in terms of percentile ranks will allow parents to compare their child's performance to that of the child's peers. When interpreting the results for the family, it is important to explain the likely cause of the child's problems, if known, and to provide realistic expectations for the future. Once the parents understand the test results, they will want to know what they can do. Recommendations presented to the family must be realistic as well. For example, the clinician should not recommend services that the family cannot access because they do not currently exist in the family's community or because they are not affordable to the family. The session ends when the child/adolescent's and parents' behavior or statements indicate that their goals have been met and when all diagnostic information has been discussed, feelings have been expressed, and concrete plans have been determined. The family should leave the session on a note of reassurance and hope.

PROCESS ISSUES

In addition to providing information, the clinician must be mindful of the interpersonal process occurring throughout the interpretive conference. At the beginning, the clinician can expect the family to be highly anxious. The clinician may continue small talk begun on the way to the conference room for a minute or two, but then it is important to end this conversation and present a clear plan for the session. The clinician should organize the information to be presented in a logical sequence but be prepared to modify the session's structure in response to the family's questions. Throughout the session, the clinician must stay closely attuned to and responsive to the child's and parents' emotions and continue to build rapport by showing respect for their ideas, responding directly to their questions, and conveying empathy with their situation. The clinician must maintain good eye contact, communicate concerns clearly, and facilitate the family's expression of feelings by reflecting their feelings and making it clear that feelings will be accepted as a normal part of the discussion. When the information presented in this session is "bad news," or not what the family wanted to hear, they may react in a number of ways. Those children and parents who are direct and vivid in their emotional expression often respond best to a clinician's accepting and normalizing their feelings and reflecting them in a gentle, supportive way. With others who do not state their feelings explicitly but show they are close to the surface, the clinician may bring their emotions out by asking direct questions about their feelings. A third pattern of response is to provide no indication of emotional reaction. The clinician may inquire directly about the reactions of a parent or child while implicitly communicating the idea that any number of responses would be understandable. If the family still does not wish to disclose their feelings in this situation, however, it is

best not to push them to do so. As long as the family is able to understand and accept the recommendations for their child's care, the important message to convey is understanding and respect for their situation and method of coping.

See also: Coping with Illness; Psychological Testing

Further Reading

Querido, J., Eyberg, S. M., Kanfer, R., & Krahn, G. (2001). Process variables in the child clinical assessment interview. In C. E. Walker & M. C. Roberts (Eds.), *Handbook of clinical child psychology* (3rd ed.). New York: Wiley.
Sattler, J. M. (1998). *Clinical and forensic interviewing of children and families: Guidelines for the mental health, education, pediatric, and child maltreatment fields.* San Diego, CA: San Diego State.
Shea, V. (1993). Interpreting results to parents of preschool children. In E. Schopler, M. E. Van Bourgondien, et al. (Eds.), *Preschool issues in autism: Current issues in autism* (pp. 185–198). New York: Plenum.

ERIN M. NEARY
SHEILA M. EYBERG

Interventions for Drug-Exposed Teenage Mothers/Infants

Interventions for drug-exposed teenage mothers and their infants are of recent origin and considerable more research must be undertaken before we can draw firm conclusions on which interventions work and which ones do not. In one of the more comprehensive/intensive intervention efforts, Field and colleagues (1998) designed an intervention to improve lifestyle, reduce drug-taking behavior, enhance educational and vocational status, and improve social skills in adolescent mothers and thereby facilitate the growth and development of their infants. The research was designed to assess a 40 hr per week Intervention/Prevention Program that was developed in a vocational training high school. It included drug prevention/rehabilitation, diploma/GED preparation, vocational training, job placement, social skills training, parenting and nutrition classes, aerobics, and free day care for their infants. Lifestyle outcome variables included drug using behavior, repeat pregnancy, high school/GED status, vocational training, employment, financial independence, suitable housing, and adequate parenting. Psychological outcome variables included the POSIT, maternal depression, parenting stress, mother–infant interactions, and infant growth and development (Bayley Scales of Mental and Motor Development and Early Social Communication Scales).

The sample included 126 young mothers (ages 16–21) who had not completed high school and who had or had not used drugs during pregnancy. Urine toxicology screens were used to assess drug exposure near the time of delivery. Specific immunoassays (EMIT, Syva) for cocaine metabolite (benzylecgonine), opiates, and marijuana were performed. Infant urine screens were limited to three assays: cocaine metabolite, cannabinoids, and opiates. Based on these urine screens, mothers and infants were assigned to a nondrug, drug control, or drug intervention group at the neonatal period. The mothers, on average, were 18 years old, had 10.3 years of education, and their socioeconomic status (SES) was 4.4 on the Hollingshead Index. Approximately 64 percent were African-American, 27 percent Hispanic, and 10 percent non-Hispanic white.

The program included educational, vocational, and parenting classes; social and drug rehabilitation; and day care for their infants while they attended school half-day. The drug-exposed infants were similar to the nonexposed infants on traditional birth measures, although they had inferior Brazelton Neonatal Behavioral Assessment Scale scores, including habituation, orientation, abnormal reflexes, general irritability, and regulatory capacity. The drug-exposed infants also spent less time in quiet sleep and more time crying and showing stress behaviors. Both the mothers and the infants in the drug groups demonstrated inferior interactions, and their dopamine and serotonin levels were significantly higher than their nondrug counterparts. As early as 3 months (following 3 months of intervention), the drug rehab mothers and their infants looked more like the nondrug group in their interactions; by 6 months, they looked similar on virtually every measure. At 12 months, the infants of drug rehab mothers (vs. the drug control group) had superior Early Social Communication Scale scores and Bayley Mental scale scores, as well as significantly greater head circumference and fewer pediatric complications. The drug rehab mothers also improved on several lifestyle variables. They demonstrated a lower incidence of continued drug use and repeat pregnancy, and a greater number continued school, received a high school or general equivalency diploma, and/or were placed in a job. Thus, a relatively cost-effective high school based intervention had positive effects on both adolescent mothers who had used drugs and their infants.

Based on these early findings, it seems likely that similar programs can be developed and evaluated for their efficacy. Assuming such programs can be developed, they hold considerable promise in reversing the insidious and negative effects associated with drug-exposed teenage mothers.

See also: Adolescence; Adolescent Parenting; Parenting Practices; Risk and Protective Factors; Substance Abuse

Further Reading

Field, T., Scafidi, F., Pickens, J., Prodromidis, M., Pelaez-Nogueras, M., Torquati, J., Wilcox, H., Malphurs, J., Schanberg, S., & Kuhn, C. (1998). Polydrug-using adolescent mothers and their infants receiving early intervention. *Adolescence, 33,* 117–143.

TIFFANY FIELD

Interviewing

Interviewing provides a forum through which information may be obtained from a client. Depending upon the purpose, this approach to information gathering is typically used in conjunction with other methods, such as questionnaires and observation. Inherent in all forms of interview is the issue that the information provided reflects the client's subjective interpretation of the question and memory and perception of the events being reported. Interviews are valuable in that they can provide material that is personal to the client, such as their thoughts, feelings, and private experiences. Information of a personal kind is not typically observable by others and thus we must rely upon subjective report, despite the potential for personal biases. However, it is generally important to obtain information from other informants in order to ensure that decisions are not based solely upon the subjective report of the client. There are many different forms of interview, each with its own strengths and limitations.

Interviews provide a valuable opportunity for the client to establish a positive relationship with the interviewer, in which the client gains sufficient trust and rapport to divulge personal information. Prior to the interview, the client must be made to feel comfortable, the purpose and process of the interview needs to be explained and issues/limits of confidentiality should be discussed. Whatever the form and purpose of the interview, the interviewer needs to demonstrate strong listening skills, empathy, and respect for the client. The interviewer signals empathic listening partly through body language, such as eye contact and body orientation, but also through verbal messages. The effective interviewer uses simple verbal responses ("mm, yes, I see") to indicate listening, in addition to more complex strategies such as reflection, paraphrasing, summarizing, and restatement to check for correct interpretation of what the client has said and feels. The interviewer also needs to be nonjudgmental in his or her responses while allowing the client to express his or her views and divulge important information. In any form of interviewing, the interviewer needs to have some form of recording the information produced in a discreet, yet adequately detailed manner. Careful, rapid note-taking is an important skill, although some interviewers prefer to tape-record the interview where this is agreed to by the client.

Interviews vary as to their purpose. In some instances it may take the form of personal history-taking or mental status examination. In other situations, the interview may explore the presenting problem(s) in sufficient detail to enable a reliable clinical diagnosis to be obtained. Interviews may also be used to gather information about the nature and parameters of a psychological problem to enable a therapist to understand the causes and maintaining factors and inform the design of a treatment program. For example, the cognitive–behavioral interview aims to obtain a detailed description of exactly what emotions, behaviors, thoughts, and physiological reactions constitute the problem. The interviewer also seeks information about when, where, and how often the problem occurs, and the events that trigger or maintain the problem. Most importantly, the interview provides an initial opportunity to observe the behavior of the client in a novel situation. In addition to the verbal material presented in the interview, a note should be made regarding the client's appearance, verbal and nonverbal social skills, language, and thought processes.

In some instances interviews have a therapeutic goal. For example, motivational interviewing as described by Miller (1983) put very simply, involves a form of questioning that is designed to highlight the advantages of change in comparison with the disadvantages of the current situation, thereby increasing the client's motivation to change. In some couple therapies, the interview may be used to elicit information that triggers positive memories and increases positive feelings between the partners.

Interview techniques may also vary according to the client characteristics and purpose of the interview. For example, there is a considerable literature relating to interviewing children following abuse and the specific techniques that must be used to elicit factual information.

Sternberg and colleagues (2002) assert that methods such as leading questions must be avoided in order to prevent the "shaping" of children's responses and the development of false memories. Similar issues apply in forensic interviewing more generally.

Interviews also vary according to their structure with varying degrees of freedom in terms of the type, order, and topic of questions asked. The following section examines three types of interviews, namely structured, unstructured, and semistructured.

STRUCTURED INTERVIEWS

In structured interviews, the interviewer is restricted to specific, predetermined questions. The interview usually takes a "tree" format with key questions which, when responded to in a particular way, lead on to "branch" questions. All interviewers follow the same question format and, given the same responses from a client, should produce the same information from the interview. The aim of the interview is generally to elicit specific information to enable some judgment to be made, such as forming a diagnosis based on strict criteria. Structured interviews are also designed to elicit information in the most efficient manner and to ensure that essential topics are covered to enable the purpose of the interview to be achieved. The question format typically includes a high number of closed (yes/no) questions and very specific questions that require only a brief response. There are many examples of structured interviews in clinical practice such as the Diagnostic Interview Schedule, developed by Robbins and colleagues (1981), and the Diagnostic Interview Schedule for Children IV described by Shaffer and colleagues (2000).

There is little opportunity for interviewers to use their subjective judgment in steering the content of the interview and decision-making based on the information produced. As a consequence, the structured interview has the advantage of producing high levels of reliability between the information produced by different interviewers when they interview the same client. Although high reliability is important in some contexts, such as making a clinical diagnosis, it can also lead to failure to obtain some key bits of information that are relevant to a client's presenting problem.

UNSTRUCTURED INTERVIEWS

In some instances, it is more important to allow the interviewer and client to use their discretion and judgment as to the direction that the interview should take. The greater flexibility in unstructured interviews means that the information obtained, and thereby the judgments that result, are likely to vary considerably if different interviewers interview the same client. This low level of inter-assessor reliability would be problematic if it is important that two or more interviewers need to draw the same conclusions from a given interview. However, unstructured interviews have the advantage of enabling the interviewer to follow particular lines of inquiry as they arise and where they seem to be leading to important, relevant information. Such material could be missed in a more structured format. There is also more opportunity for the interviewer to vary the questions from open to closed format. Thus, open-ended questions may be used to encourage a reluctant client to divulge more information where closed questions provide specific information although limited in range. The unstructured interview format is frequently required when the client divulges unexpected information that is of sufficient importance that it requires further exploration.

SEMISTRUCTURED INTERVIEWS

In practice, most clinicians are likely to use different types of interview formats in their work at different stages of the assessment process. For example, they may use a structured interview to obtain a clinical diagnosis, but use an unstructured or semistructured interview to obtain more detailed information about the parameters of the presenting problem. Most mental health professionals develop their own semistructured form of interviewing in which they have a blueprint to follow that includes the most essential areas that need to be covered during the interview. The semistructured format then enables the interviewer to follow up on significant areas in more detail when this is appropriate.

See also: *Diagnostic and Statistical Manual of Mental Disorders*; History-Taking; *International Classification of Diseases and Related Health Problems*; Mental Status Examination

Further Reading

Miller, W. R. (1983). Motivational interviewing with problem drinkers. *Behavioural Psychotherapy, 11*(2), 147–172.

Robbins, L. N., Helzer, J. E., Crughan, J. L., & Ratcliff, K. S. (1981). National Institute of Mental Health diagnostic interview schedule: Its history, characteristics, and validity. *Archives of General Psychiatry, 38*(4), 381–389.

Shaffer, D., Fisher, P., Lucas, C. P., Dulcan, M. K., & Schwab-Stone, M. E. (2000). NIMH diagnostic interview schedule for children version IV (NIMH DISC-IV): Description, differences from previous versions, and reliability of some common diagnoses. *Journal of the American Academy of Child and Adolescent Psychiatry, 39*(1), 28–38.

Sternberg, K. J., Lamb, M. E., Esplin, P. W., Orbach, Y., Hershkowitz, I. (2002). Using a structure interview protocol to improve the quality of investigative interviews. In M. L. Eisen & J. A. Quas (Eds.), *Memory and suggestibility in the forensic interview. Personality and clinical psychology series* (pp. 409–436). Mahwah, NJ: Erlbaum.

SUSAN HILARY SPENCE

Intraventricular Hematoma

See: Traumatic Brain Injury

Irritable Bowel Syndrome

DEFINITION/INCIDENCE

Irritable bowel syndrome (IBS) refers to abdominal pain and altered bowel habits without evidence of an organic disease. The syndrome is characterized by at least 12 weeks of symptoms of abdominal discomfort or pain and two or more of the following: pain is relieved by defecation, onset is associated with a change in the frequency of stool, and/or onset is associated with a change in the form or appearance of stool. Symptoms can include fewer than three bowel movements per week, more than three bowel movements per day, hard/lumpy stools, loose/watery stools, abnormal stool passage (straining, urgency, feeling of incomplete evacuation), passage of mucus, and/or bloating or abdominal distension. Clinical experience suggests that functional dyspepsia coexists in many individuals with IBS. IBS occurs in 6–14 percent of children.

ETIOLOGY

The etiology of IBS has not been established, but several interacting biopsychosocial factors likely play a role. Abnormalities in the motor responses of the intestines (dysmotility) have been documented in individuals with IBS, and several studies have shown that people with IBS have increased gut sensitivity (visceral hyperalgesia) when compared to healthy controls. A genetic predisposition has been suggested, but social learning may also contribute. A recent twin study reported that the concordance of IBS in monozygotic (MZ) twins was 17 percent, compared with 8 percent in dizygotic (DZ) twins. However, having a parent with IBS was a better predictor than having an MZ twin with IBS, which should not be the case on a purely genetic basis. This suggests that social learning plays a role. The influence of social learning is also supported by studies that have shown that children of parents with IBS make significantly more health care visits overall and significantly more health care visits for gastrointestinal symptoms than children of healthy parents.

PSYCHOSOCIAL CORRELATES

Although psychosocial correlates have been well studied in adults, only one study has investigated behavioral/emotional functioning in children with IBS. This community-based study found that children who met criteria for IBS report significantly higher levels of trait anxiety and depressive symptoms than healthy children. Among adults, individuals with IBS have significantly higher levels of anxiety symptoms than healthy adults and adults with inflammatory bowel disease (IBD), an organic disease with symptoms that can be similar to IBS. Significantly higher levels of depressive symptoms have been found in comparison to healthy individuals, but the results have been mixed when compared with depressive symptoms in individuals with IBD. Adults with IBS have significantly higher overall levels of psychological distress compared to those with IBD, and adults with IBS have higher rates of psychiatric disorders, particularly mood, anxiety, and somatoform disorders, when compared to healthy adults and those with IBD. The role of stress has been examined in IBS, and adults with IBS generally report experiencing more stressors than healthy adults and those with IBD. Research investigating if stress leads to a flare in symptoms has yielded mixed results, likely due to methodological issues, and conclusions are difficult to draw. However, clinical experience suggests that stress is associated with symptom exacerbation. Finally, past history of physical or sexual abuse is more prevalent among adults with IBS than healthy adults, with 20–67 percent of those with IBS reporting past abuse.

ASSESSMENT/TREATMENT

Diagnosis is made via history and physical examination. Laboratory screening and colonoscopy are occasionally needed to exclude diagnoses with similar symptoms. Tricyclic antidepressants and anticholinergic medications can be used to treat IBS, and increased fiber consumption may be helpful for those with constipation. However, the efficacy of these treatments has been difficult to determine in clinical trials due to placebo effects as large as 70 percent; futhermore, these treatments have primarily been studied in adults. Psychotherapy has been extensively studied in adults with IBS and has been found to be effective in improving both physical symptoms and associated psychological symptoms. Psychotherapy is more effective than waitlist control groups, symptom-monitoring control groups, and self-help support groups, and improvements have been maintained for as long as 18 months after treatment. Brief psychodynamic therapy, hypnotherapy, biofeedback plus stress management training, and cognitive behavioral therapy have all been shown to be effective. Although psychotherapy addressing IBS has not been investigated in children, these results as well as the literature on recurrent abdominal pain (RAP) suggest that psychotherapy would be beneficial for children with IBS as well.

COURSE/PROGNOSIS

As many as 94 percent of adults with IBS who participate in psychotherapy demonstrate significant improvement. Among untreated adults, studies have shown that 24–57 percent report IBS symptoms that are unchanged or worse 5 years after initial assessment. The course of IBS has not been studied in children. However, childhood RAP may be a precursor to IBS: One study reported that 18 percent of children diagnosed with RAP met criteria for IBS 5 years later, and 61 percent met criteria for IBS 20 years later.

See also: Biofeedback; Cognitive-Behavior Therapy; Functional Dyspepsia; Gastrointestinal Disorders; Inflammatory Bowel Disease; Pediatric Hypnosis; Psychodynamic Therapy; Recurrent Abdominal Pain; Relaxation Training; Stress Management

Further Reading

Blanchard, E. B. (2001). *Irritable bowel syndrome: Psychosocial assessment and treatment*. Washington, DC: American Psychological Association.
Toner, B. B., Segal, Z. V., Emmott, S. D., & Myran, D. (2000). *Cognitive-behavioral treatment of irritable bowel syndrome*. New York: Guilford.
Web sites: www.niddk.nih.gov/health/digest/pubs/irrbowel/irrbowel.htm, www.ibsgroup.org/

LAURA M. MACKNER
WALLACE V. CRANDALL

Jj

Juvenile Rheumatoid Arthritis

DESCRIPTION OF THE DISORDER

Juvenile rheumatoid arthritis (JRA) is a disease of the connective tissues of the body often manifesting as sudden and unexpected exacerbations and remissions of joint inflammation and pain. The disease process in JRA attacks the joint and adjacent supporting structures (e.g., synovium or joint lining) which become chronically inflamed, eroding cartilage, bone, and supportive tissues, producing heat, swelling, and loss of motion. High fever and rash are prominent in children with JRA. There are three subtypes of JRA, each having implications for amelioration and treatment. *Systemic onset disease* occurs in 20 percent of cases, presenting with fever of unknown origin, rash, enlarged lymph nodes, infection of the covering of the heart, pneumonia, enlarged liver and spleen and associated acute abdominal pain. Systemic manifestations include growth retardation, delayed sexual maturation, and reduced red blood cell count. Systemic symptoms may recur and subside, or develop into polyarticular arthritis, with a quarter of those children with this subtype of JRA manifesting permanent joint deformity.

The second subtype, *polyarticular disease*, affects 40 percent of all cases of JRA, with five or more joints affected. Symptoms may manifest as low-grade fever and slight enlargement of the liver and spleen, mild reduced red blood cell count, malaise, and weight loss. The cervical spine, wrists, hips, and knees may be affected by pain, decreased range of motion, and stiffness, along with symmetrical involvement of the small joints of the hands and feet.

The third and final subtype is *pauciarticular disease*, involving four or fewer joints within the first 6 months of onset of JRA. The hands and feet are rarely involved, and a preponderance of females develop this subtype of JRA. There is a subgroup of this subtype that is comprised mostly of boys over the age of 8 years, which primarily involves the lower extremities. Between 10 and 50 percent of children with this subtype of JRA will develop iridocyclitis, for example, infection of the iris of the eye, leading to permanent visual loss in one or both eyes.

ETIOLOGY

The etiology of JRA is unknown, but may result from infection, autoimmunity, trauma, or genetic predisposition. Research in the past 10 years has focused on the relationship of JRA with viruses, bacteria, immunodeficiency, stress, and trauma.

PREVALENCE

Juvenile rheumatoid arthritis is the most common joint disease of childhood, affecting between 60,000 and 200,000 children in the United States.

ASSESSMENT

There is no formal laboratory assessment for JRA. Laboratory studies typically used for adults often show

328

negative results in children with JRA. Radiological studies are able to identify articular (joint) destruction in children, but only in an advanced state. Most frequently, evaluation of JRA involves the examination of individual joints and overall functional status (e.g., degree of fatigue and length of morning stiffness). Physical and occupational therapy and assessment are important, observing posture in sitting and standing, and any abnormalities in alignment or gait. Strength, dexterity, and mobility may change as the disease progresses.

TREATMENT

JRA is a chronic, systemic disorder (bodywide), which requires intensive daily treatment regimes of medicine and specialized exercise, exacting a heavy burden on family caregiving. Currently there are no curative treatments for JRA. However, early identification and treatment serve to ameliorate the ravages of JRA. Various drugs can be used to control inflammation and systemic complications: intrajoint injection of steroids for pain or flexion; aspirin for inflammation and pain (however, this increases the risk of Reye's syndrome); and immunization against infections on an annual basis.

For acute symptoms, bed rest, splinting, and range of motion therapy can be used to facilitate recovery of the damaged joint by decreasing inflammation and preventing additional damage. Prolonged inactivity is contraindicated secondary to resultant muscle wasting.

The use of heat and light massage may promote relaxation and increased elasticity around affected joints, providing symptomatic relief. For the pauciarticular subtype of JRA, ophthalmological examinations must be regular and frequent to monitor for development of iridocyclitis. A multidisciplinary treatment team may best manage medical monitoring of a multitude of other systemic co-disorders.

Extended hospitalizations associated with the implementation of medical technology to the treatment of JRA have significant psychosocial ramifications. The use of splints, braces, or other supportive technology can also have an isolating effect in a child's social life, with predictable responses by children to someone who is "different." This can negatively impact educational functioning, as children with JRA appear to have a greater risk for academic underachievement, high absenteeism, associated fatigue, and disease-related distractibility and irritations (e.g., morning stiffness, inflammatory-related pain). These children experience difficulty with fine motor coordination and can appear awkward, adding further psychosocial stigma. Parent and peer psychoeducation and supportive psychotherapy for children maturing with such social pressures may facilitate optimal social adjustment.

PROGNOSIS

Currently there are no curative treatments and the disease impact is quite variable, often resulting in a cycle of pain, reduced activity, and more discomfort. Medications focus on reducing pain and preventing complications.

See also: Coping with Illness; Individuals with Disabilities Education Act (IDEA); Pain Assessment; Pain Management; Parenting the Chronically Ill Child; Preparation for Medical Procedures

Further Reading

Batshaw, M. L. (1997). *Children with disabilities* (4th ed.). Baltimore: Paul H. Brookes.

Koch, B. M. (1992). Rehabilitation of the child with joint disease. In G. E. Molnar (Ed.), *Pediatric rehabilitation* (2nd ed., pp. 293–333). Baltimore: Williams and Wilkins.

Web site: American Juvenile Arthritis Organization: http://www.arthritis.org

DENNIS C. HARPER

Kk

Kaspar Hauser Syndrome

See: Psychosocial Short Stature

Kidney Transplantation, Pediatric

BRIEF DESCRIPTION

The kidneys are a pair of glandular organs in the upper abdominal cavity which separate water and waste products of metabolism from the blood and excrete them as urine through the bladder. Kidney transplantation is the preferred treatment for all causes of end-stage kidney (renal) disease. This procedure involves the placement of a kidney into the lower abdomen, either from a living donor or cadaveric organ donor. Live donations may come from either living-related donors, such as a parent or sibling, or from living-unrelated donors.

In June 2001, there were 1,296 children under 18 years of age on the waiting list for kidney transplantation in the United States. This number represents 2.6 percent of the 49,860 total patients awaiting kidney transplantation. About 2–4 percent of children waiting for kidney transplantation will die because suitable donor organs will not be available in time. Waiting times are somewhat age-dependent, with older children and adolescents generally waiting 1–3 years for a cadaveric donor kidney transplant. Since 1990, there have been approximately 3,400 pediatric cadaveric and 4,200 living donor kidney transplants performed in the United States.

INDICATIONS

Children with chronic renal insufficiency and end-stage renal disease, which are not amenable to medical or surgical treatment, are considered for kidney transplantation. Glomerulonephritis (acute kidney inflammation), chronic pyelonephritis (inflammation of the kidney and pelvis), and hereditary conditions are the most frequent medical diagnoses leading to kidney transplantation. As outlined by the Pediatric Committee of the American Society of Transplant Physicians, indications for kidney transplantation in children include symptoms of uremia (excess urea—an organic compund that is the principal end product of nitrogen metabolism—and other nitrogenous waste in the blood) not responsive to standard therapy, failure-to-thrive due to limitations in total caloric intake, delayed psychomotor development, hypervolemia (abnormally increased volume of blood), hyperkalemia (a higher than normal concentration of potassium in the blood), and metabolic bone disease due to renal osteodystrophy (defective bone formation). Various factors—including delayed or impaired cognitive and academic performance, growth problems, the timing of immunizations, and disease etiology—determine the timing of transplantation. For most children with chronic renal insufficiency and end-stage renal disease, dialysis will eventually be necessary. Dialysis involves the removal of waste, salt, and extra water to prevent them from building up in the body. Kidney transplantation may allow for the discontinuation of dialysis or the preempting of dialysis altogether.

OUTCOMES

Preventing growth retardation, malnutrition, anemia, and renal osteodystrophy are primary objectives of the medical management leading up to transplantation. The age of disease onset and duration of the illness, glomerulofiltration rate, malnutrition, anemia, chronic acidosis (high blood acidity), and uremia can all contribute to growth retardation. Children may receive additional protein and growth hormones, as well as erythropoietin (to stimulate the proliferation and maturation of responsive bone marrow erythroid precursor cells), oral iron, a low-phosphate diet, phosphate binders, and vitamin D supplements.

Overall, pediatric patient survival rates are generally as good as those seen in adults and this includes a survival advantage for those who receive a living donor transplant. For cadaveric donor kidney transplants, patient survival rates are 98 percent at 1 year, 96 percent at 3 years, and 94 percent at 5 years; for living donor kidney transplants, patient survival rates are 99 percent at 1 year, 97 percent at 3 years, and 96 percent at 5 years. It is also noteworthy that transplantation affords survival advantages over dialysis, as the death rates for children on dialysis are 3.8 per 1,000 patient-years, compared to 0.4 per 1,000 patient-years for pediatric kidney transplant recipients. Infection (e.g., varicella/zoster), cardiovascular disease, hemorrhage, and malignancies are the primary causes of death after transplantation.

The growth trajectory of pediatric kidney transplant recipients is an important outcome that has considerable empirical attention. An average height deficit of about two standard deviations below the mean can be expected for most children with end-stage renal disease. Transplantation provides an opportunity for catch-up growth, especially for children who are less than 6 years old at the time of transplant.

PSYCHOLOGICAL CONSIDERATIONS

Pediatric psychologists are generally involved in the psychological evaluation of children and families at the time they are being considered for kidney transplantation. The nature and extent of these evaluations varies by transplant program, but generally includes an assessment of child development, adherence history, quality of life, psychological adaptation and coping, and family resources. For programs with living donor kidney transplantation as an option, pediatric psychologists may be called upon to provide evaluative services in determining the suitability of family members or friends to be living donors for the child. In addition to assessment-based services, psychological interventions are developed and implemented as needed to enhance both pre- and post-transplant health outcomes.

Cognitive functioning, quality of life, and adherence behaviors are frequently the focus of evaluation and intervention by the pediatric psychologist. Kidney disease, due to retention of urea, can lead to concentration, attention, memory, alertness, and perceptual-motor coordination problems in children. For many children, kidney transplantation leads to improvements in cognitive functioning, although longer disease duration, longer time on dialysis, and more severe kidney dysfunction before and after transplantation may attenuate such improvements. There is good evidence to suggest quality of life improvements with kidney transplantation, although more specific psychological benefits have not been systematically described or explicated. Nonadherence to the prescribed medical regimen is associated with significant morbidity in kidney transplant recipients, with incidence rates as high as 50 percent in some samples.

See also: Coping with Illness; Dialysis; Parenting the Chronically Ill Child; Quality of Life; Treatment Adherence: Medical

Further Reading

Fine, R. M. (1999). Renal transplantation in children: Current practices. In L. C. Ginns, A. B. Cosimi, & P. J. Morris (Eds.), *Transplantation* (pp. 312–323). Malden, MA: Blackwell Science.

Scientific Registry of Transplant Recipients Home Page. http://www.ustransplant.org (Accessed May 2002).

Tejani, A., Cortes, L., & Sullivan, E. K. (1996). A longitudinal study of the natural history of growth post-transplantation. *Kidney International, 49*(Suppl. 53), S103–S108.

United Network for Organ Sharing Home Page, http://www.unos.org (Accessed May 2002).

United States Renal Data System. (1998). *USRDS 1998 annual report*. Bethesda, MD: National Institutes of Health, National Institute of Diabetes and Digestive and Kidney Disease.

James R. Rodrigue
Willem J. van der Werf
Olivia Puyana

Klinefelter Syndrome

DESCRIPTION AND INCIDENCE

Klinefelter syndrome (KS) is a nonheritable genetic condition characterized by the presence of an extra

X chromosome. Whereas an unaffected male has a genotype of 46, XY, two thirds of males with KS possess a genotype of 47, XXY. In the remainder of cases, variant (48, XXY, 48, XXYY, and 49, XXXYY) and *mosaic* karyotypes (i.e., two or more cell types such as 46, XY/47, XXY) predominate. The phenotype (i.e., physical appearance) of individuals with KS is highly variable and features may include tall stature, disproportionately long legs, undescended testicles, poor development of the penis, and *gynecomastia* (breast development in males). Delayed puberty is seen in some cases. Infertility related to poor sperm production is a common feature, as are learning disabilities and problems with psychosocial adaptation. KS is diagnosed in approximately 1/500 to 1/1,000 male live births.

ETIOLOGY

The classic form of KS (47, XXY) is due to *meiotic nondisjunction* (failure of a pair of chromosomes to separate) of the chromosomes during development of the *gametes* (a mature germ cell capable of functioning in fertilization). About 40 percent of the responsible meiotic nondisjunctions occur during the development of sperm (*spermatogenesis*), and 60 percent occur during the production of ova (*oogenesis*). Advanced maternal age is a predisposing factor.

DIAGNOSIS

Although a KS diagnosis can be confirmed prenatally via amniocentesis or chorionic villi sampling, most patients are not diagnosed until puberty when poor development of the penis, undescended testes, and/or gynecomastia bring affected individuals to medical attention. Patients may also be diagnosed as a result of referral for mental health services, where parents express concerns about behavioral or psychosocial functioning. In all cases of KS, the diagnosis is established by documenting a characteristic karyotype. Once the diagnosis has been confirmed, concentrations of plasma testosterone are obtained to determine whether the adolescent would benefit from androgen replacement therapy.

ASSOCIATED PSYCHOLOGICAL FEATURES

Although the majority of the literature dealing with KS focuses on the physical and endocrinological features of the condition, there is a body of research devoted to addressing the cognitive and behavioral patterns commonly observed. Although most boys with KS demonstrate slightly below average intelligence, the deficits in intellectual adaptation generally derive less from impaired global intelligence than weaknesses within specific domains. In particular, boys with KS tend to have difficulty with verbal expression, verbal comprehension, verbal reasoning, and short-term auditory memory; consequently, these individuals are more likely to be diagnosed with a language-based learning disability. In thinking about this relatively common disorder, it is essential to remember that there is a wide range of variability in terms of cognitive ability; although slightly below average IQ is common among affected individuals, there are those who demonstrate above average to superior intelligence. Additionally, the limited research that has been conducted on the cognitive functioning of adults with KS suggests that intellectual capacity tends to fall within the average range.

In terms of psychosocial features, the clinical research literature indicates that individuals with KS are more likely to experience poor peer relationships, impulsivity, aggressiveness, withdrawal, apathy, and immaturity than unaffected individuals. Given that KS is a relatively common genetic disorder and one that may go undiagnosed, studies of the behavioral and emotional characteristics of this syndrome may be biased through the inclusion of those individuals who are the most severely affected. For example, early behavioral investigations detected an apparent overrepresentation of KS males in prison populations. This observation led to the speculation that men with a 47, XXY karyotype are predisposed to antisocial behavior. This hypothesis has since been disproven as more recent research has shown that learning disabilities associated with KS likely mediate the relationship between karyotype and incarceration.

TREATMENT

When a deficiency of testosterone is detected, treatment should be directed toward androgen replacement. Testosterone replacement allows for the affected individual to appear more age appropriate in terms of secondary sex characteristics. Hormone replacement therapy should initially be administered in low doses to avoid excessively rapid virilization and bone maturation. Although it is possible to receive testosterone replacement therapy orally, intramuscular injections are safer than oral preparations. Testosterone replacement therapy has recently become available in transdermal preparations (patch or gel). Eventually, patients will experience an increase in energy level, libido, and muscle strength; these changes are likely to elicit an improvement in self-image. It is noteworthy that testosterone replacement does not generally exert a salutary influence on gynecomastia; in cases where the extra breast tissue is bothersome to the patient, it can be surgically removed.

Psychoeducational counseling with the parents and affected individual should include information on the language deficits often observed in boys with KS and stress the importance of early intervention in the form of speech and language therapy. In addition, there should be an effort to involve the affected individual in organized peer activities that may prevent the social withdrawal and poor peer relations associated with KS.

As adolescents, youths with KS should be informed that infertility is a likely consequence of KS, but also that becoming a parent can be achieved through alternative routes (e.g., adoption). Infertility is not absolute, however, and the individual should be counseled regarding pregnancy prevention and safe sex practices.

PROGNOSIS

A comprehensive treatment plan should address the endocrinological, educational, and psychological needs of the affected individual. When these issues are taken into account, boys with KS can expect positive outcomes. Androgen replacement therapy is associated with an improvement in energy level and overall sense of well-being. When the specific educational needs are addressed, most boys with KS graduate from high school; some continue beyond a secondary level of education. With the current treatments available, long-term follow-up studies reveal no substantial differences in psychological and social outcomes in men with KS.

SUPPORT GROUPS

Klinefelter Syndrome and Associates, P.O. Box 119, Roseville, CA 95661-0119 USA; Web site: http://www.genetic.org; E-mail: ksinfo@genetic.org

See also: Behavioral Genetics; Gynecomastia; Turner Syndrome

Further Reading

Geschwind, D. H., Boone, K. B., Miller, B. L., & Swerdloff, R. S. (2000). Neurobehavioral phenotype of Klinefelter syndrome. *Mental Retardation and Developmental Disabilities, 6*, 107–116.

Grumbach, M., & Conte, F. A. (1998). Disorders of sex differentiation. In J. D. Wilson & D. Foster (Eds.), *Williams textbook of endocrinology* (9th ed., pp. 1303–1425). Philadelphia: W.B. Saunders.

Mandoki, M. W., Sumner, G. S., Hoffman, R. P., & Riconda, D. L. (1991). A review of Klinefelter's syndrome in children and adolescents. *Journal of the American Academy of Child & Adolescent Psychiatry, 30*, 167–172.

Rovet, J., Netley, C., Keenan, M., Bailey, J., & Stewart, D. (1996). The psychoeducational profile of boys with Klinefelter syndrome. *Journal of Learning Disabilities, 29*, 180–196.

LAUREN ZURENDA
DAVID E. SANDBERG

Ll

Language Development

DEFINITION OF THE FIELD

Language development includes the understanding of how and when children acquire both the labels that are used in speech and writing (often called "vocabulary," and technically referred to as the *lexicon*), and the rules through which such labels are ordered or marked (*syntax*) that allows one to precisely identify the agent, object, and action in a communication (e.g., subject–object or subject–verb agreement) and the time frame to which the communication refers (e.g., tense marking). In addition to the division between lexical and syntactical development, the study of language acquisition is also often segregated into *receptive development* (i.e., the understanding or comprehension of language) and *productive development* (i.e., the expression or production of spoken language).

THREE THEORETICAL MODELS

There are three fundamental theories or positions regarding language development, all of which vary most saliently on the answer to the question of whether language itself represents a qualitatively unique or separate module of human behavior in the brain. If the answer to this question is "no," then one ascribes to the *generalist* position. If the answer to this question is "yes," then one ascribes to the *modular* position. A third answer is possible, however, which holds that language

is not qualitatively unique or modular, but simply represents a quantitative extension of the superior cognitive abilities shown by humans; this is the *cognitive-interactionist* position.

The generalist, or behaviorist, position holds that language is no different than any other behavior, and is acquired through the general behavioral processes of learning, primarily reinforcement and shaping. This position is perhaps represented best in B. F. Skinner's 1957 book, *Verbal Behavior*. Although it is obvious that the environment has a critical role in the acquisition of language, and that behavioral principles can be used to promote some aspects of language development, learning theorists have been generally unsuccessful in identifying or documenting the role of fundamental learning processes that occur in language development, and as such, this position has not contributed much to basic knowledge about language in recent years.

The two other positions represent more current or productive approaches to language development. The modular position holds that language (especially syntax) does in fact represent a separate module of human behavior in the brain and likely represents a part of the human evolutionary endowment. This position is usually associated with the nativist/linguistic approaches to language development of Noam Chomsky (his book, *Syntactic Structures*, was published in 1957), although there have been major shifts and revisions to the theory since then (for an accessible and readable account, see Pinker, 1994). This approach to language is supported by the presence of clinical syndromes in which language and other intellectual functions are dissociated. For example, in the genetic condition of Williams syndrome, the general symptom of mental retardation occurs although language remains relatively intact. In Specific Language Impairment, syntactical functions are clinically impaired but other cognitive functions are not. Although in theory these syndromes would appear to provide irrefutable evidence for the modular position, the degree to which language and cognition are truly dissociated by these clinical conditions is a matter of controversy and debate.

The cognitive–interactionist position holds that language is built upon fundamental cognitive functions such as attention, memory, and representation, and is likely learned through simple "connections" that the brain naturally makes as a result of exposure to regular or predictable stimuli. This position is supported by reports that children appear to acquire language in ways that reflect underlying cognitive functions (see Bates, Bretherton, & Snyder, 1988), and that when language and cognitive deficits occur, they most often tend to occur in tandem.

LANGUAGE DEVELOPMENT MILESTONES

Language is acquired in a fairly predictable sequence. From birth, infants are sensitive to the special characteristics of human speech that are present in all languages, although by 8–10 months of age they appear to become more sensitive to speech sounds that are present in the languages spoken in their immediate environment and less sensitive to those that are not routinely heard. Infants also begin to approximate the production of words in both the form and tonal aspects of their utterances at this time. On average, however, the first word is produced at 12 months of age. The ages of 12–18 months represent a period in which only one word is typically produced at a time (the one-word, or *holophrastic stage*) and where vocabulary grows slowly, but at some point—usually halfway through the second year—there is a vocabulary "spurt" where the rate of vocabulary acquisition increases enormously. This usually coincides with the onset of the *telegraphic* stage of language development, in which utterances are usually made up of two words. During the third year, various forms of syntax typically appear in the forms of word endings (*inflections*) that mark tense, possession, or pluralization.

LANGUAGE AND THE ENVIRONMENT

Although there is considerable debate about the source or origins of the development of syntax, the acquisition of the lexicon is clearly linked to environmental exposure. In recent years, research has focused on the effects of deprived environments on children's vocabulary acquisition, and the range of those effects. This evidence clearly suggests that the amount and quality of early input from caregivers to children is related to the rate and amount of vocabulary that children acquire, and that these early differences in vocabulary acquisition have impacts on achievement and intelligence that are easily seen well into the school-age years (for a readable account of such effects, see Hart and Risley, 1995).

CLINICAL RELEVANCE

Language is a salient indicator of developmental status, and follows a roughly predictable sequence. As such, language delays are indicative of the presence of general cognitive delays, of mental retardation, and of other specific clinical syndromes such as autism and Asperger's syndrome. Indeed, language delays are often used as part of the diagnostic regime for most developmental delays.

See also: Childhood; Cognitive Development; Developmental Milestones; Infancy

Further Reading

Bates, E., Bretherton, I., & Snyder, L. (1988). *From first words to grammar.* Cambridge, MA: Cambridge University Press.
Elman, J., Bates, E., Johnson, M., Karmiloff-Smith, A., Parisi, D., & Plunkett, K. (1996). *Rethinking innateness.* Cambridge, MA: MIT Press.
Hart, B., & Risley, T. R. (1995). *Meaningful differences in the everyday experience of young American children.* Baltimore, MD: Paul H. Brookes.
Pinker, S. (1994). *The language instinct.* New York: HarperCollins.
Werker, J. (1989). Becoming a native listener. *American Scientist, 77,* 54–59.

JOHN COLOMBO

Lead Poisoning

DEFINITION

Lead poisoning refers to the harmful effects of lead on the blood, soft tissues, bones, and teeth and behavior.

In children these can result in devastating health effects such as blood disorders, cancer, and immune system effects. The greatest concern is damage to the central nervous system resulting in learning and behavior problems like Attention-Deficit/Hyperactivity Disorder (ADHD) and aggression at blood lead levels as low as 10 μg/dl. At very high levels (over 70 μg/dl) it can cause seizures, coma, and death.

Lead is the chief toxicant (poisonous agent) among 85,000 chemicals produced in the United States each year. Only 15,000 of these have been proposed for toxicity testing. Other heavy metals such as cadmium, mercury, manganese, as well as pesticides, alcohol, and environmental tobacco smoke also can be very toxic.

PREVALENCE/ETIOLOGY

Over the past 100 years, research and public health advocates have worked to reduce lead in our environment. Even so, it is estimated that there are over 890,000 children in the United States with elevated blood lead levels. Since the banning of lead in gasoline, the major exposure source is lead-based paint in old pre-1950 housing stock. Thus, hot spots tend to be in older urban areas, especially in the Northeast, but many rural areas are also not spared. However, in some states, such as Alaska, blood lead levels in children are very low. So, depending on the location, surveillance in old housing is still very important. Other point sources of exposure are living near lead smelting or recycling industries, or close to trash incinerating sites where residues of lead are burned. Many other exposures, for example, in cosmetics, paint glazes on pottery and paintings, and gunshot wounds account for fewer elevated lead levels in children.

CORRELATES

There are several important correlates of lead which tend to exacerbate its effects on learning and behavior. Nutritional deficiencies such as iron deficiency anemia, vitamin D deficiency, calcium, body fat, and nutrition tend to interact with lead metabolism to make it better or worse. Home cleanliness and caregiver practices are especially important factors among infants and toddlers at the crawling and mouthing stages. Lead in house dust or in chips of paint both indoors and outdoors can be lethal if in large quantities. The quality of the caregiving environment, parental education, and socioeconomic status are also strong correlates which combine with lead exposure to affect the child's learning and behavior. A stimulating, nurturing home environment can often offset the effects of low-level lead exposure. There are also several other covariates of lead that may interact to affect the child's development, for example, parental alcohol or substance abuse and parental smoking, which mediate the caregiving environment.

TREATMENT

Children with very high blood lead levels, usually over 30 μg/dl, are hospitalized for chelation therapy. This treatment consists of injecting the child with a chelating agent that competes with lead for protein-binding sites. The lead is then excreted in the urine. Urine and blood levels as well as diet are monitored until the lead level drops and the child can be released from the hospital. Lead also chelates other trace minerals essential for nutrition, so chelation therapy cannot be performed frequently.

By far the best treatment is primary prevention from ever being exposed to lead. Choosing a house free of lead and avoiding other risky sources, for example, location near a lead industry, unsafe drinking water, cosmetics, hobbies such as ceramics, or home remedies containing lead should be avoided.

Secondary prevention strategies involve universal screening for elevated blood lead levels, environmental assessment and monitoring, and individual risk assessment through the local county health department. These will point out the demographics, probable sources of exposure, environmental investigations needed to pinpoint the sources, and the medical interventions required to remove the risk. The Centers for Disease Control and Prevention does national monitoring and establishes guidelines for controlling risks due to lead. Lead is everywhere in our environment—in the air, the water, and the soil. We all ingest lead every day. It is therefore everybody's business to monitor its effect.

See also: Adaptive Behavior Assessment; Disruptive Behavior Disorders; Neurological Disorders; Safety and Prevention; Screening Instruments: Behavioral and Developmental

Further Reading

Centers for Disease Control and Prevention. (1997). *Screening young children for lead poisoning: Guidance for state and local public health officials.* Atlanta: Author.
Developing brain and environment. (2000). *Environmental Health Perspectives Supplements, 108*(3), 373–438.

STEPHEN R. SCHROEDER

Learning Disorders

and learning disorders will be considered interchangeable in this entry.

Learning disorders occur in persons who have at least average intelligence, but difficulty processing certain types of information; this difficulty leads to problems in learning to read, spell, write, perform math, listen, or speak. Learning disorders should be distinguished from other types of learning problems caused by such things as mental retardation, borderline intellectual ability, underachievement, primary sensory or motor disabilities, behavioral or emotional dysfunction, and/or environmental deprivation. According to *DSM-IV-TR*, the primary criterion for learning disorders is a failure to achieve at a level commensurate with one's chronological age, measured intelligence, and age-appropriate education. The learning disorder must also interfere significantly with one's academic achievement or activities of daily living. Learning disorders are commonly referred to as "learning disabilities" in school systems, and the child's eligibility for intervention services usually is determined by the presence of a severe discrepancy between the child's intellectual and academic functioning.

Children with learning disabilities comprise the largest group of children with disabilities from birth to 21 years who receive special education services in U.S. public schools. They receive 46 percent of the special education funding compared to the next largest group (speech or language impairments) that receives 17.6 percent of the funding. This corresponds to approximately 2.8 million students who have a primary diagnosis of learning disability severe enough to be eligible for special education services (U.S. Department of Education, June 2000). The terms learning disabilities

TYPES OF LEARNING DISORDERS

Early research on learning disabilities assumed that the disorder was homogeneous and possibly caused by a single underlying factor. Current researchers consider learning disabilities to be a heterogeneous set of disorders that may have several etiologies. Subtyping of learning disabilities and their underlying processing deficits has become common practice. The primary subtypes of learning disabilities are described in Table 1.

In addition to subtyping according to the academic area affected by the learning disorder, it is important to subtype also by the information processing deficits that underlie the disorder. Much of the subtyping research to date has been done with dyslexia. For instance, a child with phonological processing deficits that underlie a reading disorder may have problems remembering or discriminating between similar phonetic sounds, or have problems blending phonetic sounds together into syllables and words. A child with visual perceptual deficits may have difficulty remembering or discriminating between similar graphemes (e.g., letters such as b–d, p–q) that leads to reading errors. This child may have a poor sight-reading vocabulary. Children with sensorimotor processing problems may manifest their problems more in writing. Their written production may be slow, poorly legible, disorganized, or replete with errors of spelling. Often individuals with this type of processing problem may demonstrate their knowledge well orally, but fail to communicate this information at a commensurate level in written form.

Table 1. Primary Subtypes of Learning Disability

Reading Disorder (Dyslexia)	A disorder in one or more of the basic skills involved in reading, including basic reading skills (e.g., letter–word recognition and identification, phonetic analysis and synthesis) and reading comprehension skills.
Mathematics Disorder (Dyscalculia)	A disorder in one or more of the basic skills involved in mathematics, including computational skills (e.g., the math operations of addition, subtraction, algebra and geometry operations, etc.) and math reasoning abilities.
Disorder of Written Expression (Dysgraphia)	A disorder in one or more of the basic skills involved in written expression. This disorder may be manifest in: • Knowledge of rules for spelling, grammar, punctuation, and capitalization • Motor production of writing, including letter formation, kinesthetic-motor sequencing of letters to make words, speed of writing production, and spatial organization of written material • Semantic and syntactic abilities that underlie clear expression of ideas in written language, using age-appropriate vocabulary and correct sentence structure • Organization of ideas and themes for writing longer passages, such as themes or essays.

Accurate subtyping of learning disorders is essential for development of appropriate educational intervention strategies that will strengthen the child's information processing weaknesses while attempting to teach through their processing strengths.

DIAGNOSIS

Learning disorders are diagnosed through an individual psychoeducational evaluation that includes measures of intellectual and academic functioning, and various types of information processing abilities. Information processing refers to the brain's ability to interpret information from various types of sensory input (e.g., visual, tactile, motor), and process that information in an integrated manner to facilitate academic performance. For example, the ability to take a spelling test in class involves a complex series of processing steps, including auditory input of the spoken word, perhaps visualizing the word mentally, associating the various phonetic sounds with specific letters in the word, remembering the correct kinesthetic-motor patterns necessary for writing the letters and sequencing them correctly, as well as accessing one's knowledge of specific spelling rules that govern the irregular spelling of many words in the English language. This complex processing ability is mediated by many different parts of the brain, specific to the particular type of academic skill being performed. Psychologists are the primary professionals to conduct this type of evaluation, although educators trained in assessment may sometimes conduct the academic portion of the examination.

In addition to the intellectual, academic, and information processing assessment, individuals with suspected learning disorders should be examined medically to rule out even a subtle auditory or visual acuity deficit that could interfere with learning. A medical evaluation can also determine the integrity of the child's motor system as it supports writing skills. Often a speech/language pathologist will participate in an evaluation to examine whether receptive/expressive language, articulation, or auditory processing problems are present. Care should be taken to rule out primary sensory or motor deficits or mental retardation that could explain the individual's learning difficulty. Psychologists will also take a careful background history to determine if the child has had appropriate opportunities for learning (e.g., regular school attendance) and to rule out significant environmental deprivation and/or emotional problems as the primary cause of the child's learning problems.

COURSE OF THE DISORDER

Learning disorders typically are lifelong disabilities, although many individuals learn to compensate for the negative effects of the disorder through special education services they receive in school. A small number of children may experience a delay in maturation of functions needed for development of early academic skills, but they will typically catch up by 9 or 10 years of age. However, most individuals will continue to have some symptoms of learning disorders throughout their lives. The course of the disorder is also affected by the child's general intellectual ability and by the number of information processing areas affected by the learning disorder. For example, if a child has difficulty processing both auditory and visual information, their reading skills may be more seriously impaired than if only one processing modality is affected. A child with a learning disability who has above average intelligence will likely fare better than one with below average intelligence. Family support, and the quality and timing of special education interventions, can also affect outcome.

ETIOLOGY OF LEARNING DISORDERS

The cause of learning disorders is still under investigation, but there is wide agreement that they are neurologically based disorders that affect central learning processes. Learning disorders may be inherited, and a family history will often reveal one or more close relatives with some form of learning disorder. Often several generations will display the disorder, and the familial pattern lends strong evidence for a genetic etiology in these cases. However, researchers have explored a number of other possible etiologies as well. Culbertson and colleagues (1996) suggest that causes may include brain structural differences that underlie the information processing deficits, differences in brain activity level (e.g., glucose metabolism) during academic tasks such as reading, and even perinatal or postnatal events that affect the developing fetus or young child. At present, researchers have not determined a single cause for learning disorders, and often it is not possible to determine a specific etiology for a given individual.

TREATMENT

Learning disorders are best treated through special education provided by educators who are specially trained (usually with at least a Master's degree in special education, and certification in the area of learning disabilities). These educators are found in public school systems all across the United States, but not necessarily in every school. Special education and related services are provided free of charge to all eligible children through Public Law 101-476 (Individuals with Disabilities Education Act of 1990, or IDEA). Once a child is diagnosed with a learning disability and determined to be eligible for special education services by a multidisciplinary team of educators, ancillary professionals, and parents, the team will develop an Individualized Educational Plan (IEP) that is appropriate for the needs of the child. The type, intensity, and setting for provision of the special education services will be determined at that time. Although special education services are important in helping children learn despite their learning disability, these services should not be considered a "cure" for the disability. Often the focus in early grades is upon remedial education, but eventually the focus will shift to assisting older elementary children and adolescents to develop compensation strategies for working around their disability. In addition, modifications in the child's curriculum may be detailed in the IEP. For example, a child with a disorder of written expression may need additional time to complete written tests, or may need to request that a good "notetaker" in class share his or her lecture notes.

With the passage of the Americans with Disabilities Act of 1990 (P.L. 101-336), individuals with learning disabilities are protected from discrimination. This law has led institutions of higher learning that accept public funding to institute policies and procedures to prevent discrimination against individuals with disabilities of all types. Most colleges and universities now have programs to assist students with disabilities who are willing to identify themselves and present documentation of their disability and need for accommodations. These events have opened the door to higher education to a growing number of students with learning disabilities who have the ability and desire to undertake higher education.

See also: Adolescent Assessment; Mental Retardation; Preschool Assessment; School Age Assessment; Underachievement

Further Reading

American Psychiatric Association. (2000). *Diagnostic and statistical manual of mental disorders* (4th ed., text revision). Washington, DC: Author.

Culbertson, J. L., & Edmonds, J. (1996). Learning disabilities. In R. Adams, O. Parsons, J. L. Culbertson, & S. J. Nixon (Eds.), *Neuropsychology for clinical practice: Etiology, assessment, and treatment of common neurological problems* (pp. 331–408). Washington, DC: American Psychological Association.

Culbertson, J. L. (1998). Learning disabilities. In T. H. Ollendick & M. Hersen (Eds.), *Handbook of child psychopathology* (3rd ed., pp. 117–156). New York: Plenum.

Individuals with Disabilities Education Act of 1990, 20 U.S.C. Chapter 33, Section 1401.

U.S. Department of Education, Office of Special Education and Rehabilitative Services, Annual Report to Congress on the Implementation of the Individuals with Disabilities Education Act, June 2000.

Web Sites

Learning Disabilities Association of America (http://www.ldanatl.org)

LD OnLine (http://www.ldonline.org)

National Information Center for Children and Youth with Disabilities (http://www.nichcy.org)

National Adult Literacy and Learning Disabilities Center: Academy for Educational Development (http://www.aed.org)

JAN L. CULBERTSON

Legal Issues in Child and Pediatric Psychology

The laws regarding children's rights and their relationship with their parents are quite complex and ambiguous. In general, in the United States, parents are given the freedom to raise their children without interference from the state as long as they do not threaten children's safety and health. Parents' autonomy to make decisions about their children's well being is based on respect for the family as an institution and for protection of child welfare. However, the state is considered to have the duty and authority to protect children from serious harm when their parents are unable or unwilling to do so.

Although parents are generally given the authority to make decisions about their children, there has been a trend in law on recognizing minors' constitutional rights, such as the right to privacy. This trend has allowed minors a limited right to obtain abortions and access to mental health services without parental permission. These rights for minors remain ambiguous, as they often hinge on issues of the competence of minors to be decision-makers. Within a mental health setting, these legal issues take on significance in several areas that will be discussed below.

INFORMED CONSENT

Psychologists and other mental health providers must inform clients of the risks and benefits of psychological treatment and alternatives and obtain voluntary consent to engage in the therapy process. Similarly, researchers must obtain informed consent before individuals participate in any type of psychological research. When working with minors, psychologists should attain assent (consent) of the minor to whatever degree possible, in addition to obtaining consent from their parent or legal guardian. This requirement means that children and adolescents should be told about the evaluation and treatment process in words that they can understand. In addition, psychologists must consider the best interests of children and adolescents when treating them. Although parents and legal guardians have the legal rights to access a child's records and to know the content of therapy sessions, it is sometimes not in the best interests of the child to release all information. Some states have protections allowing mental health providers to release only summaries of therapy if it is considered in the best interests of the child. It is important to reach an agreement with parents that some information will be kept confidential between therapist and minor, while other information will be shared with parents.

There are some exceptions where minors may be able to consent to treatment independent of their parents. These exceptions can occur for emancipated and mature minors. Emancipated minors are those individuals recognized by courts as those who are sufficiently independent and separate from their parents, such as because of marriage, enlistment in the military, or financial independence. Emancipated minors are legally thought to be competent to consent to psychological treatment. Mature minors are those adolescents thought to be of a relatively mature age and can understand the nature of the procedure to which he or she is consenting. The treatments to which they consent must not be considered major and must be beneficial to the mature minor. Most states have statutes that authorize children to consent to certain treatments, such as consent to the provision of pregnancy-related services, venereal disease treatment, drug and alcohol abuse treatment, and in some cases, mental health treatment. However, to demonstrate the ambiguity of laws affecting children, these same states may require parental consent for piercing ears.

RIGHTS TO REFUSE TREATMENT

Although it is important to inform a minor about psychological treatment, a child's refusal for treatment has been seen legally to be insufficient and irrelevant so treatment can be provided even if a minor objects. Children and adolescents can enter psychiatric hospitals under voluntary or involuntary status. In most states,

parents have the right to voluntarily admit their children. However, the United Nations Convention on the Rights of the Child (1989) sets a goal that obligates anyone acting under the law to obtain the child's preferences on any matter pertaining to him or her. This document serves as a guide to mental health policy and practice. Therefore, mental health professionals should involve minors in decision-making as much as possible and seek alternatives to provide the least restrictive appropriate environment for treatment.

CONFIDENTIALITY

Confidentiality is considered the privacy right to determine who will have access to information and is granted some constitutional protection. Psychologists must discuss issues of confidentiality with their clients, including limits to confidentiality. Mental health providers have the legal and ethical duty to break this confidentiality in instances of suspected physical or sexual abuse or neglect and to report to the appropriate social services agency in order to keep minors safe and healthy. In some states, mental health professionals are required to warn known potential victims of violence by dangerous clients. Mental health providers can also break this confidentiality to protect minors thought to be in danger of hurting themselves.

Most states have provisions for "physician–patient privilege," allowing a doctor to refuse from testifying about confidential information relayed in the course of treatment. However, mental health providers are sometimes not included in these privileges. With children, this physician–patient privilege may also not be honored. Therefore, mental health providers should inform minors that they might have to testify in court about confidential material if their parents consent to it.

It is important for mental health providers to take into account not only legal but also ethical issues when providing services to children and adolescents. The United Nations Convention on the Rights of the Child (1989) provides a framework for clinicians to use in making decisions about the best mental health treatment for minors. From this Convention, Melton and colleagues (2001) have derived the following guiding principles:

1. Providing high-quality mental health services is of highest priority.
2. Children should be active participants in mental health services. Their privacy and liberty should be heavily protected.
3. Mental health services for children and adolescents should be "family-centered" and respectful of parents.

4. Children should be treated in the least restrictive environment that is appropriate. Residential placement should be made cautiously. If placement out of the home is necessary, it should be in a family setting if possible.
5. States must protect children taken into its care and protect them from harm.
6. Prevention should be the emphasis of child mental health policy.

See also: Confidentiality and Privilege; Ethical Issues; Informed Consent; Mental Health Records; Psychiatric Inpatient Treatment; Residential Treatment; Termination of Parental Rights; Training Issues

Further Reading

American Psychological Association. (1992). Ethical principles of psychologists and code of conduct. *American Psychologist, 47,* 1597–1611.

Melton, G. B., Ehrenreich, N. S., & Lyons, Jr., P. M. (2001). Ethical and legal issues in mental health services for children. In C. E. Walker & M. C. Roberts (Eds.), *Handbook of clinical child psychology* (3rd ed., pp. 1074–1093). New York: Wiley.

United Nations Convention on the Rights of the Child, U.N. Doc. A/Res/44/25 (1989). On World Wide Web: http://www.unicef.org/crc (Accessed May 9, 2002).

LISA M. BUCKLOH
MICHAEL C. ROBERTS

Leukemia

Leukemia is a malignant disorder of the blood. In children, types of leukemia include acute lymphoblastic leukemia (ALL), acute nonlymphoblastic leukemia (ANLL), and chronic myelogenous leukemia (CML). ALL accounts for the majority (about 75 percent) of childhood leukemia and will be discussed at length in this entry.

ACUTE LYMPHOBLASTIC LEUKEMIA (ALL)

Description

ALL involves production and rapid growth of malignant white blood cells (WBCs) in the bone marrow, and is diagnosed in approximately 3,000 children per year in the United States. It is the most common cancer in children less than 15 years of age and accounts for 25 percent of all childhood malignancies.

ALL is most common in children between 2 and 10 years of age, with the peak age of diagnosis at 4 years of age. It is slightly more common in boys than in girls.

Etiology

Although the cause of ALL is unknown, several associations with genetic abnormalities (trisomy 21, Bloom's syndrome, Fanconi's anemia), immunodeficiency syndromes, environmental factors (ionizing radiation), and viral infections exist.

Presentation

The signs and symptoms of ALL represent infiltration of leukemic cells into the bone marrow and extramedullary sites. Common presenting features include fever, pallor, hepatosplenomegaly (enlarged liver and spleen), bruising/bleeding, lymphadenopathy (enlarged lymph nodes), fatigue, and bone pain. ALL can be suspected by a complete blood count (CBC) with a manual differential blood count showing lymphoblasts. The majority of CBCs will have a decrease in at least one cell line (cell lines are white blood cells, red blood cells, and platelets). Only about 1 percent of patients will have a normal CBC. The definitive diagnosis is made by a bone marrow aspirate (a test in which a needle is inserted into a bone to extract the marrow).

Treatment

Treatment consists primarily of multiagent chemotherapy. It includes rapid remission induction (multiple chemotherapeutic drugs to eliminate existing leukemia cells and to prevent emergence of resistant cells), prophylactic (preventive) treatment to prevent central nervous system (CNS) relapse (with intrathecal [inserted into the spinal canal] chemotherapy), and postremission therapy with intensification (consolidation) and maintenance therapy. Therapy begins with either a 3- or 4-drug induction with vincristine, steroids (prednisone or dexamethasone), L-asparaginase, +/− doxorubicin. Treatment continues with different combinations of chemotherapy including 6-mercaptopurine, methotrexate, vincristine, steroids, L-asparaginase, cytoxan, and doxorubicin. Intrathecal chemotherapy consists of methotrexate, +/− Ara-C, and hydrocortisone. With current chemotherapy approaches, only a small percentage of patients present with CNS disease and require cranial radiation therapy (typically 18 Gy or 24 Gy). Treatment typically occurs over about a $2\frac{1}{2}$–3 year period.

Prognosis

The outcome of ALL has improved markedly over the past 25 years. Currently 70 percent of children with ALL will be cured, and children in some subgroups have a cure rate of at least 85 percent. Factors associated with a better outcome include age ≥ 1 year and < 10 years, presenting WBC count < 50,000, and cell markers consistent with a type of leukemia called precursor-B ALL. Cytogenetics, flow cytometry, and DNA evaluations help to further define therapy and outcome.

Acute complications often involve fever and neutropenia (low white cell count) after chemotherapy, which results in hospitalization. There may also be reactions to chemotherapy drugs, for example, methotrexate toxicity, mood swings and irritability from steroids, and fine motor coordination problems from vincristine. These reactions, while problematic for the patient and family, are usually reversible once the course of the drug is finished.

Long-term complications may include functional impairments, for example, leukoencephalopathy (white matter destruction), obesity, decreased bone density, cardiomyopathy (heart muscle dysfunction), and secondary malignancies.

ACUTE NONLYMPHOBLASTIC LEUKEMIA (ANLL)

ANLL is a group of diagnoses that involve blood-forming cells that are not lymphoblasts, e.g., acute myelogenous leukemia (AML) involves the granulocytes (another type of WBC). It is more common in the first years of life, then decreases until later childhood and is most common in adolescence. There is no predominance of gender. It represents about 15–25 percent of childhood leukemia. Etiology includes predisposing environmental factors (ionizing radiation and chemical exposures) as well as genetic factors (e.g., twinning, several genetic syndromes). Chemotherapy to treat ANLL is much more intensive than that used to treat ALL, and involves longer and more frequent hospitalizations. The long-term prognosis is less positive than that of ALL (event-free survival less than 50 percent overall), with about a 35 percent long-term survival rate with chemotherapy alone. Thus, bone marrow or stem cell transplants are typically done to achieve remission.

CHRONIC MYELOGENOUS LEUKEMIA (CML)

CML, found in only 2–3 percent of childhood leukemias, is comprised of an adult form and a juvenile form. In both of these forms, bone marrow transplantation is the treatment of choice.

PSYCHOLOGICAL ISSUES

Hundreds of studies have been done to examine the psychological functioning of children with cancer, and children with leukemia usually comprise the majority of participants. Relevant coping issues include coping with a potentially fatal disease, frequent painful procedures (lumbar punctures and bone marrow aspirations), side effects of medications, and issues related to having treatment for 2–3 years (those who have bone marrow or stem cell transplants also must cope with prolonged hospitalization and isolation, with several possible late effects, for example, growth, sterility, graft-versus-host disease). Studies done in the 1960s and 1970s, when the prognosis for leukemia was relatively poor, frequently found more psychological problems and family dysfunction. With increased survival rates, coupled with the ability to follow larger numbers of children and adolescents longitudinally, recent studies have found little evidence of serious psychopathology. Most children and adolescents have been found to exhibit good adjustment and adaptation over time. While the majority do not have serious psychological problems, about one-fourth to one-third may exhibit problems, such as anxiety, depression, academic, social, or family problems, at some time during or after treatment that are serious enough to warrant referral to a psychosocial professional. (Given the nature of the disease and treatment, situational and episodic anxiety and depressive symptoms are expected at times, but some show more intensive and disruptive signs and symptoms.) Research has indicated that those most at risk for coping and adjustment problems are children who are younger, have preexisting personal and family psychological problems, have fewer resources, and who have other concurrent stresses. Long-term survivors who have decreased academic functioning, or who have had CNS relapse and treatment are also at risk for coping and adjustment problems. Early child and family assessment is critical to identify problems, with early patient and family intervention to address specific coping tasks and strengthen child and family coping resources.

NEUROCOGNITIVE ISSUES

After sufficient numbers of children with leukemia who were treated on protocols, including CNS radiation, were studied, patterns of decreasing IQ, mathematical ability, memory, attention, spatial relationships, problem-solving, and processing speed were common, especially for those treated when very young (less than 4 years of age). As a result, intrathecal medication (drugs introduced into the spinal canal to prevent CNS disease) was substituted, and, while the effects are less severe, recent large institution and multisite studies have found similar, if less severe, changes in neurocognitive functioning, even 2–3 years after treatment. Thus, these children are at risk for neurocognitive problems and should be tested longitudinally, with appropriate academic interventions. It has been estimated that about 40 percent of children treated with cranial radiation and/or methotrexate are receiving some type of learning disability services. Currently, ongoing studies are being done to test the effectiveness of medical, academic, and behavioral interventions in children where attention, memory, and learning problems result after treatment.

See also: Bone Marrow Transplantation; Childhood Cancers; Coping with Illness; Parenting the Chronically Ill Child; Treatment Adherence: Medical

Further Reading

Armstrong, F. D., & Mulhern, R. K. (1999). Acute lymphoblastic leukemia and brain tumors. In R. T. Brown (Ed.), *Cognitive aspects of chronic illness in children* (pp. 47–77). New York: Guilford.

Golub, T. R., & Arceci, R. J. (2002). Acute myelogenous leukemia. In P. A. Pizzo and D. G. Poplack (Eds.), *Principles and practice of pediatric oncology* (4th ed., pp. 545–589). Philadelphia: Lippincott, Williams & Wilkins.

Kupst, M. J., Natta, M. B., Richardson, C. C., Schulman, J. L., Lavigne, J. V., & Das, L. (1995). Family coping with pediatric leukemia: Ten years after treatment. *Journal of Pediatric Psychology, 20*(5), 601–617.

Margolin, J. F., Steuber, C. P., & Poplack, D. G. (2002). Acute lymphoblastic leukemia. In P. A. Pizzo & D. G. Poplack (Eds.), *Principles and practice of pediatric oncology* (4th ed., pp. 489–544). Lippincott, Philadelphia: Williams & Wilkins.

Pui, Ching-Hon. (1995). Childhood leukemias. *New England Journal of Medicine, 332*(24): 1618–1630.

MARY JO KUPST
KELLY W. MALONEY

Licensure

In order to protect the welfare of citizens, each state or province provides regulations and laws to ensure that only those individuals with the appropriate credentials are able to provide psychological services within that state or province. The legal basis for licensure is to protect the citizens of that state or province from unqualified practitioners and to remove incompetent or/and unethical psychologists from practice. Each state or province has its own licensing board and criteria that the applicant for licensure must meet. Most states and provinces have a generic license in psychology, as opposed to specific licensure. For instance, there is no specific license to become a clinical child or pediatric psychologist. Obviously, practitioners working within the clinical child and pediatric psychology arena must not practice outside of their area of expertise as defined by training and experience. In many states, the potential licensee must first apply for licensure and be approved in order to continue with state or province-mandated requirements for licensure.

To become licensed as a psychologist, the applicant must meet requirements in three areas. In the first area, the applicant must obtain a graduate degree in an approved course of graduate study in a field of psychology from a regionally accredited institution of higher education. Applicants from American Psychological Association (APA) approved graduate programs fall into the approved status. Licensure for the independent practice of psychology requires a doctoral degree in most states and provinces. At the same time, some of the states and provinces license psychologists for the supervised practice of psychology with a minimum of a master's degree in psychology. In the second area, a majority of states and provinces require that the applicant pass the Examination for Professional Practice in Psychology (EPPP). In order to take the EPPP, the applicant must have applied through their local licensing board and must have obtained their doctoral degree, including a predoctoral internship. In addition, many states and provinces require an oral examination and/or a jurisprudence examination. Each state or provincial licensing board sets predetermined cut-off scores on the EPPP, jurisprudence exams, oral exams, and/or any additional tests they require. In the third area, the applicant must have appropriate supervised professional experience. In most cases this experience would include a one-year predoctoral internship (included in the applicant's doctoral program) and an additional one-year supervised postdoctoral experience. The specific requirements of these supervised experiences differ depending upon the state or province in which the applicant applies for licensure. Once these criteria have been met, the applicant may be issued a license, which is renewable every year as long as the licensee has followed state guidelines for renewal. Often, in order to be renewed, the licensee must obtain a certain number of continuing education credits each year.

Furthermore, the licensee must not have been convicted of ethical violations or a felony in the previous year.

Psychologists must be licensed in the state or province in which they practice. When a psychologist moves to another state or province, the psychologist must be licensed by that government entity. Because of different requirements between jurisdictions, the psychologist may find it difficult to get licensed in another state or province. According to the Association of State and Provincial Psychology Boards (ASPPB), ten states and provinces currently have agreements of reciprocity of licensure, which means that these states have determined that the procedures for licensing are similar. The licensed psychologist applying for licensure in the reciprocal state or province may benefit from streamlined procedures (e.g., can use scores from the previously taken nationally standardized written exam). Each reciprocal state or province may require its own jurisprudence exam and/or oral exam. Given the variation between the different jurisdictions, the applicant must be aware of the criteria for the state or province in which he or she wishes to be licensed. Additional information is available from the *Handbook of Licensing and Certification Requirements for Psychologists in North America* (ASPPB, 2002) that delineates the most current requirements for the various jurisdictions.

See also: Ethical Issues; Professional Societies in Clinical Child and Pediatric Psychology; Training Issues

Further Reading

American Psychological Association. (1992). Ethical principles of psychologists and code of conduct. *American Psychologist, 47,* 1597–1611.

Association of State and Provincial Psychology Boards. (2002). *Handbook of licensing and certification requirements for psychologists in North America.* Montgomery, AL: Author.

Web Sites

http://www.apa.org/ethics/code.html
http://www.apa.org/practice/licnet.html
http://www.asppb.org/exam/req.asp

WILLIAM A. RAE

Life Stress in Children and Adolescents

The term life stress is typically used to refer to cumulative life events that are experienced over a specified period of time. Examples would include major life events such as the "divorce of parents," "death of best friend," "new brother or sister," "discovering you were adopted," "unwed pregnancy," or "changing to a new school." While some view life stress as resulting from "positive" and "negative" life events, others have argued that life stress is best conceptualized in terms of events that are negative or undesirable in nature.

ASSESSING LIFE STRESS

A number of measures have been developed to assess child/adolescent life stress. Two of these, the Life Events Record (LER) and the Life Events Checklist (LEC), highlight the most popular approaches to child life stress assessment and illustrate major differences in approach.

The Life Events Record, developed by child psychiatrist Dean Coddington in the early 1970s, is based on the assumption that all major life events are stressful, as they require adaptation and social readjustment on the part of the child. Preschool, elementary, junior high, and senior high versions of this measure consist of listings of between 30 and 42 events that represent significant life changes of the type listed above. Here, parents (for young children) or children/adolescents themselves are asked to indicate life events experienced in the recent past, usually the past year. Life stress scores are obtained by summing values termed "life change units" associated with each experienced event. These values, derived from ratings of mental health professionals, are presumed to reflect the degree of social readjustment required by the event and hence its stressfulness. For example, with preschool children life change units range from a low of 21 for "change in parents financial status" to 50 for "birth of a sibling" to 89 for "death of a parent."

The LER provides only a single life stress index and makes no distinction between "desirable" and "undesirable" life events. This scale represents one of the earliest approaches to child life stress assessment, with scores from the measure having been shown to correlate with a wide range of physical health and psychological adjustment indices.

The LEC, consisting of a listing of 46 life events, was developed by Johnson and McCutcheon in the early 1980s. The LEC is based on two basic assumptions that distinguish it from the Coddington scale; that life stress is most adequately conceptualized in terms of "negative life change," and that the desirability/undesirability of events is a function of the child's unique appraisals of life changes. Consistent with these assumptions, the format of the LEC involves having the child report events they have experienced in the recent past, rate each experienced event as to whether it was a "Good" or a "Bad" event, and rate the event on a 4-point scale as to impact (0 = No Effect; 3 = Great Effect). A positive score is derived by summing impact ratings of events rated as positive, a negative score by summing impact ratings of events rated as negative and a total score by summing impact ratings of all experienced events.

Like the Life Events Record, the LEC has been widely used in child/adolescent life stress research and has proven to be of value in differentiating between desirable and undesirable life changes as they relate to problems of physical health and psychological adjustment.

In addition to life stress scales, interview methods have also been used to assess life stress. The interactive nature of an interview has the potential advantage of being able to elicit a broader range of experienced events than a structured life events scale and may yield more information about the nature, timing, and meaningfulness of individual events that have been experienced. They are, however, less economical in terms of the time required to train individuals to administer and score interview data and in terms of the administration of the measure itself.

Research comparing life stress scales and life stress interviews has suggested that the two approaches may be similar in terms of discriminating between groups (e.g., depressed and nondepressed adolescents) and that life stress scales may be preferable in obtaining a quick overall index of life stress. Interviews may, however, be preferable if the goal is to assess the full range of stressful events that precede the development of child/adolescent difficulties and for exploring the unique relevance and effects of specific life events. Each approach has advantages depending on the purpose for which it is used.

CORRELATES OF LIFE STRESS

In considering the relationship between life stress and problems of child health and adjustment, methodological issues often make it difficult to interpret the nature of the relationships formed. While it is usually assumed that life stress causes health and adjustment problems, it is possible that children with such problems experience higher levels of life stress as a result of their difficulties. Or, the stress-adjustment/illness relationship may result from the fact that both

are associated with some third spurious variable. This possibility is suggested by a 1998 twin study by Thapar, Gordon, and McGuffin that found genetic factors to be associated with *both* increased negative life changes and depression. While increased rigor is necessary to increase the interpretability of research findings, many studies have found child/adolescent life stress to be related to a range of physical health and psychological adjustment difficulties.

For example, studies have found life stress to be significantly related to increased childhood accidents, respiratory and gastrointestinal illnesses, nonorganic recurrent abdominal pain, poorer control of diabetes, greater pulmonary function impairment in children with cystic fibrosis, increased severity of symptoms in children with other types chronic illness, as well as increased frequency of visits to physicians and number of health problems reported by children.

Child/adolescent life stress has also been shown to be associated with decreased levels of psychological adjustment, poorer grades and other school-related difficulties, increased alcohol and drug use, anxiety, depression, and suicidal behavior, as well as anorexia nervosa and bulimia nervosa.

DESIRABLE/UNDESIRABLE EVENTS

As previously noted, there have been differing views as to whether life stress should be conceptualized in terms of change per se or simply in terms of negative life change. While it may be true that even positive life events require some degree of adaptation and social readjustment, studies that have separately assessed the relationships between desirable and undesirable life events and indices of health and adjustment have usually found undesirable events to be more highly associated with negative health-related outcomes. Indeed, in some instances, positive change has been found to be related to decreased levels of negative outcomes and/or increased levels of adaptive behavior. These findings fit well with commonly held views that negative events are the ones that are the most stressful and have the most deleterious effects.

MODERATORS OF LIFE STRESS

While some studies have found direct relationships between life stress and indices of health/adjustment problems, there is considerable evidence that a number of variables may serve as stress buffers, stress enhancers, or moderators of the relationship between stress and health and adjustment. Examples of factors suggested to moderate this relationship include level of social support, the presence of family routines, perceptions of controllability of events, perceptions of competence, degree of attachment to parents, as well as certain aspects of child temperament. While more work in this area is necessary, such findings strongly suggest that the link between life stress and health and adjustment is not a direct one but one that varies as a function of individual, family, and social characteristics.

MANAGEMENT OF LIFE STRESS

Given the relationship between life stress and health/adjustment outcomes, approaches to helping children and adolescents cope with heightened levels of life stress are of considerable importance. Useful approaches may involve coordinated efforts to reduce physiological arousal, develop effective problem solving strategies, modify maladaptive stress-related cognitions, and mobilize available social support networks. A more detailed consideration of treatment-related issues can be found under the listing for Stress Management.

See also: Acute Stress Disorder; Posttraumatic Stress Disorder; Stress Management

Further Reading

Duggal, S., Malkoff-Schwartz, S., Birmaher, B., Anderson, B., Matty, M., Houck, P., Bailey-Orr, M., Williamson, D., & Frank. E. (2000). Assessment of life stress in adolescents: Self-report versus interview methods. *Journal of the American Academy of Child and Adolescent Psychiatry, 34*, 445–452.
Johnson, J. H. (1986). *Life events as stressors in childhood and adolescence.* Newbury Park, CA: Sage.
Thapar, A., Gordon, H., & McGuffin, P. (1998). Life events and depressive symptoms in childhood—shared genes or shared environments. *Journal of Child Psychology and Psychiatry, 39*, 1153–1158.

JAMES H. JOHNSON
TREY A. JOHNSON

Liver Transplantation

BRIEF DESCRIPTION

The liver is a large glandular organ that secretes bile, has an important function in the metabolism of carbohydrates, fats, and proteins, and contains a substance essential to the normal production of red blood cells. Liver transplantation involves the replacement of an unhealthy or a severely damaged liver with either a liver from a cadaver organ donor or a liver segment from a healthy living donor. When a cadaveric donor is used, the entire liver may be transplanted or the donor allograft may be divided in ways that permit an adjustment for size mismatches.

In June 2001, there were 1,248 children under 18 years of age listed for liver transplantation in the United States. This number represents 6.9 percent of the 18,089 total patients awaiting liver transplantation. About 6–10 percent of children waiting for liver transplantation will die because suitable donor organs are not available. This figure is likely to decrease as the number of living donor liver transplants increases. Since 1990, there have been approximately 5,400 pediatric cadaveric and 600 living donor liver transplants performed in the United States. Nearly a quarter of all living donor liver transplants are for the benefit of children with chronic liver disease.

INDICATIONS

Biliary atresia (congenital absence or closure of the ducts that drain bile from the liver) is the most common indication for liver replacement in children, accounting for approximately 50 percent of pediatric transplants in the United States. Other indications include metabolic disorders (such as alpha 1-antitrypsin deficiency, cystic fibrosis, and glycogen storage disease), autoimmune hepatitis, and other cholestatic diseases (such as Alagille's syndrome). In addition, children affected with multisystem diseases such as cystic fibrosis may need combined liver–pancreas or liver–lung transplant. Finally, children with intestinal failure, including those with short gut syndrome, who develop chronic liver failure as a consequence of intravenous alimentation, may need a combined liver–small bowel transplant.

OUTCOMES

Overall, pediatric patient survival rates are generally as good as those seen in adults—88 percent at 1 year, 83 percent at 3 years, and 81 percent at 5 years. Initial evidence suggests that living donor liver transplantation yields a survival advantage over cadaveric donor transplantation for adults, due largely to higher quality grafts and scheduling that permits surgery to occur at a time of optimal donor and recipient health. However, survival outcomes in children appear to be comparable for both cadaveric and living donor liver transplantation.

One of the most serious complications in the immediate postoperative phase is hepatic artery thrombosis (clotting of the hepatic artery), which may lead to allograft failure and the need for retransplantation or death. Other complications following pediatric liver transplantation include primary nonfunction, bile duct problems, bowel perforation, allograft rejection, nephrotoxicity, neurotoxicity, hyperlipidemia, and lymphoproliferative disease (uncontrolled proliferation of B cells). All of these complications are potentially serious and can result in deterioration in quality of life and/or death.

At the time of liver transplantation, the average child has a height and weight deficit of about 1.4 and 0.6 standard deviations below normal, respectively. Younger children, particularly those less than 5 years old, are at increased risk for height deficits compared to adolescents. Following liver transplantation, normal weight for age and catch-up growth can be expected for most pediatric patients. However, the growth trajectory depends largely on age at time of transplantation, diagnosis, and nutritional status both before and after transplantation, among other variables.

PSYCHOLOGICAL CONSIDERATIONS

Pediatric psychologists are generally involved in the psychological evaluation of children and families at the time they are being considered for liver transplantation. The nature and extent of these evaluations varies by transplant program, but generally includes an assessment of child development, adherence history, quality of life, psychological adaptation and coping, and family resources. In addition to assessment-based services, psychological interventions are developed and implemented as needed to enhance both pre- and posttransplant health outcomes.

There is an increased risk for cognitive and academic problems among children with liver disease, and there is some evidence that such deficits may persist after liver transplantation in some patients. These neurological problems are due to the inability of the malfunctioning liver to sufficiently excrete substances that are potentially toxic to the nervous system, severe malnutrition, and vitamin E deficiency. Children with early onset of symptoms (i.e., those diagnosed during

infancy) and more significant growth delays are at highest risk for broad cognitive impairment. Regarding psychological functioning after liver transplantation, studies have highlighted the presence of social deficits and posttraumatic stress responses in some children and high stress levels in families.

See also: Cystic Fibrosis; Gastrointestinal Disorders; Liver and Pancreatic Disorder; Quality of Life, Parenting the Chronically Ill Child

Further Reading

McDiarmid, S. V., Gornbein, J. A., DeSilva, P. J., Goss, J. A., Vargas, J. H., Martin, M. G., Ament, M. E., & Busuttil, R. W. (1999). Factors affecting growth after pediatric transplantation. *Transplantation, 67*, 404–411.

Scientific Registry of Transplant Recipients Home Page. http://www.ustransplant.org (Accessed May 2002).

Stewart, S. M., & Kennard, B. D. (1999). Organ transplantation. In R.T. Brown (Ed.), *Cognitive aspects of chronic illness in children* (pp. 220–237). New York: Guilford.

Studies of Pediatric Liver Transplantation Research Group. (2001). Studies of Pediatric Liver Transplantation Research Group (SPLIT): Year 2000 outcomes. *Transplantation, 72*, 463–476.

United Network for Organ Sharing Home Page. http://www.unos.org (Accessed May 2002).

JAMES R. RODRIGUE
REGINO P. GONZÁLEZ-PERALTA
STEPHANIE TOY

Loss, Coping with

See: Bereavement

Low Blood Sugar

See: Hypoglycemia

Low Vision

See: Visual Impairment: Low Vision and Blindness

Lung Transplantation, Pediatric

BRIEF DESCRIPTION

The lung is either of the two spongelike respiratory organs that oxygenate the blood and remove carbon dioxide from it. Within the last 15 years, lung transplantation has become a feasible intervention for various end-stage lung diseases. Lung transplantation involves the replacement of unhealthy or nonfunctional lung tissue with either lungs from a cadaveric organ donor or two single lung lobes from two healthy living donors, usually relatives of the child. There is an effort to use one parent and a nonparental donor so that one parent is available for the postoperative care and that both parents and child are not at surgical risk. There are two types of lung transplants: single or double (also known as bilateral). The type that is performed depends on the child's medical status and the availability of suitable donor lungs for transplantation, although the majority of children receive a bilateral lung transplant.

In June 2001, there were 277 children under 18 years of age on the waiting list for lung transplantation in the United States. This number represents 7.3 percent of the 3,798 total patients awaiting lung transplantation. Twenty to twenty-five percent of children waiting for lung transplantation will die because suitable donor organs are not available. Waiting times are somewhat age dependent. Younger children generally have shorter waiting times, but also have higher mortality rate while on the waiting list. Wait times are approximately 1–2 years for middle aged children and 2–3 years for older children and adolescents, who compete with adults who are small for the same organs. Since 1990, there have been approximately 660 pediatric lung transplants performed in the United States.

INDICATIONS

Children with virtually any end-stage lung disease in which there are not any good medical or surgical therapeutic options are considered for lung transplantation. Cystic fibrosis with end-stage lung disease, pulmonary hypertension, pulmonary fibrosis, or retransplantation are the most frequent conditions requiring lung transplantation. The primary indications for lung transplantation vary as a function of age. In adolescent populations, 67 percent of children who undergo a transplant have a primary diagnosis of cystic fibrosis. For children under 11 years of age, no single medical condition necessitates transplantation above other diseases. In infants, however, the most common indication for transplantation is congenital lung abnormality.

OUTCOMES

Pediatric patient survival rates are generally as good as those seen in adults—81 percent at 1 year, 54 percent at 3 years, and 43 percent at 5 years. The highest mortality rate in pediatric lung recipients is noted during the first year, when graft failure, infection, rejection, hemorrhage, and cardiovascular complications can occur. Bronchiolitis obliterans (concentrically scarred or stenotic small airways in the lung periphery) and rejection become the primary cause of death after the first year.

Following transplantation, the majority of the pediatric lung recipients will be maintained on triple immunosuppressive therapy, and this relates to the development of comorbid conditions. The most common comorbid conditions are hypertension, diabetes, and renal dysfunction. Despite the use of triple immunosuppression, the majority of patients will have at least one episode of acute cellular rejection and bronchiolitis obliterans; chronic rejection will develop in the majority of survivors. Approximately 50 percent of pediatric lung transplant recipients will reenter the hospital within the first year. Despite the risk of morbidity and need for a number of medications, the functional status is excellent with more than 90 percent having a period of no functional limitation.

PSYCHOLOGICAL CONSIDERATIONS

Pediatric psychologists are generally involved in the psychological evaluation of children and families at the time they are being considered for lung transplantation. The nature and extent of these evaluations vary by transplant program, but generally include an assessment of child development, adherence history, quality of life, psychological adaptation and coping, and family resources. For programs with living-related lung transplantation as an option, pediatric psychologists may be called upon to provide evaluative services in determining the suitability of family members or friends to be living lung donors for their child. In addition to assessment-based services, psychological interventions are developed and implemented as needed, to enhance both pre- and posttransplant health outcomes.

Little research has been conducted on the psychological adjustment, cognitive functioning, and quality of life of children receiving lung transplantation. The cognitive status of such patients should be examined, as the use of corticosteroids, the presence of chronic hypoxia, and the potential for compromised nutritional status can affect cognitive functioning. It has been found that children generally cope well with their pretransplant medical status and do not report symptoms of psychological distress, but no research has yet assessed posttransplant quality of life or psychological status. Particularly noteworthy in post-transplantation is the high incidence of nonadherence with immunosuppression therapy among older children and adolescents. This is an area warranting more research and more effective clinical strategies to achieve optimal health outcomes.

See also: Cystic Fibrosis; Parenting the Chronically Ill Child; Pulmonary Disorders; Quality of Life

Further Reading

Boucek, M. M., Faro, A., Novick, R. J., Bennett, L. E., Keck, B. M., & Hosenpud, J. D. (2001). The Registry of the International Society for Heart and Lung Transplantation: Fourth official pediatric report—2000. *Journal of Heart and Lung Transplantation, 20,* 39–52.
Scientific Registry of Transplant Recipients Home Page. http://www.ustransplant.org (Accessed May 2002).
Thompson, S. M., DiGirolamo, A. M., & Mallory, G. B. (1996). Psychological adjustment of pediatric lung transplantation candidates and their parents. *Journal of Clinical Psychology in Medical Settings, 3,* 303–317.
United Network for Organ Sharing Home Page. http://www.unos.org (Accessed May 2002).
Wong, M., Mallory, G. B., Jr., Goldstein, J., Goyal, M., & Yamada, K. A. (1999). Neurologic complications of pediatric lung transplantation. *Neurology, 53,* 1542–1549.

JAMES R. RODRIGUE
GARY VISNER
OLIVIA PUYANA

Lying

Because all children lie or bend the truth at some point in their lives, some lying in childhood is generally considered developmentally normal. Lying in childhood can be broken down into two types of lies: tall tales and escape lying. Tall tales are frequently made up stories or exaggerations of the truth told to obtain attention from peers or adults. An example of a tall tale would be a 6-year-old child telling her peer that she drove the family car to school that day. Escape lying is when a child tells a lie to avoid punishment or an uncomfortable situation. For example, children may lie about having been in trouble at school to avoid being punished by their parents. Alternatively, a child may lie to a grandmother about wanting to visit her because he or she may wish to avoid or escape a situation in which the grandmother's feelings might get hurt.

While in many cases childhood lying is relatively minor and harmless, lying can be very upsetting for parents who may become concerned that the lying reflects a lack of moral values in their child. Additionally, lying may be distressing for parents and other caregivers because they may become concerned that they will not be able to trust their child to tell the truth at critical moments. Finally, while childhood lying is generally considered developmentally normal, lying is a symptom of childhood disorders such as Conduct Disorder (CD) and Oppositional Defiant Disorder (ODD).

Before problems with lying start, parents can help their child understand the difference between make believe and the truth by pointing out instances where individuals stray from the truth and the consequences of these actions. This can be done through books, such as Pinocchio, as well as through the parent's own personal stories. Parents can also encourage truthfulness by praising their child for being truthful in tough situations and by modeling truthfulness in their own behavior. Finally, parents can encourage truthfulness by establishing clear rules for lying early on.

While there are no clear-cut techniques to determine whether a child is lying or not, by paying careful attention to the child's behavior it may be possible for astute observers to pick up on possible indicators of dishonesty. For example, children who feel anxious when lying may reveal this anxiety by displaying an anxious, as opposed to relaxed, facial expression. Further, parents may be able to detect dishonesty by noticing inconsistencies in their child's stories or accounts of events. Finally, stories or accounts that appear rehearsed may indicate that a child is not telling the truth. Parents can investigate such suspicious accounts by asking the child questions about the event and observing how the child responds to such questions (i.e., whether responses are provided in a spontaneous or a rehearsed manner).

TREATMENT OF CHILDHOOD LYING

There are a number of reasons why the treatment of lying in children is difficult. A primary reason is that it is often tricky for parents and other caregivers to know just what the truth is in any particular situation. Additionally, parents may feel guilty about constantly doubting what their child has told them, and may find themselves accepting a number of lies in order to maintain a positive relationship with their child. McMahon and Wells (1998) suggest that these reasons may partially account for why there are currently no well-established treatments for lying in childhood.

Treatment for Tall Tale Telling

When children tell tall tales, they generally do so to obtain the attention of the listener and because it is enjoyable to make up stories. While some children may not know the difference between the truth and the exaggeration that they have created, others fully understand that their story does not reflect the truth. Parents and other caregivers may be able to curb tall tale telling by explaining to the child the difference between their tall tale and the truth. Additionally, parents can provide tall tale tellers the attention that they are seeking by praising the child for their creativity, while requesting that in the future the child inform the parent that they are being creative and telling a story.

Example 1: Tabitha's Tall Tales

Tabitha tells her mother that she has magical powers and can clean her room with a twitch of her nose. Realizing that her daughter is telling a tall tale, Mrs. Stevens replies, "Oh, it sounds like you are telling a really neat story and that you are being creative with your ideas! I love it when you are creative and tell stories. Next time you tell a story, please let me know that it is a story because I am so proud of you when you are creative like that!" By praising Tabitha's creativity and paying attention to her story, Mrs. Stevens can provide Tabitha with the attention that she seeks without encouraging Tabitha to insist that the story is true and real.

Treatment for Escape Lying

When dealing with escape lying, one generally agreed upon method is to have the punishment for misbehavior be less severe than the punishment for lying about the misbehavior. The goal of this method is for children to realize that they are taking a bigger risk by lying about the event than they would be by being honest about it. Additionally, it is important for parents not to reward the child in situations where lying has occurred. For example, if a child lies about their grades in order to attend a school function, the child should not be allowed to attend the school function. It is also important to consider that attention, even negative attention such as scolding and shaming, can be rewarding for some children. As such, parents should minimize the attention that they provide to a child when they discover lying. Parents can also discourage lying by increasing the extent to which they monitor their child's daily events (i.e., they can establish a school–home note system with the child's teacher). For children who lie on a frequent basis, it has been suggested that parents require the children to "prove" their truthfulness in any particular situation to avoid punishment.

Example 2: Bob's Big Booboo

In an attempt to reach the forbidden cookies, 8-year-old Bob breaks a cookie jar. Bob's parents have repeatedly explained to him that the punishment for telling a lie is immediate removal of his favorite toy truck for 3 days. The punishment for breaking a house rule, such as taking cookies without authorization, but being honest about it is a 5-minute timeout. Bob decides that the timeout is better than getting caught lying, and tells his family that he broke the cookie jar.

In general, when concerned about a child's habit of lying, parents should try to monitor the contexts in which the lying occurs so as to determine the function or purpose of the lying. If the parent notices that the lies typically occur in situations in which the child is uncomfortable and unable to speak the truth, the parent can discuss with the child ways to be assertive. Likewise, if the lying appears to serve to gain attention (e.g., tall tales), the caregiver can help the child to learn more appropriate ways to get attention from peers and adults.

See also: Behavior Modification; Conduct Disorder; Differential Social Reinforcement/Positive Attention; Oppositional Defiant Disorder

Further Reading

American Academy of Child and Adolescent Psychiatry. *Children and lying*. Retrieved May 1, 2002 from http://www.aacap.org/publications/factsfam/lying.htm
American Psychiatric Association. (2000). *Diagnostic and statistical manual of mental disorders* (4th ed.). Washington, DC: Author.

Center for Effective Parenting. *Lying*. Retrieved May 1, 2002 from http://www.parenting-ed.org/handout3/Specific%20Concerns%20and%20Problems/lying.htm

McMahon, R. J., & Wells, K. C. (1998). Conduct Problems. In E. J. Mash & R. A. Barkley (Eds.), *Treatment of childhood disorders* (pp. 111–210). New York, NY: Guilford Press.

CHERYL B. MCNEIL
CATHERINE B. MCCLELLAN

Lymphomas

DESCRIPTION

Lymphomas are malignancies of the lymphatic system. The lymphatic system involves vessels similar to veins and capillaries that convey fluid from tissues to the bloodstream. Lymph nodes (round nodules in the lymphatic system) produce lymphocytes (a type of white blood cell that is involved with immunity). This type of cancer affects the lymphocytes, spread to the lymph nodes, liver, and/or spleen, causing enlargement of the nodes or organs. Lymphomas are the third most common malignancy in childhood comprising 10–15 percent of all childhood cancers. The lymphomas that are most common in children are Hodgkin's disease and non-Hodgkin's lymphoma, which may involve similar presentations, but are usually differentiated depending upon histology.

Hodgkin's lymphomas (HD) make up 60 percent of lymphomas (850–900 cases per year), while non-Hodgkin's lymphomas (NHL) account for about 40 percent of lymphomas (750–800 cases per year). Male gender is predominant in HD and NHL. In HD the childhood form is diagnosed in children who are 14 years of age and younger; a young adult form from 15–34 years of age; and an older adult form (55 and up). In NHL, the incidence increases with age throughout life.

ETIOLOGY—HODGKIN'S DISEASE (HD)

Exposure to Epstein-Barr virus (EBV) is a risk factor in the development of HD. (EBV is a virus that is believed to cause the more common diagnosis of mononucleosis, but has also been found to be associated with the development of lymphomas.) Cases may cluster within families, suggesting a genetic predisposition to HD or a common exposure to a common toxic agent.

ETIOLOGY—NON-HODGKIN'S LYMPHOMA (NHL)

Overall, there is no single known cause of NHL. People with congenital immune deficiency syndromes, (e.g. Wiskott–Aldrich syndrome, ataxia–telangiectasia, X-linked lymphoproliferative disease), and patients who receive immunosuppressive therapy are at increased risk for NHL. EBV and ionizing radiation are also associated with the development of lymphomas.

PRESENTATION

Children with either NHL or HD typically present with painless, swollen lymph nodes. For HD, the most common sites of presentation are supraclavicular (above the clavicle) and cervical (neck) nodes. Systemic symptoms such as weight loss, fever, night sweats, and itching are seen in about 1/3 of patients with HD. At least two-thirds of patients also have mediastinal involvement (enlarged lymph nodes inside the chest near the airway and heart) that may be severe enough to cause airway compromise. Clinical presentations of NHL are more varied. Children can present with disease in the mediastinum, abdomen, or head and neck as the most common sites. They do not tend to have as many systemic symptoms. NHL includes 3 different histologic (tissue) subtypes: Burkitt's lymphoma, lymphoblastic lymphoma, and large-cell lymphoma, with treatment varying based upon subtype.

TREATMENT—HODGKIN'S DISEASE (HD)

In pediatric cases, combined-modality therapy with chemotherapy and radiation therapy is used most commonly. By combining the two therapies, decreased doses and margins of the radiation therapy can be used. Multiple combinations of chemotherapeutic agents are used. Some of the more commonly used agents include the COPP/ABVD combination: cyclophosphamide, vincristine, procarbazine, prednisone, adriamycin, bleomycin, vinblastine, $+/-$ dacarbazine, as well as etoposide and mechlorethamine (nitrogen mustard).

TREATMENT—NON-HODGKIN'S LYMPHOMA (NHL)

Chemotherapy is the mainstay of treatment. Surgery plays only a very minor role and is mainly used for diagnostic purposes (staging or categorization of the disease), with the exception of gastrointestinal tumors where complete resection (surgical removal) should be performed if possible. Chemotherapy is somewhat specific for the varying histologies and stages of NHL. Higher stage lymphomas (stage III—disease in chest with positive lymph nodes and spread; and stage IV—disease in bone marrow or central nervous system) receive more intensive therapy. For low stage disease (stage I—single tumor or single anatomic area; and Stage II—single tumor with regional node involvement on same side of the diaphragm), fewer agents and decreased intensity produce excellent outcomes. Intrathecal therapy (into the fluid surrounding the spinal cord and brain) is reserved for the low-stage patients with head and neck NHL. Chemotherapeutic agents for *Burkitt's lymphoma* include cyclophosphamide, vincristine, prednisone, +/− high-dose methotrexate, doxorubicin, cytarabine, etoposide, ifosphamide, or cisplatin. Therapeutic courses are intense but therapy time lasts only 3–8 months depending on the stage of the disease. Agents used for *lymphoblastic lymphoma* include cyclophosphamide, vincristine, prednisone, +/− doxorubicin, methotrexate, mercaptopurine, asparaginase, thioguanine, or cytarabine. Length of therapy (18 months to 3 years) depends on the stage of the disease. Chemotherapeutic agents used for *large cell lymphoma* include cyclophosphamide, vincristine, prednisone, +/− doxorubicin, methotrexate, mercaptopyrine, thioguanine or asparaginase. Therapy ranges from 3 to 24 months.

PROGNOSIS

Survival rates for HD of all stages are quite good. Event-free survival ranges from 75 percent (stage IV) to 95 percent (stage I). The overall 5-year survival rate for children with NHL is 72 percent. For low-stage disease, survival rates are greater than 90 percent.

ACUTE COMPLICATIONS OF TREATMENT—HODGKIN'S DISEASE (HD)

Although the prognosis is quite good, the treatments can be quite intensive and thus involve acute radiation effects (e.g., rash, hyperpigmentation, gastrointestinal disturbance) and acute effects of chemotherapy (e.g., nausea and vomiting, tissue damage, hair loss, fatigue). The most common acute problem is infection (e.g., bacterial infection, herpes zoster, varicella). In most cases these acute effects are reversible. The treatment, while relatively short compared to leukemia and done on an outpatient basis, may still mean some absences from

school, periods of separation from peers, and curtailment of some activities. However, most children are able to keep up with school and peer activities.

ACUTE COMPLICATIONS OF TREATMENT—NON-HODGKIN'S LYMPHOMA (NHL)

Because of the fast-growing characteristics of these tumors, life-threatening complications can develop, for example, airway obstruction, cardiac problems, renal failure, neurologic problems. Most of these can be addressed through treatment to reduce the size of the tumor. Acute problems due to chemotherapy are similar to those of HD. As in HD, most children and adolescents are able to resume normal school and activities once the intensive induction phase is over.

LONG-TERM COMPLICATIONS

Due to the excellent survival rates in HD, recent changes in therapy have been directed at decreasing the high rate of long-term complications. These complications include soft tissue and bone growth alterations, cardiomyopathy (dysfunction of heart muscle), congestive heart failure, hypothyroidism, increased infertility in males, premature menopause, and second malignancies (leukemia, solid tumors of thyroid, breast, and bone). The relative risk for breast cancer is 32.8 while the relative risk for sarcomas is 135. Thus, long-term follow-up is extremely important in those patients who were treated for HD as children.

Long-term complications of therapy for NHL, while generally less severe than those in HD, can include cardiac dysfunction (for patients who received anthracyclines [e.g., daunorubicin, doxorubicin] in large doses) and infertility. Second malignancies have not been a major issue for children who have undergone therapy for NHLs as the risk is lower largely due to lack of use of radiation in treating this form of lymphoma.

See also: Childhood Cancers; Coping with Illness; Parenting the Chronically Ill Child

Further Reading

Hudson, M. M., & Donaldson, S. S. (2002). Hodgkin's disease. In P. A. Pizzo & D. G. Poplack (Eds.), *Principles and practice of pediatric oncology* (4th ed., pp. 637–660). Philadelphia: Lippincott, Williams & Wilkins.

Magrath, I. T. (2002). Malignant non-Hodgkin's lymphomas in children. In P. A. Pizzo & D. G. Poplack (Eds.), *Principles and practice of pediatric oncology* (4th ed., pp. 661–705). Philadelphia: Lippincott, Williams & Wilkins.

Ries, L. A. G., Smith, M. A., Gurney, J. G., Linet, M., Tamra, T., Young, J. L., & Bunin, G. R. (Eds.). (1999). *Cancer incidence and survival among children and adolescents: United States SEER Program 1975–1995* (NIH Publication No. 99-4649). Bethesda, MD: National Cancer Institute, SEER Program.

Sandlund, J., Downing, J. R., Crist, W. M. (1996). Non-Hodgkin's lymphoma in childhood. *New England Journal of Medicine, 334*(19), 1238–1248.

MARY JO KUPST
KELLY MALONEY

Mm

Major Depressive Disorder

See: Depressive Disorder, Major

Mania

DEFINITION

Mania refers to a distinctly abnormal and persistently elevated, expansive, or irritable mood accompanied by several (4 or more if the mood is irritable, 3 or more if the mood is elevated/expansive) of the following symptoms: inflated self-esteem or grandiosity, decreased need for sleep, flight of ideas, increased rate or amount of speech, distractibility, increase in goal-directed activity or psychomotor agitation, and excessive involvement in pleasurable activities that have a high potential for painful consequences. According to the *Diagnostic and Statistical Manual (DSM)* of the American Psychiatric Association, to meet criteria for a manic episode, these symptoms must last at least a week, unless hospitalization is necessary; then any duration is sufficient for diagnosis of mania.

Children diagnosed with early-onset bipolar disorder (EOBD) may experience symptoms of mania differently than adults. In terms of course, children typically do not exhibit symptoms of pure mania for a week or more at a time, as many adults do. Rather, children frequently appear to cycle through manic and depressive states numerous times in one day, which is labeled "ultradian" cycling. Mixed presentations, meaning the simultaneous presence of both manic and depressive symptoms, are common. In addition, many children do not return to adequate inter-episode levels of functioning, as clear-cut episodes are less commonly seen.

The *DSM* defines hypomania as a "distinct period of persistently elevated, expansive, or irritable mood, lasting throughout at least 4 days, that is clearly different from the usual nondepressed mood" accompanied by the same number of symptoms described for mania. The two main differences between mania and hypomania are duration and intensity of symptoms. Once again, the duration distinction becomes less meaningful when applied to children, as they often do not follow the typical adult course. The lower intensity of hypomanic symptoms can be particularly difficult to discern, and requires thorough longitudinal observation (by parents, teachers, and/or clinicians) and history-taking to determine that a clinically meaningful alteration from the child's baseline has occurred.

Mania in older adolescents often appears to follow the more typical course commonly seen in adults if the mood impairment begins during adolescence. Older adolescents are more likely to demonstrate discrete manic episodes with more successful interepisodic functioning.

PREVALENCE

The true prevalence of mania in children is unknown. Some experts suggest that underdiagnosis of mania may occur in children because symptoms overlap with externalizing disorders (e.g., Attention-Deficit/

354

Hyperactivity Disorder [ADHD], Oppositional Defiant Disorder [ODD]) and because some clinicians are reluctant to diagnose bipolar disorder in prepubescent children. In adolescents, lifetime prevalence of bipolar disorders is estimated to be approximately 1 percent, although a higher percentage of adolescents have reported subthreshold manic symptoms.

ASSESSMENT

To diagnose mania, a thorough clinical interview is essential. Supplementing the clinical interview with a structured interview, such as the Children's Inventory for Psychiatric Syndromes (ChIPS) and/or a symptom severity scale, such as the Mania Rating Scale can be useful, particularly for documenting presence/absence and severity of symptoms. During the clinical interview, gathering family history information, particularly the evidence of bipolar disorder in other family members, is important. It is likewise critical to obtain a careful developmental, medical, school, and social history to understand symptom manifestation in the larger context of the child's life, to ensure that behaviors possibly resulting from poor child rearing, medication side-effects, learning disabilities, and/or developmental delays are not erroneously labeled as manic symptoms, and to determine what comorbid conditions may also be present.

DIFFERENTIAL DIAGNOSIS

When determining whether clinical manifestations are best characterized as manic symptoms rather than symptoms of other internalizing (i.e., anxiety disorders) or externalizing disorders (i.e., disruptive behavior disorders like Conduct Disorder [CD] or Oppositional Defiant Disorder [ODD]), several rules apply. First, mood symptoms must occur in clusters to warrant a diagnosis. For example, the presence of an irritable mood accompanied by aggressive behavior with no further manic symptoms is not evidence of mania. Second, manic symptoms wax and wane in intensity, often not in response to environmental triggers. Thus, a girl who becomes very upset and tearful or irritable when limits are set, but only under certain conditions, may have ODD, not mania. Third, symptoms must reflect a significant change from baseline functioning. Thus, a child who is chronically distractible and hyperactive, particularly in less structured settings, is more likely to have ADHD than mania. Fourth, the symptoms must be extreme, causing interference in

functioning at home, at school, or with peers. Thus, a child who gets very silly at the end of a school year may simply be emotionally charged, but is not manic. Finally, some behaviors that look like manic symptoms may be the result of a physical illness (e.g., a thyroid disorder) or untoward side effects of medication.

SYMPTOM DESCRIPTION

After the above-mentioned cautions have been addressed, it is important to have a template for recognizing symptom manifestation. Beginning with the mood component, the clinician must distinguish elevated, euphoric, or expansive moods from "normal" highs, and these moods must occur without a "reasonable" cause, as described above. This is particularly important in individuals with a long history of depression for whom a return to "normal" mood may be mistaken for an elevated mood. In addition, it is necessary to establish the absence of a positive stimulus that may be fueling an elevated mood. For example, a child reporting feeling "giddy, silly, and on top of the world" due to excitement about an upcoming birthday party would be very different from a child reporting those feelings "out of the blue" for no particular reason. The elevated mood needs to be clearly excessive, inappropriate, and not occurring solely under the influence of illicit substances for it to be considered a symptom of mania.

When assessing irritable mood, it is important to differentiate irritability stemming from depression from irritability stemming from mania. Discrete periods of irritability, or rages, rather than chronic irritability, can be a marker for mania. In addition, the presence of additional manic symptoms clustering with irritability is suggestive that the irritability is a manic symptom.

Decreased need for sleep in mania should be distinguished from sleep difficulties associated with depression or other causes. For example, a depressed child may have significant trouble falling asleep at night, be bothered by this, and report anxious, worrisome thoughts prior to falling asleep. Such a child is typically tired during the following day. Children with sleep apnea have restless sleep and are often chronically fatigued. By way of contrast, a child who does not want to fall asleep at night, is currently sleeping substantially less than usual, yet has the same amount of energy (or more energy) is more likely to be experiencing a manic symptom of sleep disruption.

To determine whether rapid speech is a "true" symptom of mania, the clinician must ascertain the child's baseline rate of speech. For example, some very bright and/or impulsive children speak rapidly. If rate of speech fluctuates notably with elevated mood, it is more likely to be a manic symptom. Similarly, racing thoughts must be distinguished from the rapid cognitive connections made by gifted children and the impulsive cognitive leaps sometimes observed in children with ADHD. If racing thoughts cause impairment (e.g., the teacher cannot understand why the child is on the topic he or she is loudly proclaiming), or if they wax and wane with mood, they are more likely a symptom of mania.

Inflated self-esteem or grandiosity can be obvious when extreme, but can be more difficult to detect when it occurs in a mild form, when it can be mistaken for a behavioral symptom. For example, consider a fourth grader who feels that his teacher inappropriately handled a discipline situation in the classroom and takes it upon himself to call the superintendent from the payphone in the school hallway to lodge his complaint. Although this behavior may be interpreted as defiance by school personnel, when considered in the context of additional, clustering manic symptoms, it might be better conceptualized as grandiosity.

Distractibility and psychomotor agitation can stem from anxiety, depression, ADHD, and/or mania. Once again, determining whether these symptoms are reflective of mania entails establishing a change from baseline functioning and the presence of co-occurring manic mood alteration.

Excessive involvement in pleasurable activities that have a high potential for painful consequences is the final symptom of mania. In addition to the previously stated cautions (e.g., a child with ADHD may often engage in impulsive behavior that leads to trouble), one must also consider developmentally appropriate manifestations of this symptom. Not many children have the resources to engage in excessive buying sprees or foolish business ventures. A child experiencing this symptom may give many of his or her prized possessions away to a friend and later regret it. Or, a child may become hypersexual, talking and/or acting out (e.g., by touching others inappropriately, trying to kiss adults of the opposite sex inappropriately, masturbating excessively, writing "dirty" notes to other children). In the latter case, a careful review to determine whether the child previously has been sexually abused and/or exposed to sexual content inappropriate for his or her age is in order.

TREATMENT

Treatment of childhood mania includes pharmacological and psychosocial treatments. Please see the

entry Bipolar Disorder for a detailed discussion of treatment options.

See also: Bipolar Disorder; Depressive Disorder, Major; Disruptive Behavior Disorders; Dysthymic Disorder

Further Reading

American Psychiatric Association. (2000). *Diagnostic and statistical manual of mental disorders (text revision)*. Washington, DC: Authors.
Carlson, G. A. (1996). Clinical features and pathogenesis of child and adolescent mania. In K. I. Shulman, M. Tohen, & S. P. Kutcher (Eds.), *Mood disorders across the life span* (pp. 127–147). New York: Wiley-Liss.
Geller, B., & Luby, J. (1997). Child and adolescent bipolar disorder: A review of the past 10 years. *Journal of the American Academy of Child and Adolescent Psychiatry, 36*(9), 1168–1176.
Lewinsohn, P. M., Klein, D. N., & Seely, J. R. (1995). Bipolar disorders in a community sample of older adolescents: Prevalence, phenomenology, comorbidity, and course. *Journal of the American Academy of Child and Adolescent Psychiatry, 34*(4), 454–463.
Weller, E. B., Weller, R. A., & Fristad, M. A. (1995). Bipolar disorder in children: Misdiagnosis, underdiagnosis, and future directions. *Journal of the American Academy of Child and Adolescent Psychiatry, 34*(6), 709–714.

MARY A. FRISTAD
BARBARA MACKINAW-KOONS

Marijuana, Prenatal Exposure

DEFINITION OF THE PROBLEM

Marijuana is the most common illicit drug used by women during pregnancy, with approximately 3–20 percent of pregnant women using at some point during pregnancy. Marijuana is prepared from the plant cannabis sativa that, along with other chemicals, contains the psychoactive chemical tetrahydrocannabinol (delta-9-tetrahydrocannabinol or THC). Although the amount of THC in marijuana used in the United States can vary, it has remained relatively stable for the past 10–15 years. Marijuana can be ingested orally or by smoking with effects beginning within 10–30 min. THC is rapidly absorbed into the bloodstream and metabolized by the liver. Effects can last from 2 to 3 hr and it can be detected in the urine for up to 30 days. Deficits in sensory, psychomotor, and cognitive functioning are seen when using marijuana. Street names for marijuana include weed, pot, "j," joint, blunt, herb, and crippie.

PREVALENCE

Although marijuana is the most common illicit drug used by pregnant women, it is unknown exactly how many infants and children are affected by prenatal exposure to marijuana. Identification is dependent on the self-report of the mother and/or toxicology analysis of urine, meconium, or hair. However, drug screening occurs inconsistently and is governed by local policies and procedures.

EFFECTS

During pregnancy, THC freely crosses the placenta. It can be detected in the newborn for up to 30 days after a single use by the mother. Although not considered a classic teratogenic agent (an agent causing a malformation of the fetus), as it does not produce morphological changes in newborns (e.g., Fetal Alcohol Syndrome (FAS), and thalidomide exposure), functional changes have been suggested leading to the idea of behavioral teratology. THC can also be found in breast milk with levels up to eight times higher than in the mother's bloodstream. As such, the American Academy of Pediatrics has stated that breastfeeding is contraindicated if the mother is using marijuana.

Research findings related to marijuana use during pregnancy are mixed. Studies have been confounded by a number of factors including poly-drug use by the sample, particularly alcohol and nicotine, and lack of control for environmental and socioeconomic factors such as poverty. A weak correlation appears to exist between birth weight and marijuana use, with lower birth weights more likely if marijuana is used more than four times per day. Disturbances in sleep cycling and sleep patterns are noted in children with prenatal exposure to marijuana, with these problems noted in children up to 3 years of age. Poor habituation to stimuli and visual responsiveness has also been reported in newborns. With marijuana, signs similar to nicotine toxicity such as abnormally fast heart rate (tachycardia), poor feeding, and irritability have been reported. Decreases in height, weight, and head circumference have also been noted; however, deficits do not appear to last over time. One study conducted in Jamaica found significant differences in the newborn cry. This particular study is important, as marijuana use is widespread in certain communities and variables confounding other studies, controlled. However, it should be noted that the dosages of marijuana were significantly higher than those studied in the United States. Findings indicated that cries of newborns prenatally exposed to marijuana were shorter with a higher frequency, had a higher percentage of dysphonia (loss of voice or diminished quality of vocal production), and more atypical vowel production than did babies without such exposure. The authors argue that the characteristics of a newborn's cry may be indicative of the neurophysiological status of the infant.

ASSESSMENT AND INTERVENTION

In summary, marijuana appears to produce more subtle problems in infants and children whose mothers use it during pregnancy. As such, ongoing developmental assessments are suggested. Assessments should include not only medical monitoring of growth and development, but also evaluations of cognitive, language, motor, psychosocial, and behavioral functioning. Little exists in the literature related to intervention strategies with this population.

Education with childbearing women around the issue of substance abuse is critical to reduce potential problems in their offspring. Furthermore, substance abuse treatment services for pregnant women are essential as a reduction in drug use at any point in the pregnancy can increase positive outcomes in the children. As stronger illicit drugs such as cocaine and methamphetamines have gained more attention in both the media and scientific arenas, investigations into a better understanding of the impact of marijuana use during pregnancy have diminished. Given that marijuana continues to be the most commonly used illicit substance by pregnant women, ongoing investigation into this area is essential to effectively address problems noted in children with prenatal marijuana exposure.

PROGNOSIS

As children have been followed over time, conflicting findings continue to be noted. Some studies indicate lower scores on cognitive testing in children with prenatal marijuana exposure at 4 years of age while others have noted no differences in cognitive or language functioning between children with and without exposure at 5 and 6 years of age. Several studies agree on some of the behavioral characteristics of children with prenatal exposure to marijuana, including problems of attention and vigilance as well as an increase in hyperactive and impulsive behaviors. Parental reports of behavior problems are also noted.

See also: Effects of Parental Substance Abuse on Children; Fetal Alcohol Syndrome; Nicotine, Prenatal Exposure; Substance Abuse

Further Reading

American Academy of Pediatrics Committee on Drugs. (1994). The transfer of drugs and other chemicals into human milk. *Pediatrics, 93,* 137–150.

English, D., Hulse, G., Milne, E., Holman, C., & Bower, C. (1997). Maternal cannabis use and birth weight: A meta-analysis. *Addiction, 92,* 1553–1560.

Fried, P., & Watkinson, B. (2000). Visuoperceptual functioning differs in 9- to 12-year olds prenatally exposed to cigarettes and marihuana. *Neurotoxicology and Teratology, 22,* 11–20.

Goldschmidt, L., Day, N., & Richardson, G. (2000). Effects of prenatal marijuana exposure on child behavior problems at age 10. *Neurotoxicology and Teratology, 22,* 325–336.

Lester, B., & Dreher, M. (1989). Effects of marijuana use during pregnancy on newborn cry. *Child Development, 60,* 765–771.

ROBIN H. GURWITCH

Mass Screening

See: Screening Instruments: Behavioral and Developmental

Massage Therapy

Massage therapy is older than recorded history and was considered a primary form of medicine until the advent of drugs. Drugs are sometimes ineffective and often have undesirable side effects on children because of their addictive properties. Thus, massage therapy is increasingly being used to reduce anxiety and pain in children with chronic diseases. For example, we are currently studying the effectiveness of massage therapy with children who have arthritis, asthma, autism, burns, cancer, dermatitis, diabetes, as well as infants who have been neglected, abused, exposed to cocaine and HIV in utero, and born prematurely with medical complications.

In the first published studies on massage therapy Field and her colleagues documented the positive effects of massaging preterm infants 3 times a day for 15 min over a 10 day period. The infants not only gained 47 percent more weight but also performed better on neonatal assessments and were discharged

6 days earlier at a hospital cost savings of approximately $3,000 per infant. In a more recent study on cocaine-exposed preterm infants, Field and her colleagues (1998) also found that weight gain and motor performance were significantly improved following massage therapy. We have just documented similar effects for HIV exposed preterms who were massaged on a daily basis by their mothers the first 2 weeks of life. We hope that their immune data will also reveal positive changes, not unlike the increased natural killer cells observed in the study on HIV-positive men.

In the same study on HIV-positive adults we noted increases in serotonin levels following massage therapy. Because many pain medications are serotonergic based, we hope to demonstrate the pain-relieving effects of massage therapy on children with chronic diseases. In addition, we expect to alter their anxiety and depression levels since we have been able to lower anxiety and depression and stress-related hormones (cortisol and norepinephrine), at least in children who were hospitalized for psychiatric problems.

Because we have noted the positive effects on parents administering massage therapy, we are using parents as massage therapists. We expect that actually administering the therapy would reduce their sense of helplessness and give them a more positive role in treatment. For example, the parents of diabetics can have a more positive role than simply monitoring dietary compliance and providing injections. The parents might benefit in other ways as well. For example, in a study by Field and colleagues (1998) on children with asthma preliminary data suggest not only increased peak air flow and decreased anxiety in the children but also decreased anxiety in their parents. In the case of hospitalized children and infants and children in shelters (where parental figures may not immediately available), we are employing volunteer grandparent therapists. The elderly are in fact benefiting more from giving infants and children massage therapy than from receiving it themselves. After a month of giving massages the grandparent volunteers are less depressed, are sleeping better and making fewer visits to their physicians.

Finally, we hope to alleviate some of the more common pediatric problems, namely irritability (colic) and sleep disturbances. In a study on infants of depressed mothers we noted a significant reduction in irritability and more organized sleep patterns, suggesting that these normal functions, too, can be helped by massage therapy. At the very least, massage therapy makes infants and children feel better, and the parents and therapists claim that giving the massage helps them be physically close in an acceptable way and improves their relationships.

See also: Infancy; Parenting Practices; Prematurity: Birth Weight and Gestational Age; Prematurity Outcomes; Prenatal Development; Sleep Patterns, Normal; Sleep Talking; Sleep Terrors; Sleep–Wake Cycle Problems; Sleep Walking

Further Reading

Field, T. (1998). Massage therapy effects. *American Psychologist, 53*, 1270–1281.

Field, T., Henteleff, T., Hernandez-Reif, M., Martinez, E., Mavunda, K., Kuhn, C., & Schanberg, S. (1998). Children with asthma have improved pulmonary function after massage therapy. *Journal of Pediatrics, 132*, 854–858.

Field, T., Morrow, C., Valdeon, C., Larson, S., Kuhn, C., & Schanberg, S., (1992). Massage reduces anxiety in child and adolescent psychiatric patients. *Journal of the American Academy of Child and Adolescent Psychiatry, 31*, 125–131.

Field, T., Schanberg, S. M., Scafidi, F., Bauer, C. R., Vega-Lahr, N., Garcia, R., Nystrom, J., & Kuhn, C. M. (1986). Tactile/kinesthetic stimulation effects on preterm neonates. *Pediatrics, 77*, 654–658.

Ironson, G., Field, T., Kumar, A., Price, A., Kumar, M., Hansen, K., & Burman, I. (1992). Relaxation through massage is associated with decreased distress and increased serotonin levels. Presented at the Academy of Psychosomatic Medicine.

TIFFANY FIELD

Masturbation*

DEFINITION/HISTORY

Considerable attention has been devoted in the past to the problem of childhood masturbation (self-stimulation of the genitals) because it was viewed as a deviant behavior that led to serious physical and emotional disabilities. A popular book entitled *What a Young Boy Ought to Know*, written by a minister and published in 1909, notes serious consequences from masturbation: "[Due to the shocks to the nervous system] the entire nervous system will eventually become shattered and ruined beyond all hope of complete recovery ... The bright boy that stood at the head of the class is gradually losing his power to comprehend ... His memory fails him ... The health gradually declines. The eyes lose their luster. The skin becomes sallow. The muscles become

flabby ... He complains of pain in the back; of headache and dizziness. The hands become cold and clammy ... digestion becomes poor ... The heart palpitates ... He sits in a stooping position ... and the entire body ... becomes wasted, and many signs give promise of early decline and death" (pp. 113–114). Many physicians of that era agreed that there were health risks from masturbation and a number of techniques involving mechanical devices and surgery were used to prevent boys and girls from the practice. These are some of the darkest pages of religious and medical history.

As noted by Leung and Robson (1993), childhood masturbation is now recognized as a virtually universal phenomenon in that all males and females explore their genitals as a normal part of sexual development. In addition, the majority stimulate themselves to orgasm at least once (and often very frequently) by the time they are teenagers. Masturbation does not pose a physical or mental health risk. Due to better diet and medical care, children mature physically earlier than in previous times. As a result, there may be a major time gap between reproductive maturity and opportunity to establish a relationship with a person of the opposite sex that includes sexual intimacy. Masturbation is a normal and harmless way to adjust to this circumstance.

INTERVENTION

For most parents, it is best to counsel them on the normality of masturbation and the positive aspects of the behavior while assuring them that it is not physically or mentally dangerous. For example, data suggest that men and women who have had normal masturbation experiences are better adjusted sexually in their marriages later in life. Rules and boundaries may be taught by explaining that masturbation is something one does in private. Sex education appropriate to the age of the child is an essential part of the process. There are numerous books that may be obtained from the library or local bookstore on sexual development and sex education for children and parents to read together. Parents can then answer questions and present their personal views to the child. In some families, parents may regard masturbation as inconsistent with their values. There is some movement to change these attitudes as exemplified by a very courageous pastoral counselor, Charles Shedd, who has a chapter in one of his books entitled, "Masturbation—Gift of God." Parents who maintain their opposition to masturbation should be counseled to use mild discouragement and distraction to reduce the behavior and not to overreact punitively.

*The views expressed in this article are those of the author(s) and do not necessarily reflect the official policy or position of the Department of the Navy, Department of Defense, or the U.S. Government.

Masturbation can be a problem if practiced excessively or in public. While normal children and adolescents may masturbate as often as several times a day, some children have been known to become obsessed with masturbation and to stimulate themselves to the point that the genitals are raw and bleeding. They also sometimes use dangerous instruments or methods of masturbation. Likewise, some children masturbate in public places and do not stop when encouraged by adults to do so. In all of these instances, one should immediately investigate the possibility that the child has been or is being sexually abused. If this turns out to be the case, the child should be protected and the *appropriate agencies should be notified*. It is important to note that although children who have been sexually abused often engage in excessive masturbation, many children who masturbate excessively have not been sexually abused. For these children, distraction from masturbation with an array of highly enjoyable competing activities along with cognitive therapy on rules for appropriate behavior and rewards for appropriate changes in behavior can usually decrease the excessive or inappropriate masturbation. Inappropriate masturbatory behavior sometimes is secondary to insecurity, anxiety, depression, or similar emotions in the child. In these instances, professional help may be needed to resolve the underlying problems.

See also: Differential Social Reinforcement/ Positive Attention; Sexual Abuse; Sexual Development; Sexuality Education

Further Reading

Leung, A., & Robson, W. (1993). Childhood masturbation. *Clinical Pediatrics, 32*, 238–241.
Shedd, C. (1968). *The stork is dead.* Waco, TX: Word Books.
Stall, S. (1909). *What a young boy ought to know.* Philadelphia: Vir.

DREW C. MESSER†
C. EUGENE WALKER

†I am a military service member. This work was prepared as part of my official duties. Title 17 U.S.C. 105 provides that "Copyright protection under this title is not available for any work of the United States Government." Title 17 U.S.C. 101 defines a United States Government work as a work prepared by a military service member or employee of the United States Government as part of that person's official duties.

Maternal Employment

See: Working Parents

Mayer–Rokitansky–Küster–Hauser Syndrome

DESCRIPTION AND INCIDENCE

Mayer–Rokitansky–Küster–Hauser syndrome (MRKH), also known as Müllerian Agenesis syndrome, is an uncommon congenital anomaly of the female genital tract. Its features include an absent vagina and uterine abnormalities that vary from total absence to rudimentary remnants. Affected females have functioning ovaries, normal external genitalia and a female karyotype (46, XX). Secondary sex characteristics such as breast development and growth of pubic hair are also normal. Associated renal or skeletal anomalies occur in a high percentage of cases.

MRKH syndrome is estimated to occur in approximately 1/4,000–5,000 female births. It is second only to mixed gonadal dysgenesis (malformation of the gonads due to a sex chromosome anomaly) as a pathological cause of primary amenorrhea (never having experienced menstruation). Although it has been determined that the absence of a vagina and uterus is a result of the Müllerian ducts failing to form properly early in embryonic development, its underlying cause is unknown.

ASSESSMENT

The normal appearance of the external genitalia in MRKH makes it difficult to diagnose until adolescence when a girl may present with primary amenorrhea or an inability to accomplish vaginal intercourse. Average age of diagnosis is between 15 and 18 years, although a girl may be diagnosed at birth or during early adolescence during a thorough physical examination or for various medical reasons. A diagnosis of MRKH syndrome may create significant psychological challenges for a young woman and her family.

TREATMENT

At present, although uterine transplants occur only experimentally, there are numerous options for the creation of a neovagina. Patients may choose a surgical or nonsurgical method to construct a new vagina. In the United States, the most widely used surgical method is the one described by McIndoe and Bannister in 1938. A skin graft is taken from the buttocks and used to cover a stent, which is then inserted into a surgically created space between the bladder and the rectum. Follow-up care is tedious, as the patient must use dilators to keep the newly created vagina open. As an alternative to surgery, a patient may choose the Frank method, a process of manually expanding the soft tissue between the bladder and the rectum by applying intermittent pressure to the area using a set of lucite dilators, graduated in size. The Ingram modification of the Frank method uses a stationary bicycle seat along with dilators to allow a patient to passively expand her vagina. The amount of time it takes to nonsurgically create a new vagina depends upon the commitment of the individual. It is possible for a patient to achieve a functional vagina in 4–6 months. Both the surgical and nonsurgical methods require that a young woman be comfortable with examinations by physicians and be able to touch her own body. Both methods necessitate adherence to medical recommendations and substantial effort from the patient.

PSYCHOSOCIAL ASPECTS

Follow-up studies describing the psychological health of women with MRKH are limited. Some of the following statements, particularly those regarding the early adolescent, are based primarily on clinical anecdotal reports. Age of diagnosis will determine who would likely benefit from support and what form it should take. In the case of diagnosis during the newborn period, the family must cope with the challenge of discovering that their child has a birth defect. Education about the syndrome and treatment options will facilitate the coping process. An important issue for discussion will be when and how to eventually inform the child of her condition.

A girl who learns of this diagnosis as an early teen will find it challenging to assimilate this new information about herself during the years in which she is forming a sexual identity and attitudes about sexuality. At this time, many of her friends are starting to menstruate and her lack of menstruation may make her feel different and isolated. Some of her peers will begin to engage in sexual activity causing her to question not only her desirability, but also her ability to be sexually active. Furthermore, because society places great value on a female's ability to bear children, questions about her femininity may arise. During early adolescence, she will benefit from education about her condition, support for her potential feelings of isolation, and open discussions about sexuality and her role as a female. Another significant issue for the early teen is that of privacy. Discussion should ensue as to whom and how much to

tell about her condition. She should be advised on balancing the need to share with close friends and the need for keeping personal, medical information from becoming a source of gossip. Parents who are educated about MRKH syndrome, along with its implications, and have adequate coping skills themselves, are better equipped to offer support and encouragement to their child.

Because affected females are normal in external appearance, a diagnosis may be missed until late adolescence or even early adulthood. By this time a young woman may have experienced the frustration of late menarche or an unsuccessful attempt at intercourse. She is wondering what is wrong with her. At the time of diagnosis, patients have expressed a variety of emotions from sadness and despair to shock and anger. Questions about treatment options arise soon after diagnosis because of potential problems for existing or future relationships. Counseling should include a thorough discussion of treatment options as well as what will be expected from the patient in terms of commitment to the treatment. At this time it is helpful to educate a young woman about the role of her other sex organs and reassure her that she will be able to experience sexual pleasure. Infertility becomes an even larger issue in later adolescence because young women are starting to make decisions regarding family planning. Adoption and surrogacy remain the only options at this time. An inability to conceive and bear children may result in an irresolvable sadness that needs to be expressed and recognized. Recently, different models of group support have been explored. This seems to be an efficient and practical way to provide ongoing emotional support and relevant information to affected females.

PROGNOSIS

With psychological support and proper medical intervention, an individual with MRKH syndrome can be expected to maintain relatively normal sexual relationships. Her psychological adjustment to the condition depends upon many variables including preexisting psychological health, a supportive family, care from medical advisors, and outcome of treatment. A patient and family should be reassured by this prognosis.

RESOURCES FOR AFFECTED INDIVIDUALS AND THEIR FAMILIES

The MAGIC Foundation (http://www. magicfoundation.org), a nonprofit organization providing support and education regarding growth disorders in children including genital and reproductive anomalies in children (800-362-4423); MRKH Foundation (http://www.mrkh.net), an organization that provides support and information to affected individuals and their families.

See also: Sexual Differentiation: Disorders and Clinical Management; Treatment Adherence: Medical

Further Reading

Hecker, B. R., & McGuire, L. S. (1977). Psychosocial function in women treated for vaginal agenesis. *American Journal of Obstetrics and Gynecology, 129*, 543–547

Jensen, V. K., & Reiter, S. L. (1999). Psychosocial aspects of congenital female tract anomalies. In G. Gidwani & T. Falcone (Eds.), *Congenital malformations of the female genital tract: Diagnosis and management* (pp. 223–233). Philadelphia: Lippincott Williams & Wilkins.

Laufer, M. R., & Goldstein, D. P. (1998). Structural abnormalities of the female reproductive tract. In J. Emans, M. Laufer, & D. Goldstein (Eds.), *Pediatric and adolescent gynecology* (pp. 303–362). Philadelphia: Lippincott-Raven.

Poland, M. L, & Evans, T. N. (1985). Psychologic aspects of vaginal agenesis. *Journal of Reproductive Medicine, 30*, 340–344.

Weijenborg, P. T. M., & ter Kuile M. M. (2000). The effect of a group programme on women with the Mayer–Rokitansky–Küster–Hauser Syndrome. *British Journal of Obstetrics and Gynecology, 107*, 365–368.

ELLEN BEAN

Measurement of Behavior Change

ASSESSMENT OF BEHAVIOR CHANGE

Both the clinical and research sides of clinical child psychology depend on the assessment of behavior change to increase knowledge about (1) how an individual's behavior differs across situations; (2) how behavior changes developmentally across time; and (3) how therapeutic interventions affect behavior. First, evaluating behavior in different situations helps determine what causes and maintains of behavior, which in turn can shape case conceptualizations and treatment plans. The behaviorally based field of functional assessment and analysis has been specifically developed to measure these intraindividual behavior changes, such as how a person's behavior changes when different consequences are provided for specific behaviors. For example, this

technique can be used to determine if a child's self-injurious behavior is maintained by receiving social attention or from being allowed to escape from demands. Direct observation in settings such as school and home can determine broader situational factors that may affect behavior. Examples of these factors include lack of adult supervision or a poor fit between classroom style and a child's needs.

Second, measuring developmental behavior change on a global level increases understanding of typical child development. This understanding is important in the definition of deviant behavior as behavior that is atypical for a particular developmental level. For example, wetting the bed at age 3 or 4 years might be expected developmentally, but not at age 7 years. Additionally, the developmental psychotherapy model depends on knowledge of typical behavior development, because the therapist's goal is to return the child to healthy developmental pathways.

Lastly, assessment of behavior change can be used to determine therapeutic outcome. In a clinical setting, behavior change provides an objective measure of treatment effectiveness, giving the clinician, parent, and child concrete evidence of goal achievement or failure. Research on therapeutic outcome is also important, particularly with regard to the movement in psychology (as well as other health professions) toward empirically supported treatments or evidenced-based practice. An empirically supported treatment refers to a therapeutic technique that has a strong research base demonstrating positive outcomes. Often this research literature is based on objective measures of behavior change. The empirically supported treatments movement has been fueled by scientific curiosity, the ethical obligation to provide treatments that work, and the move toward financial reimbursement by managed care systems. Increasingly, managed care companies are hesitant to provide funding for specialty clinicians (i.e., doctoral level clinical child psychologists) for treatments that cannot be justified in terms of empirical support, cost savings, consumer acceptability, and quality of care. Therefore, in a competitive health care market, measures of behavior change become increasingly important to the practice of clinical child and pediatric psychology.

DIMENSIONS OF BEHAVIOR CHANGE

In general, there are four dimensions of behavior change assessment: (1) *magnitude*, the amount of change, (2) *generality*, how much change takes place across different symptoms or situations, (3) *universality*, the percentage of children that demonstrate the same changes, and (4) *stability*, how long changes are maintained. Therefore, to adequately describe behavior change, measures need to be taken at multiple times, in multiple situations, and from multiple sources. Additionally, the depth of the behavioral information can be increased by using multiple measurement techniques. Three commonly used techniques to assess behavior change include direct observation, objective self-report measures, and tracking changes in service use. *Direct observation* can range from formal and structured (as in functional analysis, where the clinician manipulates the environment to elicit certain behaviors), to natural settings such as in home or school, to incidental observations made by the clinician during therapy. However, the most useful observation techniques contain well-defined means of measuring and tracking behavior, so that changes can be objectively documented.

Though not as individually tailored as direct observations, *objective self-report measures* have the strength of providing standardized definitions of behavior. Additionally, instead of relying on observations of a small sample of time, they are a broader measure of behavior. Because of these attributes, self-report measures provide an easy means to compare behavior change between individuals or groups, which is particularly important for research applications. Commonly used self-report measures for assessing a wide range of behavior change include the Behavior Assessment System for Children (BASC) and the Child Behavior Checklist (CBCL); both of these measures provide separate forms for children, parents, and teachers. Self-report forms to measure specific behavioral changes are also available, such as to track changes in Attention-Deficit/Hyperactivity Disorder (ADHD) symptomatology or changes in the use of appropriate social skills.

In another realm of assessment, tracking changes in service use may involve monitoring the frequency a child or family accesses medical or social services. Changes in these behaviors are considered indirect effects of treatment. For example, a child with diabetes receiving behavioral services to increase adherence to his or her insulin regimen, may have fewer short- and long-term medical complications. Therefore, demonstrating decreased service use can be an important aspect of justifying treatment services based on overall cost effectiveness.

SUMMARY

Proper measurement of behavioral change is important to the field of clinical child and pediatric psychology

for clinical and research purposes. A thorough evaluation of a treatment outcome would include a multifaceted assessment of behavior change. The assessment should include a measure of behavior before any treatment is initiated, with self-report measures gathered from parents, teachers, and the child, as well as information collected about current service use and direct observations made in multiple settings. These same procedures should be repeated at the termination of the treatment, and followed up after a sufficient amount of time (e.g., 6–12 months).

See also: Behavior and Functional Analysis; Behavior Rating Scales; Behavioral Observation; Consumer Satisfaction; Evidence-Based Treatments; Treatment Outcome Measures

Further Reading

Gresham, F. M. & Lambros, K. M. (1998). Behavioral and functional assessment. In T. S. Watson & F. M. Gresham (Eds.), *Handbook of child behavior therapy* (pp. 3–22). New York: Plenum.
Kazdin, A. E. (Ed.). (1998). *Methodological issues and strategies in clinical research*. Washington, DC: American Psychological Association.
Snyder, C. R., & Ingram, R. E. (Eds.). (2000). *Handbook of psychological change*. New York: Wiley.

MONTSERRAT C. MITCHELL
MICHAEL C. ROBERTS

Medical Hospitalization

DEFINITION

According to the U.S. Agency for Healthcare Research and Quality, over 6 million children are hospitalized annually with an average length of stay of 3.5 days. This accounts for nearly 20 percent of all medical and surgical admissions each year. Children may be hospitalized for treatment of acute or chronic conditions or for elective procedures to correct disabilities or physical malformations. The length of stay, the nature of the hospital environments experienced, and the type of procedures performed depend upon the specific reasons for admission and vary greatly according to the child's diagnosis and overall health condition.

METHODS

In the United States, most children are hospitalized in either pediatric hospitals or special units dedicated to the care of children located in general medical facilities. Pediatric hospitals and units are staffed by healthcare personnel who are sensitive to the physical, emotional, behavioral, and developmental needs of children from infancy through adolescence. These personnel include pediatricians, nurses, psychologists, social workers, educational specialists, child life professionals, and volunteers. In addition to specialized staffing, pediatric medical facilities typically offer environments that are designed to provide comfortable and stimulating physical surroundings for hospitalized children and their families. For example, playrooms for younger children and teen lounges for adolescents often are available to provide a place to relax and socialize in a developmentally appropriate manner. Additionally, many pediatric medical facilities offer accommodations in the child's hospital room for a parent to spend the night with the child.

Specialized hospital settings, such as emergency rooms, intensive care units, and isolation facilities are also sometimes required for children. These environments usually mean additional stress for the child such as immobilization, restriction of visitation by family, and exposure to frightening or unusual sensory stimulation. It is especially important for pediatric healthcare professionals and families to give the child age-appropriate information about ongoing treatment and to provide normalizing activities for children requiring this increased level of care.

PSYCHOLOGICAL CORRELATES

Emotional and behavioral adjustment difficulties have been reported in up to 30 percent of children during and following hospitalization. These difficulties may range from mildly disruptive behavior to severe withdrawal or depression. Stressors that may account for such reactions include disruption of usual activities and routines, separation from family and friends, discomfort and fear resulting from the illness and its treatment, and loss of independence.

Research has suggested several factors that may affect a child's reaction to hospitalization. Younger children appear to be at higher risk for adjustment difficulties than older children, perhaps due to their relative inability to understand illness and to accept that sometimes painful or uncomfortable treatment is intended to improve health status. Other factors that appear to influence a child's response include length of stay, previous experience during hospitalization, psychological status prior to hospitalization, the ability of the child's parents

to provide support, and the type of preparation the child receives prior to hospitalization (see *Preparation for Medical Procedures*).

TREATMENT

Psychological services in pediatric inpatient settings are an important component of the interdisciplinary care of hospitalized children. Pediatric psychologists provide consultations that range from assessment of developmental status to interventions such as pain management or assistance with coping with chronic illness. These services may be short-term in nature (e.g., designing a behavior management plan to help a child adhere to hospital routine) or require long-term follow-up care (e.g., posthospitalization family counseling to deal with issues related to death and bereavement). Regardless of the presenting problem or intervention technique, the pediatric psychologist working in a hospital setting is committed to promoting the health and well-being of children who require medical inpatient treatment.

See also: Preparation for Medical Procedures; Residential Treatment; Social Support; Treatment Adherence: Medical

Further Reading

Hamlett, K. W., & Stabler, B. (1995). The developmental progress of pediatric psychology consultation. In M. C. Roberts (Ed.), *Handbook of pediatric psychology* (2nd ed., pp. 39–54). New York: Guilford.

Siegel, L. J., & Conte, P. (2001). Hospitalization and medical care of children. In C. E. Walker & M. C. Roberts (Eds.), *Handbook of clinical child psychology* (3rd ed., pp. 895–909). New York: Wiley.

STEPHEN R. BOGGS

Medical Rehabilitation, Pediatric

Pediatric medical rehabilitation refers to comprehensive evaluation and treatment with the goal of restoring a child to the best possible level of functioning following a debilitating physical disorder or problem. A team of health professionals is usually involved including the following: physiatry, pediatrics, orthopedics, neuropsychology, psychiatry, psychology, physical and occupational therapy, social work, and education. Medical rehabilitation may be required for a variety of physical conditions including juvenile arthritis, oncology disorders, burns, respiratory disorders, spinal cord injuries, heart conditions, or any disorder or disease that interferes with the person's functioning.

                                                    DENNIS C. HARPER

Memory Development

DEFINITION

Memory is the result of a series of processes by which one forms (i.e., *encodes*), stores, and retrieves mental representations. The memory system is commonly thought to consist of two storage spaces. The *preliminary storage* space, known as short-term memory or working memory, holds information for a brief amount of time and has a limited capacity. Information may be transferred from short-term storage into long-term storage, which is thought to be relatively permanent and have unlimited storage space. *Long-term storage* holds two general types of memories: procedural memories and declarative memories. Procedural memories are memories that are retrieved without awareness, as is the case with motor skills such as riding a bicycle. In contrast, declarative memories are consciously retrieved or remembered. The declarative memory system includes semantic memory (general knowledge of facts), language, one's own personal history, and episodic memory (memory for specific episodes that are tied to a particular context). Cognitive psychologists generally agree that remembering is a constructive, rather than a reproductive, process. During encoding, individuals are thought to *construct* memory representations as they use their background knowledge to interpret to-be-remembered information and to make inferences and elaborations. The retrieval of information is seen as a similar process of *reconstruction*. Memory is a core component of children's cognitive development.

RESEARCH ON CHILDREN'S MEMORY

The earliest known empirical studies of children's memory were conducted by Alfred Binet around the turn of the 20th century. Binet's work demonstrated the phenomenon of suggestibility in children and showed that children's memory capabilities vary considerably with the meaning of to-be-remembered stimuli. It was not until the mid-20th century, however, when the attention of developmental psychologists was again turned toward an examination of memory in infants and children.

DEVELOPMENT OF MEMORY IN INFANCY

Considerable research suggests that some forms of memory are functional quite early in life. For example, shortly after birth infants prefer their mother's voices over that of other females. By 2 months of age, infants show preferences for novel stimuli over stimuli to which they have been previously exposed, suggesting that they recognize the familiar stimuli at some level. A large body of research on infant long-term memory has emerged from the use of operant conditioning procedures. By 2 months of age, infants show memories for brief periods of time (i.e., about 2 days), and the length of time over which these memories are retained increases across infancy. At later points during the first year, it can be shown that infants remember events for 2–3 weeks. This work has also led to a number of insights about the roles of reexposure and context in maintaining memories over time.

Memory for more complex information (e.g., sequences of events, knowing what to do with a particular toy) in preverbal children can be inferred from the demonstration of deferred imitation, in which infants or toddlers are shown a sequence of behaviors and then are later given the opportunity to demonstrate the sequence themselves. This *deferred imitation* is seen in infants as young as 9 months of age. Older infants are able to remember increasingly complex event sequences, and these memories have been shown to last up to several months.

DEVELOPMENT OF MEMORY IN CHILDHOOD

Memory Strategies

Until recently, most research on memory during childhood focused on the development of children's memory strategies for deliberate memory tasks. Such strategies are goal-directed operations that are adopted to facilitate memory, and they include *rehearsal* (repeating information that is to-be-remembered to oneself) or *organization* (grouping to-be-remembered items into categories). Some simple strategies are seen in preschoolers, but dramatic increases in the sophistication and effectiveness of memory strategies occur across childhood and adolescence.

Memory Scripts

Recent research on children's memory for real-life experiences suggests that, under some conditions, even very young children show considerable competence in remembering past events. For instance, children as young as 3 years readily form *scripts* (organized representations of sequences of events) for familiar or common occurrences such as going to a birthday party, getting a medical check-up, or getting ready for school. Children's scripts become more detailed, organized, and incorporate more optional or variable acts. Similarly, studies of development of episodic memory show that children as young as 2.5 years can remember specific events from the distant past (e.g., 3–6 months), but they typically require considerable prompting from adults. With age, children have more detailed and more accurate memories for past experiences, and show less forgetting over time.

Infantile Amnesia

Recent research indicates that events that occur during the first 3–5 years of life are highly susceptible to forgetting. This well-documented absence of autobiographical memories for early experiences is known as infantile or childhood amnesia. The underlying mechanisms are not completely understood. Some researchers have argued that memories are encoded differently by infants and toddlers than by older children and adults. Others have argued that the development of language is necessary for the emergence of autobiographical memory because it enables children to talk about, organize, and represent their experiences. Finally, some researchers claim that a sense of self is necessary to serve as an anchor for the retrieval of autobiographical memories, and the sense of self develops gradually over the preschool years.

FACTORS AFFECTING MEMORY

A variety of factors can have an impact on children's memory abilities. These factors can be discussed in terms of their influence on the three main phases of remembering: encoding, storage, and retrieval. First, because the human cognitive system is limited, not everything that is experienced gets attended to and encoded into memory. The encoding process can be influenced by a number of factors. For example, stress can affect what components of an event an individual attends to and encodes. Similarly, an individual's understanding of an event can also have a dramatic impact on how it is interpreted and encoded. Memories that are encoded may also vary in strength, as a function of a variety of factors such as the amount of exposure to an event or the person's age. During the second phase of storage, encoded information is transferred to and held in long-term memory until it is retrieved. Once stored, however, memory representations are subject to change, in part as a result of the passage of time, and in part as a consequence of intervening experiences such as repeated discussions or exposure to intervening events (e.g., similar experiences or information from the media). Finally, a range of cognitive and social factors can influence children's abilities to retrieve information from long term memory and report that information. For instance, strong memory representations are more easily retrieved than weak memory representations. Moreover, retrieval is generally facilitated to the extent that the conditions at the time of retrieval resemble those in place when the information was encoded. In other words, retrieval is enhanced when memory is assessed in the situation in which information was presented initially. Extending this principle to interviewing contexts, the cues offered by specific questions, as opposed to open-ended questions, aid children in retrieval. These techniques, however, also tend to lead to more errors. The retrieval of information, however, does not guarantee that it will be reported. The reports of very young children may be limited by developmental factors such as restricted language skills and poor grasp of the principles of narrative structure. There may also be some social contexts under which children are reluctant to report retrieved information. It must also be emphasized that what a child does "remember" and report may not always be retrieved from the actual memory representation. Reconstructive processes at the time of retrieval may be used to fill in gaps in memory on the basis of general knowledge and expectations, especially after long delays. Also, studies of suggestibility suggest that children's reports may sometimes be based on confusions between a particular personal experience and other "sources" of information, such as other experiences, another person's account, or information from the media.

RELEVANCE TO CLINICAL RESEARCH AND PRACTICE

Normative information about memory development in infants and children is useful to clinicians working with children suspected to have developmental disabilities or brain injuries. Research on event memory in childhood and infantile amnesia and the reliability of children's ability to remember and accurately report on various real-life events bear directly on the evaluation of children's testimony in cases of abuse and neglect.

See also: Childhood; Cognitive Development; Infancy; Language Development

Further Reading

Baker-Ward, L., Gordon, B. N., Ornstein, P. A., Larus, D. M., & Clubb, P. A. (1993). Young children's long-term retention of a pediatric examination. *Child Development, 64,* 1519–1533.

Cowan, N. (Ed.). (1997). *The development of memory in childhood.* Hove East Sussex: Psychology Press.

Nelson K., Fivush, R., Hudson, J., & Lucariello, J. (1983). Scripts and the development of memory. In. M. T. C. Chi (Ed.), *Trends in memory development research.* Basel, Switzerland: Karger.

Ornstein, P. A., Larus, D., & Clubb, P. A. (1991). Understanding children's testimony: Implications of research on the development of memory. In R. Vasta (Ed.), *Annals of child development* (Vol. 8, pp. 145–176). London: Jessica Kingsley.

Schneider, W., & Pressley, M. (1997). *Memory development between two and twenty.* Mahwah, NJ: Erlbaum.

Usher, J. A., & Neisser, U. (1993). Childhood amnesia and the beginnings of memory for four early life events. *Journal of Experimental Psychology: General, 122,* 155–165.

ALISA A. MILLER

ANDREA FOLLMEN GREENHOOT

Meningitis

DEFINITION AND SYMPTOMS

Meningitis is an inflammation of the membranes (meninges) surrounding the brain and spinal cord. The majority of cases result from viral or bacterial infections, but a few instances of meningitis stem from fungal infections, noninfectious conditions that irritate the meninges (e.g., systemic lupus erythematosus), head trauma, some types of cancer, and sensitivity reactions to medications. Symptoms in those over 2 years of age include headache, stiff neck, vomiting, high fever, lethargy, photophobia (abnormal sensitivity to light), joint pain, and seizures. In newborns and infants, fever and other typical symptoms may be absent or difficult to detect. Instead, an infant's presentation may be characterized by lethargy or irritability, poor feeding, and vomiting.

Symptom onset may be gradual, over the course of several days, or acute, with indications of systemic infection and meningeal inflammation that develops within 24 hr. The latter cases typically have a bacterial etiology, and are associated with greater risk of mortality and morbidity. If unchecked, disease progression can lead to cerebral edema and altered cerebral blood flow, elevated intracranial pressure, cranial nerve damage (e.g., hearing loss), ischemic injuries (e.g., injuries due to lack of blood supply to affected tissue or organs), and death.

INCIDENCE, ETIOLOGY, AND CONSEQUENCES OF BACTERIAL MENINGITIS

In the United States, the incidence of bacterial meningitis is 2.5–3.5 per 100,000. Prior to the 1990s, *Haemophilus influenzae type B* (*Hib*) was the most common cause of bacterial meningitis in young children. However, introduction of the *Hib* vaccine into routine childhood immunization schedules led to a 94 percent reduction in cases of *Hib* meningitis, and resulted in a shift in the median age of individuals with meningitis from 15 months in 1986 to 25 years in 1995. In neonates, *Group B streptococcus* (*GBS*) is the most common cause of meningitis. Estimates suggest that 10–30 percent of pregnant women are colonized with *GBS* in the rectum or vagina and, in a small number of cases, they pass the bacterium to the baby prior to or during delivery.

The large majority of bacterial meningitis cases in individuals over 2 months of age are caused by either *Streptococcus pneumoniae* (pneumococcal meningitis) or *Neisseria meningitides* (meningococcal meningitis). At any given time, the bacteria that cause pneumococcal and meningococcal meningitis are colonized in the throats, noses, and upper respiratory tracts of a sizeable proportion of children. They are spread through prolonged close contact and exchange of respiratory secretions (e.g., via sneezing, coughing, kissing). However, only rarely do these bacteria overcome their host's defenses, enter the bloodstream, travel to the meninges, and cause meningitis.

Focal neurologic symptoms (e.g., seizures, hearing loss, hemiparesis) are present in approximately 40 percent of patients with bacterial meningitis, and these neurologic complications persist in about 20 percent of cases at 1-year follow-up and beyond. The overall mortality rate for bacterial meningitis is 5–10 percent, but rates vary from 3–17 percent for meningococcal disease to 19–47 percent for pneumococcal disease. Risk factors include younger age at onset, rapid escalation of symptoms, and focal neurologic symptoms at the time of diagnosis.

INCIDENCE, ETIOLOGY, AND CONSEQUENCES OF VIRAL MENINGITIS

Viral meningitis is the more common form of meningitis, but is typically much less severe than bacterial disease, generally resolving itself within 7–14 days, without specific intervention. In some cases, however, headaches, fatigue, and depression may linger for a number of weeks or months. In mild cases, affected individuals may not even seek medical care, making it difficult to establish the incidence of viral meningitis.

Enteroviruses (e.g., coxsackie, echoviruses) are the most common cause of viral meningitis, accounting for up to 90 percent of cases. They are generally spread through direct contact with respiratory secretions (e.g., saliva, nasal mucus) of an infected person. These viruses also reside in the intestines of infected individuals, and can be spread as a result of poor hygiene or sewage-polluted water. Herpes simplex (HSV), measles, chicken pox, and insect-borne viruses (e.g., West Nile) are other agents that can occasionally cause meningitis. Contact with a person who has viral meningitis may result in transfer of the underlying virus, but does not significantly increase the chances of contracting meningitis, as less than 1 in 1,000 individuals hosting the virus actually develops meningitis. Viral meningitis is rarely fatal in individuals with normal immune function.

DIAGNOSIS AND TREATMENT

Diagnosis for both viral and bacterial meningitis is typically made through the analysis of cerebrospinal fluid (CSF) obtained via a lumbar puncture (spinal tap). Because the specific viral versus bacterial identity of the causative agent often cannot be determined at the time of presentation, intravenous broad-spectrum antibiotics are typically initiated while awaiting results from CSF cultures. Viral meningitis is usually treated with bed rest, hydration, and analgesics to manage fever or discomfort. In some cases (e.g., HSV), a regimen of antiviral medications also may be indicated. Bacterial disease, of the other hand, is treated with a full course of antibiotics. Other persons classified by public health surveillance methods as close contacts of index individuals diagnosed with meningococcal disease also receive prophylactic antibiotics. Corticosteroids may be administered in affected individuals who demonstrate

indications of central nervous system (CNS) swelling or inflammation, and anticonvulsants are used to prevent or treat seizures. In advanced cases, surgical intervention (i.e., shunting) may be warranted to reduce brain swelling and reduce the severity of ICP.

PSYCHOLOGICAL ASSESSMENT AND INTERVENTIONS

As with other neurological conditions, it is helpful to utilize neuropsychological assessment to establish the extent, pattern, and trajectory of recovery for any neurocognitive deficits sustained as a consequence of meningitis. The results of both baseline and follow-up evaluations conducted 6–12 months later provide a foundation for anticipatory guidance regarding appropriate expectations, direction for school and social reentry, and definition of the need for academic accommodations. Baseline assessment with developmental screening or intelligence measures alone may not be adequate—follow-up testing must be sensitive enough to pick up subtle deficits early, as well as, identify developmental delays and subtle effects that emerge or escalate later in childhood. Early identification and related environmental interventions may prevent the secondary emotional sequelae (e.g., depression) that often occur when an individual acquires new, but perhaps subtle and unrecognized, learning problems that prevent quick and easy return to prior levels of functioning. In addition, intervention may usefully target child and family adaptation to changes in the child's health status, coping strategies, and pain management.

NEUROCOGNITIVE AND PSYCHOLOGICAL SEQUELAE

Although there appears to be considerable variation in outcome as a function of differing causative agents, numerous studies of the impact of bacterial meningitis demonstrate significant effects on cognitive, behavioral, and academic functioning of survivors. For example, Bedford and colleagues' (2001) large-scale follow-up study of an index group of 5-year-olds who had bacterial meningitis during the first year of life documented their higher risk for learning and neuromotor disorders, seizures, hearing and vision problems, speech and language disorders, and behavior problems, when compared to a control group matched for sex and age. Almost 16 percent of meningitis survivors had a moderate or severe disability (versus 2 percent of controls), and more subtle deficits were also more prevalent among those with a history of meningitis. Similar elevations in risks for cognitive and academic problems were noted in other large-scale reviews. These effects are especially pronounced in those children who demonstrate acute phase neurologic complications, but sequelae are also found in those without such gross disturbances. Further, some effects emerge or become more pronounced over time. As such, follow-up assessment should be offered to all survivors and monitoring should extend across development.

Although it appears that the majority of individuals who contract viral meningitis do not suffer from long-term neurologic sequelae, congenital infections and infections in the first months of life may be related to subsequent language or developmental delays. Interestingly, the severity of acute phase viral infection does not seem to predict negative sequelae, arguing for broader monitoring of affected children even if initial symptoms of viral meningitis are mild and recovery appears complete.

See also: Neurological Disorders; Pediatric Infectious Diseases; Hospitalization—Medical; Neuropsychological Assessment; Learning Disorders; Coping with Illness

Further Reading

Anderson, V. A., & Taylor, H. G. (2000) Meningitis. In K. O. Yeates, M. D. Ris, & H. G. Taylor (Eds.), *Pediatric neuropsychology: Research, theory, and practice.* New York: Guilford.

Bedford, H., de Louvois, J., Halket, S., Peckham, C., Hurley, R., & Harvey, D. (2001) Meningitis in infancy in England and Wales: Follow up at age 5 years. *British Medical Journal, 323*, 533–536.

Centers for Disease Control and Prevention. (2001) Viral (Aseptic) meningitis. Retrieved April 14, 2002, from http://www.cdc.gov/ncidod/dvrd/revb/enterovirus/viral_meningitis.htm

Centers for Disease Control and Prevention. (1996) Prevention of perinatal group B streptococcal disease: A public health perspective. *Morbidity and Mortality Weekly Report, 45* (RR-7), 1–24.

Schuchat, A., Robinson, K., Wenger, J. D., Harrison, L. H., Farley, M., Reingold, A. L., Lefkowitz, L., & Perkins, B. A. (1997) Bacterial meningitis in the United States in 1995: Active Surveillance Team. *New England Journal of Medicine, 337*(14), 970–976.

DANIEL R. HILLIKER
J. KENNETH WHITT

Mental Care Provider

See: Health Care Professionals (General)

Mental Health Records

According to the American Psychological Association (APA) Ethical Principles of Psychologists and Code of Conduct (1992), psychologists must document the services they perform and must maintain current, accurate, and pertinent mental health records. Within these guidelines, clinical child and pediatric psychologists should maintain appropriate confidentiality in the creating, storing, accessing, disposition, and transferring of records. This includes recorded, computerized, and written records. Clinical child and pediatric psychologists should maintain and dispose of records in accordance with applicable state or provincial laws and in a manner compatible with the APA Ethics Code. In addition, a psychologist should have contingency plans to maintain confidentiality of records in the event of the withdrawal, incapacity, or death of the psychologist.

Because of their confidential nature, access to mental health records is limited. In most cases, clinical child and pediatric psychologists release mental health records only with the written consent of the parent or legal guardian of the minor patient. Depending upon the state or provincial statutes in which the psychologist practices, several situations exist where the psychologist is permitted (or required) to release records without obtaining authorization by the parent or guardian. Psychologists can release records if ordered by a court, to report suspected abuse, and to protect the patient or others from harm. In the same way, psychologists can reveal minimal information to other professionals in order to obtain appropriate professional consultations on behalf of the in patient. Clinical child and pediatric psychologists should provide mental health records to others as needed in order to serve the best interests of the child and family and to meet legal standards and mandates.

Although all mental health records should be sufficiently detailed to permit the continued provision of services by the psychologist or other professionals, only minimal intrusion into the privacy of the patient should be allowed. Records should include only that information that is germane to the purposes of the assessment or intervention. The institutional requirements for mental health records can vary widely from setting to setting. In the same way, records of private practitioners can also vary widely. Clinical child and pediatric psychologists must be cautious about retaining working notes which often contain unsubstantiated hypotheses since working notes can be revealed as part of a legal process. In general, mental health records should be written in clear, unambiguous language with a minimum of theoretical speculation. In addition, hospital-based pediatric psychologists who write chart notes in the general hospital medical record should be aware of potential conflicts between the need to be thorough and the need to reveal private information. Although other health care professionals might want confidential information available in the hospital chart so they can provide comprehensive care, the psychologist must be continually aware of the potential harm that revealing such information might have on the child and family. Although the clinical child and pediatric psychologist should strive to document as accurately and completely as possible, they should also be sensitive to the potentially harmful effects inherent in revealing confidential information.

In most circumstances, parents or legal guardians have the right to all mental health records of their minor children. Technically, parents can request and obtain copies of records during or after assessment or intervention until the child reaches the age of majority. If the clinical child or pediatric psychologist reveals sensitive information in the mental health record to parents, the trust between the child and the psychologist could be compromised. For example, information about private feelings, sexual behavior, substance use, alcohol use, and antisocial behavior should be documented with great care and sensitivity. The documentation must be in sufficient detail for the psychologist to remember the content of the session, but not be overly explicit with pejorative details that could be embarrassing and/or upsetting to the child or family. It should be noted that when the child reaches legal adulthood, he or she could also request copies of the mental health record. Since patients and parents have or can have access to mental health records, the psychologist's notes in the mental health record should be written with the assumption that the child or family will eventually read the record.

When parents of a child are divorced or are legally prohibited from custody of their child (e.g., abusive parents), special issues must be taken into account when releasing mental health records. As part of a divorce decree or other legal document, the court usually specifies who has access to the child's medical records. In some states (e.g., Texas), divorce decrees usually specify joint custody, which means that both parents have equal access to medical records regardless of who has custody of the child. In addition, some states (e.g., Texas) allow the psychologist to withhold information if release of the information would be detrimental to the well-being of the patient. For example, if the psychologist's notes indicated that the child had a preference to live with a particular parent, this information could be withheld, but the psychologist would have to provide a written explanation of why this information was withheld. Clinical child and pediatric psychologists may not withhold mental health records that are imminently needed for a child's assessment or intervention because the psychologist has not received payment for services provided. Psychologists are allowed to release minimal information to others (e.g., insurance companies) in order to obtain payment for professional services.

Clinical child and pediatric psychologists must take proper steps to retain mental health records. The professional standards vary depending on the purpose and content of the records. Out-of-date records (e.g., test protocols) should be routinely destroyed after a certain length of time since retaining this obsolete information could lead to misinterpretations. State or provincial laws usually dictate how long mental health records should be kept. Most statutes require that mental health records for children be kept for a certain number of years past the child's legal age of majority. For example, if state law requires psychological records be kept 10 years past age of legal majority, the records of a 5-year-old child should be retained for 23 years. In all cases, the psychologist is responsible for the mental health records, including the manner in which the records are retained or disposed. The clinical child or pediatric psychologist should also specify the disposition of records in the event of his or her death or incapacity.

See also: Confidentiality and Privilege; Professional Societies in Clinical Child and Pediatric Psychology; Report Writing; Training Issues

Further Reading

American Psychological Association. (1992). Ethical principles of psychologists and code of conduct. *American Psychologist, 47,* 1597–1611.

Koocher, G. P., & Keith-Spiegel, P. (1998). *Ethics in psychology: Professional standards and cases* (2nd ed.). New York: Oxford University Press.

Melton, G. B., Ehrenreich, N. S., & Lyons, P. M., Jr. (2001). Ethical and legal issues in mental health services for children. In C. E. Walker & M. C. Roberts (Eds.), *Handbook of clinical child psychology* (3rd ed., pp. 1074–1093). New York: Wiley.

Rae, W. A., Worchel, F. F., & Brunnquell, D. (1995). Ethical and legal issues in pediatric psychology. In M. C. Roberts (Ed.), *Handbook of pediatric psychology* (2nd ed., pp. 19–36). New York: Guilford.

WILLIAM A. RAE

Mental Retardation

DEFINITION

Mental retardation is a developmental disability characterized by inadequate adaptation to societal demands. This disability is typically diagnosed in childhood when a discrepancy is recognized between a child's level of functioning and that of peers of the same chronological age. The current diagnostic definition of mental retardation includes three criteria: significantly subaverage intellectual functioning, concurrent deficits or impairments in adaptive functioning, and onset before 18 years of age. General intellectual functioning includes various cognitive abilities such as attention, memory, problem solving, language, and abstract thinking. Adaptive functioning includes communication, self-care, home living, social skills, community use, self-direction, health and safety, functional academics, leisure skills, and work skills. A person must show deficits in at least 2 of the 10 adaptive functioning areas for a diagnosis of mental retardation. Significant subaverage intelligence and adaptive behavior is defined as two standard deviations below the mean on standardized measures. Such measures usually have a mean or average score of 100 points and a standard deviation of 15 points. Therefore, scores of 70 points or less are necessary on measures of general intelligence and adaptive functioning for a diagnosis of mental retardation.

Classification schemes have historically included severity levels of mental retardation. The American Psychiatric Association's *Diagnostic and Statistical Manual of Mental Disorders* (4th edition) currently uses the terms mild, moderate, severe, and profound to define severity levels. Each level corresponds to a standard deviation unit. The mild range includes scores between 56 and 70, the moderate range between 41 and 55, the severe range between 26 and 40, and the profound range corresponds to scores below 25. The mild range of mental retardation has the greatest number of people (89 percent) while the profound range has the fewest (1.5 percent). The moderate (6 percent) and severe (3.5 percent) ranges are intermediate in prevalence. A diagnosis of mental retardation, severity unspecified is appropriate when there is evidence of subaverage functioning but standardized test scores are not available.

Children with mild mental retardation are typically identified upon reaching school age. The nature and degree of their developmental delays do not become apparent until formal schooling begins. Given appropriate levels of support, these children eventually learn academic skills to approximately the sixth grade level, although at a relatively reduced rate as compared with typically developing children. They can attain adequate levels of social and vocational functioning with minimal ongoing guidance. In contrast, children with moderate mental retardation can develop language but have less adequate social awareness. Their academic attainment typically reaches the second or third grade level. They will require ongoing support to develop vocational skills.

Children with severe mental retardation acquire some communication and self-care skills but at a markedly reduced rate in comparison with typically developing children. Severe mental retardation is typically diagnosed during the preschool years. Children with profound mental retardation are usually identified soon after birth, given the likelihood of associated medical conditions and genetic etiology. Many children with profound mental retardation are nonverbal and require constant supervised care. Given the likelihood of co-occurring motor impairments, they may be nonambulatory as well.

ADDITIONAL DIAGNOSES

Many children with mental retardation have additional conditions that further affect their adaptation and development. These conditions include cerebral palsy, seizure disorders, sensory impairment (such as hearing or visual problems), and psychological disorders. Generally speaking, children with severe or profound mental retardation have a greater prevalence of cerebral palsy, seizure disorders, or sensory impairment than children with mild or moderate mental retardation. It is also possible for a person to have multiple coexisting physical conditions, such as cerebral palsy and seizure disorders, with mental retardation. Psychological disorders are four to five times more common in children with mental retardation compared to children with typical intellectual and adaptive functioning. For example, approximately 75 percent of children with autism also have mental retardation. However, oppositional behavior, conduct problems, depression, anxiety, and Attention-Deficit/Hyperactivity Disorder (ADHD) are also quite prevalent. Beyond a level of general elevated risk, some etiologies have especially high rates of particular psychological disorders. For example, children with Down syndrome often have oppositional and defiant behaviors while children with Fragile X syndrome may exhibit self-injurious behaviors or ADHD.

PREVALENCE

The exact prevalence of mental retardation in the United States is not known. It is estimated that 2 percent of children and adolescents have a formal diagnosis of mental retardation. The prevalence of mental retardation is greatest during the school-age years. During this time, many children with mild mental retardation are identified and receive services. Prevalence declines in later adolescence and young adulthood because many persons with mild mental retardation are no longer identified or receive special services. Recent studies suggest that children who meet the diagnostic criteria for mild mental retardation may actually be classified as learning disabled in the educational system. Such referral and diagnostic practices may avoid potential stigmatization but suggest that there is little value of a diagnosis of mild mental retardation in some educational settings. As a result, estimated prevalence rates of mental retardation are substantially lower than would be predicted based on hypothetical distributions of intelligence and adaptive functioning.

ETIOLOGY

Research conducted since the 1960s has substantially increased our understanding of mental retardation. The field has now begun to focus greater attention on etiologic conditions, particularly those of genetic origin (e.g., Down syndrome and Fragile X syndrome), which have mental retardation as an associated feature. There is general agreement that timing is important in determining etiology. The current American Association on Mental Retardation (AAMR) classification manual organizes etiology according to prenatal, perinatal, and postnatal causes. Prenatal causes such as chromosomal disorders, disorders associated with inborn errors of metabolism, developmental disorders of brain formation, and environmental influences such as fetal alcohol syndrome or maternal malnutrition more likely result in severe or profound mental retardation than perinatal or postnatal etiologies. Perinatal or postnatal etiologies are typically associated with mild to moderate mental retardation. Examples of perinatal causes include intrauterine disorders such as premature labor or neonatal disorders such as intracranial hemorrhage and meningitis.

Postnatal causes include various infections, head injuries, and degenerative conditions. Although many specific etiologies have been identified, the etiology of mental retardation for a particular person cannot always be determined. For example, in one study 23 percent of the group with severe mental retardation and 74 percent of a group with mild mental retardation had unknown etiology. This difference was due in large part to the number of chromosomal conditions associated with functioning levels in the severe range of mental retardation. As the field devotes greater attention to etiology determination, it is likely that the number of people with mental retardation due to unknown etiology will decline.

ASSESSMENT

General intellectual functioning is determined by an individually administered, standardized intelligence test. Measures frequently used include the Bayley Scales of Infant Development II, the Wechsler Preschool and Primary Test of Intelligence-Revised, the Wechsler Intelligence Test for Children III, the Stanford-Binet fourth edition, and the Kaufmann Assessment Battery for Children. Actual test selection is based on the chronological age of the child and general level of functioning. Given the possibility that a child may have sensory or motor impairments or be nonverbal, assessments may include specialized measures designed for these populations. Similarly the presence of significant behavioral problems or mental disorders may require that assessments be conducted by psychologists who have experience with such children.

Most theories embed adaptive behavior in a broader context of personal or social competence. Indeed, most adaptive behavior measures assess how effectively a person copes with common life demands and how well they meet societal expectations for someone of the same age, sociocultural background, and community living setting. The Vineland Adaptive Behavior Scales, the AAMR Adaptive Behavior Scale, second edition, and the Scales of Independent Behavior-Revised are commonly used instruments. Although the specific content of the measures vary, most adaptive behavior measures assess social and interpersonal skills, communication and language skills, gross and fine motor skills, and independent functioning in daily living skills.

Evaluation of psychological or behavioral disorders in children with mental retardation is a fairly specialized area that is beyond the experience and training level of many mental health professionals. Please see the entry on *Dual Diagnosis: Mental Retardation and Psychiatric Disorders* for more information.

INTERVENTION

Mental retardation is not curable. It is possible, however, that a child functioning on the border between mental retardation and borderline intelligence might not meet the definitional criteria on subsequent evaluation. Given that there is some measurement error in all psychological instruments, the *DSM-IV* and AAMR classification systems permit diagnoses of individuals with scores as high as 75 on measures of intelligence and adaptive functioning so that services can be maintained.

An elaborate system of early intervention, early childhood special education services, and school-based special education services is available. These services are mandated by federal legislation found in the Individuals with Disabilities Education Act (1997). The essence of this legislation, first enacted in 1975, is that children with disabilities deserve a free and appropriate public education. Moreover children should receive educational services in the least restrictive environment and their education should be guided by an individualized education plan (IEP). The legislation further ensures that children have the right to due process and that their educational placements should be based on nondiscriminatory testing. Children with mental retardation also qualify for Medicare reimbursement for additional services such as speech-language intervention, physical and occupational therapy, and psychological services.

It is generally believed that if children with mental retardation are provided with adequate educational and support services their level of functioning will generally improve. Early intervention has been shown to be effective in enhancing overall development. Similarly, special education services have been shown to be effective in enhancing academic achievement for children with mild to moderate mental retardation. Research has demonstrated the success of many behavioral and instructional methods in increasing functioning for children with severe or profound mental retardation. The effectiveness of behavioral interventions in reducing maladaptive behaviors is undeniable. Psychopharmacological methods are effective in minimizing maladaptive behaviors and psychopathology. Traditional methods of psychological intervention have also been shown to be effective with higher functioning persons although some modification of the techniques may be necessary. Parent groups and family education

programs may provide support to parents, siblings, and extended family members.

See also: Adaptive Behavior Assessment; Autistic Disorder; Down Syndrome; Dual Diagnosis: Mental Retardation and Psychiatric Disorders; Fragile X Syndrome; Intellectual Assessment

Further Reading

American Psychiatric Association. (2000). *Diagnostic and statistical manual of mental disorders—Text revision* (4th ed.). Washington, DC: Author.

Batshaw, M. L., & Shapiro, B. K. (1997). Mental retardation. In M. L. Batshaw (Ed.), *Children with disabilities* (4th ed., pp. 335–359). Baltimore: Paul H. Brookes.

Luckasson, R. (Ed.). (1992). *Mental retardation: Definition, classification, and systems of support.* Washington, DC: American Association on Mental Retardation: The Arc. http://www.thearc.org

WILLIAM E. MACLEAN, JR.

Mental Status Examination

The mental status examination (MSE) represents a brief examination of key areas of psychological functioning, usually administered at the point of a patient's initial contact with a mental health professional. As noted by Schogt and Rewilak (2001), the MSE typically covers key areas of functioning including general appearance and behavior, emotional expression, speech characteristics, form and content of thought, perceptual disturbances, sensorium and cognition, memory, and judgment and insight. It is an objective report based on signs that are present at the time of interview, and most information is observational. The presenting problem guides the content and depth of the interview that is necessary for a relevant and complete MSE.

The framework of the MSE provides a relatively standardized method of collecting and recording observations of the client, facilitates a thorough description of the client, and minimizes the chance of important areas being overlooked. The findings of the MSE highlight areas of psychological functioning, such as behavior, mood, language, memory, perception, and thought processes that require more in-depth assessment. The information may also indicate specific medical examinations that are warranted. The MSE has been described in various forms by many authors, with slight differences in content. One of the most well-known forms is the Mini-Mental State Exam (MMSE) developed by Folstein, Folstein, and McHugh (1975). The MSE has also been modified for use with specific populations. For example, Benham (2000) developed that Infant-Toddler Mental Status Exam for assessing young children.

GENERAL APPEARANCE AND BEHAVIOR

This section of the MSE involves an overall description of the client's appearance, nonverbal behavior, and attitude, with a particular focus on any abnormalities that may provide a clue to the nature and chronicity of a presenting problem. Visual cues such as height, weight, state of health, dress, grooming, and personal hygiene are recorded. Nonverbal behavior such as overall level of activity, gait, mannerisms, posture, movement abnormalities, facial expression, and eye contact are also observed. The client's attitude to the interviewer is described, such as degree of cooperation, responsiveness, openness, suspicion, manipulative attempts, or ambivalence. Specific examples are generally recorded. The presence of movement and posture abnormalities (e.g., psychomotor agitation, acceleration or retardation; tics; ataxia; chorea; stupor) may also assist in diagnosis.

EMOTIONAL EXPRESSION

Conventionally, emotional expression refers to the patient's mood and affect, with mood defined as the prevailing, internal emotional state; and affect as the immediate, external expression of emotion. Mood is assessed from the patient's subjective verbal report of his or her emotional state. Affect is assessed from observable emotional cues that are displayed during the interview, such as facial expression, gestures, body posture, and tone of voice. Disturbances in affect include hostility, liability (rapid shifts in affect), inappropriate affect (gross incongruence of affect with conversation content), blunted affect (minimal display of emotion), emotional flattening (absence of all emotional reactivity) and discordance between self-reported mood and behavioral indicators of affect. Both mood and affect aspects of the client's emotional state may be rated in terms of its quality, stability, reactivity, intensity, and duration.

SPEECH AND LANGUAGE

The mechanics and production of speech are the characteristics that need to be examined in this section. Observations can be recorded with reference to the

rate, volume, spontaneity, monotone, articulation, rhythm, intensity, pitch, reaction time, syntax, and vocabulary. Any abnormalities in these areas are recorded, using specific quotes and examples. In addition to the production aspects of speech, the MSE should also briefly explore the patient's ability to name objects and to comprehend simple questions.

FORM AND CONTENT OF THOUGHT

Thought form refers to the way in which thoughts are linked, whereas thought content describes the dominant themes or abnormalities of the client's ideas. Abnormalities of thought form are reflected in discourse that is illogical, incoherent, and lacking in goal direction. Some examples of formal thought disorder include derailment (loosening of associations); flight of ideas; perseveration (repetition of words); circumstantiality (overinclusion of inconsequential or extraneous information); clang association (words and ideas associated by rhyme or puns); neologism (invention of new words); tangentiality (responses that lead through associations to an unrelated area); and thought blocking (a sudden break in the flow of ideas).

Abnormalities of thought content fall under three main categories: delusions, ideas of reference, and obsessions. Delusions are false beliefs that are strongly adhered to, and are not shared by others. Identification of delusions may not always be straightforward, as some delusional beliefs may not be false beliefs (they could be correct) and some false beliefs are not delusional (they may be formed out of ignorance, inadequate information, or social circumstances). Ideas of reference are beliefs that everyday events hold some specific, personal, and unique significance to the client. Depending on the nature and rigidness of these ideas, such beliefs may also be delusional. Lastly, obsessions are repetitive, unwanted, and intrusive thoughts.

Information relating to thought form and content is recorded in response to general questions, with more specific probe questions where appropriate. General questions include reasons for attending the hospital, family background, and other topics covered in the history-taking interview. Questions regarding suicidal thought content should always be included in a MSE.

PERCEPTUAL DISTURBANCES

The presence of abnormal perceptual disturbances is determined by asking the client questions relating to the experience of illusions, hallucinations or feelings of depersonalization or derealization. Illusions refer to the misinterpretation or misprocessing of stimuli, whereas hallucinations occur in the absence of any appropriate external stimulus and can occur in any sensory modality. Anxiety, exhaustion, altered states of consciousness, delirium or a functional psychosis can all result in perceptual disturbances.

COGNITIVE FUNCTIONING

Several aspects of cognitive functioning are examined including orientation, attention, concentration, and memory.

Orientation is usually assessed through questions concerning person, time (day, week, month), and place (location, city).

Attention and concentration levels can be ascertained from observations of the client and whether he or she is focused or is easily distracted. Often, the interviewer will be required to repeat questions. Lack of cooperation and purposeful attempts to obstruct the process should be distinguished from a deficit in attention. Concentration may also be assessed with specific questions that require concentration (e.g., serial subtraction; spelling backwards). Alertness may also be included in this section, and is particularly relevant in a psychiatric or hospital setting. This factor is generally described on a range from fully awake to comatose and nonresponsive.

Memory is usually examined in terms of immediate and delayed recall and across verbal and nonverbal material. The MMSE includes several specific questions that assess the client's memory and potential deficits, including repetition of words, digits forwards and backwards, and delayed recall. Remote memory, or the ability to remember events of the remote past, can usually be evaluated when the clinician takes a history of the patient's presenting problem.

JUDGMENT AND INSIGHT

Judgment refers to the ability of the client to recognize and comply with the prevailing social norms of behavior, and to make appropriate choices between alternatives. Insight refers to the degree to which the client recognizes and understands that he or she has a problem, and is aware of the symptoms and illness of their condition.

SUMMARY

In summary, the MSE provides a descriptive, comprehensive, and mainly objective summary of the client's presenting behavior and thought processes as an indicator of psychological functioning at the time of the interview. It provides an important source of information for diagnosis and to guide further assessment requirements.

See also: History-Taking; Interviewing; Neuropsychological Assessment; Psychological Testing

Further Reading

Benham, A. L. (2000). The observation and assessment of young children including use of the infant-toddler mental status exam. In C. H. Zeanah, Jr. (Ed.), *Handbook of infant mental health* (2nd ed., p. 248). New York: Guilford.

Folstein, M. F., Folstein, S. E., & McHugh, P. R. (1975). Mini-mental state: A practical method for grading the cognitive state of patients for the clinician. *Journal of Psychiatric Research, 12,* 189–198.

Schogt, B., & Rewilak, D. (2001). The mental status examination. In D. K. Conn, N. Herrmann, A. Kaye, D. Rewilak, & B. Schogt (Eds.), *Practical psychiatry in the long-term care facility* (2nd ed., p. 17). Seattle: Hogrefe and Huber.

ANNA LOUISE STILLER
SUSAN HILARY SPENCE

Metabolic Disorder

See: Storage Diseases

Methamphetamines, Prenatal Exposure

DEFINITION OF PROBLEM

Methamphetamines are highly addictive synthetic psychostimulants that affect the central nervous system by causing the neurotransmitter dopamine to accumulate in the brain. This amphetamine analog can be inhaled, injected, smoked, or swallowed, with the effects being produced in 3–20 min. Depending on the method of use, methamphetamines remain present in the brain longer than other stimulant drugs, with effects lasting from 6 to as long as 24 hr. Effects include euphoria, increased activity, decreased appetite, enhanced concentration, and elevated blood pressure. As the use and dosage of this drug increase, aggressive behaviors and paranoia are common with an increased risk for malnutrition, possible stroke, convulsion, and death. Tolerance for methamphetamines occurs quickly, which contributes to increased dosing and addiction. In addition to cravings, shaking, and loss of energy during withdrawal, depression may present, with alcohol being sought after to alleviate its symptoms. Street names for this drug include meth, crank, ice, crystal, glass, and speed.

PREVALENCE

Methamphetamine is the most widely abused amphetamine, with annual prevalence rates increasing in many regions of the United States; users are primarily Caucasian. It is the only illicit substance with the same prevalence rate for pregnant and nonpregnant women (an estimated 0.2–5 percent), and is often concomitant with use of alcohol and other illicit substances.

EFFECTS

There are few studies examining the effects of prenatal methamphetamine exposure, with the existing literature hampered by methodological shortcomings, including small sample size, difficulty in establishing exposure status, and presence of confounding variables (e.g., other drugs and environmental effects). The available evidence, however, indicates that maternal methamphetamine use may impact children's development directly through prenatal exposure and indirectly through environmental effects. Methamphetamine use during pregnancy may result in a variety of complications, including premature delivery, separation of the placenta, cardiac anomalies, cranial abnormalities, fetal growth retardation, and altered neonatal behavioral patterns (e.g., abnormal reflexes and extreme irritability). Infants with prenatal exposure to methamphetamines may also exhibit elevated heart rates and rapid breathing, and may experience long-term difficulties including stunted growth, tremors, poor feeding habits, disturbed sleep patterns, poor muscle tone, and increased risk for Sudden Infant Death Syndrome (SIDS). The negative effects of prenatal exposure have also been reported to continue into early adolescence with social, physical, and school adjustment problems. Additional effects include cognitive, speech/language, and behavior problems.

Methamphetamine is relatively easy to manufacture using over-the-counter products and, therefore, it is often produced in homes. Children living in these homes are susceptible to a chaotic living environment, poor nutrition, and an increased risk for domestic violence and child abuse/neglect. Children residing in residential methamphetamine or "meth" labs are particularly susceptible to the toxic hazards of this drug through skin exposure, accidental ingestion of chemicals, and inhalation of fumes, with many testing positive for methamphetamine. Potential damage from exposure to methamphetamine chemicals includes anemia, neurologic symptoms, and respiratory problems. Further, the chemicals used in the manufacturing of methamphetamine are highly flammable, significantly increasing children's risk for burns, bodily injury, and death.

TREATMENT AND PROGNOSIS

Information related to effective treatment is sparse. Because of this limited knowledge, periodic developmental and physical evaluations are recommended throughout childhood with educational and psychological interventions provided as needed. It is also important to provide treatment for the parents. Cognitive-behavioral interventions have been found to be most effective for treating methamphetamine addiction. Methamphetamine recovery groups appear to be effective in addition to behavioral interventions to maximize the potential for long-term recovery. There are currently no particular pharmacological treatments for dependence on methamphetamine, but antidepressant medications may be helpful in treating the depressive symptoms often seen with withdrawal. Benzodiazepines can be used in cases of extreme excitement or panic, and short-term use of neuroleptics is successful for possible psychoses.

The emerging literature suggests that children reared in an environment in which methamphetamines are produced often require mental health interventions to address issues such as school problems, posttraumatic stress reactions, abuse and/or neglect, witnessing domestic violence, and aggressive acts. In addition, these children have to learn to deal with issues related to growing up in an unstructured, unpredictable environment. Drug Endangered Children (DEC) response teams incorporating a partnership between law enforcement, human services, medicine, and mental health agencies have been established in California and are growing in other areas of the country. These teams address the immediate needs of children removed from homes during lab seizures; evaluation of such programs are currently underway.

See also: Child Maltreatment; Effects of Parental Substance Abuse on Children; Family Assessment; Family Intervention; Posttraumatic Stress Disorder in Children; Substance Abuse

Further Reading

Heller, A. (2000). Neurotoxicology and developmental effects of meth and MDMA. *Effects of in utero exposure to methamphetamines.* Bethesda, MD: National Institute of Drug Abuse.

National Institute on Drug Abuse Research Report. (1998). Methamphetamine: Abuse and addiction. *National Institute of Health Publication No. 98-4210.*

Oishi, S. M., West, K. M., Stuntz, S., Miller, M., & Noble, A. L. (2000). *Drug endangered children health and safety manual.* California: Drug Endangered Children Resource Center.

http://www.cwcadd.org/dec

ROBIN H. GURWITCH
LAURA A. KNIGHT
ANDREA D. TURNER

Microcephaly

DEFINITION

Microcephaly is defined as a condition in which the circumference of the head is greater than two standard deviations below the population mean (third percentile) of head circumferences adjusted for age and sex. In humans, head circumference is correlated, albeit not perfectly, with the size of one's brain.

PREVALENCE AND CORRELATES

Microcephaly is often associated with developmental disabilities (DD), although there are no published studies as to its prevalence among people with DD. On the other hand, of known cases with microcephaly, 70–100 percent have DD. A greater proportion are classified as severely or profoundly retarded although some fall into the mild, moderate, or nonretarded range. Differences may be due to the heterogeneous types of disorganization of brain function caused by a particular person's neuropathology responsible for the microcephaly.

ETIOLOGY

Microcephaly is not caused by small head circumference, but rather by the numerous underlying physiological abnormalities related to small brain size. It occurs prenatally at 2–4 months of gestation during the period of neuronal proliferation when the embryo is multiplying its neurons before they migrate to their target organs. The size and number of proliferative neurons can be reduced by nongenetic causes such as teratogens (a chemical or disease that causes malformation of the fetus) like irradiation, alcohol, cocaine, phenylketonuria (PKU), infections (rubella, cytomegalovirus), and by genetic causes such as chromosomal disorders (Down Syndrome), autosomal dominant and recessive or X-linked recessive disorders, as well as a number of unspecified multiple anomalies. Thus, timing of the insult to the newly developing embryo is important. If it occurs earlier or later, the type of damage to the nervous system may be different. If it occurs later during fetal development, microcephaly may not result. There are also some environmental conditions, for example, failure-to-thrive, where microcephaly occurs due to poor nutrition and growth rate.

ASSESSMENT

Assessment of microcephaly is fairly simple. Head circumference is determined by a tape measure around the head at the level of the forehead and graphed on a normative growth chart (Nellhaus curve). This chart is age and sex specific from birth to 18 years of age.

TREATMENT

Microcephaly is treated by treating the conditions causing it. Rarely is it treated directly. There is evidence from animal research, however, that intensive and challenging operant training for a substantial period of time daily can actually increase brain weight by 15 percent. This has been demonstrated in rats prenatally exposed to the teratogen methylazoxymethanol injected into the mother at 15 days of gestation. This powerful toxin produces offspring with brains 60 percent of normal size. The effect of training is very dramatic to the extent that they catch up to the performance of normal rats by the time they are young adults.

PROGNOSIS

Research on early detection and intervention suggests that, while the effects of genetic birth defects are difficult to reverse, infants and young children at risk for biological (nongenetic) and environmental reasons are often very resilient. With appropriate intervention, they can often compensate for their early insults and grow up leading a normal life. Research suggests that the number of risks a child has may accumulate to worsen the prognosis. Reducing these environmental risks is very important to the success of early intervention programs.

See also: Alcohol-Related Neurodevelopmental Disorder; Cocaine, Prenatal Exposure; Cytomegalovirus Infection; Down Syndrome; Early Intervention; Fetal Alcohol Syndrome; Fragile X Syndrome; Mental Retardation; Prenatal Exposure to Opiates

Further Reading

Loupe, P. S., Schroeder, S. R., & Tessel, R. E. (1997). The behavior and neurochemistry of the methylazoxymethanol-induced microencephalic rat. In N. W. Bray (Ed.), *International review of research in mental retardation* (Vol. 21, pp. 187–220). New York: Academic Press.

Sameroff, A. J., Seifer, R., & Bartko, W. T. (1997). Environmental perspectives on adaptation during childhood and adolescence (pp. 507–526). In S. S. Luthar, J. A. Burack, D. Cicchetti, & J. R. Weisz (Eds.), *Developmental pathology: Perspectives on adjustment, risk and disorder.* Cambridge, UK: Cambridge University Press.

Volpe, J. J. (1995). *The neurology of the newborn* (3rd ed.). Philadelphia: W.B. Saunders.

Volpe, J. J. (Ed.). (2000). Normal and abnormal development of the CNS. *Mental Retardation and Developmental Disabilities Research Reviews, 6*(1), 1–79.

STEPHEN R. SCHROEDER

Migraines

DEFINITION

Migraines are acute recurrent headaches that are separated by pain-free intervals. The intensity, duration, and frequency of pain can be quite varying, as are the associated symptoms of nausea, vomiting, photophobia (hypersensitivity to light), and phonophobia (hypersensitivity to sound). They can occur with or without an aura (i.e., temporary neurological symptoms that precede the migraine [e.g., seeing spots or bright lights, trouble speaking]). Although adult migraneurs typically experience the pain unilaterally, children may experience it on both sides of their head. The headache pain

will often begin gradually, escalate over minutes to hours, and last from 2 to 48 hr. These migraine episodes typically occur several times a month. The International Headache Society has developed criteria to diagnose migraines, but the applicability of these criteria for children has been criticized.

EPIDEMIOLOGY

Migraine headaches are the most common neurological condition treated by pediatricians and pediatric neurologists. Migraines without auras are more prevalent than migraines with auras, with the former accounting for 60–85 percent of all migraines. The incidence of migraines without auras is approximately 1.4 percent, whereas the incidence of migraines with auras is 1 percent. Girls tend to have slightly higher rates of both types of migraines than boys. Boys are more likely to experience migraines younger (i.e., 5–10 years old), whereas girls tend to experience them more often in their teenage years.

MIGRAINE TYPES

Several different types of migraines can be identified based on their presenting symptoms.

1. Common migraine, which occurs without an aura, may last from 1 to 48 hr, and may be preceded by mood changes and physical signs of illness (e.g., pallor, lethargy, periorbital discoloration [i.e., circles under the eyes]).
2. Classic migraine is preceded by an aura of 15–30 min. The headache pain is often severe and throbbing, and may last for several hours. Associated symptoms include nausea and vomiting.
3. Complicated migraines are a group of migraine variants that present with a variety of neurological signs and symptoms, and need to be differentiated from more serious neurological conditions (e.g., brain tumor, intracranial hemorrhage).
   a. Basilar artery migraine presents as an intense attack of dizziness, vertigo, visual disturbances, ataxia (i.e., trouble walking), or double vision. These symptoms, which also co-occur with nausea and vomiting, tend to remit within 24 hr. This is the most common complicated migraine type.

b. Hemiplegic migraine is considered when the headache co-occurs with a recurrent muscle weakness or partial paralysis on one side of the body. The weakness or paralysis often abates within 24 hr. A familial form of this migraine exists.

c. Ophthalmoplegic migraine is a rare subtype that presents with a variety of visual problems (e.g., double vision, drooping eyelid, gaze directed outward) due to impairments of the third cranial nerve. The headache, which is often felt "behind the eye," remits sooner than the visual problems, which can last for days or weeks.

d. Confusional migraine's associated symptoms include confusion, disorientation, agitation, and difficulties producing or understanding speech. These symptoms, which may last from 6 to 12 hr, are often linked with mild head traumas. Given the confusional state, the actual headache may not be recalled.

e. "Alice in Wonderland" syndrome presents with a headache that is accompanied by visual illusions and spatial distortions (e.g., objects appear very small or very large or very far away).

4. Other variants of migraines also have headaches associated with a range of unusual neurological signs and symptoms.

a. Paroxysmal vertigo presents with a sudden unsteadiness (i.e., grab for a table or chair, fall to the ground) that lasts only a few minutes. The child does not lose consciousness, but may vomit forcefully.

b. Paroxysmal torticollis is present when the headache, nausea, and vomiting occur with a pronounced head tilt. These episodes may last for hours or days.

c. Cyclic vomiting is considered when unexplained abdominal pain, nausea, and vomiting occur. These episodes may lead to dehydration in the child. Headaches may or may not be present.

CAUSES

While the physiological process of rapid vascular expansion and restriction associated with migraines has been well established, the mechanisms that lead to migraine pain are unknown, but likely involve a combination of biopsychosocial factors. An individual who is genetically predisposed to migraines will be exposed to some internal or external trigger (e.g., low blood sugar, infection, toxin, stressor). Cortical and subcortical brain structures send impulses throughout the brain in response to the trigger, which cause inflammation and irritation of blood vessels within the brain. These signals will be perceived by the brain as "pain," but may be modified by unique characteristics of the individual (e.g., age, medical conditions, mood, previous experience with pain).

ASSESSMENT

Similar to the assessment of headaches, a thorough history of the events (e.g., severity, frequency, duration), medical and family history, and recent physical and neurological examinations are useful when evaluating an individual with migraines. Since serious neurological conditions present with similar symptoms, additional evaluative procedures are warranted (e.g., electroencephalogram [EEG], magnetic resonance imaging [MRI], magnetic resonance angiography [MRA]). At first occurrence, intense acute migraine pain, which is not associated with previous headaches, is the cardinal sign of intracerebral bleeding, and should be treated as an acute emergency.

TREATMENT

Psychological and nonpharmacological treatments of migraines can include changes in lifestyle (e.g., regular sleep patterns, avoidance of hectic schedules and "trigger" foods), stress management and relaxation techniques (e.g., progressive muscle relaxation, guided imagery, self-hypnosis), biofeedback, and individual or family therapy. Pharmacological interventions for migraines typically address: (1) alleviating pain and associated symptoms, (2) aborting an episode that has just started, or (3) preventing future episodes. Although a physician will oversee this aspect of treatment, a mental health professional should be aware of these additional intervention strategies. Effective management of migraines often requires a multimodal approach in which several of the above methods are incorporated into an individual treatment plan.

See also: Biofeedback; Headache; Neurologic Examination; Pain Assessment; Pain Management; Pediatric Hypnosis; Stress Management

Further Reading

McGrath, P. A., & Hillier, L. M. (2001). *The child with headache: Diagnosis and treatment.* Seattle: IASP Press.

Winner, P., & Rothner, A. D. (2001). *Headache in children and adolescents.* Lewiston, NY: B.C. Decker.

KEVIN DUFF
JAMES SCOTT

Mixed Hearing Loss

See: Hearing Impairment

Mixed Receptive–Expressive Language Disorder

DEFINITION

Mixed receptive–expressive language disorder is characterized by impairment in both language comprehension (receptive language) and language production (expressive language). Individuals with problems in receptive language may have difficulty understanding words, sentences, questions, directions, and other aspects of spoken language. Individuals with expressive language problems may have a limited vocabulary, produce errors in grammar or syntax in sentences that are inappropriate for their age, or a general difficulty expressing their ideas (American Psychiatric Association, 2000). Although an expressive language disorder can occur in the absence of receptive language deficits, it is uncommon to find a purely receptive language disorder. As young children acquire language, their expressive language skills are based upon their receptive skills. (Sign language is an appropriate means of communication, but verbal communication will be the main focus of this article.) Receptive and expressive language difficulties are distinguished from speech (phonological or articulation) difficulties, which involve the failure to use developmentally speech sounds that are appropriate for an individual's age and dialect as stated in the *Diagnostic and Statistical Manual of Mental Disorders, Fourth Edition (DSM-IV)*.

The child's cognitive development, or ability to problem-solve, reason, and otherwise use deductive skills to process information, has a major effect on language development. If there are cognitive deficits, language typically will be deficient as well. If both cognitive and language skills are delayed to a similar degree, a mixed receptive–expressive language disorder would not be diagnosed. This is because the individual's language skills are commensurate with cognitive skills. If one's cognitive abilities are average or above, and language abilities are significantly lower, then it may be appropriate to diagnose a mixed receptive–expressive language disorder.

CAUSES

Receptive and expressive language disorders have many possible causes, and can be either developmental (i.e., apparent from young childhood) or acquired (disorders that occur after some precipitating event such as an illness or accident that affects the brain). Hereditary or genetic factors may explain some cases of the developmental type of mixed receptive–expressive language disorders, as these disorders are more common in first-degree biological relatives than in the general population according to *DSM-IV*.

The developmental type occurs more often in males than in females. For acquired disorders, there is no evidence that hereditary factors are involved. Acquired disorders may result from certain types of brain trauma, stroke, or brain lesions that can occur at any age. The nature of the acquired language disorder depends upon the specific location and severity of brain pathology involved. Many individuals with the developmental type of mixed receptive–expressive language disorder have no discernable cause.

Other causes to rule out include hearing loss, behavioral concerns, psychosocial issues, auditory processing, and other such factors. Each of these factors may interfere with and/or add to receptive and expressive language challenges.

INCIDENCE

Children with language disorders represent more than one million students in the public school setting. Boys represent an increased prevalence by nearly a 2 : 1 ratio. (Retrieved April 2, 2002, from http://www.asha.org/speech/development/schools_faq.cfm) Research has clearly shown that intervention in the form of early identification, diagnosis, and therapy is the most effective method of treatment.

WARNING SIGNS AND SYMPTOMS

There are several "red flags" that may indicate that there are receptive and expressive language deficits, including speech avoidance; giving inappropriate or incorrect answers during conversation; difficulty using words to express feelings, emotions, wants, and needs; using a limited vocabulary; as well as using short phrases and sentences. Other signs include requiring frequent repetitions of instructions, displaying unresponsiveness when spoken to, and using nonverbal communication (pointing and gesturing) in response to verbally stated information.

In addition, an increase in frustration level, behavioral concerns, poor academic performance, and poor peer relations may be indicative of a language disorder.

Although all children are different and progress at different rates, an evaluation is the best way to assess if there are true concerns that put the child at risk.

APPROACHES TO ASSESSMENT

Diagnosis of a mixed receptive–expressive language disorder requires that an individual be administered standardized tests of both receptive and expressive language, and that their scores fall significantly below those obtained from standardized measures of their nonverbal intellectual functioning. If an individual has mental retardation, a hearing impairment or deafness, a motor-speech disorder, or environmental deprivation, their language difficulties must be greater than those usually associated with these problems before a diagnosis of mixed receptive–expressive language disorder is made (American Psychiatric Association, 2000). Individuals with a diagnosis of one of the Pervasive Developmental Disorders (PDD) typically have disorders in their receptive and expressive language as part of their PDD, and a separate diagnosis of mixed receptive–expressive language disorder is not made in these cases. It is important to assess whether difficulty with receptive and expressive language significantly interferes with the individual's academic or occupational achievement, or with social aspects of communication (American Psychiatric Association, 2000).

Following the administration of standardized testing, an analysis of errors can provide a map to define therapy goals. The scores determine a qualitative description of deficits. There are many different test batteries that allow for customization of the evaluation by targeting specific language concepts. Evaluation measures should be selected based upon age of the individual, suspected deficits, and the individual's current level of functioning.

Informal evaluation measures also provide valuable information. A detailed case history, language sample, hearing screening/evaluation, and the identification of other concomitant factors such as mental retardation and PDD are essential. Thus, collaboration with a psychologist to get a more comprehensive evaluation of a child's cognitive, developmental, and emotional functioning can be helpful. A skilled and credentialed clinician can also make informal inferences that aid diagnosis of communication deficits.

ACTIVITIES TO ENCOURAGE LANGUAGE SKILLS

Language is the ability to communicate our experiences. Activities such as reading to a child, providing a stimulating environment, exposure to new vocabulary and experiences, modeling appropriate language responses, and encouraging the use of communication provide the child with the tools to become a proficient language user. These activities encourage the steady development of new language concepts and ideas.

REFERRAL RESOURCES FOR ADDITIONAL INFORMATION

A speech–language pathologist is trained to perform language assessments and aid parents and other professionals in providing diagnosis, and if needed, intervention. It may be beneficial to contact the American Speech–Language Hearing Association (A.S.H.A.) to locate a therapist in one's area. A.S.H.A. recommends licensure in the state in which the speech–language pathologist is practicing. The Certificate of Clinical Competence (CCC) in Speech Pathology is awarded to a clinician with a Master's degree who has completed hands-on treatment and evaluation of clients in a variety of settings. A.S.H.A. can be reached at http://www.asha.org or at the Action Center Hotline at 1-800-498-2071. Speech–language pathologists can be found in a variety of settings such as hospitals, schools, private practices, rehabilitation facilities, state and local health departments, as well as colleges and universities.

Another resource is the National Information Center for Children and Youth with Disabilities. It provides information regarding current issues about a variety of diagnoses and can be reached at http://www.nichcy.org

See also: Adolescent Assessment; Central Auditory Processing Disorders; Cognitive Development; Hearing Impairment; Language Development; Preschool Assessment; Phonological and Articulation Disorders; School-Age Assessment; Selective Mutism

Further Reading

American Psychiatric Association. (2000). *Diagnostic and Statistical Manual of Mental Disorders, Fourth Edition, Text Revision.* Washington, DC: Author.

SHALONDA WILLIAMS

Modeling

See: Participant Modeling; Videotape Modeling

Mood Stabilizer

See: Pharmacological Interventions

Moral Development

One of the fundamental aspects of socialization and social development is the internalization of group norms and rules. This is generally reflected in the emergence of children's understanding of, and judgments about, right from wrong. This topic has been researched and theorized under the headings of *moral development* and *moral reasoning*. Moral reasoning is defined as the cognitive process by which individuals make decisions about moral issues and justify these decisions, regardless of the content of the issue. Given that every moral issue has different potential perspectives from which judgments can be derived, interest in the developmental processes at hand have not necessarily been in the solution the individual child reaches, but the processes by which the individual child comes to that solution.

EARLY RESEARCH

Research on moral development was first done through the observation of children's game-playing by Jean Piaget, who identified two stages of moral development: *moral realism* and *moral relativism*. Children in the moral realism stage view rules as fixed and absolute entities that emanate from authoritative sources (i.e., parents and teachers). As such, judgments about right and wrong are correspondingly inflexible, and based on tangible consequences, rather than on intent. For example, young children will judge intentional harm with the same moral severity as accidental harm, because the moral inference is drawn solely from the harmful consequence, not the intent.

When a child reaches the moral relativism stage, they abandon rigid obedience of rules, and instead base moral judgment more on the equity and fairness of human interactions. Children now understand that rules can be changed and moral reasoning becomes correspondingly adaptable. In addition, the circumstances and intent of the consequences are considered in the moral analysis. More recent work has shown that children are more multifaceted in their moral reasoning than was originally thought by Piaget.

KOHLBERG'S FRAMEWORK OF MORAL DEVELOPMENT

The most influential theory of moral development is that of Lawrence Kohlberg, who extended the work of Piaget. Kohlberg suggests that the development of moral reasoning can be reduced to a taxonomy of three levels, each of which is composed of two stages. Each stage represents an increase in the complexity or richness of moral reasoning, as compared to the earlier stage. Before attaining a new stage, a child or adult must achieve moral reasoning that is necessary for the current stage, but there is no requirement or guarantee that individuals will pass through lower stages or levels to higher ones.

In the first level, labeled *preconventional*, the essence of moral values lay in the external environment. In the first stage of this level, moral actions are chosen based simply on the principle of avoiding punishment. The second stage reflects a more naïve egotistic orientation, in which moral actions are chosen based on personal satisfaction.

In the second level, labeled *conventional*, moral values are determined by maintaining social values or expectations. In the first stage of this level, the child is oriented in terms of a good boy/good girl taxonomy, and moral actions are chosen based on the approval that the actions will elicit from others. It is also conformity to stereotypical images of how they should behave. The second stage of this level is oriented toward authority and the maintenance of social order, and so moral actions are chosen to the degree that they reflect respect for authority.

In the third, *postconventional* level, moral values are determined by internal values of what is right and/or wrong. The first stage of this level reflects an orientation toward the "social contract," and moral actions are based on abstract principles that are focused on larger societal goals. Laws or institutional rules are believed to have a rational basis, and emphasize equality, liberty, and justice. Thus, if conflict arises between the laws and one's internal values, the values typically prevail in forming the moral judgment. The final stage of this level (and of the framework in general) is one oriented toward universal ethics. Decisions are based on respect for universal principles and the demands of the individual's conscience. According to Kohlberg, few individuals reach this level of moral reasoning.

Kohlberg assumed that this framework of moral development reflected a universal developmental trend, although the level of attainment of moral level was believed to vary. The lasting criticisms of Kohlberg's framework have focused on this assumption, given that Kohlberg's theory was based on samples that were narrow both in terms of context and time (e.g., the subject pool was upper-class Caucasian males and all data was collected in the early 1960s).

GENDER AND MORAL DEVELOPMENT

Carol Gilligan has argued that Kohlberg's theory may have overlooked important sex differences in the definition of mature moral reasoning. Gilligan's research has suggested that moral reasoning may be based on very different principles among women than among men: women's moral judgments may be guided more by caring and maintaining relationships, whereas men's moral judgments may emphasize more rules and abstract principles of justice. Owing to differences in the way that men and women are socialized, their respective concepts of justice and morality may be different, and as such, they will exhibit important differences in the form and nature of mature moral reasoning.

CLINICAL IMPLICATIONS

The development of moral reasoning is guided by a child's cognitive development. As children develop more cognitive abilities they incorporate these abilities when they are making moral judgments. Similarly, the environment plays an essential role in the development of moral reasoning. What children experience and learn from parents, teachers, and peers influence their ability to reason about right and wrong. People who do not develop higher levels of moral reasoning do not gain awareness of the implications of their actions and as a result will engage in behavior regardless of the ultimate consequences for themselves and others or society, in general.

See also: Antisocial Behavior; Cognitive Development; Disruptive Behavior Disorders; Lying; Parenting Practices

Further Reading

Gardiner, H., Mutter, J., & Kosmitzki (1998). *Lives across cultures: Cross-cultural human development.* Needham Heights, MA: Allyn & Bacon

Newcombe, N. (1996). *Child development: Change over time.* New York: HarperCollins.

Kohlberg, L. (1994). Stage and sequence: The cognitive-developmental approach to socialization. In B. Puka (Ed.), *Defining perspectives in moral development. Moral development: A compendium* (Vol. 1, pp. 1–134). New York: Garland.

OTILIA M. BLAGA
JOHN COLOMBO

Mothers' and Fathers' Roles in Abnormal Child Development

HISTORICAL CONTEXT

Although there is a great deal known about both mothers' and fathers' roles in normal child development, research on abnormal child development has focused largely on the mother–child relationship. Research on fathers' roles in abnormal child development has lagged behind research on mothers' roles in abnormal development. There are a number of possible reasons for this imbalance, including sexist theories, mother blaming, and difficulty in recruiting fathers into clinically oriented research.

Another barrier to mother and father equity in family research has to do with family demographics. Historically, it has been the norm that children lived with both their mother and their father. Although there were many exceptions to this norm, most children were raised in two-parent families. Over the past four decades, this norm has shifted drastically. Currently, well over half of children under the age of 18 still live with their biological mother and biological father, but there are a large number of children who live in other family constellations (e.g., single-mother-headed household, stepfamily, single-father-headed household, grandparent-headed household). The prevalence of nontraditional families is even more evident in families with children who are referred for clinical services. For these reasons, it appears that fathers are often assumed to be absent from children's lives and thus they are often not invited to take part in clinical research.

Even with this caution in mind, there are some clear patterns that have emerged from the research on the roles of mothers and fathers in abnormal child development. Two primary research methodologies have been used, so these findings will be reviewed separately. Specifically, researchers interested in parents and the development of child psychopathology have explored the parents of children with psychological problems and the children of parents with psychological problems.

MOTHERS AND FATHERS OF TROUBLED CHILDREN

When the mothers and fathers of troubled children are investigated, different patterns of findings emerge depending on the type of problem exhibited by the child. In general, the mothers of children with internalizing problems (such as depression or anxiety disorders) tend to show significantly more problems themselves than do mothers of children in nonclinical control groups. Specifically, mothers of children who are depressed tend to show higher levels of depression themselves and mothers of children with anxiety problems tend to show higher levels of anxiety themselves. In contrast, fathers of children with internalizing problems do not differ significantly from fathers of children in nonclinical control groups. Thus, there are few meaningful differences between fathers of children with internalizing problems and fathers of children in nonclinical control groups.

When considering parents of children with externalizing problems (such as Oppositional Defiant Disorder [ODD] or Conduct Disorder [CD]), both mothers and fathers show more psychopathology (such as antisocial behaviors, substance abuse, and depression)

than mothers and fathers of children in nonclinical control groups. These patterns are true across family constellations, regardless of whether or not the mothers and fathers remain involved in their children's lives.

CHILDREN OF TROUBLED PARENTS

With the second type of research methodology, where children of parents with psychological problems are compared with children of well-functioning parents, clear patterns emerge. For almost every type of psychopathology that has been evaluated, children of psychologically disturbed mothers and fathers are at greater risk for developing psychopathology than are children of mothers in nonclinical control groups.

Thus, the connections between psychological problems in mothers and their children are complex and have both differences and similarities to the connections between psychological problems in fathers and their children. These patterns have clear implications for educational, medical, and clinical settings.

RELEVANCE TO PRACTICE

When considering the research literature about both normal and abnormal development, it is clear that both mothers and fathers are important in children's lives. Mothers and fathers can contribute to child development in both helpful and harmful ways. Mothers and fathers can work together with professionals to improve child and family functioning. Unfortunately, professionals often do not include mothers or fathers in their therapeutic work with children. In a recent survey of practicing clinicians by Duhig and colleagues, only 58 percent of clinicians included mothers in child-oriented therapy sessions and only 30 percent of clinicians included fathers in child-oriented therapy sessions.

Given the research findings on the connections between parents' functioning and children's functioning, it is important for day care workers, teachers, nurses, physicians, social workers, psychologists, and other professionals to consider inviting both mothers and fathers to take part in activities that enhance children's lives. Furthermore, fathers should be considered for participation in research studies. Not all mothers and fathers will agree to participate, but it is imperative to make the invitation explicit to both parents.

Overall, there are more similarities than differences between the roles of mothers and fathers in abnormal child development. It is incumbent upon professionals involved in improving children's lives to identify the helpful agents of change for that child—and sometimes fathers as well as mothers can be part of that process.

See also: Emotional Development; Fathers' Role in Treatment; Mothers' and Fathers' Roles in Normal Child Development; Parent–Child Interaction Therapy; Parenting Practices

Further Reading

Goodman, S. H., & Gotlib, I. H. (2002). *Children of depressed parents: Mechanisms of risk and implications for treatment.* Washington, DC: American Psychological Association.

Lamb, M. E. (Ed.). (1997). *The role of the father in child development* (3rd ed.). New York: Wiley.

Phares, V. (1999). *Poppa psychology: The role of fathers in children's mental well-being.* Westport, CT: Praeger.

Vicky Phares
Amy M. Duhig
Tangela R. Clark
Dimitra Kamboukos

Mothers' and Fathers' Roles in Normal Child Development

HISTORICAL CONTEXT

Current research suggests that both mothers and fathers have a role in the normative development of their children. In contrast to mothers, however, very little research has been conducted on the father–child relationship. Ironically, until the mid-1700s, parenting books were actually geared toward fathers. That practice was probably due to the fact that men (and fathers) were more likely to read than women (and mothers) and that families in Europe and America were patriarchal in structure. In the early 1800s, families became much more matriarchal in structure, partially due to men's work away from the home as a result of the Industrial Revolution. Since the mid-1800s, parenting books have been geared primarily toward mothers, and mothers have been considered the primary parent in the large majority of families.

Within the last 40 years, there has been a bit more of a focus on the father–child relationship. For example, in the mid-1970s, childrearing books began to appear that were geared specifically toward fathers. Professional research on the father–child relationship in normative development also began to flourish around that time and continues to this day. There continues to be a dearth, however, of research into the father–child relationship regarding abnormal development and psychopathology.

When both mothers and fathers are investigated in professional research, it is clear that both mothers and fathers play important roles in the development of their children. Although differences are evident, there tend to be more similarities than differences between the role and function of mothers and fathers.

DIFFERENCES

There are a number of differences as well as similarities when the mother–child relationship and the father–child relationship are compared. Regarding differences, the most salient difference that consistently emerges between fathers and mothers is the amount of time spent with their children. From birth through adulthood, mothers tend to spend significantly more time with their children than do fathers. There are debates as to whether this difference is by necessity, or choice, or some other factor (such as social expectations), but there are probably multiple and complex reasons for this pattern. Closely related to the amount of time spent with children is the issue of responsibility for children. Here again, mothers tend to have more responsibility than fathers in nearly every domain of childrearing (e.g., caretaking, homework, discipline, medical and dental appointments, dealing with teachers, etc.). These patterns of time spent and level of responsibility appear to be consistent across different family constellations (e.g., married two-parent families, single-mother families, stepfamilies).

When fathers do spend time with their offspring, they tend to be much more playful with their infants and children than are mothers. Although these group differences are not found in every family, fathers tend to spend proportionally more time playing with their children than do mothers—even when completing caretaking activities (such as changing diapers, feeding the child, or doing homework). Neither pattern of playful behavior is better or worse—they are just different. Despite these differences between mothers and fathers, there are a great deal of important similarities as well.

SIMILARITIES

In general, both mothers and fathers spend the greatest amount of time with infants and toddlers, less time with preschoolers, less time with school-aged children than preschoolers, and even less time with adolescents. These patterns are due largely to the demands of child rearing in the earlier years and to the likelihood that older children and adolescents spend increasing amounts of time with friends and in activities outside the home.

Another meaningful similarity between mothers and fathers relates to the quality of parenting. In general, the authoritative parenting style is associated with the best outcomes for children. Specifically, parents who provide warmth and affection in addition to age-appropriate and consistent limits and structure tend to have children who are well-adjusted. The authoritative parenting style appears to be advantageous whether it is used by mothers, fathers, stepmothers, stepfathers, caretaking grandparents, gay or lesbian parents, foster parents, or any other caretaking adult. Researchers believe that the combination of emotional warmth and clear guidelines (that are well-articulated in an age-appropriate manner) is the most advantageous pattern for parents to follow.

In addition, for both mothers and fathers, it appears that the quality of time spent with children is more meaningful than the quantity of time (within limits). Thus, children of mothers or fathers who are able to carve out time from their work schedule and who use the time well (e.g., playing and talking with their children, being emotionally available to the child, taking part in activities that the child enjoys, helping the child with tasks, supporting the child's development) are probably better off than children of parents who spend greater amounts of time with their child in less than optimal circumstances (e.g., yelling at the child, talking on the phone, or using the computer for long periods of the time when the child wants the parent's attention). Each family has to develop its own balance between parents' needs and children's needs, but it is interesting to point out that these patterns tend to be similar for mothers and fathers (whether the parents are married, divorced, separated, or never married).

Thus, there are both differences and similarities between mothers and fathers regarding normal child development. Interestingly, much of what we know about adaptive parenting is not only true for mothers and fathers, but is also true for any primary caretaker for children (e.g., a caretaking grandmother, a stepmother, an uncle who has primary custody, a nonbiologically related primary caretaker). The quality of parenting appears to have more of a connection to children's well-being than the actual title of the person providing the caretaking.

See also: Fathers' Role in Treatment; Mothers' and Fathers' Roles in Abnormal Child Development; Parenting Practices

Further Reading

American Academy of Pediatrics. (1998). *Caring for your baby and young child: Birth to age 5*. New York: Bantam Books.

Griswold, R. L. (1993). *Fatherhood in America: A history*. New York: Basic Books.

Parke, R. D. (1996). *Fatherhood*. Cambridge, MA: Harvard University Press.

VICKY PHARES
M. MONICA WATKINS
SHERECCE FIELDS

Motor Development

DEFINITION

The field of motor development generally studies the maturation of the child's fluency and control over the movement of the body's muscles. Motor development is an important factor in overall child development, given that the acquisition of motor skills allows the child to explore and manipulate his or her environment. This in turn allows for development in both the cognitive and social realms.

The development of motor skills proceeds in a cephalocaudal direction, with skills involving the upper parts of the body developing before skills involving the lower parts of the body. Development is also proximodistal, with control of the more proximal parts of the body (e.g., large muscles of the neck, shoulder, trunk, and thighs) emerging before control over the extremities (e.g., wrists and hands). There are several motor milestones that a child will reach during each period in development. Infants and children attain motor skills in a relatively invariant sequence. The age at which these motor skills are attained (motor "milestones") are provided in Table 1 as a guide, although the ages at which these milestones occur show a great deal of variation among infants and children.

INFANT MOTOR DEVELOPMENT

Reflexes

At birth, the infant possesses a variety of involuntary reflexes that are controlled by the more primitive areas of the brain. However, as the higher areas of the brain (e.g., in the cerebral cortex) mature, voluntary movements eventually displace the reflexes. Some of the infant reflexes appear to be adaptive for survival (e.g., the rooting and sucking reflexes made to initiate and maintain feeding). However, the purpose of other infant reflexes is not clear. Because these reflexes represent subcortical functioning, their presence can be used to evaluate maturity and neurological intactness using a scale such as the Brazelton Neonatal Behavioral Assessment.

Voluntary Motor Skills

By about 4–5 months of age, reflexes disappear and are replaced by cortex-directed voluntary movements that are more deliberate and accurately executed than the reflexes. These skills include, eye–hand coordination, head control, posture, and various types of locomotion. Table 1 lists some of the major motor developments in infancy.

Eye–Hand Coordination

The first stage in eye–hand coordination is pre-reaching, in which the infant will swat at items within the field of vision. At 7 weeks of age, the infant will begin reaching with a closed fist. Between 3–5 months of age, infants use vision to guide their reaching. Simultaneously, voluntary grasping ("prehension") emerges, with infants at first using the larger areas of the hand (e.g., palm) to pick up objects. By 9 months of age, infant acquire the use of their thumb, and at 1 year, infants can pick up items in a fully mature fashion.

Table 1. Major Motor Milestones of Infancy

Motor milestone	Age of appearance (months)
Visually directed reaching	3–5
Pick up items in mature manner	12
Control of head when held in sitting position	2–4
Rolling over	2–6
Scooting, crawling, creeping	7–9
Sit independently	5–8
Stand independently	10–13
Walking	11–15

Posture and Locomotion

Postural development begins with the improvement of head control at 2–4 months of age. This is followed by various forms of rolling, and eventually leads to locomotion. Early locomotion may take on several forms including scooting, crawling, and creeping, and these abilities begin between 7 and 9 months of age. At 8–10 months of age, the infant gains the ability to pull themselves into a standing position, and between 10 and 13 months of age the infant is able to stand alone. Soon after, the infant gains the ability to stand and walking begins, and by the second year children can climb stairs, run, and jump.

CHILDHOOD MOTOR DEVELOPMENT

Early Childhood Motor Development

Between 3 and 6 years of age, children rapidly develop a large number motor skills. Gross motor behaviors (i.e., those mediated by large muscle groups) enable children to participate in games and sports. These activities include, the ability to ascend (3 years of age) and descend (4–5 years) stairways; starting, turning, and stopping while running (4–5 years); jumping longer distances; and hopping (3–5 years). In addition, fine motor abilities (i.e., those mediated by small muscles in the hands, face, and eyes) assist them in self-help skills, games, and craft and drawing projects. Between 2 and 3 years of age, children are able to copy a straight line and build a tower of blocks. By 5 years they are able to button shirts, tie shoes, cut a straight line with scissors, and copy letters and numbers.

Middle Childhood Motor Development

Between 6 and 12 years of age, children are developing more complex motor skills, and some sex differences in motor development are beginning to emerge, although the sources of these differences are unclear. During middle childhood, children are developing the ability to shift their weight when throwing, walk on a balance beam, grip with more pressure, and run farther. In general, children are gaining more accuracy, strength, and distance in their motor skills.

Adolescent Motor Development

After the age of 13, the gap between the sexes on tests of large-muscle activities is widened, with boys making gains and girls staying the same or declining.

Before puberty, there is no need to separate girls from boys in physical activities; however, after puberty, the lighter and smaller frames of girls make them more susceptible to injury from heavier boys in collision sports.

CLINICAL IMPLICATIONS

Influences on Motor Development

Both maturation and experience contribute to the development of motor skills. Some of the influences that can affect motor development are culture, muscle strength and tone, nutrition, and practice. In the early stages of motor development, different cultural childrearing practices such as freedom from restrictive clothing, stretching exercises, and sensorimotor stimulation can advance motor development; however, these advances seem to disappear by the end of infancy. Overall, attempts to advance motor skills through training have yielded success at first, but, with age the advances disappear. In addition, motor development seems to be resilient to effects such as impoverished environments, but does not seem to be able to recover from setbacks due to malnutrition during the first year of life.

Disabilities

Although individual differences may be seen in motor development, and most delays in the acquisition of major motor milestones may not be indicative of later motor delays, some children show persistent delays that may be signs of a neuromotor disorder. Current research is seeking to refine the measurement of motor function. This will undoubtedly assist in the goal of identification and early diagnosis of physical disabilities. Disorders that generally involve motor delays include mental retardation, hypotonia in Down syndrome, cerebral palsy, and autism spectrum disorders. Although some children with mental disabilities may present persistent delays in motor development, not all children that have these disabilities show this delay.

See also: Cerebral Palsy Neurological Disorders; Muscular Dystrophy (Duchenne); Neurological Examination; Visual–Motor Assessment

Further Reading

Corbin, C. (1973). *A textbook of motor development.* Dubuque, IA: Brown.
Dennis, W. (1960). Causes of retardation among institutional children: Iran. *Journal of Genetic Psychology, 96,* 47–59.
Espenschade, A. (1960). Motor development. In W. R. Johnson (Ed.), *Science and medicine of exercise and sports.* New York: Harper & Row.
Fetters, L. (1996). Motor development. In M. Hanson (Ed.), *Atypical infant development* (2nd ed., pp. 403–450). Austin, TX: Pro-Ed.
Shaffer, D. R. (Ed.). (1998). *Developmental psychology: Childhood and adolescence* (5th ed.). Pacific Grove: Brooks/Cole.

CHRISTA J. ANDERSON
JOHN COLOMBO

Mourning

See: Bereavement

Movement Disorders

See: Chorea: Sydenham's and Huntington's; Tic Disorders: Tourette's Disorder, Chronic Tic Disorder, and Transient Tic Disorder

Mullerian Agenesis Syndrome

See: Mayer–Rokitansky–Küster–Hauser Syndrome

Multiple Sclerosis

DESCRIPTION OF THE DISEASE

Multiple sclerosis is a progressive disease of the central nervous system that destroys the insulation around the nerve fibers in the central nervous system, which includes both the brain and spinal cord. There is tremendous variability in the overall expression of multiple sclerosis depending upon where the particular degenerative process is located and the stage of such changes. Symptoms include varying combinations of dizziness, weakness, spasticity, motor unsteadiness, variable bladder control, weakness, and general fatigue. Remissions and exacerbations are very common leading to obvious mood changes. Associated mood changes include anxiety and depression, which are very common and related to both organic factors and functional impact of the disease process. Complicated changes in the motor, sensory, and cognitive system are all possible because of the wide-ranging systemic effects of multiple sclerosis.

ETIOLOGY

Causes of multiple sclerosis are unknown at this time. However, it is believed to be an autoimmune disease related to some form of virus. Onset is usually in the second to fourth decade of life; it is more common in women.

ASSESSMENT/TREATMENT

Assessment of multiple sclerosis consists of a combination of clinical neurological alternating changes, selected laboratory findings, impairments on evoked potential visual studies, EMG, and specific brain imaging findings on CT/MRI.

Currently there is no specific cure for multiple sclerosis and attention is focused on assisting with general management of associated neurological and psychological effects. A variety of muscle relaxants and antispasmodics are often utilized. Psychosocial and emotional consequences of multiple sclerosis are very significant in this chronic, lifelong condition. One of the more difficult aspects of multiple sclerosis relates to its overall unpredictability and changing physical symptoms.

PROGNOSIS

The prognosis is variable with periods of remission followed by further degeneration and limits in daily functioning.

See also: Anxiety Disorders; Coping with Illness; Depressive Disorder Major; Psychological Impact of a Parent's Chronic Illness

Further Reading

Falvo, D. R. (1991). *Medical and psychosocial aspects of chronic illness and disability*. Gaithersburg, MD: Aspen.
Livneh, H., & Antoak, R. (1997). *Psychosocial adaptation to chronic illness and disability*. Gaithersburg, MD: Aspen.
Web site: National Multiple Sclerosis Society: http://www.nmss.org

DENNIS C. HARPER

Multisystemic Therapy

DEFINITION

Multisystemic therapy (MST) is an intensive family- and evidence-based treatment for adolescents presenting serious clinical problems developed by Henggeler and colleagues (1998, 2002). Youths referred to MST programs are at imminent risk of costly out-of-home placement such as residential treatment, incarceration, group home care, or psychiatric hospitalization. The overarching goals of MST programs are to prevent out-of-home placements and maintain youths in the community by providing caregivers with the resources and support needed to attenuate those problems that are leading community stakeholders (e.g., juvenile justice authorities) to recommend or mandate placement.

METHOD

MST services are comprehensive and provided by masters' level clinicians working in teams of 3–4 practitioners. Clinicians have caseloads of 4–6 families each, which enable them to pay significant attention to family engagement in treatment and high intensity of services. Clinicians are available 24 hr a day/7 days a week to respond to crises that might lead to placment and to decrease barriers to service access. Treatment duration averages approximately 4 months, and treatment termination is based primarily on the attainment of treatment goals.

Several features are critical to the success of MST. First, interventions target known risk factors across the youth's social network (i.e., family, peers, school, and neighborhood). For example, consistent sets of risk factors have been identified for serious antisocial behavior in adolescents, including criminal activity and substance abuse. These include individual characteristics of the adolescent (e.g., poor problem solving skills, favorable attitudes toward drug use), aspects of family functioning (e.g., low supervision and monitoring, low warmth, high conflict), caregiver functioning (e.g., drug problems, untreated mental illness), association with deviant peers, poor school performance, and low levels of social support for the family. In an individualized fashion, MST examines these risk factors and determines which particular factors are applicable to an identified problem. Initial treatment plans are then developed based on this analysis.

Second, the interventions delivered by MST clinicians are based on nine treatment principles specified in two treatment manuals. Importantly, these principles guide the design of interventions that use techniques from other evidence-based treatment models, such as behavior therapy, cognitive–behavior therapy, pragmatic family therapy, and psychopharmacological interventions that have empirical support. As described subsequently, however, these techniques are used within programmatic and philosophical frameworks that differ from those used in more traditional mental health services.

Third, MST programs are committed to overcoming barriers to service access. This commitment is operationalized through the use of a home-based model of service delivery. Thus, treatment is delivered in home, school, and other community settings at times convenient to the participants. The use of a home-based model also helps to engage families in treatment and enables clinicians to gather more valid assessment data on which to base clinical decisions.

Fourth, several studies have demonstrated associations between therapist adherence to MST treatment principles and youth outcomes. Hence, MST programs include intensive and ongoing quality assurance protocols aimed at optimizing youth outcomes by promoting treatment fidelity. Components of the quality assurance system include manualization of key program features (i.e., treatment, supervision, expert consultation, and organizational manuals), site development to assure funding and interagency collaboration, training of therapists, clinical supervision following specified protocols, weekly phone consultation with an MST expert, booster training sessions, and use of an Internet-based treatment fidelity feedback system (www.mstinstitute.org).

Fifth, caregivers are viewed as the key to achieving long-term outcomes. Hence, the majority of clinical resources are devoted to determining barriers to effective parenting (e.g., parental drug abuse), and designing and implementing interventions to overcome these barriers. Together, these features are largely responsible for the favorable clinical outcomes and cost savings achieved by MST programs.

CLINICAL APPLICATIONS

MST has traditionally focused on those youths presenting very serious clinical problems (e.g., criminal violence, substance abuse, and serious emotional disturbance) that cost service systems considerable fiscal resources due to high rates of out-of-home placement. As noted subsequently, MST has been best validated in the treatment of serious antisocial behavior,

producing long-term reductions in rearrest and incarceration. As a result of this success, significant demand for the development of MST programs has emerged during the past few years. Currently, licensed MST programs are operating in 27 states and 7 nations, serving approximately 7,000 serious juvenile offenders per year (1 percent of the eligible clinical population). Although MST studies are currently examining adaptation of the model for treating a variety of other serious problems, such as physical abuse, sexual abuse, and psychiatric emergencies, these variations are not yet ready for dissemination to community-based organizations.

EFFECTIVENESS

MST has been widely cited as an effective or promising treatment by major federal entities such as the Surgeon General's Office and the National Institutes of Health. Accolades have been based on findings from eight published randomized trials of MST—three with violent and chronic juvenile offenders, one with substance-abusing delinquents, one with youths presenting psychiatric emergencies, one with juvenile sexual offenders, one with maltreating families, and one with inner-city delinquents. These findings have shown that in comparison with youths in control conditions, MST has consistently achieved:

- reduced criminal activity
- reduced out-of-home placements
- considerable cost savings
- improved family functioning
- reduced substance use
- reduced psychiatric symptomatology
- increased school attendance
- higher consumer satisfaction
- higher rates of treatment completion

Moreover, several MST randomized trials that included long-term follow-ups have shown that favorable outcomes were maintained through at least 4 years.

In addition to these published studies, approximately 15 randomized MST trials are currently in progress. Some are multisite effectiveness studies focusing on serious juvenile offenders. Others are adapting MST to different clinical populations or using additional models of service delivery.

See also: Aggression; Antisocial Behavior; Community Interventions; Delinquent Behavior; Disruptive Behavior Disorders; Substance Abuse

Further Reading

Henggeler, S. W., Schoenwald, S. K., Borduin, C. M., Rowland, M. D., & Cunningham, P. B. (1998). *Multisystemic treatment of antisocial behavior in children and adolescents.* New York: Guilford.

Henggeler, S. W., Schoenwald, S. K., Rowland, M. D., & Cunningham, P. B. (2002). *Serious emotional disturbance in children and adolescents: Multisystemic therapy.* New York: Guilford.

SCOTT W. HENGGELER

Multivariate Approach to Classification

The multivariate approach to classifying child psychopathology attempts to determine symptom patterns or syndromes through the use of multivariate statistical techniques such as factor analysis and cluster analysis. Although this approach is relatively atheoretical, it is not totally theory-free because the number and type of behaviors to be assessed need to be decided upon and entered into the analyses. The introduction of the multivariate approach was associated with the advent of computers in the 1960s and 1970s, which enable the use of multivariate analysis to identify the clustering of problems.

According to Achenbach (1995), the multivariate approach has undergone three distinct generations of research. Multivariate studies in the first generation were generally exploratory in nature, which led to the development of the ACQ Behavior Checklist, named after Achenbach, Conners, and Quay who spearheaded these efforts. The items used to tap the 12 syndromes in the ACQ were drawn largely from three existing questionnaires developed by these researchers: Achenbach's Child Behavior Questionnaire, Conners' Parent Questionnaire, and Quay and Peterson's Revised Behavior Problem Checklist. The second generation effort involved the identification of a common set of syndromes or behavioral patterns using data derived from the systematic ratings of parents. Given the findings of only a moderate relation between the child's and parent's report, the third generation effort was undertaken to examine both the similarities and differences among syndromes based on ratings from different informants. Such ratings have been obtained from different informants including the children themselves, their parents, and their teachers.

The most widely used behavior checklists are those developed by Achenbach: the Child Behavior Checklist (CBCL), the Youth Self-Report (YSR), and the Teacher's Report Form (TRF). These checklists have been used not only in a large representative population in the United States, but also in many different countries and cultural settings. They are inexpensive to administer, can be used to collect information about the children's competencies and problems within a short period of time, and have excellent psychometric properties as shown by Essau and her colleague (1997).

The CBCL is usually used to assess social competence and behavior problems in children and adolescents. It is available in two forms, one for children aged 2 and 3 years and another for the 4–18-year-olds. The social competence items of the CBCL consist of an activities scale (i.e., to measure the child's participation in sports, nonsports hobbies, activities, games, jobs, and chores), the social functioning scale (i.e., to measure the children's membership and participation in organizations, the number of friends and contacts with them, and behavior with others and alone), and the school functioning scale (i.e., to measure performance in academic subjects, placement in a regular or a special class, being promoted regularly or held back, and the presence or absence of school problems). The CBCL also contains 113 behavior problem items. Each of these items are rated by the parents on a scale ranging from 0 (not true) to 2 (very or often true), which reflect the extent to which the items are true of the child's behavior during the past 6 months.

Studies that have used the CBCL have shown the existence of two broadband syndromes: Externalizing (undercontrolled) behavior problems and internalizing (overcontrolled) behavior problems. Some characteristics associated with externalizing syndrome include temper tantrums, aggression, and destructiveness. The internalizing syndrome includes specific clusters of behaviors such as anxiety, shyness, withdrawal, and depression. Specific narrowband syndromes (e.g., schizoid, aggressive, delinquent, socially withdrawn) have been found within the two broadband syndromes of internalizing and externalizing behavior problems. Some syndromes, which do not fall within one of the two broadband categories, are listed under the "mixed" syndromes. Separate norms are available for girls and boys at ages 4–5, 6–11, and 12–16 because children make important transitions in their cognitive, physical, educational, and/or social–emotional development during these age periods.

The YSR is suitable for use with children and adolescents between the ages of 11 and 18 years. The number and types of competence and problem items are basically the same as those in the CBCL. It also has identical subscales as the CBCL, except for the school competence subscale, which is not included in the YSR.

The TRF is to be completed by a teacher who is familiar with the child. The TRF has an Academic/Adaptive Functioning section (academic performance, working hard, behaving appropriately, learning, and happy subscales, and a total adaptive score), and a Problem Item section (same subscales as CBCL). The number of items in the TRF and the CBCL are basically identical, so is its scoring and interpretation.

The main advantage of the multivariate approach is that dimensions of the constellations of behavior are obtained through empirical data. However, certain clusters of behavior are labeled differently across studies, and in some cases certain dimensions may not emerge. Additionally, the results obtained appear to be dependent on the type of statistical procedures used, the scoring format, the number and content of items, and the number of children examined in the analyses. Finally, the exclusion of rarely endorsed symptoms may limit the instrument for assessing uncommon but severe behavior problems.

See also: *Diagnostic and Statistical Manual of Mental Disorders; International Classification of Diseases and Related Health Problems*

Further Reading

Achenbach, T. M. (1995). Developmental issues in assessment, taxonomy, and diagnosis of child and adolescent psychopathology. In D. Cicchetti & D. J. Cohen (Eds.), *Developmental psychopathology. Volume 1: Theory and methods* (pp. 57–80). New York: Wiley.

Achenbach, T. M., McConaughy, S. H., & Howell, C. T. (1987). Child/adolescent behavioural and emotional problems: Implications of cross-informant correlations for situational specificity. *Psychological Bulletin, 101,* 213–232.

Essau, C. A., Feehan, M., & Üstun, B. (1997). Classification and assessment strategies. In C. A. Essau & F. Petermann (Eds.), *Developmental psychopathology: Epidemiology, diagnostics, and treatment* (pp. 19–62). London: Harwood Academic Publishers.

Weisz, J. R., & Eastman, K. L. (1995). Cross-cultural research on child and adolescent psychopathology. In F. C. Verhulst & H. M. Koot (Eds.), *The epidemiology of child and adolescent psychopathology* (pp. 42–65). Oxford: Oxford University Press.

CECILIA A. ESSAU

Munchausen's Syndrome by Proxy

See: Psychosomatic Disorders

Muscular Dystrophy (Duchenne)

DESCRIPTION OF THE DISORDER

Muscular dystrophies involve a slow progressive weakening of muscles. Eventually all muscle groups become weak, including involuntary muscles of the heart and diaphragm, ultimately leading to respiratory or heart failure. The etiology of muscular dystrophies is unknown, but it is likely that they are genetically determined or inherited illnesses, based on the current identification of a specific gene. The most common form of muscular dystrophies is Duchenne muscular dystrophy, inherited as a sex-linked disorder affecting males, with a prevalence of 2 in 10,000 cases usually beginning in childhood.

CORRELATES

Over a period of time (ranging from months to years) the child with muscular dystrophy becomes progressively weaker and less mobile. Symptoms may begin to manifest as ambulatory difficulties, a waddling gait, difficulty climbing stairs, and difficulty getting up from a supine position. Muscles nearest the torso and the legs are most affected, accompanied by pain (especially in the legs) eventually requiring the use of a wheelchair. Obesity is a common problem because of obvious inactivity, necessitating careful dietary management to control weight. Fatigue is also a problem, as well as increasing depression as the disease process continues and independence decreases. Personality changes may accompany obvious deterioration in adaptive function and contribute to negative body image. Increasing physical inactivity and subsequent limitations of immobility resulting in isolation often influence a behavioral style of extreme introversion.

ASSESSMENT

Muscular dystrophy often goes undetected until the child is approximately 3 years old. Diagnosis of muscular dystrophy is confirmed by a specific blood test and enzyme (creatine kinase), which is released by dying muscles.

TREATMENT

No specific treatments are currently available to cure muscular dystrophy. The use of steroids may slow the progression of the disease, improve lung functioning, and facilitate ambulation. Often an orthopedic surgeon collaborates with an occupational or physical therapist to assess the need for surgery (e.g., spinal fusion for scoliosis or the release of contracted tendons at elbows, heels, legs, and hips) and to determine the benefits of using assistive devices such as braces. Minimizing contractures associated with muscle weakness, and maximizing residual muscle strength are important interventions for the child with muscular dystrophy. Prescribed exercise is important, and prolonged inactivity is contraindicated. Augmentative computerized devices to assist adaptive functioning are often helpful.

The insidious nature of Duchenne muscular dystrophy often places the parent and the child in an increasing state of anxiety and ambiguity. In their later teen years, young men with Duchenne begin to demonstrate increasing weakness, cardiac-related difficulties, and other associated signs of their terminal illness. These impending signs and symptoms can create an environment focused on illness and deteriorating symptoms. These signals are often overinterpreted by parents and youth as signs of inevitable death, often resulting in a hypochondriacal attitude. Counseling with supportive medical advice, grief-focused discussions for the family and the youth, and hospice assistance is often useful.

PROGNOSIS

Children with muscular dystrophy currently do not live past their late twenties. Death for the majority of young adults is a result of complications associated with cardiomyopathy, subsequent respiratory failure, and associated pulmonary hypertension. Essentially, there is a dramatic wasting of muscle tissue, increasing weakness, anorexia nervosa, and death.

See also: Bereavement; Coping with Illness; Parenting the Chronically Ill Child; Preparation for Medical Procedures

Further Reading

Emery, A. E. H. (1994). *Muscular dystrophy: The facts.* New York: Oxford University Press.

Livneh, H., & Antonak, R. (1997). *Psychosocial adaptations to chronic illness and disability.* Gaithersburg, MD: Aspen.

Web site: Muscular Dystrophy Association: http://www.mdausa.org

DENNIS C. HARPER

Musculoskeletal Disorders

The musculoskeletal system refers to the bones, muscles, and joints, along with their associated ligaments and tendons that make movement possible. Abnormalities of the bones, joints, and muscles can lead to deformities or malformations such as club foot, developmental dislocation of the hip, scoliosis, or short-limbed dwarfism or to diseases such as muscular dystrophy and juvenile rheumatoid arthritis. Problems with the musculoskeletal system are a major source of disability in childhood.

See also: Juvenile Rheumatoid Arthritis; Muscular Dystrophy (Duchenne); Scoliosis and Spinal Curvatures

DENNIS C. HARPER

Myelomeningocele

See: Spina Bifida

Nn

Nail Biting

DEFINITION

Nail biting (onychophagia) is the eponymous term for repetitive biting and/or chewing of the finger (and sometimes toe) nails. Early research based on covert observations indicated that the following steps compose the act of nail biting: (1) placement of the hand near the mouth; (2) placing the finger against the teeth; (3) beginning biting and chewing; and (4) withdrawal and inspection of the bitten nail(s). As with other oral habits such as finger sucking, nail biting was once thought to be part of a constellation of symptoms suggestive of underlying psychopathology (e.g., oral fixation) and is now merely classified as a simple habit when its practice has not led to unhealthful consequences (e.g., cuticle damage, social problems) and a habit disorder when it has.

INCIDENCE

Nail biting begins to appear in children as young as 3 years, is most common in children between ages 6 and just after puberty, and begins to recede in adolescence. Early research estimated as many as 44 percent of children at age 13 were nail biters. More general estimates, based on all available research, are that 25–60 percent of children between the ages of 5 and 18 years will exhibit nail biting at some point and that its incidence peaks between 8 and 9 years for girls and 12 and 14 years for boys.

CORRELATES

A variety of authors have suggested an association between nail biting and a broad range of exotic psychological variables such as sociopathy, hostility, bipolarity, and suicide risk. None of these suggestions have been confirmed. A more pedestrian, plausible, and frequently reported association involves anxiety or stress, but not even this association has been confirmed consistently. Chronic nail biting, however, has been shown to be correlated with problematic social (e.g., distance, rejection) and self-perceptual (e.g., lowered self-esteem) consequences, but the supportive research was on college students and adults; whether the same correlates are present for children is currently unknown. The research on medical correlates is clearer. Nail biting can damage the cuticle, nail, and skin surface of the finger tip and can increase nail growth by as much as 20 percent. As with finger sucking, secondary bacterial infection (especially of the cuticle), diminished oral hygiene, and impaired developing dentition can result from chronic nail biting.

ETIOLOGY

Beyond a small amount of evidence suggesting that nail biting co-occurs more frequently in monozygotic than dizygotic twins, thus suggesting a genetic etiology, there is no available research directly related to cause. It is plausible that nail biting, similar to finger sucking, produces psychophysiological results such as pleasurable physical sensations and/or relief from tension and that these perpetuate the practice.

ASSESSMENT

Assessment of nail biting involves self-reports from the children who bite, direct observations and related reports from the children's caretakers and teachers, medical examination of the children's fingers, and regular measurement of their fingernails.

TREATMENT

The literature on treatments for child nail biting is limited because so little of it is devoted to children. One conclusion drawn from literature that is probably relevant for children is that aversive procedures are effective in reducing the frequency of biting but not to the point of total suppression. Typical aversive procedures include application of bitter tasting substances to the nails, loss of privileges or awards, and physical restraint. In the more effective programs, aversive procedures are accompanied by reward- or incentive-based procedures. For example, a treatment may involve a combination of bitter taste applied to target nails and a system in which children are provided rewards for extended periods (e.g., all day) for not biting their nails.

Another approach to treatment, one that has not only been shown to be successful with nail biting in children but also for a broad range of habit disorders in children and adults is habit reversal. This is a multicomponent procedure the details of which can be found in the section on Habit Reversal. A simplified version of habit reversal, one involving methods to increase awareness of biting (e.g., slow practice in front of a mirror), practice of responses incompatible with biting (e.g., holding something), and social support for progress provided by important influences (e.g., praise from parents) produced a virtual cessation of biting with children who received treatment. While again noting that the treatment literature on child nail biters is very small, best practice appears to involve package treatments that might include some combination of mildly unpleasant consequences (e.g., taste), incentives, awareness enhancement, competing responses, and social encouragement.

PROGNOSIS

As indicated, most research on nail biting has been conducted with adults and thus it is evident that it often continues well past childhood, in contrast to finger sucking, which usually ends during childhood. Additionally, although there are several published studies on treatment, data on long-term outcome is rare. However, prevalence does decline through the teen years and is believed to be well below 10 percent in persons over 35 years. The combination of minimal harmful sequelae, available effective treatment, and declining prevalence across the age suggests that the prognosis for children for whom treatment is sought is good.

See also: Behavior Modification; Finger Sucking; Habit Reversal; Interviewing

Further Reading

Addesso, V. J., & Norberg, M. M. (2001). Behavioral intervention for oral digital habits. In D. W. Woods & R. Miltenberger (Eds.), *Tic disorders, trichotillomania, and other repetitive behavior disorders: Behavioral approaches to analysis and treatment* (pp. 223–240). New York: Kluwer Academic/Plenum.
Friman, P. C., Byrd, M. R., & Oksol, E. M. (2001). Oral digital habits: Demographics, phenomenology, causes, functions, and clinical associations. In D. W. Woods & R. Miltenberger (Eds.), *Tic disorders, trichotillomania, and other repetitive behavior disorders: Behavioral approaches to analysis and treatment* (pp. 197–222). New York: Kluwer Academic/Plenum.

PATRICK C. FRIMAN

Narcolepsy

DEFINITION

In narcolepsy, sleep is disturbed across 24 hr rather than occurring in a single block at night. It involves sudden and irresistible attacks of refreshing sleep occurring during the day that are accompanied by *cataplexy* (episodes of sudden, bilateral, reversible loss of muscle tone that last for seconds to minutes). Individuals with narcolepsy frequently report *sleep paralysis*, a brief period of awakening when they cannot move or speak, and *hypnagogic hallucinations*, vivid and dreamlike experiences that begin at the start of sleep. Daily sleep episodes generally last 10–20 min, but can last up to an hour if uninterrupted. People who have narcolepsy typically experience 2–6 episodes of sleep per day.

INCIDENCE/ETIOLOGY

Narcolepsy is relatively rare, occurring in 0.03–0.16 percent of the population, with the numbers approximately equal among males and females. About 1 in 2,000 people have the disorder. For the majority of persons with narcolepsy, their first symptoms appear between the ages of 15 and 30. Specific genetic models of narcolepsy are now being studied. It appears to be a neurological disorder with a strong genetic component.

CORRELATES

Some individuals with narcolepsy experience generalized daytime sleepiness between the discrete sleep attacks. Frequent, intense, and vivid dreams may occur during nocturnal sleep, and people with narcolepsy often experience fragmented nighttime sleep as a result of spontaneous awakenings or periodic limb movements. The most common associated disorders are mood disorders, substance-related disorders, and anxiety disorders. A history of parasomnias (e.g., sleepwalking, sleep talking, nightmares, sleep terrors) and enuresis appears to be more common in individuals with narcolepsy. Significant associations in a sample of children with onset of narcolepsy before age 13 include behavioral and emotional disturbances and obesity.

ASSESSMENT

In addition to a medical history and physical examination, a diagnosis is made from polysomnogram tests in an overnight sleep laboratory to measure brain waves and body movements as well as nerve and muscle function. A diagnosis also includes the results of the Multiple Sleep Latency Test (MSLT), which measures the time it takes to fall asleep and to go into deep sleep while taking several naps over a period of time.

TREATMENT

Changes in behavior to encourage good nighttime sleep combined with medication (e.g., usually a stimulant such as methylphenidate, amphetamine, modafinil) to manage symptoms of narcolepsy can help individuals with this disorder improve their alertness. Some sleep specialists recommend a regular sleep schedule with several short daily naps along with drug treatment to help control excessive sleepiness and sleep attacks. Others report that a single, long afternoon nap works well to improve a patient's alertness. Educating parents and teachers about the medical aspects of this problem is also important.

PROGNOSIS

Although there is no cure for narcolepsy, the symptoms of narcolepsy can often be effectively managed so those individuals with this disorder can participate in the normal activities of life.

See also: Bruxism; Excessive Sleepiness; Initiating and Maintaining Sleep; Sleep Patterns, Normal; Sleep–Wake Cycle Problems

Further Reading

American Sleep Disorders Association. (1990). *The international classification of sleep disorders: Diagnostic and coding manual.* Rochester, MN: Author.

Gibbons, V. P., & Kotagal, S. (1995). Narcolepsy in children. In C. E. Schaefer (Ed.), *Clinical handbook of sleep disorders in children* (pp. 267–284). Northvale, NJ: Jason Aronson.

Mignot, E. (2000). Pathophysiology of narcolepsy. In M. H. Kryger, T. Roth, & W. C. Dement (Eds.), *Principles and practice of sleep medicine* (3rd ed., pp. 663–675). Philadelphia: W.B. Saunders.

National Sleep Foundation, 1522 K Street, NW, Suite 500, Washington, DC 20005, Phone: (202) 347-3471, Fax: (202) 347-3472, E-mail: nsf@sleepfoundation.org, http://www.sleepfoundation.org

V. Mark Durand
Kristin V. Christodulu

Natural Disasters

DEFINITION

Natural disasters include overwhelming events that cause serious injury or loss of life and property destruction as a result of natural forces that are largely beyond human control, although human activity may influence the extent of damage. Large-scale natural disasters typically affecting a wide geographic area include hurricanes, floods, wilderness fires, earthquakes, volcanic eruptions, and violent tornadoes. Acts of nature affecting individuals or single families, such as lightning strikes and smaller tornadoes, are also often viewed as natural disasters.

INCIDENCE

Natural disasters occur throughout the world, although risks for specific types of disasters vary widely.

For example, an average of five hurricanes hit the United States over a 3-year period, and most of these affect the coastal states of the South and Southeast. Western states in the United States are most vulnerable to wilderness fires and earthquakes. Tornadoes (over 800 annually) occur in all parts of the United States, but are most common in the Midwest, South, and Southeast. Cumulatively, natural disasters affect millions of children and adolescents worldwide each year. Death tolls from natural disasters of similar magnitudes are often substantially greater in less developed countries compared to industrialized nations. Overall increases in population and increased settlement in areas prone to natural disasters (e.g., coastal regions, areas with high risk for earthquakes, floods, or wildfires) lead to concerns that injuries, death, and property damage will increase in many parts of the world.

CORRELATES

Natural disasters vary in the type of traumatic exposure and adaptational challenges they pose. Hurricanes are generally preceded by a warning period of one or more days in which the population has an opportunity to prepare. However, the extent of damage over large area can lead to prolonged periods of communitywide disruption in life circumstances and economic activity. In severe hurricanes, extreme fear of serious injury or death is common. Earthquakes, unlike hurricanes, occur with little or no warning. Much of the damage and loss of life occurs from the collapse of buildings and community infrastructure (e.g., bridges, gas pipelines). Exposure to grotesque scenes, loss of life, and imminent, overwhelming threats pose risks for acute stress reactions and long-term psychological effects, including Posttraumatic Stress Disorder (PTSD). Flood disasters, with the exception of flash floods, often develop over a period of weeks or months. Buildings may remain standing, but mud, silt, mildew, and damage to electrical systems leave many families with overwhelming cleanup and restoration tasks. Damage to agriculture is often extensive, creating severe economic hardship for many in the affected areas. Wilderness fires typically do not cause large loss of life, but children and adolescents in affected areas experience a prolonged period of worry about the progression of the fire and the safety of relatives, friends, and animals that remain in affected areas.

ASSESSMENT

Evaluation of the nature of trauma exposure is a key aspect of assessment. This includes systematic inquiry regarding primary elements of trauma exposure (e.g., perceived life threat, exposure to grotesque scenes, personal injury, harm to others) and the individual's understanding of what happened and why. Important features of the postdisaster recovery environment to be assessed include ongoing disruptions and adversity since exposure (including economic hardships and physical impairments), access to supportive social relationships, and functioning of primary caregivers. Exposure-related posttraumatic stress symptoms (reexperiencing phenomena, psychic numbing or avoidance, hyperarousal) and associated features require careful assessment, including direct questioning of children rather than relying solely on adult informants. Depression, separation anxiety, and disaster-related fears or phobias are relatively common sequelae of extreme exposure involving loss of life or serious injury and should be assessed carefully.

TREATMENT

Treatment strategies vary by the point at which mental health contact is made, the severity and duration of traumatic exposure, and the extent of emotional distress shown or reported by the child or caregivers. Emergency services shortly after disasters focus on psychological first aid (e.g., support activation, debriefing or crisis-reduction counseling), information-giving, and support for adaptive functioning of the child and family. As the immediate crisis recedes, interventions for persistent trauma-related symptoms using time-limited, disaster-focused protocols are often helpful.

PROGNOSIS

Exposure-related symptoms typically diminish with time, although focused, evidence-based interventions appear to reduce the duration and intensity of psychological effects. Individual differences in reactions are well-documented, as are effects for features of the recovery environment. Trauma caused by natural forces, although potentially debilitating, is thought to be more easily reconciled than trauma stemming from intentional acts of human violence.

See also: Human-Made Disasters; Terrorism Disasters; Posttraumatic Stress Disorder in Children; Psychological Testing

Further Reading

American Red Cross Web site. Available at http://www.redcross.org/services

Federal Emergency Management Agency Web site. Available at http://www.fema.gov/kids

Gist, R., & Lubin, B. (Eds.). (1999). *Response to disaster: Psychosocial, community, and ecological approaches.* Philadelphia: Brunner/Mazel.

La Greca, A. M., Silverman, W. K., Vernberg, E. M., & Roberts, M. C. (Eds.). (2002). *Helping children cope with disasters and terrorism.* Washington, DC: American Psychological Association.

ERIC M. VERNBERG

R. ENRIQUE VARELA

Negative Reinforcement

See: Behavior Modification

Neglect

DEFINITION

Neglect is the chronic failure of a parent or caretaker to provide children with basic needs for growth and development, such as food, clothing, shelter, medical or mental health care, emotional support, education, safety, and supervision. It can also include exposure to or fostering violence or illegal behavior such as substance abuse or prostitution. Unlike other forms of child maltreatment, neglect is an act of omission rather than commission. Whether an omission is considered to be neglect depends on several factors: cultural and community standards of care, the duration of the neglect, the risk of possible harm, the age of the child, and the impact on the child.

Although there are some widely held cultural and community standards of care, these are not universal. For example, in certain areas of the United States, the failure to enroll a child in school or a structured educational program is considered to be neglectful. Neglect can be caused by chronic omissions or by momentary lapses. For example, long-term deprivation of food and nutrition can lead to enduring problems in growth and development; brief periods during which the child is not well-supervised (e.g., not watching the child near a swimming pool or a busy street), may lead to devastating injury or death. Similarly, continued failure to follow instructions for medical care of a chronic illness (e.g., diabetes) may lead to permanent

impairment (e.g., loss of eyesight, limb amputation due to poor circulation). But even a brief period of neglecting appropriate management of an illness could also lead to negative consequences such as sudden death (e.g., imbalance of certain chemicals in the blood such as glucose and sodium from diabetic ketoacidosis).

PREVALENCE

Neglect is the most common form of child maltreatment. Published statistics about the incidence and prevalence of neglect indicate that more than half of the cases of substantiated child maltreatment involve neglect. These numbers may be an underestimate for several reasons. Many instances of child maltreatment involve more than one type of maltreatment (e.g., physical abuse as well as neglect) but the concurrent neglect may not be reported. Further, the effects of other problems (e.g., poverty, general family dysfunction, environmental chaos) that have significant impact on the care of children are confounded with neglect. In spite of neglect having the highest rate of occurrence, it is the area of abuse that has received the least attention, both in service provision and research. In medical settings where visible symptoms of injury receive high rates of attention, the sometimes-subtler symptoms of neglect may be overlooked. Even in social services agencies, neglectful families may receive fewer services than abusive families. Although there has been an increase in research that focuses on neglect, a recent review of Medline and PsychINFO databases revealed over 1,500 articles pertaining to child neglect or abuse with fewer than 5 percent of these articles separating neglect from abuse or focusing on neglect alone.

RISK FACTORS

Neglect does not occur in a vacuum. It may arise as the result of or interact with other influences on the family, such as poverty, family dysfunction, parental mental illness, and child factors. In some, but not all cases, poverty is the best predictor of physical neglect: Basic survival needs can be all-consuming and leave few resources available for the care of children. Lack of knowledge about child development and age-related needs of the child can contribute to neglect. For example, a parent who does not know that a young child is not mature enough to assume care for an infant may leave both children alone in a high-risk situation that would be considered neglectful. Parental physical or mental illness can also be a significant risk factor for neglect. When a parent's needs consume all of his or her energies and resources, the child's needs can be overlooked. Substance use and abuse by parents is also a significant risk factor for child neglect. Child temperament also can affect parental responses, and poor attachment relationships increase the risk of neglect. For example, a child with an anxious or irritable temperament may be more difficult or unpleasant for the parent to spend time with, thus placing the child at risk for emotional or other forms of neglect. This effect, however, can be buffered by family support.

Thus, the context within which neglect occurs is complex. There are many risk factors that have been identified as being associated with neglect, but none are sufficient or exclusive predictors of neglect. The same risk factors are present for many other forms of maltreatment and other childhood disorders or problems.

ASSESSMENT

Assessments should address a wide variety of elements including, but not limited to: child needs and characteristics (e.g., general physical and mental health status, development, cognitive and adaptive abilities, emotional or behavior problems); parent characteristics (e.g., mental and physical health, stress and coping skills, substance use or abuse, personality, knowledge of child development and parenting skills, personal developmental history); family factors (e.g., communication styles, family composition), and community factors (e.g., availability and quality of resources and support). Information should come from several sources (e.g., self-report, reports from professionals working with the family—teachers, physicians, mental health workers), as well as from other collateral sources and direct observation. Many of the general psychological assessment techniques are also appropriate with neglectful families. See Bonner, Logue, Kaufman, and Niec (2001) for a complete discussion of measures designed specifically to assess neglect.

TREATMENT

Comprehensive reviews of projects indicate that the most effective intervention strategies include (1) group approaches, (2) the use of nonprofessional lay people, (3) skills training to supplement professional help, (4) parent education and support groups, and (5) long-term intervention and support. The least successful projects were those that lasted less than 6 months, relied solely on casework, or focused on traditional parent counseling techniques. Overall, treatment projects designed to address the problem of neglect indicate only minimal success in preventing subsequent neglect, with recidivism rates as high as 66 percent.

PROGNOSIS

Compared with nonabused children, physically neglected children may have more behavior and emotional problems, developmental delays and cognitive difficulties, poorer academic performance, and lower self-esteem. In fact, Egeland and his colleagues wrote that physically neglected children present "the least positive and most negative affect" of all types of maltreated children (Egeland, Sroufe, & Erickson, 1983, p. 469). Extreme forms of psychological neglect can lead to nonorganic failure-to-thrive, a condition that can have devastating lifelong consequences for the child. Other long-term effects include disturbances in attachment and other psychological functioning in early adulthood. Neglected children, in general, are at great risk for physical, academic, and psychological problems unless they and their families receive long-term sustained intervention services.

Long-term prognosis depends on intervention and the degree of injury the neglect has caused. If, for example, a child received appropriate services and the conditions of neglect are ameliorated, then long-term outcomes may be fairly positive. However, if neglect continues, the prognosis is poorer. The seriousness or degree of impairment resulting from neglect can have devastating effects on a child's life.

See also: Attachment; Child Maltreatment; Parenting Practices; Physical Abuse; Risk and Protective Factors; Sexual Abuse

Further Reading

Bonner, B. L., Logue, M. B., Kaufman, K. L., & Niec, L. N. (2001). Child maltreatment. In C. E. Walker & M. C. Roberts (Eds.), *Handbook of clinical child psychology* (3rd ed., pp. 989–1030). New York: Wiley.

Dubowitz, H. (1999). *Neglected children: Research, practice, and policy.* Thousand Oaks, CA: Sage.

Egeland, B. A., Sroufe, L. A., & Erickson, M. F. (1983). The development of consequences of different patterns of maltreatment. *Child Abuse & Neglect, 7,* 459–469.

Erickson, M. F., & Egeland, B. (2002). Child neglect. In J. E. B. Myers, L. Berliner, J. Briere, C. T. Hendrix, C. Jenny, & T. A. Reid (Eds.), *The APSAC handbook on child maltreatment* (pp.13–20). Thousand Oaks, CA: Sage.

US Department of Health and Human Services, Children's Bureau. (1999). *Child maltreatment 1997: Reports from the states to the national child abuse and neglect data system.* Washington, DC: US Government Printing Office.

MARY BETH LOGUE
BARBARA L. BONNER

Neonatal Assessment

The neurobehavioral and developmental assessment of the newborn infant is a relatively recent undertaking, built on the increased understanding of the unique competence and individuality of the healthy term newborn that has occurred in the past 50 years. Neonatal assessment is a highly multidisciplinary activity, with important contributions coming from the fields of neurology, pediatrics, neonatology, psychology, and physical therapy. The assessment of the newborn differs from that of the older child in a number of ways. First, there is an emphasis on delineating the behavioral organization of the individual child in contrast to obtaining a single summary score. Second, there is the need to integrate the newborn's motor functioning, including tone, posture, and reflexes into the assessment. Another crucial factor in neonatal assessment is the infant's state of arousal, which is both the matrix within which the assessment is conducted and an important variable in itself as Als points out, rather than asking where an individual child ranks in comparison to the norms for children of the same age, the neonatal assessment asks how successfully the child is handling the challenges of extrauterine life, particularly around his or her efforts to attain and maintain behavioral organization.

METHODS AND RELIABILITY/ VALIDITY ISSUES

Virginia Apgar was among the first to quantify newborn well-being. The Apgar scale gives the medical staff caring for the newly delivered infant a way of rapidly assessing how well the baby is adapting to extrauterine life through observation and scoring of five physical signs and behaviors (heart rate, respiration, reflexes, muscle tone, color). These items are scored 0–2 and the scores summed; thus the Apgar score can range from 0 to 10. It is typically repeated at 5-min intervals starting 1 min after delivery and continuing as needed. Only lower scores (≤ 3) persisting at later time periods, such as 10 and 15 min, are generally considered to be indicative of developmental risk. Thus it is often used as part of the initial stabilization process, but not as a predictor of outcome in most cases. Another assessment, authored by Dubowitz and colleagues, and adapted by Ballard, is often done as part of the physical examination of the newborn premature infant. The Dubowitz or Ballard examination as reported by Matheny combines physical and neurobehavioral indicators of maturity (such as the condition of the baby's skin, stiffness of the ears, posture, and flexibility), in order to allow medical staff to estimate gestational age, and is interpreted in light of all of the information available about a particular pregnancy and birth.

The three instruments that are currently most important for their conceptual, clinical, and research contributions to neurodevelopmental assessment of the newborn and growing premature infant are the Neonatal Behavioral Assessment Scale (NBAS) (Brazelton & Nugent, 1995), the Assessment of Preterm Infant Behavior (APIB) (Als, 1982), and the Neurobehavioral Assessment of the Preterm Infant (NAPI) (Korner & Thom, 1990). These instruments have in common a significant research base in their development and use, as well as requirements for formal, individual training and extensive practice culminating in a reliability assessment with an authorized trainer.

The NBAS has attained wide acceptance as a powerful clinical tool for understanding the unique capabilities of individual babies, sharing this understanding with new parents, and, when used repeatedly over time, possibly identifying infants at higher risk of developmental difficulties (Brazelton & Nugent, 1995). It was originally developed with and used primarily for examining the term newborn. However, it has also been used extensively in research on topics as varied as prematurity outcome, substance exposure, neurologic insult, psychosocial challenge, environmental interventions, circumcision, and cross-cultural issues; it can be found as an outcome measure, a potential predictor, and a clinical intervention tool. Work continues on the delineation of how best to organize and utilize the quantitative and qualitative data that the NBAS yields, as well as optimal timing and repetition for improved predictive utility.

The NBAS consists of the observation and elicitation of 28 behavioral items (e.g., orientation to inanimate and animate visual, auditory, and visual-auditory stimuli) and 18 reflex items (e.g., rooting, sucking), with 7 supplementary observational items (e.g., quality of alertness, general irritability) available for high-risk infants. These are administered in a relatively consistent order that can be altered to accommodate the individual infant's needs. The examiner's goal is to obtain the infant's best performance on each elicited item, so the examination is ideally timed between two feedings to maximize the chances of the infant attaining an awake, alert state. Scoring is on a nine-point scale for the behavioral and supplementary items and a four-point scale for the reflexes. However, the scores are interpreted in the context of the purposes of the assessment and the situation of the individual baby, rather than compared to a single standard. Several systems have been explored to combine and organize scores on individual items when the test is used for research purposes, though no one system is routinely used by all researchers. One of the most interesting and powerful uses of the NBAS is as an educational and interventionist tool with parents. Parents of healthy term infants and of premature or other at-risk infants have been shown to benefit in terms of both increased understanding of and connection to their infants through observing and actively participating in the administration of the NBAS.

The APIB is much more than a downward extension of the NBAS. Organized around Als's theoretical model of infant development, the "synactive formulation," it is designed to reveal in great detail the degree to which the individual subsystems of development described in this model are differentiated and modulated and how they interact with each other as the infant is challenged by both internal and external demands. While following a substantially similar set of procedures to the NBAS, handling of the baby is carefully designed to accommodate the needs of the fragile preterm infant, and the scoring system is considerably more elaborate and is organized along different dimensions. The demands of learning this examination and achieving reliability in its scoring have limited the frequency of its use, but it has played an important role in assessing the effectiveness of an innovative, research-based approach to meeting developmental and family needs in neonatal intensive care (the Newborn Individualized Developmental Care and Assessment Program or NIDCAP®) (Als, 1992).

Although there is much research demonstrating the effectiveness of both of these assessments in discriminating infants from differing risk groups, the kinds of reliability and validity studies typically available for psychological instruments is not available. This, in part, is because of the differences in their underlying structure and conceptual models, as well as the challenges of devising an appropriate standardization sample for assessments designed primarily to delineate individuality. Korner and Thom have tried to attend to these issues in the NAPI, an instrument with the primary goal of assessing the maturation of the current behavioral function of the baby. The NAPI differs from the other assessments in that it employs an invariant order of items, includes the derivation of summary scores in the scoring process, provides for scoring during the course of the examination with the help of a "scribe," and emphasizes comparing the scores obtained by an individual infant to infants of similar postconceptional ages from a medically stable standardization sample. These features have made it appealing particularly to research efforts involving large numbers of preterm infants.

The field of neonatal assessment, like the newborns it studies, is both young and rapidly evolving. The demands of sensitively and safely assessing the individual strengths, challenges, and developmental trajectories of fragile, complex, yet actively striving newborns make it perhaps inevitable that no one approach will meet all clinical and research needs. The fact that so many disciplines have contributed to the effort also adds both to the power and complexity of the effort. Continued change and progress can safely be predicted in this exciting area.

See also: Infancy; Prematurity: Birth Weight and Gestational Age; Prematurity Outcomes

Further Reading

Als, H. (1982). Toward a synactive theory of development. Promise for the assessment and support of infant individuality. *Infant Mental Health Journal, 3*, 229–243.

Als, H. (1992). Individualized, family-focused developmental care for the very low-birthweight preterm infant in the NICU. In S. L. Friedman & M. D. Sigman (Eds.), *The psychological development of low birthweight children. Advances in applied developmental psychology* (Vol. 6, pp. 341–388). Norwood, NJ: Ablex.

Brazelton, T. B., & Nugent, J. K. (1995). *Neonatal Behavioral Assessment Scale* (3rd ed.). London: MacKeith Press.

Korner, A. F., & Thom, V. A. (1990). *Neurobehavioral Assessment of the Preterm Infant Manual.* New York: The Psychological Corporation.

Matheny, A. P. (1989). Assessment of infant mental development. In J. J. Wolpe (Ed.), *Clinics in perinatology: Neonatal neurology, 16,* 565–576.

Wilhelm, I. J. (1993). Neurobehavioral assessment of the high-risk neonate. *Physical therapy assessment in early infancy* (pp. 35–69). New York: Churchill Livingstone.

MELISSA R. JOHNSON

Neonates

See: Prenatal Development

Neural Tube Defects

Neural tube defects (NTD) refer to a group of congenital malformations of the brain, spinal column, and vertebrae. Disorders resulting from these malformations vary in severity depending on the location, the extent of the bony opening, and the exposure of spinal cord or brain. The three major NTD's are spina bifida (a split in a section of the vertebrae), encephalocele (a skull malformation that allows a portion of the brain to protrude), and anencephaly (absence of the brain). The most common type of neural tube defect is the combination of spina bifida and myelomeningocele, a fluid-filled sac that protrudes from the malformed spine and contains the spinal cord.

See also: Spina Bifida

DENNIS C. HARPER

Neuroblastoma

DESCRIPTION

Neuroblastoma, an extracranial solid tumor, is derived from the neural crest cells that normally give rise to the adrenal medulla and the sympathetic ganglia. It is the most common tumor of this type in children (about 600 new cases per year in the United States) and accounts for 8–10 percent of all childhood cancers. It is the most common childhood malignancy diagnosed in infants. The median age at diagnosis is about 17 months, with most (nearly 90 percent) occurring in children less than 5 years of age (40 percent occur in children less than one year of age). It is slightly more common in boys than in girls (ratio of 1.1 : 1.0).

ETIOLOGY

There are no obvious associations with the environment, congenital or chromosomal anomalies, or immunodeficiencies. About 1–2 percent of children with neuroblastoma have a family history of the disease (familial neuroblastoma) and they are usually diagnosed earlier, have multiple tumors, and have chromosomal abnormalities.

PRESENTATION

Neuroblastoma may originate anywhere along the sympathetic nervous system. The most common site is within the abdomen (65 percent). Other sites are the paraspinal area of the thorax, the neck, and the pelvis. Approximately 5 percent of infants and 70 percent of older children present with evidence of tumor spread beyond the original site. The most common sites of metastasis are: lymph nodes, bone marrow, bone, liver, and subcutaneous tissue. Presenting symptoms depend upon the primary site and presence of metastases. These symptoms can include: a palpable mass, dyspnea (difficult or painful breathing), lethargy, anorexia nervosa, vomiting, pain, enlarged lymph nodes, pallor, weight loss, abdominal pain, weakness, and irritability.

PROGNOSIS

Over the last 30 years, the survival of young children has increased significantly (overall 5 year survival is around 65 percent). Neuroblastoma is one of the few pediatric tumors where spontaneous regression can occur in some patients (these are usually infants less than one year of age, with a small tumor and no spread). The most important predictors of survival are the age of the child (<2 years of age at diagnosis, better prognosis) and the stage of the disease (the lower, the better). Stage 1 (localized tumor with complete gross resection [i.e., surgical removal of the tumor] with a survival rate of about 90 percent), Stage 2a (localized tumor with incomplete gross resection with negative ipsilateral [same side] lymph nodes), and Stage 2b (localized tumor with incomplete gross resection with positive ipsilateral lymph nodes) have a better prognosis than Stage 3 (unresected unilateral tumor infiltrating across the midline) and Stage 4 (any primary tumor with dissemination to distant lymph nodes, bone, bone marrow, liver, skin, and/or other organs). However, Stage 4S (localized primary tumor with dissemination limited to skin, liver, and/or bone marrow in infants <1 year of age) has a better prognosis than Stage 3. These stage designations also translate into risk (severity and possibility of recurrence) categories.

TREATMENT

Treatment may include surgery, radiation, and chemotherapy and depends upon age, stage, and pathology. Surgery is done to establish staging and to resect the tumor where possible. Surgery alone is usually the only treatment for Stages 1 and 2. Surgery is usually preferable when resection is possible, but it can also be delayed in order for chemotherapy to shrink the tumor further. Neuroblastoma tumors are generally sensitive to radiotherapy. Indications for radiation include control of localized tumors that cannot be resected and that do not respond to chemotherapy, and palliative care of unresectable masses that cause pain or organ dysfunction. Chemotherapy involves multiagent combinations, for example, cisplatin, cyclophosphamide, doxorubicin, vincristine, teniposide, and etoposide. High risk (Stage 4) disease may also indicate intensive chemotherapy with autologous (from the patient) stem-cell rescue.

The risk of complications and late effects of treatment depend upon stage of disease, location and extent of surgery, type and dosage of drugs, location and amount of radiation, age, and existence of other health problems. Some of the complications and late effects of treatment include growth, cardiac malfunction, renal malfunction, and hearing problems including deafness (from cisplatin), sterility, and second malignancies. Among the psychosocial issues for the child and family are those related to coping with a life-threatening condition, preparation for treatments and procedures (surgery, radiation, and chemotherapy), dealing with complications from surgery, and long-term follow-up of treated patients. (See the entry on Osteosarcoma for further information on psychological treatment.)

See also: Bereavement; Childhood Cancers; Coping with Illness; Osteosarcoma; Parenting the Chronically Ill Child; Treatment Adherence: Medical

Further Reading

Brodeur, G. M., & Maris, J. M. (2002). Neuroblastoma. In P. A. Pizzo & D. G. Poplack (Eds.), *Principles and practice of pediatric oncology* (4th ed., pp. 895–937). Philadelphia: Lippincott Williams & Wilkins.

Granowetter, L. (1994). Pediatric oncology: A medical overview. In D. Bearison & R. K. Mulhern (Eds.), *Pediatric psychooncology* (pp. 9–34). New York: Oxford University Press.

MARY JO KUPST
ANNE B. WARWICK

Neurodegenerative Disorder

See: Multiple Sclerosis

Neurofibromatosis

DESCRIPTION

Neurofibromatosis is a genetic disorder resulting from two distinct genetic abnormalities. Both genetic disorders are characterized by multiple benign tumors of peripheral nerve sheaths but differ in the presence of associated skeletal abnormalities, learning disabilities, neuropsychological profiles, behavioral impairments, and the presence and types of brain tumors.

ETIOLOGY/INCIDENCE

The gene for Neurofibromatosis Type 1 (NF-1) is located on the long arm of chromosome 17 (17q11.2) and encodes a protein called neurofibromin while the gene for Neurofibromatosis Type 2 (NF-2) is located on chromosome 22 (22q11) and encodes a protein referred to as schwannomin. Both genetic disorders are autosomal dominant but there is great variability in both their genetic and clinical expression and in the patterns of genetic penetrance. A high mutation rate has been reported for both genotypes. NF-1 accounts for the majority of neurofibromatosis cases while NF-2 is a much rarer form (1:4,000 persons versus 1:40,000 persons respectively). There is no evidence of racial or ethnic differences in the incidence of these disorders. Atypical forms of neurofibromatosis that do not fit the characteristic features of NF-1 or NF-2 also have been reported although their exact incidence is unclear. The specific assessment, correlates, and treatment of NF-1 and NF-2 will be described in the following sections.

Neurofibromatosis Type 1

NF-1 is one of the most common single gene disorders to affect the nervous system. Although NF-1 is transmitted through autosomal dominance, spontaneous mutations are responsible for as many as half of the new cases. The disorder is characterized by abnormal cell

<table>
<tr><td colspan="2">**Table 1.** Diagnostic Criteria for NF-1</td></tr>
</table>

1. Six or more café-au-lait spots more than 5 mm in diameter in prepubertal children or greater than 15 mm in diameter postpubertal children
2. Two or more neurofibromas of any form or one plexiform neurofibroma
3. Freckling in the axillary or inguinal regions
4. Optic glioma
5. Two or more Lisch nodules (iris hamartomas)
6. A distinctive osseous lesion such as sphenoid dysplasia or thinning of long bone cortex with or without pseudarthrosis
7. A first-degree relative with NF-1 by the above criteria

Note: A definitive diagnosis requires two or more of these criteria to be met.

Table 2. Diagnostic Features and Percentages for NF-1

Feature	Percentage
Major disorder features	
Less than 6 café-au-lait spots	Less than 95%
Axillary freckling	65–84%
Cutaneous neurofibromas	as above
Lisch nodules	as above
Minor disorder features	
Short stature (height less than 3rd percentile)	30%
Macrocephaly (head circumference greater than 97th percentile)	45%
Complications	
Plexiform neurofibromas	
All lesions	25%
Large lesions of the head and neck	1–4%
Cognitive deficits	
Mental retardation	4–8%
Specific learning disability	30–60%
Scoliosis	12–20%
Surgical correction of scoliosis	5%
Optic pathway gliomas	
All lesions	15–20%
Symptomatic	5–7%
Neurologic manifestations	
Headache	10–20%
Epilepsy	3–5%
Aqueduct stenosis	2.5%
Pseudoarthrosis of the long bones	3%
Sphenoid wind dysplasia	less than 1%
Malignant peripheral nerve sheath tumors	1–4%
Renal artery stenosis	1–2%
Noonan syndrome-like facies	7%
MRI T2 hyperintensities	60–70%

From http://bcnf.bc.ca, modified from North et al. (1997).

growth and tissue differentiation that affect the central and peripheral nervous systems. The manifestations of NF-1 are variable and the diagnosis is based on criteria developed at a consensus conference sponsored by the National Institutes of Health in 1988 (National Institutes of Health Consensus Development Conference, 1988) (see Table 1). Some additional manifestations include vascular abnormalities, cosmetic disfigurement, seizures, headaches, macrocephaly, speech disturbances, and learning disabilities.

Abnormal areas of high signal intensity on brain imaging (MRI) (called Unidentified Bright Objects or UBOs) have been described. These have been interpreted to reflect aberrant myelination, gliosis, or other brain dysplasias in individuals with NF-1. A summary of associated features of the disorder and their prevalence is presented in Table 2.

Psychological Correlates

Children with NF-1 are at an increased risk of having cognitive impairments, including verbal and nonverbal learning disabilities, with a central tendency for NF-1 to be associated with impairments in visual–spatial functioning. Cognitive difficulties in NF-1 also include expressive and receptive language impairment, reading and spelling problems, lowered IQ scores, executive dysfunction, and gross and fine motor deficits pertaining to psychomotor slowing and lack of coordination. NF-1 involves a range of neuropsychological deficits that are not limited to a single domain, which is consistent with the multifocal nature of the brain involvement in this disorder.

Although behavioral manifestations in children with NF-1 have not been extensively studied, these children have the potential to develop problems given the physical, medical, and neuropsychological morbidity of the disorder. There have been some reports of increased anxiety caused by teasing, sleep disturbances, episodes of "acting out," hyperactivity, and distractibility in these children.

Treatment

Treatment for NF-1 is currently aimed at controlling symptom manifestations. Surgery can help with bone malformations and removal of tumors. Only 3–5 percent of cases develop malignant tumors, and in such cases, surgery, radiation, and/or chemotherapy may be used. However, there are no specific treatments or drug therapies for NF-1. Thus, given the variable nature and severity of NF-1, coordination of care and provision of complete medical information is the most efficient way to minimize unnecessary anxiety in patients and their family members.

Neurofibromatosis Type 2

NF-2, referred to as central or acoustic neurofibromatosis, is characterized clinically by the presence of bilateral vestibular schwannomas. Vestibular schwannomas are nonmalignant tumors of the eighth cranial nerve. These tumors may arise in childhood but most become symptomatic in the second to third decades of life. Age of onset is similar within families but differs between families. Presenting symptoms of these tumors include: problems with balance, vertigo, tinnitus (ringing or buzzing in the ears), facial nerve palsies, and hearing loss. Most NF-2 patients have bilateral vestibular tumors but some may be unilateral. Compared to children with NF-1, children with NF-2 have fewer (less than five) café-au-lait spots. Cerebral calcifications have been reported in NF-2 but their specificity to the diagnosis is unclear. Table 3 presents the criteria for the diagnosis of NF-2.

Schwannomas may also arise along the cranial nerves, especially the fifth cranial nerve, which has both sensory and motor functions. These tumors are common in NF-2 and are typically detected by MRI. Schwannomas can also appear on peripheral nerve sheaths, and overgrowth of these tumors can lead to neuropathies (loss of or diminished sensation). As a result, sensations over the face, the conjunctivae of the eye, and the mucous membranes of the nasal and oral cavities may be affected. Motor functions of the muscles of biting and chewing may also be affected.

Other tumors that may occur in NF-2 include meningiomas, ependymomas, and gliomas. Meningiomas are tumors that arise from the meninges that surround the brain and spinal cord. Although these are typically classified as benign or nonmalignant tumors, like schwannomas, they can become problematic due to their size and/or location. As these tumors enlarge, they exert pressure on nearby brain tissue causing dysfunction. Typically, once these tumors exert pressure on adjacent brain or spinal cord structures, they need to be surgically excised or treated with radiation therapy to reduce their size. Cognitive effects from meningiomas vary according to their size and location but, in general,

the smaller the tumor, the more focal the associated cognitive effects. If, however, the tumor obstructs the fluid dynamics of the cerebrospinal fluid of the brain, increased intracranial pressure will occur and more generalized effects on cognition will result.

Ependymomas and gliomas typically arise in midbrain and posterior regions of the brain, in the cerebellum and/or within the spinal cord itself. Ependymomas are nonmalignant tumors that arise from the midline linings of the brain. Gliomas are tumors of varying degrees of malignancy that can occur in many different locations in the brain and derive from glial cells. Depending upon their size and location, these tumors may be relatively asymptomatic or they may cause neurological symptoms such as seizures. If these tumors obstruct midline structures of the brainstem or cerebellum, they may cause hydrocephalus (increased intracranial pressure or ICP). Symptoms such as cranial nerve palsies, headaches, nausea and vomiting, optic disc dilation, and balance problems may also signal their presence. Surgical treatment typically is needed to relieve the ICP.

Psychological Correlates

Compared to NF-1, there have been relatively few studies of the effects of NF-2. In part, this is due to the fact that most manifestations of the disorder make their appearance in the second or third decade of life. In addition, the pathologies of the two disorders differ enough to make comparisons between NF-1 and NF-2 problematic. As a result, the cognitive and behavioral sequelae of NF-2 are more directly related to the types and locations of cranial nerve and brain tumors and their treatment than in NF-1.

Treatment

Medical treatment for NF-2 typically involves careful follow-up and brain imaging studies for children and adults with a family history of the disorder. If necessary, surgical intervention for central brain lesions may occur.

PROGNOSIS FOR NF-1 AND NF-2

The prognosis for individuals with NF-1 or NF-2 varies depending on the location of tumors of the central nervous system, the relative difficulty in surgically removing these tumors, the severity and type of cognitive impairments that result from the tumors and/or their treatment and the adjustment of the patients to the complications of these genetic disorders. As a result,

Table 3. Diagnostic Criteria for NF-2

Bilateral vestibular schwannomas or first-degree relative with NF-2 and unilateral vestibular schwannoma in patients under the age of 30 years or any two of the following:

- Meningioma
- Schwannoma of other cranial or peripheral nerve
- Ependymoma or glioma
- Posterior subcapsular cataract or cortical wedge opacity

educating the individual patient and family about specific manifestations of NF-1 or NF-2, about the educational needs of the children, and about adjustment problems that may arise due to the potential for facial and body disfigurements is an important part of the care of these patients and their families.

See also: Adjustment Disorders; Childhood Cancers; Coping with Illness; Neuropsychological Assessment

Further Reading

Korf, B. R. (2002). Neurofibromatosis. In B. L. Maria (Ed.), *Current management in child neurology* (2nd ed., pp. 400–404). Hamilton, Ontario: B.C. Decker.

Moore, B. D., & Denckla, M. (2000). Neurofibromatosis. In K. O. Yeates, M. D. Ris, & H. G. Taylor (Eds.), *Pediatric neuropsychology: Research, theory, and practice* (pp. 149–170). New York: Guilford.

National Institutes of Health (NIH) Consensus Development Conference. (1988). Neurofibromatosis: Conference statement. *Archives of Neurology, 45*(5), 575–578.

Nilsson, D. E., & Bradford, L. W. (1999). Neurofibromatosis. In S. Goldstein & C. R. Reynolds (Eds.), *Handbook of neurodevelopmental and genetic disorders in children* (pp. 350–376). New York: Guilford.

EILEEN B. FENNELL
DANIELLE A. BECKER

Neurogenetic Disorders

See: Klinefelter Syndrome; Noonam Syndrome; Prader-Willi Syndrome; Turner Syndrome

Neurologic Examination

Pediatric neurologic examination has as its goal diagnosis and localization of lesions in the central or peripheral nervous system. The central nervous system consists of the brain and spinal cord while the peripheral system consists of peripheral nerves and root ganglia exiting the spinal column. Pediatric neurologists use the principles of organization in the nervous system in conjunction with the patient history, biomedical tests (i.e., electroencephalogram [EEG], magnetic resonance imaging [MRI], etc.), presenting symptoms, and examination to diagnose and prescribe appropriate treatment for neurologic conditions affecting children.

CENTRAL NERVOUS SYSTEM ORGANIZATION

Several characteristics of the central nervous system assist pediatric neurologists in localizing lesions. The brain is divided into two hemispheres, with each hemisphere being responsible for processing sensory information and controlling motor responses from the contralateral (opposite) side of the body. The inevitable exception to this rule in sensory functioning is olfaction, which remains ipsilateral (same side). The only other uncrossed sensory and motor functions in the human brain are cranial nerve functions and cerebellar functions. The central nervous system is organized such that motor functions are represented anteriorly and sensory systems are represented posteriorly. This organization remains consistent from cerebrum to spinal cord.

Cranial nerves consist of 12 pairs of nerves, which innervate functions of the neck, face, throat, mouth, ears, and eyes. These 12 nerves are referred to as Cranial Nerves (CN) I–XII and are an integral part of the neurologic examination. They project ipsilaterally (uncrossed), with CN I–IV originating from the midbrain, CN V–XIII originating from the pons, and CN IX–VII originating from the medulla oblongata, thus offering both lateralizing and localizing information.

NEUROLOGIC EXAMINATION

The pediatric neurologic examination consists of several parts including developmental history, medical history and review of systems, physical examination, and mental status examination. This information, along with any other diagnostic tests is used to arrive at a diagnosis.

Developmental History

During this part of the examination, detailed histories of prenatal and developmental milestones are assessed. The details of gestation and delivery are elicited and any abnormalities are noted. These include any medical difficulties during pregnancy, any medication used during pregnancy, and any toxic or other substance exposure which has known impact on fetal development (i.e., alcohol, cigarette smoke). The details of the labor and birth are also elicited including the duration of labor, any fetal distress during delivery, and method of delivery (i.e., vaginal, cesarean, or vaginal with manual extraction). In addition any postdelivery complications necessitating treatment and postdelivery Apgar scores are recorded. A detailed history of subsequent developmental milestones is also taken (i.e., feeding, head raising, sitting, crawling, standing, walking, talking, etc.)

Medical History and Review of Systems

The medical history includes any diagnoses and treatments received after birth. These may well focus on infections, trauma, or known genetic abnormalities that have or are suspected to have nervous system implications (e.g., otitis media). In addition, a review of body systems is conducted with examination as necessary. These systems include, but are not limited to, respiratory, circulatory, digestive, musculoskeletal, urinary, endocrine, immune, and hepatic.

Neurologic Examination

The neurologic examination includes examination of cranial nerves, sensory function, motor function, cerebellar functioning and mental status. The cranial nerve examination tests each of the 12 pairs of cranial nerves and is summarized in Table 1. Each CN is evaluated for laterality of deficit, which would be ipsilateral to the lesion.

Sensory Functioning

Sensory testing involves establishing thresholds for vibratory, tactile, and position sensations. Sensation is evaluated for each level of the spinal cord, as well as sensation requiring cortical processing (i.e., graphasthesia, asteroagnosia, and bilateral simultaneous stimulation).

Primary sensory testing involves touch and vibratory sensation thresholds, established for each level of the body from feet to neck (recall sensation above the neck is governed by CN function). Sensation from the cervical spinal region (C2–C8) is in the upper chest and arms. The thoracic region (T1–T12) innervates from the chest to just below the umbilicus; whereas the lumbar spine (L1–L5) innervates the genitalia and legs with the exception of the dorso-lateral aspect and sole of the foot, which is innervated by the sacral region (S1–S2) of the cord.

Secondary sensation involves examination of sensory functions requiring cortical processing beyond basic perception. Such functions involve bilateral simultaneous processing of stimuli, which may indicate a lesion in the sensory cortex of the hemisphere contralateral to the body side on which the sensation was suppressed. In addition, tactile identification of objects (steroagnosia) or the ability to identify tactile information (numbers or letters) written on the palms (graphasthesia) may be impaired and typically represents right hemisphere parietal lobe lesions. In addition, examination of position sense and joint pressure can be evaluated by manipulation of joint position (toe up or down) and by asking the patient to judge weight held in the hands.

Motor Testing

Motor function is graded in terms of strength, tone, and deep tendon reflexes. In addition, cerebellar functioning and praxis are often evaluated. Motor strength is graded on a 1–5 scale where 1 is paralysis (inability to resist gravity or provide voluntary movement) and 2 through 5 range from 2 with some movement, but

Table 1. Cranial Nerves

	Cranial Nerve	Function	Abnormality
I.	Olfactory	Smell	Anosmia
II.	Optic	Vision	Prechiasmic monocular blindness
			Postchiasmic hemivisual field loss
III.	Oculomotor	Eyelid retraction	Enlarged pupil
		Pupillary constriction	Drooping eyelid
		Medial eye movement	Deviation of eye laterally (outward)
IV.	Trochlear	Rotation of eye with head tilt	Compensatory head tilt to reduce diplopia
V.	Trigeminal	Mastication muscles	Weakness in bite
		Facial sensations	Loss of sensation
VI.	Abducens	Lateral eye movement	Deviation of eye medially
VII.	Facial	Musculature of facial expression	Weakness of facial muscles
		Anterior tongue taste	Loss of taste on anterior tongue (Ageusia)
VIII.	Acoustic	Hearing	Decreased auditory sensation
IX.	Glossopharyngeal	Taste posterior tongue	Ageusia
		Gag reflex	Poor gag reflex
X.	Vagus	Motor movement of soft palate	Decreased palate movement
		Vocal cord innervation	Hoarse voice
XI.	Spinal Accessory	Neck muscles	Weakness of trapezia
XII.	Hypoglossal	Muscle of the tongue	Weakness or deviation
			Open tongue protrusion

inability to resist gravity to 5 which is normal. Scores of 2–4 represent graded degrees of paresis (weakness). Motor tone is graded on a continuum of flaccid to spastic, with muscle wasting and flaccidity being associated with peripheral (lower motor neuron) injury and spasticity being associated with central nervous system (upper motor neuron) injury. Tone is graded on a scale of 1–4, determined subjectively by muscle stretch reflexes. Hypertonicity (i.e., spastic muscle tone) is associated with central nervous system damage whereas hypotonicity (decreased muscle stretch reflex) is associated with peripheral nerve injury. In the grading system used, reflex ratings of 2 are considered normal, with ratings of 3 indicating hyper reflexia and ratings of 4 indicating hyper reflexia with clonus (repeated elicitation of stretch receptor reflex after single stimulation). These ratings are sometimes denoted with a plus sign (i.e., 2^+ or 3^+) if they are considered to be in the high end of normal or the high end of abnormal but do not elicit clonus.

Cerebellar and Praxis Examination

Examination of cerebellar functions involves performing tasks of smooth motor pursuit and balance. This is most typically evaluated by having the person perform such tasks as finger to nose in which they alternatingly touch the examiner's finger and their nose rapidly in succession. Heel-to-toe walking, walking on a straight line and raising the heel along the shinbone while seated are other common methods of assessing cerebellar function. Each activity is evaluated subjectively on a pass/fail basis.

Praxis evaluation involves performing complex, sequenced motor movements both to command and imitation. Cortical damage to the left parietal association area often disrupts such overlearned complex motor tasks and may affect such tasks as grooming, dressing, or feeding behaviors.

See also: Headache; Migraines; Neuropsychological Assessment; Traumatic Brain Injury

Further Reading

Kolb, B., & Whishaw, T. (1990). *Fundamentals of human neuropsychology.* New York: Freeman.
Victor, M., & Adams, R. D. (1989). *Principals of neurology* (4th ed.). New York: McGraw-Hill.

JAMES SCOTT

Neurological Disorders

Neurological disorders refer to a large number of disorders that involve the structures and functions of the central nervous system (brain and spinal cord) and/or the peripheral nervous system (the motor and sensory nerves outside the brain and spinal cord). These disorders can be classified as *congenital* (present at birth and arising in prenatal development) or *acquired* (arising after prenatal development). Congenital neurological disorders can include genetic disorders affecting the nervous system, infections or injuries to the child while in development or at birth, and malformations of the structures of the nervous system. Acquired disorders can include postinfectious nervous system lesions, traumatic brain and spinal cord or peripheral injuries, and toxic and anoxic brain injuries.

Neurological disorders can also be classified as primary, secondary, or tertiary in origin. Primary disorders arise within the structures of the central or peripheral nervous systems (e.g., brain tumors or vascular malformations). Secondary disorders affect the nervous system as a result of another medical disorder (e.g., hypoglycemic seizures in diabetic patients). Tertiary disorders refer to those nervous system disorders that arise as an effect of treatment of another disorder (e.g., brain calcifications resulting from chemotherapy for leukemia). In general, information about a specific neurological disorder can be obtained by looking up the disorder by its specific name.

EILEEN B. FENNELL

Neuropsychological Assessment

DEFINITION

Neuropsychological assessment is the evaluation of brain–behavior relationships using standardized tests and techniques. The goal of neuropsychological evaluation is to diagnose and/or describe neurological dysfunction through the examination of cognitive, behavioral, and emotional functioning. Standards for training and competency in the practice of neuropsychology have been established by consensus statement of the International Neuropsychological Society (INS) and the American Psychological Association. These standards require additional pre- and postdoctoral training in the foundations of neuropsychology including neuroanatomy, neurophysiology, and neuropathology and the application of standardized testing procedures to neurologically impaired populations. Neuropsychological testing has experienced phenomenal growth since 1960 as understanding of functional brain anatomy has increased. While initial studies focused on focal or lateralized brain injuries caused by penetrating injuries, neoplasms, or strokes, neuropsychological assessment has increasingly been applied to diverse populations including those with genetic abnormalities, developmental disorders, learning disabilities, and a host of chronic illnesses with potential implications for brain functioning.

METHODS

Neuropsychological assessment uses several methods of data analysis, including analysis of normative-based comparisons, patterns of performance (localization, lateralization), and evaluation of pathognomonic signs. In addition, the evaluation must be considered in the context of an individual's estimated premorbid level of functioning and his or her injury's etiological characteristics (acute, chronic, progressive, static, etc.). Accurate analysis of test performance data relies on the degree to which the normative sample appropriately represents the individual to which comparisons are being made. Test performance must be considered in the context of the demographic characteristics of the normative sample since factors such as age, gender, race, developmental level, education, and cultural experiences can play a major role in test performance. In addition to the tests' reliability and validity, neuropsychological tests must demonstrate differential effects between normal and abnormal cerebral functioning in the neurological population being assessed (e.g., Down syndrome). Further, the neuropsychological tests must be able to differentiate normal cognitive, emotional, and behavioral functioning from abnormal performance with an acceptable degree of specificity and sensitivity. For successful differentiation, the particular function under consideration must have a known distribution in the normative population (e.g., there must be data on how the normal population performs a function such as fine motor speed). Such comparisons are appropriate for those functions that are normally distributed and can

yield very precise information regarding an individual's performance relative to the normative population. However, for those functions, which are either positively or negatively skewed (e.g., visuospatial perception, where performance is often either fully intact or grossly impaired), evaluation of parametric statistical performance (standard scores) is inappropriate, and can lead to gross systematic over- or underestimation of abnormality. For example, many components of computerized attention measures expect greater than 97 percent accuracy in stimulus identification across several hundred trials thus producing a high mean and very small standard deviation. In such a case, this severe skew of the distribution allows performance to be several hundred standard deviations below the mean, but allows little room for performance above the mean, thus producing a distribution which violates the assumptions of the normal distribution. These functions must therefore be evaluated as nominal or ordinal scales (Yes/No, impaired/intact) rather than interval or ratio data. This adds the ability to not only evaluate impairment, but also to specify precisely the degree of impairment.

Neuropsychological test performance is also analyzed on the basis of cerebral localization and lateralization. Mammalian brains in general and the human brain in particular exhibit a highly specific degree of organization based on cerebral location and laterality. Although early developmental insult can result in marked deviation from typical localization and lateralization, in general, motor functions are represented anteriorly whereas sensory functions are represented posteriorly in the brain. Right-sided body sensory, motor, and language functions are primarily lateralized to the left cerebral hemisphere while visuospatial and left-sided motor and sensory functions are lateralized to the right cerebral hemisphere. While many neuropsychological functions demonstrate high degrees of laterality (i.e., sensory and motor function) and localization (i.e., expressive language and receptive language), more complex cerebral functions (e.g., rapid alternation of attentional focus, convergent and divergent reasoning) require intact integration of many cortical areas and thus by nature are less definitively localizable or lateralizing. Such functions are best understood as a culmination of constitutional prerequisite skills, all of which must be intact in order to perform adequately.

Pathognomonic signs are those which would represent cerebral dysfunction by their very presence. Examples of such signs are reemergence of previously suppressed neurologic reflexes (i.e., Babinski, root, grasp, etc.) or a loss of previously acquired skills (i.e., language, apraxia, acalculia, etc.).

DOMAINS OF FUNCTION

Several domains of functioning are included in neuropsychological assessment. While the specific tests used and domains assessed may vary depending on the reason for assessment, typical assessment includes three categories: (1) sensory, motor, and perceptual functioning, (2) cognitive functioning, and (3) behavioral/ emotional functioning. Table 1 represents domains and subdomains typically assessed in a neuropsychological evaluation. In addition, assessment must include a thorough history and interview (see the section on Neurologic Examination for elaboration).

Table 1. Neuropsychological Assessment

Sensory, Motor, and Perceptual Function
Sensory (includes Vision, Hearing, Tactile, and possibly Gustatory and Olfaction)
  Acuity/threshold
  Laterality
  Simultaneous extinction

Motor
  Fine motor speed
  Dexterity
  Strength
  Balance/Gait
  Rapid alternating movement
  Motor perseveration
  Motor disinhibition
  Cerebellar ataxia

Perceptual
  Apraxia (feeding, grooming, dressing, ideomotor, constructional)
  Agnosia (visual, auditory)
  Astereognosia
  Right–left orientation (egocentric, allocentric)
  Hemispatial neglect (visual, auditory, tactile)

Cognitive Functions
Attention/concentration
  Information processing speed
  Simple attention
  Sustained attention
  Distractibility
  Alternating/selective attention
  Dual processing

Intellectual functions
  Overall intelligence
  Verbal/nonverbal discrepancies
  Factor score discrepancies
  Subscale performance

Academic achievement
  Reading level, comprehension level, writing skill, mathematical skill

(Continued)

Table 1. *(Continued)*

Language
  Receptive language
    Auditory
    Written
    Receptive prosody
    Grapheme to phoneme conversion (phonetic processing)
  Expressive language
    Repetition, articulation
    Expressive prosody
    Rate, rhythm, volume
    Discourse (reciprocity, tangentiality)
    Naming
    Fluency (phonemic, semantic/categorical)
    Writing

Memory
  Immediate memory
  Acquisition over repeated trials
  Retention over time
  Serial/semantic clustering
  Recognition (encoding versus free retrieval)
  Verbal–nonverbal discrepancies)

Abstract reasoning/problem solving
  Inductive/deductive reasoning
  Cognitive perseveration
  Sequencing
  Verbal–visual discrepancies

Emotional functioning
  Affect
    Range/volatility
    Content (depressed/anxious)
  Thought organization
    Delusions, hallucinations, paranoia
  Behavior
    Oppositional, agitation, impulsivity
  Judgment/awareness
    Personal/social

APPLICATIONS OF NEUROPSYCHOLOGICAL ASSESSMENT

In addition to traditional applications in such populations as traumatic brain injuries, childhood cancer, and cranial surgeries (i.e., epilepsy, hydrocephalus, aneurysms), there are growing applications to genetic, hormonal, medical, and developmentally delayed populations. The application of neuropsychological assessment has added understanding to the course of cognitive, behavioral, and emotional deficits inherent in diseases with cerebral sequelae (e.g., Turners syndrome, growth hormone deficiencies). Table 2 represents a partial list of applications of neuropsychological assessment.

Table 2. Applications of Neuropsychological Assessment

Cerebral lesions
  Traumatic brain injuries (abuse, accidents, trauma)
  CNS tumors
  Vascular lesions (hemorrhagic, ischemic)
  Epilepsy
  Demylenating diseases
  Hydrocephalus
  Hypoxia/anorexia
  Neurofibromatosis

Developmental/genetic
  Turner syndrome, Williams syndrome, Downs syndrome
  Pervasive developmental disorders
  Asperger syndrome
  Learning disabilities (verbal, nonverbal)
  Toxic exposure

Medical/medical treatment
  Leukemia
  Sickle cell disease
  Radiation therapy
  Chemotherapy
  Encephalitis/meningitis
  Diabetes
  Severe asthma (hypoxia)
  Hepatic/renal disease
  Phenylketonuria
  HIV

Further Reading

Spreen, O., Risser, A., & Edgell, D. (1995). *Developmental neuropsychology*. New York: Oxford University Press.
Yeates, K. O., Ris, D., & Taylor, G. (2000). *Pediatric neuropsychology research, theory, and practice*. New York: Guilford.

JAMES SCOTT
MIKE R. SCHOENBERG

Nicotine, Prenatal Exposure

DEFINITION OF THE PROBLEM

Nicotine is highly addictive. It acts both as a stimulant and a sedative to the central nervous system. The ingestion of nicotine results in an almost immediate "kick" because it causes a discharge of epinephrine from the adrenal cortex. This stimulates the central nervous system, and other endocrine glands, which causes a sudden release of glucose. Stimulation is then followed by depression and fatigue, leading the user to seek more nicotine. Nicotine taken in by cigarette or cigar smoking takes only seconds to reach the brain but has a direct effect on the body for up to 30 min. Based on 1999 and 2000 combined data from the National Survey on Drug Use and Health (NSDUH), 18.6 percent of pregnant women aged 15–44 smoked cigarettes.

EFFECTS

As nicotine can decrease appetite, it is associated with poor nutritional status of the pregnant woman. Nicotine also freely crosses the placenta and therefore impacts the developing fetus. There is a heightened risk of fetal hypoxia (reduced oxygen supply to tissue) and fetal growth retardation. Vasoconstriction caused by nicotine leads to an increased pulse and blood pressure in the smoker resulting in fetal tachycardia (rapid heart beat) and potential hypoxia. Carbon monoxide intake also crosses the placenta by diffusion leading to problems that include fetal blood circulation and intake of oxygen and blood flow restriction to the placenta. In utero exposure to nicotine has also been reported to increase rates of spontaneous abortion.

Infants of active smokers are more likely to have lower birth weights due to fetal growth retardation occurring primarily in the last trimester of pregnancy (averaging 150–200 g less than those of nonsmokers). Low birth weight is a risk factor associated with intellectual deficits. Other infants born to smokers are at higher risk for Sudden Infant Death Syndrome (SIDS) and infant mortality than those born to nonsmokers. There is a greater incidence in respiratory distress with more hospitalizations prior to the age of five. In addition, there is an increase in ear infections in children prenatally exposed to nicotine or living in homes where smoking is present.

In infants, a decrease in motor scores and in verbal comprehension has been found on the Bayley Scales of Infant Development. There may also be an impact on sensory processing. Lower scores on overall cognitive function and receptive language as assessed by the McCarthy Scales of Children's Abilities have also been found. The behavioral effects of maternal smoking during pregnancy have been associated with a significant increase in externalizing behaviors but not internalizing behaviors. Higher scores on a measure of child behavior problems (i.e., the Child Behavior Checklist) are also associated with maternal smoking, with the exception of Anxious/Depressed and Somatic Complaints subscales. Longitudinal studies have also assessed the problems associated with maternal smoking during adolescence. Overall findings are consistent and indicate an increased incidence of Attention-Deficit/ Hyperactivity Disorder (ADHD), Oppositional Defiant Disorder (ODD), Conduct Disorder (CD), and learning disabilities.

Although there seems to be a strong association between the harmful effects of prenatal nicotine exposure and cognitive and behavioral development late in life, it is hard to separate these effects from other confounding variables. For example, children with prenatal exposure to nicotine are more likely to be exposed to second-hand smoke as they are growing up, be from families with lower socioeconomic status, and have poor nutrition during childhood. It becomes quite difficult to tease these confounding characteristics from prenatal nicotine exposure.

TREATMENT/PROGNOSIS

Pregnancy may be one of the most opportune times to introduce smoking cessation, as women are generally at a higher level of readiness to change harmful behaviors, particularly during their first trimester of pregnancy. However, reduction of nicotine exposure at any point in the pregnancy will minimize the negative impact of nicotine on the developing fetus. Researchers are mixed with respect to the use of nicotine replacement to help pregnant women quit smoking. Replacement therapy can have the benefit of removing the additional injurious substances found in smoke, however, the fetus will still be exposed to nicotine. Patches should be introduced early in pregnancy with an attempt to discontinue use after the second trimester. Smoking while wearing the patch should be heavily discouraged as this can cause more harmful effects with no benefit. The use of inhalers and nicotine gum are better means of smoking cessation therapy during pregnancy as they involve less fetal risk than steady-state systems. Cognitive behavioral approaches, including motivational enhancement therapy, have been effective in reducing smoking behaviors and should be considered as a primary avenue for treatment.

Periodic developmental and behavioral assessments may identify learning and/or social–emotional problems in young children. Behavior interventions to address externalizing problems are recommended. Medication management may also be warranted should children be diagnosed with ADHD. As learning disabilities may be subtle, a psychological evaluation for these problems may be indicated if academic problems develop. Early identification of learning problems, as well as ADHD, is important to reducing associated problems such as parental stress, decreased family functioning, and negative self-esteem in the child.

See also: Attention-Deficit/Hyperactivity Disorder; Cigarette Smoking; Effects of Parental Substance Abuse on Children; Learning Disorders

Further Reading

Abel, A. L. (1980). Smoking during pregnancy: A review of effects on growth and development of offspring. *Human Biology, 42,* 593–625.

Ernst, M., Moochan, E. T., & Robinson, M. L. (2001). Behavioral and neural consequences of prenatal exposure to nicotine. *Journal of the American Academy of Child and Adolescent Psychiatry, 40*(6), 630–641.

Eskenazi, B., & Castorina, R. (1999). Association of prenatal maternal or postnatal child environmental tobacco smoke exposure and neurodevelopmental and behavioral problems in children. *Environmental Health Perspectives, 107*(12), 991–1000.

Horwood, L. J., Mogridge, N., & Darlow, B. A. (1998). Cognitive, educational, and behavioral outcomes at 7–8 years in a national study of very low birthweight children. *Archives of Disease in Childhood: Fetal and Neonatal Education, 79,* F12–F20.

Slotkin, T. A. (1998). Fetal nicotine or cocaine exposure: Which one is worse? *Journal of Pharmacological Experimental Therapies, 285,* 931–945.

ROBIN H. GURWITCH
ERNESTINE GREEN-TURNER
FRANK L. COLLINS

Nightmares

DEFINITION

Nightmares are frightening and anxiety-provoking dreams which generally occur during the second half of the night when dreaming is most intense. Children recover alertness and orientation quickly and they are able to recall the bad dream.

INCIDENCE

About 20 percent of children experience nightmares. Girls report having nightmares more often than do boys (2–4 : 1). Nightmares frequently begin between 3 and 6 years of age, with more elementary school-age children reporting scary dreams than at other ages.

CORRELATES

Heart rate and respiratory rate may increase or show increased variability before the awakening, reflecting a fear response. Nightmares are more common in children who are under unusual stress and they are often associated with posttraumatic stress disorder. Further, the content of the nightmare reflects a developmental sequence of fears and concerns. For example, preschool children report scary dreams about imaginary creatures, personal harm, or harm to others and animals, whereas older children report dreaming about being kidnapped, as well as imaginary creatures, personal harm, and harm to others. Although nightmares are not seen as pathological, they can result in disturbed sleep and fear of going to bed.

ASSESSMENT

While no one really knows what causes nightmares, most experts feel that scary dreams develop as children resolve conflicts and fears that surface during normal child development. In addition, real-life events such as a traumatic event, scary movies, or violent television shows can precipitate nightmares. Thus, it is important to interview both the parents and the child about events preceding the nightmares that might have precipitated them. Although one is not always able to determine the cause of nightmares, the child is able to recall much of the dream content or can draw a picture of the scary dream, which can aid in formulating a treatment plan. Nightmares can be differentiated from night terrors if the child wakes up frightened but is coherent and relatively easy to comfort.

TREATMENT

It is important to provide physical contact, comfort, and reassurance to a child that has been awakened by a nightmare. After the episode, most children can tell their parents what the nightmare was about, giving parents the opportunity to reassure their child that the dream is not real. Further, staying with the child until he or she is calm, becomes drowsy, and is ready to go back to sleep on his or her own, is helpful. It is important to talk to the child in the morning to determine if anything might be bothering him or her since nightmares are more common in children who are under stress. It is important to help the child gain a sense of control over difficult situations. In some instances, the child might have been exposed to situations that are too stressful or frightening to handle. Treatment in these instances would involve removing the child from the stressful situation such as not allowing them to watch monster movies or stopping verbal or physical conflict to which he or she is exposed. Other treatment approaches could include teaching relaxation techniques, using pleasant imagery, or having the child replay the nightmare, with the child taking an active role in coping victoriously with the feared event or object in the nightmare.

PROGNOSIS

Nightmares are a normal part of growing up and most children who have nightmares outgrow the problem. However, if they are persistent and significantly interfere with the child's sleep and day-time behavior, they may be a symptom of more significant emotional difficulties.

See also: Posttraumatic Stress Disorder in Children; Sleep Patterns, Normal; Sleep Terrors; Sleepwalking; Sleep Talking

Further Reading

Halliday, G. (1995). Treating nightmares in children. In C. E. Schaefer (Ed.), *Clinical handbook of sleep disorders in children* (pp. 149–175). Northvale, NJ: Jason Aronson.

Laberge, L., Tremblay, R. E., Vitaro, F., & Montplaisir, J. (2000). Development of parasomnias from childhood to early adolescence. *Pediatrics, 106*(1), 67–74.

Mindell, J. A. (1993). Sleep disorders in children. *Health Psychology, 12*(2), 151–162.

National Sleep Foundation, 1522 K Street, NW, Suite 500, Washington, DC 20005, Phone: (202) 347-3471, Fax: (202) 347-3472, E-mail: nsf@sleepfoundation.org, http://www.sleepfoundation.org

V. MARK DURAND
KRISTIN V. CHRISTODULU

Nonverbal Learning Disability

DEFINITION

The term Nonverbal Learning Disability (NLD) was coined by researchers in the 1980s, but the syndrome described by this name has been in the literature since the 1960s, when learning disabilities pioneers Johnson and Myklebust (1967) first described children who had social perception deficits—an inability to accurately perceive the nonverbal aspects of interpersonal actions and other aspects of daily living. Johnson and Myklebust (1967) described children who had several nonverbal disorders of learning, such as problems understanding the relevance of time, size, space, direction, and various aspects of social perception. These children often failed to learn the meaning of the actions of others, and thus were unable to grasp the unspoken rules of a game. They had difficulty attending to and interpreting the meaning of gestures, facial expressions, and body language that provided important clues to a person's feelings and attitudes. As described by Johnson and Myklebust, most children learn naturally (without direct instruction) to perceive the feelings and attitudes of other persons, the meaning conveyed by their tone of voice or actions, and the significance of physical gestures and actions. However, children with social perception deficits fail to learn through experience, and may fail to attend to, or may misinterpret, nonverbal social cues. These perceptual deficits give rise to pervasive problems with social interactions and relationships that affect all aspects of a person's life.

Since Johnson and Myklebust described this syndrome, other researchers and clinicians have referred to the syndrome by such names as right hemisphere deficit syndrome, right hemisphere developmental learning disability, social-emotional learning disability, Asperger's Disorder, and nonverbal learning disability. All of these disorders have in common a pervasive and significant problem with social perception, social relatedness, and social interactions that cause significant functional impairment.

CLINICAL FEATURES

Clinical features of nonverbal learning disabilities can include such symptoms as social isolation, peer rejection, and impaired ability to engage in interactive play. Individuals with NLD may have abnormal affective expression (or poor ability to express emotional responses clearly through their body language or vocal tone), problems comprehending affective expression of others, poor eye contact, defective use of gestures, and problems with respecting interpersonal space. They may be obsessed with a narrow range of interests or topics and, coupled with their excessive talking, this may lead others to avoid interactions with them. Individuals with NLD have poor adaptation to novel situations, which

makes it difficult for them to learn from past experience. They tend to think and speak in a concrete manner, and have decreased appreciation of humor or metaphorical language. Many individuals with this disorder will also have motor coordination problems and sensory perception deficits, especially on the left side of the body (implicating problems with functioning of the right hemisphere of the brain). At a cognitive level, overall intellectual ability is in the average range but most persons with NLD will have higher verbal than nonverbal reasoning abilities on common intellectual measures. Academically, they often have a learning disability in mathematics and may have deficits in reading comprehension, especially at the upper grade levels. They also may have deficits in visuospatial skills, attention, somatosensory abilities (such as tactile perception), abstract reasoning, and complex problem-solving skills. Often, individuals with NLD are diagnosed with other psychiatric or psychoeducational disorders that pertain to some components of their deficits, but these diagnoses fail to provide an accurate and full conceptualization of the problems with social perception. These diagnoses include Attention Deficit Hyperactivity Disorder, schizophrenia, schizoid or schizotypal personality disorder, and high functioning autism. Although these disorders have some features in common with nonverbal learning disability, they do not represent the critical features of this disorder. Within the *Diagnostic and Statistical Manual of Mental Disorders*, Fourth Edition—Text Revision (*DSM-IV-R*), the closest diagnostic category is Asperger's Disorder, and this category is sometimes used synonymously with nonverbal learning disability.

CAUSES

Nonverbal learning disability is considered to be a neurologically based disorder that arises from a dysfunction either in critical right hemisphere regions of the brain or in white matter pathways leading to the right hemisphere. Research is ongoing to determine the specific underlying causes of the disorder, but most researchers agree that functions mediated by the right hemisphere of the brain are impaired. Voeller (1986) and her colleagues report neurological evidence that suggests recognition of affect in facial expressions, tone of voice (prosody), and interpretation of socially complex material is impaired in adults with right hemisphere lesions. In children with nonverbal learning disability, Voeller (1986) has reported right hemisphere abnormalities on CT scans or neurologic exam. In contrast, Rourke (1989) and colleagues propose that destruction or dysfunction of white matter—the myelinated pathways that connect regions of the brain and facilitate smooth, efficient transfer of neurological information from one part of the brain to another—underlies nonverbal learning disabilities. Rourke (1989) postulates that these neurological deficits underlie primary neuropsychological deficits that give rise to higher-level problems.

DEVELOPMENTAL PRESENTATION

Symptoms of NLD can be present from early infancy or can be acquired at later ages through illness or injury to the central nervous system. If present in infancy, parents may notice that their children have reduced sensorimotor exploration of the environment and diminished responsivity to their parents' voice or facial expressions. Parents may suspect a hearing loss or language problem initially, but typically children with NLD develop normal language abilities and often become hyperverbal. As they progress through the preschool years, they begin to show strengths in rote memory, verbal attention and memory, and language development. However, they may show relative weaknesses in motor coordination, visual attention and memory, and the social aspects of communication. As children enter school, they may show particular strengths in reading and spelling, but weaknesses in early writing skills (because of coordination problems) and mathematics. As they progress through school, their written expression skills typically improve, but they continue to have difficulties with mathematics and subjects that require reasoning and abstract thinking, such as science and reading comprehension.

Socially, children with NLD may be rejected by peers and begin to withdraw from social interaction because of repeated rejection and ostracism. In the adolescent years, the social deficits become more obvious in contrast to their maturing peer group and the expectations for more sophisticated social skills. Adolescents typically show maturing of their executive functions, or their ability to think abstractly, plan and set goals for their behavior, monitor their behavior against a standard of socially expected norms, and regulate their emotional reactions. Adolescents with nonverbal learning disabilities have core deficits with problem solving and reasoning, and with the executive functions that are expected to mature during adolescence. Thus, they have difficulty forming intimate relationships and they often struggle with the developmental task of identity formation. The distress associated with social rejection may lead to development of secondary emotional problems, including depression or anxiety. Adults with NLD have problems similar to those of adolescents, except that the expectations for social maturity and social judgment are even higher.

DIAGNOSIS

Neuropsychologists—who are trained to understand and evaluate brain–behavior relationships and assess functional impairment—are often involved in the assessment of nonverbal learning disability. This group of professionals can assess the cognitive, academic, visual/auditory perceptual and memory functions, sensory and motor skills, and social/emotional functioning, with knowledge of the research literature on nonverbal learning disabilities. Clinical, counseling, or school psychologists can assess certain aspects of NLD, but may not be trained to assess the neuropsychological assets and deficits often associated with the disorder. Neurologists or developmental pediatricians sometimes are involved in neurologic examination and/or ancillary tests such as CT or MRI. Although these tests are not necessary for diagnosis, they may add information about the possible underlying causes of NLD. Speech and language development of individuals with NLD typically is normal, but speech/language pathologists can assist with evaluating the impairment in pragmatic, or social, aspects of communication. A psychologist and/or psychiatrist may be involved in assessing the social and emotional functioning of the individual, with particular attention to the possible secondary emotional characteristics that may accompany the primary disorder. Because this disorder can have a significant impact on the family, it is very important to obtain information about siblings' and parents' reaction to, and coping with, the effects of the disorder.

TREATMENT

Treatment of nonverbal learning disability typically begins with the diagnosis, at which time providing information about the disorder can assist the child, parents, teachers, and other family members and close friends to better understand its reasons for the child's unusual behavior. A professional with knowledge about this disorder can explain the nature and characteristics of nonverbal learning disability, its developmental course, possible causes, and offer suggestions about management. Psychological intervention often involves parents and/or extended family members who can help translate nonverbal social cues in the environment to the child or adolescent with NLD. For example, a parent who witnesses a social interaction in which their child misses critical nonverbal cues may help by translating those nonverbal cues into words, so that the child can encode the information in a format that is easier for them to process. Often direct psychotherapy approaches in clinical settings may involve role-playing of social situations, teaching the child or adolescent some social "templates" for basic social skills such as introducing themselves, starting and ending a conversation, what to do with their hands, etc. Sometimes videotaping these role plays and then replaying them for discussion can help with instruction. However, a major problem with interventions such as this is the individual's difficulty with generalizing their learning to new social situations. Social situations are probably the most complex situations we encounter, and even small nuances can change the nature of an interaction. If individuals with NLD has practiced a certain way of responding socially, they may apply this method without considering and fully understanding that the context has changed in a way that makes their social interaction inappropriate. The ability to analyze and interpret each new social situation is impaired, and it is difficult to practice each and every possible scenario. Parents and teachers who work with children in everyday social situations often become the best "therapists" because they can assist with interpreting social cues or translating nonverbal cues into words right as they occur.

Much of the psychological intervention is focused on treating the secondary emotional problems that often accompany the nonverbal learning disability. Thus, attention to symptoms of depression, anxiety, somaticization, or withdrawal is important, along with positive support and regard in the relationship with the client. Social skills groups at school or in community centers can be helpful for the individual, as can bibliotherapy and parent support groups for the family.

See also: Adolescent Assessment; Asperger's Disorder; Learning Disorders; Pervasive Developmental Disorder; School Age Assessment

Further Reading

American Psychiatric Association. (2000). *Diagnostic and Statistical Manual* (4th ed., Text Revision). Washington, DC: Author.

Culbertson, J. L., & Edmonds, J. (1996). Learning disabilities. In R. Adams, O. Parsons, J. L. Culbertson, & S. J. Nixon (Eds.), *Neuropsychology for clinical practice: Etiology, assessment, and treatment of common neurological problems* (pp. 331–408). Washington, DC: American Psychological Association.

Johnson, D. J., & Myklebust, H. R. (1967). Nonverbal disorders of learning. In D. J. Johnson & H. R. Myklebust (Eds.), *Learning disabilities: Educational principles and practices*. New York: Grune & Stratton.

Rourke, B. P. (1989). *Nonverbal learning disabilities: The syndrome and the model*. New York: Guilford.

Voeller, K. K. S. (1986). Right hemisphere deficit syndrome in children. *American Journal of Psychiatry, 143*, 1004–1009.

Web Sites

http://www.asperger.org
http://www.nldontheweb.org
http://www.nldline.com

JAN L. CULBERTSON

Noonan Syndrome

DESCRIPTION AND INCIDENCE

First described in 1963, Noonan syndrome (NS) (also referred to as either Female Pseudo-Turner syndrome or Male Turner syndrome) is a genetic condition affecting 1/1,000–5,000 births. Often noted to be phenotypically similar to Turner syndrome, which only affects females, NS is distributed equally between the genders. Also unlike Turner syndrome, individuals with NS exhibit a normal karyotype (46, XX or 46, XY). Although symptoms and their severity are highly variable, common features of NS include widely spaced, downwardly slanting eyes, low-set ears, a short neck with webbing, and *cubitus valgus*, an arm deformity where the forearm deviates laterally. Short stature is also common among affected individuals; height is typically below the third percentile for norms. Perhaps the most serious features, affecting 85 percent of individuals with Noonan syndrome, are the cardiac anomalies that accompany the condition. The most commonly seen heart defect in NS patients is pulmonary stenosis, the narrowing of the opening into the pulmonary artery from the right cardiac ventricle.

In boys, delayed and/or arrested pubertal development is common. Cryptorchidism (undescended testicles) is a related feature affecting approximately 60 percent of boys with NS; this condition, if left untreated, can contribute to reduced fertility. In both sexes, additional features include specific cognitive deficits, motor delays, and the increased prevalence of behavioral problems.

ETIOLOGY

Approximately half of the cases of NS appear to be sporadic in nature, stemming from a "spontaneous mutation." In these cases, a change is thought to have occurred in a once normal sperm or egg cell, resulting in a "Noonan syndrome genotype." However, a family history of NS is reported in approximately 50 percent of cases, and the condition is thought to be transmitted via an autosomal dominant gene. While a sperm or an egg cell can transmit this gene, it appears that the majority of inherited cases result from the maternal contribution. Although the responsible gene has yet to be identified, there is some indication that NS may result from a mutation on chromosome 12.

ASSESSMENT

Because the clinical features of NS resemble those associated with several other syndromes (fetal alcohol syndrome, Leopard syndrome, primidone teratogenicity syndrome, Turner syndrome, and Williams syndrome), diagnosis can be difficult; there are data to indicate the mean age of diagnosis is as late as 9 years old. Although there is no diagnostic test for NS, laboratory studies can be used to rule out those conditions with overlapping characteristics that feature genetic abnormalities. Having excluded other candidate syndromes, the diagnosis is made when an individual exhibits characteristic features of NS. Because of their high incidence in NS patients, heart defects, growth delay, and cubitus valgus are typically the features most relevant to diagnosticians.

PSYCHOLOGICAL FEATURES

As is true for any genetically based syndrome, it should not be assumed that accompanying psychological features stem directly from the condition. Environmental factors, including parenting style that may be influenced by knowledge of the diagnosis, along with psychosocial stresses that can accompany any chronic health condition, must also be considered. It is recommended that the psychosocial functioning observed in NS patients be conceptualized as deriving from an interaction between genes and the environment.

Studies designed to identify psychological features associated with NS indicate that affected individuals are more likely than others to display clumsiness, communication problems, stubbornness, and mood problems.

While it has been reported that 90 percent of children with NS attend regular school, there are data to suggest that 25 percent show some degree of mental retardation, usually mild. However, because NS is associated with deficits in *specific* cognitive domains that may be responsible for the decreased IQ scores, such data can be misleading. Delayed motor skills and deficits in specific verbal and praxic (visual-constructional) abilities have been associated with NS. Motor delays are likely to contribute to clumsiness, while verbal or praxic deficits may exacerbate communication problems. These communication problems, in turn, may lead to the described stubbornness and mood problems.

In addition, children with NS are at heightened risk for stigmatization by peers related to their short stature and delayed puberty. These children may also experience the psychosocial stresses associated with any chronic health condition requiring repeated visits to the medical setting.

TREATMENT

Because of the mixture of medical and psychological aspects of NS, a multifaceted approach to treatment is indicated. Depending on the individual case, the individual with NS may require cardiac intervention, hormone therapy, special education services, and psychotherapeutic intervention to address problems of psychosocial adaptation.

Cardiac Correction

Upon diagnosis, it is essential that the affected child's heart status be carefully assessed. In cases in which a cardiac defect is detected, the child is referred to a pediatric cardiologist where an electrocardiogram and echocardiogram will be obtained. Depending upon the severity and type of heart problem, surgery may be necessary. In the most frequently observed heart defect, pulmonary stenosis, a partial valvectomy is the procedure typically performed. A well-tolerated surgical procedure, mortality, or major cardiac morbidity is extremely rare. In all cases where a heart defect is detected, regular follow-up visits to the cardiologist are indicated.

Growth Hormone Therapy (GHT)

Although children with NS are not generally growth hormone deficient, it has been suggested that the short stature characteristic of this population is a result of an abnormality of the growth hormone axis. A preliminary study of the benefits of growth hormone therapy (GHT) in NS suggests that, at least in the short term, growth velocity and relative height can be increased. One major concern relating to the administration of GH for children with NS is a possible risk alteration of cardiac function (associated with left ventricular hypertrophic cardiomyopathy). For this reason, NS children with particular heart defects have been excluded as candidates for GHT.

In addition to GHT, androgen therapy might be necessary to initiate puberty in boys who experience a significant delay in pubertal onset.

Psychological Intervention

Knowledge of the heightened risk of developmental delays among children with NS creates the opportunity for early detection and remediation once the diagnosis has been made. Anticipatory guidance for families regarding emotional and behavioral problems believed to be associated with NS also offers the hope of minimizing or eliminating the risk for developmental delays. To date, however, there are no studies of the effectiveness of such interventions. Furthermore, the benefits of syndrome-specific knowledge of the behavioral and cognitive characteristics of NS must be balanced against the risk of creating circumstances for a "self-fulfilling prophecy." Finally, because NS is a potentially heritable condition, genetic counseling is recommended for all affected youths and their families.

PROGNOSIS

Because of the wide variability in phenotype of individuals with NS, and the limited number of long-term behavioral outcome studies that have been conducted, no general statement regarding prognosis can be made.

SUPPORT GROUP

The Noonan Syndrome Support Group, Inc., P.O. Box 145, Upperco, MD 21155, U.S.A. Web site: http://www.noonansyndrome.org/home.html; E-mail: info@noonansyndrome.org

See also: Genetic Counseling; Parenting the Chronically Ill Child; Prenatal Development; Short Stature: Psychological Aspects; Turner Syndrome

Further Reading

MacFarlane, C. E., Brown, D. C., Johnston, L. B., Patton, M. A., Dunger, D. B., Savage, M. O., McKenna, W. J., & Kelnar, C. J. (2001). Growth hormone therapy and growth in children with Noonan's syndrome: Results of 3 years' follow-up. *Journal of Clinical Endocrinology & Metabolism, 86,* 1953–1956.

Mendez, H. M., & Opitz, J. (1985). Noonan syndrome: A review. *American Journal of Medical Genetics, 21,* 493–506.

Sharland, M., Burch, M., McKenna, W. M., & Paton, M. A. (1992). A clinical study of Noonan syndrome. *Archives of Disease in Childhood, 67,* 178–183.

Wood, A., Massarano, A., Super, M., & Harrington, R. (1995). Behavioural aspects and psychiatric findings in Noonan's syndrome. *Archives of Disease in Childhood, 72,* 153–155.

LAUREN ZURENDA
DAVID E. SANDBERG

Norms and Normative Data

Most assessment techniques provide some objective index of a child's performance that is called the child's raw score (e.g., sum of the items on a rating scale, number of errors on a measure of sustained attention, number of aggressive responses on a projective storytelling technique). These raw scores do not indicate how a child's performance compares to other children of a similar age, gender, ethnicity, or other characteristics. "Norm-referenced" scores are designed to provide such information. As described by Anastasi and Urbina (1997), these scores involve converting a child's raw score to a standardized score, reflecting where the child's score falls in the distribution of scores from some comparison sample of children. One of the most commonly used metrics for standard scores is the T-score, which has a mean of 50 and a standard deviation of 10. Using the T-score metric, if a child receives a standard score of 60 this indicates that his or her score falls at one standard deviation above the mean of the comparison sample (a standard deviation is based on the variability of scores around the mean).

STANDARD SCORE CONVERSIONS

As we have noted elsewhere, there are a number of important considerations for interpreting standard scores. For example, there are a number of variations in how the standard scores are computed from the distribution of scores in the comparison sample. One of the most common techniques is to create a distribution that approximates a normal curve. Since most assessors have some experience with interpreting normal distributions, such transformations can enhance the ease of interpretation of the norm-referenced scores. Furthermore, if a test provides multiple norm-referenced scores (e.g., multiple subscales on a personality inventory), forcing scores to conform to a common distribution allows for greater comparability across subscales. However, basing standard scores on a normalized distribution rests on the assumption that the psychological construct being assessed is a normally distributed trait, and this assumption may not be appropriate for many psychopathological constructs that tend to have positively skewed distributions in the general population (i.e., the vast majority of persons in the population having very low levels of the trait; see Kamphaus and Frick [2001] for a discussion of this issue). By forcing a normal distribution onto these traits, standard scores can make a child's score seem more deviant from the comparison sample mean than they actually are, especially when the score is slightly to moderately higher than the comparison sample's mean.

In response to this issue, some tests have chosen to use linear transformations to form norm-referenced standard scores. These transformations maintain the skewed shape of the raw score distribution in the comparison sample rather than trying to force the scores to approximate a normal distribution. The advantage of this procedure is that the standard scores are based on the actual distribution of scores from the comparison sample. However, the disadvantage is that, if multiple scores from the same technique have different distributions, then the standard scores may be difficult to compare. For example, a score of one standard deviation above the mean on one subscale of the test may be associated with a different percentile rank than a score of one standard deviation above the mean on another subscale.

QUALITY OF THE NORMATIVE SAMPLE

The usefulness of norm-referenced scores rests on their ability to provide an index of how a child's score on the test compares to the scores obtained from persons in some reference group. Therefore, it is critical to consider the quality and appropriateness of the reference group from which the standard scores were derived when interpreting norm-referenced scores. Obviously, the reference group should be large enough to ensure that the distribution of scores is not significantly influenced by a few very deviant or unusual scores. However,

the importance of other characteristics of the normative sample depends on the specific interpretations that will be made from the standard scores.

One of the most common interpretations an assessor wishes to make from norm-referenced scores is how "normative" or typical a child's score is compared to other children of the same age. In this case, the sample on which the scores are based should be representative of the general population and large enough within a given age group to provide a distribution of scores that are representative of children of that age. There is great variation in how large and representative standardization samples are for assessment techniques used with children and adolescents. For example, some standard scores are based on large samples (e.g., $n = 3,483$ children between the ages of 4 and 18) that were collected to approximate the U.S. census on variables such as gender, race, and socioeconomic status, whereas other scores are based on relatively small samples ($n = 200$ children between the ages of 6 and 15) with very questionable representation of children from diverse backgrounds (e.g., children from three school districts in southern California). Because of such substantial variations in the samples on which norm-referenced scores are based, assessors must evaluate these comparison samples and determine if they are appropriate for the interpretations one wishes to make from the standard scores.

NORMAL VERSUS NORMATIVE SCORES

Another important issue for interpreting norm-referenced scores is determining whether or not the comparison group is a "normative" sample or a "normal" sample. A normal sample is one that excludes children with significant emotional, behavioral, or learning problems. If children with potential problems in adjustment are excluded, it is quite likely that the upper end of the distribution of scores on the assessment technique is eliminated or at least severely reduced. A normative sample, however, is representative of the general population, not only on demographic variables (i.e., ethnicity, socioeconomic status, gender, community size, parental occupation), but also attempts to include children with problems in adjustment at a rate that is "typical" for the population of children of interest. This issue is important when interpreting standard scores because a child's score may appear more deviant when compared to a "normal" sample in which the upper end of the distribution is eliminated but may appear less deviant when compared to a "normative" sample in which the upper end of the distribution is maintained.

NORM-REFERENCED SCORES AND SEX OF THE CHILD

A related issue is whether norm-referenced scores should be based only on children of the same sex as the child being tested. This is a critical issue because many types of emotional and behavior problems experienced by children and adolescents show clear sex differences in their prevalence. Although basing standard scores only on single-sex samples is common, the theoretical rationale for such sex-specific norms is debatable. For example, if one has a scale assessing impulsive and overactive behaviors in children, boys are quite likely to be rated higher on these behaviors than girls. Using sex-specific norms, this difference in prevalence is "removed" because a child is considered to have an elevated level of behavior if his or her scores are deviant compared to others of the same sex. If these differences reflect true sex differences in the trait being assessed in the normal population, the rationale for removing such differences may be unclear.

See also: Cultural Influences on Assessment; Gender and Psychopathology; Psychometric Properties of Tests; Test Bias

Further Reading

Achenbach, T. M. (1991). *The Child Behavior Checklist—1991*. Burlington, Vermont: University of Vermont.

Anastasi, A., & Urbina, S. (1997). *Psychological testing* (7th ed.). New Jersey: Prentice Hall.

Frick, P. J., & Cornell, A. H. (in press). Child and adolescent assessment and diagnosis research. In M. C. Roberts & S. S. Ilardi (Eds.), *Methods of research in clinical psychology*. London, UK: Blackwell.

Kamphaus, R. W., & Frick, P. (2001). *Clinical assessment of children's personality and behavior* (2nd ed.). New York: Allyn & Bacon.

AMY H. CORNELL
PAUL J. FRICK

Nursing

BACKGROUND

The nursing profession is the center of health care and it is found in the majority of all health care settings. Once thought to be a hospital based or public health provider, the nurses' care responsibilities have expanded beyond the traditional hospital patient care role, school nursing, community health nursing, and military nursing to a variety of settings and specialized roles. These include clinical nurse specialists (e.g., dialysis nurses; breastfeeding nurses; operating room nurses); medical care team coordinators (e.g., transplant team; trauma team; palliative care team); and physician partners (e.g., nurse practioners; nurse clinicians). Others specialize in a certain clinical area or with a certain patient population (e.g., pediatric nurse clinician; geriatric nurse clinician). Some have become more specialized in the business of health care (e.g., nursing administrators; third party case managers; health care consultants; legal consultants). These are a few of the roles nurses work in with the potential for individual nurses to design their own roles as the environment dictates.

Because of the variety of nursing roles, fewer people going into nursing, and the patient population increasing, the nursing shortage has become worse in the 21st century than ever before in the history of nursing. Women, the predominate gender for nursing, are now going into other professions including the traditional male professions, such as medicine, law, and business. At the same time, men and minorities are entering the nursing profession but not at the rate that had been predicted. The 21st century is faced with a major nursing shortage.

REGISTERED NURSE

Registered Nurse (RN) refers to the license a nurse earns upon successful completion of a national licensure examination. Often the term is confused with a degree a nurse earns. An individual earning a diploma, an associate degree, or a baccalaureate degree in nursing has to pass the same examination to qualify as a registered nurse.

NURSING EDUCATION PROGRAMS

Diploma Nursing Education

Historically, programs that were located in hospitals taught nursing education. Students took classes there and received the majority of their clinical experience in that hospital. This 3-year program still exists but is being phased out throughout the nation. Students successfully completing this program are awarded a diploma in nursing. Usually their coursework does not count for college credit.

Associate Degree Nursing Education

The students choosing to enter a junior or community college for their nursing studies will achieve an associate degree in nursing after completion of 2 years in nursing courses and other related courses. The clinical practicum is conducted in community hospitals and a variety of other health agencies. Many of these programs provide coursework that is accepted into baccalaureate programs should the nurse choose to further her education.

Baccalaureate Nursing Education

The student choosing to attend a college or university offering a Baccalaureate in Nursing (BSN) will attend for 4 or 5 years to complete this degree. Some students begin their nursing program at the beginning of their college studies, while others start after they complete their sophomore year of prenursing requirements. Students applying at this time generally have to have a high grade point average for admission. There are some programs that accept students after they have completed their bachelors in science or another major. They are placed on a track that may be an intense 1-year program or a more common 2-year program.

Graduates of a BSN program are referred to as graduate nurse (GN) prior to the successful completion of the national board exam at which time they are referred to as a registered nurse.

GRADUATE DEGREE IN NURSING

Masters Nursing Education

Presently there are masters programs in nursing leading to either a Masters in Science in Nursing (MSN) or a Masters in Nursing (MN). These programs last 1–2 years and result in the nurse having a clinical specialty. Graduates are referred to as a clinical nurse specialist, nurse clinician, or clinical nurse practitioner. These nurses are qualified for an Advanced Registered Nurse Practitioner (ARNP) license. The individual state boards of nursing determine this license.

Nurse Practitioner

The nurse practitioners are nurses that have specialized in certain areas of health care. These nurses are responsible for a number of tasks that traditionally have been done by physicians (e.g., physical examinations, surgical procedures, invasive tests, diagnosing and treating health problems, and writing prescriptions, etc.). They practice under the supervision of a physician and in some cases as a solo practitioner. Their education is usually a part of a nursing masters program. There are still a few certificate programs that nurses take after they complete their basic education.

Doctoral Nursing Programs

Nursing now offers PhD programs in nursing. There are a few Doctorates of Nursing (ND) and Doctorates in Science in Nursing (DSN) but the majority are PhD programs. These programs usually focus on research in nursing. There are some that have combined the research with advanced nursing practice.

PRACTICAL NURSING

The individual entering the practical nurse program may do so after completing a high school diploma, or for some, the graduate equivalency diploma (GED). The program usually lasts 1 year and is usually taken through vocational schools. After passing a board examination the practical nurse is referred to as a licensed practical nurse. Additional training is usually required for them to be eligible to administer medications.

NURSING ORGANIZATIONS

There are two major professional nursing organizations, The National League for Nursing (NLN) and the American Nurses Association (ANA). Both can be queried about concerns and questions related to the nursing profession. In addition, each state has a State Board of Nursing, which regulates nursing and acts as a resource for questions pertaining to nursing in the individual states.

THE NATIONAL INSTITUTE OF NURSING RESEARCH

The National Institute of Nursing Research (NINR) supports "clinical and basic research" to answer research questions as they relate to patient care throughout the life span. Studies supported by the NINR have focused on "promotion of healthy life styles, care during illness, reduction of risks for disease and disability, and care for at-risk and underserved populations" (National League of Nursing, 2002, p. 3).

See also: Health Care Professionals (General); Health Care Use; Physician Assistant

Further Reading

National League for Nursing. (2002). Tri-council testimony (pp. 1–5). Washington, DC.: Author.

MARTHA UNDERWOOD BARNARD

Nutritional Assessment

DEFINITION

Nutritional assessment is critical for understanding and treating all types of feeding and growth disorders. Nutritional assessment provides information on the adequacy of food intake in relation to weight, height, and age. This type of assessment yields information on deficiencies or excesses in vitamins, minerals, or calories.

TYPES OF ASSESSMENT

Nutritional assessment can take many forms. The most immediate and simple assessment involves 24-hour food recall reports made by caregivers or completion of retrospective food frequency questionnaires. Prospective diaries completed over a 1–2 week period provide more details and are more accurate. Caregivers are instructed to record everything the child eats and drinks during the identified time period. Reports can be exceptionally rigorous accounts involving weighing and measuring all foods before and after meals or less exact estimates (e.g., approximately 8 ounces of milk, a half-cup of peaches). Trained nutritionists, sometimes aided by dietary software programs, analyze the information.

USES OF ASSESSMENT

Nutritional assessment helps to determine the place of treatment (i.e., inpatient versus outpatient). For example, children with excessive weight loss or significant growth failure are likely to be treated as inpatients where ongoing monitoring of nutritional and medical status is possible. Nutritional assessment also helps to determine treatment goals. Children with identified deficiencies, such as vitamin deficiencies due to food selectivity, will have treatment goals that include consumption of types and amounts of foods to address the deficiencies. In contrast, children with identified excesses (e.g., carbohydrates, salt) will have treatment goals aimed at reducing consumption of some foods. As treatment of feeding disorders has evolved, attention has changed from simply increasing amount or type or texture of foods to insuring that children are eating foods that contribute to a nutritionally ideal diet. Careful nutritional assessment is needed to meet this goal of treatment.

See also: Anorexia Nervosa; Failure-to-Thrive; Food Refusal; Obesity

Further Reading

Linscheid, T. R., & Rasnake, L. K. (2001). Eating problems in children. In E. Walker & M. Roberts (Eds.), *Handbook of child clinical psychology* (4th ed., pp. 523–541). New York: Guilford.

Linscheid, T. R., Budd, K. S., & Rasnake, L. K. (in press). Pediatric feeding disorders. In M. Roberts (Ed.), *Handbook of pediatric psychology* (3rd ed.). New York: Wiley.

Stark, L. J. (1999). Commentary: Beyond feeding problems: The challenge of meeting dietary recommendations in the treatment of chronic diseases in pediatrics. *Journal of Pediatric Psychology, 24,* 221–222.

THOMAS R. LINSCHEID
L. KAYE RASNAKE

Oo

Obesity

DEFINITION

Obesity is generally defined as excessively high ratio of fat tissue to lean body mass. This is differentiated from being overweight, which refers to high weight to height based on normative or criterion-referenced standards. There is no consensus operational definition of pediatric obesity. An adult body mass index (BMI) above certain levels has been significantly correlated with later health problems. These criteria have not been established in pediatric populations. Thus, most operational definitions of pediatric obesity have been normative, based on height/weight/age or BMI/age data in specific pediatric populations. Many research studies define pediatric obesity as children with a BMI at or above the 95th percentile for their age. Clinically, the 95th percentile on growth charts, for example, weight to height, for given age ranges is often used as a cutoff for pediatric obesity.

INCIDENCE/PREVALENCE

Recent data suggest that about 13 percent of children and adolescents are seriously overweight (BMI equal to or greater than the 95th percentile). This number has more than doubled since the early 1970s. Adolescent obesity has tripled since 1980. Increased availability and consumption of energy-dense and micronutrient-poor foods, decreased physical activity, and increased sedentary habits have been targeted as possible contributory trends to explain the increases in pediatric obesity. Higher rates of pediatric obesity are also associated with specific genetic, metabolic, and physiological conditions, such as Prader–Willi Syndrome, Cushing's Disease, hypothyroidism, pseudotumor cerebri, and hypotonia, among many others. Obese children have higher rates of abnormalities such as hyperlipidemia, high blood pressure, and problems with glucose tolerance. Obese children are also more likely to become obese adults, who are at increased risk for cardiovascular, endocrine, gastrointestinal, respiratory, sleep, orthopedic, reproductive, and psychosocial problems, as well as for some types of cancer.

ETIOLOGY

Pediatric obesity occurs when food intake is greater than energy use. However the factors that contribute to this equation are complex and their relation remains unclear. There are many environmental and psychosocial factors thought to be associated with the development of eating behaviors and habits. These can include early eating experiences, learning as a result of physiological experiences associated with eating, and modeled behaviors, among others. Similarly, there are many ecological and psychological factors associated with the development of physical activity behaviors. Some factors that have been studied include geography and seasonality, safety, availability of facilities, competing interests, school programs, and modeled behaviors. Physiological and genetic factors also contribute to the development of, and changes over time in, eating behavior and physical activity patterns. Some of these include developmental and growth-related changes, heritability, and

423

health and constitutional factors. Research continues on identifying genes associated with pediatric obesity and on the role of specific hormones, such as leptin, in weight regulation and body fat levels.

ASSESSMENT

A comprehensive medical history, physical examination, and family history are important steps in the assessment process. It is important to rule out endogenous factors that may contribute to pediatric obesity. Child and family eating and activity habits should also be carefully evaluated. Growth charts can be used to plot the child's weight to height for age. BMI can also be calculated and plotted on BMI–age charts. It is also important to rule out comorbidities that can be associated with pediatric obesity.

TREATMENT

Attempts to treat pediatric obesity have generally been more effective than adult obesity treatment programs. Successful treatment of pediatric obesity involves attainment of a more appropriate weight or BMI, and long-term maintenance of these changes. Most effective pediatric obesity treatment programs have focused on modification of diet and activity. Some approaches focus on weight maintenance, taking advantage of natural patterns of growth, while others focus on weight loss. Dietary interventions generally use operant approaches to reduce caloric intake and teach eating habits that better conform to current nutritional guidelines. Interventions aimed at decreasing sedentary behavior and increasing physical activity, and maintaining these changes, are also part of effective programs. Ecobehavioral changes, such as family involvement, training, and support, are considered important for the successful treatment of pediatric obesity. Pharmacological and surgical interventions for pediatric obesity have been studied but, to date, have not been found as efficacious as behavioral and systemic approaches. There have also been concerns about deleterious side effects associated with drug and surgical interventions.

PROGNOSIS

Although child weight loss is typically less significant than that found in adults, maintenance of that weight loss is often more long-term. Prognosis is better for younger children than with older children. After age three the likelihood of becoming an obese adult increases steadily with age, with an estimated 70–80

percent of obese adolescents becoming obese adults. Family involvement and support are important components of successful intervention programs.

See also: Behavior Modification; Differential Social Reinforcement/Positive Attention; Health Education/Health Promotion; Treatment Adherence: Behavioral

Further Reading

American Academy of Pediatrics. (1998). Supplement: The causes and health consequences of obesity in children and adolescents. *Pediatrics, 101*(3), 497–570.
Barlow, S. E., & Dietz, W. H. (1998). Obesity evaluation and treatment: Expert Committee recommendations. The Maternal and Child Health Bureau, Health Resources and Services Administration and the Department of Health and Human Services. *Pediatrics, 102*(3), E-29.
Epstein, L. H., Roemmich, J. N., & Raynor, H. A. (2001). Behavioral therapy in the treatment of pediatric obesity. *Pediatric Clinics of North America, 48*(4), 981–993.
Goldstein, G. S., Raynor, H. A., & Epstein, L. H. (2002). Treatment of pediatric obesity. In T. A. Wadden, & A. J. Stunkard (Eds.), *Handbook of obesity treatment* (pp. 532–555). New York: Guilford.
Jelalian, E., & Saelens, B. E. (1999). Empirically supported treatments in pediatric psychology: Pediatric obesity. *Journal of Pediatric Psychology, 24*(3), 223–248.
Kedesdy, J. H., & Budd, K. S. (1998). *Childhood feeding disorders: Biobehavioral assessment and intervention*. Baltimore: Paul H. Brooke.
Linscheid, T. R., & Rasnake, L. K. (2001) Eating problems in children. In C. E. Walker & M. C. Roberts (Eds.), *Handbook of clinical child psychology* (pp. 523–541). New York: Wiley.
Nationwide weight loss program directed specifically for children. www.shapedown.com
Web site of American Academy of Family Physicians, article by Rebecca Moran, M. D. (1999) about pediatric obesity. http://www.aafp.org/afp/990215ap/861.html

THOMAS R. LINSCHEID
BERNARD METZ

Observation

See: Behavioral Observation

Obsessive Compulsive Disorder

DEFINITION/CLINICAL PRESENTATION

Obsessive Compulsive Disorder (OCD) is defined as the presence of distressing, time consuming, and/or interfering obsessions or compulsions. Obsessions refer to recurrent or persistent intrusive or inappropriate thoughts, impulses, or images that cause marked anxiety or distress. Compulsions are repetitive behaviors or mental acts that are performed in response to an obsession or according to some other rigidly applied rules. Compulsions are meant to reduce anxiety and distress or prevent some dreaded event from occurring but are clearly excessive and not realistically connected with the triggering stimulus. Among children and adolescents, the most common OCD symptoms tend to focus on fear of germs or contamination, followed by fears of harm to self or others, concerns with symmetry, and excessive moralization or religiosity. The most common compulsions include excessive washing and bathing, repeating, checking, touching, counting, and ordering or arranging.

The vast majority of youngsters with OCD experience both obsessions and compulsions. However, not all obsessions are anxiety-related, with some children describing intrusive thoughts or feelings related to disgust, discomfort, or an otherwise vague sensation that something is not right (the so-called "just-right" phenomenon). Similar to adult-onset OCD, the pattern and type of OCD symptoms in childhood typically shift over time, although the absolute number of symptoms generally remains constant. Children may be somewhat more likely than adults to engage in compulsive reassurance-seeking and involve family members in their rituals.

Childhood OCD is reactive to stress and many children experience acute symptom exacerbations during times of psychosocial challenge (e.g., start of school year, moving to a new home, death of or separation from a family member). Many youngsters with OCD are able to inhibit or control symptoms for short periods of time and with substantial effort, for example, while at school or in social situations. In some cases, parents, teachers, and others close to the child may remain unaware of the child's problem for significant periods of time, learning of it only after the child is no longer able to control his or her symptoms or becomes too overwhelmed to cope.

OCD is a highly comorbid disorder in childhood with up to 80 percent of affected youngsters meeting diagnostic criteria for another mental health disorder, most commonly another anxiety disorder, depressive disorder, tic disorder, or behavioral disorder. Moreover, over half of adults with OCD report that their symptoms began during childhood or adolescence and evidence suggests that pediatric OCD may predict adult morbidity.

INCIDENCE

OCD is a relatively common disorder with 1–3 percent of children and adolescents meeting diagnostic criteria. Subclinical OCD, or obsessions and compulsions occurring in the absence of significant distress or impairment, is more common, occuring in up to 20 percent of the child population. The average age of onset for childhood OCD is between 6 and 11 years of age, with some suggestion that boys may experience an earlier onset of symptoms than girls.

ASSESSMENT

The successful diagnosis and treatment of OCD require careful and systematic evaluation. Initially, a thorough diagnostic evaluation is necessary to accurately establish a diagnosis of OCD, to rule out phenomenologically similar conditions, and to identify comorbid conditions that could influence treatment planning. The assessment of baseline symptom severity and illness-related functional impairment also allows for the systematic evaluation of treatment response over time, and can guide the development of exposure and response prevention exercises for cognitive-behavioral treatment. The Children's Yale-Brown Obsessive Compulsive Scale (CYBOCS) is the most widely recommended measure for assessing OCD severity in children and adolescents. The CYBOCS is a comprehensive clinician-rated checklist covering the most commonly endorsed obsessions and compulsions and provides an overall severity score derived from global ratings of time spent, interference, distress, resistance, and control associated with the OCD symptoms. The assessment of childhood OCD can be hampered by the embarrassing nature of symptoms and resultant efforts to keep them secret. This difficulty can often be overcome by taking the time to establish rapport with the child, providing adequate psychoeducation, normalizing the content of symptoms, and ensuring confidentiality.

TREATMENT

Current evidence supports the efficacy of exposure-based cognitive-behavior therapy and pharmacotherapy with the selective serotonin reuptake inhibitors (SSRIs) for the treatment of OCD across the age span. Cognitive–behavioral therapy for OCD is based on the behavioral conceptualization of obsessions as intrusive and unwanted thoughts, images, or behaviors, which trigger a significant and rapid increase in anxiety or distress, and compulsions as overt behaviors or cognitions (covert behaviors), which are designed to reduce these negative feelings. The most effective form of behavior therapy consists of systematic in vivo exposure to the feared situations and objects paired with supervised response prevention of the relevant compulsion (i.e., exposure plus response prevention, or ERP). In ERP, treatment progresses in a gradual fashion according to a symptom hierarchy with milder symptoms exposed first followed by more difficult exposures as treatment progresses. Although exposures are typically developed and initially practiced in session, most treatment gains accrue from repeated practice in the natural environment. The most commonly proposed mechanism for ERP effectiveness is that over repeated exposures, associated anxiety dissipates through the process of autonomic habituation (i.e., the graduated reduction of physiological symptoms). In addition, successful completion of exposure facilitates the development and storage of corrective cognitive information pertaining to the feared situation. Controlled trials using this treatment have yielded response rates of 75–90 percent for adult OCD with impressive maintenance of gains over long-term follow-up. Although current data for childhood OCD is limited, CBT has yielded impressive and durable results in this age range with response rates ranging from 60–100 percent, mean symptom reduction rates ranging from 50–67 percent, and gains maintained for up to 18 months.

Controlled multisite trials with children and adolescents have demonstrated the efficacy and tolerability of antiserotonergic agents for OCD in this age range. Large multicenter trials of the selective serotonin reuptake inhibitors (SSRIs), sertraline (Zoloft), fluvoxamine (Luvox), and fluoxetine (Prozac), have established the efficacy of these medications for childhood OCD with the first three compounds currently approved by the FDA for use in children and adolescents with the disorder. Controlled data also supports the use of the tricyclic antidepressant and serotonin reuptake inhibitor, clomipramine (Anafranil), although safety concerns have relegated this medication to second-line status. Given concerns regarding medication use in children as well as the significant relapse potential associated with medication withdrawal, consensus treatment guidelines agree that CBT, when available, should be considered as the initial treatment choice for OCD in this age range.

PROGNOSIS

Longitudinal studies attest to the chronicity of OCD in childhood, with 50–70 percent of youths with OCD from community and clinical samples meeting diagnostic criteria for OCD at 2–14 year follow-up. It is likely, however, that the relatively negative outcomes associated with childhood OCD in the past have been at least partially due to the lack of effective interventions for this condition. As effective treatments, especially cognitive behavior therapy, become more widely available, it is reasonable to expect that the long-term outcome for children with OCD will improve.

See also: Anxiety Disorders; Cognitive–Behavior Therapy; Exposure and Response Prevention; Evidence-Based Treatments

Further Reading

Albano, A., March, J., & Piacentini, J. (1999). Cognitive behavioral treatment of obsessive-compulsive disorder. In R. Ammerman, M. Hersen, & C. Last (Eds.), *Handbook of prescriptive treatments for children and adolescents* (pp. 193–215). Boston: Allyn & Bacon.

Grados, M., Scahill, L., & Riddle, M. (1999). Pharmacotherapy in children and adolescents with obsessive-compulsive disorder. *Child and Adolescent Psychiatric Clinics of North America, 8,* 617.

Obsessive-Compulsive Foundation (OCF). http://www.ocfoundation.org/

Piacentini, J., & Bergman, R. L. (2000). Obsessive-compulsive disorder in children. *Psychiatric Clinics of North America, 23,* 519–533.

JOHN PIACENTINI
AUDRA LANGLEY

Obstructive Sleep Apnea

DEFINITION

Obstructive sleep apnea (OSA) is a breathing disorder characterized by brief interruptions of breathing during sleep which can last from 10 s to 3 min, with an average of 30–40 s and can occur up to several hundred times per night. Obstructive sleep apnea occurs when air cannot flow into or out of the person's nose or mouth although efforts to breathe continue. In some people, the airway is too narrow, while in others some abnormality or damage interferes with the ongoing effort to breathe. Children with sleep apnea present with very restless sleep, characterized by loud snoring, snorting, or gasping for breath, and intervening silences. These children can arouse frequently during the night, toss and turn, sweat, and fall asleep during the day at inappropriate times. OSA is not the same disorder as Sudden Infant Death Syndrome (SIDS) where the stopping of breathing does not involve airway obstruction, rather the baby simply stops breathing.

INCIDENCE/ETIOLOGY

Sleep apnea occurs in all age groups in both sexes, but is more common in males. It is thought to occur in 1–2 percent of the population with the average age for diagnosis in children at 7 years. Although once thought to be rare in children, reports of up to 14 percent of children seen in sleep disorders clinics have a primary diagnosis of OSA. Obstructive sleep apnea is most common in prepubertal children with enlarged tonsils and adenoids. Sleep apnea seems to run in some families, suggesting a possible genetic basis. Other risk factors are obesity, oral or facial abnormalities such as a markedly recessed chin or repaired cleft palate, Down Syndrome, and cystic fibrosis.

CORRELATES

Agitated arousal and unusual sleep postures, such as sleeping on the hands and knees, commonly occur in children with obstructive sleep apnea. Nocturnal enuresis is also common and may be a sign of this sleep difficulty, especially in a child who was previously dry at night. Children may have morning headaches, and they are at risk for the development of hypertension. Complaints of lethargy, daytime fatigue, and extreme difficulty waking in the morning are also common. Daytime mouth breathing, difficulty in swallowing, and poor speech articulation are also common features in children. Due to frequent nocturnal arousals, excessive daytime sleepiness, and hypoxia, the child can suffer from inattention, decreased academic achievement, oppositionality, and restlessness.

ASSESSMENT

In addition to the primary care physician, pulmonologists, neurologists, or other physicians with specialty training in sleep disorders may be involved in making a definitive diagnosis and initiating treatment. Several tests are available for evaluating a person for sleep apnea including *polysomnography* (evaluation where a person spends one or more nights sleeping in a sleep laboratory, being monitored on a number of measures that include respiration and oxygen desaturation—a measure of airflow; leg movements; brain wave activity; eye movements; muscle movements; and heart activity) and the *Multiple Sleep Latency Test*, which measures the time it takes to fall asleep and to go into deep sleep while taking several naps over a period of time. Diagnostic tests usually are performed in a sleep

disorders center, but new technology may allow some sleep studies to be conducted in the child's home.

TREATMENT

The specific treatment for sleep apnea is tailored to the individual patient based on medical history, physical examination, and the results of polysomnography. For mild or moderate cases of obstructive sleep apnea, treatment usually involves either *medication* (e.g., medicines that help stimulate respiration, such as medroxyprogesterone, or the tricyclic antidepressants, which affect REM sleep) or a *mechanical device* (e.g., a device that repositions the tongue or lower jaw during sleep) that improves breathing. Severe breathing problems may require *surgery* to help remove blockages in parts of the airways, such as tonsillectomy and/or adenoidectomy, which relieve 70 percent of all cases. In more severe cases, tracheostomy, in which a tube is inserted into a hole made through the neck below the vocal cords and into the windpipe, is performed. *Behavioral changes* are an important part of the treatment program, and in mild cases behavioral therapy may be all that is needed. For example, excessive weight (e.g., obesity), smoking (e.g., which causes swelling of the mucus membranes in the nose, swelling of the tissue in the throat, blockage of the small vessels in the lung), and alcohol (e.g., causes too great a relaxation of the airway during sleep) are all factors that greatly contribute to the development of apnea. Weight management, smoking cessation, and avoidance of alcohol and sedatives at bedtime are often enough to achieve the desired results.

PROGNOSIS

With treatment, the prognosis is good in most cases. For some individuals with obstructive sleep apnea, behavioral changes may eliminate the problem without further treatment.

See also: Excessive Sleepiness; Narcolepsy; Sleep Patterns, Normal; Sleep–Wake Cycle Problems

Further Reading

Gozal, D. (1998). Sleep-disordered breathing and school performance in children. *Pediatrics, 102,* 616–620.
Palasti, S., & Potsic, W. P. (1995). Managing the child with obstructive sleep apnea. In C. E. Schaefer (Ed.), *Clinical handbook of sleep disorders in children* (pp. 253–266). Northvale, NJ: Jason Aronson.

Standards of Practice Committee of the American Sleep Disorders Association. (1995). Practice parameters for the treatment of snoring and obstructive sleep apnea with oral appliances. *Sleep*, *18*, 511–513.

National Sleep Foundation, 1522 K Street, NW, Suite 500, Washington, DC 20005, Phone: (202) 347-3471, Fax: (202) 347-3472, E-mail: nsf@sleepfoundation.org, Web site: http://www.sleepfoundation.org

V. MARK DURAND
KRISTIN V. CHRISTODULU

Oncology

See: Cancers, Childhood

Opiates, Prenatal Exposure

DEFINITION OF PROBLEM

Opiates are highly addictive narcotics that affect the central nervous system (CNS), acting as depressants as well as painkillers. Opium is derived from the poppy plant which when processed, produces morphine that is synthesized to produce heroin. It can be inhaled, smoked, injected, or consumed orally. Depending on the method of use, the effects can begin in as short as 10–20 s and last up to 6 hours. Street names for heroin include: smack, junk, bags, black tar, horse, tar, and bundles.

Approximately 5,000–10,000 babies are born each year with prenatal exposure to heroin. Heroin freely crosses the placenta and produces withdrawal symptoms in 55–94 percent of babies born to mothers using heroin. Methadone, a synthetic drug used in the treatment of heroin addiction, also produces withdrawal symptoms in as many as 60 percent of affected neonates. A new medication, buprenophine, is being used for treating pregnant women with opiate addiction. Early findings suggest a decrease in neonatal withdrawal symptoms.

EFFECTS

Neonatal Abstinence Syndrome (NAS) is the term applied to the withdrawal of neonates from prenatal exposure to opiates. Infants generally will begin to show signs of withdrawal within 1–3 days of life; however, signs may take as long as 7–10 days with methadone exposure. Therefore, the hospital stay for infants with prenatal exposure must be increased in order to observe for symptoms as well as to provide

treatment. Symptoms of withdrawal in the neonate are very similar to that of the adult opiate user. Signs can be seen in dysfunction of the autonomic nervous system, the gastrointestinal system, and the respiratory system. Infants may have convulsions; tremors and jitteriness are common as is increased muscle tone and unprovoked muscle jerks. Babies may be inconsolable with crying lasting upward of 3 hr. In general, they are more irritable and more easily aroused. Persistent or projectile vomiting over a 12 hr period may be present and multiple episodes of explosive diarrhea are also common. Other symptoms of NAS include abnormally fast heart rate (tachycardia), fever, weight loss of >10 percent, and water loss in the stool. Treatment of NAS and weaning from the opiate is based on observed infant behaviors, weight change, and feeding. Morphine solution, Phenobarbitol, and Diazepam are used in the treatment for NAS.

In addition to NAS, infants with prenatal exposure to opiates are often born with low birth weight, intrauterine growth retardation, and with increased risk for fetal distress and death. An increased number of platelets in the peripheral blood may occur in the second week of life and continue for several months. Infants with opiate exposure, including methadone, are also at increased risk for Sudden Infant Death Syndrome (SIDS). Many of the mothers who abuse opiates also abuse a variety of other drugs (polysubstance abusers), making attributions regarding the negative effects to the opiates alone difficult. Furthermore, environmental risk factors related to opiate use may also be responsible for findings in this population. Most opiate users are in the lower socioeconomic status category, have poor or absent prenatal care, and poor nutrition, all of which are risk factors for poor developmental outcome. In addition, opiate use is associated with increased maternal psychopathology, insensitivity in parenting, increased risk for abuse/neglect in children; again, these environmental risk factors may be responsible for problems observed in neonates. Interestingly, studies have found little difference on the Bayley Scales of Infant Development in babies with opiate exposure compared to those without such exposure; however, a decrease on this measure was noted in babies with exposure by the age of 2 years. It should be noted that although findings were significant, scores continued to be within the normal limits of functioning.

TREATMENT AND PROGNOSIS

As with other substances used by women during pregnancy, reduction or abstinence in use at any time during gestation improves the potential outcome of the infant. Pregnancy should be considered a significant window of opportunity to intervene via substance abuse treatment since readiness to change may be heightened. For babies exposed prenatally to opiates, the likelihood of NAS is high, so close observation in the hospital is warranted and an extended stay for treatment is common. Current research indicates that long-term outcome of these infants is not significantly impaired as with children with Fetal Alcohol Syndrome (FAS). Subtle problems with sustained attention and distractibility have been noted and, thus, periodic developmental evaluations are recommended, particularly as these children enter school. Further, the environmental risk factors may severely impact the growth and development of youngsters remaining in homes where opiate or other substance abuse is present. Evaluation of these risk factors appears crucial to gain a better understanding of risk to the children and improve their outcomes.

See also: Effects of Parental Substance Abuse on Children; Infant Assessment; School Age Assessment; Substance Abuse

Further Reading

American Academy of Pediatrics Committee on Drugs. (1998). Neonatal drug withdrawal. *Pediatrics, 101,* 1079–1088.

Aylward, G. P. (1992). The relationship between environmental risk and developmental outcome. *Developmental and Behavioral Pediatrics, 13,* 222–229.

Hans, S. L., & Jeremy, R. J. (2001). Postneonatal mental and motor development of infants exposed in utero to opioid drugs. *Infant Mental Health Journal, 22,* 300–315.

Kaltenbach, K. A. (1994). Effects of in-utero opiate exposure: New paradigms for old questions. *Drug and Alcohol Dependence, 36,* 83 87.

Wagner, C., Katikaneni, L., Cox, J., & Ryan, R. (1998). The impact of prenatal drug exposure on the neonate. *Obstetrical and Gynecological Clinics of North America, 23,* 169–194.

ROBIN H. GURWITCH

Oppositional Defiant Disorder

DEFINITION

Oppositional Defiant Disorder (ODD) is listed in the *Diagnostic and Statistical Manual of Mental Disorders, 4th Edition (DSM-IV)* as one of the disruptive disorders under the heading "Disorders Usually First Diagnosed in Infancy, Childhood, or Adolescence." Children with ODD have a recurrent and long-standing pattern of negativistic, defiant, disobedient, and hostile behavior toward authority figures (e.g., parents, teachers) that is developmentally inappropriate and which leads to impairment. For example, children with ODD frequently argue with adults, defy rules, blame others for their own mistakes, and annoy others more than other children their age. Because the majority of children with Conduct Disorder (CD) display ODD symptoms, the ODD diagnosis is not given concurrently with a CD diagnosis.

PREVALENCE

The prevalence of ODD in child and adolescent community samples ranges from 2 percent to 16 percent depending on the diagnostic criteria employed, the informants, and the age range, gender and geographical location of the sample. For example, prevalence rates of ODD are higher when parental reports are employed than when boys' self-reports are used. The prevalence of ODD as a function of age is unclear as results across studies are inconsistent. Data on gender differences in the prevalence of ODD are more consistent, with the majority of studies indicating a higher rate of ODD in boys compared to girls, especially in younger samples.

CORRELATES

Studies that compare children with ODD to non-problem children have found that ODD is associated with child, familial, and environmental factors. In terms of child factors, ODD is associated with higher levels of attention problems, thought problems, aggressive or delinquent behavior, social problems, academic problems, and teen pregnancy. Familial factors associated with ODD are higher levels of coercive parenting, less parental monitoring, and other problematic family interactions. Finally, children with ODD tend to come from homes that have lower socioeconomic status and higher rates of adverse life experiences.

COMORBIDITY

There is a paucity of research examining comorbidity in ODD samples where children with ODD and CD are not combined into a single group. The studies that have identified children with ODD (without comorbid CD) have reported rates of Attention-Deficit/Hyperactivity

Disorder (ADHD) ranging from 14 to 93 percent. Other disorders that tend to co-occur with ODD are anxiety disorders, depressive disorders, and conduct disorder. As noted before, most boys with CD would also meet diagnostic criteria for ODD (84–96 percent), bringing into question the distinctiveness of the ODD diagnosis from CD. Whether ODD is a milder form of CD, a precursor to CD, or a separate disorder altogether has been the subject of much debate and is an issue which remains unresolved.

ASSESSMENT

Assessment of ODD often begins with a clinical interview with the parent that covers information such as developmental history, social functioning, school behavior and performance, and family/parental functioning. Although the value of a child interview has been debated, frequently it is recommended if only to establish a relationship prior to initiation of treatment. Structured interviews that assess diagnostic criteria as outlined in the *DSM-IV* and yield a categorical diagnosis also are recommended. Given the relatively common nature of oppositional behaviors such as noncompliance among all children, the use of standardized measures that provide appropriate age and gender norms are essential. Among the many appropriate questionnaires would be the Child Behavior Checklist and Teacher Report Form or the Revised Conners' Parent Rating Scale. Such measures yield dimensional assessments of oppositional behavior and their norms allow comparison of the child's level of oppositional behavior to other children of the same age and gender. Finally, because ODD is frequently correlated with parental dysfunction and family disturbance, parenting practices, family and marital functioning, parental psychological functioning, as well as parent/family stress and social support should be assessed. The relation between ODD and family problems also highlights the potential for factors such as stress or depression to negatively influence parental ratings of the child. For this reason, information from teachers or peers and observational measures of the child's behavior are important adjuncts to parental reports of ODD.

TREATMENT

As with all disruptive disorders, agreement exists that prevention and early intervention are the most effective courses of action. In fact, the treatment of ODD in young children has been viewed as an important opportunity in the prevention of more serious conduct and antisocial problems later in life. Beyond prevention efforts, treatments for children with ODD are commonly based on the evidence of an association between ODD and parenting difficulties. Several parent management training programs that focus on teaching parents skills such as monitoring child behavior, giving clear instructions, and using consistent feedback have demonstrated efficacy in reducing child oppositional behaviors and increasing compliance . All forms of behavioral parent training appear to be most helpful with younger children and successful treatment is inversely related to the presence of family or parental problems. School-based programs focusing on teaching children anger management or social interaction also have shown treatment efficacy, although these treatments appear to be most useful for older elementary-school-aged children. Finally, pharmacotherapy is occasionally used in the treatment of ODD, but this form of treatment has an extremely limited base of supportive evidence.

PROGNOSIS

Longitudinal studies demonstrated that, among children referred to clinics, approximately half to two-thirds of those with ODD progress to having more serious conduct problems, while for the remaining children the problems desist with age. In contrast, in the general population of children there is less continuity from oppositional to conduct-disordered behavior. Severity, early onset, a wide range of ODD behaviors, and perhaps co-occurring attentional problems are predictors of continuity of problems into adolescence. Because most studies of ODD have been conducted with boys, less is known about the stability and prediction of continuing conduct problems in girls with ODD. However, some data suggest that stability may be as likely in girls as in boys.

See also: Aggression; Conduct Disorder; Disruptive Behavior Disorders; Parent Training; Temper Tantrums

Further Reading

Brestan, E. V., & Eyberg, S. M. (1998). Effective psychosocial treatment of conduct-disordered children and adolescents: 20 years, 82 studies, and 5,272 kids. *Journal of Clinical Child Psychology, 27*, 180–189.
Carlson, C. L., Tamm, L., & Hogan, A. E. (1999). The child with oppositional defiant disorder and conduct disorder in the family. In H. C. Quay & A. E. Hogan (Eds.), *Handbook of disruptive behavior disorders* (pp. 337–352). New York: Kluwer Academic/ Plenum.

Kazdin, A. E. (1997). Parent management training: Evidence, outcomes, and issues. *Journal of the American Academy of Child and Adolescent Psychiatry, 36*, 1349–1356

Loeber, R., Burke, J. D., Lahey, B. B., Winters, A., & Zera, M. (2000). Oppositional defiant and conduct disorder: A review of the past 10 years, Part I. *Journal of the Academy of Child and Adolescent Psychiatry, 39*, 1468–1484.

CHARLOTTE JOHNSTON
CANDICE MURRAY

Oral Health Behavior

See: Behavioral Dentistry

Orthopedic Disabilities

This term refers to disabilities or disorders relating to the bones or joints; common examples include scoliosis, juvenile rheumatoid arthritis, and neuromuscular disorders which effect movement because of damages to the spinal cord (e.g., spinal cord injury, spina bifida). Orthopedic disabilities can be the result of congenital (present before or at the time of birth), developmental (a condition that appears later in life), genetic, traumatic (sports injuries, accidents), infectious-inflammatory, metabolic, and neoplastic (tissue growth) problems.

See also: Injury Prevention; Juvenile Rheumatoid Arthritis; Spina Bifida; Spinal Cord Injury;

DENNIS C. HARPER

Osteosarcoma

DESCRIPTION

Osteosarcoma (OS), arises from bone-forming tissue and involves rapid proliferation of osteoid (bone) tissue or immature bone. It is the most common bone tumor in children. The incidence in the United States is about 8.7 cases per million children and adolescents under 20 years of age with about 400 cases diagnosed per year. It is more common in boys than in girls with the peak incidence occurring in adolescence.

ETIOLOGY

Etiology is generally unknown, but there is an association with ionizing radiation, and the disease may not occur for many years after radiation. Other associations are with alkylating agents (e.g., cyclophosphamide cisplatin, melphalan), in patients with Paget's disease, and possibly familial factors (higher incidence in the hereditary form of retinoblastoma, genetic mutations of the p53 gene, Li-Fraumeni syndrome).

PRESENTATION

Presentation often includes pain sometimes accompanied by a soft-tissue mass. The child or adolescent may have had the symptoms for several months before diagnosis. The average duration of symptoms is about 3 months, although it can be much longer. Common diagnostic procedures include biopsy, and imaging studies, such as CT and bone scans. Osteosarcoma is found most often in the long tubular bones (distal femur, proximal tibia, and humerus), although it may also occur in the pelvis and skull. Metastasis (spread of cancer to other tissues or organs) is present in 15–20 percent of cases at the time of diagnosis, most with pulmonary involvement.

TREATMENT

Surgery is the treatment of choice for control at the primary site; without surgery, the survival rate is poor. Surgery, however, is not sufficient, with metastases likely to occur if there is no other treatment, such as, chemotherapy. Surgery is usually amputation or limb salvage (removal of the affected bone and tissue but not the entire limb) and depends upon location, size, presence of metastases, age, skeletal development, and lifestyle preference. Osteosarcoma is not very responsive to radiation therapy. Chemotherapy is used to treat systemic disease (cancer cells that may be present elsewhere in the body). It is also used to shrink the tumor before local surgery. A common combination of chemotherapy drugs includes doxorubicin, cisplatin, and high-dose methotrexate, but the effectiveness of the latter is debated. Recent studies have included the addition of ifosfamide and/or immunological agents. After treatment, the patient must undergo physical therapy and either additional surgeries to fit prostheses or additional grafting after limb salvage.

When metastatic disease is present at diagnosis, treatment is similar to that of localized primary tumors.

Resection (surgical removal) of all tumours is the best hope for cure—but patients with tumours that cannot be fully removed or lung metastases have a poor prognosis. Aggressive surgery (thoracotomy) is indicated for pulmonary disease, except when there are too many lesions in the lungs or where the disease has metastasized to other areas of the body and cannot be removed. In those cases, aggressive chemotherapy may still be indicated in the hope of shrinking the tumours and providing a chance for long-term disease control. Prognostic factors for metastatic disease include: presence at diagnosis or within 6 months of surgery (worse prognosis) and having a large number of pulmonary nodules. If curative treatment is not possible, palliative care to provide comfort and decrease pain or drugs still being tested may be used. Radiation therapy may also be used as a palliative measure.

It is important for patients and their families to receive adequate preparation for amputation and limb salvage procedures and to have emotional support before, during, and after the procedures. In general, adolescents have been found to adapt well, and there has been a lack of evidence favoring either amputation or limb salvage in terms of functional or psychological adaptation. However, long-term effects of amputation or limb salvage surgery as well as effects of intensive chemotherapy have not been well-studied.

PSYCHOSOCIAL ISSUES

Coping with the real or threatened loss of a limb, disfigurement, and loss of functioning are major issues. A multidisciplinary pain team should be involved early to assess and treat surgical pain and later phantom pain if it occurs. Side effects of chemotherapy, such as nausea and vomiting, can often be decreased with newer effective antiemetic medications and behavioral interventions, which are helpful in promoting relaxation and reducing anxiety. Prolonged and intermittent separation from family and friends, absence from school and activities, inability to use previously helpful coping mechanisms, (for example, exercise, sports, and frequent social contacts) can stress the adolescent's coping resources. At a time when adolescents typically become more independent from their parents and family, they are forced to assume a more dependent role, sometimes resulting in anger and resentment towards family members and staff as well as withdrawal and depressive thoughts and behaviors. There may be great difficulty in reassessment of identity and future goals. Given developmental and cognitive level, previous adjustment and coping, as well as family functioning, psychosocial staff

can help the adolescent and family to process these issues and to begin to deal with them as part of the recovery process. In addition to cognitive-behavioral therapy focused on specific coping tasks in recovery, it can be helpful to introduce children or adolescents to others who have had the same procedures and who are doing well, but this is dependent upon the desires of the individual. Groups and camps for adolescents and young adults, as well as organized activities and outings (frequently coordinated by child life) are often effective ways of helping them to resume social contacts, as well as to share feelings and experiences with peers who have undergone similar treatments.

Effects from the cancer treatment itself can occur later, for example, problems in cardiac function after anthracycline chemotherapy, hearing loss from cisplatin, infertility, growth problems, and second malignancies. Long-term follow-up, both medically and psychosocially, is crucial for optimal long-term survival of these patients. In the past, many adolescent and young adult patients have not been followed adequately once they are no longer patients in a pediatric oncology service, however, efforts are being made in the cooperative group (COG; groups of clinical researchers providing data on large numbers of children in a timely fashion) to provide better coordination and continuity of care between pediatric and adult oncology centers.

PROGNOSIS

The overall survival rate for patients with osteosarcoma is about 66 percent. Favorable prognostic factors include extent of disease at diagnosis (lesser, better), histology (parosteal and intraosseous well-differentiated OS, better), no diagnosis of Paget's disease, DNA content, primary site (more distal, better), small tumor size, absence of "skip" lesions (areas of tumor away from the primary tumor), duration of symptoms (longer, better), age (older, better), female gender, low levels of serum LDH and/or serum/tumor alkaline phosphatase, and, once in treatment, response to chemotherapy.

See also: Childhood Cancers, Coping with Illness; Parenting the Chronically Ill Child; Preparation for Medical Procedures; Treatment Adherence: Medical

Further Reading

Granowetter, L. (1994) Pediatric oncology: A medical overview. In D. Bearison & R. K. Mulhern (Ed.), *Pediatric psycho-oncology* (pp. 9–34). New York: Oxford University Press.

Helligenstein, E. & Holland, J. C. (1989) Malignant bone tumors. In J. C. Holland & J. Rowland (Eds.), *Handbook of psycho-oncology* (pp. 250–253). New York: Oxford.

Link, M. P., Gebhardt, M. C., & Meyers, P. A. (2002). Osteosarcoma. In P. A. Pizzo, & D. G. Poplack (Eds.), *Principles and practice of pediatric oncology* (4th ed., pp. 1051–1089). Philadelphia: Lippincott Williams & Wilkins.

Smith, M. A., & Ries, L. A. (2002). Childhood cancer: Incidence, survival, and mortality. In P. A. Pizzo & D. G. Poplack (Eds.), *Principles and practice of pediatric oncology.* (4th ed., pp. 1–12). Philadelphia: Lippincott Williams & Wilkins.

Tyc, V. (1992). Psychosocial adaptation of children and adolescents with limb deficiencies: A review. *Clinical Psychology Review, 12,* 275–292.

Mary Jo Kupst
Anne B. Warwick

Otitis Media

DEFINITION

Otitis media (OM) is a bacterial or viral infection of the middle ear that results from failure of the eustachian tube to drain middle ear fluid. Acute OM may be accompanied by ear pain, fever, sudden hearing loss, and other signs of an acute infection (e.g., irritability, lethargy, diarrhea, vomiting, nasal congestion, headache, sore throat); perforation of the ear drum may occur. Recurrent OM (i.e., three or more acute infections in 6 months) or OM with effusion (i.e., presence of middle ear fluid for 2–3 months without acute infection) may be associated with sustained hearing loss, and, if hearing loss is bilateral and greater than 20 dB, the young child may be at risk for developmental problems.

INCIDENCE

OM occurs in approximately 70 percent of children younger than 3 years of age and approximately 20 percent of children have recurrent OM.

CORRELATES

A complication of recurrent OM is sustained hearing loss, which may be associated with delay in language development and possibly later learning and attention problems. Developmental problems, however, occur in a minority of children with recurrent OM. A number of risk or predisposing factors have been identified for OM, including exposure to passive smoke, family history of OM, congenital disorders (e.g., cleft palate, trisomy 21), exposure to allergens, recurrent episodes of sinusitis, excessive use of a pacifier, and exposure to recurrent infections through contact with ill children.

ASSESSMENT

Children with OM require diagnosis and treatment by a health care provider. This involves a history of the child's health, development, and environmental conditions, and a physical examination including the use of pneumatic otoscopy (which allows for the delivery of puffs of air to observe movement of the eardrum). Lack of movement indicates the presence of middle ear fluid. Diagnostic tests are not usually ordered.

TREATMENT

The most common treatments include pain relievers (e.g., acetaminophen) and antibiotics (e.g., amoxicillin). The current trend is to use antibiotics sparingly to reduce the likelihood of bacterial resistance; antibiotic treatment has been shown to have a relatively minimal effect on clinical outcome of OM. Adherence to the prescribed medical regimen and scheduled follow-up visits should be promoted to assure that the infection is resolved, the middle-ear fluid has cleared, and normal hearing has returned. Other recommendations include modifying risk factors (i.e., avoid exposure to passive smoke, control exposure to allergens, appropriate treatment of sinusitis, limit young children's use of a pacifier, reduce situations in which recurrent infections are likely such as group day care). Recurrent OM may be treated by the insertion of tympanostomy tubes to prevent accumulation of middle ear fluid and to restore normal hearing. Antihistamines and decongestants are indicated only for concomitant symptoms (e.g., upper respiratory congestion). For recurrent OM, parents may benefit from supportive counseling to enhance adherence with treatment regimens, assist with modifying risk factors, and promote language development in children at risk due to sustained bilateral hearing impairment.

PROGNOSIS

OM resolves without complication in most children. Recurrent OM with effusion (fluid in the ear) requires monitoring by a health care provider to address sustained hearing loss that may compromise language development and may lead to later learning and attention problems. If there are signs of developmental problems, referral for developmental evaluation and treatment should be made.

See also: Hearing Impairment; Pediatric Infectious Diseases; Speech and Language Assessment; Treatment Adherence: Medical

Further Reading

Graham, M. V., & Uphold, C. R. (1999). *Clinical guidelines in child health* (2nd ed.). Gainesville, FL: Barmarrae Books.

Petersen-Smith, A. M. (2000). Ear disorders. In C. E. Burns, M. A. Brady, A. M. Dunn, & N. B. Starr (Eds.), *Pediatric primary care: A handbook for nurse practitioners* (2nd ed., pp. 783–807). Philadelphia: W.B. Saunders.

JACK W. FINNEY

Outcome Measures

See: Measurement of Treatment Outcome

Overanxious Disorder

See: Generalized Anxiety Disorder

Overcorrection

Overcorrection is a widely researched behavior management procedure involving a number of principles of behavior change. Overcorrection is a reductive procedure that aims to decrease the future occurrence of a problem behavior. However, unlike other reductive techniques such as time out and response cost, in which the individual loses access to reinforcement or is fined, overcorrection involves the application of a corrective or educative consequence to misbehavior.

Overcorrection typically consists of two components: restitutional overcorrection and positive practice overcorrection. The restitutional overcorrection component is a punitive component in that it requires the child to correct the consequences of his misbehavior by restoring any damage to the environment he may have caused. For example, if a student upon entering the classroom rushes down the aisle and knocks books and papers off desks as he goes, he would be required to return the scattered books and papers to their proper place. Positive practice overcorrection is an educative component in that it provides the child with an opportunity to repeatedly practice an alternative appropriate behavior, contingent on the occurrence of problem behavior. In the example described above, the positive practice overcorrection component would require the child to leave the classroom, enter in an orderly manner, and sit gently in their chair. Typically, this behavior is repeated several times, with the clinician providing manual guidance. This guidance is then progressively faded through the course of treatment.

It is important to note that not all behaviors lend themselves to the use of both restitutional overcorrection and positive practice overcorrection. Specifically, if the environment is not altered by an inappropriate act, then only positive practice overcorrection can be used. An example of such an instance is self-stimulatory behavior, whereby no disruption to the environment occurs and where only positive practice overcorrection can be used.

Overcorrection has been used extensively to treat disruptive behaviors, particularly those of children with a developmental disability, although its popularity as a behavior change technique has waned in recent years. This could be due to the fact that the positive practice component often involves physically forcing the child to engage in the behavior, and this has been perceived to be unnecessarily aversive.

See also: Applied Behavior Analysis; Positive Reinforcement; Response Cost; Time Out

Further Reading

Cole, G. A., Montgomery, R. W., Wilson, K. M., & Milan, M. A. (2000). Parametric analysis of overcorrection duration effects: Is longer really better than shorter? *Behavior Modification, 24*, 359–378.

Jones, M. L., Eyberg, S. M., Adams, C. D., & Boggs, S. R. (1998). Treatment acceptability of behavioral interventions for children: An assessment by mothers of children with disruptive behavior disorders. *Child & Family Behavior Therapy, 20*, 15–26.

Rhymer, K. N., Dittmer, K. I., Skinner, C. H., & Jackson, B. (2000). Effectiveness of a multi-component treatment for improving mathematics fluency. *School Psychology Quarterly, 15*, 40–51.

Shapiro, E. S., Barrett, R. P., & Ollendick, T. H. (1980). A comparison of physical restraint and positive practice overcorrection in treating stereotypic behavior. *Behavior Therapy, 11*, 227–233.

SOPHIA XENOS
ALAN HUDSON

Pp

Pain Assessment

DEFINITION

Pain is a complex and highly subjective phenomenon containing both sensory and affective components. Accurate assessment of multiple aspects of children's pain is critical for ensuring that proper management strategies are delivered to children with acute, recurrent, and chronic pain. Pain in children can be measured by self-report, overt observation of behaviors, or recording of physiological measures suggestive of pain. Because pain is a highly individualized and subjective event, a child's self-report has generally been considered to be the "gold standard" for pediatric pain assessment, despite its limitations.

METHODS

Self-report measures rely on children reporting their own subjective pain experience through words, numbers, colors, pictures, or manipulating objects. For example, faces pain scales, which provide a series of facial expressions depicting gradations of pain, are appealing and have become the most popular format to elicit children's self-reported pain intensity. Because children must have adequate cognitive and communicative skills to use these measures, the lower age limit has been reported to be 3–5 years. Behavioral measures, on the other hand, rely on trained observers who document specific distress behaviors (e.g., motor movement, facial expression, vocalizations) that are typically associated with pain. For example, facial coding systems have been developed to measure the pain experience of infants and children. Behavioral observation tools serve as the primary measure when evaluating pain in the infant or child with limited communication skills.

Table 1 describes examples of selected measurement tools aimed at assessing core dimensions of a child's pain experience. Because *acute pain* is of a relatively brief duration, measures of pain intensity, location, and affect are primary dimensions assessed by these pain instruments. The majority of validated measures have been developed to describe pain intensity or the amount of subjective pain or hurt experienced by children. Measuring aspects of *recurrent and chronic pain* requires tools that also measure the duration, time course, and activity interference due to pain. These measurements are considered to be more valid if collected in a prospective manner (e.g., a daily diary) versus in a retrospective report (e.g., interview questions about pain over the prior month). For a more complete overview of specific pain assessment tools in children, the reader is referred to Finley and McGrath (1997).

RELIABILITY/VALIDITY

Obtaining reliable and accurate measures of children's pain experience has presented challenges to researchers and clinicians. Pain measures may be influenced by a child's cognitive or language skills, or the positive or negative consequences that their own pain reports may produce (e.g., fear that a high pain rating

Table 1. Description of Core Pain Domains and Assessment Methods

Domain	Description	Example of instrument	Age/Population for use
	Pain intensity		
Numerical pain intensity	Child selects a number on a scale that best describes amount of pain or hurt, typically 0–10 scale	Numerical pain scale	School-age to adolescence
Visual analog scales	Usually consists of a 10-cm line with anchors that describe pain or affect Child places mark along line to indicate intensity of pain or affect and this is then measured to determine score	Varni-Thompson Pediatric Pain Inventory; Children's Comprehensive Pain Questionnaire	Lower age limit 5–7 years
Faces rating scales	Pain scale with pictures of faces or cartoon drawings of faces with anchors (typically 5–7 categories). Child chooses the face that best describes pain at present or how he or she is feeling	Wong-Baker Faces Rating Scale; Bieri faces	Lower age limit 3–4 years
Behavioral observation scales	A trained observer uses categories of behaviors (e.g., grimacing, torso movement) to score pain complaints	Children's Hospital of Eastern Ontario Pain Scale	Infants, toddlers. Specific scales are available for the cognitively or physically impaired child
	Pain location		
Body maps	Outline of human figure. Child marks areas where he or she is experiencing pain.	Adolescent Pediatric Pain Tool	Typically older school-age to adolescence
	Multiple dimensions		
Daily diary records	Child reports on his or her pain each day or multiple times a day (e.g., morning, noon, bedtime) and may record location, duration, mood, activity interference	Headache Diary	Typically older school-age to adolescence; recurrent and chronic pain
	Functional impact		
Functional status and disability	Child rates impact of pain on important everyday activities including school, peers, and physical activities	Functional Disability Inventory; PedsQL	Typically school-age to adolescence; recurrent and chronic pain

may lead to an injection). Perhaps due to these challenges, measures of children's pain intensity have received ample research attention and subsequently have been more thoroughly validated than those of adult pain intensity. On the other hand, assessment of other aspects of pain such as affect and activity interference or functional impact of pain need much more research in order to develop reliable and valid measures.

A number of valid and reliable measures of children's pain intensity have been developed. Several of the more widely used instruments are listed in Table 1. Validity has been demonstrated through correlations between different types of measures and informants. For example, child's self-report of pain intensity has been found to correlate with direct overt behavioral signs of pain and with adult observer ratings of the child's pain intensity.

There has been an emerging interest in comparing the validity of different forms of child's self-report of pain intensity. This interest has arisen from a debate in the literature concerning which format of the faces pain scales provides the most reliable and valid measure of a child's self report of pain intensity. Faces scales with a smiling face as the "no pain" anchor may confuse affective states with pain (e.g., children who are not in pain are not necessarily happy). Investigators have documented that children do in fact overestimate pain intensity in situations that involve negative emotions and pain when using faces scales with a smiling "no pain" anchor compared to a neutral "no pain" anchor. One suggestion that has been proposed is to first ask children to rate their anxiety on a separate scale and then to ask children to rate their pain intensity.

CLINICAL APPLICATIONS

Pain assessment is critical for understanding a child's experience of pain in acute situations such as a venipuncture or bone marrow aspiration as well as the more complex pattern of pain and behaviors that may accompany recurrent and chronic pain. Accurate pain assessment allows the clinician to individualize pain treatment strategies to the child and family's needs and to assess treatment progress in achieving important goals of pain reduction or increasing function.

The majority of pain assessment tools have been developed for use with children presenting with a variety of pain complaints due to medical procedures, injuries, or from chronic health conditions. Several daily diaries have been developed specifically for children with recurrent or chronic pain. For example, daily diaries have been validated for use in children with headaches. There are general measures of disability and quality of life that may be useful for documenting the impact of pain on children's functioning and well-being, but there has been inadequate study to assess their usefulness. Several measures of function and quality of life have been tailored to specific pain syndromes or chronic health conditions. For example, in juvenile chronic arthritis, disease-specific measures of function and quality of life include the Childhood Health Assessment Questionnaire and the PedsQL. Investigators believe that one advantage of disease-specific measures is that they may be more sensitive to changes in a child's health and functional status with treatment, such as pain management interventions.

See also: Coping with Illness; Pain Management; Preparation for Medical Procedures; Quality of life

Further Reading

Chambers, C. T., Giesbrecht, K., Craig, K. D., Bennett, S. M., & Huntsman, E. (1999). A comparison of faces scales for the measurement of pediatric pain: Children's and parents' ratings. *Pain*, *83*, 25–35.

Finley, G. A., & McGrath, P. J. (1997). *Measurement of pain in infants and children.* Seattle: IASP Press

Tonya M. Palermo
Chantelle Nobile

Pain Management

DEFINITION

Pediatric pain management refers to intervention strategies designed to reduce pain sensations, increase comfort, and/or reduce associated disability and dysfunction in children from infancy to adolescence. These intervention strategies may include either pharmacological strategies alone, nonpharmacological strategies alone, or a combination of the two. Nonpharmacological pain management strategies will be the focus of this entry.

The International Association for the Study of Pain defines pain as "an unpleasant sensory and emotional experience associated with actual or potential tissue damage, or described in terms of such damage" (IASP, 1979, p. 249). Acute pain refers to pain associated with a brief episode of tissue injury or inflammation such as pain related to medical procedures. Recurrent pain alternates with pain-free periods such as in recurrent headaches or abdominal pain, while chronic pain persists beyond the usual time period required for healing (usually 6 months) or develops and persists without obvious physical damage such as in reflex sympathetic dystrophy (i.e., chronic neuropathic pain).

DESCRIPTION OF TREATMENT

There are a number of nonpharmacological treatment approaches designed to reduce children's pain. The reader is referred to Kuttner (1996) for a comprehensive review of pain management strategies. A subset of the more commonly used cognitive–behavioral, rehabilitation, and physical modalities are described in Table 1. Distraction and relaxation strategies can be taught to a variety of health care professionals (e.g., nurses, physicians) for use with children. A psychologist, on the other hand, typically is responsible for working with a child or family on cognitive–behavioral strategies such as stress inoculation training.

CLINICAL APPLICATIONS

Much of the research efforts to manage pain in children have focused on children who undergo medical, surgical, or dental procedures. Specific clinical populations who experience *acute pain* include

Table 1. Examples of Specific Pain Management Strategies

Intervention strategy	Description	Indications for use	Ages/Populations
Cognitive–Behavioral Techniques			
Cognitive strategies	Helping the child develop a sense of mastery over anxious or distressing thoughts through strategies such as positive self-statements and challenging irrational thoughts	Maladaptive or anxious thoughts are interfering with pain management	Typically school-age children and adolescents; across types of pain (acute, recurrent, chronic)
Distraction	Focusing the child's attention on unrelated internal (e.g., breathing) or external (e.g., music, books) processes to the exclusion of pain sensations	Anxiety/distress is interfering with coping	Older infancy to adolescence; acute pain (especially procedural pain)
Relaxation training	Teaching the child a skill that produces a sensation incompatible with negative emotional and/or physiological arousal through deep breathing, imagery, or progressive muscle relaxation	Negative emotions or physiological arousal are contributing to the pain experience	Most often used with children ages 7 and above; across types of pain
Biofeedback	Electronic monitoring, measurement, and display of physiological processes such as body temperature or muscle tension, which can come under voluntary control through training and observation	Often used to facilitate relaxation training	Most often used with children ages 7 and above; typically for recurrent and chronic pain
Stress inoculation training	Regimen involving education, skills training (i.e., relaxation and positive self-statements), and application training using in vivo or imagined exposure to the painful event	Self-control strategies are needed for managing anxiety or pain	School-age children and adolescents; typically for acute procedural pain
Activity pacing	Helping children control pain by learning to pace and then gradually increase their activity level	Fear or avoidance of activities is present and/or functional status is impacted by pain	School-age children and adolescents; primarily for recurrent or chronic pain
Rehabilitation approaches	Interdisciplinary approach to treatment, may include pharmacotherapy, relaxation training, exercise, hydrotherapy	Significant disability is present requiring multiple treatment modalities	Across developmental levels; primarily for chronic pain
Physical modalities	Strategies such as heat, cold, massage, stretching, exercise used to relieve pain typically under the supervision of a physical or occupational therapist	Typically considered for musculoskeletal pain	Across developmental levels; across types of pain

otherwise healthy children undergoing medical procedures or presenting to emergency departments with injuries, as well as children with chronic health conditions such as cancer or HIV who must undergo medical procedures as part of treatment.

Although estimates of as many as 30 percent of children experience pain at least once a week, much less research attention on pain management has focused on recurrent and chronic pain in children. *Recurrent pain* populations include children with recurrent pain syndromes in which pain itself is the syndrome or disease process such as recurrent abdominal pain and headaches. *Chronic pain* populations typically include children with diseases in which pain is a common associated complication such as in sickle cell disease or juvenile rheumatoid arthritis. In addition, children may experience chronic pain following physical trauma or injury such as in reflex sympathetic dystrophy (i.e., chronic neuropathic pain).

EFFECTIVENESS

Acute Pain

Of the types of pain that children may experience, nonpharmacological approaches for acute pain have been the best researched. Cognitive–behavioral treatment approaches are well-established approaches for treating acute procedure-related pain. Included under the rubric of cognitive–behavioral approaches are relaxation strategies such as deep breathing and imagery, cognitive approaches such as distraction, and behavioral approaches such as filmed modeling, behavioral rehearsal, and contingent reinforcement programs. These strategies have typically been used with preschool to school age children. There are also specific comfort measures (e.g., pacifier, swaddling) that have been found to be useful for reducing behavioral signs of pain in infants.

Recurrent Pain

The recurrent pain condition that has received the most research attention is pediatric headache, where the use of relaxation strategies and self-hypnosis have been found to be effective treatments for reducing the frequency and severity of headache pain in children in a small number of studies. The use of thermal biofeedback in pediatric headache has also received some support. Cognitive–behavioral strategies for reducing pain and increasing function have been effective in children with recurrent abdominal pain.

Chronic Pain

Due to the lack of research on pain management strategies for chronic disease-related pain, it is unknown whether nonpharmacological treatments are effective for these children. However, in small, uncontrolled studies, cognitive–behavioral treatment strategies have been found to be promising techniques for treating pain across a number of disease conditions such as juvenile rheumatoid arthritis, fibromyalgia, and sickle cell disease. For example, use of pain coping skills including deep breathing relaxation, pleasant imagery, and calming self-talk are associated with increased function (e.g., attending school) on days with pain in children with sickle cell disease. Similarly, although modalities such as splinting, ice, heat, paraffin baths, massage, active exercise, and stretching have been shown to be useful for pain management in adults with chronic pain from arthritis, there have not been rigorous evaluations of their potential benefit in children with chronic pain. However small studies have demonstrated some pain reduction benefits from massage therapy and stretching exercises in children with chronic musculoskeletal pain.

See also: Behavior Modification; Biofeedback; Coping with Illness; Hypnosis; Preparation for Medical Procedures; Relaxation Training; Stress Management

Further Reading

American Academy of Pediatrics. (2001). *Policy statement: The assessment and management of acute pain in infants, children, and adolescents (0793)*. Retrieved on April 25, 2002 from: http://www.aap.org/policy/9933.html

Dahlquist, L. M. (1999). *Pediatric pain management*. New York: Kluwer Academic/Plenum.

International Association for the Study of Pain, Subcommittee on Taxonomy. (1979). Pain terms: A list of definitions and notes on usage. *Pain*, 6, 249–252.

Kuttner, L. (1996). *A child in pain: How to help, what to do*. Point Roberts, WA: Hartley & Marks.

McGrath, P. J., & Finley, G. A. (1999). *Chronic and recurrent pain in children and adolescents*. Seattle: IASP Press.

Pediatric Pain—Science Helping Children Web site: http://is.dal.ca/~pedpain/

Powers, S. W. (1999). Empirically supported treatments in pediatric psychology: Procedure-related pain. *Journal of Pediatric Psychology*, 24(2), 131–145.

TONYA M. PALERMO
CHANTELLE NOBILE

Pancreas Transplantation, Pediatric

BRIEF DESCRIPTION AND INDICATIONS

The pancreas is a large elongated gland situated behind the stomach; it secretes a digestive juice into the small intestine and also produces insulin. Pancreas transplantation is the preferred treatment for patients with renal (kidney) failure secondary to insulin-dependent diabetes mellitus. By conducting simultaneous pancreas–kidney transplantation, renal failure and endocrine pancreatic failure can be treated at the same time. Transplantation of a pancreas into an adult who already has a functional kidney transplant is done to treat the complications associated with diabetes, which may include diabetic retinopathy, neuropathy, nephropathy, and accelerated vascular disease. For patients with diabetes who do not respond to conventional therapy, pancreas-only transplantation may be done. In virtually all cases, the pancreas is obtained from a cadaveric organ donor, although there are a few cases involving live donors of pancreatic segments.

In June 2001, there were 24 children under 18 years of age on the waiting list for pancreas transplantation in the United States. This number represents less than 1 percent of the 3,600 total patients awaiting pancreas or pancreas–kidney transplantation. Since 1990, there have been fewer than 100 pediatric pancreas transplants performed in the United States, although there have been over 15,000 pancreas transplants performed in adults worldwide. One-year patient survival rates are 98 percent for pancreas transplant alone, 95 percent for simultaneous pancreas–kidney transplantation, and 94 percent for pancreas-after-kidney transplantation.

OUTCOMES

Historically, pancreas transplantation has been associated with a higher complication rate than other solid organ transplants. However, with improvements in technique and immunosuppressant medication, the complication rate has been reduced to 20–30 percent. Other complications related to pancreas transplants occur within the first month and include graft thrombosis, acute rejection, pancreatic leak, infection, postoperative bleeding, and wound dehiscence (i.e., split along surgical site). Late complications include chronic rejection, small bowel obstruction, pseudocyst, and incisional hernias. Bladder-drained pancreas transplants are also associated with urological complications such as hematuria, urethritis, urethral stricture or disruption, urinary tract infection, reflux pancreatitis, and late pancreatic leak.

There appears to be higher morbidity following pancreas–kidney transplantation, when compared to kidney transplantation alone. Hospitalization length is longer, the readmission rate is higher, and complete recovery occurs over a more prolonged period.

However, a successful pancreas transplant normalizes hemoglobin A_1c levels and eliminates the need for insulin therapy.

Given the small number of pediatric pancreas transplants performed to date, it follows that little is known about the pre- and postoperative cognitive functioning, quality of life, and psychological status of children who have undergone this procedure. As with other solid organ transplants, it is important to monitor the child's development, adherence history, quality of life, psychological adaptation and coping, and family resources throughout the transplant process. An improvement in quality of life is inferred from the elimination of blood glucose monitoring and insulin therapy; however, systematic studies that provide convincing empirical evidence of quality of life benefits are lacking.

See also: Coping with Illness; Cystic Fibrosis; Diabetes Mellitus (Type 1, Type 2); Endocrine Disorders; Quality of Life; Treatment Adherence: Medical

Further Reading

Auchincloss, H., & Shaffer, D. (1999). Pancreas transplantation. In L. C. Ginns, A. B. Cosimi, & P. J. Morris (Eds.), *Transplantation* (pp. 395–421). Malden, MA: Blackwell Science.
International Pancreas Transplant Registry Home Page. http://www.iptr.umn.edu (Accessed May 2002).
Scientific Registry of Transplant Recipients Home Page. http://www.ustransplant.org (Accessed May 2002).
United Network for Organ Sharing Home Page. http://www.unos.org (Accessed May 2002).

JAMES R. RODRIGUE
WILLEM J. VAN DER WERF
OLIVIA PUYANA

Panic Attacks/Panic Disorder

CLINICAL PRESENTATION

Panic Attacks (PAs)

A panic attack (PA) is an acute anxiety episode in which the child, in the absence of real danger, experiences emotional, cognitive, and somatic symptoms similar to those triggered by objective threatening situations. Specifically, the child experiences intense fear and at least 4 of the 13 symptoms described in the American Psychiatric Association's *Diagnostic and Statistical*

Manual of Mental Disorders, Fourth Edition (DSM-IV). Often the PA peaks in intensity within a few minutes (i.e., 5–10 min) before it gradually subsides. The child feels that something is wrong or that something bad is going to happen but does not know what is going to happen, when it will happen, where it will happen, and, perhaps most frightening of all, why it will happen. As a consequence, the child may believe that he or she is going to lose control, faint, have a severe illness (e.g., a heart attack), or even die or go crazy. The above-noted symptoms by themselves can increase the child's level of anxiety and create a vicious circle, which worsens and maintains PA frequency, intensity, and duration. PAs can and do occur in a variety of anxiety disorders in addition to Panic Disorder (PD).

There are three types of PAs: (1) *uncued* (unexpected, spontaneous, "out of the blue"); (2) *cued* (situationally bound); and (3) *situationally predisposed* (likely to occur in certain situations but not necessarily so). Situationally bound PAs almost always occur immediately upon exposure to, or in anticipation of, a triggering event (e.g., the presence of a phobic object). Situationally predisposed PAs are also triggered by certain situations (e.g., a threatening or embarrassing situation); however, the attacks do not always occur immediately after exposure to the external trigger. For example, a child may experience an attack at school or in a restaurant, but does not always do so. It is important to note that a PA may initially be *uncued* but, over time, becomes paired with specific stimuli (e.g., elevator, shopping center, school) and results in *situationally bound* or *situationally predisposed* attacks. Frequently, regardless of the type of PA, avoidance behaviors follow. Ollendick (1995) reported a wide variety of agoraphobic situations endorsed by adolescents with PD: churches, malls, parties, grocery stores, restaurants, theaters, auditoriums, and schools. Avoidance of such situations precludes the adolescent from engaging in a host of normative experiences and socializing events.

Panic Disorder

PD is characterized by recurrent *uncued* PAs which last for at least one month and present persistent concern about having another PA (anticipatory anxiety), worry about the implications and consequences of the PA, and impairment in functioning. In addition, for a diagnosis of PD, the PA should not be accounted for primarily by other physical or psychiatric illnesses.

Clinical studies by Moreau and Follet (1993), among others, have shown that most referrals for pediatric PD are adolescents, Caucasian, female, and middle class.

However, these results need to be viewed with caution because the demographics of the referred patients reflect the socioeconomic status, geographical area, and clinical settings where the studies took place. Similar to the adult literature, more than half of the pediatric patients report palpitations, tremors, dizziness, shortness of breath, faintness, sweating, chest pressure/pain, and fear of dying.

Although PD has been reported in children, it appears that this disorder is less frequent in this age range. It has been suggested that children have less PD because they do not have the cognitive ability to make internal, catastrophic misinterpretations of the somatic symptoms associated with PD (e.g., thoughts of losing control, going crazy, or dying in response to the somatic symptoms associated with PD). However, these notions have not been supported empirically. On the contrary, although children of varying ages do tend to make non-catastrophic interpretations of these symptoms (e.g., "I am catching a cold or the flu"), they are *capable* of making internal, catastrophic cognitions (e.g., "I must be dying like my grandfather"), as demonstrated by Mattis and Ollendick (1997). Rarely, however, do young children attribute the somatic symptoms to "going crazy"; rather, they are more likely to think something is wrong and that they might die.

INCIDENCE

The prevalence of PD in child and adolescent unselected community samples has been reported to range between 0.5 and 5.0 percent and in pediatric psychiatric clinics from 0.2 to 10 percent, with most cases occurring in female adolescents. Retrospective investigations in adults have found that up to 40 percent of patients with PD report that their disorders began before they were 20 years old. The peak prevalence of PD in these studies has been shown to be between 15 and 19 years of age, with 10–18 percent of the youths experiencing their first PA before they were 10 years of age. These prevalence rates, together with preliminary evidence that there is a decrease in age of onset of PD in successive generations, indicate the need to study the clinical characteristics, course, and treatment of PD in both children and adolescents.

CORRELATES

PD is a disabling condition accompanied by psychosocial, family, peer, and academic difficulties.

Moreover, PD is associated with increased risk for major depressive disorder (MDD), substance abuse, and, in some instances, suicide. Such adverse outcomes are more prevalent in persons whose PDs start early in life (≥ 17 years of age). Despite this, it takes on an average 12.7 years from the onset of symptoms to initiate treatment and, unfortunately, it appears that very few youngsters with PD actually seek help.

ASSESSMENT

A variety of diagnostic interviews, clinician rating scales, self-report instruments, self-monitoring forms, and behavioral observations tools are available to assess both PAs and PD. In brief, these interviews, questionnaires, and forms can be used to evaluate specific progress in treatment as well as continued treatment response following discontinuation of treatment. Given the frequent presence of comorbid disorders and associated features in PD, it is important to evaluate the presence of other psychiatric disorders that require different interventions such as depressive, bipolar, and disruptive disorders. Finally, it is recommended to assess anticipated side effects before starting any pharmacological treatment. Many parents and the children themselves may mistakenly attribute somatic symptoms as side effects to the medications, when in fact these somatic symptoms may be manifestations of the PD or other anxiety and mood disorders. Careful and ongoing assessment is a prerequisite to effective, evidence-based practice, as noted by Birmaher and Ollendick (2003).

TREATMENT

Both psychosocial and pharmacological treatments have been examined in the treatment of PD, more so with adults than children or adolescents. Most of the studies in adults and all the studies in youth address the acute treatment of PD. Studies evaluating the effects of continuation (to avoid relapses) and maintenance (to avoid recurrences or new episodes) are scarce in the adult literature and nonexistent in the youth literature.

Effective psychosocial treatment models for the treatment of PD have been based largely on cognitive–behavioral theories. The primary proponent of the cognitive–behavioral model has been David Barlow, and the treatment evolving from this perspective has come to be called Panic Control Treatment (PCT). Although empirical support for the treatment of PD with PCT in

adults is robust, only two studies have examined its use with adolescents. In both of these studies, treatment consisted of information about panic, relaxation training and breathing retraining, cognitive restructuring, interceptive exposure (e.g., exposure to the internal sensations and cues of panic), participant modeling (e.g., therapist and then parent demonstrating approach behavior in agoraphobic situations), in vivo exposure, and praise and social reinforcement. In addition, parents of the adolescents were enlisted to assist in treatment implementation and follow-up. Treatment varied in length but lasted between 10 and 15 sessions. The treatment program was effective. No studies have as yet examined the efficacy of PCT with preadolescent children, however.

To date, there are no randomized controlled trials (RCT) for the psychosocial and pharmacological treatment of childhood or adolescent onset PD. In adults, RCTs comparing the following classes of medications with placebo have been found effective in the treatment of PD: the selective serotonin reuptake inhibitors (SSRI) (60–80 percent vs. 36–60 percent), the tricyclic antidepressants (TCA) (45–70 percent vs. 15–50 percent), and the high potency benzodiazepines (55–75 percent vs. 15–50 percent). The SSRIs have been the first choice due to their easier administration and side effects profile, and they are much less dangerous in case of an overdose. On the basis of the adult literature, clinical experience, results of several open studies, and the fact that SSRIs have been found to be effective in the treatment of children and adolescents with other anxiety disorders and major depressive disorder, it appears that the SSRIs are a safe and promising treatment for children and adolescents with PD. However, as noted by Birmaher and Ollendick (2003), these medications should be initiated with low doses (e.g., fluoxetine 5 mg/day, fluvoxamine 12.5 mg/day, paroxetine 10 mg/day, sertraline 25 mg/day) to avoid the potential exacerbation of panic symptoms that sometimes have been observed in adult patients with PD. Starting with low doses also diminishes the risk of producing negative side effects, especially in children who already are highly sensitive to experiencing somatic symptoms and whose parents usually also have anxiety disorder and may be overanxious about the appearance of any minor side effect.

PROGNOSIS

Although the study of PAs and PD in children is largely in its own early stages of development, the prognosis for these conditions in children and adolescents is good if effective psychosocial and pharmacological treatments are used. In the absence of such treatments, the long-term course of these conditions is more protracted and resistant to subsequent interventions. Early intervention and prevention are recommended.

See also: Anxiety Disorders; Cognitive–Behavior Therapy; Evidence-Based Treatments; Pharmacological Interventions

Further Reading

American Psychiatric Association. (1998). Practice guidelines for the treatment of patients with Panic Disorder. *American Journal of Psychiatry, 155,* 1–34.

Birmaher, B., & Ollendick, T. H. (2003). Childhood onset Panic Disorder. In T. H. Ollendick & J. S. March (Eds.), *Phobic and anxiety disorders: A clinician's guide to effective psychosocial and pharmacological interventions.* Oxford, UK: Oxford University Press.

Mattis, S. G., & Ollendick, T. H. (1997). Children's cognitive responses to the somatic symptoms of panic. *Journal of Abnormal Child Psychology, 25,* 47–57.

Moreau, D. L., & Follet, C. (1993). Panic disorder in children and adolescents. *Child and Adolescent Psychiatric Clinics of North America, 2,* 581–602.

Ollendick, T. H. (1995). Cognitive-behavioral treatment of panic disorder with agoraphobia in adolescents: A multiple baseline design analysis. *Behavior Therapy, 26,* 517–531.

THOMAS H. OLLENDICK

Parent Training

DEFINITION

Parent training is a behavior management intervention in which parents are taught skills for interacting more effectively with their children. This intervention has been used to address a variety of childhood disorders including habit, conduct, internalizing, developmental, and parent–child relationship problems. Although the majority of this work has concentrated on parents of children with externalizing behaviors (e.g., hyperactivity, aggression, defiance), parent training has also been employed with parents of children with internalizing behavior problems in recent years (e.g., anxiety, depression, social withdrawal). The focus of parental training is often on behavior modification, relationship enhancement, or some combination of these two strategies. Behavior modification is grounded in social learning and conditioning principles, whereby parents are taught to alter the antecedents and consequences of their children's behavior to increase adaptive and decrease maladaptive behaviors. Relationship enhancement concentrates more on reducing maladaptive behaviors by strengthening the parent–child relationship, placing particular emphasis on effective communication skills.

There are many advantages to training parents as co-therapists. One advantage is that it allows parents to quickly acquire and utilize new skills, leading to a sense of control and competence. Another benefit is that this approach makes the parent the agent of change. Because the parent spends more time with the child than other adult figures (including the therapist), it is logical that the parent would be the most effective agent in implementing a behavior modification program.

EFFECTIVENESS

Empirical research suggests that parent training is an effective treatment for managing behavior problems in children. Further, results from parent training have been found to generalize over time to other behaviors and to untreated siblings. Parent training has also been demonstrated to have social validity, indicating that parents are accepting of this approach.

HISTORY

Early parent training models instructed parents how to modify their child's behavior using basic behavioral principles such as positive reinforcement (e.g., praise, star charts), extinction (ignoring), and response cost (time-out). Later models placed more emphasis on the interaction between the parent and child, such as the two-stage operant conditioning model developed by Constance Hanf. During the first stage, parents are taught to follow their child's lead during play, provide attention for positive behaviors, and withdraw attention (i.e., use ignoring) for negative behaviors. In the second stage, parents learn to give effective commands, praise compliance, and punish noncompliance with the use of time-out. Many researchers and clinicians have adapted this two-stage model for use with varying populations.

APPLICATIONS

One of the first applications of the Hanf model was Forehand and McMahon's program, *Helping the Noncompliant Child.* This program begins with a differential-attention phase (Phase 1) during which parents are taught to attend to their children's appropriate behavior and describe it without using questions, criticisms, or commands. Parents are instructed to let their child lead the play and provide reinforcement (e.g., specific praise) for behaviors they would like to see increase while actively ignoring behaviors they wish to decrease. Ignoring consists of avoiding eye contact and physical contact, as well as avoiding verbal and nonverbal communication. Ignoring also may include having parents turn their back to the child or walk out of the room. Parents are asked to practice these skills at home during 10-min daily practice sessions. Once these skills have been mastered, parents move on to Phase 2 where they are taught to give direct and concise commands. The parent issues a command and waits for 5 s to give the child an opportunity to comply. If the child does not comply, they are given a warning that there will be a consequence for noncompliance. If the child does not begin to comply within 5 s, the parent implements a time-out procedure.

The Barkley training program was developed for children with Attention-Deficit/Hyperactivity Disorder (ADHD). This program is similar to those developed by Hanf and Forehand, but is tailored to meet the unique needs of children with ADHD. Aspects of the program are based on the theory that ADHD is in large part, biologically based. The Barkley training program is completed in 9 to 12 therapy sessions and is often provided as part of a multimodal treatment package, which may also include medication, family therapy, and social skills training. Throughout the program, parents are educated about ADHD, parent–child relations, and the principles of behavior management. Parents are instructed on using attending skills with their children to increase compliance and positive behavior. They learn to implement a token economy whereby the child earns tokens for appropriate behavior and loses tokens for inappropriate behavior. Parents then learn the process of time-out for noncompliance and later learn to use time-out for other misbehaviors. Finally, parents are taught to manage their child's behavior in public places and learn problem-solving skills for handling future behavior problems that may arise.

Parent–Child Interaction Therapy (PCIT), developed by Eyberg (1988), is another parent training program based on the Hanf model. During sessions, the therapist observes parent–child interactions from behind a one-way mirror while parents wear a bug-in-the-ear device that allows the therapist to communicate with them throughout the session. Parents are given immediate feedback on the use of parenting skills. In the first phase of treatment (Child-Directed Interaction [CDI]),

parents are taught to use differential reinforcement to modify child behavior by providing positive attention for appropriate behavior (e.g., reflecting children's appropriate verbalizations) and withdrawing attention for inappropriate behavior (e.g., ignoring whining). Once parents have mastered the CDI skills, Parent-Directed Interaction (PDI) skills are introduced. During PDI, parents are directed to lead the play and are taught three basic skills to manage misbehaviors, particularly noncompliance: (a) giving effective commands, (b) praising the child for exhibiting compliant behavior, and (c) using time-out to punish noncompliant behavior. Webster-Stratton's (1987) program uses similar treatment phases and skills aimed at providing early intervention for conduct problems, but it is unique in that skills are taught in a parenting group format using discussion of videotaped parent–child interactions rather than direct coaching of individual families.

Patterson developed a family-based intervention program focusing on antisocial children. He based this program on the theory that a child's level of aversive behavior is related to her or his interactions with other family members. Patterson's coercion hypothesis states that children may be negatively reinforced by their parents for behaviors such as noncompliance. For example, when a parent gives a child a command such as, "Please put your shoes away," the child may respond with noncompliance—refusing to complete the task. If the child persists and the parent gives up, the child has, in effect, learned that they do not need to comply with parental requests. A second component of Patterson's theory suggests that parents may escalate their own level of coercion as well by engaging in explosive discipline and nattering (i.e., nagging the child). As a result, the child responds with aversive behavior until a cycle of increasingly coercive behavior is established. This program places less emphasis on teaching parents positive parenting skills. Instead, the program begins with a focus on compliance and noncompliance by teaching parents the effective use of commands. Parents are then taught to use positive reinforcement to increase appropriate behavior and time-out to decrease inappropriate behavior. Patterson and colleagues use an individualized training format lasting approximately 18 sessions.

More recently, research has examined the effectiveness of parent training for internalizing disorders, particularly anxiety disorders (e.g., school refusal, separation anxiety disorder). Dadds, Barrett, and Rapee have found promising results indicating that parent training may be an effective addition to the more traditional cognitive–behavioral treatments for child anxiety, which focus on teaching children coping skills. Parents are taught to reinforce their child by using verbal praise, tangible rewards, or privileges when the child faces up to feared situations. When the child exhibits anxious behavior, the parent is taught to use planned ignoring. When using planned ignoring, the parent may respond empathetically to their child's first complaint and if the child continues to complain, the parent prompts the child to use a coping strategy learned in an earlier part of the program. If the child still continues to complain, the parent ignores the child. In addition, parents are taught to be aware of their own anxiety responses they may unintentionally be modeling for their children. Parents are then taught to model proactive responses. This is a promising beginning for research in the area of parent training with internalizing disorders

See also: Behavior Modification; Differential Social Reinforcement/Positive Attention; Disruptive Behavior Disorders; Parent–Child Interaction Therapy

Further Reading

Barkley, R. A. (1987). *Defiant children: A clinician's manual for parent training.* New York: Guilford.

Briesmeister, J. M., & Schaefer, C. E. (Eds.). (1998). *Handbook of parent training: Parents as co-therapists for children's behavior problems* (2nd ed.). New York: Wiley.

Eyberg, S. (1988). Parent–child interaction therapy: Integration of traditional and behavioral concerns. *Child and Family Behavior Therapy, 10,* 33–45.

Webster-Stratton, C. (1987). *The parent and child series.* Eugene, OR: Castalia.

CHERYL B. MCNEIL
LISA M. WARE

Parental Psychopathology

Research has documented a cross-generational link for many forms of psychopathology, including anxiety disorders, major affective disorders, antisocial personality disorder (APD), substance use disorders, attention deficit disorders and schizophrenia. Understanding the mechanisms involved in this link is difficult because parents and children share both genes and environment. As a result, this link can be due to hereditary influences (e.g., a shared biological predisposition for the disorder), social learning factors (e.g., problems in adjustment disrupting a parent's ability to be an effective parent), or a combination of genetic and environmental influences.

Research on the link between parent and child substance abuse illustrates the potential complex interplay of genetics and environmental influences in the transmission of risk for disorder from parent to child. Research has documented a strong relationship between drug use and abuse in parents and drug use and abuse in their children, irrespective of gender, for a wide variety of drugs. For example, alcoholism in parents is one of the strongest risk factors for alcohol abuse in their offspring. While heritability studies have documented a substantial contribution of genetics, parents who abuse substances can also contribute to their child's development of substance abuse by providing an environment more conducive to the child's own development of problem behavior. As recently noted by both Beardslee and colleagues (2002) and Marikangas (2002), parents with substance abuse disorders are more likely to expose the child to drugs at an early age, express more positive attitudes towards drugs, act as a negative role model in terms of promoting the benefits of drug use, and allow for illicit substances to be more readily available to the child.

A number of behavioral genetics methods are used to study the relationship between parent and child psychopathology. These include family, twin, and adoption studies. These methods allow for an investigation of the rates of disorder in relatives of individuals with psychopathology (family studies), the difference in concordance rates for disorder between monozygotic and dizygotic twins (twin studies), and the difference in associations on measures of psychopathology between adopted children and their biological parents and between adopted children and their adoptive parents (adoption studies). These methods allow for an estimation of the relative strength of genetic and environmental influences on the development of psychopathology. Further, new behavioral genetic methodology even allows for a determination of the types of environmental influences that may be contributing to the familial link to a disorder, such as those shared by members of the families and those that are unique to individuals within the family.

However, in addition to determining the relative strength of environmental and genetic influences, it is also important to investigate the mechanisms through which these influences operate across generations. One important issue in this research is that the mechanisms, both genetic and environmental, can be specific or nonspecific to a certain disorder. For example, parental depression appears to be a nonspecific risk factor, placing the child at risk for many different types of problems in adjustment, including anxiety, conduct problems, and depression. Similarly, parents with substance abuse disorders seem to also provide a more generalized risk to their children, whereby their children show more aggression and conduct problems, affective disorders, attention disorders, and difficulties in social relationships. In contrast, Frick and Loney (in press) recently suggested that parental Antisocial Personality Disorder appears to show a more specific association with childhood adjustment, being related to an increased risk for conduct problems and aggression but being less strongly related to other problems in adjustment.

Importantly, not all children of parents with problems in adjustment develop problems themselves. Therefore, it is important to consider what factors contribute to a child's resiliency in families in which a parent has a psychiatric disorder. For example, research has documented that high intelligence, an internal locus of control, adaptability, involvement in extracurricular activities, strong social networks, and a consistent and stable family environment are just a few of the factors that can protect children from showing problems in adjustment when their parents have some form of psychopathology. In addition, it is important to consider that in some cases the link between parent and child adjustment can involve bidirectional effects in which the child's problems in adjustment cause or worsen parental problems through a cyclical transactional process. For example, Barkley has noted that there is some evidence that the stressors associated with raising a child with Attention-Deficit/Hyperactivity Disorder (ADHD) can increase the level of depression in the child's parents.

See also: Depressive Disorder, Major; Disruptive Behavior Disorders; Life Stress in Children and Adolescents; Risk and Protective Factors; Substance Abuse

Further Reading

Barkley, R. A. (1998). *Attention-deficit hyperactivity disorder: A handbook for diagnosis and treatment*, (2nd ed.). New York: Guildford.

Beardslee, W. R., Versage, E. M., Van de Helde, P., Swatling, S., & Hoke, L. (2002). Preventing depression in children through resiliency promotion: The preventative intervention project. In R. J. McMahon & R. D. V. Peters (Eds.), *The effects of parental dysfunction on children* (pp. 71–86). New York: Kluwer Academic/Plenum.

Frick, P. J., & Loney, B. R. (2002). Understanding the association between parent and child antisocial behavior. In R. J. McMahon & R. D. Peters (Eds.), *The effects of parental dysfunction on children* (pp. 105–126). New York: Kluwer Academic/Plenum.

Jackson, Y. K., & Frick, P. J. (1998). Stress and resilience in children: Testing protective models. *Journal of Clinical Child Psychology, 27*, 370–380.

Merikangas, K. R. (2002). Familial factors and substance use disorders. In R. J. McMahon & R. D. Peters (Eds.), *The effects of parental dysfunction on children* (pp. 17–40). New York: Kluwer Academic/Plenum.

EVA R. KIMONIS
PAUL J. FRICK

Parental Substance Abuse

See: Effects of Parental Substance Abuse on Children

Parent–Child Interaction Therapy

DEFINITION

Parent–Child Interaction Therapy (PCIT), developed by Eyberg and her colleagues, is an evidence-based treatment for behavior problems in young children, which is based on principles of attachment theory and social learning theory. In PCIT, parents are taught skills to establish a nurturing and secure relationship with their child while increasing their child's prosocial behavior and decreasing their child's negative behavior. Treatment progresses through two distinct phases. Child-Directed Interaction (CDI) resembles traditional play therapy and focuses on strengthening the parent–child bond, increasing positive parenting, and improving child social skills; whereas Parent-Directed Interaction (PDI) resembles clinical behavior therapy and focuses on improving parents' expectations, ability to set limits, consistency and fairness in discipline, and reducing child noncompliance and other negative behavior.

METHOD

PCIT sessions are typically conducted once a week and are 1 hr in length. The principles and skills of each phase of treatment are first taught to the parents alone in a teaching session, and in subsequent sessions parents are coached in the skills as they play with their child. The parents practice the CDI skills at home during daily 5-min play sessions. Families continue in treatment until the parents demonstrate mastery of the skills and their child's behavior comes within the normal range. The average length of treatment is 13 sessions.

During the Child-Directed Interaction phase, the parents learn to follow the child's lead in play by using the nondirective PRIDE skills: *P*raising the child, *R*eflecting the child's statements, *I*mitating the child's play, *D*escribing the child's behavior, and using *E*nthusiasm in the play. They learn to change child behavior by directing the PRIDE skills to the child's appropriate play and consistently ignoring undesirable behaviors. During CDI coaching sessions, therapists coach parents in their use of the PRIDE skills until parents meet criteria for skill mastery, as assessed during a 5-min observation at the start of each session. It is through the CDI coaching that therapists convey important developmental expectations for child behavior and point out specific effects of the parents' behavior on the child. Coaching may also teach stress-management or anger-management skills to parents as they interact with their child.

During the Parent-Directed Interaction, parents learn to direct the child's behavior, when necessary, with effective commands and specific consequences for compliance and noncompliance. In PDI coaching sessions, parents work toward meeting the mastery criteria of PDI skills that serve as an indicator of their consistency. Throughout the PDI phase of treatment, the therapist guides the parents in applying the principles and procedures of CDI and PDI to the child's behavior at home and in other settings. Initially, parents are instructed to practice the PDI skills in brief 5- to 10-min practice sessions after the daily CDI play session. Homework assignments proceed gradually to use of the PDI procedure only at times when it is important that the child obey a specific command. In the last few sessions, parents are taught variations of the PDI procedure to deal with aggressive behavior and public misbehavior, as they approach mastery of the PCIT skills and assume increasing responsibility for applying the principles creatively to new situations that arise.

CLINICAL APPLICATIONS

PCIT research has focused on the treatment of young children with Oppositional Defiant Disorder, many of whom have comorbid Attention-Deficit/ Hyperactivity Disorder. The children studied to date have been primarily from lower socioeconomic status, single-parent Caucasian families, although several clinical trials with primarily Hispanic and African American families are in progress. More recently, PCIT has been successfully applied to families experiencing child physical abuse, where the parent is typically the referred patient.

EFFECTIVENESS

PCIT has demonstrated statistically and clinically significant improvements in children's behavior at the end of treatment on parent and teacher rating scales and direct observations in the clinic and at school. Important changes in parents' interactions with their child include increased reflective listening, physical proximity, prosocial verbalization, and decreased criticism and sarcasm at treatment completion. Studies have also shown significant changes on parents' self-report measures of psychopathology, personal distress, and self-efficacy. The changes in children's oppositional behaviors seen during treatment have been shown to last, both at school and at home. Hood and Eyberg (submitted) reported 3- to 6-year maintenance of treatment gains in children's behavior and parents' confidence in their ability to manage their children's behavior.

See also: Attachment; Attention-Deficit/Hyperactivity Disorder; Behavioral Observation; Disruptive Behavior Disorders; Oppositional Defiant Disorder

Further Reading

Herschell, A., Calzada, E., Eyberg, S. M., & McNeil, C. B. (2002). Parent–child interaction therapy: New directions in research. *Cognitive and Behavioral Practice, 9*, 9–16.

Herschell, A., Calzada, E., Eyberg, S. M., & McNeil, C. B. (2002). Clinical issues in parent–child interaction therapy. *Cognitive and Behavioral Practice, 9*, 16–27.

Hood, K. K., & Eyberg, S. M. (2002). *Outcomes of parent–child interaction therapy: Mothers' reports on maintenance three to six years after treatment.* (submitted for publication).

Neary, E. M., & Eyberg, S. M. (2002). Management of disruptive behavior in young children. *Infants and Young Children, 14*, 53–67.

Schuhmann, E., Foote, R., Eyberg, S. M., Boggs, S., & Algina, J. (1998). Parent–child interaction therapy: Interim report of a randomized trial with short-term maintenance. *Journal of Clinical Child Psychology, 27*, 34–45.

SHEILA M. EYBERG

Parenting Practices

PARENTING AND DEVELOPMENT

Parenting practices play a critical role in the development of children. Parent behavior enables children to develop and use coping skills that make them more resilient, or, conversely, that can place children at increased risk for problems. Each period of development places different demands on parents. Table 1 summarizes key issues of development and the associated parenting tasks from infancy through school age.

DETERMINANTS OF PARENTING

The interaction of multiple factors influence how parents behave with their children. These include

Table 1. Issues of Normal Development and Associated Parental Tasks

Area of development	Infancy 0–1 years	Toddlers 1–2 years	Preschoolers 2–5 years	School-aged 5–12
Physical/motor	• Brain develops rapidly • Weight triples, height doubles • Develops capacity for self-regulation	• Stands and walks alone • Imitates motor actions • Goes up and down steps holding on to hardrailing	• Hops, skips, and jumps • Throws ball • Dresses	• Slow and steady growth • Increased hand–eye coordination • Sense of body position and gross motor function permit participation in organized sports
	• Physiological regularity increases • Becomes oriented to external world: sensory integration, visual and auditory acuity • Motor skills develop: (rolling, sitting, crawling, standing, walking, reach and grasp, pincer grasp, hand to mouth, hand–eye coordination	• Stands on one foot • Uses implements (crayons, spoons)	• Undresses • Ties shoes • Copies shapes	
Cognitive	• Needs environmental stimulation and exploration	• Intense interest in exploring the world	• Memory capacity develops (processing and storage in place, good recognition memory, increase in ability to use retrieval strategies)	• Attention, persistence, and goal-directedness allow formal schooling
	• Engages in sensorimotor actions and experiences	• Explores properties and functions of objects	• Uses verbally mediated thinking	• Increased capacity to store, retain, and retrieve new information
	• Learns about contingencies	• Observation and imitation are key to learning	• Understands real vs. not real	• Improved memory skills: uses retrieval strategies
	• Develops object permanence	• Develops expectations based on memory of past	• Engages in pretend play	• Increasingly accurate perception of reality
	• Imitates adult behavior	• Symbolic play and thinking begin	• Understands consequences and rules	• Reversibility—can analyze events by thinking about them
	• Repeats pleasurable experiences • Anticipates familiar events	• Conscious goals and plans • Views the world egocentrically	• Views the world egocentrically • Uses magical thinking	• Understands cause and effect • Spurt in cognition at 7 years: Spatial and visual organization, time orientation, seriation, auditory processing

(Continued)

Table 1 *(Continued)*

Area of development	Infancy 0–1 years	Toddlers 1–2 years	Preschoolers 2–5 years	School-aged 5–12
	• Begins goal-directed behavior			• Increase in executive processes: problem-solving, sustained attention
Language	• Cries or smiles to communicate	• Imitates single words	• Rapid development of grammar, syntax, and pronunciation	• Expression in written language begins
	• Orients to sound	• Uses single words to communicate needs	• Uses language to understand the world	• Vocabulary continues to increase
	• Babbles and vocalizes	• Combines words and gestures	• Asks questions	• Uses language to express ideas and feeling, to plan for the future and remember the past, and to solve problems
	• Imitates vocalization	• Vocabulary of 10–100 words	• Follows 3-step commands	
	• Learns turn-taking	• 2–3 word sentences	• Uses 4-word complex sentences	
	• Looks and points		• Relates long stories and experiences	
	• Understands single words and labels		• By age 5: 1,500–2,000 word vocabulary, grammar similar to adults	
	• Follows simple directions by end of 1st year			
Social/emotional	• Attachment develops	• Balances desire for closeness with caregiver and independence, exploration	• Group play begins	• More consistent sense of self
	• Uses strategies to maintain proximity	• Plays independently and in parallel	• Develops friendships	• Increased sense of identity based on gender, race, ethnicity, and personal characteristics
	• Uses caregiver to decrease arousal and regulate affect	• Imitates others and role plays daily events	• Follows rules	• Self-esteem based on sense of competence and status in peer group
	• Smiles responsively	• Becomes self-assertive	• Plays cooperatively	• Uses cognition to regulate internal arousal, to delay action, to attain goals, and to control behavior
	• Initiates play interactions	• Bites or hits peers	• Internalizes parental standards	• Internalizes values, norms, and rules
	• Cooperates in simple games (peekaboo)	• Expresses needs and feelings in gestures and words	• Interacts appropriately with adults and peers	• Can see conflicting viewpoints and tolerates ambivalence
	• Joint attention	• Has limited internal control	• Uses language to express feelings	• Identifies with parents as role models
	• Beginning sense of self	• Recovers quickly from upset	• Uses words to control impulses	• Increased identification with same-sex peers
	• Cautious with new people	• Begins to understand social expectations		

(Continued)

Table 1 *(Continued)*

Area of development	Infancy 0–1 years	Toddlers 1–2 years	Preschoolers 2–5 years	School-aged 5–12
Parenting tasks	• Responds to parents limit setting by end of 1st year • Scaffold or support child's development • Adapt to child's ongoing development • Be sensitive and responsive to child's cues • Provide appropriate stimulation and experiences • Follow child's lead/joint attention	• Provide opportunities for exploration and motor activities • Talk to and describe child's actions • Ensure child's safety • Start setting limits • Use distraction to discipline	• Be an authoritative parent • Be a good role model for appropriate behavior, expression of feelings, and relationships • Provide consistent daily routines and expectations • Be a good listener • Describe child's actions and feelings	• Be an authoritative parent • Be a good role model • Encourage and model independent problem solving • Provide consistency • Be a good listener • Monitor and supervise child's activities and friendships

Source: C. S. Schroeder and B. N. Gordon, *Assessment and treatment of childhood problems: A clinician's guide*. Copyright 2002 Guilford Publications. Reprinted by permission.

Table 2. Predictors of Parenting Practices and Components of Dysfunctional and Optimal Parenting

Predictors of parenting styles	Components of dysfunctional parenting	Components of optimal parenting
• Attitudes and expectations • One's own parenting models • Education • Characteristics of the child—temperament, conduct problems, activity level, and developmental changes • Parental mental health, depression • Marital status, discord • Social support: insularity—few friends and frequent, highly aversive contact with relatives and helping agencies • Socioeconomic status, poverty	• Uninvolved and not responding to child with sufficient warmth and stimulation • Overly harsh and controlling • Unable to set reasonable expectations and limits • Attends to and reinforces inappropriate behavior while *not* attending to appropriate behavior • Vague or attacking in communication with child • Does not listen to child • Inconsistent and/or inept in handling situations that require punishment • Too gentle, lengthy, or delayed in dealing with misbehavior	• Enforces rules consistently • Has age-appropriate expectations • Reinforces appropriate behavior • Accepts and nurtures child • Models appropriate behavior • Assigns age appropriate responsibilities • Provides developmentally appropriate stimulation • Monitors child's activities • Provides reasons for rules/limits

Source: C. S. Schroeder and B. N. Gordon, *Assessment and treatment of childhood problems: A clinician's guide*. Copyright 2002 Guilford Publications. Reprinted by permission.

(1) characteristics of the parents, including their genetic and environmental origins and personal psychological resources; (2) characteristics of the child, especially his or her unique temperamental profile; (3) characteristics of the environmental context of the parent–child relationship, especially levels of stress and/or social support; and (4) attitudes and beliefs about childrearing. Table 2 summarizes factors that predict parenting practices.

OPTIMAL PARENTING PRACTICES

Considerable research has addressed the question "What can parents do to ensure more optimal development for their children?" Table 2 summarizes the major components of optimal and dysfunctional parenting. It is important to note that parenting practices must change as the child grows and develops. In infancy, cognitive and motivational competence and healthy socioemotional development are promoted by parents' attentive, affectionate, stimulating, responsive, and nonrestrictive caregiving. Authoritative parenting (warm, reasonable, nonpunitive, and firm) is associated with positive child behavior during the preschool years. By school age, inductive reasoning, consistent discipline, and expressions of affection are positively related to self-esteem, internalized controls, prosocial orientation, and intellectual achievement.

Across all developmental periods, parental monitoring is emerging as a critical skill for parents. Parental monitoring is defined as "a set of correlated parenting behaviors involving attention to and tracking of the child's whereabouts, activities, and adaptations" (Dishion & McMahon, 1998, p. 61). Monitoring enhances parent's awareness of children's activities and communicates to children that their parents are concerned about and interested in what they are doing. Monitoring in infancy is reflected in sensitive and responsive parenting, as well as joint attention to play activities. During the preschool years, monitoring ensures the child's safety and is also seen in joint attention, with verbal descriptions of the child's activities. Monitoring the school-aged child involves keeping track of school achievement, homework, and activities, knowing who the child's friends are, and attending extracurricular activities. During adolescence, monitoring means knowing where the child is and who he or she is with, tracking school achievement, and attending extracurricular events.

PHYSICAL PUNISHMENT

Nonabusive corporal punishment is extremely common among US parents; almost all parents have hit their children at some time during childhood. The prevalence of corporal punishment peaks during the preschool years at 94 percent of parents but over half of parents hit their 12-year-old children and as many as 13 percent hit their 17-year-olds. Parents of clinic-referred children are more likely to use corporal punishment than parents of nonreferred children. Reviews

of research indicate some inconsistency regarding the effects of corporal punishment on children's development; some studies find an association with a variety of adverse effects such as aggression, depression, and later spousal abuse, whereas others find no negative effects, at least when the punishment occurs in the context of a warm, supportive parental relationship. Nonetheless, many children experience corporal punishment as highly stressful and for some, it is associated with adjustment problems. Moreover, the risk of escalation from corporal punishment to severe physical aggression is high for parents who rely on physical discipline tactics to control their children, especially when those children are difficult to manage. In addition corporal punishment may lead to a coercive cycle that is seen in parents and children with conduct problems.

The critical question is whether corporal punishment accomplishes what parents want it to accomplish. That is, does it teach children to behave in a more appropriate manner? Research suggests that although spanking certainly gets a child's attention and may stop inappropriate behavior initially, it is not effective over time. The more it is used, the less effective it becomes, in part because children habituate quickly, forcing parents to punish more frequently and more harshly. Spanking does not teach children acceptable alternative behaviors; it simply teaches them what not to do. Moreover, physical punishment models an aggressive way of dealing with problems and indicates that it is okay for a bigger person to hit a smaller one.

See also: Adolescence; Attachment; Childhood; Developmental Milestones; Emotional Development; Identity Development; Infancy

Further Reading

American Academy of Pediatrics. (1998). Guidance for effective discipline. *Pediatrics, 101,* 723–728.

Dishion, T. J., & McMahon, R. J. (1998). Parental monitoring and the prevention of child and adolescent problem behavior: A conceptual and empirical formulation. *Clinical Child and Family Psychology Review, 1,* 61–75.

Mahoney, A., Donnelly, W. O., Lewis, T., & Maynard, C. (2000). Mother and father self-reports of corporal punishment and severe physical aggression toward clinic-referred youth. *Journal of Clinical Child Psychology, 29,* 266–281.

Schroeder, C. S., & Gordon, B. N. (2002). *Assessment and treatment of childhood problems: A clinician's guide.* New York: Guilford.

Straus, M. A., & Stewart, J. H. (1999). Corporal punishment by American parents: National data on prevalence, chronicity, severity, and duration, in relation to child and family characteristics. *Clinical Child and Family Psychology Review, 2,* 55–70.

BETTY N. GORDON

Parenting the Chronically Ill Child

DEFINITION

Parenting the chronically ill child involves caring for the complicated needs of the child and siblings, as well as attending to one's own needs as the parent. Approximately 20 percent of children in the United States are living with a chronic illness. Due to medical advances in recent years, improved treatments have been developed for illnesses that were previously fatal. Thus, greater numbers of children are living longer with their diseases, increasing the need for attention to the issues families face when coping with childhood chronic illness.

Parents experience the child's illness directly, and the impact of the illness creates shifts in parenting demands and priorities. Upon diagnosis, parents are typically consumed with the day-to-day demands of learning about their child's disease and its treatment, as well as managing the daily life stressors that do not abate and may be exacerbated by the illness. As treatment progresses and the family acclimates to the illness, it is common for parents to begin dealing with the emotional issues concomitant with having a chronically ill child.

ISSUES SPECIFIC TO THE ILL CHILD

Due to the medical demands of illness, it is easy to focus only upon the child's physiological functioning and lose sight of other areas of development. However, it is essential for the parent to be aware of, and to attend to, all aspects of their child's functioning.

Parents should strive to maintain a sense of normalcy and continuity in the midst of this nonnormative life event. Many parents allow structure and discipline for the ill child to fully lapse, and behavioral difficulties often ensue. Siblings may feel left out and unimportant in comparison to the ill child, and may experience anger and guilt about their sibling's illness and their reactions to it. Parents should involve siblings when possible by bringing them to the hospital and allowing them to help with their brother's/sister's care. It is equally important to check in with siblings regarding what is happening (separate from the illness) in their own lives.

Illness is no longer perceived as an impediment to normal development. Rather, in some instances, the challenges of illness can enhance the emotional and social development of the child. To optimize developmental opportunities and to increase awareness of potential difficulties associated with a chronic illness, parents must be aware of common issues that arise for children and families dealing with a chronic illness. Prominent issues include emotional, social, cognitive, and educational concerns.

Emotional Concerns

There is controversy in the childhood chronic illness literature as to whether illness actually increases the risk for emotional difficulties in children. However, it is well known that certain situations that occur with illness are distressing and anxiety-provoking for children. These situations include (among others) needle pricks, pill swallowing, hospitalization, missing school, and side effects of treatment (such as loss of hair from chemotherapy). Pediatric psychology has developed effective techniques for management of many of these issues, and therefore referral is often beneficial to the child. It is of obvious importance to note when a child's mood or affect changes in a significant manner for a sustained period of time, and to then refer the child for assessment of depression, anxiety, or other psychological distress.

Social Concerns

Due to the practical constraints of illness, it can be difficult for chronically ill children to have the social contact that is developmentally appropriate for them. Hospitalization, homebound education, and need for isolation (in cases of immunosuppression) all compound the effect of children having reduced interactions with their peers. Parents can find creative ways to help their children maintain social connections with existing friends, and make new contacts, in spite of the constraints of their children's illness. Children in isolation can chat with one another in new online chat rooms designed to facilitate communication between children with illness. Pediatric hospitals often encourage supportive friendships between children on inpatient units via group meetings and social times with videos, games, etc. Parents and teachers can speak to the child's classmates and explain the illness so that the other children are not anxious or afraid. This type of education can encourage the ill child's friends to visit him or her at home and in the hospital, which can be invaluable for maintaining social connections.

Homebound education is often necessary due to the child's physical condition. However, returning to school can be very anxiety-provoking for the child, and thus parents need to attend to specific school refusal behaviors. If the child is physically well enough to return to the mainstream classroom, it is very important for reasons of social and educational development to do so. Pediatric psychologists can offer school reintegration programs for the child and his/her classmates to facilitate this process.

Cognitive Concerns

Assessment is vital to track the child's cognitive performance throughout the course of the illness. Routine assessment will allow problem areas to be identified early so that appropriate interventions can be put into place for the child. Certain treatments dispose the child to particular areas of cognitive challenge and decline (such as late effects of radiation therapy), so it is essential to track the child's cognitive patterns before, during, and after treatment.

Educational Concerns

The parent is often required to serve as the child's educational advocate in obtaining necessary services for the child. It is the child's right to be provided with education tailored for the special needs that may accompany his/her illness. The parent should request an individualized educational plan (IEP) which will provide the structure in which the school system will meet the child's needs. These needs may include individualized attention via a teacher's aide, structural design in the classroom for specific handicaps, and a behavioral plan, as well as any specialized teaching methods that may be needed.

ISSUES RELATED TO THE FAMILY SYSTEM

In the course of caring for a chronically ill child, parents often neglect their own physical and emotional needs. A child's illness places immense strain upon the marital relationship as well as the whole family (brothers, sisters, and extended family). It is essential for the parents to enlist social support for themselves. This may be in the context of the family, but it is also immeasurably helpful for parents to get linked to societal support structures (e.g., other parents of ill children, stress management support groups, religious groups). Parents often feel guilty when caring for themselves, and should be reminded that they can best care for an ill child when they themselves are healthy.

HONESTY

"What do I tell my child about being sick?" This is a question asked by the majority of parents upon learning of their child's diagnosis. The information sharing process is a balance between maintaining a positive focus as well as being honest with the child. Information should be relayed in a developmentally appropriate manner, and should also be shared with the siblings. It is important for children to understand their treatment (i.e., "what is going to happen to them") as it occurs and why it is being done. For example, needle sticks and bone marrow aspirations should be described as medical procedures that can help them get better. Often, the optimal explanation of these procedures may come from other children who have received the procedure or treatment. It has been demonstrated in the research literature that "hiding" a diagnosis from a child or not being honest with a child about his/her illness is related to poorer adjustment on the part of the child. It is therefore not protective to choose full nondisclosure with a child. Rather, parents need to facilitate an environment of openness and discussion with their child (and siblings) so that the children feel comfortable voicing concerns and fears, as well as asking questions about the illness and treatment and taking an age-appropriate active role in coping with the illness.

See also: Coping with Illness; Endocrine Disorders; Neurological Disorders; Oncologic Disorders; Parenting the Handicapped Child

Further Reading

"BandAides and Blackboards." http://www.faculty.fairfield.edu/fleitas/contents.html

Thompson, R. J., Jr., & Gustafson, K. E. (1996). *Adaptation to chronic childhood illness.* Washington, DC: American Psychological Association.

Woznick, L. A., & Goodheart, C. D. (2002). *Living with childhood cancer: A practical guide to help families cope.* Washington, DC: American Psychological Association.

C. Alexandra Boeving
Jack W. Finney

Parenting the Handicapped Child

With the anticipated birth of a child, many parents dream about the personal qualities and upcoming life of the new addition to their family. Parents may discuss potential child characteristics such as sex, attractiveness, personality, and intelligence. Such speculation may extend to their child's choice of college, spouse, and career. Parents do not typically expect the birth of a child with a handicapping condition—nor the accompanying limitations that may result. Parental adjustment to such circumstances has been likened to a period of mourning as they cope with the loss of their idealized child.

Although increasing numbers of genetic diagnoses are made prenatally, most parents are informed of their child's handicapping condition in early childhood. For children with a mild handicap, a formal diagnosis may not be offered until after the child enters school. Common parental reactions to the presence of a handicapped child in the family include shock, denial, sadness, anger, anxiety, projection of blame, fear of the diagnosis, guilt, a strong sense of loss, and social isolation. In rare cases, parents respond by devaluing, abusing or neglecting the child, setting unrealistic goals, minimizing the child's positive qualities, or escaping from the parental role. Over time, most families move toward accepting their child and the diagnosis. These parents are able to integrate their child's strengths and weaknesses, set realistic developmental goals, and find joy in raising their child. Nonetheless, feelings of emptiness and sorrow may occasionally resurface for even the most accepting of parents. As children progress through life, certain developmental/social milestones (i.e., being invited to parties, obtaining a driver's license, going to the prom, graduating from high school, going to college, getting married, and having children of their own) may not be met resulting in distress for children with handicapping conditions and their parents.

Research suggests that some families of children with handicapping conditions experience high levels of parenting stress for extended periods of time. These parents are often faced with numerous physical demands associated with providing personal care, managing problem behaviors, or coping with children who have irregular sleep patterns. Additionally, they may have difficulty finding babysitters or accepting respite care for their children. As a result, parents of children with handicapping conditions are at increased risk for depressive symptoms, physical illnesses, and/or burnout.

In addition to the physical demands of caring for a child with a handicapping condition, parents may have frequent contact with various professionals. Children with handicapping conditions may require services from numerous professionals, all of which typically require regular parent meetings. Thus, parents may find it difficult to balance the needs of their disabled child with personal and career goals. Additional everyday stressors include health problems, arranging transportation for appointments, financial difficulties, advocating for specialized programs, interacting with state agencies, and hiring legal assistance when necessary. Family accommodations may be necessary to cope with these stressors. In general, families with strong marital relationships, healthy family cohesion, good parenting skills, adept problem-solving skills, financial stability, and ample social support tend to exhibit less stress and more family satisfaction. Additionally, strong religious beliefs, supportive community affiliations, and effective home-based behavioral interventions have also been associated with positive family functioning. Parent support groups and family education programs can provide a forum for additional growth and adjustment.

Children often have mixed feelings about their siblings with handicapping conditions. Children may have difficulty integrating their desire to be well-liked and their perceived duty to protect their sibling from being teased. At times, children may experience anxiety when out in public with their sibling. Persistent anxiety may lead to an active avoidance of the child with a handicapping condition. Children may also experience anger toward their parents and/or sibling, especially when they are overburdened with childcare responsibilities. Nonetheless, most siblings of children with a handicapping condition do not experience significant psychological distress. In fact, many children display increased maturity, self-confidence, independence, and tolerance for individual differences. In general, siblings of children with a handicapping condition have better outcomes when their parents have a stable and supportive marriage, when their feelings can be addressed openly, when they are educated about their sibling's condition, and when they are not assigned excessive childcare responsibilities. These children may benefit from participation in sibling support groups with other children who have brothers or sisters with handicapping conditions.

Extended family members and close friends may experience emotions quite similar to parents following the birth of a child with a disability. Although extended family members and close friends are often a strong source of support, they may initially have difficulty dealing with their own reactions to the child's handicapping condition. Close friends and extended family members grieve their own loss, as well as that of their loved ones. Grandparents may have difficulty accepting the diagnosis, deny that the child has a handicapping condition, or place blame on the unrelated parent for the child's difficulties. When present, these responses can interfere with the family's adaptation to the condition and place an additional strain on the parents. With time, close friends and extended family members can become a strong source of emotional support. They may also provide greatly needed respite care and/or financial assistance that may be invaluable toward meeting the needs of the child with a handicapping condition.

In summary, parenting a child with a handicapping condition can be a significant challenge. Parents may endure extended periods of uncertainty regarding the nature of their child's difficulties while securing an accurate diagnosis and its associated features. Accommodation and adaptation takes time and may be facilitated by involvement of knowledgeable helping professionals who can assist the family. Other parents of children with handicapping conditions can be effective in educating parents about their legal rights and helping them advocate for their children.

See also: Group Psychotherapy; Mental Retardation; Parenting Practices; Siblings

Further Reading

Batshaw, M. L. (Ed.). (2001). *When your child has a disability: The complete sourcebook of daily and medical care* (Rev. ed.). Baltimore, MD: Paul H. Brookes.

Naseef, R. A. (2001). *Special children, challenged parents: The struggles and rewards of raising a child with a disability* (Rev. ed.). Baltimore, MD: Paul H. Brookes.

Stoneman, Z. (1997). Mental retardation and family adaptation. In W. E. MacLean, Jr. (Ed.), *Ellis' handbook of mental deficiency, psychological theory and research* (3rd ed., pp. 405–437). Mahwah, NJ: Lawrence Erlbaum.

Trachtenberg, S. W., & Batshaw, M. L. (1997). Caring and coping: The family of a child with disabilities. In M. L. Batshaw (Ed.), *Children with disabilities* (4th ed., pp. 743–756). Baltimore, MD: Paul H. Brookes.

MICHAEL L. MILLER
WILLIAM E. MACLEAN, JR.

Parent's Chronic Illness

See: Psychological Impact of a Parent's Chronic Illness

Partial Hospitalization

See: Day Treatment

Participant Modeling

DEFINITION

Modeling procedures facilitate learning through the observation of another individual performing a specific action or behavior. As described earlier by Bandura (1971), all modeling procedures are based on the principles of vicarious or observational conditioning. Children can acquire new responses, both appropriate (e.g., dressing oneself) and inappropriate (e.g., hitting a sibling), through observing others on a regular basis. In addition, Bandura described how already acquired responses can be facilitated, inhibited, or disinhibited through vicarious learning or modeling procedures. For example, a child who observes his/her parent engage in fearful behaviors toward dogs may inhibit approach behavior toward dogs. Likewise, a child who is fearful of snakes and observes a peer engaging in nonfearful interactions with a snake may disinhibit avoidant responses and engage in approach behavior to the previously feared snake. With fearful children, this disinhibiting effect is believed to play a critical role. That is, as the child observes appropriate positive interaction with the feared stimuli without any negative consequences, extinction of the child's fear is facilitated, thus making approach possible.

Several different types of modeling have been employed in the treatment of childhood fears and phobias. *Videotape modeling* consists of having the child view a filmed version of a model (with similar characteristics as the child) demonstrating successively greater interactions with the feared stimuli. The same procedures are followed with *live modeling*; however, the child observes the interactions directly (but is not asked to participate in them). *Participant modeling* combines live modeling procedures along with therapist-guided interaction with the feared object, first with the model serving as a guide and then directly with the feared stimulus.

METHOD

Prior to initiating treatment, fearful or avoidant children are often assessed using a behavioral avoidance task (BAT). The BAT consists of predetermined and progressively intimate interactions with the feared stimulus or situation. The child's ability to progress through the tasks is assessed and oftentimes the child is asked to indicate his/her subjective distress or discomfort (e.g., on a 0–10 scale) during each of the interactions. These tasks are then incorporated into treatment with the goal of having the child progress through the BAT without significant distress or anxiety.

Participant modeling generally consists of three stages: observation of live modeling, therapist-guided interaction, and unaccompanied interaction. Since participant modeling is most often used for the treatment of childhood fears and phobias, these procedures will be described with regard to a dog-fearful child. During the first stage, the therapist or model demonstrates gradually successive nonfearful approach behavior (usually the same or similar tasks to those assessed on the BAT) toward the feared stimuli. For a dog-phobic child, this might entail the following successive steps: having the model walk toward the dog with an out-reached hand, letting the dog sniff the model's hand, petting the dog on the back and then head, and sitting on the ground and playing with the dog. During this stage of live modeling, it is important that the child observe only positive consequences and appropriate coping skills. In the second stage, the therapist-model uses physical contact to guide the child through the behavioral approach tasks previously demonstrated. Continuing with the example of a dog-phobic child, this process might involve having the therapist hold the child's hand while they approach the dog together, having the child place his/her hand on top of the therapist's while they pet the dog, and sitting next to the therapist on the ground while the therapist plays with the dog. During this stage, the therapist-model offers encouragement and support while physically assisting the child approach the feared stimulus. Finally, the third stage consists of the child performing the same behavioral approach tasks without the physical assistance of the therapist-model. During this stage, the therapist would again accompany the child through the dog-approach and interaction tasks; however it would be requested that the child perform these tasks alone. Furthermore, throughout these procedures, the child is reinforced profusely or praised for initiating nonfearful approach and imitation behaviors.

CLINICAL APPLICATIONS

Participant modeling has primarily been used to treat children and adolescents with fears and/or phobic avoidance of specific stimuli. As indicated by Bandura, the goals of participant modeling with such cases are to reduce fear and facilitate new skill acquisition. Although participant modeling has been described herein with regard to the reduction of phobic avoidance and fearful behaviors, modeling procedures have also been used with children who are socially withdrawn, autistic, mentally retarded, and distractible. In addition, participant modeling is often combined with other behavioral treatment strategies (e.g., systematic desensitization, reinforcement). Empirical studies employing participant modeling have been conducted with individuals of all ages including children of preschool and early elementary school grades. Despite the use of participant modeling with a diverse array of childhood fears, research is lacking regarding the long-term maintenance of treatment gains attained with this approach as well as its utility with clinically phobic children and adolescents.

EFFECTIVENESS

Ollendick and colleagues (1991, 1998) have provided detailed description of studies demonstrating the effectiveness of modeling in general, and participant modeling in particular. Overall, significant improvements in approach behavior along with reductions in fearful avoidance have been reported in research and clinical case studies that have employed participant modeling procedures. To illustrate these findings, two prominent studies will be described.

Ritter (1968) conducted an early study of treatment effectiveness with 44 elementary school-age children identified as snake-avoidant. A 29-item BAT was constructed and only those children who were unable to hold a snake for a few seconds with gloved hands were selected for treatment. Children were matched based on their level of snake-avoidant behavior and randomly assigned to one of three groups. The modeling-only treatment group simply observed an adult and five peers demonstrate progressive interactions with a harmless snake. The participant-modeling treatment group observed the same modeling procedures, were then assisted by the adult in completing the interactive tasks, and finally completed the interactions with the snake alone. The control group of children completed only the pre- and posttreatment BAT. At posttreatment, children from both the modeling-only and participant-modeling groups indicated less fear of the snake than the control group. In addition, the children who were treated with participant modeling demonstrated superior gains than those in the modeling-only group. That is, at posttreatment, 80 percent of the children from the participant-modeling treatment condition were able to complete the entire 29-item BAT compared with 53 percent of children from the modeling-only condition, and none of the control children.

Lewis (1974) also provided support for the superior efficacy of participant modeling by comparing modeling-only, participation-only, and participant-modeling (a combination of the previous two) treatment groups with a control condition. Forty African-American boys (aged 5–12) who displayed water-avoidant behaviors were individually assessed using a 16-item BAT of progressively greater interactions in a pool. Children were matched based on their level of water-avoidance and randomly assigned to one of the four conditions. In the modeling-only treatment group, children observed a videotape of three peers modeling each of the approach behaviors from the BAT and then played a game with an adult model. The participation-only group of children viewed a neutral videotape and were subsequently accompanied to the pool by an adult who physically aided them in performing the behavioral approach tasks. The participant-modeling group of children viewed the videotape of peers performing the BAT task and were then physically assisted in completing the tasks by an adult. Finally, the control group of children viewed the neutral videotape and then played a game with an adult.

Results from Lewis's (1974) study revealed less fearfulness and greater involvement regarding water activities for all three treatment groups when individually compared to the control condition. Furthermore, greater changes were reported for children who received the participation component in their treatment as compared with those from either the modeling-only or control conditions. Finally, comparison of the participant-modeling treatment and participation-only treatment revealed greater changes for the former, suggesting that the combination of modeling and assisted participation is superior to either of these conditions alone.

Finally, Ollendick and Cerny (1981) reported overall percentages of treatment efficacy (i.e., the percentage of subjects performing the final BAT or approach response), clearly demonstrating the superior successes achieved with participant modeling. That is, efficacy for filmed modeling was reported to range from 25 to 50 percent, live modeling from 50 to 67 percent, and participant modeling 80–92 percent. Based on these empirical findings, childhood treatment of fears and phobias with participant modeling has received "well established" status according to the guidelines set forth by the Task Force for Promotion and Dissemination of Psychological Procedures.

See also: Anxiety Disorders; Systematic Desensitization; Videotape Modeling

Further Reading

Bandura, A. (1971). *Psychological modeling: Conflicting theories.* Chicago: Aldine-Atherton.

Lewis, S. (1974). A comparison of behavioral therapy techniques in the reduction of fearful avoidance behavior. *Behavior Therapy, 5,* 648–655.

Ollendick, T. H., & Cerny, J. A. (1981). *Clinical behavior therapy with children.* New York: Plenum.

Ollendick, T. H., & King, N. J. (1998). Empirically supported treatments for children with phobic and anxiety disorders: Current status. *Journal of Clinical Child Psychology, 27,* 156–167.

Ritter, B. (1968). The group desensitization of children's snake phobias using vicarious and contact desensitization procedures. *Behaviour Research and Therapy, 6,* 1–6.

AMIE E. GRILLS
THOMAS H. OLLENDICK

Pediatric Human Immunodeficiency Virus-1 (HIV)

Human Immunodeficiency Virus-1 (HIV) is an infectious agent (retrovirus) that infects and destroys specific blood cells (i.e., CD4 "T-cells") in the human immune system, causing a breakdown of an individual's ability to defend against other infections. At the severe end of the spectrum of HIV-infection, Acquired Immune Deficiency Syndrome (AIDS) is a chronic disease that is technically defined by the following conditions: (1) a CD4 T-cell count of less than 200 cells per cubic millimeter of blood, and (2) the presence of a number of opportunistic infections, such as those listed in Table 1.

Table 1. Common AIDS-Defining Conditions for Children Younger than 13 Years Old in the United States ($N = 8908$), Reported Through December 2000

Condition	% cases	N
Pneumocystis carinii pneumonia (PCP)	33	2940
Lymphoid interstitial pneumonitis	24	2138
Recurrent bacterial infections	21	1871
HIV wasting syndrome	18	1604
HIV encephalopathy	17	1515
Candida esophagitis	16	1425
Cytomegalovirus disease	10	891
Mycobacterium avium infection	8	713
Severe *herpes simplex* infection	5	445
Cryptosporidiosis	5	445
Pulmonary candidiasis	4	356

Note: More than one diagnosis reported was for some children. Thus, the sum of the percentages does not equal 100%.
Source: Centers for Disease Control and Prevention (CDC), National Center for *HIV, STD,* and *TB* Research, Division of HIV/AIDS Prevention, Surveillance Division. http://www.cdc.gov/hiv/dhap.htm

Opportunistic infections are diseases that the healthy immune system usually successfully overcomes, but that a compromised immune system cannot.

According to the Centers for Disease Control and Prevention (CDC), HIV is generally passed from one person to another through blood-to-blood and sexual contact. In addition, infected pregnant women can pass HIV to their babies during pregnancy or delivery, as well as through breast-feeding.

ETIOLOGY, INCIDENCE, AND PREVALENCE

The first case of pediatric AIDS was reported to the scientific and medical communities in 1982, just prior to the identification of the virus that causes AIDS (HIV) in 1983. During the early 1980s, the most common route of pediatric HIV-infection was transfusion- or hemophilia-related. In fact, approximately 60 percent of individuals with hemophilia (including children) became infected with HIV prior to 1985 due to HIV-tainted blood products. Since 1985, however, methods of identifying HIV-tainted blood and blood products have all but eliminated transfusion-related transmission of HIV. Currently, less than 2 percent of new pediatric AIDS cases are believed to be transfusion- or hemophilia-related. The vast majority (90 percent) of new pediatric AIDS cases are the result of vertical transmission (i.e., mother to child) during the pre- or perinatal period.

The prevalence (i.e., number of *total* cases) and incidence (i.e., number of *new* cases) of pediatric *HIV-infection* are hard to estimate, because of national reporting standards. However, the prevalence of pediatric AIDS in the United States, including all cases reported to the CDC through the year 2000, was just under 10,000. The incidence of pediatric AIDS increased each year until 1992, but has been declining since that time. In the year 2000, 196 new cases of pediatric AIDS were reported to the CDC. African-American children were 17 times more likely, and Hispanic children were 3 times more likely than Caucasian children to develop AIDS. The discrepant incidence rates across racial groups reported among children in 2000 reflect a similar pattern of prevalence among women of childbearing age.

TREATMENT

Prevention

Given that the majority of new cases of pediatric AIDS are the result of vertical transmission, control of

the disease among adults of childbearing age stands the greatest chance of reducing the incidence of pediatric HIV infection. However, even if the rate of new cases of adult HIV infection remains stable, medical management of HIV infection among pregnant women significantly reduces the chance of vertical transmission. In 1994, the Public Health Service (PHS) published guidelines for the use of zidovudine (ZDV) by pregnant women to reduce the risk of pre- and perinatal transmission of HIV. Estimates suggest that the rate of vertical transmission among HIV-infected women dropped from near 30 percent (untreated women) to less than 10 percent (ZDV-treated women). These guidelines, and the 1995 PHS-recommended HIV counseling and testing of pregnant women may have helped to reduce the incidence of pediatric HIV-infection over the past 10 years.

Detection and Treatment

HIV can be reliably detected in most infected infants by age 1 month, and in virtually all infected infants by age 6 months. However, initial testing is recommended within 48 hr of birth, because almost 40 percent of infected neonates can be identified at this time. Unlike HIV-infected adults, who may not present symptoms for several years post-infection, infants who acquire HIV at birth typically demonstrate some symptoms within the first 18–24 months of life if they remain untreated. The CDC recommends initiation of antiretroviral therapy (ART) for all infected infants (<12 months) regardless of disease status because of the likelihood of disease progression.

For infected children older than 1 year, two approaches for treatment have been offered. The first approach is to initiate therapy regardless of symptom presentation or status. This approach ensures treatment of infection as early as possible, and before deterioration of the immune system. The second approach is to defer treatment in HIV-infected children who do not yet demonstrate symptoms of illness. This approach minimizes the risk of drug resistance when adherence is likely to be low. Active treatment would then be initiated when changes are observed in viral load or symptom status.

Combination therapy is usually recommended for all infected infants, children, and adolescents. Combination therapy generally involves two nucleoside analog reverse transcriptase inhibitors (NRTIs; e.g., ZDV, lamivudine, stavudine) and one highly active protease inhibitor (e.g., ritonovir, indinavir). The specific mechanisms of these drugs are beyond the scope of this entry, but each drug type (protease inhibitor, NRTI) operates to reduce the ability of the virus to reproduce and spread throughout the body. Treatment with a single drug is not recommended because of the likelihood of the virus developing resistance. However, in cases where nonadherence (i.e., noncompliance) with combination therapies is suspected, monotherapy may be prescribed for a period of time.

PSYCHOSOCIAL ISSUES

Adherence

As suggested by the above discussion of pharmacological therapy for HIV-infection, adherence to therapy is of utmost importance. Unfortunately, among children, adherence is often difficult to achieve: Published estimates of child adherence to ART hover around 50 percent. That is, children in study samples take, on average, about 50 percent of the medications that they are prescribed, or take their prescribed medications "well" about 50 percent of the time. Such adherence is problematic because of the likelihood of the virus developing resistance to the drugs if they are not taken as prescribed. Nonadherence is thought to be a significant reason for treatment failure and disease progression.

Several factors have been reported as predictors of nonadherence to ART, including child depressive symptoms, difficult dosing regimens, and environmental stressors (e.g., housing instability, negative life events). Parental factors, such as parental depressive symptoms and poor social support have also been implicated as predictors of child nonadherence. Such factors should be addressed by competent mental heath professionals in the context of a multidisciplinary team effort (i.e., physicians, nurses, psychologists, social workers) to ensure adequate adherence to therapy.

Neuropsychological and Behavioral Consequences of HIV Infection

Several behavioral or neuropsychological consequences of pediatric HIV infection have been identified, including encephalitis, cognitive and developmental delays or deficits, and behavioral deficits, such as hyperactive or impulsive behaviors. Studies that have focused on neurological implications of the disease have suggested a higher rate of short-term memory problems, poorer performance on verbal and arithmetic reasoning tasks, and delayed motor development. Similarly, poorer attention and concentration have been

identified among children with HIV. In most cases, children who developed AIDS-defining criteria prior to age 2 years evidence the most severe deficits. However, at least some of these deficits may be ameliorated by an enriched and stimulating environment and good prenatal health of the mother. Other research suggests that approximately 25 percent of school-aged children with HIV evidence clinically significant anxious/depressive or aggressive/impulsive behavioral symptoms.

Disclosure of Illness

Because of the stigma associated with HIV infection, issues surrounding the disclosure of health status deserve clinical attention. At issue are both disclosure of the illness to the child and disclosure of the child's illness to extended family, friends, and potential support people. With regard to disclosure to the child, questions regarding *when* and *how* to disclose become paramount. There is little empirical research to guide such decisions, other than findings that school-aged children who had *not* been told of their HIV-status evidenced more behavior problems than those to whom HIV-status had been disclosed. Rather than a discrete "disclosing event," a gradual disclosing process may be therapeutically advantageous. That is, a continuing, age-appropriate dialogue about illness and health that culminates (after weeks or months) in specific disclosure of the child's illness may be most appropriate. Prior to such disclosure, the child should possess cognitive and emotional skills sufficient to discern "private" versus "public" information.

Support may also be necessary to establish timelines for disclosure of the child's illness to extended family, friends, and other relevant parties (e.g., teachers). Advantages of disclosure to extended support networks include the potential for help with adherence or behavioral issues (particularly at school), and emotional support for family members. Clearly, the potential advantages of disclosure to extended family and community members should be weighed against potential disadvantages and the child's right to privacy.

Emerging Issues for HIV Infection in Adolescence

Regardless of the route of transmission, children with HIV are living longer than in previous decades, and are more likely to live to see their adolescent years. As a result, a number of issues must be addressed as *children* with HIV become *adolescents* with HIV, such as safer sexual practices, responsible behavior regarding drug and alcohol use, and adherence to medication. These emerging issues lie at the intersection of several of the issues described above (i.e., development, adherence, disclosure). Clearly, disclosure of HIV status should occur prior to the onset of adolescence, preferably with sufficient time for the adolescent to incorporate healthy lifestyle decisions into her or his behavioral repertoire.

Beyond healthy lifestyle decisions, adolescents with HIV may be at significant risk for symptoms of depression. The presence of a serious chronic illness, the stigmatization that may accompany that illness, and the behavioral demands to cope with the illness are all issues that may need to be addressed with the adolescent to minimize the likelihood of adjustment difficulties.

See also: Bereavement; Children with Parents or Siblings with HIV-Infection; Health Care Use; Parenting the Chronically Ill Child; Pediatric Infectious Diseases; Treatment Adherence: Medical

Further Reading

Armistead, L., Forehand, R., Steele, R., & Kotchick, B. (1998). Pediatric AIDS. In T. H. Ollendick & M. Hersen (Eds.). *Handbook of Child Psychopathology* (3rd ed., pp. 463–481). New York: Plenum.

Boyd-Franklin, N., Steiner, G. L., Boland, M. G. (1995). *Children, families, and HIV/AIDS: Psychosocial and therapeutic issues.* New York: Guilford.

Centers for Disease Control and Prevention. (1998). Guidelines for the use of antiretroviral agents in pediatric HIV-infection. *Morbidity and Mortality Weekly Report; 47*(No. RR-4), 1–51. (http://www.cdc.gov/mmwr/PDF/rr/rr4704.pdf).

RIC G. STEELE

Pediatric Hypnosis

INTRODUCTION

Hypnosis as an adjunct to treatment in pediatrics has increased in use since the 1960s. Today, hypnotherapy is offered at many pediatric institutions for treating different problem behaviors. In addition, it is an adjunct in the treatment of some physical disorders. For example, pediatric hypnosis has become an acceptable tool in assessing as well as in managing pain, as noted by Kohen and Olness (1993). Contributing to this acceptance are the positive findings of ongoing pediatric hypnosis research demonstrating the effectiveness of hypnotherapy in helping children with diverse problems

such as juvenile migraine headaches, cancer-related pain, and the strengthening of self-control in the management of behavior problems.

The history of hypnosis has been erratic, popular one day, in disrepute the next. Currently, it is viewed positively. The earliest reports of hypnosis as a tool for sick children can be traced to ancient times, where sick children were given suggestion and faith as a healing tool. It was in the 18th century that Anton Mesmer used "animal magnetism" for healing. His treatment of several children was reported, but after an international commission observed his technique and theory, they concluded that improvement happened not because of animal magnetism, but because of the placebo effect. Nevertheless, hypnosis continued to be used sporadically until 1900 with some successful reports, but it was not until the 1960s when hypnosis began to be studied scientifically. The modern studies, as reviewed by London (1963), demonstrated that children were good hypnotic subjects and that hypnosis techniques were effective with diverse medical and psychological problems of children.

DEFINITION

Many pediatric hypnotherapists define hypnosis as an alert state of awareness characterized by heightened and focused attention. This alternative state of awareness, in contrast to the normal state of awareness, permits the child to strongly focus on a particular goal, such as controlling pain or increasing self-control. Children at play frequently alternate between an experience of play and fantasy, even without a hypnotic induction. Thus, children may sometimes enter a hypnotic state while playing or daydreaming. In these spontaneous states, they can interact with the doctor, learn, and understand. The children display signs of hypnosis such as absorption in fantasy, focused attention, and heightened suggestibility. The health care worker who can use hypnotic suggestion with the child in this focused state can tap the inner resources of the child in three major ways: helping the child (1) to gain control, (2) to feel more comfortable, and (3) to be more motivated to participate in the treatment. The benefit of these positive outcomes, as noted by Gardner and Olness (1981), is to provide "an attitude of hope in the context of mastery" (p. 89).

A number of other definitions of hypnosis offer explanations which clarify particular hypnotic activity such as: (1) the social–cultural theory which highlights motivation and role playing, (2) learning theories which emphasize conditioning and behavior, (3) physiological theories which describe alterations of neural connections, and (4) combinations of these theories working together. Most hypnotherapists concur that in hypnosis (1) awareness is more focused, (2) suggestibility is tapped, and (3) hypnosis permits some access to unconscious and physiological processes.

METHOD

Children are taught self-hypnosis in individual sessions. Generally, the training begins with discussion of hypnosis and relaxation so that the child understands what to expect. Then, the child is taught relaxation of the body, sometimes using a doll to demonstrate the floppiness of relaxation. Once the child is relaxed, fantasy and imagery are introduced to deepen the relaxation, and imagery is used to focus the child on a specific goal such as pain reduction or comfort. For example, the child may focus on being at his or her favorite place, like the beach, with a favorite toy where he or she is having fun. A child's susceptibility to hypnosis can be tested by London's *Children's Hypnotic Susceptibility Scale.* The scale contains 22 items in two parts, tapping sensory (seeing and hearing), imaginative (fantasy), and motor response ("Your arm is becoming stiff") to hypnosis. Morgan and Hilgard (1979) developed a second measure of hypnotic responsivity in 1979, which has two forms, one for children 6–16 and another form for children 4–8. The latter is based on an active imagination induction because young children have difficulty responding to suggestions to close their eyes. Hypnotic susceptibility measures can be useful to clarify a diagnosis and to provide information about hypnotic skills. While these tests tell us that children are more responsive to hypnosis than adults, there is much more research that needs to be done.

CLINICAL APPLICATIONS

Pediatric hypnosis has been used to treat a variety of disorders, syndromes, and mental conditions. It is particularly helpful when discomfort is recurrent or when behaviors are undesirable and need modification. For example, children with pain, whether it is cancer pain or some other type of repeated painful experience, demonstrate successful use of hypnosis by diminishing their perception of pain. Behavior problems can be modified with hypnosis by setting realistic goals such as building self-control, supporting the self with positive

interaction by the therapist, and uncovering conflict by working through the emotions. Table 1 lists the problem areas that showed a positive response to pediatric hypnosis. While most of the disorders are based on case studies, increasingly, controlled research has been undertaken to confirm these results.

Generally, a play therapy situation provides a natural environment for children to use hypnosis. To the child, hypnosis is a form of play and the play helps the child to develop (1) of physical reactions such as pain; (2) of psychological reactions such as anxiety, and (3) of external actions such as movement and behavior. As a form of play, self-hypnosis reinforces the hypnosis augmented by the therapist, and as we have noted elsewhere, such play enables the child to improve, by degrees, because of the daily practice. The world of play and imagination is so natural to the child because his or her pretend world is more under control than the world of reality, which is often a mystery.

Hypnosis is best used when the child is motivated, the problem is treatable by hypnosis, and the child responds to hypnotic induction. The starting point is for both child and parents to agree to the use of hypnosis because agreement by the parents permits the child freedom to explore hypnosis. However, hypnosis is not a panacea. It is not indicated when the use of an altered state of awareness could lead to physical danger such as the risk of serious infection when possible infection is ignored.

Table 1. Disorders Treated by Hypnosis

Disorders	Outcome
Allergies	Less medication
Asthma	Self-control
Dermatological	Tissue healing
Burns	Reduction of pain
Warts	Regression of wart
Diabetes	Self-control
Hemophilia	Relaxation, control
Abdominal pain	Pain reduction
Neurological pain	Pain reduction
Surgery	Preparation
Behavior disorders	Self-control
Anxiety disorders	Relaxation
Phobic disorders	Mastery of symptoms
Sleep disorders	Improved sleep
Resistance	Improves rapport
Postoperative pain	Lower pain ratings
Cancer pain	Pain relief
Nausea	Decreased nausea
Dysphagia	Self-management

Second, it is not indicated when using hypnosis could aggravate emotional problems. For example, if independent behavior leads to less attention from the family, the child may become depressed. Finally, hypnosis is not indicated if the problem can be more effectively treated by some other approach.

EFFECTIVENESS

While many examples of pediatric hypnosis are descriptive, increasing numbers are being studied methodically. Many of the disorders listed in Table 1 have been studied, and the results demonstrated statistically and clinically significant improvements in at least one of several factors: changes in the presenting problem; changes in the child's self-control; and changes in parent behavior. Such changes can be significant in helping the child to feel more control, to experience more comfort, and to become an active participant in the treatment. However, some of the disorders have only case study information and lack long-term study making it difficult to generalize.

While children are more susceptible to hypnosis than adults, not every child can be hypnotized. Evaluation is necessary to determine if hypnosis is appropriate.

Usually, hypnosis is not used as the primary tool in pediatrics, but it is frequently used as an adjunct to ongoing medical treatment. As such, studies have not found any significant side effects other than perhaps sleepiness or a slight headache in a few studies. Nonetheless, as can be seen from Table 1, many physical and behavioral problems are affected in a beneficial way by pediatric hypnosis. Today it is viewed as a most promising adjunct to treatment.

See also: Behavior Modification; Behavior Therapy; Pain Assessment; Pain Control; Relaxation Training; Self Management

Further Reading

Gardner, G. G., & Olness, K. (1981). *Hypnosis and hypnotherapy with children.* New York: Grune & Stratton.

Kohen, D. P., & Olness, K. (1993). Hypnotherapy with children. In J. W. Rhue, S. J. Lynn, & I. Kirsch (Eds.), *Handbook of clinical hypnosis* (pp. 357–381) Washington, DC: American Psychological Association.

London, P. (1963). *Children's hypnotic susceptibility scale.* Palo Alto, CA: Consulting Psychologists Press.

Morgan, A. H., & Hilgard, J. R. (1979). The Stanford hypnotic susceptibility scale for children. *The American Journal of Clinical Hypnosis, 21,* 148–155.

SHIRLEY SANDERS

Pediatric Infectious Diseases

Infectious or contagious diseases are the leading cause of death in the world. The most common types of germs responsible for infectious diseases are viruses and bacteria. A virus comprises a central core of either DNA or RNA, surrounded by a protein coating called a capsid. Once a virus has infected an organism, the virus inserts its DNA or RNA into the nucleus of a cell and begins to replicate, or create copies of itself. The normal protein synthesis of the host cell is typically disrupted, and the host cell is usually destroyed either by the virus or by the immune system in order to neutralize the virus. Replicated copies of the virus are released from the infected cell and move to infect other cells. Infection of host cells is the only means of replication available to the virus. Symptoms associated with a viral infection include those associated with the virus itself, and those caused by the person's immune response (e.g., fever, body aches). Some infectious diseases caused by viruses include colds, influenza, measles, chicken pox, HIV-infection, herpes, and rubella.

Bacteria are generally more biologically complicated than viruses. A bacterium is a single-celled organism that may live in or on the tissue of a larger organism. Unlike viruses, bacteria can carry on all necessary activities for life (e.g., DNA synthesis, replication) and can reproduce independently. However, bacteria must have a host to supply nourishment and a supportive environment for reproduction. Bacterial infections occur when a harmful species of bacteria invades the body and begins cell replication. A disease state exists when the consequences of this bacterial replication (e.g., bacterial toxins) disrupt the normal functioning of the person's body. Beyond the direct effects of the bacteria, symptoms associated with bacterial infections also include those caused by the person's immune response (e.g., fever, inflammation, localized swelling). Some infectious diseases caused by bacteria are acute otitis media, bacterial pneumonia, enteritis, bacterial meningitis, urinary tract infections, impetigo, and scarlet fever.

INCIDENCE AND CORRELATES

Infectious diseases are among the most common childhood illnesses. Children are thought to be more susceptible to infection because of transmissions from mother to child during the birth process, breast-feeding, and greater vulnerability of the child's developing immune system.

Several factors are related to the incidence of infectious diseases in children. Research indicates that the child's environment, socioeconomic status, and general health are important mediators of the impact of the disease. For example, a child of lower socioeconomic status may be at increased risk of infection due to crowded living conditions, the presence of an increased concentration of germs in the environment, poor nutrition, or poor access to adequate medical care. For example, despite the improved available medical treatment for *tuberculosis* (TB), children from lower socioeconomic groups (particularly those from urban environments) are at increased risk for contracting this illness.

Beyond environmental and socioeconomic factors, parental values and beliefs may influence a child's risk of infection. For example, some cultural groups may hold health beliefs that reduce the likelihood of adequate preventative measures for many pediatric infectious diseases (e.g., vaccinations). Culturally sensitive education regarding the risks and benefits of health-related behaviors may be one mechanism by which health care professionals may impact the quality of care provided to children.

ETIOLOGY

Although some bacteria are capable of independent movement, the most common means of transmission is via contact with a contaminated surface or individual. Some bacteria are capable of person-to-person contagion via airborne droplets of mucus (e.g., sneeze, cough). It is worth noting that bacterial infections may be more likely when an individual's immune system is weakened (e.g., because of viral infection, poor nutrition, fatigue, etc.).

Similar to bacterial infections, viral infections may be transmitted through skin-to-skin contact, via airborne virus particles, contaminated surfaces, or through direct communication of bodily fluids. However, because of their minute size, viruses may permeate filters that withhold the relatively larger bacteria. Childhood infectious diseases are most commonly transmitted via contact with mucus membranes and airborne viral particles (e.g., through sneezing and coughing). Because of this, the best behavioral defenses against both bacterial and viral infections are: (1) limiting children's contact with people with known viral or bacterial illnesses, and (2) frequent handwashing.

TREATMENT

Natural Defenses

The body's primary defenses against viral and bacterial infections are specialized white blood cells (lymphocytes), natural chemicals that interfere with viral reproduction, and antibodies that the individual has acquired to the specific virus or bacteria.

Immunizations

Current medical technology has helped many children to avoid infections that were much more common in the past. Whereas previous generations of children were more likely to be infected with measles, chicken pox, and mumps, most children today receive a complete series of vaccinations against 10 major diseases before the age of 2. In brief, immunizations work by giving the child an injection that contains weakened or killed viruses or bacteria. This stimulates the body to produce antibodies against those specific bacteria or viruses. These antibodies then protect the child against the disease, should he or she come in contact with it in the future. Consequently, the natural defenses against infection are strengthened, and children who receive a complete set of vaccinations are protected from many childhood infectious diseases.

Antibiotics

Beyond vaccinations, the advancement of antibiotics has also helped decrease the number and severity of many childhood bacterial infections. One issue with antibiotics, however, is that the course of the antibiotic often lasts longer than the abatement of symptoms. Frequently, children begin to feel better, their symptoms diminish, and they no longer wish to take their medication. However, complete adherence to the prescribed course of antibiotics is necessary to reduce the likelihood of continued infection and the development of antibiotic-resistant bacterial strains.

Antiviral Medications

A more recent development in the treatment of viral infectious diseases is the use of medications designed to disrupt the replication and dissemination of viruses. Although the most well-known of these treatments are designed to treat HIV infection (antiretroviral therapy), pharmacological agents (e.g., neuraminidase inhibitors) recently have been developed to disrupt the replication of viruses such as *Influenza A* and *B*. As with other medications, strict adherence is necessary for maximum benefit.

PSYCHOSOCIAL FACTORS

A number of psychosocial sequelae to pediatric infectious diseases have been documented, but these consequences are generally due to unresolved symptoms of the infection, rather than the infection itself. For example, unresolved *otitis media* may result in compromised hearing sensitivity, delayed speech production, and compromised cognitive development, particularly when the affected child is very young and the infection very severe or recurrent. Behavioral and cognitive changes have also been diagnosed in children with *encephalitis*, although these changes are usually transitory.

Secondary effects of bacterial or viral infections may include isolation, excessive school absences, and compromised self-esteem. Serious and long-term infections may require that the child be quarantined, which may disrupt social and academic pursuits. Further, infections that require long-term treatment (e.g., *hepatitis C*) may cause a child to feel that she or he is "different," which may impact subsequent social functioning. Further, some treatments (e.g., interferon injections) may themselves place a child at risk for depressive symptoms. Finally, the risk of relapse or of treatment failure may place some children at risk for adjustment difficulties. For example, while 30–35 percent of patients with *hepatitis C* improve medically with interferon injections, about half of them relapse if removed from the treatment program.

PSYCHOSOCIAL INTERVENTIONS

Pain

Although the pain is often considered relatively mild, many treatments and immunizations for infectious diseases involve subcutaneous or intramuscular injections. For many children this pain is associated with significant distress. Research has demonstrated that children who are unaware of the immunization process fare much better during the injection than children who are forewarned of the immunizations. That is, children who are "warned" ahead of time often exhibit more concern and greater reports of pain than children who are not warned. Further, research has suggested that

distraction (e.g., watching a cartoon, reading a book, telling a story) and "coping statements" made by the medical professional and/or parents (e.g., "You're doing a great job!") are more effective at reducing child (and parent) distress than apologies or words of comfort (e.g., "I know it hurts, but it won't last long").

Adherence

As noted above, adherence to antibiotic or antiviral therapies for infectious diseases is of utmost importance. Thus, strategies for insuring optimal adherence should be used. When possible, simple dosing regimens should be employed. When this is not possible, daily reminders, "daily pill boxes" (i.e., unit dosings), or behavioral reinforcements may be necessary to help improve adherence. Education to address parental or child health beliefs that do not support good adherence may also be useful in improving adherence. Finally, some research has suggested that poor adherence may be occasioned by depressed mood. As such, symptoms of depression or distress should be monitored and addressed.

Adjustment to Illness

For children with a severe or chronic infection, such as *TB* or *hepatitis C*, the professional cooperation of an interdisciplinary team (e.g., psychologists, social workers, nurses, physicians, educators) may help ease the emotional and physical burdens experienced by the child and the family. Beyond symptoms of distress and adherence issues, families of children with a chronic infectious illness may be required to navigate behavioral limitations or lifestyle changes. Changes in the educational or social environments may also be required, which may be proactively addressed by the members of the treatment team.

See also: Coping with Illness; Health Care Use; Parenting the Chronically Ill Child; Pediatric Human Immunodeficiency Virus-1 (HIV); Treatment Adherence: Medical

Further Reading

Alcock, K. J. & Bundy, D. A. (2001). The impact of infectious disease on cognitive development. In R. J. Sternberg & E. L. Grigorenko (Eds.), *Environmental effects on cognitive abilities* (pp. 221–254). Mahwah, NJ: Erlbaum.

Palumbo, D. R., Davidson, P. W., Peloquin, L. J., & Gigliotti, F. (1995). Neuropsychological aspects of pediatric infectious diseases. In M. C. Roberts (Ed.), *Handbook of pediatric psychology* (2nd ed., pp. 342–361). New York: Guilford.

Rice, C. A., & Pollard J. M. (Eds.). (2001, December). *Colds, flu and other respiratory infections*, 5. [On-line]. Available: http://fcs.tamu.edu/health/Health-Education_Rural_ Outreach/Health_Hints/2001/december/december-2001.htm#6

MARGARET MARY RICHARDS
RIC G. STEELE

Pediatric Psychology

In 1995, the American Psychological Association (APA) established the Commission for the Recognition of Specialties and Proficiencies in Professional Psychology (the acronym is CRSPPP, pronounced "crisp"). This Commission provided official recognition for existing specialties and recognized some new ones. In each case, the APA Council acted on its recommendations, and an archival document was created describing the specialty.

Pediatric psychology, which has existed for over 30 years, is clearly a specialty in professional psychology, although it has not yet been officially recognized as such by CRSPPP. On the APA Web site (www.apa.org), the Society of Pediatric Psychology is listed as Division 54, and its self-description is as follows:

> Founded in 1968, the Society of Pediatric Psychology provides a forum for scientists and professionals interested in the health care of children, adolescents, and their families. The field of pediatric psychology is defined by the concerns of psychologists and allied professionals who work in interdisciplinary settings such as children's hospitals, developmental clinics, pediatric or medical group practices, as well as traditional clinical child or academic arenas. We focus on the rapidly expanding role of behavioral medicine and health psychology in the care of children, adolescents, and their families.

Sometimes, this field is referred to as "child health psychology" to emphasize its scientific rather than its professional facets. There are a certain number of psychologists doing important research in child health psychology but who are not clinically trained. Of the three founders of the Society of Pediatric Psychology (Logan Wright, Lee Salk, and Dorothea Ross), Dorothea Ross was such an individual. The "Bobo Doll" study of children's imitation of aggression (published with her mentor, Albert Bandura, and her sister, Sheila Ross, as coauthors) is a classic in the psychological literature. She also published important work on educational strategies that are effective with

children with intellectual disabilities, on children's pain, and on Attention-Deficit/Hyperactivity Disorder (ADHD).

Perhaps the best way to describe pediatric psychology (the specialty area within professional psychology) in more detail is to portray it as a combination of clinical child psychology and clinical health psychology. Let us therefore examine the CRSPPP archival descriptions of these two specialties:

> Clinical Child Psychology is a specialty of professional psychology which integrates basic tenets of clinical psychology, developmental psychopathology, and principles of child and family development. Clinical child psychologists conduct scientific research and provide psychological services to infants, toddlers, children, and adolescents. The research and services in Clinical Child Psychology are focused on understanding, preventing, diagnosing and treating psychological, cognitive, emotional, developmental, behavioral, and family problems of children. Of particular importance to clinical child psychologists is an understanding of the basic psychological needs of children and the social contexts which influence child development and adjustment.

These words would be equally accurate, at least as far as they go, in describing pediatric psychology.

According to the CRSPPP archival document,

> the specialty of Clinical Health Psychology applies scientific knowledge of the interrelationships among behavioral, emotional, cognitive, social and biological components in health and disease to the promotion and maintenance of health; the prevention, treatment and rehabilitation of illness and disability; and the improvement of the health care system. The distinct focus of Clinical Health Psychology is on physical health problems. The specialty is dedicated to the development of knowledge regarding the interface between behavior and health, and to the delivery of high quality services based on that knowledge to individuals, families, and health care systems.

These words also apply to pediatric psychology.

The knowledge base of pediatric psychology is very broad. It includes normal development, normal family processes, developmental psychopathology, assessment principles and methods, theory and research concerning the treatment of childhood mental disorders, ethical and legal issues, and knowledge of cultural context. In addition, this knowledge base includes the biological, cognitive, affective, and social bases of health and disease. It includes pharmacology, anatomy, human physiology and pathophysiology, and psychoneuroimmunology. Pediatric psychologists need to know how children's experiences and behavior are affected by physical illness, injury, and disability, and how their behavior in turn affects children's health.

The populations of interest to pediatric psychologists include infants, children, adolescents, and their families. Some pediatric psychologists work in primary care medical settings, where they end up dealing with the broad range of developmental issues and with garden variety child psychopathology as well as with health-related issues. The health problems addressed by pediatric psychologists include asthma, pain, physical disability, headache, hemophilia, diabetes, arthritis, terminal illness, cardiovascular disease, cancer, acquired immune deficiency syndrome (AIDS), sickle cell disease, injury, obesity, and dental disease, as well as with individuals at risk for these problems and those who wish to develop a healthy lifestyle. Patients' family members and health care providers also benefit from the services of pediatric psychologists.

Procedures used by pediatric psychologists include interviews, observations, age-normed psychological tests, personality and family assessment measures, and also health assessment procedures including psychophysiological measures. Interventions include the usual behavioral and cognitive–behavioral approaches, play therapy, individual psychotherapy, family therapy, and counseling. They also include on occasion biofeedback, relaxation training, crisis intervention at the time of medical diagnosis or a change in the child's health status, methods for improving compliance, preparation for stressful medical procedures, and training in coping skills. Collaboration with pediatricians and other health care personnel is a crucial part of their work.

The diversity and complexity of pediatric psychology research and practice is considerable. Each particular physical illness, such as asthma, diabetes, or cancer, has its own extensive medical knowledge base that must be mastered by the psychologist who hopes to be of help to children with that type of chronic or life-threatening illness. A division of labor is necessary, since no one could be an expert on the psychosocial aspects of every illness that might affect a child. In a tertiary care medical center, pediatric psychologists often work with more narrowly defined populations and acquire detailed knowledge concerning a particular medical specialty—for example, hematology–oncology—that is sufficient to cooperate in the research activities and clinical service delivery of a team working at the frontier.

Training in pediatric psychology typically occurs in a specialized track within an APA-approved doctoral program in clinical psychology. Such training would necessarily include significant amounts of practicum and internship work in medical settings with children and their families. Alternatively, the pediatric psychologist may have originally been trained in an APA-approved program in clinical child psychology or clinical health psychology, and then receive additional training in pediatric psychology in a postdoctoral program. Some excellent pediatric psychologists have also begun with training in APA-approved programs in counseling or school psychology and proceeded on to pediatric psychology training at the postdoctoral level.

The prospects of pediatric psychology seem to be bright. Logan Wright, my internship supervisor, at one time noted only some children have mental health problems. He went on to say that all of them have health problems during their lives. Such health problems routinely have psychosocial aspects that need to be dealt with, so the future of Pediatric Psychology looks very good indeed.

See also: Clinical Child and Adolescent Psychology; Clinical Psychology; Professional Societies—Clinical Child and Pediatric Psychology; School Psychology; Training Issues

DONALD K. ROUTH

Pediatric Psychology Organizations

See: Professional Societies in Clinical Child and Pediatric Psychology

Pediatrician

A pediatrician is a physician, doctor of medicine (MD) or doctor of osteopathy (DO), who specializes in the physical, emotional, and social health of infants, children, and adolescents. After completion of medical school training, a pediatrician undergoes 3 years of residency training. During residency training, the physician gains clinical experience in many aspects of pediatrics and pediatric subspecialties including normal child development and behavior. After completion of the pediatric residency, the physician is qualified to practice as a general pediatrician. Some pediatricians decide to pursue 3 years of fellowship training to subspecialize in an area such as neonatology, pediatric pulmonology, cardiology, development, and behavior, to name a few.

All physicians, including resident physicians, require a medical license granted by the state in which they practice. After completion of residency and/or fellowship training, many pediatricians or pediatric subspecialists seek certification from the American Board of Pediatrics (ABP). This requires the pediatrician to have graduated from an accredited medical school, completed 3 years of residency training, attained a valid, unrestricted state license to practice medicine, and completed a comprehensive two-day examination covering all aspects of health care of infants, children, and adolescents. Since 1988, recertification is required every 7 years. Many pediatricians and pediatric subspecialists are members of the American Academy of Pediatrics (AAP). The AAP is a professional organization whose mission is to help all infants, children, adolescents, and young adults achieve optimal physical, mental, and social health and well-being. Full members of the AAP are called "Fellows" and require certification by the ABP. Fellow of the AAP is designated as FAAP and may be seen after a pediatrician's name, that is, John Smith, MD, FAAP.

The role of the general pediatrician is to provide comprehensive care of infants, children, and adolescents, which includes the diagnosis and management of acute and chronic illness, as well as preventive health care. Acute illnesses that are commonly seen in the pediatrician's office are infections, such as ear infections, strep throat, and pneumonia, sports or musculoskeletal injuries, such as fractures and sprains, and exacerbations of chronic illness. Some of the chronic illnesses seen in pediatrics are asthma, diabetes, constipation, seizure disorder, and Attention-Deficit/Hyperactivity Disorder (ADHD). Preventive health care or well-child care is a general health maintenance visit in which acute and chronic illness may be discussed but the focus of the visit is the overall well-being of the patient. During the well-child care visit, the pediatrician obtains a history by interviewing a parent and the child, conducts a physical exam of the child, administers vaccinations, and orders screening laboratory tests (such as blood counts and lead levels) when appropriate. Disease and injury prevention is often discussed with patients and their families. With improved disease prevention through the use of multiple vaccinations, the pediatrician has more time to use the health maintenance visit to discuss growth, development, and psychosocial concerns. The pediatrician recognizes that the home and family environment are crucial to the patient's well-being and may contribute to some of the somatic complaints that a patient may have, for example, abdominal pain in a 6-year-old child may be a result of marital discord between the parents. The health maintenance visit is a time to address any concerns about behavior or psychological concerns in the home or school environment. The pediatrician may

individually or in collaboration with a child or school psychologist begin the evaluation of these behavior concerns. Upon diagnosis of a psychological problem such as ADHD or depression, the pediatrician may offer therapeutic intervention (e.g., counseling or medications) and/or recommend a referral to a child psychologist or psychiatrist.

The general pediatrician serves as the coordinator of the health care for infants, children, and adolescents. Insurance companies often mandate the pediatrician, as the primary care provider, to serve as the "gatekeeper" for access to subspecialty services. The pediatrician is often the first to address medical, behavioral, and psychosocial concerns of the pediatric patient and then determines the need for subspecialty care. The pediatrician continues to provide follow-up care of ongoing medical needs in conjunction with subspecialists, while monitoring the child's growth and development and serving as a stable health care provider until young adulthood.

See also: Family Physician; Health Care Professionals (General)

Further Reading

American Academy of Pediatrics. (2002). AAP fact sheet. http://www.aap.org/visit/facts.htm

American Board of Pediatrics. (1996). What is pediatrics? http://www.abp.org/pedsinfo/peds.htm

Drotar, D. (1995). *Consulting with pediatricians: Psychological perspectives for research and practice.* New York: Plenum Press.

Sugar-Webb, J. (2000). *Opportunities in physician careers* (pp. 76–78). Chicago, IL: VGM Career Horizons.

TERRY STANCIN
SUSAN K. SANTOS

Peptic Ulcer Disease

DEFINITION/INCIDENCE/ETIOLOGY

Peptic ulcers are deep ulcers in the stomach or duodenum. Peptic ulcer disease is divided into two major categories: primary and secondary peptic ulcer disease. Most cases of primary peptic ulcer disease are caused by infection with the organism *Helicobacter pylori*, and in children, symptoms include episodic epigastric pain that may be associated with vomiting and/or nocturnal awakening. Secondary peptic ulcer disease is associated with medical stressors such as burns, severe head injury, major surgical procedures, medications such as aspirin and nonsteroidal antiinflammatory drugs, and diseases such as Crohn's disease. This entry will focus on primary peptic ulcer disease.

The organism that causes primary peptic ulcer disease, *H. pylori*, is most often acquired in childhood, and poverty, poor sanitation, and crowding are major risk factors for infection. The overall prevalence of *H. pylori* infection is 10 percent, but the prevalence in people living in poverty can be as high as 50 percent. Only 15 percent of those infected with *H. pylori* develop ulcers, and the reasons for this are unclear. Peptic ulcer disease is rare in children, who are more likely to display chronic, active gastritis. Prevalence rates range from 5 to 10 percent in adults.

ASSESSMENT/TREATMENT/PROGNOSIS

In children, endoscopy and urea breath tests are most commonly used for diagnosis. Treatment consists of eradicating the *H. pylori* infection via a 1-week treatment regimen of at least two antibiotics and an acid suppressive medication. Successful treatment of *H. pylori* results in complete healing of the ulcer and resolution of symptoms. Adherence to treatment is particularly important in eradicating *H. pylori*, given that antibiotic resistance can develop.

PSYCHOSOCIAL CORRELATES

Prior to the discovery of *H. pylori*, peptic ulcer disease was considered to be a classic psychosomatic illness that was caused by an interaction of a stressor with an unconscious personality conflict. As a result, a great deal of early research investigated personality factors associated with peptic ulcer disease. Much of this research was poorly designed, and no consistent results emerged. More recent research has focused on life stressors and emotional symptoms, primarily in adults. Results in the area of major life stressors have been mixed, but three studies found that chronic stressors were associated with the onset of peptic ulcer disease in adults. Research on anxiety and depressive symptoms in adults with peptic ulcer disease compared to healthy adults has been mixed, and no conclusions can be drawn. Very little well-designed research has examined psychosocial issues in children with peptic ulcer disease, and no studies published after the discovery of the etiological contribution of *H. pylori* were found.

See also: Gastrointestinal Disorders

Further Reading

Ernst, P. B., & Gold, B. D. (1999). *Helicobacter pylori* in childhood: New insights into the immunopathogenesis of gastric disease and implications for managing infection in children. *Journal of Pediatric Gastroenterology and Nutrition, 28*, 462–473.

Gold, B. D., Colletti, R. B., Abbott, M., Czinn, S. J., Elitsur, Y., Hassall, E., Macarthur, C., Snyder, J., & Sherman, P. M. (2000). *Helicobacter pylori* infection in children: Recommendations for diagnosis and treatment. *Journal of Pediatric Gastroenterology and Nutrition, 31*, 490–497.

Lewin, J., & Lewis, S. (1995). Organic and psychosocial risk factors for duodenal ulcer. *Journal of Psychosomatic Research, 39*, 531–548.

LAURA M. MACKNER
WALLACE V. CRANDALL

Perceptual Development

See: Sensory and Perceptual Development

Perinatal Development

DEFINITIONS

The perinatal period involves the birth and the period closely surrounding the time of the birth. Perinatal development is affected by biologic risks, meaning that the infant is subject to many conditions that may negatively affect central nervous system (CNS) functioning. The spectrum of CNS disorders following perinatal insults is determined by the brain's maturational stage at the time of the insult, as well as the nature and severity of the insult. As a result, the effects of a particular type of perinatal CNS event will differ in preterm and full-term infants. Preterm infants in particular are faced with many clinical factors such as chronic lung disease (need for oxygen at 36 weeks postconceptual age), recurrent apnea and bradycardia (reduction in breathing and heart rate), exposure to glutocorticoids, hyperbilirubinemia (excess bilirubin), and hypothyroxemia (reduced thyroid hormone)—all of which have negative consequences on brain development. Moreover, issues encountered in the newborn nursery such as high noise levels, bright lights, disruption of diurnal rhythms, and stressed maternal–infant interactions further exacerbate the potentially negative effects of biomedical factors.

Hypoxemia is a reduction of oxygen in the blood (brain hypoxia is a reduction of oxygen to brain tissue); *ischemia* is reduced blood flow to the brain, while *asphyxia* is a disturbed exchange of oxygen and carbon dioxide due to an interruption in respiration. Asphyxia is accompanied by multisystem organ dysfunction, and results in decreased blood pressure and loss of autoregulation in the brain. *Hypoxic–ischemic encephalopathy* (HIE) refers to a deprivation of oxygen to the brain, due to the combined effects of hypoxemia and ischemia. Asphyxia is the precipitating event for HIE and perinatal HIE is the major cause of neurodevelopmental problems in the neonatal period. Hypoxemia and ischemia are thought to trigger a "neurotoxic biochemical cascade" that produces permanent cell death over a period of hours to days. This cascade then causes synaptic dysfunction and overactivation of excitatory brain receptors (due to the release of glutamate).

STAGE OF DEVELOPMENT AND PROBLEMS

The major CNS developmental events that occur during the perinatal period (depending on gestational age) include establishment and differentiation of subplate neurons, proper alignment and layering of cortical neurons, development of dendrites and axons with resultant synapse formation, programmed cell death, pruning, and proliferation of glial cells. The developing brain of the newborn is vulnerable to injury secondary to HIE, intraventricular/periventricular white matter hemorrhage (IVH/PVH), disruption of brain organizational events, and specific vulnerabilities of certain brain areas to excitotoxic neurotransmitters (e.g., basal ganglia and glutamate) or hypoxia (e.g., hippocampus).

In full-term infants, HIE causes cell death in the cerebral cortex, diencephalon, brain stem basal ganglia, and cerebellum. Moderate and severe HIE in term infants is associated with microcephaly, mental retardation, epilepsy, and cerebral palsy. Mild HIE (Stage I) lasts <24 hr and the infant displays hyperalertness, uninhibited reflexes, irritability, and jitteriness. Cognitive sequelae are minimal. Moderate HIE (Stage II) is characterized by lethargy, stupor, hypotonia, depressed primitive reflexes, seizures, and decreased movements; this persists for approximately one week and 20–40 percent of these babies will have sequelae. Severe HIE (Stage III) involves coma, flaccid tone, seizures, increased intracranial pressure, and suppressed brain stem function. Virtually all survivors have significant cognitive and psychoeducational sequelae.

In the preterm infant, HIE causes cell death deeper within the brain, namely in the white matter behind and to the side of the lateral ventricles (*periventricular leukomalacia*; PVL). There is less effect on gray matter and

this insult is more often associated with spasticity and neurosensory and motor problems than with cognitive deficits per se. PV/IVH involves bleeding into the subependymal germinal matrix (site of cell proliferation) and this occurs in 35–45 percent of infants <32 weeks gestational age. IVH is graded (I–IV) based on the amount of blood in the ventricles and degree of distention, with grades III (bleeding in >50 percent of the ventricular area, with distension of the lateral ventricle) and IV (intracerebral involvement with death of periventricular white matter, typically large and asymmetric infarction) being considered severe. The risk of later disability increases directly in relation to the grade of IVH: 5–10 percent with Grade I, 15–20 percent with Grade II, 35–50 percent with Grade III, and >90 percent with Grade IV.

More recently, there is increased interest on the combination of prenatal maternal infections and perinatal hypoxia–ischemia as being a two-component model of brain damage in infants. Both hypoxia–ischemia and maternal bacterial and viral gestational infections produce inflammatory cytokines (polypeptides) which have particularly devastating effects on the preterm infant's brain because of an underdeveloped blood–brain barrier, high rate of migration and proliferation, and lack of developed, endogenous protective factors ("neurotrophins"). The inflammatory cytokines cause cell death (necrosis). Even in full-term infants, the combination of HIE and maternal infection can increase the likelihood of cerebral palsy 70-fold.

SUMMARY

Hence, in the perinatal and neonatal (newborn) period, there is a complex interplay of biomedical conditions, stressful environmental factors, and vulnerable brain regions. While major brain pathways in the infant are specified in the genome, the connections between brain and behavior are fashioned by the effects of disruption of CNS organization due to prematurity, actual CNS damage, recovery, and social experience. Social experience, which begins in the neonatal period, can affect the very structure of the brain, and subsequent experience (activity) selects out synapses that will persist, while lack of experience (inactivity) will produce regression and apoptosis (cell death). Intervention will need to incorporate both biomedical and environmental stress-reducing strategies during the perinatal period and postnatal hospitalization.

See also: Neonatal Assessment; Prematurity: Birth Weight and Gestational Age; Prematurity Outcomes; Prenatal Development

Further Reading

Aylward, G. P. (1997). *Infant and early childhood neuropsychology.* New York: Plenum.

Dammann, O., & Leviton, A. (1999). Brain damage in preterm newborns: Might enhancement of developmentally regulated endogenous protection open a door for prevention? *Pediatrics, 104,* 541–550.

Eisenberg, L. (1999). Experience, brain and behavior: The importance of a head start. *Pediatrics, 103,* 1031–1035.

Perlman, J. M. (2001). Neurobehavioral deficits in premature graduates of intensive care—Potential medical and neonatal environmental risk factors. *Pediatrics, 108,* 1339–1348.

GLEN P. AYLWARD

Pervasive Developmental Disorder—Not Otherwise Specified (PDDNOS)

DEFINITION

Pervasive Developmental Disorder—Not Otherwise Specified (PDDNOS) is the diagnostic category used for individuals who present with severe impairments in social relating and reciprocity, but who do not meet the diagnostic criteria for any of the other pervasive developmental disorders. In addition to social deficits, individuals with PDDNOS must demonstrate either impairments in communication development or restricted, repetitive interests and activities. Relative to autism, individuals with PDDNOS typically have a later age of onset, milder symptoms, and/or atypical symptoms.

PDDNOS is the most prevalent of the pervasive developmental disorders, occurring in approximately 36 per 10,000 births. The etiology is presumed to be neurobiological, though no definitive medical tests or biological markers have yet been identified. The diagnosis of PDDNOS is based primarily on behavioral observations and developmental history.

TREATMENT/OUTCOME

Educational and behavioral treatments are essential for promoting optimal functioning for persons with PDDNOS. In most cases, treatment approaches designed for children with autism are also appropriate for children with PDDNOS. Early intervention, individualized educational plans, home–school collaboration,

and access to collateral therapies as appropriate (e.g., speech–language therapy, occupational therapy) are necessary to optimize social, communicative, and cognitive functioning. Just as educational supports are needed for children, family supports such as informational resources, case coordination, and respite care can enhance the functioning and well-being of the family. Prognostic indicators for autism spectrum disorders are average cognitive functioning and the acquisition of functional language by age 5. To the extent that individuals with PDDNOS have milder symptomatology, they would be expected to have more positive outcomes, as a group, relative to those with the more pervasive or severe impairments seen in autism.

See also: Autistic Disorder; Pervasive Developmental Disorders

Further Reading

American Psychiatric Association. (2000). *Diagnostic and statistical manual of mental disorders* (4th ed., text revision). Washington, DC: Author.

Cohen, D., & Volkmar, F. R. (1997). *Handbook of autism and other pervasive developmental disorders* (2nd ed.). New York: Wiley.

Committee on Educational Interventions for Children with Autism. (2001). *Educating children with autism.* Washington, DC: National Academy Press.

WENDY L. STONE
SUSAN L. HEPBURN

Pervasive Developmental Disorders

DEFINITION

The term Pervasive Developmental Disorders (PDDs) refers to a superordinate category used in *DSM-IV* to refer to a class of neurodevelopmental disorders that emerge in childhood and involve significant impairments in the development of social reciprocity, communicative functioning, and/or a restricted range of interests and behaviors. According to current conceptualizations, five disorders are included within this diagnostic category: autistic disorder, Asperger's disorder, Rett's disorder, childhood disintegrative disorder, and pervasive developmental disorder—not otherwise specified (PDDNOS). These conditions are also referred to as

"Autism Spectrum Disorders," a term that recognizes the continuous nature, overlapping symptomatology, and variations in symptom severity among this class of disorders. Diagnostic distinctions between the PDDs are made on the basis of age of onset, course, and individual patterns of symptom expression (see Table 1).

ETIOLOGY

The PDDs are considered to be neurobiological disorders with organic etiology. Research has been directed toward identifying genetic, neuroanatomical, neurochemical, and environmental contributions to the pathogenesis of these disorders. With the exception of Rett's disorder, for which a specific gene has been identified, no single causal factor has been found to be uniquely or universally associated with any of the PDDs. Rather, these disorders are thought to be the common end result of a broad range of different pathologic events.

EPIDEMIOLOGY

Recent epidemiological studies suggest that the prevalence of PDDs is about 60 cases per 10,000 children. This prevalence rate represents a substantial increase over estimates from the recent past. The reason for this increase is unknown, and may reflect substantive changes in clinical practice (e.g., broader clinical criteria, increasing diagnostic expertise, improved assessment methods), and/or an actual rise in incidence. The largest proportion of individuals with PDD consists of those functioning at the milder end of the spectrum (i.e., Asperger's disorder and PDDNOS); these milder forms represent about 70 percent of the PDD population. In contrast, the more severe regressive

disorders (i.e., childhood disintegrative disorder and Rett's disorder) are much less prevalent, representing only about 2 percent of the PDD population.

SYMPTOM PRESENTATION

The manifestation of the three behavioral features of PDD (i.e., social deficits, communication deficits, and restricted/repetitive activities) differs according to the specific disorder. In addition, each symptom cluster can vary in severity and nature as a function of an individual's developmental level and overall impairment (see Table 2). Social impairments are considered to be a core feature of PDDs and may include significant impairments in social responsivity (e.g., aloofness, isolation), social initiation (e.g., awkward or inappropriate overtures), and/or social reciprocity (e.g., difficulty understanding the thoughts or feelings of others). Communication impairments can range from a failure to acquire functional spoken language to demonstration of unusual language features, such as pedantic language or echolalia (i.e., repeating phrases heard elsewhere). Restricted and repetitive activities can include stereotyped sensorimotor behaviors (e.g., hand-flapping, spinning), restricted play patterns, development of circumscribed interests, and/or a rigid adherence to routines and/or rules. Cognitive functioning in individuals with PDDs can range from above average levels of intelligence to severe levels of mental retardation.

ASSESSMENT/TREATMENT

With the exception of Rett's disorder, PDDs are behaviorally defined diagnoses for which there are no biological markers or medical tests. Because the pattern

Table 1. Comparison of Pervasive Developmental Disorders

Disorder	Relative impairment	Relative prevalence	Behavioral regression?	Onset before 3 years?
Autistic disorder	Variable	Higher	Variable	Yes
Asperger's disorder	Milder	Intermediate	No	Variable
Rett's disorder	More severe	Lower	Yes	Yes
Childhood disintegrative disorder	More severe	Lower	Yes	No
Pervasive developmental disorder—not otherwise specified	Milder	Higher	No	Variable

Table 2. Examples of Variability in Symptom Expression of PDDs

Symptom	Mild impairment	Severe impairment
Social relating and reciprocity	Shows social interest and initiative; seeks interactions; has difficulty understanding the perspective and feelings of others	Shows limited awareness of or interest in others; appears aloof and unresponsive to the initiations of others
Language and communication impairment	Has conversational language; engages in one-sided conversations that focus on topics of particular interest; fails to monitor the interest of others in conversational topics	Does not develop functional language; may learn to communicate basic needs using augmentative communication system
Restricted and repetitive activities	Has circumscribed areas of interest that are pursued intently; shows some behavioral rigidity and/or resistance to unexpected changes in schedules or routines	Engages in stereotyped sensory and/or motor behaviors; uses toys and other objects in a repetitive and nonfunctional manner

of behavioral features spans many areas of development, diagnoses are usually made by multidisciplinary teams using information gathered through behavioral observations and parental report. There is no known cure for PDDs; treatment is directed toward improving social, communicative, and behavioral functioning across settings. The most effective treatments are behaviorally and educationally focused. Medication can be a useful adjunct to other therapies for amelioration of attentional and behavioral problems, or comorbid symptoms of anxiety or depression. Psychotherapy with a cognitive–behavioral focus can be helpful for some individuals with PDDs. Provision of support to families is also critical. Long-term outcomes for individuals with PDDs are variable, and are generally dependent on the level of cognitive, language, and social impairments.

See also: Asperger's Disorder; Autistic Disorder; Childhood Disintegrative Disorder; Pervasive Developmental Disorder—Not Otherwise Specified; Rett's Syndrome

Further Reading

American Psychiatric Association. (2000). *Diagnostic and statistical manual of mental disorders* (4th ed., text revision). Washington, DC: Author.

Cohen, D., & Volkmar, F. R. (1997). *Handbook of autism and other pervasive developmental disorders* (2nd ed.). New York: Wiley.

Committee on Educational Interventions for Children with Autism. (2001). *Educating children with autism.* Washington, DC: National Academy Press.

WENDY L. STONE
SUSAN L. HEPBURN

Pharmacological Interventions

ISSUES IN PEDIATRIC PHARMACOLOGY

Significant advances in pediatric psychopharmacology have paralleled monumental developments in the neural sciences, coupled with our understanding of both the structural and functional differences of the central nervous systems (CNS) in children identified with learning disorders and emotional difficulties. Despite these recent advances, many have observed that clinical use of psychotropic drugs in children far outweighs our knowledge with regard to their safety and efficacy. Unfortunately, there is no database available to provide specific statistics regarding the number of children and adolescents receiving psychotropic medications for specific disorders. However, there have been some surveys with specific psychotropic agents (e.g., stimulants) to suggest an increase in the use of these medications. Specific psychiatric disorders for which psychotropic agents have been used most widely include Attention-Deficit/Hyperactivity Disorder (ADHD), mental retardation, autism spectrum disorders, mood disorders, enuresis, and Tourette's syndrome.

A rationale for distinguishing between adult and pediatric psychopharmacology includes those factors that separate medical and psychological practice between the two populations. These include physiological factors (e.g., differences in body weight, absorption of medication, and medication interactions) and psychological factors (children, adolescents, and adults typically have different means to describe both positive and adverse effects of medication). In addition, children almost always rely on caregivers for medication administration and for reporting beneficial as well as adverse effects. Further, psychotropic medication is only one treatment modality of many that children may be receiving (e.g., special education, family psychotherapy).

For pediatric populations, assessment of psychotropic drug effects is monitored in the areas of learning, psychosocial functioning, as well as physical functioning. For this reason, it is essential that assessment be conducted across informants (e.g., caregivers, teachers, and clinicians) and from a variety of sources (e.g., home and school). Assessment domains typically include physical effects, structured interviews, behavioral rating scales, direct observations of behavior, and in some cases specific laboratory measures of psychological performance (e.g., attention and concentration). Although the search for an ideal assessment battery that may predict response to psychotropic medication continues, to date no instrument has been developed to predict response to any class of psychotropic agent. The reader is referred to Brown and Sammons (2002) for a review of this important topic.

DISORDERS FOR WHICH PSYCHOTROPICS ARE EFFECTIVE

Although specific data pertaining to the prevalence of children being treated with psychotropic agents is not available, those disorders that have accounted for the majority of psychotropic use include: ADHD, autism spectrum disorders, mental retardation, developmental disabilities, seizure disorders, mood disorders, enuresis, and Tourette's syndrome.

Attention-Deficit/Hyperactivity Disorder (ADHD)

ADHD, the most common behavioral disorder encountered by pediatricians, has been generally responsive to stimulant medication. In recent years, there has been concern regarding possible "overuse" and increase in the use of stimulants. Increases have been attributed to children being managed on stimulants for long periods of time, enhanced identification of children diagnosed with ADHD-inattentive type, a higher frequency of females receiving treatment, and more children receiving medication during the summer months. Notwithstanding their

increasing incidence, the stimulants have been the most meticulously documented treatment in child psychiatry.

Autism Spectrum Disorders

While little is known regarding the etiology and cure of the autism spectrum disorders, some psychotropic medications have been successfully employed to improve target behavioral symptoms, including overactivity, aggression, obsessions, and stereotypical behaviors. In fact, in a recent survey, it has been suggested that nearly one-third of a state's population of children with autism were receiving psychotropic agents, the most common of which are antipsychotics and stimulants. The selective serotonin reuptake inhibitors (SSRIs) have been prescribed for the management of symptoms related to obsessions and ritualistic behaviors in this population.

Tourette Syndrome

Characterized by involuntary, repetitive, and stereotyped motor or vocal productions, Tourette's, syndrome is a comorbid condition associated with a number of developmental and psychiatric disorders (e.g., learning disabilities, obsessive compulsive disorder [OCD], ADHD). Although antipsychotic agents such as haloperidol were the mainstay of management at one time, due to concerns associated with adverse effects, agents with a more favorable side-effect profile ("atypical" antipsychotics such as risperidone, olanzapine, or ziprasodone) have been the medications of choice. Although their efficacy and safety are promising, additional controlled trials are clearly needed.

Enuresis

Although behavioral methods are the treatment of choice for children with enuresis, there has been some interest in the use of pharmacotherapy with this disorder. Pharmacotherapies available for the management of enuresis include the antidiuretic hormone desmopressin (DDAVP) and the tricyclic antidepressants, although high relapse rates have been reported for both drugs. Cardiac toxicity has been well-documented as an adverse effect of tricyclic antidepressants.

Affective and Mood Disorders

Relative to the aforementioned disorders, there are few clinical trials addressing the management of affective and mood disorders with psychotropic agents. It is our impression that the use of both antidepressant and anxiolytic agents far exceeds the data that are available pertaining to efficacy and safety for pediatric populations. However, some recent preliminary studies attest to the efficacy and safety of the SSRIs in the management of mood disorders in children and adolescents.

Mental Retardation

Use of psychotropic agents in individuals with developmental disabilities and mental retardation continues at high levels, including the antipsychotic and stimulant agents. The concern among professionals has been the limited ability of these individuals to report adverse effects that frequently may be deleterious.

CLASSES OF PSYCHOTROPIC AGENTS

Most have found it useful to categorize psychotropic agents according to a classification system. These classes include the stimulants, antidepressants, antipsychotics, anxiolytics, and finally the mood stabilizers and anticonvulsants. They are reviewed in this order.

Stimulants

Stimulants are the first line of pharmacological treatment for ADHD. Stimulants do not affect the natural course of the condition, but assist in managing target symptoms of the disorder. There are many types of stimulants available to practitioners and include dextroamphetamine (i.e., Adderall and Dexedrine), methylphenidate (Ritalin, Concerta, Medadate CD, and Focalin), and magnesium pemoline (Cylert). These drugs are believed to exert their effect by increasing the reuptake of norepinephrine or dopamine at the synapse. Because of the severe side effect of liver toxicity, magnesium pemoline is no longer recommended for management of the disorder.

Methylphenidate and dextroamphetamine compounds come in both short- and long-acting preparations. The short-acting forms of methylphenidate are Ritalin and Focalin, and the short-acting forms of dextroamphetamine are Dexedrine and Adderall. One advantage of the long-acting preparations is that less-frequent doses may be administered, and these agents (e.g., Concerta, Metadate CD, Adderall XR) are gaining increasing popularity with the ease of once-daily dosing. Most commonly reported adverse effects of the stimulants include appetite suppression, abdominal pains, insomnia, headaches, irritability, rebound phenomena, and tics.

Antidepressants

Antidepressant medications traditionally are used to treat symptoms of depression in children and adolescents. In addition they have been shown to improve symptoms of ADHD, OCD and enuresis. The first line of management for depression is the SSRIs. These exert their effects by selective blockade of serotonin reuptake. The SSRIs currently available are fluoxetine (Prozac), Sertraline (Zoloft), Paroxetine (Paxil), Fluvoxamine (Luvox), and Citalopram (Celexa). Sertaline is the only SSRI that has received Food and Drug Administration (FDA) approval for use in pediatric populations. Fluvoxamine is also approved in adults and children for the management of OCD. Common adverse side effects for the SSRIs include nausea, restlessness, weight gain, and dry mouth, although generally reported to be mild and transient. Less common adverse effects include dermatitis, sexual dysfunction, and blurred vision. Serotonin syndrome caused by excess serotonin in the CNS (i.e., symptoms that include hyperthermia, CNS irritability, coma, seizures, and death) can be a complication of treatment with SSRIs and research regarding efficacy and safety with the SSRIs is still in its infancy.

Buproprion (Wellbutrin) is an atypical antidepressant that has also shown some efficacy in the treatment of ADHD, having its main effects on norepinephrine and dopamine reuptake. It is also approved for use in smoking cessation (Zyban). Buproprion may be a viable alternative particularly when children have been refractory to stimulant medication, when there is a remarkable family history for tics where stimulants might be contraindicated, or when a family member is at risk for abusing or selling stimulant medication. Side effects include insomnia, agitation, confusion, irritability, and possible hypertension. Use of buproprion is contraindicated in patients with a history of a seizure disorder or an eating disorder.

Tricyclic antidepressants have not been shown to be effective in the management of depression or enuresis when compared to placebo in pediatric populations. In addition, their side-effect profile can be severe, with the possibility of cardiac complications including sudden death. As a result, these medications are not recommended for the management of depression in children and adolescents.

Antipsychotics

Historically, Haloperidol (Haldol) has been the treatment of choice for childhood psychosis, with its efficacy well-established, although the incidence of extrapyramidal side effects is high. As a result, the atypical antipsychotics including olanzapine (Zyprexa), risperidol (Risperidone), ziprasidone (Geodon), quetiapine (Seroquel), and clozapine (Clozaril) are more frequently prescribed due to their more favorable side effect profile. Adverse events include sedation, weight gain, elevated prolactin levels, and anticholinergic effects (e.g., dry eyes, mouth, throat, constipation). Clozapine is associated with severe, possibly fatal side effects (e.g., agranulocytosis and cardiotoxicity) and should only be used as an agent of last resort.

Anxiolytics

The majority of empirical data support the use of behavioral therapy for the treatment of childhood anxiety disorders; there are few studies examining the efficacy of anxiolytic agents in children. Buspirone (Buspar) has been shown to be efficacious for the treatment of generalized anxiety disorder in children. Its side effect profile is mild, although potential drug–drug interactions may occur. Although there is no evidence that Buspirone may lead to tardive dyskinesia, occasional extrapyramidal side effects have been reported. Clomipramine (Anafranil) has been shown to be effective in the management of OCD, however its side-effect profile may be severe, as it is structurally similar to the tricyclics. Clonazepam (Klonipin) also has been found to be effective for anxiety as well as panic attacks, however, as with any benzodiazepine, the risk of long-term dependence is possible and for this reason, these agents are recommended only when other treatments have failed.

Anticonvulsants and Mood Stabilizers

Lithium carbonate may be effective in the management of bipolar disorder in adolescents. To date no studies have been identified that evaluate the use of lithium in younger children.

Anticonvulsant agents such as phenobarbitol, phenytoin (Dilantin), carbamazepine (Tegretol), and valproate (Depakote, Depakene) in addition to managing seizure disorders can also be effective in treating behavioral disorders such as manic episodes and aggressive behaviors. The newer anticonvulsants, including gabapentin (Neurontin), tiagabine (Gabitril), and lamotrigine (Lamictal) require further investigations prior to endorsing their use for cyclical mood disorders in pediatric populations.

Alpha-Adrenergic Agents

Clonidine (Catapress), an alpha-adrenergic agent used in the treatment of hypertension, has also been found to be effective in the treatment of ADHD, specifically overactivity and impulsivity. Guanfacine (Tenex) is a longer acting agent than clonidine and is associated with fewer adverse effects. Adverse events of alpha-adrenergic agents include hypotension and sedation.

ATTITUDES, CONSUMER SATISFACTION, AND LEGAL ISSUES

Relative to behavioral therapies or other forms of psychotherapy, psychotropic medication may be rated less favorably as a treatment option by caregivers and teachers. Research typically has indicated that caregivers are more accepting of psychotropic medication when it is combined with a psychological therapy and when its efficacy is assessed in a systematic clinical trial. Children's and adolescent's attitudes regarding psychotropic medication are also important and have been found to predict adherence to treatment. Notwithstanding the aforementioned issues, the well-informed practitioner must also consider critical issues including informed consent, children's and adolescent's right to refuse treatment, issues of custody, confidentiality, and the best interest of the child or adolescent.

See also: Anxiety Disorders; Attention-Deficit/Hyperactivity Disorder; Depressive Disorder, Major; Mental Retardation; Tic Disorder

Further Reading

Brown, R. T., & Sammons, M. T. (2002). Pediatric psychopharmacology: A review of new developments and recent research. *Professional Psychology Research and Practice, 33*, 135–147.

Brown, R. T., & Sawyer, M. G. (1998). *Medication in school-age children: Effects on learning and behavior.* New York: Guilford.

Kutcher, R. (1997). *Child and adolescent psychopharmacology.* Philadelphia: W. B. Saunders.

Phelps, L., Brown, R. T., & Power, T. (2002). *Pediatric psychopharmacology: A collaborative approach.* Washington, DC: American Psychological Association.

Safer, D. J., Zito, J. M., & Fine, E. M. (1999). Increased methylphenidate usage for attention deficit disorder in the 1990s. *Pediatrics, 98*, 1084–1088.

Werry, J., & Aman, M. (1998). *Practitioner's guide to psychoactive drugs for children and adolescents* (2nd ed.). New York: Kluwer Academic/Plenum.

RONALD T. BROWN
ANGELA LAROSA

Phenotype

See: Behavioral Genetics

Phenylketonuria

DEFINITION

Phenylketonuria (PKU) is an autosomal recessive disorder that results in an inborn error of metabolism in which several mutations in the phenylalanine hydroxylase (PAH) gene lead to an elevation in blood phenylalanine (Phe), a liver enzyme. The elevation in Phe happens within 48 hr after birth. If not treated within 2 weeks with a low Phe diet to bring the Phe levels down, the infant is likely to have microcephaly, severe mental retardation, delayed speech, seizures, eczema, behavior problems, negative mood, and motor disturbance. Since the PKU diet is so successful in prevention, all states do newborn screening. Women with PKU must also maintain the diet throughout pregnancy, or their fetus will be at high risk for neurotoxicity due to PKU. A person with complete lack of enzyme activity will have classic PKU with high Phe levels (>20 mg/dl). A partial deficiency of PAH results in a less severe form called non-PKU hyperphenylalaninemia in which the neurotoxic symptoms are reduced.

INCIDENCE AND PREVALENCE

Even though newborn screening has been conducted for over 40 years in the United States, we still only have estimates of incidence and prevalence of PKU. States vary in their definitions and in their reporting of demographic data, but the range for classic PKU is from 1 per 13,500 to 1 per 19,000 of newborns. For non-PKU hyperphenylalaninemia, it is 1 per 48,000. Incidence is higher in Whites and Native Americans than in African Americans, Hispanics, and Asians. These two forms of PKU account for the vast majority of cases.

ETIOLOGY

There may be over 400 mutations at the PAH gene locus, so many genotypic combinations can lead to a heterogeneous expression of a given clinical behavioral phenotype. Different behavioral expression among siblings who share the same genotype may be due to other genetic and environmental factors affecting their expression. In fact, a small number of people with PKU have no mental retardation, even without dietary treatment. The neuropathological mechanism is only partially understood.

Phe is a toxin which inhibits transport of large amino acids (LNAA) into the brain. This causes inhibition of protein and neurotransmitter synthesis and leads to lower levels of dopamine and serotonin, two essential brain neurotransmitters linked to learning and emotional regulation. There are two hypotheses as to the cognitive deficit produced by PKU: (1) high Phe competes with tyrosine at the blood–brain barrier, preventing the metabolism of dopamine; (2) high Phe inhibits the oligodendrocytes, the glial cells in the central nervous system that assemble and maintain myelin, which sheaths the neuron and affects its conductivity. Myelin is essential for neuronal function. Loss of myelin leads to decreased dopamine levels and to cognitive deficits in PKU. Both of these hypotheses have merit and their relative importance is being researched with animal models of PKU, which may lead to gene therapy as a treatment.

ASSESSMENT

Since the early 1960s assessment strategies in the United States have concentrated on newborn screening. Neonatal blood samples using a few drops of blood on special filter paper during the first days of life are evaluated for the presence of high Phe levels. Infants with high levels are referred for further evaluation, treatment, and care. Effective screening is complex, involving specimen collection, transport, tracking laboratory analysis, data collection and analysis, locating and tracking families with diagnosis, treatment, long-term follow-up. Older laboratory tests, while extremely useful for mass screening, also resulted in many false positives. Newer methods, especially tandem mass spectroscopy, are much more precise. Occasionally, the complex screening procedures fail and an infant is missed. Parents can also refuse the screening test in all but four states.

TREATMENT

Treatment involves long-term management of the diet and family compliance with psychological and medical treatment, nursing, social services, nutrition therapy, genetic counseling, and family counseling. Medical foods and modified protein foods are expensive (up to $300,000 over one's lifetime), but they are necessary to maintain a low Phe level. There is no consensus as to optimal levels. In the United States and British Commonwealth, infants and young children are maintained between 2 and 6 mg/dl. Levels may be less restricted between 10 and 15 years (up to 15 mg/dl) and after 15 years (up to 20 mg/dl). In some other countries, higher Phe levels than 20 mg/dl may be tolerated for adults. Monitoring is done once weekly for the first year, twice monthly from 1 to 12 years, monthly after 12 years of age, and twice weekly during pregnancy of a woman with PKU, beginning 3 months before pregnancy. Before the 1990s, it was considered acceptable to stop the diet after 6 years of age; however, recent studies agree that children regress when Phe levels increase and they improve when the diet is reinstated. Metabolic control can be difficult to achieve and maintain because the diet is distasteful and very restrictive. If it is liberalized, however, a significant decline in mental and behavioral performance can result. Even for those who have been missed at birth and are put on the diet later, while their cognitive performance may not improve measurably, their social, emotional, and nondestructive behaviors do improve.

Research on other treatments for PKU focus on gene therapy and drugs that might control Phe levels. While not available at present, these strategies show promise for future treatment.

PROGNOSIS

If PKU is detected at birth and dietary treatment is begun within 7 or 8 days, the child is likely to grow up without a disability. Cognition and performance are highly correlated with Phe levels, so compliance with the diet is always an issue. If the diet is begun later than two weeks after birth, serious impairments are likely to occur and may not be reversible. Even in children detected early and kept on the PKU diet, recent neuropsychological research has shown that they may have subtle deficits related to prefrontal lobe function resulting in learning disabilities.

See also: Behavioral Genetics, Genetic Counseling; Mental Retardation; Microcephaly; Speech and Language Assessment, Epilepsy

Further Reading

American Academy of Pediatrics. (2001). National Institutes of Health Consensus Development Conference Statement: Phenylketonuria: Screening and management, October 16–18, 2000. *Pediatrics*, *108*, 972–982.
Diamond, A., Prevor, M. B., Callender, G., & Druin, D. P. (1997). Prefrontal cortex cognitive deficits in children treated early and continuously for PKU. *Monographs of the Society for Research in Child Development, 62*(4), 1–207.
Koch, R., & De La Cruz, F. (Eds.). (1999). Phenylketonuria. *Mental Retardation and Developmental Disabilities Research Reviews, 5*(2), 101–161.

STEPHEN R. SCHROEDER

Phobia

See: Specific Phobia

Phonological and Articulation Disorders

DEFINITION AND CLINICAL SYMPTOMS

Phonological abilities include phonological production (i.e., articulation)—defined by the way that speech sounds, or phonemes, are produced—as well as cognitively based phonological abilities (e.g., ability to correctly categorize speech sounds, or determine which sounds relate to a difference in meaning) (American Psychiatric Association, 2000). Intelligibly, or clarity of speech, may be affected by either type of phonological problem. According to *Diagnostic Statistical Manual of Mental Disorders (4th ed., Text Revision) (DSM-IV-TR)*, the essential feature of a phonological disorder is the inability to use developmentally expected speech sounds that are appropriate for the person's age and dialect.

The *DSM-IV-TR* (2000) lists three criteria that must be met for diagnosis of a phonological disorder. First, the individual must demonstrate delayed acquisition or inability to produce age-appropriate speech sounds. These problems could include such things as omission of necessary speech sounds in words, substitution of the correct speech sound for an incorrect one, distortion of the speech sound, or errors in correct sequencing of speech sounds in words or a series of words. Second, the problems in speech sound production must be severe enough to have a functional impact on the individual's academic, occupational, and/or social functioning. In this regard, one would expect that intelligibility would be affected to the degree that there were difficulties with understanding the individual's speech. Third, in individuals with mental retardation, sensory deficits, motor-speech disorders, or environmental deprivation, the problems in speech sound production would need to be in excess of those usually associated with these problems.

CAUSES OF PHONOLOGICAL DISORDERS

Articulation or phonological disorders can be either functional or organic. When the cause of the articulation disorder is not known, it is assumed to be functional in nature. In these cases, it is possible to find a family history of other close relatives who had speech delays early in development, but often there may be no specific medical or developmental cause identified for these problems. In other cases, there may be an organic, or physical, cause of a phonological disorder that can be identified. For instance, sensory deficits such as hearing loss, or structural problems with the "articulators" (i.e., tongue, lips, palate, etc.) can cause problems with speech sound production. (Roth and Worthington, 1996). Another possible cause of articulation problems is cognitive impairment (such as mental retardation).

INCIDENCE

One in ten children entering the first grade have speech disorders that are significant enough to require intervention (Retrieved April 4, 2002, from http://professional.asha.org/resources/factsheets/speech_voice_language.cfm). Articulation or phonological problems typically are evident during the preschool years when children fail to meet developmental expectations for producing certain sounds. School-age children represent the majority of the targeted population of therapeutic intervention. It is estimated that 16 out of every 1,000 children have a chronic speech disorder (Retrieved April 4, 2002, from http://professional.asha.org/resources/factsheets/speech_voice_language.cfm).

Girls often acquire and master phonemes earlier that boys, but mastery of all phonemes by age 7 is considered to be developmentally appropriate for both genders.

TYPICAL ACQUISITION OF SOUNDS

An infant begins communicating with others initially through the production of vowels. Pitch variations add dimension and also provide information about the urgency and nature of the communicative intent. For example, a vowel produced with increased intensity and pitch may indicate a more pressing need than a softly produced vowel during playtime. Consonants are produced later in varying orders.

Although many different reference charts can be used, all phonemes should be in place and produced correctly in the child's native language by the age of 7 years. Bilabials, or sounds made with the compression of the lips, such as /p/, /b/, and /m/ are among the first to be produced and mastered. Liquids, or sounds made during fluid movements of the tongue, such as the /r/ are mastered last.

EVALUATION

A speech–language pathologist will use several evaluation measures and procedures to assess the nature of the articulation disorder.

A thorough oral motor exam is essential. An oral motor exam consists of gauging the child's ability to move the articulators (tongue, lips, cheeks, jaw, etc.) on command. It is important to rule out concerns regarding oral dyspraxia (oral apraxia). Dyspraxia involves the inability or difficulty moving the articulators on command. A thorough examination of the oral cavity, or mouth and other structures, is also essential. It must be established that the child's anatomical structures are within normal limits. Concerns that negatively impact articulation include: microcheilia (abnormally small lips), poor velopharyngeal closure (inadequate movement and closure of the soft palate during speech), microglossia (abnormally small tongue), misalignment of teeth, as well as other features (Nicolosi, Harryman, & Kresheck, 1996). A collaborative relationship should be established with other professionals such as physicians (e.g., plastic surgeon, pediatrician, radiologist), psychologists, dental specialists (orthodontics and prosthetic physicians) as well as social workers, nutritionists, and others to determine if intervention in the form of surgery, dentistry, or other means would benefit the child to improve articulation (Shprintzen & Bardach, 1995).

A full audiological evaluation should also be performed. If a child cannot hear speech sounds accurately, then production of these sounds is compromised.

The speech–language pathologist would include several aspects of the comprehensive exam prior to diagnosis. The exam will include a speech sample of both single word productions and conversational, or connected speech. It is also important to conduct formal testing that targets which sounds the child has mastered, which sounds are still developing (emerging skills), or which sounds are produced incorrectly. Following this evaluation, an analysis of errors can be conducted to decipher if the articulation model or phonological model would best suit the client.

Other considerations to include involve factors such as: is the phoneme in error one that is produced frequently? (e.g., such as the one in the child's name), can the child produce the sound with instructions regarding placement of the tongue, lips, and cheeks? (stimulatibility), or is the mispronunciation of the target sound a concern for the child? (e.g., is the child discouraged from communicating because of fear of ridicule).

Informal tools such as parental reports, medical history, and informal observations also provide valuable information that helps clinicians gain a clear picture of deficits.

IMPACT OF PHONOLOGICAL AND ARTICULATION DISORDERS

Individuals with phonological and articulation disorders may be affected in various aspects of their lives, depending upon their age and the severity of the problem. At almost any age, there are potential social and self-esteem issues associated with poor intelligibility of speech. Depending upon the severity of the phonological problems, an individual's expressive language functioning could also be affected. For instance, if a child has difficulty producing multisyllabic words, he/she may substitute easier or shorter words instead. This may appear to indicate a delay or deficiency in the child's vocabulary knowledge, whereas the problem actually lies in the ability to correctly produce speech sounds and connect them together to produce the longer words. Finally, severe phonological problems can also interfere with acquisition of early reading, spelling, and writing abilities in young children. As these children attempt to learn phonetic sounds associated with the symbols of our language (i.e., letters), their speech sound distortions, substitutions, or omissions can interfere with this type of learning. This speaks to the need to identify phonological disorders early—during the preschool years, if possible—in order to provide early intervention prior to entering school and being confronted with symbol-associative learning tasks.

APPROACHES TO INCREASING INTELLIGIBILITY

The two main approaches for improving intelligibility are the articulation therapy model and the phonological approach.

Articulation therapy focuses on single phoneme (sound) production and remediation. Single sounds are targeted and remediated. Articulation therapy is considered to be the most traditional approach to intervention.

Another approach to improving clarity of speech is the phonological approach. The phonological approach to therapy focuses on remediation of a pattern of speech errors. This approach was introduced in the 1970s and 1980s (Stoel-Gammon, Sotne-Goldman, & Glaspey, 2002) and continues to be beneficial in improving speech intelligibility. When speech errors are analyzed, a pattern can be established and used as a way to attack more than one sound at a time. When considering which approach to therapy should be used, it is important to conduct a full speech battery, as described in a previous section.

See also: Central Auditory Processing Disorders; Hearing Impairment; Mixed Receptive–Expressive Language Disorder; Selective Mutism

Further Reading

American Psychiatric Association. (2000). *Diagnostic and statistical manual of mental disorders* (4th ed., text revision). Washington, DC: Author. http://professional.asha.org/resources/factsheets/speech_voice_language.cfm

Nicolosi, L., Harryman, E., & Kresheck, J. (1996). *Terminology of communication disorders* (4th ed.). Baltimore, MD: Williams & Wilkins.

Roth, F., & Worthington, C. (1996). *Treatment resource manual for speech–language pathology.* San Diego: Singular.

Shprintzen, R., & Bardach, J. (1995). *Cleft palate speech management.* St. Louis: Mosby.

Stackhouse, J., Wells, B., Pascoe, M., & Rees, M. (2002). *Seminars in Speech and Language, 23,* 27–39.

Stoel-Gammon, C., Stone-Goldman, J., & Glaspey, A. (2002). *Seminars in Speech and Language, 23,* 3–12.

SHALONDA WILLIAMS
JAN L. CULBERTSON

Physical Abuse

DEFINITION

Physical child abuse is typically defined as a non-accidental act by a parent or caregiver involving beatings or some other form of overt physical violence that results in injuries to a child that may include fractures, bruises, lacerations, burns, or internal injuries.

INCIDENCE

In 1999, a total of 826,000 children suffered from abuse or neglect, and just over 20 percent (21.3) of these children were physically abused. After neglect, physical abuse is the most common form of maltreatment with a rate of 2.5 per 1,000 children. National estimates of the rates of physical abuse indicate an increase of 42 percent between 1986 and 1993, with the incidence rate increasing from 4.3 to 5.7 children per 1,000. Approximately equal numbers of boys and girls are physically abused. In 1999, parents were identified as the perpetrators in approximately 85 percent of the cases, with 36 percent being the mother only and 27 percent being the father only. Physical abuse, either alone or in combination with neglect or other factors, accounted for more than half of the child abuse-related fatalities reported in 1999. Younger children and children with disabilities appear to be at a higher risk for physical abuse.

RISK FACTORS FOR PHYSICAL ABUSE

Some of the characteristics found to be associated with physical abuse are: parent's own history of child abuse, being young parents, beliefs about discipline, lack of knowledge about child development, negative attributions toward the child and the child's behavior, life stressors, and psychiatric problems (e.g., depression, substance abuse). Certain child characteristics may also be related. Younger children are seen to be more at risk for physical abuse, as are children with disabilities.

EFFECTS OF PHYSICAL ABUSE

Children who have been physically abused have been found to have more psychosocial problems than children in the general population. Problems include academic and behavioral difficulties in school, deficits in receptive and expressive language, conduct problems, aggression, hyperactivity, delinquency, poor problem-solving skills, decreased self-esteem, social withdrawal, poor peer interactions, lower social competence, depression, and anxiety. These children are also at risk for developing Posttraumatic Stress Disorder (PTSD).

In some cases, the child's problems are directly related to the physical abuse, such as permanent developmental and cognitive problems due to head trauma. In other instances, the physical abuse and the dynamics in the family—such as a poor parent–child relationship or other factors of the home environment—lead to the child's difficulties.

ASSESSMENT OF CHILDREN AND CAREGIVERS

There are two types of assessments in child abuse cases. First, the investigation of the alleged incident by Child Protective Services (CPS) or law enforcement takes place to determine if abuse occurred and, if so, the specific details of the abusive act, and to make recommendations regarding the safety of the child, for example, out-of-home placement. The second type of assessment involves a mental health professional examining the impact of the abuse on the child and determining if treatment is necessary.

No specific disorder or "syndrome" is associated with physical abuse. A child can experience a wide array of difficulties after being physically abused and, therefore, a broad mental health assessment covering multiple domains of functioning and using multiple informants is necessary. The goal of the assessment is to determine if the child needs treatment, and if so, to establish the goals of treatment.

Typically, an assessment will include gathering information from CPS about the abuse the child experienced, an interview with the child and caregiver(s), and obtaining collateral information from the school or day care provider. The assessment should address the child's understanding of the abusive behavior, a description of the home environment and family relationships, and the child's past and current emotional and behavioral difficulties. Strengths of the child and family should be assessed as well as weaknesses. The assessment may include psychological tests to assess cognitive, behavioral, and affective functioning.

Assessment of the caregiver(s) who physically abused the child focuses on specific areas including: parenting skills, knowledge of child development, the adult's history and childhood experience with discipline, anger/impulse control issues, parent–child relationship, behavior of the child, current discipline techniques, and current social supports and stressors for the family. Specific information about the caregivers' current level of depression, anxiety, or other mental health disorder, as well as current and past substance use and abuse should be evaluated.

Self-report and standardized instruments can be used in the assessment of caregivers. Specific areas to be evaluated include personality characteristics and disorders, psychopathology (e.g., depression, anxiety), parental stress, parental perceptions of child behavior problems, problem-solving abilities, and anger. Some assessment tools are specific to abuse and include an evaluation of violence in the family, opinions on child-rearing, and the level of risk of an adult committing a violent act against a child. For example, parents may be asked to complete the Child Abuse Potential Inventory, the Parent Opinion Questionnaire, and/or the Conflict Tactics Scale.

TREATMENT FOR CHILDREN

Historically, treatment of physical abuse has focused on the parent, not on the child. Therapy for physically abused children, however, can be utilized to reduce the negative impact of the abuse, teach the child coping skills, and help with adjustments to being removed from the family or other significant changes and losses that may occur. It is important to note that not all children who experience physical abuse have adverse psychological effects. If a child is not having difficulty adjusting, therapy is not warranted, and may actually be disruptive to the child. Thus, it is important to do a careful assessment prior to beginning treatment.

Few specific treatments for children who have been physically abused have been evaluated. However, the symptoms that often emerge as a consequence of physical abuse (e.g., depression, anxiety, impulse-control, etc.) can be treated by techniques that are supported by research. Treatment typically involves the use of cognitive–behavioral techniques which focus on learning and rehearsing coping skills, relaxation techniques, and self-talk. Social skills groups and peer social support can also be beneficial for the child who has been physically abused. If the child is experiencing PTSD, exposure-based therapy, where the child talks about the experience in a controlled setting using relaxation techniques when becoming distressed, may be necessary to reduce the impact of the trauma. On average, most abused children are seen for about 12 sessions. Longer-term treatment may be necessary when the physical abuse has been severe or the effects of the abuse continue to interfere with the child's functioning and development.

TREATMENT APPROACHES FOR CAREGIVERS

Treatment goals for caregivers typically include the termination of any current maltreatment and the prevention of future occurrences. Thus, the targets of treatment need to address the precursors to abuse, such as reducing family stressors, increasing knowledge of child development, developing realistic expectations of the child, learning nonphysical discipline techniques, and

having an adequate repertoire of appropriate parenting skills. Other goals include the parent(s) obtaining the necessary treatment and/or medication for any psychiatric disorders they may be diagnosed with, as well as addressing any issues related to substance abuse.

Typical approaches used with caregivers include psychoeducational groups and/or individual therapy focusing on child development, parenting skills, problem solving, anger and stress management, and increased support networks. Cognitive–behavioral techniques such as parent–child interaction therapy (PCIT) and in-home therapy, which tries to address parenting stressors and education as well as increasing the family's social support have been utilized. It appears that these approaches lead to the acquisition of skills, but not necessarily to improvements in family interactions. Very little, if any, research has been done to follow these families to see if they have a future report of child abuse.

PROGNOSIS

Some children who have experienced physical abuse experience few if any difficulties later in life. Other adults who have a history of physical abuse are more likely to have continued problems with aggressive and violent behavior, nonviolent criminal behavior, substance abuse, suicidal and self-injurious behavior, emotional problems (e.g., depression and anxiety), interpersonal problems, and academic and vocational difficulties. Thus, the impact of physical abuse can have long-lasting effects that extend beyond childhood into the adult years.

See also: Cognitive–Behavior Therapy for Children, Group Psychotherapy; Parent–Child Interaction Therapy; Parenting Practices; Parent Training; Risk and Protective Factors

Further Reading

Bonner, B. L., Logue, M. B., Kaufman, K. L., & Niec, L. N. (2001). Child maltreatment. In C. E. Walker & M. Roberts (Eds.), *Handbook of clinical child psychology* (3rd ed.). New York: Wiley.

Kolko, D. J. (2002). Child physical abuse. In J. E. B. Myers, L. Berliner, J. Briere, C. T. Hendrix, C. Jenny, & T. A. Reid (Eds.), *The APSAC handbook on child maltreatment* (2nd ed., pp. 21–54). Thousand Oaks, CA: Sage.

U.S. Department of Health and Human Services, Administration on Children, Youth and Families. (2001). *Child maltreatment 1999.* Washington, DC: U.S. Government Printing Office.

Warner-Rogers, J. E., Hansen, D. J., & Hecht, D. B. (1999). Child physical abuse and neglect. In V. Van Hasselt & M. Hersen (Eds.),

Handbook of psychological approaches with violent physical offenders: Contemporary strategies and issues (pp. 329–355). New York: Kluwer Academic/Plenum.

DEBRA B. HECHT
BARBARA L. BONNER

Physician Assistant

A physician assistant (PA) is a health care professional licensed to practice medicine under the supervision of a physician. Acceptance into most PA programs requires some college education (minimum of 2 years in science or health profession program) and previous health care experience. Many applicants are nurses, emergency medical technicians (EMTs), and paramedics. PA programs last approximately 2 years (25 months). The first year is spent on classroom and laboratory instruction in the basic medical and behavioral sciences. The second year consists of clinical rotations in internal medicine, pediatrics, family medicine, obstetrics and gynecology, emergency medicine, and surgery. Some PAs pursue postgraduate education (residencies or fellowships) in medical specialties such as emergency medicine, surgery, and neonatology.

After graduation, PAs take a certification exam to become certified by the National Commission on Certification of Physician Assistants (NCCPA). Maintenance of national certification is accomplished by completing 100 hr of continuing medical education every 2 years and taking a recertification exam every 6 years. PAs who successfully complete these requirements may use physician assistant–certified (PA–C) after their name. State licensure requires the PA to have graduated from an accredited program and to have passed the national certifying exam. Many PAs belong to the American Academy of Physician Assistants (AAPA), a national professional society.

The PA's clinical role includes primary and specialty care in medical and surgical specialties. Most PAs work in primary care settings such as pediatrics, internal medicine, family medicine, and obstetrics and gynecology. Specialty areas in which PAs may work include dermatology, radiology, psychiatry, infectious disease, and geriatrics. Some PAs work in surgical subspecialties where they assist in major surgical procedures. In the emergency department, the PA may perform suturing and wound care and help manage trauma and other life-threatening situations. The PA is responsible for obtaining medical histories, performing physical exams, developing and implementing patient management plans, ordering and interpreting laboratory tests and performing procedures under the direction of a physician. In the primary care setting, the PA is also involved in preventive health care, including counseling about injury and disease prevention and administration of vaccinations. Many states authorize the PA to write prescriptions. The PA may be involved with research and administrative activities. PAs work in a variety of practice settings and are considered an integral part of the health care team.

See also: Family Physician; Health Care Professionals (General)

Further Reading

American Academy of Physician Assistants. (2002). About PAs and AAPA. http://www.aapa.org/00aboutpas.html

Snock, I. D., & D'Orazio, L. (1998). *Opportunities in health and medical careers* (pp. 26–27). Chicago, IL: VGM Career Horizons.

Swanson, B. M. (2000). *Careers in health care* (pp. 205–210). Chicago, IL: VGM Career Horizons.

TERRY STANCIN
SUSAN K. SANTOS

Physician, Family

See: Family Physician

Physician (General, Specialty)

Physicians are medical doctors who prevent, diagnose, and treat diseases and conditions. A physician must obtain a doctor of medicine (MD) or doctor of osteopathy (DO) degree from an affiliated university or free-standing medical school before obtaining a license from the state in which he or she will be permitted to practice. DOs and MDs are considered to have comparable professional skills. Table 1 lists educational and credentialing steps involved in becoming a primary care physician or specialist. During medical school, a physician receives an education in the basic sciences and clinical medicine. The first 2 years are spent in classroom and laboratory instruction in the basic sciences (e.g., anatomy, physiology, and pharmacology) and the second 2 years are spent rotating through a variety of medical specialties (i.e., pediatrics, family practice, surgery, and obstetrics and gynecology).

After completing necessary coursework and clinical experience, a physician then pursues a residency in an

Table 1. Physician Education and Credentials

Educational or credentialing step	Credential conferred upon completion	Description or typical program
Undergraduate education	Baccalaureate degree (e.g., BA, BS, AB)	4 years of education at a college or university with some premedical course preparation.
Medical school	Doctor of Medicine (MD) or Doctor of Osteopathic Medicine (DO) degree	4 years at an accredited medical school or school of osteopathic medicine. Includes preclinical courses (e.g., human anatomy, pharmacology) and clinical rotations (e.g., rotations in medicine, psychiatry, surgery, pediatrics).
Medical license	License # issued by each state	A physician must apply for and obtain a medical license in the state of his/her practice. License must be renewed periodically.
Residency		3–8 years (depending on specialty) at a medical facility residency program under the supervision of senior physicians and other health care faculty members. Residencies in pediatrics and family medicine are usually 3 years.
Board certification	Two levels: general medical specialties (e.g., pediatrics) and subspecialties (e.g., developmental–behavioral pediatrics)	Process of evaluating a physician's knowledge and experience in a specialty area and determining that s/he is qualified to provide patient care in the specialty. Board certification in pediatrics involves successful completion of written tests. Most certifications must be renewed every 6–10 years by written examinations.
Fellowship		1–3 years of additional training in a subspecialty (e.g., pediatric gastroenterology).
Continuing medical education (CME)	CME credits	To remain current in medical knowledge, physicians are required to receive credits for continuing education through seminars, courses, and reading. Often required for state license renewal.

area of medical practice such as pediatrics, family medicine, internal medicine, obstetrics and gynecology, surgery, ophthalmology, or psychiatry. Depending on the area of practice, residency training may last from 3 to 8 years. After residency, some physicians pursue further specialization within their area by completing a fellowship, which usually includes learning advanced clinical techniques as well as conducting research.

Primary care physicians focus on providing general medical treatment and refer patients to other specialists when additional skills are needed. In the United States, primary care specialties include *internal medicine* (general medical needs of adults), *pediatrics* (children and adolescents), and *family practice* (all members of a family). In Canada, family practice is the only primary care specialty, and pediatricians and internists are considered specialists. In the United Kingdom, primary care doctors are called *general practitioners*.

See also: Health Care Professionals (General)

Further Reading

American Medical Association. (2002, March 29). Becoming an MD. http://www.ama-assn.org/ama/pub/category/2320.html

Pace, B. (2000). Your doctor's education. *Journal of the American Medical Association, 284,* 1198.

Sugar-Webb, J. (2000). *Opportunities in physician careers* (pp. 76–78). Chicago, IL: VGM Career Horizons.

TERRY STANCIN
SUSAN K. SANTOS

Pica

DEFINITION

Pica is a condition in which inedible substances are ingested. This behavior is common in the first year of life and usually disappears spontaneously by 2 years of age. Common substances associated with pica include cigarettes, dirt, paint, chalk, and plaster. The level of danger associated with pica varies according to the specific item consumed. Ingestions can result in lead or nicotine toxicity, surgical interventions, or parasitic infestation.

PREVALENCE

Pica is most often diagnosed in individuals with mental retardation. Prevalence estimates in populations of persons with mental retardation range from 4 percent to 26 percent. Individuals with mental retardation living in institutions are more likely to display pica (9–25 percent) than those living in the community (0.3–14.4 percent). Individuals with more severe mental retardation are more likely to exhibit pica and do so across all age ranges.

ETIOLOGY AND TREATMENT

A specific etiology for pica has not been identified. The common explanations are nutritional, psychological, environmental, and pharmacologic. Pica may be a manifestation of obsessive–compulsive disorder, particularly in persons with mental retardation. Most individuals with mental retardation appear to engage in pica behaviors for nonsocial reasons (i.e., automatic reinforcement). However, pica behaviors may be maintained through social reinforcement. Given that there is no agreed upon etiology for pica, most clinicians view it as a learned behavior and a variety of behavioral treatments have been shown to be effective in reducing or eliminating pica. Discrimination training in which a collection of medically approved nonfood items are used to help establish the connection between inedible substances and punishment has been shown to be an effective strategy. Differential reinforcement of alternate behaviors, negative reinforcement, and habit reversal have also been used to effectively treat pica behaviors. A creative treatment using a pica box filled with both edible and nonharmful, inedible items was shown to successfully reduce pica behavior. In persons with intractable pica, preventive measures (e.g., environmental control, restraints) may be necessary.

Further Reading

Ali, Z. (2001). Pica in people with intellectual disability: A literature review of aetiology. *Journal of Intellectual and Developmental Disability, 26,* 205–215.

Kedesdy, J. H., & Budd, K. S. (1998). *Childhood feeding disorders: Biobehavioral assessment and intervention.* Baltimore: Paul H. Brookes.

Linscheid, T. R., and Rasnake, L. K. (2001). Eating problems in children. In E. Walker & M. Roberts (Eds.), *Handbook of child clinical psychology* (4th ed., pp. 523–541). New York: Guilford Press.

Matson, J. L., & Bamburg, J. W. (1999). A descriptive study of pica behavior in persons with mental retardation. *Journal of Developmental and Physical Disabilities, 11,* 353–361.

Pizza, C. C., Fisher, W. W., Hanley, G. P., LeBlanc, L. A., Worsdell, A. S., Lindauer, S. E., & Keeney, K. M. (1998). Treatment of pica through multiple analyses of its reinforcing functions. *Journal of Applied Behavior Analysis, 31,* 165–189.

Thomas R. Linscheid
L. Kaye Rasnake

Platelet Abnormalities—Thrombocytopenia

DEFINITION

Bleeding problems may occur because of platelet abnormalities (called thrombocytopenia), usually resulting from destruction of platelets as part of an immune response, or impaired production of platelets in the bone marrow. In both cases, the result of the platelet abnormality is some sign of bleeding, most commonly seen as some type of bruising or prolonged bleeding from trauma.

The most common type of destructive thrombocytopenia is idiopathic thrombocytopenic purpura (ITP), which occurs when the immune system is triggered to attack and destroy platelets. Many times, ITP follows a viral illness or immunization. Besides ITP, there are multiple immunologic and nonimmunologic causes for platelet destruction, including allergies, posttransfusion reactions, use of catheters, and heart disease.

INCIDENCE

Because there are so many factors, known and unknown, that cause thrombocytopenia in children, incidence figures are not clear. In children, there is no gender difference in occurrence, but in older adolescents and adults, females are three times more likely to have the disorder. In the majority of cases, thrombocytopenia resolves within a month of onset, but ITP generally persists for a longer period of time and may be either acute or chronic. The acute form of ITP usually occurs between 2 and 4 years of age; ITP diagnosed after age 10 is usually chronic.

DIAGNOSIS

Thrombocytopenia is diagnosed on the basis of clinical symptoms, a blood count indicating low platelet count, and a bone marrow aspiration to determine if platelets are being produced, and to rule out malignant disease such as leukemia.

CLINICAL SYMPTOMS

The clinical symptoms of thrombocytopenia include tiny red spots on the skin (patechiae) and bruising. In limited cases, bleeding from the nose, mouth, or gastrointestinal tract may occur.

TREATMENT

In many cases, thrombocytopenia will resolve without treatment, or with the discontinuation of use of any medication associated with its occurrence. In those cases where it does not resolve quickly, corticosteroids and intravenous immune globulin may be used. For more severe cases, surgical removal of the spleen, which is the primary site of platelet destruction, may be necessary. Removal of the spleen is successful in 70–80 percent of cases, but also results in an increased, lifelong risk for infection. Immunosuppressant medications used in the treatment of malignancies or following organ transplantation may be used in some very severe cases, but these are limited because of undesirable side effects.

Behavioral support for children may be helpful, as lifestyle changes are sometimes necessary to lessen the risk of accidental injury that might produce a bleeding event. Assistance with these modifications, and with the psychological aspects of more chronic disease management, is often helpful to children and their families.

PROGNOSIS

In most cases, thrombocytopenia can be successfully treated or managed (if chronic). The primary threat to life is bleeding in the brain, which fortunately is a rare occurrence.

See also: Bleeding Disorders; Bone Marrow Failure and Primary Immunodeficiency; Hereditary Coagulation Disorders; HIV; Leukemia; Orthopedic Disabilities; Pediatric Human Immunodeficiency Virus-1; Self-Management

Further Reading

Beardsley, D. S., & Nathan, D. G. (1998). Platelet abnormalities in infancy and childhood. In D. G. Nathan & S. H. Orkin (Eds.), *Nathan and Orkin's hematology of infancy and childhood* (5th ed., pp. 1585–1630). Philadelphia: W.B. Saunders.

Montgomery, R. R., & Scott, J. P. (2000). Hemorrhagic and thrombotic diseases. In R. E. Behrman, R. M. Kliegman, & H. B. Jenson (Eds.), *Nelson textbook of pediatrics* (16th ed., pp. 1504–1525). New York: W.B. Saunders.

F. DANIEL ARMSTRONG

Play Therapy

Play is used in therapy with children by many therapists today. Therapists use play because children naturally communicate through play, especially pretend play. Pretend play involves the use of fantasy, make-believe, and symbolism. Play has been utilized in therapy from a variety of theoretical traditions. As of 1992, play in some form was used in child therapy by a majority of clinicians, as reported by Koocher and D'Angelo.

Play is a tool that can be used in therapy for a variety of purposes. Whether or not play is used with a child depends on the child's ability to play, developmental level, ability to verbalize, and the overall treatment approach. Play therapy is generally used with children from 4 to 10 years of age. Most therapists agree that unstructured toys and materials are best to use. Toys that leave much room for individual expression are best. Examples of relatively unstructured toys are puppets, dolls and dollhouses, trucks, Legos, crayons, and clay.

HOW PLAY HELPS

In the child therapy literature, four broad functions of play emerge as important in therapy. First, play is a natural form of expression in children. Chethik (2000) refers to the language of children's play. Children use play to express feelings and thoughts. Chethik states that play emerges from the child's internal life and reflects the child's internal world. Therefore, children use play to express affect and fantasy and, in therapy, to express troubling and conflict-laden feelings. The expressions of feelings itself, sometimes termed catharsis, is thought to be therapeutic. The therapist facilitates this process by giving permission for feelings to be expressed and by labeling the affect. By labeling the affect, the therapist helps to make the feelings less overwhelming and more understandable.

Second, the child uses this language of play to communicate with the therapist. The therapist actively labels, empathizes, and interprets the play, which, in turn, helps the child feel understood. For many children, this feeling of empathy from the therapist facilitates change in their interpersonal world.

A third major function of play is as a vehicle for the occurrence of insight and working through conflicts. Psychodynamic theory views the emotional resolution of conflict or trauma as a major mechanism of change in psychotherapy. Children reexperience major developmental conflicts or situational traumas in therapy. Many of these conflicts and traumas are expressed in play. The expression of the negative affect associated with the event, at the child's own pace in the play and with the support of the therapist, helps the child resolve and integrate the negative affect and, to use Erikson's term, gain mastery over these issues.

A fourth major function of play in therapy is that of providing opportunities to practice with a variety of ideas, behaviors, interpersonal behaviors, and verbal expressions. Because play is occurring in a safe environment, in a pretend world, with a permissive, nonjudgmental adult, the child can try out and rehearse a variety of expressions and behaviors without concern about real-life consequences. In some forms of play therapy, the therapist is quite directive in guiding the child to try new behaviors. For example, Knell developed a cognitive behavioral play therapy approach that actively uses modeling techniques and a variety of cognitive behavioral techniques.

It is important to point out that although these major functions of play occur in normal play situations, the therapist builds on these normal functions by enhancing the play experience. The therapist creates a safe environment, gives permission for play to occur, actively facilitates the play, and labels the thoughts and feelings expressed. The psychodynamic therapist interprets the play. Because there are so many individual differences in play skills and abilities in children, and differences in theoretical orientations of therapists, there are many different kinds of play therapy techniques that are utilized.

PSYCHODYNAMIC PLAY THERAPY AND NONDIRECTIVE PLAY THERAPY

Play was first used in therapy by psychoanalysts such as Anna Freud and Melanie Klein in the 1920s and 1930s. One of the key techniques used by psychodynamic therapists is interpretation. The therapist interprets the play and ties the interpretation to what is happening in the child's daily life. Interpretation helps the child gain insight or an understanding of internal conflicts and fears. For example, the therapist might interpret the play to mean that the doll does not want to go to school because she is afraid the mother will be lonely, and wonder if the child might feel that way sometimes. Some psychodynamic therapists such as Messer and Warren do not think that insight is always necessary for change to occur. They believe that the child can often work through and master problems by playing, experiencing the emotion, and re-experiencing memories in the therapy.

Non-directive play therapy approaches also have a long history, beginning with the work of Axline in the 1940s. The client-centered and person-centered approaches focus on play as a form of communication for and with the child. A key technique would be empathizing and understanding what the child is expressing. There would be little or no interpretation of underlying dynamics or conflicts about which the child was unaware. The therapist follows the child's lead in the play and labels feelings expressed in the play. The therapist trusts the child's developmental process and striving for self-development. Genuineness in the relationship is an important ingredient in the therapy.

RESEARCH IN PLAY THERAPY

Somewhat surprisingly, there are no empirical studies that have investigated and supported play therapy with clinical populations. These studies need to be carried out. However, there are some play intervention studies with specific types of problems and child populations that have found that play sessions have reduced fears and anxiety in children. Fears have been reduced around medical procedures and around issues of separation. Several of these studies suggest that the imagination and fantasy components of play are key factors in reducing the anxiety.

There is a large body of research in child development that shows that pretend play relates to and facilitates creativity and relates to coping, emotional understanding, and adjustment. Play training studies in a recent review by Dansky found that children can be taught to improve their play skills.

Future play therapy studies must build on the research in the child development area. A fruitful area of research will be to investigate exactly how play helps with the processing of negative emotions and the balance between negative and positive emotions. The research should also build on the long history of clinical scholarly writing in this area.

See also: Child Psychotherapy; Client-Centered Therapy; Cognitive–Behavioral Play Therapy; Evidence-Based Treatments; Family Intervention

Further Reading

Chethik, M. (2000) *Techniques of child therapy: Psychodynamic strategies* (2nd ed.). New York: Guilford.
Russ, S. (1998). Play therapy. In A. Bellack, M. Herson (Editors-in-chief), & T. Ollendick (Vol. Ed.), *Comprehensive Clinical Psychology. Children and adolescents: Clinical formulation and treatment* (Vol. 5, pp. 221–243). Oxford: Elsevier Science.

Singer, D. L., & Singer, J. (1990). *The house of make-believe.* Cambridge, MA: Harvard University Press.

SANDRA W. RUSS

Positive Attention

See: Differential Social Reinforcement/ Positive Attention

Positive Practice

See: Overcorrection

Positive Reinforcement

The term positive reinforcement is used in two ways. First, it is used to describe the process involved when a behavior occurs more often as a result of its occurrence being followed by a desirable consequence. Second, it is used to describe an intervention procedure that is used by clinicians in an attempt to strengthen an existing behavior or teach a new behavior. Here the term is used in the latter sense.

Positive reinforcement as a procedure has been developed as part of applied behavior analysis. It is one of the simplest methods of strengthening existing behaviors and teaching new behaviors. To use positive reinforcement effectively, the clinician waits for the desired behavior to occur and then immediately provides the reinforcer. It is important to note that a reinforcer is defined by its effect on the behavior that it follows. It is only a reinforcer if the behavior increases as a result of its presentation. What is reinforcing for one person may not be reinforcing for another. Therefore, the parent/teacher/ clinician needs to tailor the selection of reinforcers for the child, and this can only be done after careful assessment of the child. Often, a variety of reinforcers are identified and used for each individual. This ensures that the recipient does not become satiated with the single reinforcer to the extent that it no longer serves as a reinforcer.

Reinforcers can be categorized in a number of ways. First, reinforcers can be described as being primary and secondary reinforcers. Primary reinforcers have a biological importance that makes them reinforcing in themselves, without any prior learning. Things such as food, water, and warmth are considered to be primary reinforcers. Secondary reinforcers are those things that have developed reinforcing properties through pairing with primary reinforcers. For example, praise that is paired with the presentation of food for an appropriate behavior will become reinforcing in itself. The clinical use of primary reinforcers can be controversial as they are considered basic necessities to which children should always have access. However, some forms of primary reinforcers that are not necessary for survival can be used with success (e.g., use of candy).

Second, reinforcers can be categorized according to the form they take, for example, social, activity, food, and token reinforcers. Social reinforcers include affection, praise, and attention from significant others (e.g., parents, teachers, peers). Activity reinforcers involve the child having access to things he/she likes to do, such as games, outings, and watching television. Food reinforcers are things that the child likes to eat, generally treats that the child does not have on a regular basis. Token reinforcers are things that in themselves do not have value, but can be used to access other desirable reinforcers. An example is using plastic chips that can be traded in for social, activity, and food reinforcers once a certain number of chips have been obtained. Money, of course, is a token reinforcer that all people are familiar with (and for the most part respond to).

A third way reinforcers are categorized is according to whether they are intrinsic or extrinsic to the behavior being reinforced. For some behaviors (e.g., eating ice cream or masturbation) the reinforcement is part of the behavior. In other words, the behavior itself is reinforcing. For other behaviors (e.g., doing homework, doing household chores) there is likely to be little intrinsic reinforcement and the continuation of these behaviors will rely on extrinsic reinforcement (e.g., parent and teacher praise, pocket money).

What is reinforcing for a particular child can be identified through a number of methods. The simplest way is to ask the child what he or she would like. This can be effective if the child identifies realistic reinforcers that are easy to access and are of a size appropriate for the behavior. Of course, if a child asks for a new bicycle for washing the dishes, more realistic reinforcers will need to be identified.

A second method of selecting reinforcers is to observe the child to see what he or she chooses to do in his or her free time. For example, watching television may be an activity that a child chooses to do on a regular basis. This could be used as a reinforcer for a less preferred behavior, such as homework. The use of high preference behaviors to reinforce low preference behaviors is often referred to as the Premack Principle.

Finally, reinforcer sampling can be used to select a reinforcer. This involves allowing the child to have access to several types of reinforcers and observing which one he or she prefers.

Whichever method is chosen to select a reinforcer, it is important to closely monitor the behavior that is followed by the selected reinforcer to determine if this specific behavior increases in frequency. If it does increase in frequency, one can be confident that an appropriate reinforcer has been selected. If not, another reinforcer may need to be tried.

Some basic principles of reinforcement should be followed to maximize the effect of positive reinforcement in strengthening the desired behavior. Reinforcement should occur immediately following the desired behavior (or as soon as is possible thereafter). The importance of reinforcement occurring as close as possible to the desired behavior cannot be overstated. If the reinforcer occurs following a delay, the child may forget why he or she is receiving the reinforcer. Alternatively, another behavior may occur between the desired behavior and the reinforcer, resulting in this second behavior becoming the one that is reinforced.

Initially, reinforcement should occur every time the behavior occurs (continuous schedule) in order to have the greatest strengthening benefit. Once the behavior occurs frequently, the schedule of reinforcement should gradually be spread across occurrences (intermittent schedule) so that the behavior is less likely to weaken once reinforcement no longer occurs every time.

It is interesting to note that while reinforcement has been shown to be one of the simplest and most effective strategies for strengthening behavior, it is not often used in classrooms. Recent research indicates that punishment is far more frequently used in the classroom to change behavior. Strategies such as time-outs, reprimands, and response costs are favored consequences for dealing with student misbehavior. It is important to ensure that these strategies are paired with reinforcement of appropriate behavior, as it is only through reinforcement and other positive procedures that children will learn appropriate behaviors to replace inappropriate ones.

See also: Applied Behavior Analysis; Extinction; Token Economies

Further Reading

Grant, L., & Evans, A. (1994). *Principles of behavior.* New York: HarperCollins.
Hudson, A. (1998). Applied behavior analysis. In A. Bellack, M. Hersen (Series Ed.), & T. Ollendick (Vol. Ed.), *Comprehensive clinical psychology. Children and adolescents: Clinical formulation and treatment* (Vol. 5, pp. 107–129). New York: Pergamon.
Lattal, K. A., & Neef, N. (1996). Recent reinforcement-schedule research and applied behavior analysis. *Journal of Applied Behavior Analysis, 29,* 213–230.
Maag, J. W. (2001). Rewarded by punishment: Reflections on the disuse of positive reinforcement in schools. *Exceptional Children, 67,* 173–186.
Premack, D. (1959). Toward empirical behavioral laws: I. Positive reinforcement. *Psychological Review, 66,* 219–233.

EMMA LITTLE
ALAN HUDSON

Posttraumatic Stress Disorder in Children

In recent years, media reports of devastating natural disasters, school shootings, and terrorist activities have drawn attention to the significant trauma that children and adults experience following such events. In fact, it has become apparent that children's exposure to traumatic events can lead to reactions that may interfere with their day-to-day functioning and cause them and their families significant distress. Specifically, exposure to natural disasters (e.g., hurricanes, tornadoes, fires, earthquakes, floods), as well as to man-made disasters (e.g., terrorist bombs, sniper shootings, plane crashes), represent traumatic events that frequently result in the emergence of a specific set of symptoms—those of Posttraumatic Stress Disorder (PTSD). Moreover, exposure to life-threatening health conditions or medical treatments, and exposure to violence of a personal nature, such as through rape, kidnapping, physical and sexual abuse, and community violence, may also precipitate symptoms of PTSD.

PTSD DIAGNOSTIC CRITERIA AND RELATED SYMPTOMS

The diagnostic category of PTSD was introduced in the third edition of the American Psychiatric Association's *Diagnostic and Statistical Manual of Mental Disorders* (*DSM*). At that time, PTSD was primarily considered to be an adult disorder. However, in recent years, there has been an increased awareness that children and adolescents also experience PTSD, and this is reflected in the fourth edition of the *DSM*, published in

1994. In *DSM-IV*, PTSD refers to a set of symptoms that develop following exposure to an unusually severe stressor or event; one that causes or is capable of causing death, injury, or threat to the physical integrity of oneself or another person. To meet criteria for a diagnosis of PTSD, a child's reaction to the traumatic event must include intense fear or helplessness; this may be expressed by agitated or disorganized behavior. Moreover, specific criteria for three additional symptom clusters must be met: reexperiencing, avoidance/numbing, and hyperarousal. *Reexperiencing* symptoms include recurrent or intrusive thoughts or dreams about the event and intense distress at cues or reminders of the event. For young children, reexperiencing may be reflected in repetitive play with traumatic themes or by reenactment of traumatic events in play, drawings, or verbalizations. *Avoidance* or *numbing* symptoms include efforts to avoid thoughts, feelings, or conversations about the traumatic event, avoiding reminders of the event, diminished interest in normal activities, and feeling detached or removed from others. *Hyperarousal* symptoms include difficulty sleeping or concentrating, irritability, angry outbursts, hypervigilance, and an exaggerated startle response; these behaviors must be newly occurring since the onset of the precipitating event. For a diagnosis of PTSD, the above symptoms must be evident for at least one month, and be accompanied by significant impairment in the child's functioning (e.g., problems in school, or in social or family relations). In addition, "types" of PTSD can be specified as follows: acute (duration of symptoms < 3 months), chronic (duration of symptoms ≥ 3 months), or delayed (onset of symptoms at least 6 months after the stressor).

Community studies suggest that reexperiencing symptoms are most commonly reported by child trauma victims; for example, Vernberg and colleagues found that 90 percent of children exposed to a catastrophic hurricane reported symptoms of reexperiencing 3 months after the disaster. In contrast, symptoms of avoidance and numbing are far less commonly reported by children, although Lonigan and colleagues found that their presence is a good indicator of the full PTSD diagnosis.

Diagnosing PTSD is especially difficult in very young children, such as infants, toddlers, and early preschoolers, in part due to their limited verbal capacity. With young children, generalized anxiety and fears, avoidance of certain situations that may be linked to the traumatic event, and sleep disturbances may be useful indicators of PTSD.

PTSD may be present or comorbid with other psychological difficulties. Following trauma, many children also report high levels of anxiety and/or depression.

When trauma leads to the loss of loved ones, symptoms of bereavement may also be present.

PREVALENCE AND DEVELOPMENTAL COURSE

It is difficult to estimate the prevalence of PTSD in children and adolescents. Studies have been extremely diverse with respect to the type of trauma evaluated, assessment methods and sampling procedures used, and the length of time passed since the traumatic event occurred. Community studies suggest that approximately 24–39 percent of children and adolescents exposed to trauma (e.g., community violence, a natural disaster) meet criteria for PTSD. However, when subclinical levels of PTSD are considered, up to 55 percent of the children in large community samples have reported at least moderate levels of symptoms during the first 3 months following a traumatic event. Thus, PTSD symptoms are common among children exposed to trauma, although fewer youth will meet criteria for a PTSD diagnosis.

Little is known about the developmental course of PTSD in children over time. However, PTSD symptoms may emerge in the days or weeks following a traumatic event and can take months or years to dissipate. In the absence of reexposure to trauma or of the occurrence of other traumatic events, the typical developmental course of symptoms appears to be one of lessening frequency and intensity over time. For example, 3 months after a devastating and highly destructive natural disaster (Hurricane Andrew), La Greca and associates (2002) indicated that 39 percent of the children in one community sample informally met criteria for PTSD, but this was reduced to 24 percent at 7 months postdisaster, and to 18 percent by 10 months postdisaster. A subgroup of children reporting moderate to severe PTSD symptoms was followed 42 months postdisaster, revealing that 40 percent continued to report moderate or more severe symptoms, as well as impairment in functioning; yet, almost none of the children who had mild or no symptoms at 10 months postdisaster reported any symptoms later on.

These data suggested a steady reduction in the frequency and severity of PTSD symptoms over time (with no further exposure to similar disasters), although a significant minority (approximately 7–10 percent) did not "recover" and continued to report substantial difficulties almost 4 years postdisaster. These findings also suggested that it may be highly unusual for children to report significant PTSD symptoms a year or more after a traumatic event, if they did not experience or report symptoms within 3 months of the event. Although there may be a brief period of "shock" or numbing, or sometimes elation and relief at still being alive, it is unusual to find a child reporting high levels of PTSD symptoms a year after the trauma, if no signs of distress were evident within the first few months after the traumatic event occurred.

With respect to the persistence of PTSD symptoms, findings suggest that children's reactions to disasters and other traumatic events are not merely transitory events that quickly dissipate. On the contrary, they appear to linger and persist and, thus, are likely to cause distress to children and their families for some time. One factor that contributes to the persistence of PTSD symptoms over time is the occurrence of other significant life stressors. For example, La Greca and colleagues (2002) found that children who encounter major life stressors, such as a death or illness in the family or parental divorce, in the months or first few years following a traumatic event, do not appear to recover quickly, and report persistently high levels of PTSD over time.

DEMOGRAPHIC TRENDS

Several studies suggest that PTSD appears more frequently among girls than boys, although this has not consistently been the case. In addition, it is difficult to draw generalizations regarding children's vulnerability to PTSD at different ages, as findings on age-related differences have been inconsistent and are probably influenced by diverse developmental manifestations of PTSD (see the report of the American Academy of Child and Adolescent Psychiatry published in 1998).

PTSD occurs across diverse ethnic and cultural groups. Community studies suggest that some minority youth exposed to severe natural disasters report more symptoms of PTSD and have a more difficult time recovering from such events than nonminority youth. It is possible that, at least in part, socioeconomic factors might account for such findings, in that children and families from minority backgrounds may have less financial resources or less adequate insurance to deal efficiently with the rebuilding process. This, in turn, could prolong the period of life disruption and loss of personal possessions that typically ensures after destructive natural disasters.

FACTORS THAT CONTRIBUTE TO PTSD IN CHILDREN

A wide range of traumatic events has been linked to the emergence of PTSD in children. However, first and foremost of these factors is children's *exposure to the traumatic event*. Two aspects of exposure that are important are: (1) the presence or perception of *life threat*, and (2) *personal loss or disruption* of everyday events. In fact, the presence or perception of life-threat is considered to be essential for the emergence of PTSD. Children who witness or are exposed to acts of violence, such as sniper shootings or severe physical abuse, understandably may feel that their life is in danger (i.e., life-threat). It is also the case, however, that catastrophic natural disasters or personal disasters (e.g., residential fires, motor vehicle accidents) can elicit perceptions of life-threat in children, *even if no one is injured or hurt*. For example, although relatively few lives were lost in South Florida as a result of Hurricane Andrew, the extensive destruction of homes and property that occurred during the storm was terrifying to many children and adults. In a study conducted by Vernberg and colleagues, 60 percent of the children interviewed "thought they were going to die" during the storm. Thus, perceptions of life-threat can occur in the absence of actual loss of life or serious injury. In addition to life-threat, the experience of loss (of family and friends, of personal property) and disruption of everyday life (displacement from home, school, community) also contribute to PTSD in children. The life-changes that result from this aspect of exposure to trauma also predict PTSD symptoms in children.

A second factor that contributes to PTSD in children following traumatic events is the presence of prior psychological difficulties. Children with preexisting psychological problems, especially anxiety, seem to be more vulnerable to PTSD reactions following trauma. For example, in another study conducted by La Greca and associates (2002), children's anxiety levels 15 months *before* a traumatic event were found to predict their levels of PTSD symptoms 3 and 7 months postdisaster, even when controlling for children's exposure to the event. In addition, children who had greater levels of exposure to the disaster showed an increase in anxiety symptoms following the disaster. These findings are interesting in that the current conceptualization of PTSD, as reflected in *DSM-IV*, suggests that trauma must be present for PTSD to emerge. However, anxious children may have a vulnerability to PTSD, even if their degree of exposure to a trauma is relatively low.

Other factors that predict the severity and persistence of PTSD symptoms in children following trauma are the occurrence of intervening life events and reexposure to the traumatic event. On the other hand, factors that have been found to mitigate the impact of trauma include the availability of social support and the types of coping skills children use. Following traumatic events, children with higher levels of social support from significant others (especially parents, teachers, friends, and classmates) report fewer symptoms of PTSD than those with low levels of social support. Some community studies have found that children with more negative coping strategies for dealing with stress (e.g., anger, blaming others) show greater persistence in their PTSD symptoms over time. Because of these findings, efforts to enhance the social support of children exposed to trauma, and to encourage adaptive coping skills, may be useful for strategies for interventions with children following traumatic events.

See also: Acute Stress Disorder; Anxiety Disorders; Child Maltreatment; Cognitive-Behavior Therapy; Eye-Movement Desensitization and Reprocessing; Specific Phobia

Further Reading

American Academy of Child and Adolescent Psychiatry. (1998). AACAP Official Action: Practice parameters for the assessment and treatment of children and adolescents with posttraumatic stress disorder. *Journal of the American Academy of Child and Adolescent Psychiatry, 37* (Suppl.), 4S–26S.

American Psychiatric Association. (1994). *Diagnostic and statistical manual of mental disorders, 4th edition (DSM-IV)*. Washington, DC: Author.

Hamblen, J. (date unknown). *PTSD in children and adolescents: A National Center for PTSD fact sheet*. http://www.ncptsd.org/facts/specific/fs_children.html Retrieved on 6/7/02.

La Greca, A. M., Silverman, W. K., Vernberg, E. M., & Roberts, M. C. (2002). *Helping children cope with disasters and terrorism*. Washington, DC: American Psychological Association.

ANNETTE M. LA GRECA

Prader–Willi Syndrome

DESCRIPTION AND INCIDENCE

Prader–Willi syndrome (PWS) is a multisystem disorder featuring mental retardation or learning disability, infantile *hypotonia* (i.e., weak muscle tone and poor suck reflex), growth failure, short stature, delayed sexual development, and characteristic physical features (i.e., narrow face, almond-shaped eyes, small mouth with thin upper lip, downturned corners of the mouth, fair skin and hair compared to that of family members, small hands, and small feet). Hypothalamic endocrine dysfunction, including *hypogonadotropism* (i.e., reduced secretion of gonad stimulating factors) with associated osteoporosis, is also

characteristic of this disorder. Common behavioral characteristics associated with PWS include childhood onset of *hyperphagia* (i.e., excessive eating) with obesity, skin-picking, and other compulsive behaviors. Temper tantrums and a tendency to be argumentative are also associated with this condition. However, when considering those features associated with PWS, as well as with other neurogenetic disorders, it is essential to remember that there is a great deal of variability among individuals in terms of symptoms and severity.

Between 1 in 10,000 and 15,000 people are diagnosed with PWS. This condition affects individuals of all races and both sexes equally.

ETIOLOGY

PWS is the first recognized human disorder resulting from parent-of-origin differences in gene expression, or *genomic imprinting*. Genomic imprinting is the reversible process by which the expression of some genes is modified as a function of the gender of the parental provider. The majority of PWS cases (75 percent) are caused by a small deletion in the paternally contributed chromosome 15. The remaining 25 percent of cases are caused by other abnormalities in the maternally or paternally contributed chromosome 15. In general, linkages between the specific origin of PWS and its clinical manifestations are unknown; however, it is important to ascertain the cause of the disorder during assessment for genetic counseling purposes.

DIAGNOSIS

In the early 1990s, laboratory technology was developed allowing for the detection of defects in chromosome 15. Presently, there are several laboratory tests that can be used to verify the diagnosis and to characterize the particular genetic etiology. *Methylation analysis* is considered to be the most effective of these tests. *High-resolution chromosome analysis* and *microsatellite repeated sequences* on chromosome 15 are other techniques that can be used to confirm a diagnosis of PWS. All of these tests are effective for prenatal as well as postnatal diagnosis.

Before modern medical technology allowed for accurate analysis in the laboratory, diagnosis was based upon the identification of associated clinical features. Therefore, the ability of a clinician to accurately diagnose a person with PWS depended largely on his or her experience and familiarity with the disorder. As a result, many individuals who carried a diagnosis of PWS did not actually have PWS as a cause of their mental retardation or obesity; an even larger number of people with PWS went undiagnosed. Since then, thorough diagnostic criteria have been developed in addition to the laboratory tests. However, because genetic testing is the only definitive way to confirm a PWS diagnosis, these criteria currently serve only to suggest a diagnosis and indicate the appropriate laboratory tests.

ASSOCIATED PSYCHOLOGICAL FEATURES

Clinical features of PWS include behavioral characteristics such as hyperphagia and food foraging, obsessive–compulsive behavior, skin-picking, stealing, lying, and frequent temper tantrums, as well as a tendency to be argumentative, possessive, and manipulative. Individuals with PWS may also exhibit attention-deficit problems (with or without hyperactivity), and many exhibit sleep disorders. Deficits in "social cognition" are also thought to characterize PWS. Specifically, similar to children with other disorders associated with mental retardation, many children with PWS have trouble reading social and affective cues, and interpreting other's behavior as compared with healthy comparison groups. Thus, it is believed that this type of faulty interpretation (likely stemming from the cognitive deficits associated with PWS), may contribute to the social isolation and poor interpersonal relationships that are common among affected individuals. This isolation may, in turn, contribute to the increased incidence of depressed mood observed within the PWS population.

Individuals with PWS tend to have deficits in broader areas of cognitive functioning as well. In terms of overall intelligence, this condition is associated with a wide range of IQs, spanning from severe retardation (20–34) to average intelligence (85–115). The mean IQ for children with PWS approximates 70 (i.e., the lower third percentile for the general population) and is higher than that seen in other syndromes featuring mental retardation (i.e., *Down syndrome*, *Fragile X syndrome*). Most individuals with PWS have mild to moderate mental retardation; few have IQ scores falling within the severe range (less than 40).

In addition to the increased rates of mental retardation, PWS is associated with a particular pattern of cognitive strengths and weaknesses. Typically, affected individuals demonstrate relative strengths in reading and writing, spatial-perceptual processing, and visual processing. Commonly noted weaknesses include mathematical ability, sequential processing, and short-term

memory tasks. One study distinguishes between cases where the condition results from a deletion on chromosome 15 versus other abnormalities on chromosome 15; results indicate that the deletion subtype is more closely associated with low verbal IQ scores than were other subtypes.

Many children with PWS begin their schooling in a mainstream primary school, with varying levels of support. Others are placed in settings for people with moderate learning difficulties. Although some older children are able to progress to a mainstream secondary school, others transfer to a special needs school or a residential program. When appropriate educational services are rendered, individuals with PWS can be expected to achieve a satisfactory level of schooling.

TREATMENT

Because of the wide range of symptoms featured in individuals with PWS, a multimodal approach to therapy is recommended. Studies suggest that a combination of behavioral, supportive, and pharmacological treatments is imperative to maintaining the affected individual's maximal potential for functioning. A limited number of hospitals have created specialized inpatient programs aimed at the treatment of behavior problems and/or morbid obesity in children and adults with PWS. The treatment program that has been found to be the most successful features a highly structured schedule with minimal free time, allowing for a high degree of predictability. In general, patients are verbally praised for appropriate behaviors, while inappropriate behaviors are ignored. In addition to the behavioral component of this type of program, patients are expected to attend group psychotherapy twice weekly. During these sessions, patients are encouraged to speak freely about the difficulties they encounter in living with the syndrome.

When the structured program and group therapy are not sufficient to curb the troublesome behavioral symptoms, patients are prescribed psychotropic medications as an adjunctive treatment. *Selective Serotonin Reuptake Inhibitors* (SSRIs) have been found to be useful in curtailing depression, stubborn oppositionality, rigidity, impulsivity, temper tantrums, and aggression. Antipsychotic medication can be helpful for patients with psychotic symptoms, and mood stabilizers are used in cases where there is persistent mood instability.

There are also treatments available for some of the physical symptoms of PWS. Growth hormone therapy is the most common treatment and has been shown to benefit children with PWS in terms of increased height and growth rate, as well as overall improved body composition (i.e., reduced adipose tissue and increased lean body mass). In addition, growth hormone therapy may result in improvements in respiratory function and physical performance.

Typically, growth hormone therapy is prescribed until the growth plates near the ends of the bones have closed (i.e., until the bones have "fused"). However, because there are data to indicate that a deficiency in growth hormone during adulthood may cause problems (including poor body composition, reduced energy and physical performance, osteoporosis, and disorders of sleep and mood), it has been suggested that low doses of growth hormone may be helpful for growth-hormone deficient adults with PWS.

Although there are few documented safety risks associated with growth hormone therapy, there is a need for long-term safety studies, especially with regard to its effects on glucose metabolism.

PROGNOSIS

Earlier diagnosis, made possible by recent advances in medical technology, along with an increased emphasis on coordinated care, have allowed for an improved quality of life for many living with PWS. Because of the multidimensional nature of the condition, it is essential that there is cooperation among endocrinologists, geneticists, primary care physicians, nutritionists, psychologists, psychiatrists, teachers, and families. When both medical and psychological needs are met, many individuals with PWS are able to become gainfully employed or participate in volunteer work. Higher education is an additional possibility for some. Given the severe nature of the hyperphagia that is so commonly associated with PWS, along with the serious health concerns that accompany obesity, most people with this disorder will need some degree of dietary assistance throughout their adult lives. A combination of dietary supervision, caloric restriction, behavioral therapy, exercise, and pharmacological treatment can significantly increase the life expectancy of this population.

SUPPORT GROUP

The Prader–Willi Syndrome Association (USA), 5700 Midnight Pass Rd. Sarasota, Florida 34242 USA; Web site: www.pwsausa.org, E-mail: national@pwsausa.org.

See also: Short Stature: Psychological Aspects

Further Reading

Cassidy, S. B. (Ed.). (2001). Prader-Willi syndrome in the new millennium [Special issue]. *Endocrinologist, 10*(4, Suppl. 1).

LAUREN ZURENDA
DAVID E. SANDBERG

Prematurity: Birth Weight and Gestational Age

PREMATURITY

Prematurity is defined as being born <37 weeks gestational age, and babies born prematurely comprise 11 percent of births. The limit of viability with respect to prematurity is 23–24 weeks gestation. Babies born low birth weight (LBW) and smaller make up 7.4 percent of births; LBW infants are those born at <2500 g (5.5 lbs), very low birth weight (VLBW) babies are born <1500 g (3.3 lbs), while extremely low birth weight (ELBW) infants are born <1000 g (2.2 lbs).

LBW children comprise a heterogeneous group that includes preterm infants as well as babies born at term but who are below normal in weight due to abnormal maternal or fetal conditions. Prior to the 1990s, infants were primarily grouped by birth weight versus gestational age because of the uncertainty of the obstetric estimation of gestational age and the questionable utility of the postnatal assessment, particularly in very small infants. However, with the improvement in fetal ultrasound techniques, estimation of gestational age has become more precise. Gestational age is a stronger determinant of organ/system maturation and viability than is birth weight. Moreover, infants of very low birth weight may be: (1) extremely premature babies with average-for-gestational-age (AGA) birth weights; (2) less premature babies with small-for-gestational-age (SGA; <3rd percentile) birth weights; or (3) older preterm and term infants with extreme SGA birth weights. This distinction is necessary because the ultimate survival and outcome of infants included in these groups can vary markedly. SGA infants often are at higher risk for developmental problems than AGA infants.

DEVELOPMENTAL ISSUES

Much of the improvement in survival of these smaller, more premature infants is attributable to increased use of antenatal and postnatal steroids (to enhance lung maturation), more aggressive approaches to delivery room resuscitation, and surfactant replacement (to enhance oxygen exchange in the lungs). These children are at biologic risk and therefore the baby's admission status (degree of sickness measured with variables such as birth weight, gestational age, Apgar scores), medical response to intervention (ventilation, secondary/tertiary level of care), and sequelae at discharge (need for oxygen, chronic illness, neurosensory deficit) are important considerations. Various risk scores and neonatal admission severity scores for physiologic status and intensity of therapeutic intervention have been developed and these often prove helpful in clarifying an infant's medical course. Intracranial events, pulmonary immaturity, and infections are the major sources of morbidity in premature infants.

CORRECTION FOR PREMATURITY

A related issue is that *correction for prematurity* (chronologic age minus the number of weeks of prematurity) must be considered when preterm infants are followed longitudinally. However, correction is controversial. The general consensus is that correction should occur up to 2 years of age. However, some investigators suggest that correction not be utilized, correction continue throughout childhood, or that it be applied in an incremental fashion (e.g., half correction) depending on the infant's gestational age, age at time of measurement, and area of function being assessed. Correction reflects a biological/maturational perspective, while use of chronologic age represents an environmentally based orientation. Adjustment for prematurity is assumed to differentiate transient effects of preterm birth from more persistent deficits, although some contend that it simply masks these deficits. Arguments for incremental correction or total lack of correction are unconvincing at this point.

See also: Infant Assessment; Neonatal Assessment; Perinatal Development; Prematurity Outcomes; Prenatal Development

Further Reading

Aylward, G. P. (2002). Methodological issues in outcome studies of at-risk infants. *Journal of Pediatric Psychology, 27,* 37–45.
Blasco, P. A. (1989). Preterm birth: To correct or not to correct. *Developmental Medicine and Child Neurology, 31,* 816–826.
Hack, M., & Fanaroff, A. A. (1999). Outcomes of children of extremely low birthweight and gestational age in the 1990s. *Early Human Development, 53,* 193–218.

GLEN P. AYLWARD

Prematurity Outcomes

There is increased interest in the outcome of infants born prematurely, particularly those born at low birth weight (LBW; < 2,500 g or 5.5 lbs), very low birth weight (VLBW; < 1,500 g or 3.3 lbs), and extremely low birth weight (ELBW; < 1,000 g or 2.2 lbs). Improved survival rates have raised the concern of a corresponding greater prevalence of neurodevelopmental deficits, particularly in terms of cognitive and neuropsychological outcome.

A gradient of developmental sequelae in children exists that is inversely related to decreasing birth weight (i.e., the lower the birth weight, the higher the risk for developmental problems); however, birth weight must be considered in conjunction with other biomedical and environmental risks. Initially, the primary emphasis was on the incidence of major disabilities that include moderate/ severe mental retardation, sensorineural hearing loss/ blindness, cerebral palsy, and epilepsy. LBW babies have a 6–8 percent incidence of these major handicaps, VLBW infants have a 14–17 percent incidence, while ELBW babies have a 20–25 percent rate of occurrence. In comparison, major handicaps occur in 5 percent of full-term infants. These rates of handicap have remained relatively consistent over the last decade, although the nature of impairment may be changing, with significant problems frequently being found in "non-disabled" survivors. These high prevalence/ low severity dysfunctions appear to be increasing and include learning disabilities, borderline mental retardation, Attention-Deficit/Hyperactivity Disorder (ADHD), specific neuropsychological deficits (e.g., visual motor integration), and behavioral problems. It is estimated that these high prevalence/low severity dysfunctions occur in as many as 50–70 percent of VLBW infants, with an inverse birth weight gradient again being found. However, social, ethnic, and educational backgrounds of parents may also influence the prevalence of these disabilities. Moreover, while major disabilities are often identified during infancy, the more subtle problems become more obvious as the child grows older (i.e., reaches school age). There has also been increased interest on a broader, multidimensional conceptualization of outcome and health, including functional and health-related quality of life.

In an earlier metaanalysis, IQ scores in LBW children were 5–7 points less than full-term controls. More recent comparisons of VLBW and ELBW babies reveal a 0.3–0.6 *SD* decrement, generally ranging from 3.8 to 9.3 points. In nonhandicapped VLBW and ELBW infants, mean group IQs generally fall in the borderline to average range, with low average scores being the mode.

The majority of ELBW and VLBW infants appear to manifest some type of visual motor problem in copying, perceptual matching, spatial processing, finger-tapping, pegboard performance, visual memory, or visual-sequential memory. Estimates of visual perceptual and visual motor integration problems are in the 11–20 percent range, with fine motor problems occurring in as many as 71 percent in ELBW children.

Language functions such as vocabulary and receptive language are generally normal; however, more complex verbal processes (understanding syntax, abstract verbal skills, verb production) often are deficient.

More than one half of VLBW and 60–70 percent of ELBW children require special assistance in school. By middle school age, ELBW children are 3–5 times more likely to have a learning problem, particularly in reading and mathematics. An inverse gradient of learning difficulties is found: a 50–63 percent rate in those born <750 g (66 percent in those born <28 weeks gestational age), 30–38 percent in those 750–1499 g, and 7–18 percent in full-term infants. Many of these children display non-verbal learning disabilities (NVLD), and a higher prevalence of weaknesses in executive functions such as organization, planning, problem solving, and abstracting. Symptoms of ADHD are reported to occur 2.6 times more frequently in VLBW/ELBW infants than in controls, with some estimates indicating almost a 6-fold increase. Conduct disorders, shyness, unassertiveness, withdrawn behavior, and social skill deficits occur more frequently in LBW children than in their normal birth weight peers. It is hypothesized that prematurity and its effects act indirectly through the association with health, cognitive, and neuromotor function to explain behavioral and emotional problems at school age.

Perhaps one of the most alarming trends is the worsening outcome of ELBW and VLBW children as they become older, with rates of "normalcy" in some studies decreasing from 39 to 75 percent at 6 years to 14–26 percent by age 8. In summary, the spectrum of sequelae found in nonhandicapped children who were born prematurely does not differ dramatically from the array of problems found in the general school-aged population. However, what is different is the disproportionately greater incidence and complexity of these problems and the specific profiles of deficits.

See also: Infant Assessment; Neonatal Assessment; Perinatal Development; Prematurity: Birth Weight and Gestational Age; Prenatal Development

Further Reading

Aylward, G. P. (1992). The relationship between environmental risk and developmental outcome. *Journal of Developmental and Behavioral Pediatrics*, *13*, 222–229.

Aylward, G. P. (2002). Cognitive and neuropsychological outcome: More than IQ scores. *Mental Retardation and Developmental Disabilities Research and Reviews*, *8*, 234–240.

Aylward, G. P., Pfeiffer, S. I., Wright, A., & Verhulst, S. J. (1989). Outcome studies of low birth weight infants published in the last decade: A metaanalysis. *Journal of Pediatrics*, *115*, 515–521.

Breslau, N. (1995). Psychiatric sequelae of low birth weight. *Epidemiologic Reviews*, *17*, 96–106.

Taylor, H. G., Klein, N., & Hack, M. (2000). School-age consequences of birth weight less than 750 g: A review and update. *Developmental Neuropsychology*, *17*, 289–321.

GLEN P. AYLWARD

Prenatal Development

DEFINITIONS

Prenatal development refers to the development before birth; neonates are newly born infants through the first month of life. There are numerous causes for developmental problems in neonates and many have prenatal origins. These include infections and genetic, nutritional, metabolic, traumatic, intoxicant, maternal disease-related, or idiopathic factors. The timing of exposure to these potentially damaging agents is important. A *critical period* is the time during which the action of a specific internal or external influence is necessary (critical) for normal development. A *sensitive period* is the time during which the central nervous system (CNS) is highly susceptible to the effects of harmful conditions. A critical period occurs when certain conditions are necessary for the CNS to develop normally: a sensitive period is the time in which damage to the CNS can lead to alterations, reorganization, and potential disruptions in the infant. Critical periods generally are very circumscribed, while sensitive periods are more variable. A primary malformation refers to an anomaly that results from disruption of normal developmental events, resulting in failure in formation of an anatomic structure; a secondary malformation results from the breakdown of a previously formed structure because of a destructive event such as infection, or a later perinatal injury.

STAGES OF DEVELOPMENT AND PROBLEMS

The first stage of prenatal CNS development is the *dorsal induction phase* (3–4 weeks gestational age). This involves development and closure of the neural tube. Problems in this phase result in neural tube defects such as anencephaly (open skull with missing parts of the brain), encephalocele (protruding brain tissue), myelomeningocele (spina bifida; incomplete closure of the spinal cord), or congenital hydrocephalus (increased pressure and enlarged ventricles due to fluid backup).

The second stage is the *ventral induction phase* (5–6 weeks gestation), where the major portions of the brain and face are formed. Problems during this period cause the brain to not make proper cleavages and result in abnormalities of the face or brain that include holoprosencephaly (single-lobed brain), or Dandy Walker malformation (agenesis of cerebellar hemispheres).

In the *proliferation phase* (2–4 months), there is production of nerve cells; proliferation increases exponentially during the first 20 weeks of gestation and continues into the second and third postnatal year before leveling off. The principal neurons are generated in the germinal matrix—the area deep inside the brain surrounding the ventricles. Disruptions may result in too many or too few neurons being produced, causing conditions such as microcephaly or megalencephaly (macrocephaly).

The *migration phase* (3–5 months of gestation) involves movement of nerve cells from their sites of origin (ventricular zone) to their final positions. These events transform the fetus's brain into the six-layered structure of the adult cerebral cortex. The earliest generated neurons occupy the deep cortical layers, while those generated later will reside in more superficial (outward) layers. Migration is vulnerable to genetic disturbances, viral infections, and vascular disruptions. During the fifth month of gestation, the sulci (groovelike depressions) and gyri (elevations or ridges) appear. Disruptions produce anomalous formation of the cortical plate and result in disorders such as schizencephaly (thickened cortical mantle with seams or clefts), lissencephaly (absence of gyri, resulting in a smooth brain), polymicrogyria (small gyri with shallow convolutions), heterotopias (neuronal migration to wrong locations), or agenesis of the corpus callosum.

Once neurons reach their destination, they begin to grow and differentiate; this occurs during the *organization/differentiation phase* (6 months gestation–5 years). Dendritic, axonal, and synaptic development occur. Problems during this stage result in disorders in neural differentiation or the development of synapses, causing aberrant cortical circuitry.

The final phase is *myelination* (6 months–adulthood). Glial cells produce myelin, a fatty sheath, that eventually covers and insulates many axons. Disruptions result in nerve conduction problems and include cerebral white matter hypoplasia (underdevelopment). Amino acid deficits (e.g., phenylketonuria), inborn errors of metabolism, degenerative diseases (e.g., adrenoleukodystrophy), and early malnutrition can affect myelin development.

Dorsal and ventral induction and proliferation occur prenatally, while migration may occur postnatally in preterm infants. Organization/differentiation and myelination occur prenatally and postnatally in all babies. As a general rule of thumb, brain growth varies by region, and regions are most vulnerable when they are most rapidly growing. Because of its prolonged period of development, the brain is the most vulnerable of all embryonic/fetal organs to teratologic insult.

See also: Perinatal Development; Prematurity: Birth Weight and Gestational Age; Prematurity Outcomes

Further Reading

Aylward, G. P. (1997). *Infant and early childhood neuropsychology.* New York: Plenum.

Capone, G. T. (1996). Human brain development. In A. J. Capute & P. J. Accardo (Eds.), *Developmental disabilities in infancy and childhood.* (2nd ed., Vol. 1, pp. 1–22). Baltimore, MD: Paul H. Brookes.

Geidd, J. N. (1997). Normal development. In B. S. Peterson (Ed.), *Neuroimaging: Child and adolescent clinics of North America, 6,* 265–282.

GLEN P. AYLWARD

Prenatal Exposure to Cocaine

See: Cocaine, Prenatal Exposure

Prenatal Exposure to Marijuana

See: Marijuana, Prenatal Exposure

Prenatal Exposure to Methamphetamines

See: Methamphetamines, Prenatal Exposure

Prenatal Exposure to Nicotine

See: Nicotine, Prenatal Exposure

Prenatal Exposure to Opiates

See: Opiates, Prenatal Exposure

Prenatal Exposure to Psychotropic Drugs

See: Psychotropic Drugs, Prenatal Exposure

Preparation for Dental Procedures

See: Behavioral Dentistry

Preparation for Medical Procedures

DEFINITION

Prevention of child anxiety and behavioral distress is the primary goal of interventions designed to prepare children psychologically for medical procedures. Preparation programs typically involve a combination of educational and cognitive-behavioral strategies designed to assist children to cope with a medical situation (such as hospitalization or surgery) or with an invasive procedure (such as injection or lumbar puncture). These programs are offered to children prior to an upcoming medical experience in order to provide knowledge and to teach skills that may help to minimize negative experiences and promote adaptive functioning.

METHODS

Preparation for medical procedures involves multicomponent treatment packages that may include providing information to the child and family regarding what to expect during the procedure, modeling by a peer of successful coping with the procedure, and teaching active coping skills or distraction techniques for use during a procedure. Information can be provided using age appropriate play materials or demonstrations. For example, a doll might be used to show a young school-aged child where and how an area on the body will be cleansed prior to an injection. In providing such information, it is helpful to discuss or present the sights, sounds, smells, and other environmental correlates of the situation that the child may experience. This provides an opportunity for desensitization to potentially anxiety producing stimuli that may be associated with the medical event.

Giving the child an opportunity to observe a peer model coping successfully with a procedure is another common component of preparations. This helps to consolidate information provided previously and gives a concrete example of any coping or distraction technique that may be suggested. Models can be presented through audiotapes, slides, videotapes, or films. In a classic study of preparation for hospitalization and surgery, Melamed and Siegel (1975) showed children the film *Ethan Has an Operation* in which a boy experiences going to the hospital, getting blood tests, having anesthesia and surgery, recovering from the procedure, and being discharged. Children in the study who observed the film prior to hospitalization experienced less anxiety and behavioral distress than children who viewed a nature film instead.

Most preparation programs for medical procedures include not only information and peer models but also teach the child a specific coping strategy or distraction technique for use when feeling anxiety or discomfort. Training in muscle relaxation strategies, breathing techniques, use of cognitive imagery, and positive self-instruction have been helpful for some children in decreasing distress and improving cooperation during procedures. Distraction techniques that have been used to assist with painful procedures include using a party blower for young children and allowing older children and adolescents access to favorite music through headphones. Practice prior to experience with the medical event is essential for successful implementation of such strategies. During the procedure the child will often benefit from a coach who prompts the child to use the specific techniques learned. This coach can be a psychologist, another healthcare professional, or the child's parent (the parent must be able to interact with the child in a calm supportive manner).

EFFECTIVENESS

Critical reviews of intervention studies that evaluate protocols for preparing children for hospitalization and for painful medical procedures consistently conclude that providing children with preparation experiences can help to reduce anxiety and behavioral distress. Children who are appropriately prepared for medical events have more knowledge of their illness and associated treatment procedures, and there is evidence that they experience less discomfort and negative emotional reactions during and after the procedures than unprepared peers.

Determining what preparation procedure may be most effective for which child has received some attention in the treatment outcome literature. Important considerations include the child's developmental status, previous experience with hospitalization, and timing of the preparation activities. Very young children (below age 7) may not benefit from extensive or detailed preparation procedures because they have not yet developed the cognitive skills necessary to understand illness, they may remember less of the preparation information, and they may be less able to implement strategies effectively during anxiety-producing situations. For these children the best approach is to encourage the parents to describe the medical environment that the child will experience in simple terms and to answer any questions that the child may have using language that can be easily understood. Parents may also play with the child using medical toys to familiarize the child with common instruments and to elicit questions. Preparation should begin no earlier than one or two days prior to the procedure or hospitalization. Children who have previous negative experiences with hospitalization or surgery also may not benefit from

standard preparation procedures and may require more individualized programs to assist with their distress. In addition, it appears that timing of preparation programs may affect outcome. For example, some studies have suggested that for same day surgeries, preparation may be helpful the day before surgery but may actually increase anxiety if provided immediately before the procedure.

Because preparation programs have demonstrated effectiveness for many children, it is important that healthcare professionals continue to incorporate such procedures into standard pediatric practice. It is also important that researchers in this area continue to explore such issues as what components of the procedures are most effective, how such procedures should be modified for individual children, and how to assure that children continue to use these strategies in future stressful medical situations.

See also: Cognitive–Behavior Therapy; Medical Hospitalization; Pain Management; Relaxation Training; Videotape Modeling

Further Reading

Harbeck-Weber, C., & McKee, D. H. (1995). Prevention of emotional and behavioral distress in children experiencing hospitalization and chronic illness. In M. C. Roberts (Ed.), *Handbook of pediatric psychology* (2nd ed., pp. 167–184). New York: Guilford.
Melamed, B. G., & Siegel, L. J. (1975). Reduction of anxiety in children facing hospitalization and surgery by use of filmed modeling. *Journal of Consulting and Clinical Psychology, 43,* 511–521.
Powers, S. W. (1999). Empirically supported treatments in pediatric psychology: Procedure-related pain. *Journal of Pediatric Psychology, 24,* 131–145.
Siegel, L. J., & Conte, P. (2001). Hospitalization and medical care of children. In C. E. Walker & M. C. Roberts (Eds.), *Handbook of clinical child psychology* (3rd ed., pp. 895–909). New York: Wiley.

STEPHEN R. BOGGS

Preschool Assessment

INTRODUCTION

Preschool assessment typically refers to the assessment of children aged 2–6. The need for preschool assessment has been addressed with amendments to the legislation of 1975, the Education for All Handicapped Children Act (PL 94-142). Under the amendments

(PL-99-457 and PL 101-476), all children are entitled to appropriate free education and related services. The purpose of evaluating preschool children is to determine which children need early educational services and what those services should be. Assessment typically involves cognitive, motor, and speech and language components, and can also include preacademic and social components. Preschool assessments take several forms, depending on their purpose. Screening assessments are typically brief and are used to identify potential areas of delay. Diagnostic evaluations are more comprehensive and go into greater depth of the problems for which the child has been referred. Progress or follow-up evaluations are done to determine if interventions are effective or if they need to be changed.

REASONS FOR REFERRAL

There are a myriad of reasons why a child may be referred for an evaluation. Pregnancy and birth complications or conditions (e.g., maternal use of alcohol or other drugs during pregnancy, maternal smoking during pregnancy, oxygen deprivation during birth, being born small or with low birth weight for gestational age, having congenital or genetic problems) put a child at risk for developmental problems. A child may be referred due to failure to meet developmental milestones at appropriate times (e.g., walking, manipulating objects with the hands, talking). He/she may be referred because major developmental problems, such as mental retardation or autism, are suspected. A child may also be referred if there has been abuse or physical trauma that may have caused head injury, thus impacting development. Finally, a child may be referred if he or she is having social or emotional difficulties that are interfering with normal functioning.

PROFESSIONALS WHO DO PRESCHOOL ASSESSMENT

In larger communities, preschool assessment is often done at a child development center and includes assessment by a number of professionals who are qualified to administer and interpret tests specific to a particular developmental area. Typically, these centers have a clinical or school psychologist, a developmental pediatrician, a speech and language pathologist, and a physical and/or occupational therapist. Some centers also have social work and nutrition specialists. Children are often seen by several professionals during one visit and information from each professional is considered in making joint recommendations for the child and his or her family. In smaller communities that may not have a child development center, the child is often referred specifically to the professional who can evaluate the referral problem. For example, a pediatrician may refer a child to a psychologist if cognitive delays are suspected, to a physical therapist if motor delays are suspected, or to a speech and language pathologist if language delays are suspected. The team approach is ideal, as it allows information about the child to be considered from several perspectives and often results in the most appropriate and comprehensive recommendations.

Knowledge of normal development is essential for evaluators of preschool children so that deficits or delays may be identified. Knowledge of the medical conditions related to high-risk pregnancy or birth complications, genetic conditions (e.g., Down Syndrome), metabolic conditions (e.g., phenylketonuria [PKU]), and neurological problems (e.g., microcephaly) is also necessary so that predictions about the development of children who have these problems may be made. Knowledge of environmental/social conditions is also imperative to make appropriate recommendations. For example, professionals who evaluate preschool children need to be aware of the typical effects that neglect, abuse, or divorce, to name a few, may have on a child's development. Evaluators also need to be aware of the psychometric properties and the limitations of the tests or techniques that they use to make diagnoses. They also need to ensure that the tests are appropriate for the referral questions.

Input from parents is essential in preschool assessment, and the reason for this is twofold. First, parents are usually the best reporters about their children's abilities and behaviors. They typically have the most experience with the child and they are aware of when the child met specific developmental milestones and how the child typically functions. They are also important because preschool children are often timid or noncompliant when brought for an assessment. Often, children have not been put into the structured situation that the evaluation requires. They may be fearful of the professionals who are seeing them, they may have problems adjusting to the new setting or separating from their parents, and they may refuse or have difficulties completing items on the assessment. The parent can facilitate the evaluation by helping the child become more comfortable and compliant or by reporting on the specific skills the child has that he/she may not be displaying during the evaluation (e.g., running, catching a ball, counting, drawing a circle, etc.).

DEVELOPMENTAL ABILITIES THAT NEED TO BE ASSESSED

Cognitive Abilities

When referred for an evaluation of cognitive abilities, preschool children are typically administered an intelligence test, such as the Wechsler Preschool and Primary Scales of Intelligence, Revised (WPPSI-R) or the Stanford Binet, Fourth Edition (SB-IV). These tests measure broad cognitive abilities ("IQ" or "g"), including verbal and nonverbal reasoning, crystallized intelligence, fluid intelligence, short-term memory, quantitative reasoning, and/or abstract visual reasoning. The Differential Ability Scales-Preschool Level (DAS) is also used to measure "g," verbal intelligence, and nonverbal intelligence. Brief screeners of cognitive abilities may be administered, including the Kaufman Brief Intelligence Test (K-BIT) or the Test of Nonverbal Intelligence-2 (TONI-2).

Motor Abilities

Assessment of motor skills is typically done by a physical therapist, although psychologists who have training in the administration of motor tests may also administer these tests. Three areas are usually evaluated, including fine motor skills, gross motor skills, and sensorimotor functioning. Fine motor skills include holding a pencil, drawing, stacking blocks, building puzzles, using scissors, or opening doors. Gross motor skills include walking, running, going up and down stairs, throwing or catching a ball, jumping, and balancing. Tests that are often used to assess motor skills in preschool children include the Peabody Developmental Motor Scales or the Bruininks-Oseretsky Motor Test. Sensorimotor functioning is typically assessed in preschoolers through interview of the parents. It involves examining the child's tolerance for sensory information and stimulation, and then determining how problems may be affecting the child. Psychologists are also likely to administer a perceptual-motor test, such as the Beery Developmental Test of Visual Motor Integration (VMI), to evaluate the child's visual and fine motor ability. The VMI is a drawing task that requires the child to reproduce two-dimensional shapes that become increasingly complex.

Speech and Language Abilities

Preschool assessment of speech and language skills is typically done by a speech and language pathologist, although a psychologist may also do the assessment. It usually involves evaluating two main areas of language development, expressive and receptive communication. Expressive communication refers to the child's ability to use words and gestures to communicate his or her thoughts with others. Receptive communication refers to the child's ability to understand and interpret what is said to him/her. Briefly, assessment of these skills typically is made with a standardized test such as the Peabody Picture Vocabulary Test or the Preschool Language Scale—Third Edition. Articulation tests are usually administered to determine if the child is having difficulty saying particular sounds. The speech and language pathologist may also undertake audiological screenings to determine if the child has hearing problems that may be interfering with the ability to talk or to hear what is said.

Social/Emotional Functioning

Assessment of preschool children usually involves some measure of emotional or behavioral functioning. There are many different tests that provide information about a child's emotional functioning, and most of these rely on the parent's report because the evaluator is interested in learning about what the child does outside of the structured clinic setting. Emotional and behavioral assessment is typically done by a psychologist who is trained in early childhood development. Emotional problems are often evaluated through interview of the parent, direct observation of the child in the testing setting and in interactions with the parent, and, when possible, through information provided by others who are familiar with the child (i.e., preschool teachers). The psychologist is interested to know the child's typical range of emotions, how he/she responds to changes in schedule or environment, how he/she responds to other children and what his/her interactions with them are like, and how he/she responds to authority figures such as parents or teachers. They are also interested to learn about the child's sleeping and eating habits and if he/she is toilet trained.

Assessment of behavior is done to determine if the child exhibits particular behaviors that are characteristic of psychological problems. Behavior rating scales that the parents and others who are familiar with the child complete are most often used. Popular scales include the Achenbach scales—the Child Behavior Checklist and the Teacher Report Form—and the Behavior Assessment System for Children, Parent and Teacher Rating Scales. Each of these provides a behavioral profile, based on national norms, that is used to compare the child's behavior to that of other children his age.

Adaptive Abilities

Another area that is often assessed in the evaluations of preschoolers is adaptive functioning—a measure of what the child does in daily life, regardless of the child's assessed level of functioning. The Vineland Adaptive Behavior Scales is most commonly used, and with it, four domains of functioning are assessed. The Communication Domain provides an estimate of the child's receptive, expressive, and written language. The Daily Living Skills Domain provides an estimate of the child's self-help and personal skills, as well as his typical activities within the home and community. The Socialization Domain provides an estimate of his typical interactions with peers and others, how he plays and conforms to the rules of play, and the strategies he uses to cope with everyday situations. The Motor Skills Domain provides an estimate of the fine and gross motor skills the child uses in daily life.

SUMMARY

The main purpose of preschool assessment is to determine the need for early intervention for the 2- to 6-year old child. Once it is determined that a child needs early intervention, the professionals who work with the child make recommendations and referrals. It is important to understand the child's functioning in all of the areas described above so that appropriate recommendations can be made and opportunities for remedial services are not missed. Many preschoolers have significant delays in several areas, which affect the priority of the interventions that are suggested. Each child must be considered individually, but there are some common guidelines that professionals use to make referrals. When cognitive delays are revealed, the child is often referred to an early intervention preschool or for a special education classroom, depending on the severity of the delays. When motor delays are revealed, the child is referred for physical or occupational therapy. When communication delays are revealed, the child is typically referred for speech and language therapy or for special education to learn alternative ways of communicating. Most referrals can be made to professionals within the school system due to current laws that provide for such services. Occasionally, the child will be referred to external professionals who provide services such as psychological therapy.

See also: Adaptive Behavior Assessment; Developmental Milestones; Intellectual Assessment; Language Development; Language Disorders; Speech and Language Assessment

Further Reading

Bracken, B. (1991). *The psychoeducational assessment of preschool children* (2nd ed.,). Boston: Allyn & Bacon.
Culbertson, J. L., & Willis, D. J. (1993). *Testing young children*. Austin, TX: PRO-ED.

Web Sites

http://www.childpsychologist.com/
http://www.ncld.org/advocacy/fedlaws.cfm

Tracy Hopkins-Golightly
Jan L. Culbertson

Prescreening

See: Screening Instruments: Behavioral and Developmental

Prevention

See: Early Intervention; Safety and Prevention

Primary Care

See: Physician (General, Specialty)

Primary Care Physicians

See: Physician (General, Specialty)

Primary Immunodeficiency

See: Bone Marrow Failure and Primary Immunodeficiency

Primary Prevention

See: Safety and Prevention

Problem-Solving Assessment

See: Social Problem-Solving Assessment

Problem-Solving Training

Problem-solving training is a therapeutic intervention that aims to assist children to improve their ability at general problem-solving, although the focus tends of be on problems of an interpersonal nature. This technique discourages children from responding rashly to problem situations, and instead encourages them to follow a problem-solving routine that involves several steps and is more likely to result in a successful outcome. Problem-solving training can be aimed at a single individual or can involve a group of people. When a group is involved, the training may be limited to the interactions within that group, for example, those between adolescents and their parents.

The key objective of problem-solving training is not for the clinician to help the child solve a particular problem. In contrast, it is for the clinician to teach the child to use a problem-solving routine that can then be used to solve any presenting problem. As such, it is a complex process.

Problem-solving training typically begins with some form of general orientation in which the clinician explains the rationale for problem-solving. The clinician encourages the children to view their difficulties as problems to solve, and discourages them from using maladaptive responses, such as ignoring the problems or viewing them as insoluble.

Following the general orientation, children are introduced to the problem-solving routine that can be used with most problems. This routine comprises of five steps, the first of which is problem definition and formulation. The child is encouraged to define the problem in specific, objective terms. This involves breaking down the problem into more manageable parts, and seeking out all available facts about the problem in an effort to answer the who, what, when, where, why, and how of the situation.

The second step of the problem-solving routine involves actively brainstorming multiple solutions to the identified problem. An important part of this stage is to identify as many alternative solutions as possible, which means that seemingly "silly" or "impossible" solutions

count equally as potential solutions. Although there is no required number of solutions, the client is instructed that having more alternatives will increase optimism about their ability to solve problems.

The third step of the problem-solving routine is decision-making. After having generated several options, the child is encouraged to consider the potential consequences and positive outcomes of each alternative solution and weigh the costs and benefits of each before proceeding with implementation. Each alternative is rated in terms of its feasibility, the likelihood of the solution yielding a positive outcome, the perceived fit between the solution and the selected problem, and the ability of the child to cope with obstacles that may arise. The child then decides on the strategy with the most reinforcing and the fewest punishing consequences. Consideration is then given to specific behaviors that are needed to carry out the chosen solution.

The fourth step of the problem-solving routine is that of implementing the selected solution to the problem.

The fifth step is to systematically review the outcome of the implementation of the solution selected and to assess its success. Children are encouraged to evaluate how effective their solution was in solving the problem and to identify the effects and consequences for each individual involved in the problem situation. If success has not been achieved, children are encouraged to either modify the implemented solution or try one of the options previously considered. This process continues until a satisfactory solution is achieved.

When teaching a child to use the problem-solving routine, the clinician helps the child client work through several problem situations. At first the clinician is quite directive and leads the child through each of the steps of the routine. As the child becomes more confident and competent, the clinician plays a less directive role and the child implements the routine more independently.

Throughout the total process of problem-solving training, the clinician and child deal with a number of the child's problems. It is important that the problems chosen for the early trials of using the problem-solving routine are not the most difficult ones in the child's life. These should be saved for when the child becomes more able to successfully implement the routine.

Problem-solving training is an intervention with generalized applicability. It has been used successfully for resolving parent–adolescent conflict, for marital and relationship counseling, for anger control, for overcoming social skill deficits, as well as for other disorders of childhood and adolescence. Effective problem-solving can yield a variety of additional benefits, including warding off negative emotions such as anxiety and anger that hamper problem-solving efforts, promoting positive emotional experiences and a sense of competency and self-efficacy that facilitate future problem-solving and positive mental well-being.

From a theoretical perspective, problem-solving training, like behavior contracts, is related to the establishment of rule-governed behavior. Rule-governed behavior involves individuals engaging in particular behaviors because they have been informed of the reinforcement that will be earned by that behavior. Unlike behavior contracts, however, these rules are not command rules but more advisory as the clinician is unlikely to control the relevant reinforcers.

See also: Applied Behavior Analysis; Behavior Contracts; Positive Reinforcement; Rule-Governed Behavior

Further Reading

Barkley, R. A., Edwards, G. Laneri, M. Fletcher, K., & Matevia, L. (2001). The efficacy of problem-solving communication training alone, behavior management training alone, and their combination for parent-adolescent conflict in teenagers with ADHD and ODD. *Journal of Consulting & Clinical Psychology*, 69, 926–941.

Blechman, E. A. (1980). Family problem-solving training. *The American Journal of Family Therapy*, 8, 3–21.

Nangle, D. W., Carr-Nangle, R. E., & Hansen, D. J. (1994). Enhancing generalization of a contingency management intervention through the use of family problem-solving training: Evaluation with a severely conduct-disordered adolescent. *Child & Family Behavior Therapy*, 16, 65–76.

SOPHIA XENOS
ALAN HUDSON

Table 1. Professional Societies Relevant to Clinical Child and Pediatric Psychology

Society Name & Web Site	Mission/Description	Publications
American Psychological Association (APA) http://www.apa.org/	Largest scientific and professional organization representing psychology in the United States; the world's largest association of psychologists.	*American Psychologist, Monitor on Psychology*
APA Division 53—Society of Clinical Child and Adolescent Psychology http://www.clinicalchildpsychology.org/	Represents teaching, research, clinical services, administration, and advocacy in clinical child psychology. Supports task forces on the development and evaluation of effective treatments for childhood disorders; coordinates efforts for dissemination of information about evidence-based services.	*Journal of Clinical Child & Adolescent Psychology; Clinical Child & Adolescent Psychology Newsletter*
APA Division 54—Society of Pediatric Psychology http://www.apa.org/divisions/div54/	Dedicated to research/practice issues, addressing the relationship between children's physical, cognitive, social, and emotional functioning and their physical well-being, including maintenance of health, promotion of positive health behaviors, and treatment of chronic or serious medical conditions, including the behavioral and developmental aspects of acute and chronic diseases. Sponsors task forces on empirically supported treatments, health-related treatment outcomes, and collaborating with pediatricians.	*Journal of Pediatric Psychology;* Newsletter: *Progress Notes*
APA Divison 12—Society of Clinical Psychology http://www.apa.org/divisions/div12/homepage.html	Practice, research, teaching, administration, and/or study in the field of clinical psychology. Has several subsections, including the Society for a Science of Clinical Psychology, Clinical Psychology of Ethnic Minorities, and the Association of Medical School Psychologists.	*Clinical Psychology: Science and Practice;* Newsletter: *The Clinical Psychologist.*
APA Division 7—Developmental Psychology http://classweb.gmu.edu/awinsler/div7/homepage.html	Promotes and fosters the development of researchers; facilitates exchange of scientific information about developmental psychology; promotes high standards for the application of scientific knowledge on human development to public policy issues.	Newsletter: *Developmental Psychology*
APA Division 37—Child, Youth, and Family Services http://www.apa.org/divisions/div37/	Promotes application of psychological knowledge to advocacy, service delivery, and public policies affecting children, youth, and families. Advances research, education, training, and practice. Activities have focused on such topics as: divorce and custody, child abuse prevention, pediatric AIDS, drug-exposed infants, latchkey children, homelessness, and systems of care, as well as having a subsection on child maltreatment.	Newsletter: *The Child, Youth & Family Services Advocate*

(Continued)

Table 1. (*Continued*)

Society Name & Web Site	Mission/Description	Publications
Association for Advancement of Behavior Therapy (AABT) http://www.aabt.org/	Interdisciplinary organization regarding application of behavioral and cognitive sciences to understand human behavior, developing interventions to enhance the human condition, and promoting the appropriate utilization of these interventions.	*Behavior Therapy; Cognitive & Behavioral Practice;* Newsletter: *the Behavior Therapist*
Society for Research in Child Development (SRCD) http://www.srcd.org/	Multidisciplinary, international association of researchers and practitioners. Purposes: to promote multidisciplinary research in the field of human development, to foster the exchange of information, and to encourage applications of research findings.	*Child Development; Monographs of SRCD; Social Policy Report*
American Academy of Pediatrics (AAP) http://www.aap.org/	Promote optimal physical, mental, and social health and well-being for all infants, children, adolescents and young adults. Dedicated to enhancing health, safety, and well-being of infants, children, adolescents and young adults.	*Pediatrics; Pediatrics in Review,* Newsletter: *AAP News*
Society for Developmental and Behavioral Pediatrics (SDBP) http://www.dbpeds.org/	Promote multidisciplinary research in the field of human development, to foster the exchange of information among scientists and other professionals of various disciplines, and to encourage applications of research findings. Promote better care and outcomes for children and families affected by developmental, learning, and behavioral problems.	*Journal of Developmental and Behavioral Pediatrics*
American Psychological Society (APS) http://www.psychologicalscience.org/	Dedicated solely to scientific psychology. Promote, protect, and advance the interests of scientifically oriented psychology in research, application, and the improvement of human welfare.	*Psychological Science; Current Directions in Psychological Science; Psychological Science in the Public Interest*
American Academy of Child and Adolescent Psychiatry (AACAP) http://www.aacap.org/	Professional medical organization comprised of child and adolescent psychiatrists trained to promote healthy development and to evaluate, diagnose, and treat children and adolescents and their families who are affected by disorders of feeling, thinking, and behavior.	*Journal of the American Academy of Child and Adolescent Psychiatry*
Society of Behavioral Medicine http://www.sbmweb.org/	Interdisciplinary field concerned with the development and integration of behavioral, psychosocial, and biomedical science knowledge and techniques relevant to the understanding of health and illness, and the application of this knowledge and these techniques to prevention, diagnosis, treatment, and rehabilitation.	*Annals of Behavioral Medicine*
National Association of School Psychologists http://www.nasponline.org	Promotes educationally and psychologically healthy environments for all children and youth by implementing research-based, effective programs that prevent problems, enhance independence, and promote optimal learning.	*School Psychology Review* and *Communiqué* official newspaper

Professional Societies in Clinical Child and Pediatric Psychology

Membership in professional societies is an important component of professional practice in clinical child and pediatric psychology. Societies provide a forum for clinicians, researchers, educators, and students to participate in salient issues within the field. Communication is facilitated through regular newsletters and Internet list discussions regarding up to date legislative and policy issues, legal and ethical issues in professional practice, in addition to state of the art science and clinical practice. These organizations often sponsor publications of journals, newsletters, and clinical workshops for continuing education credit. Membership also facilitates collaboration among colleagues within one's own discipline, as well as providing an avenue for extending beyond one's own practice into alternative realms (e.g., working with pediatricians). Societies foster future collaboration and consultation between groups of professionals who are dedicated to a similar cause, namely, the promotion of health and well-being among children and families in society and enhance professional identity.

Table 1 provides a list of professional societies that are relevant to clinical child and pediatric psychology. Within this area, there are a number of broad and specific organizations with a variety of missions. For example, the American Psychological Association (APA) acts as the umbrella institution to a number of more specific interest Divisions, several with child, family, and health interests. Divisions 53 and 54 of APA are specific to Clinical Child and Adolescent Psychology and Pediatric Psychology, respectively, with their focus on relevant issues to research, practice, and advocacy within the field. APA Division 37 focuses on child, youth, and family service issues, integrating public policy issues and child advocacy. This Division also has a focused section on child maltreatment. Division 38, Health Psychology, addresses a variety of health-related issues across the lifespan, although it emphasizes topics often related more to adults than to children. Similarly, the Association for the Advancement of Behavior Therapy (AABT) represents professionals interested in behavior therapy and now cognitive therapy as a whole, but also has Special Interest Groups where those with more specific interests can communicate on issues of greater interest and in greater depth (e.g., Child and School-Related Issues, Child and Adolescent Anxiety). Another broad-based organization important to clinical child and pediatric psychology is the Society for Research in Child Development (SRCD), which is focused on normative human development and has a strong scientific orientation.

Professionals often find a "professional home" from society membership, in that they relate with colleagues dedicated to similar interests and values within the profession. Annual meetings are one way to stay in touch with dispersed colleagues or friends from graduate school. Access to information through membership is effective, convenient, and often provides practical information that can be applied to daily practice. One is able to stay in touch with state-of-the-art research and practice. Communication between clinicians, researchers, and academicians is also facilitated through membership, and a sense of professional identity is established and maintained. These organizations frequently have special student membership dues and programs to foster development of a professional identity early in a career.

See also: Child and Adolescent Psychiatry; Clinical Child Psychology; Family Physician; Health Care Professionals (General); Nursing; Pediatrician; Pediatric Psychology

SARAH T. TRANE
MICHAEL C. ROBERTS

Projective Techniques

The term "projective" derives from the traditional psychoanalytic concept of projection. This concept describes the process of organizing and giving meaning to our sensory perceptions, which are based largely on our individual attributes and life experiences. When presented with something that is clear and unambiguous, for example, a pencil, the interpretation of it tends to be fairly consistent among observers. However, when presented with something unclear and ambiguous, for example, a light or shadow in the dark, there is a fairly wide range of interpretations among observers. These interpretations reflect the unique attributes of each individual observer. In reacting to such an ambiguous stimulus, the person organizes the perception and "projects" outwardly from within to shape and give meaning to the "reality" perceived. This unique interpretation or "projection" can potentially reveal something meaningful about the person. This is the "projective hypothesis" that underlies the use of "projective techniques" in psychological assessment.

The development of projective techniques originated in the early 20th century with strong ties to the clinical traditions of psychoanalysis. The use of a projective technique involves presentation of a standard set of ambiguous stimuli (e.g., pictures, words, inkblots) to a person, requesting the person to respond to these stimuli, and recording the person's responses to them. These responses are then examined in a systematic way for content and patterns of response, which can reveal important facets of psychological functioning. A wide variety of measures have evolved over time, which make use of visual and auditory stimulus materials to elicit primarily verbal and writing/drawing responses. These measures are usually categorized as one of three types: (1) drawing methods, (2) apperceptive methods, and (3) inkblot methods.

1. *Drawing methods* (e.g., Draw-a-Person, Human Figure Drawing, Kinetic Family Drawing, House-Tree-Person) employ a strategy of providing a standard set of materials and instructions for the person to draw certain objects and/or people. The person has a free rein to draw the figures however he/she chooses, in true projective fashion. In the long history of drawing methods, there have been numerous attempts to establish a standard scoring system and normative data by which drawings can be evaluated and interpreted with some degree of scientific rigor. These efforts have not been very successful and, to date, there is no one system for scoring

drawing responses that has strong empirical support for its use. The current state of the art for the use of drawing methods involves the impressionistic evaluation of a drawing for signs that a given clinician, based on clinical experience, determines to be meaningful and related to different aspects of psychological functioning.

2. *Apperceptive methods* (e.g., Thematic Apperception Test [TAT], Children's Apperception Test, Roberts Apperception Test for Children) are composed of a standard set of pictures that are presented to a person, with a standard set of instructions for responding. For each picture, the person is asked to tell a story about the picture, after which the clinician typically asks a number of questions to clarify details of the story. As with drawing methods, there have been attempts to develop standard scoring procedures and normative data, but these have proven to be cumbersome and few clinicians make use of such approaches to evaluating the data gathered. Additionally, there is limited empirical support for these scoring procedures. The current state of the art for the use of apperceptive methods involves the impressionistic evaluation of the stories produced, to identify prominent themes related to the thinking style, emotional experience, interpersonal relations, and other important facets of experience for the subject.

3. *Inkblot Methods* (e.g., Rorschach) rely on the presentation of a standard set of printed inkblots with instruction to respond verbally to the question, "what might this be?" The person's responses are written down and evaluated by the clinician in one of two ways. It is fairly common for clinicians to use the Rorschach much like the other projective methods, impressionistically, based on their clinical experience. However, there is a standard scoring system available, the Comprehensive System, for which there is fairly strong empirical support and normative data available for a more systematic approach to interpretation.

From the beginning, the use of projective techniques has been controversial, and these techniques have been the target of criticism regarding their reliability and validity. In recent years, the controversy has centered primarily upon the Rorschach Inkblot Method and the scientific merit of the Comprehensive System for Scoring the Rorschach. With passionate arguments from proponents and opponents, the controversy continues without resolution. For a more thorough review of this controversy, the reader is referred the references that follow.

Despite the controversy surrounding their reliability and validity, projective techniques, including the Rorschach, Human Figure Drawings, and TAT, remain among the most frequently used psychological assessment tools in the mental health professions. In the hands of a talented and experienced clinician, these methods can yield rich clinical data which can greatly enhance the assessment and understanding of complex psychological processes. As with any good tool, however, in the hands of an amateur, the potential for misuse is great. The key to appropriate use of projective techniques is recognition of and respect for their limitations, and confining their use within those limits to enrich and enhance a comprehensive psychological evaluation that employs multiple methods to gather data from multiple sources of information.

Projective techniques are especially well-suited for use with children, adolescents, and others who, for various reasons, are unable or unwilling to fully express the thoughts, emotions, and issues relevant to understanding the psychological difficulties they experience. They afford a vehicle to access such material that otherwise might not be accessible through other means. In the context of criticisms of the reliability and validity of projective techniques and their known limits, they may best be reserved for use at the early stages of the assessment process, to generate hypotheses, identify potentially relevant issues, and uncover otherwise inaccessible material for further evaluation with other assessment tools. Thus, many projective techniques can be used appropriately and effectively for initial exploration to discover issues or areas of functioning requiring more thorough assessment. Yet, within the scope of standardized administration, scoring, and interpretation, some methods such as the Rorschach can be used reliably and validly in the later stages of assessment as a component of a comprehensive, empirically sound evaluation.

See also: Psychometric Clinical Utility; Interviewing Mental Status Examination; Properties of Tests

Further Reading

Finch, A. J., Jr., & Belter, R. W. (1993). Projective techniques. In T. H. Ollendick & M. Hersen (Eds.), *Handbook of child and adolescent assessment* (pp. 224–236). Boston: Allyn & Bacon.

Rabin, A. I. (Ed.). (1986). *Projective techniques for adolescents and children*. New York: Springer.

Weiner, I. B. (1996). Some observations on the validity of the Rorschach Inkblot Method. *Psychological Assessment, 8,* 206–213.

Wood, J. M., Nezworski, T., & Stejskal, W. J. (1996). The comprehensive system for the Rorschach: A critical examination. *Psychological Science, 7,* 3–17.

RONALD W. BELTER

Pseudoseizures

See: Epilepsy

Psoriasis

See: Dermatology: Dermatitis and Psoriasis

Psychiatric Inpatient Treatment

DEFINITION

Psychiatric inpatient treatment provides 24-hr care to children and adolescents with serious emotional disturbances. Although there are no widely accepted criteria for hospitalization, inpatient care is generally reserved for children who are in acute crisis and are seen as dangerous to themselves or others. Common presenting problems include highly aggressive or destructive behavior, suicide attempts or threats, acute psychotic episodes, and severe self-harming behaviors (e.g., cutting self, anorexia). Psychiatric inpatient units may be self-contained facilities or special wards in a general medical hospital. Some families voluntarily admit their children to inpatient care; other children are committed by the state. State laws vary as to criteria and procedures for involuntary admission.

Due largely to general fiscal trends over the past 20 years, such as the rising cost of health care and the emergence of health maintenance organizations (HMOs), the average length of child inpatient stay has declined in the United States from at least a month (and often longer) to slightly over a week. Children are usually discharged as soon as it is felt that they no longer pose an acute danger to themselves or others. At present, psychiatric inpatient care is commonly seen in the United States as the equivalent of medical intensive care—as a brief, expensive intervention that should be undertaken only when absolutely necessary and whose goal should be crisis stabilization and transition of the child to less restrictive outpatient services.

METHODS

Methods of inpatient treatment vary according to the facility and the needs of the individual child. Unit staffs generally include nurses, psychiatric aides, psychiatrists, social workers, and teachers. Psychologists, art therapists, and recreational therapists are commonly employed as well. Children are almost always seen for brief individual therapy, although the amount of therapy, the provider, and the theoretical orientation vary widely. Children generally also attend the group therapy of the unit. Group therapy may take the form of general groups that allow for appropriate emotional expression and review of problems or progress. Some units include specialized group therapy that targets children with specific problems, such as a history of abuse or substance use. Children may attend art therapy or recreational groups, as well. Brief family therapy is frequently offered, as are parent support and educational groups. Inpatient treatment also allows for trials of psychotropic medications in a controlled environment where the child's reactions can be closely monitored. A major component of treatment is in ensuring that the family will have adequate aftercare services after the child is discharged, such as individual and family therapy and medication management. For children who have been removed from their home environment by the state, aftercare planning normally includes finding appropriate residential or therapeutic foster care, and these children at times experience prolonged inpatient stays until these services can be put into place.

Inpatient care is frequently seen as an opportunity for intensive behavioral intervention, because children are observed at all times by unit staff. Most inpatient units have in place a level or point system in which the child's behavior determines what privileges he or she is allowed. Levels and points are often discussed at community group meetings involving patients and nursing staff, allowing children to receive feedback about their behavior from their peers and staff members. Children who demonstrate good behavior usually earn special treats such as time playing with special toys or video games, picking from a prize box, or going outside the unit with family members. Time out and loss of points or privileges are common interventions for disruptive behavior.

Staff members intervene individually when children become distressed or aggressive, providing support and limits. Children who become uncontrollably aggressive or self-injurious are dealt with in various ways. Some hospitals place out-of-control children in unlocked or locked seclusion rooms or in mechanical restraints (e.g., to a mattress with leather cuffs) until they calm down. Other hospitals use therapeutic holding, in which the out-of-control children are physically held in a safe position by unit staff until the child regains self-control. Sedating medication is sometimes used instead of, or in addition to, the above interventions.

Some psychiatric hospitals include a day treatment program, in which children arrive in the morning and go home every evening. Day treatment is often used (if the child's insurance will cover it) as a transitional level between inpatient care and discharge to the home environment. This transition allows children's behavior at home in the evenings to be closely monitored, with a transition back to inpatient care easily facilitated if necessary.

CLINICAL APPLICATIONS

Child and adolescent inpatient care had been studied with patient populations ages 3–17. Studies have included patients from a wide range of socio-economic and ethnic backgrounds. Reviews of inpatient studies show that the most common diagnoses are non-psychotic mood and conduct disorders, often with comorbid attention-deficit hyperactivity disorder (ADHD). A smaller percentage of children receive diagnoses of psychotic disorders. Children with pervasive developmental disorders (e.g., autism, mental retardation) can also be treated in an inpatient setting if they are severely aggressive or self-injurious.

EFFECTIVENESS

A major review of treatment outcome studies conducted in 2000 by Pottick and colleagues showed that all follow-up studies demonstrated some positive treatment outcome, with more than half reporting long-term improvements. In general, healthier children responded better to inpatient treatment, especially children with adequate intelligence, pure anxiety or affective disorders, later onset of symptoms, nonpsychotic and nonorganic diagnoses, and absence of antisocial features or bizarre symptoms. The level of parent and family pathology appears to be a strong factor in treatment outcome because, while the child's symptoms may improve during hospitalization, he or she usually returns to an unchanged home environment.

It is important to note that the outcome studies in the 2000 review all had longer mean lengths of stay than is currently the norm. No study to date has examined treatment outcome for the short-stay, continuum of care model that is now widespread in the United States. In 1988, psychiatrists John Jemerin and Irving Philips warned that the trend in shortened inpatient stays was resulting in less intensive child and family interventions, increased use of physical restraints, and a "revolving door" pattern in which children with severe emotional disturbances cycle between one hospitalization to the next without adequately resolving the issues that brought them into inpatient care in the first place. Between the years 1988 and 1995, the median length of psychiatric inpatient stay in U.S. general hospitals declined further from 20 to 11 days for children ages 6–12 and from 12 to 8 days for adolescents. It is clear that this new model of care warrants further research before it can be considered an effective intervention.

See also: Child Psychotherapy; Cognitive–Behavior Therapy; Group Psychotherapy; Residential Treatment

Further Reading

Blanz, B., & Schmidt, M. (2000). Practitioner review: Preconditions and outcome of inpatient treatment in child and adolescent psychiatry. *Journal of Child Psychology and Psychiatry, 41*(6), 703–712.

Jemerin, J., & Philips, I. (1988). Changes in inpatient child psychiatry: Consequences and recommendations. *Journal of the American Academy of Child and Adolescent Psychiatry, 27*(4), 397–403.

Pottick, K., McAlpine, D., & Anderson, R. (2000) Changing patterns of psychiatric inpatient care for children and adolescents in general hospitals, 1988–1995. *American Journal of Psychiatry, 157*, 1267–1273.

MARY BRINKMEYER
SHEILA M. EYBERG

Psychiatric Interview

See: Interviewing

Psychodynamic Therapy

Psychodynamic therapy focuses on underlying cognitive, affective, and interpersonal processes from a developmental perspective. The level of development of these processes and the interaction among them determines the child's behaviors, relationships, and internal feelings and thoughts. The therapist works with these internal processes in order to bring about changes in symptoms and the child's overall functioning.

Psychodynamic approaches evolved from psychoanalytic theory and therapy. Psychodynamic therapy has more focused goals, is less intense (weekly sessions versus more frequent sessions), and is more flexible in terms of types of intervention techniques and theoretical perspectives than psychoanalytic therapy. For example, the therapist might include modeling techniques, role-playing, or family sessions with a particular child, but always within a psychodynamic conceptualization of the case.

TYPES OF PSYCHODYNAMIC THERAPIES

In most forms of psychodynamic therapies, the child and therapist meet individually once a week for 40–50 min sessions. The mutual agreement between the child and the therapist is that the therapist is there to help the child express feelings and thoughts, understand causes of his or her behavior, and form a relationship with the therapist. Traditionally, the child structures the therapeutic hour by choosing the topics, forms of play, and, in general, determines the pace of the therapy. For children from 4 to 10, play is usually an important part of the therapy. In most cases, individual work with the child is only part of the treatment program.

Different types of psychodynamic therapies have different treatment goals and utilize different intervention techniques and mechanisms of change. The psychodynamic framework views childhood disturbance within a developmental context. Through the assessment process, one identifies which underlying processes have developed problems or deficits and need to be addressed in therapy. Three major types of therapy emerge in the current child psychotherapy literature. Discussions of these types of therapies can be found in commentaries by Chethik (2000) and Russ (1998).

Insight-Oriented Therapy

The form of therapy most associated with the psychodynamic approach is insight-oriented therapy, and it is most appropriate for the child with anxiety and internalized conflicts. This approach is appropriate for children who show evidence of internal conflicts and unresolved fears, can trust adults and form relationships, and are verbal or can use play as a form of communication. Many of the anxiety disorders, post-traumatic stress disorders, and depressive disorders are appropriate for insight-oriented therapy.

The goals of insight-oriented therapy are to help the child resolve internal conflicts and master developmental tasks. The major mechanism of change is insight and working through these conflicts. Through the use of play and interpretation from the therapist, the child expresses negative emotion and frightening thoughts and learns to understand those feelings and to manage them. The therapist labels, clarifies, and interprets what the child expresses. The therapist helps the child re-experience the conflict or situational trauma in therapy. Cognitive insight into origins of feelings and conflicts, causes of symptoms, and links between thoughts, feelings, and actions is the goal of therapy. Verbal labeling of unconscious impulses, conflicts, and causes of behavior helps lend higher order reasoning skills to understanding problems. However, in many cases, especially with young children, this cognitive insight does not occur. Rather, as Messer and Warren (1999) pointed out, emotional reexperiencing, emotional working through, and conflict resolution do occur and result in symptom reduction and healthy adjustment.

Structure Building Approaches

Structure building approaches are used with children who have deficits in internal representations (i.e., problems with having clear, steady, and positive mental images and expectations of others). These children typically have problems forming attachments to others, empathizing with others, differentiating fantasy from reality, and modulating emotions and impulses. These problems are evident in children with psychotic disorders and characterological disorders.

The growing theory on the development of internal representations, attachment, and the self reflects a new phase in psychodynamic theory. In this form of therapy, empathy and understanding on the part of the therapist (a general relationship factor) is a much more important technique than interpretation. The therapist empathizes and validates the experience of the child and this helps with relationship building and self-development. Kohut and Wolfe have discussed the importance of communicating understanding of the pain of empathic failures in the past. The therapist also helps differentiate fantasy from reality. Chethik (2002) provides an excellent discussion of treating borderline children and narcissistically disturbed children. Therapy with these seriously disturbed children is usually long-term (1–2 years).

Supportive Therapy

Supportive therapy is most appropriate for children with externalizing disorders. These children frequently act out, have antisocial tendencies, and are impulse-ridden. Theoretically, psychodynamic theory views these children as having major developmental problems in processes that would help them control impulses and empathize with others. Supportive therapy focuses on the here and now, and on the development of problem-solving and coping skills. A psychodynamic understanding informs the use of role-playing or self-talk to manage impulses.

CURRENT TRENDS IN PSYCHODYNAMIC THERAPY

Short-term therapy and more active therapeutic approaches are a growing trend in psychodynamic therapy. Messer and Warren (1995) point out that short-term therapy (6–12 sessions) is a frequent form of psychodynamic intervention. The practical realities of health maintenance organizations (HMOs) and of clinical practice in general have led to briefer forms of treatment. Messer and Warren (1995) conclude that children with less severe psychopathology are more responsive to brief intervention than children with chronic developmental problems. Chethik (2000) also discussed a short-term approach, "focal therapy," which deals with specific stressful events in the child's life such as divorce or illness. The therapist is very active in these brief interventions in that she is active in interpreting play, may be directive in suggesting topics or toys, uses modeling and role-playing, and integrates techniques from other theoretical approaches.

RESEARCH WITH PSYCHODYNAMIC APPROACHES

Unfortunately, there is little empirical support for the effectiveness of broad-based psychodynamic approaches with specific populations at this time. Fonagy and Moran in 1990 pointed out that the main reason for this lack of research is that the rather global approach and broad goals of psychodynamic approaches do not lend themselves easily to carefully controlled outcome studies. However, some studies do exist. Fonagy and Moran (1990) themselves have carried out different types of studies that are well-suited to psychodynamic therapy. For example, they used a time-series analysis and found a relationship between major

themes in therapy and diabetic control in a diabetic teenager. There is also empirical support in the play intervention literature that the use of fantasy play decreases anxiety and fear in children. These new research approaches should be used to empirically investigate psychodynamic approaches.

See also: Child Psychotherapy; Cognitive–Behavioral Play Therapy; Family Intervention; Play Therapy

Further Reading

Chethik, M. (2000). *Techniques of child therapy: Psychodynamic strategies*. (2nd ed.). New York: Guilford.
Fonagy, P., & Moran, G. S. (1990). Studies on the efficacy of child psychoanalysis. *Journal of Consulting and Clinical Psychology, 58*, 684–695.
Messer, S. B. & Warren, C. S. (1995). *Models of brief psychodynamic therapy*. New York: Guilford.
Russ, S. W. (1998). Psychodynamically based therapies. In T. H. Ollendick & M. Hersen (Eds.) *Handbook of child psychopathology* (3rd ed., pp. 537–556). New York: Plenum Press.

SANDRA W. RUSS

Psychoimmunology

DEFINITION

Psychoimmunology refers to the effects of psychological variables on the immune system and vice versa. Thus, influences are bidirectional. Deficiencies in the immune system may lead to psychological disorders, for instance in a subset of children diagnosed with autism. Alternatively, some environmental toxins, such as endotoxins, may be inhaled in dust inflaming the lungs resulting in respiratory problems and "sickness" behaviors. Very little of this research has been done on children. Although most of research has been done on the effects of negative emotions on health among adults and the aging population, many of these studies are also relevant to infants and children.

There is now substantial evidence, mostly gathered over the last decade, that severe depression, anxiety, and hostility or anger negatively affect physical health by affecting the nervous system, the immune system, and the cardiovascular system. A key mechanism appears to be the failure of proinflammatory cytokines, especially interleukin-6 (IL-6), to respond properly when the immune system responds to infections or trauma. Prolonged failure leads to several diseases in later life, such as cardiovascular disease, osteoporosis, arthritis, type 2 diabetes, cancer, Alzheimer's disease, atherosclerosis, and periodontal disease. Cytokines are protein substances that regulate the immune response to injury and infection. A key concept is allostatic load, that is, the cumulative effects of prolonged exposure to stress due to poor immune function. The immune system is also directly related to the release of pituitary and adrenal hormones and both are affected by emotional stress. People with emotional stress also often have other bad habits, for example, sleep disorders, drug and alcohol abuse, poor nutrition, lack of exercise, all of which make their situation worse.

CLINICAL APPLICATIONS

The main treatments that have been successful have to do with the promotion of developing and maintaining positive emotion through personality and coping styles and close personal relationships. Positive emotions help to reduce risk due to adverse life events, for example, outcome of surgery. They might also undo the effects of negative emotional risks during physiological recovery. In addition, they may reduce social isolation, a major risk factor for mortality and morbidity. Specific techniques used have been hypnotic suggestion, relaxation training, and classical conditioning of immune function. These interventions have been done mostly on middle-aged adults with low levels of stress, so their generality may be limited.

EFFECTIVENESS

Psychosomatic medicine has a history going back at least two millennia, but it is only recently that psychoimmunology, a sub-discipline of psychosomatic medicine, has gained momentum. Only a few well-controlled studies are available on children, but this is likely to be an area of substantial growth in the future.

See also: Anger; Anxiety Disorders; Cognitive–Behavior Therapy; Depressive Disorder, Major; Pediatric Hypnosis; Rage; Stress Management

Further Reading

Kiecolt-Glaser, J. K., McGuire, L., Robles, T. F., & Glaser, R. (2002). Psychoneuroimmunology and psychosomatic medicine: Back to the future. *Psychosomatic Medicine, 62,* 15–28.

Kiecolt-Glaser, J. K., McGuire, L., Robles, T. F., & Glaser, R. (2002). Emotions, morbidity, and mortality: New perspectives from psychoneuroimmunology. *Annual Review of Psychology, 53,* 83–107.
Solomon, G. F. (2002). *From psyche to soma and back: Tales of biopsychosocial medicine.* Philadelphia: Xlibris.

STEPHEN R. SCHROEDER

Psychological Consultation with Physicians

Psychological consultation is defined as the application of psychological knowledge to the medical management of children and adolescents in the context of a relationship with a physician or another professional. While the primary purpose of psychological consultation is to facilitate the management of clinical problems that present to pediatricians, consultation can also be conducted concerning research and teaching. The process of consultation concerning clinical problems includes collaborative communication about the child's problem, providing new information to the physician and facilitating clinical management by means of collaborative problem-solving.

MODELS OF PSYCHOLOGICAL CONSULTATION

Multiple models of psychological consultation are currently used in practice that vary with respect to the level and depth of shared responsibility as well as their scope (e.g., how many people are involved). Each of the following models has utility depending on the clinical problem and setting.

Independent Consultation Model

The independent consultation model is most familiar to pediatricians because of its similarity to medical consultation. In this model, the psychologist functions as a specialist who provides an assessment and, in some instances, treatment for patients who are referred by pediatricians.

Indirect Consultation Model

In the indirect psychological consultation or process-educative model, the pediatrician retains sole responsibility for clinical management while the psychologist assumes the role of teacher or colleague who provides advice about diagnosis and clinical management of clinical problems or protocols for patient management.

Collaborative Team Model

A third model of psychological consultation, the collaborative team model, is characterized by shared responsibility and joint decision-making among psychologists, pediatricians, and/or other professionals. Collaborative team models can involve a diverse range of programs such as interdisciplinary care of children with developmental disabilities in university-affiliated centers, comprehensive care programs for children and adolescents with chronic physical illness, etc. Effective collaborative team consultation involves sharing of information and expertise across different disciplines in clinical management, research, or teaching.

Systems-Oriented Consultation

The models of consultation described thus far emphasize individual interactions and relationships among the psychologist, pediatrician, and/or other professionals. A final model, the systems-oriented approach, considers the impact of the broader context in which collaborative relations occur. Systems-oriented consultation can involve multiple professionals in different settings and deals with change at a broad level. For example, a systems approach to consultation might address how psychological services in pediatric settings can be modified to be more responsive to families by increasing their access to care.

SETTINGS IN WHICH PSYCHOLOGICAL CONSULTATION TAKES PLACE

Each of the above models can be adapted to specific settings, which influence the kind of consultation that is optimal for that setting.

Outpatient Settings

Psychologists typically provide consultation to pediatricians who are in practice in community settings. As primary health care professionals, pediatricians provide preventive care to children with a wide range of behavioral and developmental problems that might otherwise develop into more serious mental health problems.

Pediatricians' referrals are made by phone, letter, or the parent directly. A broad range of behavioral, developmental, and learning problems are typically referred to psychologists from pediatricians in primary care. Psychologists typically provide feedback concerning their assessments and ongoing intervention to pediatric practitioners by phone, letter, and/or report.

Many parents are especially receptive to psychological services that are offered to their children in the context of a pediatric office because this avoids the stigma often associated with attending a mental health practitioner's office or clinic. Moreover, the frequency of contacts between psychologist, child, and family that generally occur within private pediatric offices usually is often less costly than psychological interventions provided in other settings. Finally, the ready availability of a psychologist within the pediatric office facilitates the referral process as well as continuity and integration of physical and mental health care between pediatricians and psychologists.

Inpatient Settings

Psychological consultation for hospitalized children generally follows a traditional medical model in which the consultant's primary responsibilities involve assessment and communication to referring physicians about diagnostic findings and advice concerning management. Communication of findings from consultation is accomplished by face-to-face contact, notes in the body of the medical chart and/or on a consultation sheet that includes a brief description of presenting problems, history, and procedures, a brief appraisal of the child's problem, and recommendations for management.

RESEARCH ON CONSULTATION

Studies of the effectiveness of psychological consultation services delivered by psychologists in a range of settings have indicated improvement in behavioral problems in response to brief, targeted, psychological interventions and a high level of satisfaction of parents who received the services and for pediatricians who made the referral. Moreover, responsive services that provide timely access for children and families and rapid, clear feedback to practitioners are associated with pediatricians' satisfaction with psychological consultation (see Drotar, 1995, for more detail).

See also: Family Physician; Health Care Professionals (General); Pediatrician; Physician (General, Specialty)

Further Reading

Drotar, D. (1995). *Consulting with pediatricians: Psychological perspectives.* New York: Plenum Press.

Drotar, D., & Zagorski, L. (2001). Providing psychological services in pediatric settings in an era of managed care: Challenges and opportunities. In Hughes, J. N., LaGreca, A., & Conley, J. C. (Eds.), *Handbook of psychological services for children and adolescents* (pp. 89–107). New York: Oxford University Press.

Roberts, M. C., & Wright, L. (1982). The role of the pediatric psychologist as consultant to pediatricians. In J. M. Tuma (Ed.), *Handbook for the practice of pediatric psychology.* New York: Wiley.

Schroeder, C. S. (in press). Collaborative practice in primary care: Lessons learned. In Wildman, B. W., & Stancin, T. (Eds.), *New directions for research and treatment of pediatric psychosocial problems in primary care.* Westport, CT: Greenwood.

DENNIS DROTAR

Psychological Dwarfism

See: Psychological Short Stature

Psychological Factors Affecting Physical Conditions

See: Psychosomatic Disorders

Psychological Impact of a Parent's Chronic Illness

DESCRIPTION

Chronic conditions describe a broad range of illnesses and disabilities that affect adults such as cancer, asthma, diabetes, hemophilia, chronic pain, multiple sclerosis, muscular dystrophies, heart and coronary disease, sensory impairments, and physical disabilities. Frequently these conditions co-occur and complicate the situation, for example, multiple sclerosis and an inability to ambulate. These physical conditions potentially interfere with or strain the normal challenges of parenthood. Although there has been considerable work examining differences in adjustment and development among chronically ill children and adults, far less attention has been devoted to developmental outcomes for children whose parents experience illness and disability.

Parental illness and disability may disrupt developmental pathways for children similar to other adverse events including divorce, financial stress, or alcoholism. Illness-related demands such as restrictions on activities or hospitalizations, and inadequate financial, social, and physical resources for meeting these demands may negatively affect the child and strain his or her coping resources. In contrast, such demands actually may have a positive effect for some children that also should be explored.

APPROACHES

Attempts to understand the effect of parental illness on child development have considered different models and mechanisms by which chronic conditions affect children. Parental illness may challenge family roles. For example, adolescent daughters of ill mothers may take on additional caretaking roles in the family, which increases the child's stress. Other models have approached parental chronic illness as a source of increased stress that challenges family members' coping. For example, parental illness also has been conceptualized as disrupting parenting in many ways such as illness-related stigma, loss of social support, and stress.

FACTORS AFFECTING ADJUSTMENT

The relative severity of an illness (e.g., fatal versus chronic) has not been shown to be a strong predictor of child outcomes. Family members' perceptions of stress and coping styles, however, are associated with child adjustment. Similarly, children's perceptions of illness severity are associated with more distress and less effective coping than objectively measured disease severity; and, the child's perceptions of illness-related demands (e.g., more responsibility in the home) also predict his or her distress. Ineffective coping by parents is associated with more child behavior problems and with ineffective coping by their children.

Parenting behavior and relationships between parents and children also may be affected by chronic conditions. For example, an inability for the ill parent to provide adequate supervision, increased parent–child conflict, and a lack of cohesion in the family all predict poorer child outcomes. Moreover, parental illness occurs in a social context and families may face illness-related reductions in social, financial, and emotional support, such as loss of income when a parent stops working or the other parent cuts back on work to give care. Age and gender are also associated with developmental outcomes in that girls seem to pick up more caregiving roles with ill parents, as do older children generally, than boys and younger children. Unfortunately, far too few studies have carefully examined the effects of parental physical or sensory disabilities to draw definitive conclusions regarding child adjustment.

RESPONDING TO PARENTAL CHRONIC ILLNESS

Clinical child and pediatric psychologists are likely to be called upon to help families attempting to adjust to or live with a parent's chronic condition, or when it appears to be negatively affecting child development. Unfortunately, at this time, research studies offer only general guidance for clinical interventions. To facilitate understanding of families experiencing parental illness, clinicians should be informed about the objective illness severity and illness-related demands as well as family members' perceptions of the illness or condition. Information about conditions can be obtained from several national support organizations such as the National Multiple Sclerosis Society or the American Diabetes Association.

A careful assessment of both the family's and child's past and current level of functioning is needed to plan interventions that will meet the needs of the individual family and child. Family assessment should focus on parenting behavior, family members' perception of illness severity, additional demands placed on the family by the illness, family members coping strategies and changing family roles. The child's functioning should be assessed in multiple settings (e.g., school, home, friends) and from multiple perspectives (e.g., self-report, parent-report, teacher-report). Attention should also be given to the effects of the parent's condition on social roles and social support. For example, the condition may have led to job loss or prevented full participation in children's community activities, which may have contributed to social rejection.

Intervention strategies could include family therapy and cognitive-behavior therapy dealing with coping with the changed situation for the child and his or her increased demands.

SUMMARY

Research has shown that parental chronic illness is associated with increased emotional, social, and financial stress for families and children. Child outcomes in the context of parental illness are influenced by many factors including parenting behavior, family members' perceptions of illness severity, additional demands and stressors, family members coping strategies and changing family roles. Many of the factors influencing adjustment interact with other factors and scientifically supported explanatory models are greatly needed to guide future studies.

See also: Bereavement; Coping with Illness; Family Assessment; Family Interventions; Parental Psychopathology; Stress Management

Further Reading

Armistead, L., Klein, K., & Forehand, R. (1995). Parental physical illness and child functioning. *Clinical Psychology Review*, 15, 409–422.

Champion, K. M., & Roberts, M. C. (2001). The psychological impact of a parent's chronic illness on the child. In C. E. Walker & M. C. Roberts (Eds.), *Handbook of clinical child psychology* (3rd ed., pp. 1057–1073). New York: Wiley.

KELLY M. CHAMPION
MICHAEL C. ROBERTS

Psychological Maltreatment

DEFINITION

Psychological maltreatment is currently defined as a recurrent pattern or extreme instance(s) by a caregiver that communicates to the child that he or she is worthless, flawed, unloved, unwanted, endangered, or of value only if meeting another's needs. It can occur alone or in association with other forms of abuse and neglect. Psychological maltreatment can be evidenced by acts of commission (displays of hostility and aggression) and acts of omission (emotional unavailability), and has been divided into six types: (1) spurning; (2) terrorizing; (3) isolating; (4) exploiting/corrupting; (5) denying emotional responsiveness; and (6) unwarranted withholding of medical care, mental health services, or education. While these categories provide a framework for research, the lack of a consistent definition of psychological maltreatment across disciplines continues, due to several factors: (1) psychological maltreatment occurs in both acts of commission and omission; (2) a lack of physical evidence exists; (3) it may exist alone or in tandem with other forms of maltreatment; (4) it can be identified only within an interpersonal context; and (5) it is often dependent on the developmental stage of the child.

PREVALENCE

Accurate estimates of the incidence rates of psychological maltreatment are unattainable due to the lack of definitional clarity and the difficulties of obtaining clear evidence of its occurrence. According to the U.S. Department of Health and Human Services, in 1999, 6 percent of substantiated child maltreatment cases were purely psychological in nature, distinct from other types of abuse. Retrospective studies examining adults' reports of childhood psychological maltreatment have ranged from 10 to 15 percent. There are no reliable data on the prevalence of psychological maltreatment across socioeconomic levels and different ethnic backgrounds.

RISK FACTORS

Although there are no well-documented risk factors for psychological maltreatment, given its frequent occurrence with other abuse, many of the risk factors for neglect and physical abuse might apply to psychological abuse, for example, heightened levels of parental distress and inappropriate parenting strategies, as well as childhood characteristics such as temperament.

SHORT- AND LONG-TERM EFFECTS

Research examining the short- and long-term effects of psychological maltreatment on children and adolescents has been conducted. Empirically supported short-term effects include: (1) insecure attachment to caregivers; (2) lower levels of social competence and adjustment; (3) higher rates of peer aggression; (4) intellectual deficits such as academic problems, lower academic achievement, and deficits in cognitive ability and problem-solving; and (5) affective-behavioral problems, such as aggression, delinquency, disruptive classroom behavior, self-abusive behavior, hostility, anger and anxiety. Retrospective studies with adults have found evidence of low self-esteem, anxiety,

depression, dissociation, and interpersonal sensitivity. Most notably, in instances of multiple forms of abuse, the presence and severity of psychological maltreatment has been found to be the strongest predictor of maladaptive outcomes and may represent the most important cause of problematic adjustment.

ASSESSMENT OF CHILDREN AND CAREGIVERS

The American Professional Society on the Abuse of Children (APSAC) established a framework for evaluating psychological maltreatment in children and caregivers entitled, *Guidelines for the Psychosocial Evaluation of Suspected Psychological Maltreatment in Children and Adolescents.* According to these guidelines, psychological maltreatment should be assessed when evaluating other forms of maltreatment. The clinical assessment should remain separate from any forensic assessment, and a developmental psychopathology model should be used to assess the child's developmental functioning and abilities. A comprehensive and ecological assessment would include: (1) interviews with the child, family, and other caregivers, such as school personnel; (2) the use of self-report questionnaires; and (3) structured observations to assess the overall functioning, adaptation, and level of symptomatology of the child, family, and parents, as well as the quality of parent–child interactions. There are several instruments in addition to the standard measures used to assess cognitive behavior patterns that are available to evaluate psychological maltreatment. For example, the Trauma Symptom Checklist for Children can be used to assess the child's behavior and symptomatology, the Family Environment Scale can be used to assess family factors, and parental factors can be assessed with the Child Abuse Potential Inventory.

TREATMENT APPROACHES FOR CHILDREN AND CAREGIVERS

Research on treatment effectiveness for children and adolescents who have experienced psychological maltreatment remains sparse due in part to the inconsistency in the definition and recognition of psychological maltreatment. Empirically based treatment approaches that are utilized with various affective and behavioral problems of maltreated children are recommended, as are treatments that (1) incorporate prevention; (2) are available to all families; and (3) continue throughout the child's developmental stages. Fraiberg's clinical infant mental health program and the University of Minnesota's STEEP Project have been shown to be effective for families with infants. Moderate success has been found for play therapy with preschool-aged children, while group therapy and behavioral programs that target relationship problems and promote social competence have evidenced some success with older children. Other recommended treatments for children and adolescents include fostering supportive relationships to resolve the effects of trauma, addressing developmental delays, promoting social competencies, and developing significant positive relationships.

Behavior and cognitive-behavior therapies have proven effective in treating abusive parents when the following techniques have been applied: parent–child management; communication skills training; social skills training; problem-solving skills training; perspective-taking skills training; and independent living skills training (such as money management and assertiveness with social agencies). Other recommended treatments include: (1) a comprehensive treatment model, which emphasizes problem-solving skills, interpersonal relationships, and the resolution of past trauma through crisis intervention; (2) addressing unmet cognitive and emotional developmental needs of the parent to enhance empathy and protection of the child; (3) marital and substance abuse treatment; and (4) emphasizing the family's resources and strengths.

PROGNOSIS

Without intensive child and caregiver treatment, children who are victims of psychological abuse are at high risk for emotional and behavioral problems that can affect their relationships and functioning throughout their lifetimes.

See also: Neglect; Parenting Practices; Physical Abuse; Risk and Protective Factors

Further Reading

American Professional Society on the Abuse of Children (APSAC). (1995). *Guidelines for the psychosocial evaluation of suspected psychological maltreatment in children and adolescents.* Chicago: author.
Bonner, B. L., Logue, M. B., Kaufman, K. L., & Niec, L. N. (2001). Child maltreatment. In C. E. Walker & M. C. Roberts (Eds.), *Handbook of clinical child psychology* (3rd ed., pp. 989–1030). New York: Wiley.
Friedrich, W. N. (2002). An integrated model of psychotherapy for abused children. In J. E. B. Myers, L. Berliner, J. Briere, C. T. Hendrix, C. Jenny, & T. A. Reid (Eds.), *The APSAC handbook on child maltreatment* (2nd ed., pp. 141–158). Thousand Oaks, CA: Sage.
Hart, S. N., Brassard, M. R., Binggeli, N. J., & Davidson, H. A. (2002). Psychological maltreatment. In J. E. B. Myers, L. Berliner, J. Briere, C. T. Hendrix, C. Jenny, & T. A. Reid (Eds.), *The APSAC handbook on child maltreatment* (2nd ed., pp. 79–104). Thousand Oaks, CA: Sage.
U.S. Department of Health and Human Services, Children's Bureau. (1999). *Child maltreatment 1998: Reports from the States to the National Child Abuse and Neglect Data System (NCANDS).* Washington, DC: U.S. Government Printing Office.

BARBARA L. BONNER
MARIANN SUAREZ

Psychological Testing

DEFINITION

In general, psychological testing can be defined as an objective and standardized measure of a sample of behavior administered to assess the cognitive and emotional functioning of children and adults. For example, how quickly a person can arrange a set of colored blocks to match a particular design is a behavior that is measured on many tests of intelligence. Copying marks on a piece of paper followed by spelling words such as cat, hat, horse, and hieroglyphics are behaviors that reflect a measure of a person's ability to spell words. Reading a passage and answering questions about the passage is a behavior that is used to indicate the level of a person's reading comprehension. Endorsing statements such as, "I enjoy learning about new developments in space," may reflect a person's vocational interests. Agreeing or disagreeing with statements such as, "I believe that most people are truthful" or "I am happy most of the time" reflect personality characteristics. The common element in these examples is that a person's behavior is being measured. Psychologists use these samples of behavior to measure abstract attributes such as intelligence, personality, organic pathology, etc. The key word here is "sample." If you want to know about a person's reading ability you ask them to read a sample of words—not the entire dictionary. When the teacher sends home a list of 50 spelling words for Johnny to learn by Friday, the teacher is probably going to test Johnny's spelling by giving him a sample of 15 words from the list, not the entire list.

PSYCHOLOGICAL TESTS VERSUS OTHER TESTS

Several factors differentiate psychological tests from other tests such as a spelling test, tests of intelligence, compatibility tests, relationship tests, health tests, vocational interest tests, and others that can be found on the Internet. First, psychological tests are carefully constructed tests that use samples of behavior to represent the domain of interest. The test developer does not assume that because the questions on the test appear to reflect intelligence, personality, or spelling ability that the test does in fact measure those attributes.

Second, psychological tests are reliable and valid measures. Reliability means consistency—that is, the test results are consistent over time. Validity refers to what the test measures and how well it measures it. A test that consists only of addition problems may be a very valid and reliable measure of addition skills but would not be considered a valid measure of overall math ability. You can have a reliable measure of something without that measure being valid. For example, suppose you weigh yourself and you weigh 125 pounds. Tomorrow, next week, next month, you weigh yourself again and you still weigh 125 pounds give or take a few ounces. You would conclude that the scale was very reliable (consistent) but not accurate (valid) with respect to your weight.

Third, psychological tests are standardized in their administration and scoring to ensure that different examiners administer and score the test in the same manner. Interpretation of scores should also be done in a standardized manner. This requires a normative group to establish a frame of reference for the interpretation of scores.

Fourth, psychological tests are normed on a large group of people. The normative group should represent the people that you expect to take the test. For example, if you wish to measure vocational ability, you would not include young children in the normative sample. Without a normative group as a frame of reference it is not possible to make inferences about a particular score relative to other people. For example, if you score 80 percent on a math test, you might be patting yourself on the back thinking that this score was excellent. And, if the next highest score was 75 percent, you might be correct. However, if the next lowest score was 85 percent your score of 80 percent takes on an entirely different meaning. The normative group establishes the "norm" or average score for psychological tests and the absolute value can vary across tests. For example, the average or mean IQ score is 100, while the average

or mean depression score on the Minnesota Multiphasic Personality Inventory (MMPI) is 50.

COMMON TYPES OF PSYCHOLOGICAL TESTS

Psychological tests are used to assess a variety of abilities and traits, including but not limited to academic achievement, intelligence, personality, vocational skills, and neurological functioning.

Intellectual and achievement tests are most often used to answer questions about school placement or educational needs of a child. These tests are used to diagnose the individual with a variety of disorders or conditions—for example, learning disability, mental retardation, developmental delays being gifted. In addition, for adults, these tests are often used in career counseling or determining the appropriateness for certain types of jobs.

There are many types of personality tests, ranging from tests that measure only one specific trait, for example, depression, to tests that measure the basic dimensions of personality or temperaments such as introversion/extroversion, to tests that aid in diagnosing psychopathology (e.g., anxiety, depression, or a personality disorder) by measuring multiple personality traits. Other uses of personality tests include screening job candidates for positions requiring certain attributes, for example, workers in nuclear power plants or police officers.

The purpose of vocational tests is to help individuals identify occupations that they are well suited for as indicated by their interest and ability. The tests are designed so that the results will help an individual to reach his or her highest level of vocational achievement. These typically include formal psychometric approaches such as occupational interest inventories and aptitude batteries. In general, measures assess an individual's vocational potential for a wide variety of potential jobs.

Neuropsychological tests are used to assess the mental functioning of individuals who have had a traumatic brain injury, or who have dementia, or some other illness known to affect cognitive functioning. The tests are also used to evaluate the progress of patients undergoing rehabilitation for a brain injury or severe illness.

WHAT SHOULD YOU BE AWARE OF WHEN CONSIDERING PSYCHOLOGICAL TESTING?

All psychological tests should be administered, scored, and interpreted by a clinically trained examiner with expertise in the particular area being evaluated.

For example, a person conducting a learning disability evaluation should have training and experience in the administration, scoring, and interpretation of tests of intelligence, academic achievement, and areas related to cognitive and academic skills. This person would not have to have extensive training in the administration and interpretation of personality measures, however. The reverse would be true for someone doing a personality assessment.

PSYCHOLOGICAL TESTING DOES NOT EQUAL PSYCHOLOGICAL ASSESSMENT

Tests are only one part of a comprehensive psychological assessment and test results should never be used alone as the sole basis for decision-making. Test results are influenced by many factors such as cultural and language differences, motivation level of the examinee, or the examinee's motive for taking the test. For example, a person who is being asked to take a battery of tests in relation to a job interview might perform quite differently than a juvenile delinquent who has been court-ordered to undergo psychological testing.

See also: Academic Achievement; Adolescent Assessment; Intellectual Assessment; Preschool Assessment; Psychometric Properties of Tests; School Age Assessment

Further Reading

Internet sources for information about psychological tests and testing: http://www.apa.org/science/testing.html, http://www.ericae.net
Sattler, J. M. (2001). *Assessment of children: Cognitive applications* (4th ed.). San Diego: Jerome M. Sattler.

JEAN SPRUILL
LAURA STOPPELBEIN

Psychology

See: Counseling Psychology; Clinical Psychology; Clinical Child and Adolescent Psychology; Pediatric Psychology; School Psychology

Psychometric Properties of Tests

DEFINITION

As Kamphaus has noted, the term "psychometric" is dated. It emanates from the early days of the modern human testing movement of the 20th century when the enterprise was dominated by individuals who identified themselves as psychologists, at least in the United States, including luminaries such as E. L. Thorndike, Henry Goddard, Arthur Otis, James McKeen Cattell, Lewis Terman, Arthur Pintner, Robert Yerkes, and Florence Goodenough. These influential individuals, among numerous others, created the forerunners of modern cognitive ability tests (intelligence or IQ test would be the dated term to use in reference to these measures) and multilevel survey academic achievement test batteries, more commonly known as group administered achievement tests. Now the field of human measurement is far more diverse and is influenced by statisticians and measurement scientists who would more likely describe the field as "measurement" rather than psychometrics. Further evidence of the breadth of the field and its diverse contributors is provided by the latest version of the *Standards for Educational and Psychological Testing* (AERA, APA, NCME, 1999), where only a single chapter is devoted to "psychological testing" and the term "psychometrics" is not to be found in the index.

Psychological testing, however, may refer to the assessment of cognitive function, neuropsychological assessment, personality testing and temperament assessment, vocational testing, family systems assessment, adaptive behavior assessment, behavior problem assessment, and the assessment of medical coping strategies, among others (AERA, APA, NCME, 1999).

The range of measures used by psychologists is staggering and expanding at an extraordinary rate, as indicated by Kamphaus and colleagues (2000). For example, while the assessment of cognitive function is still dominated by the Wechsler Scales, there are at least 17 alternatives available that are also widely used. In addition, Kamphaus and Frick (2002) note that more than 30 widely used measures of child behavior problems or psychopathology are also in use.

METHODS

This diverse range of measures, however, contains measurement commonalities. Some of these common characteristics include norm-referencing, use of standard score scales, and evidence of reliability and validity. The use of norms is central to most psychological testing because of the need for diagnosis. Inherent in the logic of diagnosis is the concept of deviance from some norm—typically considered to be the typical standard of a population of interest. With regard to intelligence testing, for example, the psychologist may be concerned with ruling out a significant cognitive deficit such as mental retardation. In order to do so, a norming sample based on the population to which the individual is to be compared must be available to make this comparison. Similarly, if a psychologist concludes that a child is "anxious," a norm-referenced statement has been made; the psychologist makes the conclusion that the patient is anxious in comparison to some other normative group or standard such as the population of 6-year-old children, other boys, or girls in treatment for anxiety disorders, for example. For this reason, the creation of adequate norming samples is a central issue in the test development process. When a norm-referenced conclusion is made, it is only as good as the norm sample on which it is based.

Since psychologists are often concerned with diagnosis, they are similarly concerned about comparing individuals. A standard score scale is needed for this purpose. For example, it is often not adequate to determine simply that a child is anxious. For diagnostic purposes it is equally important to determine how anxious he or she is, or the severity of the anxiety. Psychological tests are particularly well-suited for determining the severity of a difference, disability, or disorder since standard scores are offered based on norm samples. While use of history and symptom information is adequate to make a diagnosis based on systems such as the *Diagnostic and Statistical Manual of Mental Disorders (DSM-IV)*, psychologists seek to go further and determine the severity of the disorder or problem domain using psychological tests. Hence, a psychological test may be used to say that the child is not only anxious, but that she is more anxious than 98 percent of the children her age. In addition, her standard score of 75 on the anxiety scale indicates that she is significantly more anxious than she was 6 months ago when her standard score was 60 on the same anxiety scale. Psychological tests, because of their use of norms and standard score scales, allow for the assessment of deviance and severity in a scientific manner.

APPLICATIONS

Psychological testing is ubiquitous and highly variable by country and culture. Practitioners in the United States, for example, have always made great use of psychological testing, although the Chinese are usually credited with having created the forerunners of modern tests of human abilities about 3,000 years ago. Traditionally, psychological tests have been commonly used in many cultures for the assessment of the cognitive abilities of school children and the diagnosis of behavior problems and disorders. Some newer and expanding uses of tests include the assessment of behavioral sequelae of medical disorders, and the health-related behaviors of patients undergoing medical procedures.

See also: Behavioral and Functional Analysis; Intellectual Assessment; Psychological Testing; Projective Techniques; Reliability; Validity

Further Reading

American Educational Research Association, American Psychological Association, & National Council for Measurement in Education. (1999). *Standards for educational and psychological testing.* Washington, DC: Author.

DuBois, Philip H. (1970). *A history of psychological testing.* Boston: Allyn & Bacon.

Kamphaus, R. W. (2001). *Clinical assessment of children's intelligence* (2nd ed.). Needham Heights, MA: Allyn & Bacon.

Kamphaus, R. W., & Frick, P. J. (2002). *Clinical assessment of child and adolescent personality and behavior* (2nd ed.). Needham Heights, MA: Allyn & Bacon.

Kamphaus, R. W., Petoskey, M. D., & Rowe, E. W. (2000). Current trends in psychological testing of children. *Professional Psychology: Research and Practice, 31*, 155–164.

RANDY W. KAMPHAUS

Psychopharmacology

See: Pharmacological Interventions

Psychosocial Short Stature

DEFINITION

Psychosocial Short Stature (PSS), also known as Psychosocial Dwarfism or Kaspar Hauser syndrome, involves otherwise unexplained childhood growth failure or delayed puberty in the context of emotional deprivation and/or a pathological psychosocial milieu. Three distinct subgroups of PSS have been identified and studied. These vary by age of occurrence, association with parental rejection, presence of bizarre behavior, decreased secretion of growth hormone, and response to growth hormone treatment. PSS Type I occurs in infancy, and is not associated with parental rejection, bizarre behavior, and decreased growth hormone. There may be variable response to growth hormone treatment. Failure-to-thrive may be present and parents may be depressed. Type II, or Classic PSS, is the most severe manifestation. It occurs at age 3 or older and is associated with bizarre behavior, decreased growth hormone, and parental pathology or rejection. There is also minimal response to growth hormone treatment. PSS Type III can occur in infancy and beyond, and is associated with normal growth hormone secretion and response to growth hormone. Bizarre behaviors, failure-to-thrive, and parental rejection are not present. It is thought that children with PSS Type III often have co-morbid depression and/or attachment disorders. Parents of these children typically have insight into the problem, and may have feelings of depression and/or guilt.

PREVALENCE/ETIOLOGY

There is little data on the prevalence or etiology of this rare disorder. It is thought to occur most often in Caucasian families. PSS Type I occurs most frequently in families with many young children, with parents who are disorganized, have many other responsibilities, and/or are depressed. Given the bizarre behaviors associated with PSS Type II, it has been the most studied and this type of PSS will be the focus of this entry. Classic PSS is thought to be the result of extreme and prolonged psychosocial stress and emotional deprivation resulting in decreased hormone secretion and abnormal growth and development. Inadequate nutrition is insufficient to account for this phenomenon. Thus, classic PSS is typically found in children with histories of abuse, neglect, and/or emotional deprivation.

DIAGNOSIS

The diagnostic assessment of classic PSS is often performed on an inpatient basis. Diagnosis involves first ruling out other organic causes that could explain the short stature, including primary and idiopathic (unknown etiology) growth hormone deficiencies, congenital abnormalities, cystic fibrosis, and heart defects, among others. Neurological examinations must also be performed to rule out other possible organic causes for bizarre behaviors. A physical examination for signs of abuse is usually part of the diagnostic protocol, as are a detailed psychosocial history and a family assessment. Children with classic PSS typically have a history of abuse with abnormal parent–child relationships. Caregiver pathology is often present and can include mood disorders, substance abuse, and personality disorders, among others.

CORRELATES

There are a number of behaviors, developmental patterns, and psychological factors typically associated with classic PSS. Most striking are bizarre behaviors, which can include preoccupation with food, hoarding, polydipsia (excessive ingestion of water), eating non-food items, drinking from toilets, rapid eating and vomiting, encopresis, enuresis, stealing food, and eating from garbage cans. Other behavior problems can include tantrums, aggression, depression, withdrawal, irritability, and self-injury. These children are often found to display developmental delays, with specific delays in language development, motor development, learning, and/or intellectual functioning. Sleep disturbances and pain agnosia (lack of response to pain) may also be present. These children may also be diagnosed with an attachment disorder.

TREATMENT

Treatment of classic PSS usually involves a team that includes medical, mental health, and casework professionals. The primary intervention is removal of the child from his or her current unsafe or nonnurturing environment. Upon placement in a safe and nurturing environment, catch-up growth and reduction or elimination of behavior problems is usually observed. In addition, abnormal endocrine function that is common in classic PSS is also resolved when they are removed from their nonnurturing or abusive environment. Caregiver treatment may be a component of intervention, although children with classic PSS can display growth deceleration upon return to their former environments. Mental health, medical, and developmental follow-ups constitute an important part of treatment.

PROGNOSIS

When placed in a safe and nurturing environment, the prognosis for catch-up growth is good, with better outcomes associated with early diagnosis. Similarly, better developmental outcomes are associated with early intervention although the data is limited. There is better data to suggest that prognosis for stable emotional functioning in adulthood is poor, especially for children diagnosed late in childhood. As adults, they typically are at higher risk for other psychiatric diagnoses and emotional problems, and have significant difficulty parenting appropriately.

See also: Child Maltreatment; Failure-to-Thrive; Family Assessment; Family Intervention; Psychological Maltreatment; Short Stature: Psychological Aspects

Further Reading

Blizzard, R.M., & Bulatovic, A. (1992). Psychosocial short stature: A syndrome with many variables. *Baillieres Clinical Endocrinology and Metabolism, 6*(3), 687–712.

Bowden, M. L., & Hopwood, N. J. (1982). Psychosocial dwarfism: Identification, intervention, and planning. *Social Work in Health Care, 7*(3), 15–36.

Gohlke, B. C., Khadilkar, V. V., Skuse, D., & Stanhope, R. (1998). Recognition of children with psychosocial short stature: A spectrum of presentation. *Journal of Pediatric Endocrinology and Metabolism, 11*(4), 509–517.

Money, J. (1992). *The Kaspar Hauser syndrome of psychosocial dwarfism: Deficient statural, intellectual, and social growth induced by child abuse.* New York: Promethean Press.

Sirotnak, A. (2002). Child abuse and neglect: Psychosocial dwarfism. *EMedicine Journal, 3*(1). http://www.emedicine.com/PED/topic566.htm

THOMAS R. LINSCHEID
BERNARD METZ

Psychosomatic Disorders

DEFINITION

Psychosomatic disorders broadly refer to illnesses or symptoms with both a significant physical and psychological component. These may emerge or be exacerbated during times of crisis or stress and may ameliorate when stressful periods end. The *Diagnostic and Statistical Manual of Mental Disorders, Fourth Edition (DSM-IV)* divides psychosomatic disorders into three categories: specifically, somatoform disorders, factitious disorders, and psychological factors affecting physical conditions. Psychological and emotional factors appear to mediate the relationship between stressful situations and the occurrence of physical symptoms, particularly one's interpretation of stressors.

Somatoform disorders are involuntary physical manifestations of psychosocial stress that can mimic a medical condition but are not fully explained by a medical condition. Symptoms of these disorders are present during emotional distress and are notable for their high intensity and persistence for long periods of time. Specific types of somatoform disorders that affect children are conversion disorder and chronic pain. Somatization disorder and hypochondriasis also are somatoform conditions, but these typically occur during adulthood and will not be discussed further here. Conversion disorder has been reported in children as young as 10 years of age and is a physical expression of a psychological conflict or need that enables an affected individual to remove or avoid discomfort from conscious awareness of the conflict while concomitantly receiving support from others. Symptoms are associated with voluntary motor and sensory functioning (e.g., paralysis, blindness). Chronic pain disorders are characterized by an obsessive preoccupation with pain despite an inadequate explanation for the pain or its level of intensity. Pain complaints often are localized to the head (i.e., headache), abdomen, limbs, or chest.

Factitious disorders such as malingering and Munchausen's disorder, unlike somatoform disorders, involve an illness that is not real. Physical symptoms suggestive of organ system involvement are simulated or induced voluntarily to deceive medical professionals and to elicit medical treatment. Secondary gain in either attention or monetary compensation is often the motivation for adopting a "sick" role. Factitious disorder by proxy, often referred to as Munchausen's syndrome by proxy (MSBP), involves a parent or a caregiver who intentionally induces illness in a child. Similar to factitious disorder, the motivation for the perpetrator's behavior is often to gain attention or fulfillment of other psychological needs (i.e., to serve as a martyr, rescuer, etc.).

Psychological factors that affect physical conditions refers to the presence of psychological or behavioral factors that can adversely affect a medical condition. Such factors can influence the course of, interfere with the treatment of, or exacerbate a true medical condition. This diagnosis is made when psychological or behavioral factors have a clinically significant impact on the course or outcome of a medical condition. For example, a child with Type 1 diabetes who does not adhere to his or her insulin regimen due to depression (feeling hopeless about his or her future) or anxiety (fear of needle sticks) is at risk for complications related to poor metabolic control.

INCIDENCE

The incidence rates of somatoform disorders vary. The diagnosis of conversion disorder in children ranges from 0.5 to 10 percent, is three times more prevalent in adolescents than preadolescents, and is rarely seen in children under 5 years of age. Onset usually does not occur before age 10 or after age 35. Conversion disorder is seen more often in adolescent females than adolescent males, whereas in younger children the gender ratio is equal. Higher rates of conversion disorder have been reported in rural populations of low socio-economic status, especially those with lower levels of education. Recurrent pain complaints are far more common among children and adolescents than conversion disorder, with a 7–30 percent incidence rate documented in both clinical and community settings.

Factitious disorder typically emerges in early adulthood, but cases of malingering and Munchausen's syndrome have been reported in some older children and adolescents. While individuals diagnosed with factitious disorders are typically adults, victims of MSBP tend to be children under the age of 16 and most often are of preschool age. Siblings are also victimized in approximately 8.5–25.8 percent of the reported cases. Incident reports for cases within specific pediatric diagnostic groups indicate that about 1 percent of asthmatic patients have been reported as victims of MSBP, as well as 0.27 percent of infants on apnea monitors, and 5 percent of children presumed to have food allergies or intolerance. Two to four cases per million have been reported in the general population, and about 1,000 out of 2.5 million cases of child abuse are related to MSBP. About 90 percent of the perpetrators are biological mothers, and 5 percent are fathers, grandmothers, or babysitters. The fatality rate of children victim to MSBP is approximately 10 percent. Both genders are equally affected and there is no correlation between the prevalence of the disorder and socioeconomic status.

The incidence of psychological factors affecting physical conditions spans all ages. Given the inherent involvement of psychological and behavioral factors in physical or medical conditions, the potential for such factors to significantly impact the course or outcome of an illness is high; however, the likelihood of occurrence is determined by the individual's ability to cope with psychosocial factors.

CORRELATES

Until recently, psychosomatic disorders of childhood were regarded as physical manifestations of unresolved psychological conflict. The etiology, diagnosis, and treatment of these disorders in children and adolescents were considered analogous to those of adults with similar diagnoses. Increasingly, the importance of developmental considerations has become apparent. For example, children's perceptions of illness and the knowledge of physical symptoms vary according to their level of cognitive development. Young children do not understand the origins of illness, nor do they comprehend the relationship between illness and treatment. With further development, their concrete way of conceptualizing illness and its symptoms evolves more logically, and then they can meaningfully link concepts such as illness, pain, and treatment.

Psychosocial factors such as parental attitudes and coping styles can influence children's perceptions of and reactions to physical symptoms and illness. Young children are dependent upon their parents for both physical care and emotional support when they are ill. Parental attitudes about their child's illness and treatment are observed and imitated by children. Parental expectations also affect children's level of independence, such that a child may be more or less reluctant to assume responsibility for aspects of their care.

Coping styles, or the management of pain and distress, also are important aspects of psychosomatic response. Children who have a lower threshold for pain may report more somatic symptoms on a consistent basis. Further, symptoms are perceived to be more adverse and reactions are more negative, including anxiety, depression, and hopelessness. In contrast, children who have adaptive coping styles report fewer physical symptoms, report lower levels of pain, and tend to understand more about the source of their pain.

Correlates of factitious disorders include personality disorders and, in the case of Munchausen's disorder, neuropsychological impairment, including deficits in conceptual organization and complex information processing. The parent/caregiver perpetrator of MSBP has a pathologic attachment to the child victim and a personality profile which includes personality disorder, somatizing behaviors, and significant family dysfunction.

ASSESSMENT

Assessment of somatoform disorders requires a comprehensive approach that includes the patient and family, in addition to medical and mental health professionals. It is important for professionals to acknowledge a patient's suffering and familial concerns, and to evaluate previous assessment and treatment experiences in an effort to establish and maintain rapport and a working partnership. Patient records should be reviewed so that a legitimate, but unrecognized, physical disease is not inadvertently ruled out; however, excessive and unnecessary tests and procedures should be avoided to minimize a worsening of somatic symptoms.

MSBP is very difficult to detect and diagnose, which makes assessment and treatment more challenging. Assessment may include detailed investigation of the child's medical history focusing on detection of frequent, unexplained medical illnesses or hospitalizations, which may help in discerning a pattern of behavior. Covert video surveillance in the hospital also may be initiated in cooperation with local law enforcement to monitor parent–child interactions.

Factors affecting a physical condition may include mental illness, stress-related physiological responses, psychological symptoms, maladaptive coping styles, or particular personality traits. Evaluation requires a continuous process that involves frequent monitoring by a professional trained to assess cognitive, personality, and behavioral change. Assessment of a child's intellectual and cognitive functioning can be used to determine a child's level of understanding of his or her medical condition. Evaluation of a child's personality or behavioral style may identify traits with a predisposition to particular psychosomatic conditions, and detect emotional problems that might contribute to or aggravate a condition.

TREATMENT

Cognitive–behavioral interventions, including coping skills training, relaxation therapy, and reinforcement of healthy behaviors, have proved useful in the treatment of somatic symptoms. A rehabilitation approach can help patients and their families to cope with and overcome a distressing physical symptom by encouraging a return to regular activities and responsibilities, and discouraging behaviors that inadvertently reinforce symptomatology. Psychopharmocalogical interventions, such as antidepressant medications, may prove useful for treatment of persistent medically unexplained pain, headaches, and gastrointestinal symptoms, or

when psychotherapeutic interventions have been unsuccessful.

Successful management of factitious disorder includes reinforcement of positive health behaviors, emphasis on psychotherapy, and maintenance of a consistent relationship with a primary physician regardless of whether or not the individual responds to medical intervention. Combining psychotherapy and psychiatric drug treatment can also be an effective treatment approach.

Treatment of MSBP requires a multimodal approach focused on family intervention and individual cognitive–behavioral treatment for parents. MSBP has the best outcome if detected when a victimized child is still young and if the child's contact with the caregiver is limited or prevented. Typically, this medical abuse is deemed pathological enough to warrant removal of a child from the home. Return of a child to the home environment should be considered only if circumstances are conducive to a child's well-being and supervision will occur. This procedure may require temporary separation of the caregiver and child, assisting the caregiver in recognizing and taking responsibility for his or her harmful actions, and long-term therapy for the victimized child. A permanent separation may be necessary if it becomes clear that the child would be in danger if returned to the caregiver's custody.

Treatment of psychological factors affecting a medical condition may typically involve traditional psychotherapy techniques such as cognitive–behavioral interventions, relaxation and hypnotic techniques, behavior therapy, family therapy, individual play therapy, and reinforcement of healthy behaviors.

PROGNOSIS

The prognosis of somatoform disorders varies with the specific diagnosis. Symptoms of conversion disorder can abate within 2 weeks but recurrence is common and 20–25 percent of individuals experience recurrent symptoms within 1 year. Prognosis is better for those who have acute symptom onset, a clearly identifiable stressor at the time of diagnosis, remediation of symptoms shortly after treatment begins, and above average intelligence. A better prognosis is predicted with the presentation of paralysis, aphonia (inability to speak), and blindness, whereas tremor and seizure suggest a poorer prognosis.

A child victim of MSBP is at risk for poor psychological health. An estimated 49 percent of such children exhibit conduct or emotional disorders as well as concentration and attention difficulties. The prognosis for individuals diagnosed with psychological factors affecting physical conditions is dependent upon remediation of the psychosocial factors contributing to the disorder or the acquisition of adequate and effective coping skills necessary to manage life stressors.

See also: Adjustment Disorders; Adolescent Health; Cognitive–Behavior Therapy; Life Stress in Children and Adolescents; Psychological Impact of a Parent's Chronic Illness; Stress Management

Further Reading

American Psychiatric Association. (2000). *Diagnostic and statistical manual of mental disorders* (4th ed., Text Revision). Washington, DC: Author.
Campo, J. V., & Fritz, G. (2001). A management model for pediatric somatization. *Psychosomatics, 42*(6), 467–476.
Davis, P., McClure, R. J., Rolfe, K., Chessman, N., Pearson, S., Sibert, J. R., & Meadow, R. (1998). Procedures, placement, and risks of further abuse after Munchausen syndrome by proxy, non-accidental poisoning, and non-accidental suffocation. *Archives of Disease in Childhood, 78*(3), 217–221.
Kenny, T. J., & Willoughby, J. (2001). Psychosomatic problems in children. In C. E. Walker & M. C. Roberts (Eds.), *Handbook of clinical child psychology* (3rd ed., pp. 359–372), New York: Wiley.
Klykylo, W. M., Kay, J., & Rube, D. (1998). *Clinical child psychology.* Philadelphia: W.B. Saunders.
Larson, D. E. (Rev. ed.). (1996). *Mayo clinic family health book.* New York: William Morrow.
Walker, L. S., Garber, G., & Greene, J. (1994). Somatic complaints in pediatric patients: A prospective study of the role of negative life events, child social and academic competence, and parental somatic symptoms. *Journal of Consulting and Clinical Psychology, 62*(6), 1213–1221.

DONNA MARSCHALL
TASHYA EKECHUKWU
ROSARIO GOMEZ-LOBO
CARLA L. MESSENGER
CLARISSA S. HOLMES

Psychotropic Drugs

See: Pharmacological Interventions

Psychotropic Drugs, Prenatal Exposure

Women with a history of chronic psychiatric conditions must make difficult decisions regarding the continuation

Table 1. Food and Drug Administration Ratings

A—Controlled studies show no risk. Adequate, well-controlled studies in pregnant women have failed to demonstrate risk to the fetus.
B—No evidence of risk in humans. Either animal findings show risk, but human studies do not, or if no adequate human studies have been done, animal findings are negative.
C—Risk cannot be ruled out. Human studies are lacking, and animal studies are either positive for fetal risk or lacking as well. However, potential benefits may justify the potential risk.
D—Positive evidence of risk. Investigational or postmarketing data show risk to the fetus. Nevertheless, potential benefits may outweight potential risk.
X—Contraindicated in pregnancy. Studies in animals or humans, or investigational or postmarketing reports have shown fetal risk that clearly outweighs any possible benefit to the patient.

Source: From the American Academy of Pediatrics, 2002.

of psychotropic medication treatment during pregnancy. Unfortunately, because of practical and ethical barriers, few controlled studies that investigate the effects of psychotropic drugs on the developing fetus are available in the literature. As a result, most psychotropic drugs are classified by the Food and Drug Administration as Category B (i.e., either evidence of risk from animal studies or no human studies have been completed) or Category C (i.e., risk cannot be ruled out) for use during pregnancy (see Table 1).

Concerns about the adverse effects of prenatal exposure to psychotropic medications include the possibility of miscarriage, fetal malformation, or damage to the unborn infant's developing central nervous system (CNS) that may result in subsequent learning or behavioral problems throughout childhood. Additionally, some neonates born to women taking psychotropic medications may display symptoms of withdrawal in the days and weeks after birth.

There are four primary categories of psychotropic medications where evidence is available with regard to the teratogenic effects of these agents: antidepressants, anxiolytics, antimanic agents including anticonvulsants, and antipsychotics. The literature regarding the safety of use during pregnancy for each of these agents will be reviewed.

ANTIDEPRESSANTS

Specific serotonin reuptake inhibitors (SSRIs) (e.g., fluoxetine [Prozac]) are the most commonly prescribed antidepressants. To date, no studies indicate that SSRIs have been associated with spontaneous loss of pregnancy or with major fetal anomalies. However,

Ahluwalia and Meyer (1998) showed that infants exposed during the third trimester of pregnancy were more likely to be born premature and had a higher rate of admission to high-risk nurseries. With regard to tricyclic antidepressants, Craig and Abel (2001) report that there is no evidence linking the use of these agents during pregnancy with congenital abnormalities, miscarriage, or premature births. With regard to the atypical antidepressants (e.g., monoamine oxidase inhibitors) that are sometimes used for individuals who are refractory to other antidepressant agents, there are no data available to support their safety during pregnancy.

ANXIOLYTICS

Occasionally benzodiazepines (e.g., diazepam) are used when an immediate anxiolytic effect is desired. The use of benzodiazepines during pregnancy has been associated with "floppy infant syndrome" (i.e., hypotonia, lethargy, sucking difficulties, cyanosis, and hypothermia) and symptoms associated with withdrawal (i.e., tremors, irritability, mypertonia, and hyperflexia). Although, as reported by Ahluwalia and Meyer, studies to date have been inconclusive, some evidence links the use of diazepam (Valium) during pregnancy to an increased incidence of cleft lip and palate.

ANTIMANIC AGENTS

Lithium carbonate is typically used to manage individuals with bipolar disorder. Use of lithium during the first trimester of pregnancy has been associated with Epstein's anomaly, a congenital malformation of the triscuspid valve of the heart, as shown by Ernst and Goldberg (2002). Moreover, use of lithium during the second and third trimesters of pregnancy has been associated with premature delivery, thyroid abnormalities, nephrogenic diabetes insipidus, and floppy baby syndrome.

Anticonvulsant agents are frequently used as antimania treatments as well as for the management of seizure disorders. The use of valproate (Depakote) and carbomazepine (Tegretol) during pregnancy is associated with increased risks for major congenital malformations such as skeletal abnormalities, spina bifida, congenital heart defects, developmental disabilities, and intrauterine growth retardation. Ernst and Goldberg (2002) report that risks can be minimized by using supplements of folic acid and vitamin K. Finally, although the newer anticonvulsants have offered some possibility of hope of fewer teratogenic effects, animal studies have

not been particularly encouraging with regard to safety, suggesting fetal toxicity and possible birth defects.

ANTIPSYCHOTICS

The antipsychotic agents are frequently employed for schizophrenia, severe aggression, and Tourette's disorder. In managing women with schizophrenia, the use of antipsychotic agents poses a significant dilemma. However, Craig and Abel (2001) indicate that there is evidence that there are no specific teratogenic effects associated with low doses of traditional antipsychotic agents including chlorpromazine (Mellaril, Thorazine) and haloperidol (Haldol). More recently, there has been a trend for increased use of the atypical antipsychotic agents because they are associated with fewer adverse effects such as tardive dyskinesia and extra pyramidal effects. However, animal studies have suggested potential teratogenic effects of these agents on the developing fetus including pup death, stillbirths, and developmental delays. Although studies with humans are needed with these agents, given the associated adverse effects in animals, cautious use of these medications with pregnant women is clearly warranted. A case registry of infants born to mothers taking olanzapine is available (Zyprexa) and to date there have been few reported teratogenic effects suggesting the possible viability of this medication for pregnant women in need of antipsychotic agents.

Decisions about the use of psychotropic medication during pregnancy must be made on a case-by-case basis after carefully weighing the risks associated with an untreated psychiatric disorder against the risks associated with medication use. Any woman who is pregnant or is planning to become pregnant should discuss medication use with her health care provider. The American Academy of Pediatrics has made two specific recommendations for cases in which psychotropic medication must be used during pregnancy. First, the mother should be prescribed the lowest dose possible to manage her symptoms. Second, exposed newborns should be monitored for "evidence of persistent drug effect or development of an abstinence syndrome" (American Academy of Pediatrics, 2000: 886).

In many cases, nonpharmacological interventions may be effective in managing psychiatric symptoms in pregnant women. For example, a vast literature supports the effectiveness of psychotherapy for individuals with various psychiatric diagnoses such as depression and anxiety. It has also been noted by O'Grady and Cohen (1992) that in some cases where pharmacotherapy may be clearly contraindicated, electroconvulsive therapy (ECT) may serve as a safe, alternative treatment for affective and psychotic symptoms occurring during pregnancy.

See also: Effects of Parental Substance Abuse on Children; Infant Assessment; Pharmacological Interventions; Prenatal Exposure to Opiates; Preschool Assessment; School Age Assessment; Substance Abuse

Further Reading

Ahluwalia, Y. K., & Meyer, B. E. B. (1998). Psychiatric disorders. In N. Gleicher (Ed.), *Principles & practice of medical therapy in pregnancy* (pp. 1417–1425). New York: Appleton & Lange.

American Academy of Pediatrics, Committee on Drugs. (2000). Use of psychoactive medication during pregnancy and possible effects on the fetus and newborn (RE9866). *Pediatrics, 105,* 880–887.

Craig, M., & Abel, K. (2001). Prescribing for psychiatric disorders in pregnancy and lactation. *Best Practice and Research in Clinical Obstetrics and Gynecology, 15,* 1012–1030.

Ernst, C. L., & Goldberg, J. F. (2002). The reproductive safety profile of mood stabilizers, atypical antipsychotics, and broad-spectrum psychotropics. *Journal of Clinical Psychiatry, 63,* 42–53.

O'Grady, J. P., & Cohen, L. M. (1992). Drug treatment and the use of electroconvulsive therapy. In J. P. O'Grady (Ed.), *Obstetrics: Psychological and Psychiatric Syndromes* (pp. 333–345). New York: Elsevier.

LAURA ARNSTEIN
RONALD BROWN

Puberty, Delayed

DESCRIPTION AND INCIDENCE

Puberty is the transitional period between the onset and completion of sexual maturation during which sexual organs develop and secondary sex characteristics emerge. Pubertal changes also include a rapid rate of linear growth (the "growth spurt") and the development of secondary sex characteristics. Although there is a wide range of variability among individuals in terms of the normal age of onset, puberty is considered delayed if the process has not begun by age 13 in girls and by age 14 in boys. A diagnosis of delayed puberty (DPUB) is also given to girls when the entire process is not complete over 4 years (4–5 years for boys), or if *menarche* (first menses) has not occurred by age 16. These age boundaries are based on norms derived from studies of healthy children in the general population. Descriptive standards for the assessment of pubertal advancement have also been developed in order to allow for the objective recording of the maturation of sexual characteristics. This system distinguishes

among sequential stages of development, known as "Tanner stages." Tanner stages are assigned to the appearance of the external genitalia and pubic hair distribution in boys, and to pubic hair distribution and breast development in girls. Tanner Stages 1 and 5 refer to the prepubertal and the fully sexually mature states, respectively.

Although a diagnosis of DPUB may be indicative of an underlying medical problem, most affected children are physically healthy. *Constitutional growth delay* (CGD) is the most common cause of pubertal delay and short stature and is a variant of normal growth. In children with CGD, velocity and weight gain is slow during the first year of life and continue in this manner until 2 or 3 years of age. Subsequently, linear growth follows the lower growth channels of the pediatric growth curve, or beneath the curve but parallel to it for the remainder of the prepubertal years. The onset of puberty and the pubertal growth spurt (associated with catch-up growth) occur later than average, resulting in adult stature commensurate with family background.

While it is known that boys are referred to pediatric endocrinologists for CGD more often than girls, there are no precise estimates regarding the incidence of this condition in the general population.

ETIOLOGY

CGD represents a delay in biologic development that affects the entire body. The proximal cause of CGD is a delay in the activation of the hypothalamic–pituitary–gonadal axis. Although a specific genetic mode of inheritance has not been identified, CGD has been shown to run in families.

DPUB can also result from *hypogonadism*, which refers to a state of inadequate production of sex hormones (estrogen or testosterone) by the gonads (ovaries or testes). Hypogonadism can stem from insufficient stimulation of the gonads by pituitary-derived stimulating factors (*hypogonadotropic hypogonadism*), such as that commonly associated with brain tumors and Kallmann syndrome. Hypogonadism can also be secondary to a problem with the ovary or testis itself (*hypergonadotropic hypogonadism*), such as that which is observed as a feature of Klinefelter syndrome, Turner syndrome, or other instances of primary testicular or ovarian failure.

ASSESSMENT

The goal of medical evaluation is to rule out pathological causes of pubertal delay. The diagnostic workup includes a family history, physical examination, radiograph of the hand and wrist to determine bone age (i.e., skeletal maturation), and laboratory tests of sex hormone and thyroid hormone levels. The evaluation should also include a detailed assessment of the individual's psychosocial and educational adaptation, as adolescents with DPUB are at risk for stigmatization related to their condition.

ASSOCIATED PSYCHOLOGICAL FEATURES

Individuals with DPUB are no more at risk for the development of clinically significant mental health problems than are youths with on-time pubertal development. However, like those with *precocious puberty*, children with DPUB show a discrepancy between physical appearance and chronological age. Consequently, the misperceptions of others, and associated psychosocial stress, may place them at risk for problems of psychosocial adaptation such as teasing by peers, disturbed body image, and poor self-concept. These children may be self-conscious about their lack of secondary sexual characteristics and avoid certain activities accordingly (e.g., swimming, gym class). Regarding the achievement of psychosocial milestones (e.g., age at first hand-holding, kissing, etc.), there is some evidence to suggest that these may occur at a later age in affected youths.

As DPUB is often associated with Short Stature, please see "Short Stature: Psychological Aspects" entry for further details.

TREATMENT

Because DPUB is not a disorder in most cases, medical treatment is usually unnecessary. However, short-term treatment with sex hormones is an option for those individuals who experience emotional distress as a result of their condition. This type of treatment has been successful in terms of the acceleration of pubertal onset and growth velocity. Importantly, this effect can be achieved without compromising adult height attainment. Psychoeducational counseling may be useful as an alternative, or adjunct, to medical treatment.

In cases where DPUB is attributable to hypogonadism (hypogonadotropic or hypergonadotropic hypogonadism), lifelong hormone replacement therapy is recommended.

PROGNOSIS

Adults with a history of CGD are largely indistinguishable in their psychosocial adaptation from individuals who had experienced on-time puberty. In contrast, the psychological prognosis for those with pathological causes of DPUB is more guarded. Syndromes responsible for hypogonadism (e.g., Klinefelter syndrome, Turner syndrome, Kallmann syndrome) are associated with specific psychosocial and educational features.

See also: Klinefelter Syndrome; Puberty, Normal; Puberty, Precocious; Short Stature; Psychological Aspects; Turner Syndrome

Further Reading

Bancroft, J., & Reinisch, J. M. (Eds.). (1990). *Adolescence and puberty.* New York: Oxford University Press.
Lee, P. A. (1996). Disorders of puberty. In F. Lifshitz (Ed.), *Pediatric endocrinology* (pp. 175–193). New York: Marcel Dekker.
Mazur, T., & Clopper, R. R. (1991). Pubertal disorders: Psychology and clinical management. *Endocrinology and Metabolism Clinics of North America, 20,* 211–227.

LAUREN ZURENDA
DAVID E. SANDBERG

Puberty, Normal

DESCRIPTION

Often confused with *adolescence*—a time of social, cognitive, and emotional growth—*puberty* refers to a biologic process during which sexual organs mature and secondary sex characteristics become apparent. Other aspects of pubertal development include a rapid rate of linear growth (*growth spurt*), and the emergence of reproductive fertility. Puberty begins with activation of the hypothalamic–pituitary–gonadal axis and typically occurs during adolescence; however, it may occur either very early (*precocious puberty*) or relatively late (*delayed puberty*).

For many years it was thought that typical puberty in girls commenced between ages 9 and 13 years, with most beginning the process at age 11 years (Figure 1). Signs of puberty (breast development) appearing younger than 8 years were considered abnormally early or *precocious*. However, a recent study suggests that a more appropriate cutoff for precocious puberty is age 7 years for white girls and age 6 years for African-American girls. The average age for this first sign of puberty for African-American and white girls is 8.87 years and 9.96 years, respectively. The average age

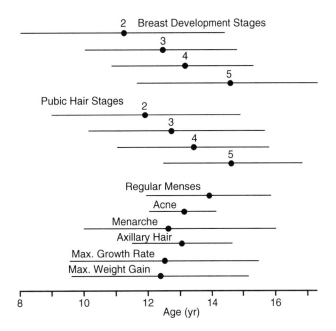

Figure 1. Mean ages (dots) and ranges (horizontal lines) of onset of pubertal development in girls. (From P. A. Lee, Disorders of puberty. In F. Lifshitz (Ed.) (1966), *Pediatric endocrinology* (3rd ed., p. 176). New York: Marcel Dekker. Copyright by Marcel Dekker, Inc. Reprinted with permission.)

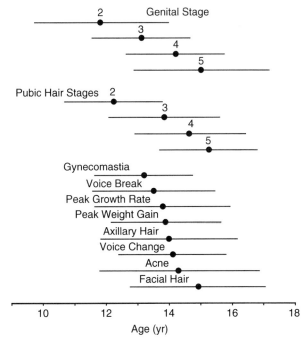

Figure 2. Mean ages (dots) and ranges (horizontal lines) of various pubertal changes in boys. (From P. A. Lee, Disorders of puberty. In F. Lifshitz (Ed.) (1966). *Pediatric endocrinology* (3rd ed., p. 178). New York: Marcel Dekker. Copyright by Marcel Dekker, Inc. Reprinted with permission.)

for onset of menses is 12.16 years for African-American girls and 12.88 years for white girls. For boys, the age range for the onset of puberty is between 12 and 16 years, with an average age of 13 years (Figure 2). Pubertal onset before age 9 years in boys is considered precocious. Determined by cross-sectional or longitudinal studies of healthy youths in the general population, these age cutoffs provide a standard against which the pubertal onset of individual children can be classified. Descriptive standards for the assessment of pubertal advancement have also been developed to allow for the more objective "staging" of physical sexual maturation (*Tanner staging*). Tanner stages are assigned to the appearance of the external genitalia and pubic hair distribution in boys, and to pubic hair distribution and breast development in girls. Tanner Stages 1 and 5 refer to the prepubertal and the fully sexually mature states, respectively (Figures 1 and 2).

PHYSICAL CHANGES

Puberty is marked by pronounced changes in multiple aspects of physical appearance in both boys and girls. Although the physiological process is orderly in terms of the sequence of events, there exists a wide range of variability among individuals in other aspects of pubertal development (Figures 1 and 2).

Secondary Sex Characteristics

Whereas *primary* sex characteristics involve the genitals and reproductive function, *secondary* sex characteristics are physical features that are not directly related to reproduction, but serve to physically distinguish males from females. For girls, secondary sex characteristics include breast development and the growth of pubic hair and leg hair. In males, these characteristics include facial, pubic, and body hair, as well as muscle development. Boys also experience an increase in vocal cord length that eventually leads to the development of a deeper voice. Though generally more pronounced in males than in females, individuals of both sexes experience changes in oil- and sweat-producing glands. These changes often result in acne of varying degrees.

Gonadal Development/Function

In girls, ovarian development leads to *menarche*, or the onset of menses. Occurring at an average age of 12.5 years (with small racial differences), menarche marks the beginning of menstrual cycles during which ova (egg cells) are released. Although girls are commonly anovulatory (i.e., do not release an egg) immediately after menarche, ova are released with regularity approximately 18 months after the first menstruation.

In boys, the first sign of pubertal onset is an increase in testicular volume. This occurs, on the average, between 11.5 to 12 years and may occur normally as early as 9.5 years. *Spermarche* is the male's first ejaculation, usually resulting from masturbation or experienced as a nocturnal emission. During ejaculation, sperm transported in semen produced by the seminal vesicles and prostate is released. As with menarche for girls, there is variation among individuals regarding the age of spermarche. For both physiological milestones, genetic factors seem to influence age of onset.

Pubertal Growth Spurt

Resulting from a complex interaction among several hormones (namely growth hormone, sex hormones, and thyroid hormone), the *growth spurt* refers to a marked increase in growth rate that is characteristic of the pubertal process. For both males and females, this period of accelerated growth typically spans approximately two years; however, whereas boys begin their growth spurt during midpuberty, girls achieve their peak growth velocity relatively earlier in the process. On average, boys will grow an average of 7–13 cm (3–5 inches) throughout puberty and girls will grow from 6–11 cm (2.5 to 4.5 inches). For individuals of both sexes, normal growth ceases when the growth plates at the ends of bones (epiphyses) fuse. This typically occurs between the ages 14–17 years for boys, and 13–15 years for girls.

Body Composition/Shape

Along with major increases in height, the body composition of boys and girls undergoes distinct changes during puberty as well. Although there are no differences in lean body mass, skeletal mass, or body fat between males and females prior to puberty, postpubertal males have approximately one and a half times greater the amount of lean body and skeletal mass than postpubertal females. Meanwhile, postpubertal females have approximately twice as much body fat as postpubertal males. These changes in body composition are accompanied by a redistribution of body fat that also differs between males and females. Whereas males tend to store adipose tissue around the torso, fat deposition in females occurs predominantly in the hips, thighs, and buttocks. Overweight has been found to be associated

with an acceleration of pubertal onset, in particular among girls. While moderate obesity is associated with earlier menarche, morbid obesity is associated with later onset of menses.

Hormones

In terms of their influence on the pubertal process, the major hormonal players include the gonadotropins (gonad stimulating factors) and sex hormones (testosterone and estradiol). A complex process of hormonal stimulation not only serves to activate the process of physical pubertal changes, but may also exert an influence on the cognitive, emotional, and behavioral life of the individual. One area where data consistently indicate an effect of hormones concerns sexual interest and behavior. These effects are noted below.

Associated Psychological Features

Although popular culture leads one to believe that pubertal changes (and hormonal influences, in particular) are responsible for the stereotypical image of the moody and irritable adolescent, relatively few adolescents exhibit severe difficulties in adjusting to the physical and social changes that occur during this period of development. In a recent unique study in which the level of sex hormones (estrogens and testosterone in girls and boys, respectively) was experimentally manipulated in adolescents, investigators detected minimal effects of the hormones on either the emergence of behavior problems or altered mood states.*

The influence of sex hormones upon the initiation and maintenance of sexual behavior has drawn substantial research attention. This is a particularly challenging area for investigation, largely due to strong societal taboos against the expression of sexual behavior by youths together with restrictions placed on its scientific study. Further complicating research is the co-occurrence, in the vast majority of youths, of rising levels of sex hormones during puberty and the developmental stage of "adolescence" which is associated with changes in societal norms, age-dependent experiences, and skills typically acquired by teens in our culture. Researchers have attempted to disentangle these influences by conducting studies in which both sexual

---

*Because it would be unethical to manipulate the levels of sex hormones in physically healthy children, this particular study was conducted in adolescents with abnormally low hormone levels due to various medical conditions or constitutionally delayed puberty.

behavior and sex hormones are measured while simultaneously statistically controlling for chronological age. This research has revealed that testosterone levels in males are directly related to masturbation, noncoital sexual experience, and sexual intercourse. In females, androgens (originating from the adrenal gland) have an influence on the expression of noncoital sexual behavior but not on sexual intercourse. It appears that social processes are more potent regulators of sexual intercourse in girls than in boys.

See also: Adolescence; Adolescent Sexuality; Puberty, Precocious; Puberty, Delayed; Sexual Development

Further Reading

Bancroft, J., & Reinisch, J. M. (Eds.). (1990). *Adolescence and puberty.* New York: Oxford University Press.

Becker, J. B., Buchanan, C. M., & Eccles, J. S. (1992). Are adolescents the victims of raging hormones: Evidence for activational effects of hormones on moods and behavior at adolescence. *Psychological Bulletin, 111,* 62–107.

Herman-Giddens, M. E., Slora, E. J., Wasserman, R. C., Bourdony, C. J., Bhapkar, M. V., Koch, G. G., & Hasemeier, C. M. (1997). Secondary sexual characteristics and menses in young girls seen in office practice: A study from the Pediatric Research in Office Settings network. *Pediatrics, 99,* 505–512.

Lee, P. A. (1996). Disorders of puberty. In F. Lifshitz (Ed.), *Pediatric endocrinology* (pp. 175–193). New York, NY: Marcel Dekker.

Offer, D., & Schonert-Reichl, K. A. (1992). Debunking the myths of adolescence: Findings from recent research. *Journal of the American Academy of Child and Adolescent Psychiatry, 31,* 1003–1014.

LAUREN ZURENDA
DAVID E. SANDBERG

Puberty, Precocious

Puberty is the transitional period between the onset and completion of sexual maturation. As there has been a trend toward a declining age of normal pubertal onset for both boys and girls in the past century, the standards used to distinguish between normal and precocious puberty have changed. Current evidence suggests that breast budding—the initial signs of normal puberty in girls—commences as early as 7 years among White girls and 6 years among black girls. In boys, testicular development is the initial physical evidence of normal puberty and may occur as early as 9.5 years. By these standards, girls who begin puberty before age 6, and boys who begin puberty before age 9 are said to have *precocious puberty* (PPUB). These age cutoffs have been determined by cross-sectional and longitudinal studies of healthy children. Descriptive standards for the assessment of pubertal progression have also been developed to allow for the objective recording of the maturation of sexual characteristics. This system distinguishes among sequential stages of development, known as "Tanner stages." Tanner stages are assigned to the appearance of the external genitalia and pubic hair distribution in boys, and to pubic hair distribution and breast development in girls. Tanner Stages 1 and 5 refer to the prepubertal and the fully sexually mature states, respectively.

DESCRIPTION AND INCIDENCE

PPUB is associated with the normal physical signs of pubertal onset, including the maturation of sexual organs, development of the secondary sexual characteristics, accelerated growth, and in some cases, fertility. Though affected children tend to be taller than their age-mates, affected individuals ultimately end up as adults with short stature if the condition is left untreated. This occurs because the hormones responsible for the early sexual development and growth spurt also cause the growth plates at the ends of the bones (epiphyses) to fuse, thereby marking the end of linear growth.

The incidence of PPUB in children is reported inconsistently within the research literature, largely because of changing standards of age of onset. Based on the most current standards, an estimated 4–5 percent of White and Black girls are considered to show precocious pubertal maturation and should be referred to a specialist for evaluation. Further, any child who exhibits a rapid progression of pubertal milestones, or any girl who menstruates before age 9 years should receive a similar evaluation. Although population-based prevalence estimates of PPUB in boys are currently lacking, clinical experience suggests the rates of referrals of boys to pediatric specialists for evaluation are between a fifth to a tenth as many as girls.

It is critical that PPUB not be confused with two common variants of normal puberty: *premature thelarche* and *premature pubarche*. Premature thelarche refers to the isolated appearance of breast development, usually in girls younger than age 3 years; premature pubarche refers to the appearance of pubic hair (without other signs of puberty) in girls or boys younger than age 7–8 years. Although they resemble

PPUB in isolated respects, both conditions are benign and do not progress to development of other aspects of pubertal development. Because treatment varies substantially according to diagnosis, it is extremely important to differentiate between these forms of early sexual development. A thorough medical history, physical examination, and assessment of the child's growth curve can help distinguish these normal variants from true pubertal precocity.

ETIOLOGY

PPUB can be caused by several different factors. In some cases, early activation is caused by an underlying pathological condition, such as a central nervous system malfunction; however, most cases are *idiopathic*, or without known cause. In girls, 90 percent of cases are idiopathic. In contrast, pathological causes of PPUB are far more common in boys, accounting for a significant number of cases. For both boys and girls, the likelihood of an underlying pathological cause of PPUB declines with increasing age of the child.

ASSESSMENT

Children who show signs of premature pubertal onset should be referred to a pediatric endocrinologist. This evaluation features a detailed family history and a thorough physical examination. Laboratory studies include the measurement of sex hormones and gonadotropins (gonad stimulating factors). Because affected children typically show advanced skeletal maturation, a radiograph is typically ordered to determine bone age. Imaging studies of the head such as magnetic resonance imaging (MRI) are often ordered in an effort to detect abnormalities. As already noted, the likelihood of detecting abnormalities varies according to sex and age of onset.

ASSOCIATED PSYCHOLOGICAL FEATURES

Although children with PPUB are no more likely to experience clinically significant emotional or behavioral disturbances, they remain at risk for disturbances in social and emotional functioning. As it is common for adults to overestimate the age of the affected child, teachers and parents may hold expectations that are beyond the child's emotional and cognitive capacities. As a result, these children may be perceived as socially immature or intellectually slow.

The incongruence between physical age and chronological age may place the child at risk for problems with peer relations as well. Because of their advanced physical appearance and abilities, affected children may be less desirable companions for age-mates and may experience teasing related to the physical signs of early maturation. Meanwhile, forming friendships with older children may present difficulties as well, as the social skills of affected children tend to correspond more closely to their chronological age rather than their physical age.

With respect to sexual interest and behavior, parents and teachers of children with PPUB often express concern that affected children will seek out sexual experiences before their peers. While children with PPUB may be vulnerable to inappropriate sexual interest of others because of the physical signs of early maturation, research indicates that the psychosexual maturation of affected children typically matches social age rather than physical age. Achievement of psychosexual milestones (e.g., age at first hand-holding, kissing, and breast petting) has been shown to fall within the normal range when compared with matched control subjects, though affected males and females may engage in masturbation at a younger age.

In terms of intellectual potential, idiopathic PPUB is associated with IQ scores falling within the average to high average range. The slight increase in scores is likely attributable to the tendency for teachers and parents to place greater expectations on affected children because of their mature appearance.

TREATMENT

In cases where PPUB is the consequence of premature activation of the hypothalamic–pituitary–gonadal axis, a gonadotropin-releasing hormone (GnRH) agonist is an effective intervention strategy for children with PPUB, and early treatment is associated with the best outcomes in terms of preventing further pubertal development and achieving the maximal potential for adult height. Importantly, treatment does not adversely affect later pubertal development and fertility.

Affected children and their families should also be provided psychoeducational counseling designed to inform them about the pubertal process. Individual counseling may be helpful for the child who requires support in the development of coping skills to address psychosocial challenges. This type of support may serve to avoid emotional and behavioral difficulties that might otherwise arise.

Further, school acceleration has been a successful strategy for affected children who socialize better with older children than with agemates. Acceleration can help children develop a psychosocial age closer to their physical age, and thus blend in with their peers.

PROGNOSIS

Early treatment with GnRH is an effective strategy for slowing down (or arresting) pubertal progression and does not adversely affect later development or fertility. Furthermore, once peers catch up with the child's physical development, blending in with agemates is not a problem. In light of the success demonstrated in the endocrine and psychological management of PPUB, long-term prognosis is excellent.

See also: Puberty, Delayed; Puberty, Normal; Sexual Development

Further Reading

Herman-Giddens, M. E., Slora, E. J., & Wasserman, R. C. (1997). Secondary sexual characteristics and menses in young girls seen in office practice: A study from the Pediatric Research in Office Settings Network. *Pediatrics, 99*, 505–512

Kaplowitz, P. B., & Oberfield, S. E. (1999). Reexamination of the age limit for defining when puberty is precocious in girls in the United States: Implications for evaluation and treatment. Drug and Therapeutics and Executive Committees of the Lawson Wilkins Pediatric Endocrine Society. *Pediatrics, 104*, 936–941.

Lee, P. A. (1996). Disorders of puberty. In F. Lifshitz (Ed.), *Pediatric endocrinology* (pp. 175–193). New York: Marcel Dekker.

Mazur, T., & Clopper, R. R. (1991). Pubertal disorders: Psychology and clinical management. *Endocrinology and Metabolism Clinics of North America, 20*, 211–227.

LAUREN ZURENDA
DAVID E. SANDBERG

Pulmonary Disorders

Pulmonary disorders are among the most common and complex chronic diseases of childhood. Treatment of respiratory diseases in children accounts for the greatest proportion of visits to the pediatrician and emergency room, and is the leading cause of hospitalization for children. Asthma, for example, is currently the most prevalent chronic illness affecting children and adolescents, with nearly five million children diagnosed in the United States, and its incidence is on the rise. Other common pediatric pulmonary disorders include cystic fibrosis (CF), chronic bronchitis, and sleep apnea.

Most chronic pulmonary disorders are challenging to manage, requiring adherence to a variety of medication regimens that can be time-consuming, complex to administer, and difficult to fit into daily routines. Rates of adherence vary greatly depending on the medical condition and demands of the treatment regimen, however for both asthma and CF, average rates of adherence are below 50 percent. Poor adherence is the leading cause of treatment failure and is associated with a number of serious health consequences, including increased morbidity and mortality, the emergence of resistant strains of bacteria, reduced quality of life, and higher health care costs. Efforts to identify the major barriers to good disease management and the development of interventions (e.g., behavioral family systems therapy; school based interventions) that are successful in improving adherence are beginning to increase the rates of adherence.

Children with chronic conditions are also at increased risk for adjustment difficulties, such as social, emotional, and behavioral problems. However, there is little evidence that children with chronic pulmonary disorders display substantially greater rates of psychopathology (e.g., severe depression or anxiety) than nonaffected children. In general, the literature suggests that most children and families cope fairly successfully with the additional stressors of managing chronic illnesses, such as asthma and CF. Thus, makes more sense to assess the impact of chronic illness on daily functioning and health-related quality of life rather than traditional psychiatric indices.

See also: Asthma; Cystic Fibrosis; Family Intervention; Medical Hospitalization; Quality of Life; Treatment Adherence

Further Reading

American Lung Association. (2002). Retrieved May 2, 2002, from http://www.lungusa.org/

Cadman, D., Boyle, M., Szatmari, P., & Offord, D. R. (1987). Chronic illness, disability, and mental and social well-being: Findings of the Ontario Child Health Study. *Pediatrics, 79*, 805–813.

Dozor, A. J. (2001). *Primary pediatric pulmonology*. Armonk, NY: Futura.

Quittner, A. L., Davis, M. A., & Modi, A. C. (in press). Health-related quality of life in pediatric populations. In M. Roberts (Ed.), *Handbook of pediatric psychology*.

Quittner, A. L., Drotar, D., Ievers-Landis, C., Seidner, D., Slocum, N., & Jacobsen, J. (2000). Adherence to medical treatments in adolescents with cystic fibrosis: The development and evaluation of family-based interventions. In D. Drotar (Ed.),

Promoting adherence to medical treatment in childhood chronic illness: Interventions and methods. Hilsdale, NJ: Erlbaum Associates.

ALEXANDRA L. QUITTNER
AVANI C. MODI
MELISSA A. DAVIS

Punishment

A key aspect of learning theory approaches to explaining human behavior is that behavior is affected by the events that precede it (antecedents) and those that follow it (consequences). The likelihood that a particular behavior will be exhibited again in the presence of the prevailing antecedent events depends on the consequences of that behavior. If the behavior is followed by reinforcement, it is more likely to occur again. If it is not followed by reinforcement, or if it is followed by punishment, it is less likely to occur again.

The term punishment is used here in a technical sense. A consequence is considered to be punishment if and only if it results in a reduction in the likelihood of the behavior it follows occurring again. This is different from the meaning of punishment in common usage where it might be intended to have some deterring affect, but it also has an element of retribution.

The technical form of punishment occurs frequently in a child's life. If he touches the hot stove and burns himself, he is less likely to touch that stove in the future. Similarly, if he falls off his bicycle and hurts himself, he may not want to ride his bicycle again.

Punishment has been used by parents and teachers in order to eliminate problem behaviors in children. The punishments used, however, tend not so much to involve the use of aversive procedures such as slaps, but rather less intrusive procedures such as time out and response cost.

The use of punishment has always been controversial. It is generally accepted that it is better to use positive procedures such as the frequent use of positive reinforcement to encourage children to develop appropriate behaviors. The use of punishment has probably been most controversial in the field of developmental disability where aversive procedures have been used for the treatment of serious problems such as self-injurious behavior. Even with these serious behaviors, however, contemporary research is showing that the use of aversive procedures is not necessary.

See also: Applied Behavior Analysis; Positive Reinforcement; Response Cost; Time Out

Further Reading

Hudson, A. (1998). Applied behavior analysis. In A. Bellack, M. Hersen (Series Ed.), & T. Ollendick (Vol. Ed.), *Comprehensive clinical psychology (Vol. 5). Children and adolescents: Clinical formulation and treatment* (pp. 107–129). New York: Pergamon.

Lucyshyn, J. M., Dunlap, G., & Albin, R. W. (Eds.). (2002). *Families and positive behavior support: Addressing problem behaviors in family contexts.* Baltimore, MD: Paul H. Brookes.

Repp, A. C., & Singh, N. N. (Eds.). (1990). *Perspectives on the use of nonaversive and aversive interventions for persons with developmental disabilities.* Sycamore, IL: Sycamore.

The Association for Behavior Analysis. http://www.wmich.edu/aba

The Institute for Applied Behavior Analysis. http://www.iaba.com

ALAN HUDSON

Qq

Quality of Life

DEFINITIONS AND CONCEPTUALIZATION

Quality of life is defined as a sense of contentment, happiness, and satisfaction with one's life and surroundings, and integrates the individual's health, values, culture, and basic life conditions (Department of Health and Human Sciences, 2000). In fact, the World Health Organization (WHO) has deemed quality of life to be an important component of healthy functioning and has developed a measure to assess global quality of life. Quality of life is emerging as an increasingly important construct in pediatric populations as many children and adolescents with chronic illnesses are living longer lives due to medical advances in treatment efficacies. However, this increase in quantity of life is often associated with late effects of treatments, as well as continued physiological and psychological challenges. Thus, increasing quality of life has been identified as one of two overarching goals of *Healthy People 2010*, emphasizing the importance of incorporating quality of life into conceptualizations of overall healthy functioning. Further, the definition regarding quality of life is made more specific to illness populations in the construct health-related quality of life (HRQOL). HRQOL is conceptualized as the child's perception of the influence of disease and treatment upon multiple domains, including physical, mental, and social functioning.

Eiser and Morse (2001) have cogently reviewed the extant literature related to quality of life and issues with regard to quantification of this construct in childhood

populations. They present quality of life as having both objective and subjective components. Objective components include the child's functional capacities, while subjective components reflect the individual's perceptions of their well-being. More importantly, there is a hypothesized discrepancy between self-reported quality of life and objective measures of physical functioning. This underscores the importance of obtaining information about overall well-being directly from the child.

MEASUREMENT ISSUES

One major problem in the assessment of quality of life is that various experts conceptualize the construct, and hence its measurement, differently. Due to the abstract nature of the construct, development of measurement tools to assess quality of life have been fraught with difficulty in adult populations, and this problem has been exacerbated for pediatric populations. It is imperative that valid assessments of the construct be developed and implemented across health care settings so that clinical trials and health care systems will attend to this important ingredient in the care of children's health. As Cella (2001) has astutely observed, quality of life has posed more measurement challenges than predicting quantitative elements of health, however, it is of equal importance in examining treatment efficacy related to both the economic and emotional impact of illness.

Consistent with the psychopathology literature, the issues of cross-informant and cross-situational assessment are likely to influence the assessment of quality of life. It also should be noted that quality of life is a dynamic construct that is fluid across time and settings. We are not aware of any empirical data to suggest that assessment of quality of life across informants actually yields more informative data than the report of the child. Clearly, further investigation in this area is warranted.

A review of the numerous quality of life measurement tools is not possible within the scope of this entry. However, it is desirable for the assessment paradigm to incorporate cross-domain functioning (e.g., physiological, cognitive, emotional). In addition, some measurement tools also incorporate reports on the child's quality of life from various informants including caregivers, physicians, teachers, and the children themselves.

It is well recognized that in pediatric populations there is great heterogeneity with regard to symptom display. For example, a child undergoing treatment for cancer will likely experience significantly more pervasive adverse effects than a child with mild to moderate reactive airway disease (asthma). However, there is some controversy as to whether a quality of life measurement scheme should actually capture these specific disease- and treatment-related effects. Typically, research has addressed heterogeneous illnesses as a single group and has compared the quality of life of these children to normally developing comparison controls. While this seems to represent a preliminary stage in this area of investigation, it is also important to consider the differential effects of various diseases and their associated treatments on quality of life.

Assessment of Quality of Life

Following the various conceptualizations previously noted, numerous measurement schemes have been developed for the purpose of quantifying quality of life in children and adolescents. In general, the measures fall into two primary categories of assessment: generic quality of life and disease-specific quality of life. The reader is directed to work by Eiser and Morse (2001) for further discussion of the available instruments for the assessment of quality of life. Based on several criteria including reliability and validity, the availability of both self- and proxy reports, and the clinical utility of the instrument (i.e., that the assessment be brief and appropriate for a clinical setting), Eiser and Morse have identified three generic measures (Child Health Questionnaire, Pediatric Quality of Life Inventory [PedsQL], and Health Utilities Index, as well

as two disease specific instruments: Pediatric Asthma Quality of Life Questionnaire and Pediatric Oncology Quality of Life Questionnaire).

As a final note, it is important that quality of life research be integrated into medical decision-making. This is especially true since medical treatment choices are driven by their impact upon both quality and quantity of life. Thus, accurate examination of treatment effects upon quality of life has assumed increasing prominence in the medical literature. Given recent movement in the field toward defining health as the presence of well-being (both physical and psychological), quality of life is an increasingly salient variable in recommending treatment options. For example, in a clinical trial examining the efficacy of various pharmacotherapies for children, given equivalent effects upon symptom presentation and a favorable side effect profile, and then the medication impact upon the child, quality of life would be the deciding factor. Thus, with an increasing emphasis on evidenced-based medicine and empirically validated treatments, issues pertaining to quality of life will assume a prominent role in medical decision-making.

See also: Child Self-Reports; Interviewing; Medical Hospitalization; Global Functioning; Evidence-Based Treatments

Further Reading

Cella, D. (2001). Quality of life measurement in oncology. In A. Baum & B. Andersen (Eds.), *Psychosocial interventions for cancer* (pp. 57–76) Washington, DC: American Psychological Association.

Department of Health and Human Services. (2000, January). *Healthy people 2010*. Washington, DC. Available online: http://www.health.gov/healthypeople/

Eiser, C. & Morse, R. (2001). The quality of life in children: Past and future perspectives. *Journal of Developmental and Behavioral Pediatrics, 22*(4), 248–256.

Power, M., Bullinger, M., Harper, A., & World Health Organization Quality of Life Group. (1999). The World Health Organization WHOQOL-100: Tests of the universality of quality of life in 15 different cultural groups worldwide. *Health Psychology, 18*(5), 495–505.

Varni, J. W., Seid, M., & Rode, C. A. (1999). The PedsQL: Measurement model for the pediatric quality of life inventory. *Medical Care, 37*(2), 126–139.

Wallander, J. L., Schmitt, M., & Koot, H. M. (2001). Quality of life measurement in children and adolescents: Issues, instruments, and applications. *Journal of Clinical Psychology, 57*(4), 571–585.

C. ALEXANDRA BOEVING
RONALD T. BROWN

Rr

Rage

DEFINITION

Rage is defined by the American Psychiatric Association as a sudden and violent outburst of uncontrolled and severe anger usually preceded by increased arousal and tension and followed by a feeling of relief, regret, and fatigue. The increase in arousal is often characterized by feeling trapped, criticized, rejected, and insecure and includes heightened verbal aggression moments before the loss of control. The uncontrollable outbursts of anger are often referred to as temper outbursts, anger/rage attacks, or episodic dyscontrol, and may include serious assaultive behavior or destruction of property. The destruction of property is often purposeful and can include injury to self and others. In each instance, the outburst of anger is disproportionate to the environmental factors that seemingly precipitated the event.

Although rage can be associated with various medical and psychological disorders (e.g., alcohol abuse and Conduct Disorder [CD]), rage is one of the defining characteristics and a criterion for a diagnosis of an impulse control disorder and, more specifically, is a primary symptom of Intermittent Explosive Disorder in both children and adults. Rage attacks are distinguishable from more ordinary temper tantrums by their magnitude and serious destructive properties. Episodes of rage typically range from a few minutes to up to an hour or more, and the recipient of the rage is typically a family member, especially when perpetrated by children.

INCIDENCE/CORRELATES

Research on rage attacks and Intermittent Explosive Disorder (IED) is scarce, and although the prevalence of the disorder is unknown, it is considered to be rare. Although a diagnosis of rage is rare, there are multiple disorders in which explosions of anger are quite prominent such as CD. Anger explosions are also found in almost half of all children and teenagers diagnosed with Tourette's syndrome. In addition, mood and anxiety disorders are frequently comorbid with IED. Certain personality disorders are also associated with a diagnosis of IED, including narcissistic, schizoid, paranoid, and obsessive personality disorders.

Rage, like aggression, is much more common in males than females and has a typical age of onset from childhood to early adulthood. Many adults with a diagnosis of IED were characterized as difficult children and typically displayed what is often referred to as temper tantrums.

ETIOLOGY

Much of the literature on the etiology of rage focuses on neurobiological factors. A subgroup of adolescents that exhibits explosive episodes of rage may have a predisposition for violent or explosive behavior as an innate characteristic of their central nervous system and have similar electroencephalogram (EEG) patterns to those of criminals and psychopaths, as suggested by Bars and colleagues (2001).

Neurotransmitters and the limbic structures of the temporal lobe and the cerebrum have also been

536

targeted in the incidence of rage outbursts. Rage attacks, particularly in children with Tourette's, may be the consequence of a variety of imbalances in neurotransmitter systems. Research by McElroy suggests that because serotenergic neurons are involved in the regulation of the ability to tolerate delay before acting, serotenergic neurons might play a significant role in explosive episodes of rage. Finally, when areas of the brain that regulate impulse control, such as the limbic structures of the temporal lobe and cerebrum, are damaged, rage outbursts become much more likely. Consistent with distinctions made between two types of anger responses, Lochman and colleagues (1997) suggest that rage may be more associated with amygdala activation, in the limbic system, and less immediate anger reactions may be more associated with cortical processing.

ASSESSMENT

The first step toward assessment of rage or impulse control should include a structured clinical interview that assesses psychopathology to rule out other disorders and to assess for comorbid conditions. In addition, because rage is a more explosive kind of anger, many of the assessment techniques used for anger and anger control are also appropriate in the assessment of rage outbursts.

TREATMENT

There is some evidence in the literature to suggest that psychopharmacological treatment is effective in reducing outbursts of rage. Serotonin reuptake inhibitors (SRIs) and mood stabilizers have been effective treatments in the reduction of rage outbursts, as noted by McElroy (1997), and lithium carbonate has been shown to reduce the frequency and severity of aggressive behavior in children and adolescents, but long-term side effects are currently unknown.

Cognitive-behavioral techniques in combination with psychopharmacological treatment have been the preferred treatment for rage in both children and adolescents. Cognitive-behavioral therapy appears to be effective—perhaps due to the sense of tension relief that typically follows the rage episode. The sense of relief can serve as negative reinforcement, and can increase the likelihood for rage responses to occur in the future to escape or reduce tension.

Although the literature suggests that psychopharmacological treatments are effective in reducing rage and severe aggression in children and adolescents, there is a lack of research on the potential side effects of many of the medications that are currently administered. As a result, Lochman and colleagues (1997) suggest that medication should be monitored closely and combined with cognitive behavioral interventions to address the problematic rage outbursts.

See also: Anger; Behavior Therapy; Cognitive–Behavior Therapy; Pharmacological Interventions

Further Reading

American Psychiatric Association. (2000). *Diagnostic and statistical manual of mental disorders (DSM-IV-TR)* (4th ed., Text Revision). Washington, DC: Author.

Bars, D. R., Heyrend, F. L., Simpson, C. D., & Munger, J. C. (2001). Use of visual evoked-potential studies and EEG data to classify aggressive, explosive behavior of youths. *Psychiatric Services, 52*, 81–86.

Gordon, N. (1999). Episodic dyscontrol syndrome. *Developmental Medicine and Child Neurology, 41*, 786–788.

Lochman, J. E., Dunn, S. E., & Wagner, E. E. (1997). Anger. In G. Baer, K. M. Minke, & A. Thomas (Eds.), *Children's needs II: Development, problems, and alternatives*. Bethesda, MD: National Association of School Psychologists.

McElroy, S. L. (1999). Recognition and treatment of DSM-IV intermittent explosive disorder. *Journal of Clinical Psychiatry, 60*, 12–16.

HEATHER K. MCELROY
JOHN E. LOCHMAN
NANCY PHILLIPS

Rational Emotive Behavior Therapy

DEFINITION

Rational emotive behavior therapy (REBT) is a form of cognitive–behavioral psychotherapy that is based on social learning theory, operant conditioning, and instrumental conditioning principles. Originally founded in the late 1950s and 1960s by Albert Ellis, REBT is built on the premise that the way children and adolescents interpret events shape their emotional and behavioral reactions. Ellis maintains that people are born with a biological predisposition to irrational thinking and that social learning experiences exacerbate as well as maintain this vulnerability. Moreover, Ellis believes cultural contexts influence thought content as well as perceptual processes. The capacity and motivation for self-initiated change is fundamental to REBT. In short, people are seen as purposeful and goal-oriented.

DiGiuseppe (1999) notes that cognitive errors are central to psychological distress in REBT. For Ellis (1994), cognitive errors and irrational beliefs are either empirically false or unverifiable. Additionally, DiGiuseppe and Bernard (1990) emphasize that emotions are also important in REBT. Distressing emotions prompt maladaptive behavior, which in turn prevents people from achieving their goals. Accordingly, rational thinking is seen as the path for goal attainment.

METHOD

REBT makes use of the classic ABCDE paradigm. (*A*) signifies an environmental event, which triggers beliefs (*B*). These beliefs, if irrational, set in motion distressing emotions and dysfunctional behavioral consequences (*C*). The therapist's job is to first identify these problematic events, thoughts, feelings, and behaviors. DiGiuseppe (1999) recommends therapists look for four major cognitive patterns. One theme is *awfulizing* which is a cognitive set where negative outcomes are seen as catastrophic rather than simply unwanted. A second major cognitive tendency is *emotional intolerance or frustration intolerance* where youngsters "can't stand" unpleasant emotional states. *Personal imperatives*, which are demanding and contain "must", "should", and "ought" commands are a third trend. The fourth pattern is *harsh critical labeling of oneself and others*, which includes self-condemnation and blaming. Once these patterns are uncovered, therapists work to dispute (*D*) the irrational thoughts via various methods. *E* reflects the emotional consequence associated with the new rational thinking pattern. DiGiuseppe (1999) notes that throughout the therapeutic process, REBT attends to developmental and cultural vicissitudes. Therapists regularly use homework or self-help exercises which are completed outside of the office between sessions. Homework makes the therapy become more generalizable.

Disputation includes multiple procedures and processes including Socratic dialogues, problem-solving methods, stress inoculation training, pleasant activity scheduling, attribution training, relaxation, and rational-emotive imagery. Disputations involve, "detecting illogical, unrealistic, and irrational beliefs, debating irrational beliefs, showing why they are irrational, and reformulating irrational beliefs into rational ones" (DiGiuseppe & Bernard, 1990, p. 272). Behavioral

experiments or experiential learning exercises are frequently constructed where clients empirically analyze their illogical/irrational thoughts. Children make hypotheses based on their irrational beliefs, collect data, and then compare the obtained results to their predictions. In sum, the goal of disputation is developing more productive, adaptive, and rational inferences. Bernard (1990) suggests that REBT can be made more effective by including concrete teaching aids, applying diagrams, inviting the child to take the lead in disputation, therapist enthusiasm and animation, and working on one problem at a time.

CLINICAL APPLICATIONS

REBT has been applied to a myriad of emotional and behavioral problems experienced in childhood and adolescence. In general, children with low frustration tolerance, highly self-critical thinking, and high levels of emotional insecurity are good candidates for REBT. More specifically, DiGiuseppe (1990) wrote that REBT has been applied to depression, low self-esteem, anxiety, fears, phobias, stealing, bullying, vandalism, aggression, underachievement, obesity, and social isolation. Additionally, REBT may be used with individuals, families, and groups. Finally, DiGiuseppe and Bernard found REBT education programs have been employed in multiple school programs.

EFFECTIVENESS

Overall, REBT is a promising approach to treat children, adolescents, and their families. Empirical investigations and case studies demonstrate positive and enduring results with the populations listed above. DiGiuseppe (1999) stated that REBT could be advanced further by greater specificity of its methods and theory as well as by increasing the number of empirical studies examining its effectiveness.

See also: Behavior Modification; Behavior Therapy; Cognitive–Behavioral Play Therapy; Cognitive–Behavior Therapy; Evidence-Based Treatments

Further Reading

Bernard, M. E. (1990). Rational emotive therapy with children and adolescents: Treatment strategies. *School Psychology Review, 19*, 294–303.
DiGiuseppe, R. (1999). Rational emotive behavior therapy. In H. T. Prout & D. T. Brown (Eds.), *Counseling and psychotherapy*

with children and adolescents: Theory and practice for school and clinical settings (pp. 252–301). New York: Wiley.

DiGiuseppe, R., & Bernard M. E. (1990). The application of rational-emotive theory and therapy to school-age children. *School Psychology Review, 19*, 268–286.

Ellis, A. (1994). *Reason and emotion in psychotherapy: A comprehensive method of treating human disturbance* (Revised and updated). New York: Birch Lane Press.

Friedberg, R. D., & McClure, J. M. (2002). *Clinical practice of cognitive therapy with children and adolescents: The nuts and bolts.* New York: Guilford.

ROBERT D. FRIEDBERG

Reactive Attachment Disorder of Infancy and Childhood

DEFINITION

The attachment between an infant and caregiver has long been considered of critical importance to a child's social and emotional development. When a child does not experience emotionally sensitive care and comes to lack trust in the responsiveness of the caregiver, the child is said to have an insecure attachment. An extreme subgroup of children with insecure attachments has a clinical disorder referred to as Reactive Attachment Disorder (RAD) of infancy and childhood. RAD of infancy and childhood is a severe developmental disturbance in social relatedness that in most contexts that begins before the age of 5 years.

ETIOLOGY

Certain life events, such as extended separation and inconsistent care, have the potential to disturb the formation of a secure infant–caregiver attachment. Much of the research on attachment disorders has focused on children raised in institutions and on case reports of children raised in abusive and neglectful environments. Although these populations constitute extremes, a range of risk factors may contribute to the experience of separation or inconsistent care for the child. Caregiver risk factors include parental depression, isolation, lack of social support, and experiences of abuse or neglect in the parent's own upbringing. Child risk factors include difficult temperament, disability, chronic illness, extended hospitalizations, and multiple

changes in his or her primary caregiver early in life. RAD is the only diagnosis in which the presumed etiology, "pathogenic" care, is part of the criteria for diagnosis.

DIAGNOSTIC CRITERIA

Although the reliability of the diagnosis of RAD has improved with changes in the criteria over time, concerns about the validity and reliability of this diagnosis remain. The *Diagnostic and Statistical Manual for Mental Disorders, Fourth Edition* (*DSM-IV*), published by the American Psychiatric Association, distinguishes between two types: (1) inhibited, characterized by a failure to initiate or respond to social interactions in a developmentally appropriate manner and (2) disinhibited, characterized by a marked inability to show developmentally appropriate selectivity in attachments. In the inhibited type, the child may be withdrawn, overly cautious, avoidant, hypervigilant, or highly ambivalent toward primary caregivers. This type tends to be associated with children who have been maltreated. In the disinhibited type, the child makes little or no distinction between strangers and primary caregivers. The child exhibits "indiscriminate sociability," responding to strangers with inappropriate familiarity or friendliness. This type tends to be associated with children who have had frequent changes in caregivers (e.g., multiple foster care placements) or an absence of a primary caregiver (e.g., institutionalized children). The *DSM-IV* criteria for RAD currently includes grossly "pathogenic" care, evidenced by persistent, extreme emotional or physical neglect, maltreatment, or repeated changes in primary caregivers.

The first appearance of attachment disorders in the official nosologies was in the *DSM-III* in 1980. In the *DSM-III*, RAD included failure-to-thrive in terms of growth and development and required an onset of symptoms before 8 months of age. In 1987, criteria were substantially changed in the *DSM-III-R*. Failure to thrive was eliminated as a central feature of the disorder and the age of onset was extended to within the first 5 years of life. In addition, the two clinical subtypes of "inhibited" and "disinhibited" were introduced. These subtypes were preserved in the *DSM-IV*. In addition, the *DSM-IV* was the first edition to require evidence of "pathogenic" care.

PREVALENCE

The *DSM-IV* describes RAD as a fairly uncommon disorder. However, epidemiological data are limited and the prevalence data are inconsistent at this time.

CHARACTERISTICS OF CHILDREN WITH RAD

Children with RAD often do not believe that adults can keep them safe. They frequently have experienced adults as uncaring, rejecting, cruel, unreliable, incompetent, inconsistent, hurtful, or neglectful. They may have a sense of themselves as being "bad" and "unlovable." One moment they may show intense self-hatred and, at another moment, intense rage at and blame toward caregivers. They often develop a very negative sense of self, as this is better than believing that their own parents did not want or love them. Because increased intimacy with primary caregivers may elicit intense fear of being discovered as "bad" and "unlovable," these children often have intensely ambivalent relationships. One moment they may be indiscriminately and superficially affectionate. At another moment, they may create emotional distance from their caregivers by being angrily provocative, challenging, or callously disregarding. They may also unexpectedly or seemingly unintentionally "spoil" a positive experience with their caregivers. These children may be very bossy, interpersonally exploitative, demanding, clingy, or defiant. They may be prone to engage in power struggles with caregivers. They often have great difficulty maintaining positive peer relationships. They also may show little capacity for empathy and little remorse for their negative behavior. In addition, they may lie when there does not appear to be any motive to avoid getting in trouble. They may have impulse control problems and aggression toward self, others, or property. Given the wide range of characteristics observed among children with RAD, it can be difficult to distinguish RAD from behavior, attention, and mood disorders.

STATUS OF THE CURRENT DIAGNOSTIC CRITERIA

In recent years, there has been a proliferation of developmental research on attachment; however, the results of this research have not been integrated into the diagnostic criteria for RAD. In addition, the concern has been raised that the clinical usefulness of the current diagnostic criteria is limited by its focus on maltreatment. It has been suggested that the criteria should be broadened to include children who may not have experienced overt maltreatment but who are in disordered attachment relationships. Further, the current diagnostic criteria have been criticized for requiring that disordered attachment be present across social contexts. This requirement does not acknowledge that a child may express attachment in a variety of ways in different relationships.

In response to critiques of the current diagnostic criteria, Zeanah (1996) has set forth an alternative system of classification that attempts to better reflect the developmental research. This system identifies three major types of attachment disturbances: nonattached (show no preferred attachment to anyone), disordered (do not use the caregiver as a secure base of exploration), and disrupted (grief in response to loss of a primary caregiver). This system reduces the emphasis on pathogenic caregiving history and focuses on current behavior. As a result, the classification system applies to a broader range of children in disturbed relationships with their primary caregivers.

ASSESSMENT

Because of similarities in symptom presentation, it is important to distinguish RAD from other disorders, such as Attention-Deficit/Hyperactivity Disorder (ADHD), Oppositional Defiant Disorder (ODP), Conduct Disorder (CD), Mood Disorders (MD), Intermittent Explosive Disorder (IED), and Posttraumatic Stress Disorder (PTSD). It is not unusual for a child with RAD to have a comorbid diagnosis of learning or communication disorders or any of the previously mentioned disorders. Some investigators have suggested that RAD may predispose an individual to or be a precursor CD later in childhood or adolescence and of antisocial, borderline, or narcissistic personality disorders in late adolescence or adulthood. An assessment for RAD requires that the evaluator spend time with the child and parents or primary caregivers separately and together and observe interactions (i.e., the quality of emotional and behavioral exchanges and contrasts between interactions with caregivers versus interactions with the evaluator). The evaluator takes a thorough developmental, social, and family history, including as much information as possible on maltreatment, neglect, and changes in caregivers. Collateral sources of information include social services records, pediatric examinations, prior treatment or psychiatric records, and prior developmental, educational, or psychological evaluations. If possible, an assessment may include a home visit to observe interactions in the natural family context.

Formal assessment methods and instruments for RAD are underdeveloped and underresearched. One instrument in current use is the Randolph Attachment Disorder Questionnaire (RADQ), developed at the Attachment Center in Evergreen, Colorado. It is a 30-item screening instrument for differential diagnosis of children between ages 5 and 18 and for determining the severity of RAD. However, there is little information on its reliability and validity. The Parent–Infant Relationship Assessment Scale has been used in research to measure the overall relationship functioning without regard to whether impairments arise from the infant, caregiver, or the fit between the two. However, as noted by Boris and colleagues (1998), the reliability and validity of this scale has not been established in a large sample.

TREATMENT

Wilson (2001) has indicated that children with RAD often do not respond well to individual psychotherapy because they lack the trust that is necessary to establish a therapeutic relationship with a therapist, often have limited ability to benefit from experience, may show little motivation to change, have little regard for authority, and have poor impulse control.

Therapies for these children usually are directed at both the family (especially, the parents) and the child with RAD. Family-directed efforts may include: (1) providing support to the parents to ensure consistency and responsiveness toward the child, (2) teaching parenting strategies and techniques to manage the child's extreme and seemingly contradictory reactions, (3) teaching the parents to balance consistent limit-setting with a sense of genuine concern, (4) helping the parents to support each other in limit-setting and parenting tasks so as to prevent one parent from becoming "the good parent" and the other becoming "the bad parent," and (5) helping the parents to provide emotional and behavioral containment to aid the child in developing emotional and behavioral regulation.

Therapy must address the unique symptom presentation for each child with RAD; however, a core treatment emphasis for all such children is fostering trust. Therapy may focus on helping the child to develop a more positive sense of the environment in which primary caregivers are genuinely caring and competent, capable of protecting children, able to deal effectively with the child's intense and ambivalent feelings toward caregivers, and equipped to provide a nurturing, consistent, and predictable home environment. This requires that the child's immediate environment (usually with his family but sometimes in a psychiatric hospital unit or residential treatment setting) demonstrate to the child that the negative environment which he or she previously experienced is different from the environment in which he or she now lives. Treatment usually involves a tandem process of immediate environmental change (creating a safe and positive home environment) and therapeutic work with the child to recognize the change

in environment. The therapist may also work with the child to develop a new array of behaviors to effectively function and get needs met in this new environment. With the disinhibited type of RAD, efforts may be directed at helping the child to relinquish his or her parental, controlling stance and to accept being parented by a genuinely caring adult. Socially indiscriminate children may be taught to be more discriminating of adults in their world. Psychotropic medications, preferably prescribed by a child and adolescent psychiatrist, may target specific symptoms in a particular child (e.g., depression, unstable mood, rage reactions, hyperactivity, or impulsivity) and may be an important adjunct to psychological interventions.

A controversial intervention advocated by some residential treatment settings and attachment centers is called "holding therapy." Holding therapy, which involves physical holding to elicit the child's rage, is intended "to recreate the bonding cycle that the infant experiences with a parent" (Wilson, 2001, p. 47). Another approach aimed at enhancing attachment is called "Theraplay." Munns (2000) indicates that Theraplay involves developing an inventory of a child's positive features, rocking a child in a blanket, putting lotion or powder on the child, and engaging in mutual feeding. However, evidence is lacking on the benefits or risks of either holding therapy or Theraplay.

See also: Attachment; Child Maltreatment; Disruptive Behavior Disorders; Foster Care; Residential Treatment

Further Reading

American Psychiatric Association. (1994). *Diagnostic and statistical manual of mental disorders (DSM-IV)* (4th ed.). Washington, DC: Author.

Boris, N. W., Zeanah, C. H., Larrieu, J. A., Scheeringa, M. S., & Heller, S. S. (1998). Attachment disorders in infancy and early childhood: A preliminary investigation of diagnostic criteria. *American Journal of Psychiatry, 155*(2), 295–297.

Munns, E. (Ed.). (2000). *Theraplay: Innovations in attachment-enhancing play therapy*. Northvale, NJ: Jason Aronson.

Wilson, S. L. (2001). Attachment disorders: Review and current status. *Journal of Psychology, 135*(1), 37–51.

Zeanah, C. H. (1996). Beyond insecurity: A reconceptualization of attachment disorders in infancy. *Journal of Consulting and Clinical Psychology, 64*(1), 42–52.

Web Site

The Center for Mental Health Services Knowledge Exchange Network http://search.mentalhealth.org/default.asp?q1=reactive+attachment+&ct=KEN&advanced=&q2=&language=

Luis A. Vargas
Jennifer M. Stein

Recurrent Abdominal Pain

DEFINITION

Recurrent abdominal pain (RAP) refers to chronic abdominal pain with no demonstrated underlying physical disease. By definition, the syndrome is characterized by three or more episodes of abdominal pain over a 3-month period severe enough to interfere with routine functioning, and separated by asymptomatic (i.e., symptom free) periods. RAP varies widely in frequency, duration, intensity, location, and associated symptoms with pain episodes tending to cluster, alternating with pain-free episodes of variable length. Commonly associated symptoms are headache, pallor, nausea, dizziness, limb pain, and fatigue.

INCIDENCE/PSYCHOLOGICAL CORRELATES

Between 10 and 20 percent of school-age children experience repeated episodes of abdominal pain and in only about 10 percent of these cases is an organic etiology discovered. Thus, nonorganic recurrent abdominal pain is the most common presenting physical symptom in childhood. The typical age of presentation is between 5 and 14 years but it may occur as early as 3 years with the highest incidence between ages 8 and 10 years. The ratio of girls to boys is 5:3. Prevalence rates for boys show little variation across ages, but for girls the prevalence increases dramatically to about 30 percent at age 9 and then drops back to 10–15 percent in 11–12-year-old girls. Prevalence rates are similar in European and North American countries and RAP occurs across all socioeconomic levels.

Somatic complaints and emotional distress is similar for patients with RAP and those with organically based pain, although RAP patients report greater parental encouragement of illness behavior, more models for pain behavior, and more positive consequences of pain. Further, higher levels of somatization symptoms in parents of children with RAP are associated with higher levels of somatization symptoms in children with RAP but not for children with organic based pain. Similarly, children of parents with chronic pain reported more frequent abdominal pain and used more medication than children of parents without pain. In general, the number of somatic complaints

increases if the onset of RAP is prior to age 6 and persists for over a year. RAP appears to persist longer than organically based pain with over 50 percent of children with RAP reporting pain over a period of several years.

In addition to high levels of somatic complaints, children with RAP are also reported to have high levels of anxiety and symptoms of depression. Although negative life events do not appear to be more frequent for children with RAP, they do appear to increase the maintenance of symptoms, particularly if the child has low social competence.

ETIOLOGY

There is no established etiology for RAP. There appear to be a variety of subtypes of RAP and, therefore, the symptoms associated with RAP can have various etiologies. The developmental pathways could include physiological mechanisms (constipation, lactose intolerance, musculoskeletal abnormalities), psychological factors (higher levels of anxiety, stress and somatization, deficient or ineffective coping styles), and environmental factors (reinforcement for pain complaints and poor coping strategies, stress and negative life events, and modeling). Thus, RAP appears to be neither solely organic nor functional but rather the result of multiple environmental, psychological, and biological factors.

ASSESSMENT

Diagnosis of RAP should be based on integration of information from history, a complete physical exam including routine laboratory tests, and an understanding of the emotional and social context in which the pain occurs. Approximately 10 percent of the cases presenting with chronic abdominal pain are found to have an underlying physical disease including cholelithiasis, peptic ulcer, carbohydrate malabsorption, obstipation, and bowel dysmotility (see Gastrointestinal Disorders for a description of these diseases). A diary should be kept that includes dietary intake, the time, severity, location, and length of the pain episode, as well as its antecedents and consequences. The parents' views of the illness, the family's and extended family's experiences with somatic complaints, and their coping strategies should be assessed. The child's developmental status, perception and interpretation of the illness, stress and anxiety level, negative life events, and coping strategies should also be assessed. Coping strategies are particularly important to assess since they have been related to the number of reported somatic, anxious, and depressive symptoms in children with RAP. Walker and colleagues (1997) have developed a reliable and valid instrument for the assessment of coping with RAP, The Pain Responses Inventory. Both parent and child (8 years or older) can also complete another instrument developed by Walker's group, the Child Somatization Inventory, which lists 36 psychophysiological symptoms and gives an intensity as well as frequency score.

TREATMENT

Given the heterogeneity of RAP and its varying etiologies, effective treatment will depend on a careful assessment of the individual child's presenting symptoms, the possible etiological factors, the antecedents of the pain, and the consequences for both the child and the family. This will help determine the processes contributing to RAP and to other problem areas in the child's life so that the treatment strategies can be matched to the problem. Although there is no well-established treatment for RAP, a number of treatments have proven to be effective. Fiber therapy has been found effective for treating RAP in children that have symptoms of constipation. Dietary fiber is increased by 5–10 g per day through the consumption of high fiber cookies or wafers and has been found to decrease the number of RAP incidents by 50 percent.

Currently, the most promising treatment is cognitive–behavioral therapy. This intervention strategy has a combined focus on the parents and child that includes educating parents about RAP and the rationale for pain management techniques, teaching the parents behavioral management strategies including distraction techniques, and how to prompt and reinforce appropriate coping skills. Fewer somatic complaints and symptoms of anxiety and depression have been reported with coping strategies that are directed toward adapting to and engaging pain by regulating attention and cognition. The child can be taught effective coping strategies through self-monitoring, relaxation and imagery, and in self-talk control strategies. Eighty-seven percent of RAP children treated with this approach have been reported to be pain-free 3 months after treatment. Treatment of other problem or deficit areas such as

academic problems or social incompetence can also be helpful interventions.

PROGNOSIS

Many children with RAP will become symptom-free without treatment but a significant number will experience recurrent pain for years and are at increased risk for future health-related problems such as irritable bowel syndrome. High levels of abdominal pain, somatic symptoms, and functional disability, including school and work absence, have been reported 5 years after the initial diagnosis of RAP.

See also: Cognitive–Behavior Therapy; Coping with Illness; Encopresis; Gastrointestinal Disorders; Relaxation Training

Further Reading

Janicke, D. M., & Finney, J. W. (1999). Empirically supported treatments in pediatric psychology: Recurrent abdominal pain. *Journal of Pediatric Psychology, 24,* 115–127.

Sanders, M. R., Shepherd, R. W., Cleghorn, G., & Woolford, H. (1994). The treatment of recurrent abdominal pain in children: A controlled comparison of cognitive–behavioral family intervention and standard pediatric care. *Journal of Consulting and Clinical Psychology, 62,* 306–314.

Thomsen, A. H., Compas, B. E., Colletti, R. B., Stanger, C., Boyer, M. C., & Konik, B. S. (2002). Parent reports of coping and stress responses in children with recurrent abdominal pain. *Journal of Pediatric Psychology, 27*(3), 215–226.

Walker, L. S. (1999). The evolution of research on recurrent abdominal pain: History, assumptions, and a conceptual model. In P. J. McGrath & G. A. Finley (Eds.), *Chronic and recurrent pain in children and adolescents. Progress in pain research and management* (Vol. 13, pp. 141–172). Seattle, WA: IASP Press

Walker, L. S., & Greene, J. W. (1989). Children with recurrent abdominal pain and their parents: More somatic complaints, anxiety and depression than other patient families? *Journal of Pediatric Psychology, 14,* 231–243.

Walker, L. S., Smith, C. A., Garber, J., & Van Slyke, D. A. (1997). Development and validation of the Pain Response Inventory for children. *Psychological Assessment, 9,* 392–405.

CAROLYN S. SCHROEDER

Reflux

See: Gastroesophageal Reflux Disease

Relaxation Training*

DESCRIPTION

Relaxation refers to reducing electrical activity in the muscles and thus producing a feeling of physical and emotional calmness. By practicing specific exercises, one can learn to do this at will. Relaxation exercises increase an individual's ability to tolerate stress and to remain calm in the face of life's pressures and problems by interrupting the feedback loop that causes anxiety to spiral. Instead of allowing anxiety to steadily increase, the individual returns periodically to a calm, resting state and starts over. If practiced with regularity, relaxation exercises can significantly reduce levels of tension and anxiety. Common relaxation techniques include progressive muscle relaxation, meditation, breathing exercises, and differential relaxation.

METHODS

Progressive muscle relaxation is one of the simplest techniques for learning to relax. Teenagers and adults can be taught to do this by sitting in a comfortable chair or lying on a couch or bed and focusing on relaxing all of the muscle groups, saying something like the following to themselves: "I am going to relax completely. I will relax my forehead and scalp. I will let all the muscles of my forehead and scalp relax and become completely at rest. All of the wrinkles will smooth out of my forehead and that part of my body will relax completely. Now I will relax the muscles of my face. I will just let them relax and go limp. There will be no tension in my jaw. Next I will relax my neck muscles. Just let them become tranquil and allow all of the pressure to leave them. My neck muscles are relaxing completely. Now I will relax the muscles of my shoulders. That relaxation will spread down my arms to the elbows, down the forearm to my wrist, hands, and fingers. My arms will just dangle from the frame of my body. I will now relax the muscles of my chest. I will take a deep breath and relax, letting all of the tightness and tenseness leave. My breathing will now be normal and relaxed, and I will relax the muscles of my stomach. Now I will relax all of the muscles up

*The views expressed in this article are those of the author(s) and do not necessarily reflect the official policy or position of the Department of the Navy, Department of Defense, or the U.S. Government.

and down both sides of the spine and let that relaxation spread throughout my back. Now I will relax the waist, buttocks, and thighs down to my knees. Now the relaxation will spread to the calves of my legs, ankles, feet, and toes. I will just stay here and continue to let all of my muscles go completely limp. I will become completely relaxed from the top of my head to the tips of my toes."

If one has trouble doing this exercise at first, they can try deliberately tensing the muscles a few times and then letting them relax completely following the forced tension. This teaches discrimination between tensed and relaxed states and trains one to produce relaxation at will. If one still has trouble learning to relax, it is possible to see a professional therapist who can help. Some professionals may choose to use biofeedback to help clients learn to relax. The basic strategy with biofeedback is to arrange for the individual to receive some type of recognizable feedback (a sound that changes in volume or a visible meter reading) when muscle activity is changing in the direction that will produce relaxation.

For younger children, a parent can talk to them gently and instruct them to relax the muscles in the same sequence given above. Some parents find that it helps if they rub the child's head or back as they give the instructions. Massaging the arms and legs also helps, as does preceding the relaxation session with a warm bath. Some parents record the instructions and have the child listen to the tape as they relax. Commercial tapes can also be purchased. Tapes are available for all age levels from 4 or 5 years of age to adult. While there has not been extensive research in this area, some data suggest that having children practice relaxation before going to sleep at night has benefit in terms of reduced anxiety, fewer behavioral problems, and better overall adjustment.

There are numerous approaches to *meditation*, most of which derive from Eastern philosophy and religion. Older children and teenagers who practice meditation are able to achieve a considerable degree of bodily relaxation and calmness. Meditation exercises are best performed for half an hour to an hour on a daily basis. Regular use brings the best results. Meditating to a certain sound, such as a piece of music, may be of help. Others find meditating on a poem or a passage from a book rewarding. There are numerous books for the general reader that may be obtained in the library or from a local bookstore that provide meditation exercises for personal use.

Breathing exercises are also very useful and can be taught to children of all ages. When one is tense, breathing tends to be shallow and rapid. If one finds a comfortable place to sit and practices slow, deep breathing, this process tends to induce relaxation. Many people find it helpful to take a few deep breaths before entering a stressful situation. This helps one to relax before starting the activity. A useful technique with young children is to have them take a deep breath and imagine that they are a balloon being filled with air. They can then let the air out with a small hissing sound.

Differential relaxation is also a very important concept. The basic point of this is that when one is sitting, standing, walking, running, or whatever, some muscle groups can be relaxed while the others work. Many people tend to tense and work numerous muscles throughout the day that could otherwise be in a state of relaxation. This is because people typically involve themselves totally in what they are doing. To practice differential relaxation, one should first analyze their daily activities and identify muscles than can be relaxed rather than tense, and then discipline themselves to keep the muscles relaxed when possible. Teenagers can paint a small red dot on the crystal of their watch. Then, every time they look at their watch they will be reminded to check for any muscles that can be relaxed at that moment and to relax them. Younger children can carry a rubber or fur stress ball, make a pet rock to carry in their pocket, or even just squeeze a piece of their clothing. They can be encouraged to do this any time they feel anxious or "wound up."

CLINICAL APPLICATIONS

Just as regular physical exercise is the way to develop physical strength, regular practice of relaxation exercises can help one relax and reduce anxiety. Relaxation training has been found to be useful in treating all types of disorders caused or made worse by stress and anxiety, as well as in the prevention of problems such as the preparation for medical procedures. It has also been widely used in systematic desensitization procedures. Relaxation is most effective if practiced as a lifestyle to prevent development of problems, though it also works in crises. More information on this topic can be found in *The Relaxation Response* by Herbert Benson and *Learn to Relax* by C. Eugene Walker. Both of these are available in paperback editions.

See also: Acute Stress Disorder; Anxiety Disorders; Life Stress in Children and Adolescents; Pain Management; Preparation for Medical Procedures; Systematic Desensitization

Further Reading

Benson, H. A. (2000). *The relaxation response—updated and expanded.* New York: Avon.
Ollendick, T. H., & Cerny, J. A. (1981). *Clinical behavior therapy with children.* New York: Plenum.
Walker, C. E. (2000). *Learn to relax.* New York: Wiley.

C. EUGENE WALKER
DREW C. MESSER†

†I am a military service member. This work was prepared as part of my official duties. Title 17 U.S.C. 105 provides that "Copyright protection under this title is not available for any work of the United States Government." Title 17 U.S.C. 101 defines a United States Government work as a work prepared by a military service member or employee of the United States Government as part of that person's official duties.

Reliability

DEFINITION

Reliability refers to the consistency of measurements when a testing procedure is repeated on a population of groups or individuals (AERA, APA, NCME, 1999). Estimates of relevant reliabilities should be reported for each total score, subscore, or combination of scores that is to be interpreted.

METHODS

The more common types of reliability coefficients reported in test manuals include internal consistency, interrater, and test–retest. Internal consistency coefficients, for example, assess the average correlation among the items, or the homogeneity of the test item pool. Data are accumulated from a single administration of a test and the coefficients are based on the relationships among the scores derived from individual items or subsets of items with a test. These coefficients are valuable for the test construction process because they only require one administration of a test, they serve as good estimates of test–retest or stability coefficients, and they are inexpensively produced. Internal consistency reliability coefficients are also useful in comparing tests or measurement procedures. According to Kamphaus, popular computational procedures and formulas for internal consistency coefficients include split-half coefficients, Kuder Richardson 20, and Coefficient or

Cronbach's alpha. Internal consistency coefficients should not be considered equivalent to alternate-form, test–retest, and generalizability coefficients because each may have a distinct definition of measurement error.

Interrater, interjudge, or interobserver reliability coefficients are important for assessing the accuracy of certain assessment methods, especially history taking, observational, or other "nontest" assessment procedures. For example, while application of diagnostic criteria is not a "test" per se, it is nevertheless important to know if the diagnostic criteria are explicit enough to be applied consistently by different clinicians. A typical study of interdiagnostician reliability may be used to construct the diagnostic criteria for a disorder. First, diagnostic criteria are stated and then clinicians are asked to collect information via history, interview, or other means and make a diagnosis based on the criteria. Then, a statistic such as Cohen's kappa may be used to compare the diagnoses of several clinicians who have seen the same patient or otherwise have the same patient information.

Test–retest reliability refers to the consistency of measurements when a testing procedure is repeated on a population or groups of individuals (AERA, APA, NCME, 1999). Said another way, this method is the one that clinicians and the public usually consider to be the exemplar of the term "reliability," meaning the stability of test scores over time. A test–retest reliability estimate is obtained by correlating pairs of scores from the same groups of individuals on two independent administrations of the same test. Test–retest reliability coefficients may fail, however, to reflect measurement error associated with changes in an individual's health, efficiency, or motivation. As time between administrations of a test increase, the correlation between scores on that test for a particular individual decreases. The longer the time interval, the more likely the test–retest reliability coefficient will be low (AERA, APA, NCME, 1999).

See also: Psychometric Properties of Tests; Validity; Psychological Testing

Further Reading

American Educational Research Association, American Psychological Association, & National Council for Measurement in Education. (1999). *Standards for educational and psychological testing.* Washington, DC: American Educational Research Association.

RANDY W. KAMPHAUS
ERIN DOWDY
ANNA P. KRONCKE

Report Writing

Psychological reports document the process and outcome of assessment, facilitate appropriate intervention, ensure accountability, and meet legal and institutional requirements. Reports will typically reflect the standards of the institution and/or the individual clinician; however, several elements will be common to all reports that meet the APA Ethics Code. The clinical child or pediatric psychologist must rely on scientific and professional judgments that take into account human differences. Assessment tools (e.g., standardized tests, clinical interviews) must be used for the purposes for which each was intended. Interpretation of assessment results must take into account the individual's characteristics as well as assessment conditions that may impinge upon the accuracy of the results. The results must be reported in a way that is understandable to the client (or parent/legal guardian in the case of minors). The report must be maintained, stored, and destroyed in a manner that keeps confidentiality and meets legal requirements. In short, the report must be ethical, legal, and useful.

Reports will typically have specific elements that are dictated by the institution, pertinent laws (e.g., Individuals with Disabilities Education Act, 1997), and the needs of the patient. Most reports will contain a referring question, which is the reason that the assessment is occurring. Assessment tools used are listed, and outcomes will be reported. Conclusions of the clinical child or pediatric psychologist, diagnostic impressions, and specific recommendations will typically be included. In addition, reports must be written and disseminated in a timely manner.

Reports may contain some variations of the following elements, which will be adapted and guided by specific institutional expectations and the referral question.

IDENTIFYING INFORMATION

This includes name, age, gender, grade in school, dates of assessment, date of report, and may include address and telephone number.

REFERRAL QUESTION

This includes who is the source of the referral, specific concerns that are to be addressed in the assessment process, and a brief summary of the conditions that led to the referral.

ASSESSMENTS USED

This is a listing of the tools used in the assessment process, which includes both informal (e.g., observations) and formal (e.g., clinical interview, standardized measures) tools.

BEHAVIORAL OBSERVATIONS

These are descriptions of the patient and the patient's behaviors that occur throughout the assessment process. Typically these observations will include a physical description of the child, general behavior, activity level, communication style, mood and affect, motor skills, and unusual mannerisms. In some behavioral observations, both the descriptions and the interpretation of the behaviors are included.

CASE HISTORY INFORMATION

This is generally information that is obtained from others (e.g., parents, teachers) that includes a history of development, health, family situation, school performance, living situation, and mental health. Other history may be reported as well, such as past abuse or encounters with the legal system. Typically both past and present information is reported.

ASSESSMENT RESULTS

Typically, standardized assessment tools (e.g., Wechsler Intelligence Scale for Children, Third Edition [WISC–III]) are described in terms of purpose and scores that are reported. Results of the assessment process are reported, and as appropriate, specific test scores are included. Scores are typically reported in ranges and percentiles, and charts include specific numerical outcomes, including standard scores and confidence intervals.

CLINICAL IMPRESSIONS

The clinician evaluates validity and reliability of the information and presents his or her hypotheses about the overall functioning of the child. These impressions are based on the preponderance of the evidence guided by valid and reliable professional and scientific judgment. Often this is the section where specific diagnostic impressions (e.g., *DSM-IV* diagnoses) are presented.

SUMMARY

The summary is not always included, but when it is, it is a precise and concise summarization of the report, where no new material is presented.

RECOMMENDATIONS

The recommendations must address the referral question, and must take into account the consumers of the report. For example, a report to the schools should not include specific placement recommendations (see Individuals with Disabilities Education Act, 1997). Recommendations ideally involve all those who may be instrumental in carrying them out (e.g., parents, teachers, the child), take into account resources that are available (e.g., a recommendation for therapy four times a week may not be feasible given family finances and insurance coverage), and are useful to all concerned (e.g., recommending further counseling that emphasises anger management is more helpful than simply recommending counseling).

SIGNATURE

This includes written and printed signature block with the clinician's name, professional title, and degree.

Reports have both ethical and legal constraints. Applicable ethics include those outlined in the APA Ethics Code, those of other organizations that are pertinent to the clinician (e.g., National Association of School Psychology), and those of the institutional setting (e.g., hospitals and schools). Legal considerations include both federal and state statutes as well as case law (e.g., Family Education Rights and Privacy Act, 1974; state statutes that accompany special education law). The clinical child and pediatric psychologist must know and practice within the ethical guidelines and legal constraints that pertain to each case.

The ethical, legal, and useful report should include only pertinent information, provide definitions of abbreviations and acronyms (e.g., not "the child is LD according to IDEA and *DSM-IV* standards"), avoid theoretical bias (e.g., defining all behaviors as "reaction-formation defenses"), avoid jargon (e.g., "manifests overt hostile behaviors resulting in subsequent injury to others" vs. "hits others"), ensure correct grammar and spelling, and be written in a language easily understood by the consumer.

See also: Confidentiality and Privilege; Ethical Issues; Individuals with Disabilities Education Act; Legal Issues in Child and Pediatric Psychology; Mental Health Records

Further Reading

Kamphaus, R. W. (2001). *Clinical assessment of child and adolescent intelligence* (2nd ed.). Needham Heights, MA: Allyn & Bacon.
Koocher, G. P. (1998). Assessing the quality of a psychological testing report. In G. P. Koocher, J. C. Norcross, & S. S. Hill III (Eds.), *Psychologists' desk reference* (pp. 169–171). New York: Oxford.
Sattler, J. M. (1998). *Clinical and forensic interviewing of children and families: Guidelines for the mental health, education, pediatric, and child maltreatment fields.* San Diego, CA: Jerome M. Sattler.
Wolber, G. J., & Carne, W. F. (1993). Writing psychological reports: A guide for clinicians. Sarasota, FL: Professional Resource Press.

Web Sites

http://www.apa.org/ethics/code.html
http://www.ed.gov/offices/OSERS/OSEP

WILLIAM A. RAE

Residential Treatment

DESCRIPTION

Residential treatment of children and adolescents with behavioral and/or emotional problems encompasses those forms of treatment that involve the removal of the child from the home. It is estimated that over 50,000 children and adolescents in the United States are served by some form of residential treatment each year. The diagnoses or presenting problems of children treated in such settings range from schizophrenia to Conduct Disorder (CD). Often, children for whom residential treatment is indicated have exhibited dangerous behaviors (e.g., violence; self-injurious behaviors) and/or lack of an intact, functional family environment. Residential treatment is further indicated if the child is considered to be at risk of harm in the present home environment or if the family is geographically isolated to the extent that nonresidential treatment options are not feasible. The duration of treatment can range from as brief as

one night (i.e., for crisis intervention/stabilization) to a lifetime (i.e., for severe mental disturbance). It is important to emphasize that residential treatment is an extremely invasive intervention that involves disruption of virtually every aspect of a child's life. Therefore, residential treatment should be viewed as only one option for intervening with children and adolescents with behavioral and/or emotional difficulties. The ideal form of treatment for a particular child would be one that is least disruptive of his or her natural environment while still allowing for effective intervention.

CLINICAL APPLICATION

The specific types of services that could be considered under the term "residential treatment" vary considerably in their structure, duration of treatment, and theoretical approach to treatment. Respite care is a term often used to describe treatment provided for short periods of time (e.g., 12 hr to 3 weeks) with its focus on providing relief and support for caregivers. Shelter care describes placements that primarily serve to protect and comfort the child during crises such as abuse, abandonment, or parental incapacitation. These treatment settings may or may not provide formal therapeutic interventions for a child.

Group homes and residential treatment centers comprise two models that provide formal treatment services to children and adolescents for one month up to several years. Group homes are differentiated from traditional foster care in that they are located in facilities owned and operated by a child care agency and provide services to a number of children (e.g., 10–12) at one time, as opposed to providing services in a private single family home for a very small number of children. In such programs, children typically attend public schools and are cared for at home by trained staff members. Residential treatment centers provide services whereby children are even more isolated from their communities, as school services and other activities, including individual and group therapy are provided at the center, and children live in a group home type of setting located at the treatment center. These centers often include staff trained in various disciplines, including psychology, medicine, education, social work, nutrition, and nursing. Formal interventions (e.g., individual therapy) are provided by trained professionals in these settings, and day-to-day behavioral management strategies are implemented by direct-care staff.

Such programs are differentiated from inpatient hospitalization in that inpatient treatment is often used in circumstances where the child's problems appear to have some significant somatic or organic causal component, pharmacological interventions and monitoring seem indicated, or a child/adolescent is in a state of significant crisis (e.g., active suicidal ideation or recent attempts). Inpatient settings are typically not oriented to provide intervention for school or family-based problems because of the deemphasis on educational programming and limited contact between the child and his or her family in these settings.

Although psychodynamically oriented models characterized early residential treatment programs that emphasized intervening through isolating the child from a dysfunctional family environment and providing psychoanalytically based treatment, current models are more behaviorally oriented or based more firmly on attachment theory. Attachment-based programs seek to give youths an opportunity to form more trusting, positive relationships with adults through positive experiences with residential staff. Behavioral programs view maladaptive behaviors as resulting largely from past learning experiences, and thus, the residential environment is structured to encourage more adaptive behaviors through the consistent delivery of positive consequences for desired behaviors and negative consequences for targeted maladaptive behaviors. In such environments, direct-care staff have a primary treatment responsibility by administering the consequences and working with children to ensure that they understand the behavioral expectations of the residential and classroom environments.

For example, children may be allowed to earn "points" on target behaviors specific to their referral concerns for daily (e.g., free time) and/or weekly privileges (e.g., group outings). To reduce maladaptive behaviors, residential treatment programs may employ some form of withholding of privileges or "time out," a procedure through which a child exhibiting disruptive behaviors such as aggression or refusing to comply with a staff member's instructions is removed from the situation for a certain period of time, often depending on when the child's behavioral or emotional reaction decreases. Anger management and social skills programs also are often included in residential treatment with some demonstrated success. Peer culture programs, which utilize group therapy and peer and staff feedback regarding target behaviors, are increasingly being implemented as the central component of residential treatment or as an additional aspect of behaviorally oriented programs. Another component that has recently been added to many residential

treatment programs, particularly for adolescents, is that of formal work training and actual work experience at the treatment center.

In summary, residential treatment options for child and adolescent emotional and behavioral problems vary considerably in the degree to which the client is removed from his or her natural environment, the physical setting of the treatment facility, and the major emphasis of treatment. In addition, programs vary in the type and number of direct-care staff who are employed, the age, sex, and presenting problem of the children who are served, the role of psychotherapy in treatment, the degree of involvement of the family in the child's treatment, the specific management strategies employed in the treatment environment, the steps taken to maintain the child's involvement with his or her community, and the procedures taken for reintegrating the child into the community at the time of discharge. Practical issues such as these should be considered by professionals and families if they determine that a child's difficulties might warrant some form of residential treatment.

EFFECTIVENESS

Because of the greatly varied interventions that could be considered under the term "residential treatment" and the varied presenting problems that such programs are designed to treat, methodologically sound, controlled research on the outcomes associated with residential treatment has been difficult to conduct. The existing treatment outcome literature suggests that most children placed in residential treatment show improvements, particularly shortly after discharge. However, this research also indicates that the long-term improvement of children treated in residential programs may not be significantly greater than untreated control groups. Some general findings have emerged from this research. For example, behaviorally oriented programs have been shown to be more effective in improving emotional and behavioral functioning than more psychodynamically oriented programs. Children with conduct disorders or psychotic disorders have shown less improvement than children with other types of mental health complaints, whereas higher child intelligence has been associated with better outcomes. In addition, family involvement in residential treatment has been positively correlated with treatment effectiveness.

Interestingly, the outcomes reported from research on day treatment and in-home intervention programs are comparable to those reported for residential treatment programs. These findings suggest that such programs should be considered as viable alternatives to residential treatment, particularly when the lower cost of nonresidential treatment is considered. Lastly, the outcome research on residential treatment has largely failed to investigate possible interactions among child characteristics, family characteristics, program characteristics, and outcome to determine which programs might be most effective for which clients. Research suggests that children can benefit from residential treatment programs; however, more research is needed to determine which children might best benefit from these alternatives to more community-based intervention. At that point, better informed cost–benefit analyses of treatment options for children and their families can be conducted.

See also: Behavior Contracts; Day Treatment; Foster Care; Hospitalization—Medical; Time Out

Further Reading

Lyman, R. D., & Campbell, N. R. (1996). *Treating children and adolescents in residential and inpatient settings.* Thousand Oaks, CA: Sage.
Lyman, R. D., Prentice-Dunn, S., & Gabel, S. (Eds.). (1989). *Residential and inpatient treatment of children and adolescents.* New York: Plenum Press.
Pardek, J. T. (2002). *Children's rights: Policy and practice.* New York: Haworth Press.
Web address: http://www.nationalyouth.com/residentialtreatment.html

ROBERT D. LYMAN
CHRISTOPHER T. BARRY

Respiratory Diseases

See: Pulmonary Disorders

Response Cost

Response cost is a behavioral procedure that has been developed within the framework of applied behavior analysis. It involves a previously earned or awarded reinforcer being removed, contingent upon the occurrence of an inappropriate behavior. The aim of response cost is to remove positive reinforcers in order to decrease the probability of the future occurrence of a problem behavior. There are many examples of response cost in the lives of children. The teacher who reduces the length of the usual lunchtime contingent upon disruptive behavior is using a response cost procedure. Similarly, the parent who removes a child's usual access to television upon failure to complete homework is also using a response cost procedure. Each occurrence of the inappropriate behavior results in the loss of a specific amount of positive reinforcement already held by the individual.

Response cost has been shown to be highly effective in classroom settings, and can be combined with other procedures, such as behavior contracts, reinforcement, and time out, in a comprehensive behavior change program. Students know beforehand via classroom rules or behavior contracts what behavior will produce "fines." Each fine that is levied indicates that a positive reinforcer has been lost and serves to remind the student that future occurrences of the same behavior will result in the same consequence.

It should be noted that response cost should not be used as the sole approach to changing behavior because this procedure is not able to teach new behaviors. It should be combined with the use of positive reinforcement for appropriate behavior whenever possible.

See also: Applied Behavior Analysis; Behavior Modification; Positive Reinforcement; Token Economies

Further Reading

Carlson, C. L., & Tamm, L. (2000). Responsiveness of children with attention deficit-hyperactivity disorder to reward and response cost: Differential impact on performance and motivation. *Journal of Consulting and Clinical Psychology, 68,* 73–83.
Grant, L., & Evans, A. (1994). *Principles of behavior.* New York: HarperCollins.
McGoey, K. E., & DuPaul, G. J. (2000). Token reinforcement and response cost procedures: Reducing the distruptive behavior of preschool children with attention-deficit/hyperactivity disorder. *School Psychology Quarterly, 15,* 330–343.
Stein, D. B. (1999). Outpatient behavioral management of aggressiveness in adolescents: A response cost paradigm. *Aggressive Behavior, 25,* 321–330.
Truchlicka, M., McLaughlin, T. F., & Swain, J. C. (1998). Effects of token reinforcement and response cost on the accuracy of spelling performance with middle-school special education students with behavior disorders. *Behavioral Interventions, 13,* 1–10.

SOPHIA XENOS
ALAN HUDSON

Retinoblastoma

DESCRIPTION

Retinoblastoma is a malignant tumor of the eye, more specifically of the embryonic neural retina. It is usually diagnosed before the age of three, and occurs in 1/18,000 births. About 200 children per year develop retinoblastoma in the United States. Thus, it is a relatively rare disease.

ETIOLOGY

In contrast to other pediatric tumors, about 40 percent of the cases of retinoblastoma are hereditary and are caused by a gene mutation. In these cases, the tumor is often bilateral (occurring in both eyes). Children of patients with hereditary retinoblastoma have about a 45 percent chance of developing the tumor. Children with the hereditary type of retinoblastoma are also at risk for developing other cancers. In addition, about 10 percent of children with bilateral retinoblastoma will develop osteosarcoma, with which it may share a genetic basis. Research in the biology and genetics of retinoblastoma has increased understanding of the genetics and heredity of childhood cancer.

PRESENTATION

The signs and symptoms depend on the size and position of the tumor. It may be recognized when the child is squinting or has a "white pupil," that is, there is no red reflex in the eye (leukocoria). Another sign is strabismus. Ophthalmic (eye) examination is usually followed by ultrasound and computed tomography (CT), and may also be followed by magnetic resonance imaging (MRI).

PROGNOSIS

Prognosis in unilateral retinoblastoma for maintaining vision in the unaffected eye is excellent, but the prognosis for vision in bilateral form depends on the extent of tumor and effectiveness of treatment. The overall survival rate is about 90 percent. Metastatic disease (spread beyond the primary tumor) has a less favorable prognosis and varies with the extent of spread or invasion from 20 to 90 percent.

TREATMENT

Treatment depends on tumor size and the extent of the disease. Many modalities are used: enucleation (removal of the eye), radiotherapy, laser photocoagulation (light to destroy blood supply), cryotherapy (cold), themotherapy (heat), systemic chemotherapy (common drugs are vincristine, cyclophosphamide, doxorubicin, cisplatin, etoposide, and carboplatin), and radiation.

Late effects may include abnormalities in bone growth around the eye, inflammation of the cornea, retinal damage, altered facial appearance, and secondary malignancies. Where there is a family history of retinoblastoma, all children should receive genetic screening shortly after birth, with regular follow-up exams. The psychosocial team is important in helping the family deal not only with cancer but also potential or real loss of an eye and vision. Cognitive–behavioral therapy can help the child and family cope with rehabilitation issues.

See also: Behavioral Dentistry; Bone and Soft Tissue Tumors; Childhood Cancers; Coping with Illness; Preparation for Medical Procedures

Further Reading

Granowetter, L. (1994). Pediatric oncology: A medical overview. In D. Bearison & R. K. Mulhern (Eds.), *Pediatric psychooncology* (pp. 9–34). New York: Oxford.

Hurwitz, R. L., Shields, C. L., Shields, J. A., Chevez-Barrios, P., Hurwitz, M. Y., & Chimtagumpala, M. M. (2002). Retinoblastoma. In P. A. Pizzo & D. G. Poplack (Eds.), *Principles and practice of pediatric oncology* (4th ed., pp. 825–846). Philadelphia: Lippincott Williams & Wilkins.

MARY JO KUPST
ANNE B. WARWICK

Rett's Syndrome

DEFINITION

Rett's syndrome is a Pervasive Developmental Disorder (*DSM-IV*) almost exclusively affecting females. The syndrome was first described in 1966 by an Austrian physician named Andreas Rett. It is characterized by a period of apparent normal development until 6–18 months of age followed by deteriorating motor development, declining social interaction, and diminishing cognitive and language abilities. A loss of purposeful hand movements leads to stereotypic hand clasping, hand-washing movements, and hand-mouthing. These stereotypic hand movements have become the behavioral hallmark of the syndrome. Affected children typically function within the severe to profound range of mental retardation. Mobility, if achieved, is characterized by a very stiff and shaky gait. Deceleration of head growth (acquired microcephaly) presumably reflects diffuse brain atrophy and deterioration. Other commonly associated symptoms are breathing dysfunction, including breath holding, apnea or air swallowing, seizures, scoliosis, chewing and swallowing difficulties, growth retardation, and sleep abnormalities. Eighty-five percent of those affected are considered to have classic Rett syndrome. The remaining 15 percent manifest a milder form of the disorder.

PREVALENCE AND COURSE OF THE DISORDER

Prevalence is estimated to be 1 per 10,000–22,800 females. Although there may be as many as 10,000 girls with Rett's syndrome in the United States, only a small percentage has been identified. A four-stage system has been developed to describe the typical clinical presentation and course of Rett's syndrome. Before 6 months of age the child appears to be healthy and develops normally. Stage 1 (6–18 months) is characterized by deterioration or general slowing of motor development. Prominent features include hypotonia, failure to develop postural adjustment skills, and delayed attainment of motor milestones. During Stage 2 (1–3 years) there is significant degeneration that results in the primary characteristics listed above. During Stage 3 (2–10 years) some of the symptoms can actually lessen, including irregular or restless sleep, autistic features, and irritability. Stage 4 (10 years and older) is marked by gradual decrease in ambulatory ability, if it is present. Other cognitive abilities such as social interaction, communication, and hand-use abilities remain relatively stable.

ETIOLOGY

Rett's syndrome appears to be a sex-linked genetic disorder. Approximately 80 percent of females with classical Rett's syndrome have a mutation of the gene for methyl-CpG-binding protein 2 (*MECP2*) located on the X chromosome, as established by Amir and

colleagues (1999). MECP2 protein inactivates genes that are no longer needed or which are only active at particular points during development. Mutations of the *MECP2* gene are thought to occur spontaneously within the father's gametes thus accounting for transmission to female children almost exclusively. The very few cases of males with Rett's syndrome have occurred with concurrent diagnoses of Klinefelter syndrome—a male who has two X chromosomes and a Y chromosome. Females with less severe symptoms may have a bias in X chromosome activation. Specifically, the X chromosome containing the *MECP2* mutation may not be activated in as many cells as the non-mutated chromosome, thus resulting in fewer deleterious effects.

ASSESSMENT

Although Rett's syndrome has a distinctive clinical course, presentation during Stage 1 is fairly nonspecific—thus hampering early detection. Diagnosis begins with a complete developmental history and review of findings from primary care well-child visits. If there is evidence of slowed head growth, decreased motor capability, or developmental delay, then a more thorough evaluation should take place. This evaluation should include cognitive, communication, and motor assessments. If Rett's syndrome is suspected, then a test for a *MECP2* gene mutation would be appropriate.

TREATMENT

There is no cure for Rett's syndrome. The discovery of the gene mutation may lead to gene therapies such as selective activation of the nonmutated X chromosome or the development of a synthetic MECP2 protein. In the absence of such genetic treatments, current treatment options include medications and procedures to treat some of the effects of Rett's syndrome. Regular medical care is recommended to monitor health problems that may develop. Also, seizures and electroencephalogram (EEG) irregularities are often treated through the use of anticonvulsant medication. Physical therapy may mitigate the effects of apraxia and loss of muscle tone. Assistive devices may enhance mobility and communication. Applied behavior analysis may be employed to manage behavioral concerns that may develop. Finally, parent groups and family education programs may provide support to parents, siblings, and extended family.

See also: Applied Behavior Analysis; Autistic Disorder; Childhood Disintegrative Disorder; Mental Retardation; Pervasive Developmental Disorder—Not Otherwise Specified (PPDNOS)

Further Reading

Amir, R. E., Van den Veyver, I. B., Wan, M., Tran, C. Q., Francke, U., & Zoghbi, H. Y. (1999). Rett syndrome is caused by mutations in X-linked MECP2, encoding methyl-CpG-binding protein 2. *Nature Genetics, 23*(2), 185–188.

International Rett Syndrome Association (n.d.). http://www.rettsyndrome.org/

Van Acker, R. (1997). Rett's syndrome: A pervasive developmental disorder. In D. J. Cohen & F. R. Volkmar (Eds.), *Handbook of autism and pervasive developmental disorders* (2nd ed., pp. 60–93). New York: Wiley.

ERIC L. CANEN
WILLIAM E. MACLEAN, JR.

Reye's Syndrome

DEFINITION AND SYMPTOMS

Reye's syndrome is a rare but severe neurological disorder characterized by encephalopathy and fatty degeneration of the liver. Typically, Reye's syndrome has a rapid onset, appearing about a week (1–14 days) following a viral illness, such as varicella (chicken pox), upper respiratory infection, or influenza. Symptom progression (from persistent or recurrent vomiting and listlessness, to "personality changes" such as irritability, combative behavior, disorientation or confusion, agitation, and delirium) is a manifestation of the rapid, and potentially life-threatening, swelling of (and pressure on) the brain. As the condition progresses, the child becomes semiconscious or stuporous. Ultimately seizures and coma may develop, followed by death in as many as one-third of the patients.

INCIDENCE

Although adults are not invulnerable, Reye's syndrome predominantly affects children between 4 and 16 years of age. It is more frequent during winter months when viral diseases are epidemic, or following an outbreak of chicken pox or influenza. Reye's syndrome was not always as infrequent as current incidence figures (1:1,000,000) indicate. Since the peak incidence of 555 cases documented by the Centers for Disease Control and Prevention (CDC) in 1980, the annual number of cases has declined rapidly; since 1987, fewer than 37 cases have been reported each year.

ETIOLOGY

Over 20 years of research has failed to elucidate the etiology of Reye's syndrome. However, early investigations focused attention on the condition and demonstrated a statistical association between using aspirin or aspirin-containing medications to treat viral illness symptoms, and the subsequent increased risk of developing Reye's syndrome.

As a result, the CDC began cautioning physicians and parents about a possible connection between Reye's syndrome and the use of aspirin to treat children with chicken pox or influenza-like illnesses. The U.S. Surgeon General issued a formal advisory about salicylates (specifically aspirin and aspirin-containing products) in 1982, and, since 1986, the Food and Drug Administration has required that aspirin manufacturers add a health warning to all product labels.* The efficacy of this public health education strategy appears to be confirmed by the marked decrease in the use of aspirin among children with viral illness, accompanied by a sharp decline in reported cases of children, especially those 5–10 years of age, with Reye's syndrome.

MEDICAL TREATMENT

In the absence of a specific lesion or underlying pathophysiological mechanism, there is no known medical cure for Reye's syndrome. Early diagnosis and procedures designed to manage symptoms and reduce their impact on the brain and other body organ systems are vital for survival. Currently available treatment, typically provided in a medical center intensive care unit, involves careful monitoring, often via an indwelling brain pressure gauge; titrating medications that seek to reduce brain swelling and protect the central nervous system (CNS) against irreversible damage; repairing metabolic injury; preventing complications in the lungs; and anticipating cardiac arrest.

PSYCHOLOGICAL ASSESSMENT
AND INTERVENTIONS

It is helpful to define the extent, pattern, and trajectory of recovery for any neurocognitive deficits sustained as a consequence of Reye's syndrome. Affected areas may include attention and concentration, speech articulation, language processing, memory,

*Surgeon General's prescribed warning label: "Children and teenagers should not use this medicine for chicken pox or flu symptoms before a doctor is consulted about Reye's syndrome, a rare but serious illness reported to be associated with aspirin."

visual–perceptual–motor skills, and planning and organizational abilities. Baseline neuropsychological screening conducted around discharge, and a comprehensive assessment within 3–6 months of diagnosis (and repeated, as clinically indicated), should help define any neurocognitive deficits. Early identification and related environmental interventions may prevent the secondary emotional sequelae (e.g., depression) that often occur when an individual acquires new, but perhaps subtle and unrecognized, learning problems that prevent quick and easy return to prior levels of functioning. In addition, intervention may target child and family adaptation to changes in the child's health status. Particular attention may be paid to patterns of entrenchment in the sick role, contrasted with a return to usual family routines that serve to maintain an appropriate developmental trajectory and facilitate a child's relationships, play interactions, explorations, and quality of life.

PREVENTION

Despite its unknown cause, Reye's syndrome illustrates a model for effective illness prevention, with public health interventions focused on: (1) early recognition and treatment of symptoms; (2) accommodations for subtle CNS effects experienced by some child survivors; and (3) reduction in incidence accomplished via an international effort to educate physicians and the public at large about the association between use of aspirin in the management of children's symptoms of influenza or viral illness and subsequent development of Reye's syndrome. Recent CDC data and a historical review published in the *New England Journal of Medicine* demonstrate the dramatic impact that these public education and surveillance programs have had. Ongoing efforts will be necessary, given the continuing availability of salicylate-based products, to keep new generations of parents and physicians, who may not have had direct experience with Reye's syndrome, alert to the potential for a secondary resurgence of this disease.

PROGNOSIS

Despite the sharp drop in incidence, the life threatening nature of Reye's syndrome is no less severe. Unless an individual is promptly diagnosed with Reye's syndrome and treated successfully, death is common and may occur after only a few days. In a recent series of cases, the overall fatality rate was 31 percent, with the highest mortality rate among children under 5 years of age and in those whose serum ammonia reaches very high levels (above 45 μg/dl).

Morbidity among pediatric patients varies. It is possible for a child with Reye's syndrome to recover completely with no aftereffects or observable sequelae. However, survival may be accompanied by brain damage and dysfunction ranging from very subtle motor and/or learning disabilities, to profound neuromuscular problems and mental retardation. Outcome, especially the incidence of permanent neurological complications, seems related to the severity, rate of progression, and duration of swelling experienced by the brain. Poorer outcome occurs more often when the disorder progresses rapidly and the patient lapses into a coma, compared with those with a less severe course.

See also: Coping with Illness; Hashimoto's Encephalopathy; Hospitalization—Medical; Learning Disorders; Neurological Disorders; Neuropsychological Assessment

Further Reading

Belay, E. D., Bresee, M. D., Holman, R. C, Khan, A. S., Shahriari, A., & Schonberger, L. B. (1999). Reye's syndrome in the United States from 1981 through 1997. *New England Journal of Medicine, 340,* 1377–1382.

Hurwitz, E. S., Barrett, M. J., Bregman, D. et al. (1987). Public Health Service Study of Reye's syndrome and medications: Report of the main study. *Journal of the American Medical Association, 257,* 1905–1911.

National Center for Infectious Diseases, Centers for Disease Control and Prevention, Atlanta, GA. Online URL: http://www.cdc.gov/ncidod/diseases/reye.htm

National Reye's Syndrome Foundation, Inc. Online URL: http://www.reyessyndrome.org

Whitt, J. K. (1984). Children's adaptation to chronic illness and handicapping conditions. In M. G. Eisenberg, M. Jansen, & L. Sutkin (Eds.), *The impact of chronic disabling conditions on self and family: A life span perspective.* New York: Springer.

J. KENNETH WHITT

Rhabdomyosarcoma

DEFINITION/INCIDENCE

Rhabdomyosarcoma (RMS) is the most common soft tissue sarcoma in childhood and is the third most common extracranial solid tumor after neuroblastoma and Wilm's tumor. The incidence in those under 20 years of age is about 4.3 cases per million children, with about 350 new cases diagnosed annually in the United States. Two-thirds of the cases are in children less than 6 years of age with a smaller incidence peak in early to mid-adolescence.

ETIOLOGY

RMS is slightly more common in males than in females. It may be associated with several genetic syndromes (Li–Fraumeni syndrome, Beckwith–Wiedemann syndrome, and neurofibromatosis type I), and therefore with abnormalities of the p53 tumor suppressor gene. Environmental factors may include toxic environmental agents.

PRESENTATION

RMS may be discovered clinically either by the appearance of a mass lesion in a body region without history of trauma or disturbance of a bodily function by an otherwise enlarging tumor. Head and neck tumors are most common in children less than 8 years of age, while extremity tumors are more common in adolescents and tumors of the bladder or vagina are most common in infants. Fewer than 25 percent have metastases (spread of tumors beyond the primary site) at diagnosis, and these sites include lung, bone marrow, bone, lymph node, and visceral organs.

PROGNOSIS

Prognosis depends upon risk status: low risk, around 90 percent; intermediate risk, around 75 percent; and high risk, around 20 percent. Prognostic factors depend upon stage and include presence or absence of distant metastases, site (orbit most favorable), surgical resectability, that is, removal (total, better), histology (embryonal vs. alveolar), and age (less than 10 years of age, better prognosis). Based on the Intergroup Rhabdomyosarcoma Studies-III (IRS-III) data, overall 5-year event-free survival was about 65 percent. Most patients with nonmetastatic disease are now considered to be cured, although recurrence can occur years after treatment has ended (usually 3–4 years).

TREATMENT

Treatment is multimodal and involves surgery (to remove the tumor if possible), radiation therapy, and systemic chemotherapy. The type and intensity of chemotherapy depends upon risk assignment. IRS-III used different dosing variants of vincristine, actinomycin D, and cyclophosphamide, sometimes alternating with cisplatin. Later surgery is often done to increase function or to provide an improved appearance.

LATE EFFECTS

Late effects are related to the site of disease and to treatment. For nearly all patients, there will be scarring and tissue loss. Lymphedema may occur if lymph nodes are removed. Radiation treatment may result in irregular or asymmetrical growth in the affected areas; if to the central nervous system, it can result in cognitive problems. Some of the effects of treatment are infections, anemia, bleeding, leukoencephalopathy, white matter changes (rare), fibrosis, infertility, organ dysfunction (heart, kidney, bladder), and development of a second cancer.

Psychological issues are similar to those in cancers where bone or tissue is removed (see *Osteosarcoma*). As many of these tumors are visible, body image is an important concern. Children may become more withdrawn because of their appearance, and psychosocial professionals can help through gradual exposure techniques, as well as in social skills training, to address dealing with reactions of others. Interaction with others who have similar late effects can be helpful through groups, camps, and activities sponsored by the center. School liaison is important to help the child reintegrate into the class and peer activities.

See also: Childhood Cancers; Osteosarcoma; Parenting the Chronically Ill Child; Coping with Illness; Bereavement

Further Reading

Lawrence, W. Jr., Anderson, J. R., Gehan, E. A., & Maurer, H. (1999). Pretreatment TNM staging of childhood rhabdomyosarcoma. A report of the Intergroup Rhabdomyosarcoma Study Group. *Cancer, 80*, 1165–1166.

Ruymann, F. B., & Grovas, A. C. (2001). Progress in the diagnosis and treatment of rhabdomyosarcoma and related soft tissue sarcomas. *Cancer Investigation, 18*, 223–241.

Wexler, L. H., Crist, W. M., & Helman, L. J. (2002). Rhabdomyosarcoma and the undifferentiated sarcomas. In P. A. Pizzo & D. G. Poplack (Eds.), *Principles and practice of pediatric oncology* (4th ed., pp. 939–971). Philadelphia: Lippincott, Williams & Wilkins.

MARY JO KUPST
ANNE B. WARWICK

Risk and Protective Factors

DEFINITION

Risk factors present in persons or environments result in a heightened probability for the subsequent development of a disease or disorder. Conversely, protective factors are "those attributes of persons, environments, situations and events that appear to temper predictions of psychopathology based upon an individual's 'at risk' status" (Garmezy, 1983, p. 73). Risk factors can be categorized as: (1) established risk, such as a frank genetic disorder (e.g., Fragile X Syndrome, Down Syndrome); (2) biological risk such as poor prenatal care, drug and/or alcohol abuse by the mother during pregnancy, prematurity, anoxia, and low birth weight; and (3) environmental risk, such as poor responsivity or lack of sensitivity by the mother to her child, low level of language stimulation, or poverty. Protective factors can be grouped in these three categories.

SPECIFIC RISK AND PROTECTIVE FACTORS

Research in developmental psychopathology has identified many factors that directly or indirectly affect children's resistance or vulnerability to stress. These are summarized in Table 1. The clinician must also understand the complex interplay between and among these risk and protective factors. Chronic life stress, for example, is associated with increased adjustment problems among children who have few protective factors available to them, but has little effect on children who have greater numbers of protective factors. Moreover, the association between risk and protective factors and adjustment appears to be stronger for boys than girls.

A multivariate, cumulative, and dynamic approach to risk and resilience, in which various factors interact over time to exacerbate or moderate the effects of adversity at any given time, is most helpful in explaining why children with similar histories will have different outcomes, and why those with similar outcomes may reach them by different developmental pathways. Rutter (1996) points out that it is not the isolated life event or stressor but rather the aggregated accumulation of stressful events that contributes to psychological vulnerability for the individual child. Similarly, it is recognized that protective factors are also

Table 1. Risk and Protective Factors in Child Development

Risk factors	Protective factors
Child characteristics	
Medical problems	Good physical health
Genetic disorders	Absence of genetic disorder
Birth complications	Uncomplicated birth
Being male	Being female
Difficult temperament	Easy temperament
Low intelligence	High intelligence
Uneven development	Even development
Extremes of activity level	Moderate activity level
Attention deficit	Developmentally appropriate attention
Language disorder or delay	Normal language development
External locus of control	Internal locus of control
Physical unattractiveness	Physical attractiveness
Being first-born	Being later-born
Poor coping strategies	Flexible coping strategies
Social skills deficits	Good social skills
Insecure attachment	Secure attachment
Poor academic achievement	High academic achievement
Poor self-esteem	High self-esteem
Family/environment characteristics	
Single parent	Two parents
Many children	Fewer children
Marital conflict	Family cohesiveness
Disagreement over child rearing	Consistent discipline
Chronic poverty	Higher socioeconomic status
Poor social support network	Good individual and agency support
Unemployment or underemployment	Stable employment
Inadequate child care resources	Adequate child care resources
Stressful life events	Low stress
Urban environment	Rural environment
Chaotic home environment	Consistent, stable home environment
Parent characteristics	
Depression or schizophrenia	Good psychological adjustment
Low intelligence	High intelligence
Fewer years of education	More years of education
Teenage mother	Mature mother
Insensitive/unresponsive parenting	Sensitive/responsive parenting
Unavailability	Availability
Low self-esteem	High self-esteem
Poor parenting models	Good parenting models
Avoidance coping style (denial)	Flexible coping style
Hypercritical	High nurturance/warmth
Inappropriate developmental expectations	Knowledge of developmental norms
Overly harsh or lax discipline	Authoritative discipline
Poor supervision of child	Close supervision and monitoring
Poor physical health	Good physical health
Low expectations for child behavior and academic performance	High expectations for child

Source: C. S. Schroeder and B. N. Gordon (2002). *Assessment and treatment of childhood problems: A clinician's guide*. Copyright 2002: The Guilford Press. Reprinted by permission.

on a continuum, and when accumulated and present across time these factors can increase the probability of a positive outcome for children in high-risk situations. Thus, the accumulation and interaction of risk and protective factors, and the identification of areas of strength and vulnerability at any specific point in time, are the critical foci for assessment and treatment.

SOCIOCULTURAL RISK

The socioeconomic context of growing up plays an important role in determining the vulnerability or resilience of children. Socially and economically disadvantaged children, for example, are exposed to many more negative life events, and also are more adversely affected by these negative life events, than are children from more affluent families. On the other hand, a number of child and parent characteristics help buffer the effects of stress, even for those children who grow up in poverty. Masten and Coatsworth (1998), in a summary of the research on resilence in children, state that the two variables most consistently found to differentiate resilient from vulnerable children are good intellectual functioning and a close relationship with a caring parental figure. Other related factors included an easy-going, sociable temperament, connections to an extended family support system, supportive contacts with adults outside the family, and participation in socially acceptable extracurricular activities. Parenting that involves consistent, highly structured, age-appropriate discipline combined with warmth and sensitivity, high expectations for behavior and academic achievement, and a strong sense of parenting efficacy have also been shown to buffer the effects of risk.

The parent–child relationship is a critical component in determining risk and resilience among children. Viewed in a broad context, this relationship is influenced by characteristics of the child, such as sex, intelligence level, temperament, and biological status, which interact with parental, familial, and environmental characteristics to predict the path of development for individual children. The childrearing practices of parents are certainly an important component of this configuration. Parent behavior can set the stage for children to develop and use coping skills that make them more resilient, or, conversely, can place children at increased risk for problems.

See also: Attachment; Emotional Development; Identity Development; Parenting Practices; Temperament Assessment

Further Reading

Ackerman, B. P., Kogos, J., Youngstrom, E., Schoff, K., & Izard, C. (1999). Family instability and the problem behaviors of children from economically disadvantaged families. *Developmental Psychology, 35,* 258–268.

Cowen, E. L., Wyman, P. A., Work, W. C., Kim, J. Y., Fagen, D. B., & Magnus, K. B. (1997). Follow-up study of young stress-affected and stress-resilient urban children. *Development and Psychopathology, 9,* 565–577.

Garmezy, N. (1983). Stressors of childhood. In N. Garmezy & M. Rutter (Eds.), *Stress, coping and development in children* (pp. 43–84). New York: McGraw-Hill.

Greenberg, M. T., Lengua, L. J., Coie, J. D., Pinderhughes, E. E., & The Conduct Problems Prevention Research Group. (1999). Predicting developmental outcomes at school entry using a multiple-risk model: Four American communities. *Developmental Psychology, 35,* 403–417.

Masten, A. S., & Coatsworth, J. D. (1998). The development of competence in favorable and unfavorable environments. *American Psychologist, 53,* 205–220.

Rutter, M. (1996). Stress research: Accomplishments and tasks ahead. In R. J. Haggerty, C. R. Sherrod, N. Garmezy, & M. Rutter (Eds.), *Stress, risk and resiliency in children and adolescents: Processes, mechanisms, and interventions.* New York: Cambridge University Press.

BETTY N. GORDON

Risk Assessment and Risk Management

RISK ASSESSMENT: OVERVIEW

The term risk assessment is used in different ways by different disciplines from different frames of reference (e.g., statistics, economics, biology, engineering, toxicology, systems analysis, operations research, health care). In the broadest context, risk assessment is seen as one of several interrelated activities that fall under the more general heading of risk analysis, which includes risk assessment, risk characterization, risk communication, risk management, and risk-related policy issues. Risk assessment can focus on risks to the environment as well as risks to the health, safety, and well-being of individuals that result from both naturally occurring and human factors. From the more general perspective, risk analysis focuses on risks of concern to both individuals and society.

ASSESSING RISK IN CHILDREN AND ADOLESCENTS

Pediatric and clinical child psychologists have long been interested in factors that place children and adolescents at risk for various types of negative outcomes, whether these outcomes relate to physical health difficulties or problems of psychological adjustment. This interest has resulted in their involvement in research that has focused on outcomes associated with various types of risk factors in addition to their frequent involvement in conducting risk assessments within the context of applied clinical work.

Examples of research in this area include studies investigating the health/safety risks associated with variables such as the failure to properly use infant seats or seat belts, child/adolescent tobacco use, alcohol use, drug use, unsafe sexual practices, and childhood obesity, among others. While some working in this area have focused primarily on research designed to highlight risks associated with these types of variables, others have been more interested in the implications of risk research findings for the development of prevention programs to reduce negative outcomes.

Although the research examples cited above relate primarily to behavioral and lifestyle risk factors, other approaches to risk assessment have focused on biological markers such as immune responses and genetic variations to assess risks of developing specific types of physical disease. An example especially relevant to pediatric psychology is the use of islet-cell antibody testing to assess risk for developing Type I diabetes in children with a family history of this disorder. This approach makes it possible to determine (with some degree of error) increased risk of developing diabetes well in advance of initial symptom development and highlights issues commonly associated with risk assessment. One of these issues relates to the effects of being given risk-related information. Here, research suggests that learning a child is at risk for future development of diabetes can result in significant levels of anxiety and family-related stress, making it important for those conducting risk screenings to provide counseling in those instances where positive findings are obtained. An additional issue relates to the fact that screening can sometimes result in "false positives," where testing suggests increased risk in error. As false positive results can unnecessarily result in increased family stress without concurrent benefit, providing risk/benefit counseling *prior* to screening is also important. Given that ongoing work in the biotechnology arena promises to dramatically increase the number and popularity of a range of genetic screening methods, issues related to the cost/benefits of such approaches will become an increasingly important consideration when using these types of screening measures in clinical practice.

Other approaches to clinical risk assessment relate to the identification of those children who are at increased risk for negative outcomes due to the potential dangerousness of their behavior. While a number of examples might be cited here, two that are especially noteworthy relate to the assessment of suicidal risk and the potential for violent behavior in children and adolescents.

With suicide being the third leading cause of death in individuals between the ages of 15 and 24 and the sixth leading cause of death in children between the ages of 5 and 14, assessing suicidal risk is not uncommon in clinical child/pediatric psychology practice. Likewise, the number of school shootings and other acts of physical violence perpetrated by children and adolescents that have recently received national attention emphasize the importance of clinical risk assessment in identifying those individuals at greatest risk for engaging in this type of behavior. While space does not permit a full consideration of the range of issues involved in risk assessment of problems such as these, examples of features thought to signify increased risk for child/adolescent suicide and violence are presented in Table 1.

In assessing risk with problems such as these it is important to recognize that the costs of failing to identify those at highest risk are great, as inaccurate assessment can result in actual loss of life, whether it be through violence toward self or others. Likewise, classification errors, whereby a child as judged to be at high risk for, say school violence, when he/she is not can also have potential consequences, as under some circumstances such a child might be singled out by school personnel for differential treatment that could itself result in negative outcomes. The difficulty in making judgments in this type of situation is influenced by the fact that problems like school violence have very low base rates (occur infrequently), making it likely that the large majority of children assessed for these problems are not likely to engage in such behavior. This fact, along with the serious nature of the consequences for being wrong make the assessment of this type of risks especially complex.

ON THE RELEVANCE OF RISK MANAGEMENT

In clinical work it is difficult to separate issues of risk assessment from those of risk management. While the term risk management, like risk assessment, is used differently across disciplines, for psychologists it can perhaps best be thought of in terms of quality assurance. This refers to the process of assuring that clinical services meet basic ethical and legal standards and are consistent with generally accepted standards of practice.

Table 1. Examples of Characteristics Suggestive of Increased Risk for Suicide and Youth Violence*

Suicide

- Past suicide attempts
- Involvement in alcohol or drug use
- Telling others of thoughts about suicide, death, or dying
- Becoming more moody and more withdrawn or isolated
- Displaying changes in eating or sleeping habits
- Expressing feelings of hopelessness, worthlessness, or guilt
- Showing a loss of interest in usual activities
- Giving away important possessions
- Talking about not being around in the future or saying goodbye to others

Signs such as these may be more significant in the context of a recent death or suicide of a friend or family member, a recent break-up with a boyfriend/girlfriend, major conflict with parents, or other suicides by children/adolescents in the same school or community.

Violence

- Having a history of aggressive behavior
- Recently losing ones temper on a daily basis
- Making threats or telling others about plans to hurt others
- Showing enjoyment in hurting animals
- Involvement in alcohol or drug use
- Carrying a weapon
- Having access to or a fascination with weapons
- Being a gang member or wanting to be in a gang
- Decreased interest in usual activities and withdrawal from friends
- Showing feeling of rejection and isolation
- Having a history of being bullied by others

*Note that this listing of characteristics suggestive of increased risk for child/adolescent suicide and violence is not exhaustive. Clinical risk assessment in these areas will, of necessity, involve looking at a range of features other than these, within the context of a full clinical evaluation by a qualified professional.

Although aspiring to meet the highest professional standards is important in all clinical care, an understanding of the basic principles of risk management is especially relevant where issues of dangerousness are concerned. Here, the consequences of errors in judgment, resulting from the failure to follow accepted standards of practice (or to document them), can be costly in terms of potential harm to patients and society, professionally and from a legal standpoint.

While space does not permit a detailed discussion of risk management principles, it can be noted that these have to do with such important issues as having a basic understanding of ethical and legal standards, practicing within the boundaries of one's competence, taking the time and engaging in all the activities necessary to obtain all the information needed to form good clinical judgments, consulting with colleagues if necessary, documenting decisions in writing, maintaining

clear boundaries with patients, and following accepted standards of practice. A more comprehensive discussion of this issue has been provided by Doverspike (1999) in his excellent book, *Ethical Risk Management: Guidelines for Practice.*

See also: Aggression; Ethical Issues; Legal Issues in Child and Pediatric Psychology; Mental Health Records; Suicide

Further Reading

American Psychological Association. (2002). *APA Help Center: Warning signs of teen violence.* Washington, DC: Author. http://helping.apa.org/warningsigns/violence.html

Doverspike, W. F. (1999). *Ethical risk management: Guidelines for practice.* Sarasota, FL: Professional Resource Press.

UCLA School Mental Health Project Center for Mental Health in Schools. (2002). *School Mental Health Project: Child and adolescent suicide prevention.* Los Angeles, CA: Author. http://smhp.psych.ucla.edu/qf/p3002_02.htm

JAMES H. JOHNSON
TREY A. JOHNSON

Risk-Taking Behavior

See: Adolescent Health

Rule-Governed Behavior

According to learning theory approaches to explaining human behavior, the likelihood that a behavior will be repeated in the future depends on the current consequences of the behavior. If the behavior is followed by reinforcement, it is more likely to occur again. If it is not followed by reinforcement, or if it is followed by punishment, it is less likely to occur again.

Much of human behavior is developed and maintained by the reinforcement that occurs naturally in the environment. For example, if a child does a painting and this is followed by praise from a parent, the child is more likely to want to paint in the future. The praise is reinforcement for the behavior of painting.

Unfortunately, the reinforcement that occurs naturally in the environment does not always serve to strengthen behaviors that parents and teachers are happy with. Take for example the child who makes a noise in class and all the other children laugh at him. Here the classmates' laughter is likely to be reinforcement for the bad behavior, and the child is more likely to do this sort of thing in the future.

In the examples given above, the behavior occurs, then the reinforcement occurs, and hence the behavior is then more likely to occur again. This type of learning is called "contingency shaped" learning, because the reinforcement is contingent on the occurrence of the behavior. As the behavior becomes well-established it is referred to as contingency shaped behavior.

Not all behavior of humans is contingently shaped behavior. Much human behavior, possibly even most, is what is described as rule-governed behavior. This type of behavior is able to occur because humans can use language. With rule-governed behavior, a person does not have to exhibit a behavior first and then have it reinforced for the behavior to become a regular, predictable behavior of that person. Someone else tells the person that if he exhibits the behavior he will be reinforced. Take, for example, the case of a child who has never been ice skating. His friend tells him that if he accompanies him to the rink he will have a good time. The child goes and has a great time (i.e., is reinforced for going). The behavior of going to the rink is rule-governed, not contingency shaped.

This type of behavior is called rule-governed because it results from the person following a sort of rule. "If you go to the rink, you will have a good time." Or more generally, "If you do X, then you will get Y." More technically, it can be stated, "If you exhibit a prescribed behavior, you will receive a prescribed reinforcement." The rules involved in rule-governed behavior can be divided into two types, command rules and advice rules.

A command rule is one where the person stating the rule is in control of whether or not the other person will receive the reinforcement. Take the situation of a mother saying to her child "Eat your dinner and then you can have some dessert." If the child eats his dinner the mother can give him the dessert. Alternatively, if the child does not eat his dinner, the mother can withhold his dessert.

An advice rule is one where the person stating the rule does not control the availability of reinforcement. Take the situation of a teacher who says to her student "Work very hard and you will pass your test." The student might work hard but not pass his test. He could also not work hard and yet pass the test. What the teacher was doing here was only giving advice to the student. She did not really control if the student passed

the test or not. She thought that if the student worked hard he would be likely to pass, but she could not guarantee it.

Understanding the operation of rule governed behavior can be quite important in therapy. For example, when working with families of children with conduct problems, the objective is often to establish compliance by the child to command rules given by parents. This is done by systematically reinforcing compliance by the child to parental requests and not reinforcing noncompliance.

Alternatively, many behavioral counselors use advice rules when making suggestions to children as part of a treatment program. For example, the counselor treating an anxious and withdrawn child might say to the child "If you ask your teacher for help when you need it, your teacher will assist you." The counselor does not control how the teacher will respond, but is advising the child about what the teacher is likely to do.

See also: Applied Behavior Analysis; Behavior Contracts; Positive Reinforcement

Further Reading

Grant, L., & Evans, A. (1994). *Principles of behavior.* New York: HarperCollins.

Hayes, S. C. (Ed.). (1989). *Rule-governed behavior: Cognition, contingencies, and instructional control.* New York: Plenum Press.

Hudson, A. (1998). Applied behavior analysis. In A. Bellack, M. Hersen (Series Eds.), & T. Ollendick (Vol. Ed.), *Comprehensive clinical psychology (Vol. 5). Children and adolescents: Clinical formulation and treatment* (pp. 107–129). New York: Pergamon.

ALAN HUDSON

Rumination

DEFINITION

Rumination is the voluntary act of regurgitating food or liquid, often accompanied by reswallowing the food. The behavior can persist for long periods after food ingestion and can occur hundreds of times per day. If significant food or liquid is lost during rumination, weight loss and dehydration occur and the disorder is potentially life threatening. It is primarily seen in two populations, normal infants, and adults with severe to profound mental retardation. The diagnosis is made after medical etiologies have been ruled out (e.g., gastroesophageal reflux), but the diagnosis should be suspected when the infant or adult ruminating appears to do so with pleasure rather than with distress, as is usually noted during regurgitation.

INCIDENCE AND ETIOLOGY

The incidence of this disorder is rare in modern society. Historically, infants living in large orphanages with little stimulation or individuals with mental retardation living in institutions were at increased risk. With the deinstitutionalization movement has come a reduction in the incidence of rumination. There are two theories of etiology. The first is psychodynamically based and suggests psychopathology in the caregiver leading to lack of stimulation for the infant. The infant finds comforts through rumination as a re-creation of the nurturing feeding situation. The alternative etiological mechanism is behavioral and proposes that ruminating is a form of self-stimulation reinforced by the act itself or by attention given to the individual when rumination occurs.

ASSESSMENT

Rumination is a diagnosis made by exclusion. Medical assessment is needed to rule out organic causes of vomiting and direct behavioral observation is necessary to determine the rate of the behavior and the mood of the individual during rumination. The absence of physical or emotional distress during rumination episodes points to the voluntary nature of the act and aids in diagnosis.

TREATMENT

The treatment of rumination has two components. The first component is an increase in the stimulation in the ruminator's environment. For infants this may require replacement of the primary caregiver and an increase in environmental stimulation. For individuals with mental retardation, it may mean moving the individual to a community or workshop setting that provides increased interactions with peers and activities. Behavioral techniques designed to decrease attention paid to the act of ruminating are also appropriate in the treatment package. If rumination is severe and has resulted in serious health risks, a more aggressive

approach may be warranted. Aversive conditioning procedures (e.g., contingent electric shock, aversive tastes) have resulted in rapid and dramatic reductions in rumination and should be considered in medically serious situations.

PROGNOSIS

Rumination, in almost all cases, can be treated effectively and rapidly by environmental changes and intense behavioral treatment. The prognosis is excellent.

See also: Failure-to-Thrive; Feeding Disorders; Vomiting—Psychogenic

Further Reading

Cunningham, C. E., & Linscheid, T. R. (1976). Elimination of chronic infant ruminating by electric shock. *Behavior Therapy,* 7, 231–234.
Kanner, L. (1957). *Child psychiatry* (3rd ed.). Springfield, IL: Thomas.
Linscheid, T. R., & Rasnake, L. K. (2001). Eating problems in children. In C. E. Walker & M. C. Roberts (Eds.), *Handbook of clinical child psychology* (3rd ed., pp. 523–541). New York: John Wiley & Sons.

THOMAS R. LINSCHEID

Running Away

DEFINITION/CLINICAL PRESENTATION

Running away has been defined several ways over the years. Presently, the *Diagnostic and Statistical Manual of Mental Disorders, Fourth Edition* (*DSM-IV*), includes running away as one of the characteristics of Conduct Disorder (CD). Core components of CD include a persistent pattern of behavior that breaks societal rules and/or violates of the basic rights of others. There are four main groupings of conduct problems and running away falls under the category of "serious violations of rules," which includes children with persistent patterns of staying out at night without permission, running away from home, and/or truancy from school. The *DSM-IV* mentions a caveat, however; namely, if the running away occurs as a direct result of physical or sexual abuse, the running behavior would not meet this criterion. Those children who run away and meet criteria for CD are more likely to have developed the behavior earlier, to remain on the run longer, and to exhibit a range of problematic behaviors that gets them into legal trouble.

This information suggests that running away may describe a wide range of behaviors that might not all be captured within the diagnosis of CD. Research regarding runaways has shown that many types of children evidence this behavior. Most children run away for short distances for short periods of time; however, some children run away for long periods of time and may end up living on the streets. Some clinicians have described different types of runaways, including those that are "running from" situations, those that are "running to" something, and "throwaway youth" who have been "pushed from" their homes. The most consistent finding across runaways is problematic parent–child relationships.

INCIDENCE

Approximately 1.3 million or 2 percent of the juvenile U.S. population runs away from home each year. Ninety percent of these youths run fewer than 50 miles from home and 70 percent of runaway episodes are brief (lasting from 1 to 6 days). No gender differences have been noted in the incidence of runaway behavior.

CORRELATES

Children who run away represent a heterogeneous group, and therefore may have different correlates to their behavior. Running away is often a sign that there are more severe difficulties in the family or with the youth. Correlates of running away include physical and sexual abuse, substance abuse, depression and suicidality, as well as learning disabilities, Communication Disorder (CD), Attention-Deficit/Hyperactivity Disorder (ADHD), and a history of conduct problems. In addition, there are strong correlations between runaway behavior and family difficulties, including a history of family violence, parental rejection, and poor parental monitoring.

As much as possible, a distinction should be made between characteristics of youth before they run away from home and characteristics of youths that may develop after they have been on the run. Statistics have shown worsening outcomes for children the longer they stay on the streets, because of the heightened exposure to drugs, prostitution, HIV and other sexually transmitted diseases, as well as the threat of aggression from others.

ASSESSMENT

The clinician will want to do a comprehensive assessment of risk factors that may be associated with the running behavior. These may include the cause of the running away, family dynamics, individual dynamics, sociocultural variables, age of the youth, and the length of time they are away. In order to assist in addressing these factors, Sells (1998) proposes questions that should be asked of the family before treatment begins, including "What is happening within the household that is potentially poisonous to the teenager?" and "What are all the things that would need to change to make your teenager want to come back and stay at home?" These questions help to assess the range of environmental and individual factors that will need to be addressed during treatment. Family factors such as family violence, marital violence, parental rejection, poor parental monitoring, and physical and/or sexual abuse are often related to running away and will need to be identified and addressed for a child to remain safely in the home.

TREATMENT

For youths that display a range of conduct problems that lead to contact with the law, Multisystemic Treatment has been shown to be effective. Interventions that are systemic, or that include multiple areas such as family, peers, school, and neighborhood, tend to be more successful at addressing family and environmental issues that impact the youth.

Sells (1998) describes intensive interventions for runaways who have not responded to traditional behavioral methods. He cautions, however, that these interventions are short-term fixes while the family can work on more long-term changes. These strategies include "atom bomb interventions" such as selling, pawning, or removing prized possessions if the youth runs away, instituting a 24-hr watch on the youth, or removing all the youth's clothing except for what they are wearing. Other strategies include the "Gandhi strategy" where the youth and adult sit for a day and look at each other without talking, "poisoning the youth's safe house" where the adult makes sure the youth is not welcome at alternate homes by alerting adults at those homes of the situation and consequences of hiding the child. Other traditional approaches include using positive reinforcers to counteract negative interactions, building trust between the family members, and predicting and planning for relapse behavior.

The above treatment interventions assume that the youth is reunited with his or her family. If reunification is not an option, individual cognitive–behavioral treatment to build coping skills for depression and suicidal symptoms as well as skill building around daily life skills may be effective.

PROGNOSIS

The prognosis for a runaway youth may be correlated with the reasons for running and the amount of time that she or he spends on the streets. The longer that youths stay separated from regular society that may include friends, social interactions, academic instruction, and occupations, and adopt the style of the street counterculture, the worse their outcomes. In addition, those youths with early behavior difficulties and more chronic conduct problems are more likely to have a worse prognosis.

See also: Aggression; Anger; Conduct Disorder; Depressive Disorder, Major; Multisystemic Therapy

Further Reading

American Psychiatric Association. (2000). *Diagnostic and statistical manual of mental disorders* (4th Edition, Text Revision). Washington, DC: Author.
Hagan, J., & McCarthy, B. (1997). *Mean streets: Youth crime and homelessness.* New York: Cambridge University Press.
Sells, S. P. (1998). *Treating the tough adolescent.* New York: Guilford.
Tomb, D. A. (1991). The runaway adolescent. In M. Lewis (Ed.), *Child and adolescent psychiatry: A comprehensive textbook* (pp. 1066–1071). Baltimore: Williams & Wilkins.
Whitbeck, L. B., Hoyt, D. R., & Bao, W. (2000). Depressive symptoms and co-occurring depressive symptoms, substance abuse, and conduct problems among runaway and homeless adolescents. *Child Development, 71,* 721–732.

JULIANNE M. SMITH
DANIEL J. KRALL

Ss

Safety and Prevention

DEFINITIONS

Prevention is a multidisciplinary science designed to identify and eliminate undesirable problems that may occur in the future. That is, preventive actions are taken to avoid the development of a problem or disorder before one occurs and to minimize negative effects should any problems develop. Historically, three types of prevention approaches have been described: primary, secondary, and tertiary. *Primary prevention* seeks to prevent problems from appearing within general populations. For example, immunizations protect children before any diseases can affect them. *Secondary prevention* programs focus on populations identified as having a problem, or the potential for one, in order to prevent the difficulties from progressing. Targeting Attention-Deficit/Hyperactivity Disorder (ADHD) children for classroom behavior self-control training is an example of a secondary preventive strategy. *Tertiary prevention* strategies attempt to lower the intensity or severity of existing problems. Recently, there has been difficulty differentiating between tertiary prevention and traditional treatment or rehabilitation, reducing the development of tertiary programs within a prevention framework.

TARGETED POPULATIONS

In a somewhat similar framework, the selection of target populations for preventive interventions is organized using three primary approaches: universal, high-risk, and transition. A *universal approach* focuses on recruiting individuals from entire populations, such as all preschool children receiving a preventive intervention. The *high-risk* tactic incorporates populations who have been previously identified as being at-risk for problem development, yet currently show no problems. Examples of at-risk populations might include low socioeconomic status families or teenage mothers with parenting difficulties. The *transition* approach encompasses populations that are experiencing major life change events such as divorce, movement from junior high to high school medical traumas, or medical hospitalization and surgery (Durlak, 1997).

INTERVENTIONS

Prevention interventions can occur at the individual or environmental level. The individual approach focuses solely on the individual person in order to prevent particular problems (e.g., teaching a young child to walk safely around traffic or teaching social skills to a child). An environmental approach attempts to change the person by changing aspects of his or her surroundings to be more supportive and growth enhancing. Interventions implemented around the family, the peer group, the school, or community would be considered environmental.

A variety of preventive programs addressing a number of child- and adolescent-related issues have been developed and implemented, including child maltreatment, behavioral and social problems, drug use, health related issues, and injury prevention. Physical abuse and neglect preventive efforts focus on providing social support and teaching effective parenting strategies. Although some evidence exists to support the effectiveness of reducing child physical abuse, there is little evidence demonstrating the actual reduction of child sexual abuse through skills training.

Prevention programs for behavioral and social problems have shown success through empirical measurement. For example, interventions in schools have been shown to be effective in improving academic performance and psychological functioning. Increasing social supports and reducing stressful environmental factors have been identified as key components in improving prevention outcomes.

Drug prevention efforts have been most heavily implemented within schools under the program entitled Drug Abuse Resistance Education (DARE). Unfortunately, research studies on DARE demonstrated poor efficacy in the reduction of drug use, both immediately after the program and during long-term follow-ups. However, other drug prevention programs have been shown to reduce drug use when they emphasized systematic skills training and focused on positive social and environmental factors.

Injury prevention has been shown to be successful in many settings. Traditional methods of preventing injuries have reduced environmental hazards, integrated behavior training, and provided intensive education. Programs which incorporate incentives, social reinforcement, and community involvement have increased the amount of safety related behaviors in children and parents.

Public policy remains integral to prevention efforts. Presently, very little funding is dedicated to preventive efforts, although research indicates that prevention has the potential to provide widespread influence on behavior. The American Academy of Pediatrics suggests incorporating preventive strategies in multiple health care settings.

CONCLUSION

Psychology remains the primary discipline towards furthering mental health prevention research. Although prevention research is relatively young when compared to other fields, many programs have been shown to be successful. However, education-alone preventive programs have been ineffective; therefore multiple component interventions should be implemented. Positive results have been obtained for different aspects of mental and physical health, drug use, academic performance, childhood injuries, and physical abuse and neglect.

See also: Accidental (Unintentional) Injuries; Health Education/ Health Promotion; Injury Prevention; Preparation for Medical Procedures

Further Reading

Durlak, J. A. (1997). *Successful prevention programs for children and adolescents.* New York: Plenum.

Mrazek, P. J., & Haggerty, R. J. (1994). *Reducing risks for mental disorders: Frontiers for preventive intervention research.* Washington, DC: National Academy Press.

Roberts, M. C., Brown, K. J., Boles, R. E., & Mashunkashey, J. O. (in press). Prevention of injuries: Concepts and interventions for pediatric psychology in the schools. In R. T. Brown (Ed.), *Handbook of pediatric psychology in school settings.* Mahwah, NJ: Erlbaum.

Web Site

http://www.cdc.gov

RICHARD E. BOLES
JOANNA O. MASHUNKASHEY
MICHAEL C. ROBERTS

Schizophrenia

See: Childhood-Onset Schizophrenia

School Age Assessment

Assessment of school age children typically refers to children aged 6–12 years, prior to the time they enter adolescence. Conducting assessments of children during the school age range provides information about their learning abilities and disabilities, need for educational interventions, prediction of school success, social and emotional functioning, and behavioral functioning. The laws guaranteeing a free, appropriate public education to all children (currently, P.L. 101-476, Individuals with Disabilities Education Act, 1990) provide the basis for assessment to determine if the child has a disability and to facilitate decisions regarding an appropriate individualized educational plan for that child. Assessments may involve cognitive, academic, adaptive, perceptual, motor, speech/language, behavioral, and social/emotional components. The scope of the assessment depends upon the specific referral question(s) or types of problems suspected, and also the purpose for which the information will be used (e.g., to assist with planning psychotherapy interventions, or to assist with special education placement and programming, etc.).

DEVELOPMENTAL TASKS AND COMMON REASONS FOR REFERRAL

During the school age range, children have numerous developmental tasks to accomplish on their path to adolescence. They seek to master new academic and learning skills, although their cognitive abilities are tied to concrete thought processes. Their social world is beginning to expand beyond their nuclear family to a wider circle of social contacts and relationships, and their understanding of emotions in other people is improving. Children at this age are more self-reflective than before, and have increased capability for taking the perspective of others. However, they may only be able to consider one point of view at a time during the early part of this age range.

Several types of problems may emerge and provide a reason for referral during this age range. Coinciding with beginning school, children with learning disabilities, mild mental retardation, attention problems, hyperactivity, speech/language disorders, or motor disorders may first come to the attention of professionals who note their difficulties in the school environment. Children with serious disabilities, such as moderate to severe to profound mental retardation, will often receive diagnosis and treatment well before entering school. However, children with problems such as learning disabilities may appear to be developing normally until they encounter a formal educational environment. Their specific learning deficits may not be apparent until they are exposed to formal instruction in reading, mathematics, spelling, and writing. Likewise, children with attention problems and/or hyperactivity may not be diagnosed during the preschool years because the symptoms of their disability may not interfere with their day-to-day activities until they enter the classroom environment with its many expectations and rules. Problems with articulation, receptive and/or expressive language, and motor skills will likely interfere with academic functioning, and they may also be reasons for referral. Finally, entrance into school provides an opportunity, and a challenge, for children to broaden their social contacts. Moreover, peer relationships take on a new importance in their lives. Sometimes problems with social skills and peer interactions may surface in the early elementary years and may lead to behavioral or emotional adjustment problems. Stresses related to academic or peer problems may also result in emotional or behavioral disorders. The assessment procedures will help to differentiate the primary problems that are present, and evaluate their impact on the child's social/emotional adjustment.

PROFESSIONALS WHO CONDUCT SCHOOL AGE ASSESSMENTS

The public schools provide an opportunity for all children who are suspected of having a disability to be evaluated at public expense. School systems typically hire or contract with school psychologists, speech/language pathologists, occupational therapists, physical therapists, and sometimes nurses, who are trained and qualified to conduct assessments of school age children. Psychologists can evaluate children's cognitive or intellectual functioning, adaptive functioning, academic skills, and to some extent, their language and motor skills as they relate to school functioning. Psychologists can also assess the child's behavioral and social/emotional functioning, conduct observations of the child's behavior in the classroom, and offer suggestions for classroom educational and/or behavioral interventions to teachers. Most often, the psychologist works collaboratively with other professionals (occupational, physical, or speech/language therapists) to provide a comprehensive assessment of the child's strengths and weaknesses. Special education teachers often conduct educational assessments at the beginning and end of the academic year to facilitate setting educational goals and measuring the child's progress toward those goals. Medical professionals such as pediatricians, family medicine physicians, and nurse practitioners provide essential screenings of a child's sensory functions (e.g., auditory and visual acuity), motor functioning, and general health issues. Finally, parents often provide very important information about the child's behavior and symptoms that is essential to an evaluation.

ABILITIES THAT NEED TO BE ASSESSED

Cognitive Abilities

School age children who are having difficulty with some aspect of learning will probably be referred to a school psychologist or clinical child psychologist for intellectual and academic assessment. Common intellectual measures, such as the Wechsler Intelligence Scale for Children—Third Edition (WISC-III), will typically provide measures of verbal reasoning as well as nonverbal reasoning and performance abilities. The WISC-III also yields a profile of 10–12 separate abilities that provide specific information about a child's cognitive strengths and weaknesses. Other cognitive measures commonly used with school-age children include the Stanford–Binet Intelligence Scale—Fourth Edition, Kaufman Assessment

Battery for Children (K-ABC), and Differential Ability Scales (DAS)—School Age Level. For children who have hearing or severe language deficits, it is important to assess their intelligence in a manner that allows them to understand the test instructions and provide responses without the use of spoken language. Measures such as the Leiter International Performance Scale—Revised or Test of Nonverbal Intelligence-3 (TONI-3) allow the examiner to pantomime or use nonverbal instructions, and allow the child to respond by pointing, moving test items, or make other nonverbal responses without the use of spoken language. For children who do not use English as their first language, it is required by law that the cognitive testing be administered in the child's first language. A translator may be used to assist with testing in these cases.

Much concern has been raised about the possible biases inherent in testing culturally and linguistically diverse children. According to Sattler (2001a, b), various empirical studies have investigated the issue of cultural bias in intelligence testing, and generally this research has failed to support the contention that culturally and linguistically diverse groups are at a disadvantage on these measures. For example, validity studies with the most commonly used intelligence tests for children indicate that these tests are equally good predictors of African American, Hispanic American, and Euro American children's abilities. These tests have large standardization groups in which the representation of minority groups parallels that of the U.S. population. Only in those cases where children's language backgrounds differ from the standardization group will the test results likely be invalid. For these children, verbal tests alone should never be used to determine their cognitive ability if English is not their native language. Measures of nonverbal cognitive ability, as well as measures of adaptive functioning, must be included in the assessment process to provide a more culture-fair approach to assessment. Adaptive information is often provided by the child's parents or others who have opportunities to observe the child's behavior in his/her natural environment over time. This information can provide an important perspective about the abilities of many children that may not be apparent from their performance on formal clinical measures of intelligence.

Academic Achievement

Measures of academic achievement and knowledge will typically accompany cognitive testing in a psychoeducational evaluation. These tests often include measures of basic reading (using phonics to decode words, recognizing sight words), reading comprehension, math

computation (e.g., performing operations of adding and subtracting), math reasoning, spelling, and written expression (writing sentences or themes). The child's performance on these measures of academic achievement is compared to his/her "predicted" achievement level, using a regression formula that is based on the child's intellectual ability. This formula provides an estimate of the child's expected level of performance compared to his/her own ability to learn. Thus, a child with delayed or deficient intellectual ability who is achieving at a similar level would be achieving at an appropriate level for his/her ability even if this performance is below the grade level at which the child is placed. Children who perform significantly lower than their expected achievement level may have a learning disability and may be eligible to receive special education services to address their disability. Many of the common achievement tests for children have been normed on the same group of persons as the associated intelligence test. For example, the WISC-III may be given with the Wechsler Individual Achievement Test—Second Edition (WIAT-II). The K-ABC may be given with the Kaufman Test of Educational Achievement (K-TEA), and the Woodcock Johnson Psychoeducational Battery—Third Edition (WJ-III) Tests of Cognitive Ability may be given with the WJ-III Tests of Achievement. These co-normed measures increase the sensitivity with which one can determine discrepancies between a child's ability to learn and his or her actual achievement.

Over and above the use of these tests, other important information should be gleaned from an assessment that would help others understand a child's primary style of learning (e.g., does the child process information better through the visual or auditory modality?), the procedures that facilitate the child's learning (e.g., rehearsal strategies, analysis of errors), the speed of information processing (e.g., does the child need additional time to process questions and/or complete written assignments, even though he or she knows the information), and the types of rewards (intrinsic or extrinsic?) that impact the quality of the child's performance. An assessment should also provide information about the quality of the child's memory, attention, perceptual-motor skills, and speech/language abilities as they relate to learning. This qualitative information facilitates the development of intervention strategies that are individualized to a child's specific learning style and learning needs.

Assessment of Attention and Activity Level

Attention-Deficit/Hyperactivity Disorder (ADHD) often is first diagnosed during the early school age years. Children with the predominantly hyperactive/impulsive subtype of ADHD will often show significant symptoms during the preschool years, whereas children with the predominantly inattentive subtype may not show significant symptoms until the demands of the classroom environment and academic curriculum are present. Details of assessment for ADHD are discussed under a separate entry, and will not be elaborated here. However, school age assessment must consider ADHD as a common disorder emerging during this age range.

Social/Emotional Functioning

According to Campbell (1998), several large-scale studies of children's social and behavioral adjustment during the school age years indicate that achievement and behavioral problems tend to occur together. Children with poor achievement are more likely to be viewed by parents and teachers as more uncooperative, disruptive, and prone to having impaired relationships with teachers and peers. Other studies have found an association between the child's adjustment and the presence of family discord, parental separation and divorce, and other family stressors. Research has also provided a link between children's social competence with peers and their emotional adjustment. Although some behavioral and emotional symptoms in the school age child are transient and related to identifiable stressors at a given time, other symptoms may herald a more long-term course of adjustment problems and risk for psychiatric disturbance in the future. For example, children with early externalizing problems (such as significant oppositional/defiant behavior, problems with anger regulation, impulsivity, overactivity, aggression) are at high risk for more serious and pervasive externalizing disorders later. Internalizing problems (such as anxiety, psychosomatic complaints, and mood disturbance) may be less persistent over time than externalizing problems, but they often are a focus of evaluation and treatment during the school age years.

Assessment methods will typically include a clinical interview with parents or other caretaking adults to obtain information about the nature, frequency, and severity of current behavioral or emotional symptoms. School age children can also provide their own perceptions and information about the nature of their symptoms. Use of age-normed behavioral rating scales that survey a broad range of internalizing, externalizing, and adaptive behaviors can provide extremely useful data about the severity of a given child's problems compared to their age group and gender. Scales such as the Behavior Assessment System for Children (BASC) and the Child Behavior Checklist (CBCL) have empirically derived factor scales that are based on large normative populations. They also have parent, teacher, and youth self-report versions of the scales that allow for cross-informant comparisons of ratings. These broadband scales can be supplemented by more specific, narrow-band behavioral rating scales that examine symptoms of a certain disorder (such as attention, hyperactivity, or impulsivity symptoms).

In addition to obtaining reports from others who observe the child's behavior and social functioning, a psychologist may also conduct direct observations of the child's behavior in such settings as the classroom or the clinic (e.g., observing parent–child interaction or peer interaction with a group of youth). Finally, projective assessment methods may provide a window into the child's thinking, feelings, and relationships with significant others through storytelling, sentence completion, or drawings that elicit the child's responses. The indirect nature of the projective methods may facilitate information exchange from children who are reluctant to discuss their own behavior or feelings, but may be willing to express themselves in a more indirect manner. The psychologist who conducts the evaluation will choose from among these various approaches to obtain the most appropriate types of information regarding a child's social/emotional functioning. Ideally, the evaluation should provide important information about differential diagnosis and intervention approaches that could benefit the child and family. Interventions may be done in the school setting, within the family, or with the child individually. The advancement of psychotherapy research in recent years has led to many empirically validated, developmentally appropriate, and culturally appropriate approaches to treatment for common social, behavioral, and emotional problems in the school age years.

See also: Adolescent Assessment; Attention-Deficit/Hyperactivity Disorder; Learning Disorders; Preschool Assessment; Underachievement

Further Reading

Campbell, S. B. (1998). Developmental perspectives. In T. H. Ollendick & M. Hersen (Eds.), *Handbook of child psychopathology* (3rd ed., pp. 3–36). New York: Plenum.

Sattler, J. M. (2001a). *Assessment of children: Cognitive applications* (4th ed.). San Diego, CA: Jerome M. Sattler.

Sattler, J. M. (2001b). *Assessment of children: Behavioral and clinical applications* (4th ed.). San Diego, CA: Jerome M. Sattler.

JAN L. CULBERTSON

School Psychology

In 1995, the American Psychological Association (APA) established the Commission for the Recognition of

Specialties and Proficiencies in Professional Psychology (the acronym is CRSPPP, pronounced "crisp"). This Commission provided official recognition for existing specialties and recognized some new ones. In each case, its recommendations were acted on by the APA Council, and an archival document was created describing the specialty. The specialty of School Psychology dates its origins to the work of Lightner Witmer, also considered the founder of Clinical Psychology. Witmer founded a "Psychological Clinic" at the University of Pennsylvania in 1896, but his work resembled the activities of modern School Psychologists more than they did those of today's Clinical Psychologists. He was primarily interested in understanding and helping children with academic retardation or deviant behavior. Thus, in effect, School Psychology is over a century old, though not by that name. School psychology also has roots in the Child Study Movement started by G. Stanley Hall, who is also known as the founder of developmental psychology in America, and in educational psychology, based on the work of such pioneers as Edward L. Thorndike. The field could hardly have developed as it did without Alfred Binet's invention of the intelligence test in France in 1905. The Division of School Psychology in APA was one of its original 19 divisions in 1944. The consensus as to the definition of School Psychology was stabilized by the Thayer Conference in West Point, New York, in 1954. The federal Education of All Handicapped Children Act in 1975 and its successors provided a strong impetus for School Psychology. In any case, School Psychology was the first specialty reaffirmed by CRSPPP in February, 1998. To state what this specialty involves, one can therefore do no better than quote the corresponding archival document (obtainable on the APA Web site, http://www.apa.org). This is done selectively below, together with some elaboration and the addition of historical context to clarify how this specialty came to be what it now is. According to the archival document:

> School Psychology is a general practice and health service provider specialty of professional psychology that is concerned with the science and practice of psychology with children, youth, and families; learners of all ages; and the schooling process. The basic education and training of School Psychologists prepares them to provide a range of psychological diagnosis, assessment, intervention, prevention, health promotion, and program development and evaluation services with a special focus on the developmental processes of children and youth within the context of schools, families, and other systems.

The archival statement goes on to say:

> School Psychologists are prepared to intervene at the individual or system level and develop, implement, and

evaluate preventive programs. In these efforts, they conduct ecologically valid assessments and interventions.

The term "general practice specialty" distinguishes School Psychology from more specialized areas such as Clinical Child Psychology or Pediatric Psychology. The words "health service provider" apply to School, Clinical, and Counseling Psychology to set them apart from areas such as Organizational and Industrial Psychology, whose clients tend to be businesses rather than individuals.

As the archival definition makes clear, the central topic in School Psychology is work within a particular setting, the school. It shares this interest with related fields such as school guidance, counseling, and special education. The CRSPPP definition applies to doctoral level School Psychologists. Increasingly, these psychologists are those who received their PhD or PsyD degrees from one of approximately 50 APA-approved programs in School Psychology. It is true that many persons who legitimately carry the title of School Psychologist were instead trained at the Master's or Specialist's level in programs accredited by the National Council for the Accreditation of Teacher Education and the National Association of School Psychologists (NASP) and are certified by state Departments of Education. The umbrella professional organization of such School Psychologists is the NASP rather than APA. Unlike Clinical and Counseling Psychology, School Psychology was never provided with federally funded doctoral positions in organizations such as the Veterans Administration. State and county government budgets have often not permitted the hiring of many doctoral personnel in school settings.

What domains of knowledge must School Psychologists possess? According to the archival document:

> School psychology has evolved as a specialty with core knowledge rooted in psychology and education. School psychologists have advanced knowledge of theories and empirical findings in developmental and social psychology, developmental psychopathology within cultural contexts, and in the areas of learning and effective instruction, effective schools, and family and parenting processes. School Psychologists conceptualize children's development from multiple theoretical perspectives and translate current scientific findings to alleviate cognitive, behavioral, social, and emotional problems encountered in schooling. A strong foundation in measurement theory and applications of advanced statistical methodology support efforts by school psychologists to design or evaluate standardized and nonstandardized measures in emerging assessment areas for individuals from culturally or linguistically diverse backgrounds and to design and evaluate

innovative classroom programs, comprehensive and integrated service systems, and educational and psychological interventions.

Thus, the knowledge base of School Psychology comprises elements of clinical, developmental, and educational psychology but combines them in a unique way. There are still those who conceptualize School Psychology as either Clinical Psychology carried out in a school setting, as applied Educational Psychology, or primarily as consultation. It is all of these and more.

What populations are served by School Psychology? The archival document distinguishes four groups:

1. Individuals from birth to young adulthood presenting learning or behavior problems.
2. Families who request diagnostic evaluations of learning disabilities and social problems and assistance with academic problems at home and at school.
3. Teachers, parents, and other adults to enhance their ability to provide healthy relationships and environments that promote learning and development.
4. Organizations and agencies to promote contexts that are conducive to learning and development.

There was a time when many School Psychologists were coerced by their role of gatekeepers for special education into giving one intelligence test after another—Binet jockeys or Wechsler jockeys, so to speak. This time is fading fast. At present, the field has begun to see the emergence of intervention procedures with a strong empirical as well as theoretical basis. The watchword in special education is "inclusion," and consultants such as School Psychologists are in high demand to help ordinary classroom teachers and families deal with diverse student problems in academic, emotional, social, and health domains.

See also: Child and Pediatric Psychology; Clinical Child and Adolescent Psychology; Clinical Psychology; Counseling Psychology; Health Psychology; Pediatric Psychology; Professional Societies in Clinical Child and Pediatric Psychology

DONALD K. ROUTH

School Refusal/School Phobia

DESCRIPTION/CLINICAL PRESENTATION

The term "school phobia" is reflective of the terminological and conceptual confusion that has plagued the problem of excessive school absenteeism since it was first introduced as a "phobia," by Johnson and colleagues in 1941. Most investigators currently working in the area have come to view school phobia as a subset of school refusal behavior. As a consequence, the more comprehensive term, "school refusal behavior" (SRB), has come to be preferred over school phobia. Even the term SRB has its difficulties as it may be taken to imply a conscious decision on the part of the child to refuse to go to school—a perspective that is not appropriate in all cases. Truancy usually is characteristic of children who are absent from school on an intermittent basis, usually without parental knowledge. Children with SRB are absent for extended durations, such as consecutive days, weeks, or months, and usually with parental knowledge. Truancy also is usually associated with other externalizing child behavior problems (e.g., conduct problems) as well as poor academic performance.

There is no one picture of the "school-refusing child." Some children who display SRB fail to attend school fully and completely. Other children may initially attend school in the morning but call their parents to be picked up early, frequently because they have somatic complaints (e.g., nausea, headaches). Another group of children who display SRB may attend school and even manage to stay there all day. However, it is a chore each morning to get these children to school because of their severe problem behaviors (e.g., temper tantrums, crying, pleading). Another group of children with SRB similarly attend school, but they experience high levels of distress while in school, leading to regular pleas to remain home in the future. These are not distinctive patterns of SRB, and it is not uncommon for children to display more than one such pattern at a given time. Nor is it uncommon for children to "move in and out" of varying patterns over time.

PREVALENCE AND CORRELATES

Research evidence suggests that the most common age of onset for SRB is generally in early adolescence, though this may simply reflect age at the time of referral. In terms of gender, SRB occurs fairly evenly across boys and girls as indicated in several studies. According to the U.S. National Center of Education Statistics, 5.5 percent of students are absent from school on a typical school day. Only a small number of studies have examined cultural/ethnic or race variations in SRB. Although there is evidence that school dropout rates are substantially higher among Hispanic American (29.4 percent) than African American (13.0 percent) or

Euro-American students (7.3 percent) (see http://www.nces.ed.gov for recent updates), some studies have shown that absence from school is higher among African-American students and families of lower family income as indicated by survey data of Berg and colleagues. It is not clear however whether families of diverse minority and socioeconomic status were well represented in these studies.

Kearney (2000) indicated in his book *School Refusal Behavior in Youth* that several factors have been found to be associated with SRB. Such factors include homelessness, maltreatment, school victimization, teenage pregnancy, divorce, and child self-care. Homelessness in youth also has been linked to educational problems such as school dropout, severe absenteeism, expulsion, school failure, and poor achievement in reading and arithmetic specific family factors also have been linked with SRB, including birth order, family size, marital problems, and family status, as well as parental psychopathology. In terms of birth order, several studies indicate that children with SRB tend to be the youngest in two-child families. For example, in a study conducted on a sample of 100 youth with SRB, 55 percent of the children were either an only child or the youngest child, and the average number of children in these families was 2.93. Another study conducted on a sample of 177 fourth-grade students reported that boys from single-parent families were absent from school significantly more than boys from two-parent families. In terms of parent psychopathology, another study conducted on clinic-referred children with SRB found that 57.1 percent of the mothers met *DSM* diagnostic criteria for an anxiety disorder and 14.3 percent met criteria for an affective disorder.

ASSESSMENT

A variety of semistructured and structured diagnostic interviews are useful for assessing the various psychiatric disorders that might be presented by the child with SRB. The Anxiety Disorders Interview Schedule for *DSM-IV*: Child and Parent Versions contain a module specific to SRB. A specific measure for assessing SRB is the School Refusal Assessment Scale (SRAS) by Kearney and Silverman (1999), which is used to assess "why" a child is refusing school based on motivating conditions that seem to maintain this behavior (e.g., to obtain positive reinforcement, to avoid negative situations).

When assessing SRB, it is important to conduct a thorough and comprehensive assessment to identify the presence of comorbid disorders including anxiety, mood, and externalizing disorders.

TREATMENT

Generally, all psychosocial treatment approaches stress the importance of getting the child back to school, and thus, in parents taking an active approach in returning the child to school. Controlled clinical trials provide empirical evidence for the efficacy of using exposure-based cognitive–behavioral treatments in reducing SRB. However, because some studies have indicated that children in the comparison control condition displayed significant improvements as well, further treatment research is needed.

Kearney and Silverman provided preliminary evidence in a study conducted in 1999 that treatment for SRB may be improved if treatment is matched or prescribed in accordance with the motivating condition(s), specific to a particular child as assessed with the SRAS. For example, for children whose SRB is maintained by attention-getting behavior, emphasis in treatment might be placed on parent training in contingency management, establishing clear parent commands, regular evening and morning routines, and consequences for noncompliance.

The pharmacological literature for treating SRB is sparse, as noted by Stock and colleagues (2001). The available literature consists of a small number of open label trials and case studies. Although there is research showing that benzodiazapines, selective serotonin reuptake inhibitors, and tricyclic antidepressants may be effective in treating SRB in youth, firm inferences cannot be drawn in light of methodological limitations of many of the studies. In addition, although early studies found that children with SRB showed improvement upon receiving tricyclic antidepressants (i.e., imipramine), subsequent studies have failed to yield positive results.

See also: Behavior Rating Scales; Behavior Therapy; Cognitive–Behavior Therapy; Interviewing; Separation Anxiety Disorder

Further Reading

Johnson, A. M., Falstein, E. I., Szurek, S. A., & Svendsen, M. (1941). School phobia. *American Journal of Orthopsychiatry, 11,* 702–711.

Kearney, C. A. (2000). *School refusal behavior in youth.* Washington, DC: American Psychological Association.

Kearney, C. A., & Silverman, W. K. (1999). Functionally based prescriptive and nonprescriptive treatment for children and adolescents with school refusal behavior. *Behavior Therapy, 30,* 673–695.

Stock, S. L., Werry, J. S., & McClellan, J. M. (2001). Pharmacological treatment of pediatric anxiety. In W. K. Silverman & P. D. A. Treffers (Eds.), *Anxiety disorders in children and adolescents: Research, assessment and intervention* (pp. 335–367). Cambridge, U.K.: Cambridge University Press.

XIMENA FRANCO
WENDY K. SILVERMAN

School-Based Treatments

DESCRIPTION OF SCHOOL-BASED TREATMENTS

School-based treatments have developed in response to growing awareness of the unmet mental health needs of students. The adverse effect of behavioral and emotional problems on students' academic and social achievement at school has been well established. In addition, there is widespread recognition of the amount of time children and adolescents spend in school and thus, the potential for school-based treatments to influence behavior on and off school grounds. Traditional mental health services within schools have consisted of special education programs and student guidance services, with support services pieced together from outside agencies to address more severe mental health needs. School-based interventions take a variety of forms, from within-classroom behavior management, to pulling out individual students for services, to providing school-wide violence prevention programs. Issues addressed by staff in schools may have a direct influence on academic achievement such as drug or alcohol use and dropout risk, but school staff members have also found themselves addressing child abuse and other home-based crises. In recent years, the focus of school-based interventions has widened to include behaviors that influence students' social development such as anger management, body image distortions, dating violence, social skills, and bullying.

A number of sociopolitical factors and philosophical shifts have spurred the development of comprehensive, coordinated mental health services housed within schools. Parents, teachers, and even therapists have shown an interest in seamless, comprehensive, school-based interventions. Possible explanations for this shift can be explained by reduction in the number of different people closely connected to the child's treatment, increased use of consultative services by mental health professionals, and enhanced communication between providers, parents, and teachers. Programs which have developed out of this shift toward school-based services range from a solitary, idea-specific skills training program in an individual school, to comprehensive programs that offer a variety of services such as psychological testing, group therapy, and intensive individual therapy. School districts may have a more narrowly focused intervention group in each school or a team of mental health professionals that provide an array of services to every school in the district. Innovations and unique designs appear to be as numerous as there are schools. One such innovative program is the Intensive Mental Health Program (IMHP) in which students showing severe emotional and behavioral problems spend half of each school day in their neighborhood school and the other half in a therapeutic classroom staffed by a certified special education teacher, a paraprofessional, and a masters level psychologist. The students receive assessments, individual therapy, group therapy, individualized behavior programs, specialized academic instruction, home visits, and service coordination. The ultimate goal of comprehensive programs such as the IMHP for severely emotionally disturbed youth is to help students develop the skills they need for full-time successful transition back to their neighborhood school.

ADVANTAGES

Comprehensive mental health services within schools reduce many of the barriers to children and adolescents utilizing traditional clinic-based services. By offering services in a location where children naturally spend much time, school-based treatments do not have the barrier of transportation. As many school-based treatments receive federal funding, the cost of these programs is not a barrier to children and families in accessing these services. Finally, there is still an unfortunate social stigma associated with going to a mental health center; a stigma of which older school-aged children and adolescents are particularly aware. Children and families may feel more comfortable accessing mental health services in a more natural setting such as the school. In addition to their appeal to clients, school-based treatments have several features that make them attractive to service providers. Being based within a school allows mental health professionals greater access to information on their clients' behaviors such as through direct observation. Communication with others involved in children's lives is important in providing effective services. Schools are locations where one might gather academic information from teachers, health information from the school nurse, and behavioral information from parents with greater ease. The increased knowledge of and involvement in an important child environment also has the potential to lead to greater generalization of treatment effects. It appears that school-aged children may accomplish as much or more when housed within and integrated into the school system than when confined to mental health centers or removed to residential centers.

EFFECTIVENESS

Research on the effectiveness of school-based treatments is still in its infancy, but the initial findings are encouraging. In addition to examinations of clinical effectiveness and cost considerations, research is needed comparing the outcomes of school-based mental health interventions to traditional clinic- and community-based services. Some studies do indicate that school-based interventions are at least as effective as interventions from community-based mental health centers. Concerns arising with respect to school-based treatments such as coordinating services between clinical staff hired for a specific school-based treatment program and the traditional mental health staff already established within the schools and confidentiality also need further exploration. In terms of implementation, communication between concerned adults, ease of behavioral observations, and generalizability of treatment effects, school-based treatments have the potential to show great success.

See also: Community Interventions; Community Mental Health Centers; Day Treatment; Multisystemic Therapy; Residential Treatment; Social-Skills Training

Further Reading

Adelman, H. S., & Taylor, L. (1993). School-based mental health: Toward a comprehensive approach. *The Journal of Mental Health Administration, 20,* 32–45.

Evans, S. W. (1999). Mental health services in schools: Utilization, effectiveness, and consent. *Clinical Psychology Review, 19,* 165–178.

Vernberg, E. M., Roberts, M. C., & Nyre, J. (2002). School-based intensive mental health treatment. In D. Marsh & M. Fristad (Eds.), *Handbook of serious emotional disturbance in children and adolescents* (pp. 412–427). New York: Wiley.

Weist, M. D. (1998). Mental health services in schools: Expanding opportunities. In H. S. Ghuman & R. M. Sarles (Eds.), *Handbook of child and adolescent outpatient, day treatment and community psychiatry* (pp. 347–357). Philadelphia, PA: Brunner/Mazel.

Weist, M. D., Evans, S. W., & Lever, N. A. (Eds.). (2003), *Handbook of school mental health.* New York: Kluwer Academic/Plenum.

ANNE K. JACOBS
NOEL J. JACOBS
MICHAEL C. ROBERTS

Scoliosis and Spinal Curvatures

Spinal curvature deformities include scoliosis, a lateral spinal curvature; kyphosis, a spinal hump; and kyphoscoliosis which is essentially a combination of both conditions. Scoliosis is the most common of these deformities; it is generally congenital or may develop in later childhood. A developmental scoliosis is a result of general muscle imbalance often related to paralysis in the chest–thoracic region. There are numerous screening programs for such problems in public schools. Spinal curvatures are reported to occur in approximately 90 percent of the children with spina bifida–myelomeningocele.

If spinal deformities are not treated they may interfere with sitting and walking. Bracing and surgical correction is utilized. Surgical procedures usually involve spinal fusions and in more serious cases, placement of rigid steel rods next to the vertebrae in the back.

An obvious and significant problem with scoliosis relates to general deformity of the body and children's reactions to such deformities. Although surgical correction is designed primarily for improving positioning and maintaining lung capacity, cosmetic benefits are obvious. Prognosis for independent function as an adult is very good when treatment (physical or surgical) is completed early.

See also: Muscoskeletal Disorders; Preparation for Medical Procedures; Spina Bifida

Further Reading

Batashaw, M. L. (1997). *U* (4th ed.). Baltimore, MD: Paul H. Brookes.

Mayfield, J. K. (1991). Comprehensive orthopedic management in myelomeningocele. In H. L. Rekate (Ed.), *Comprehensive management of spina bifida* (pp. 113–163). Boca Raton, FL: CRC Press.

Web Site: National Scoliosis Foundation. http://www.scoliosis.org

DENNIS C. HARPER

Scratching

See: Dermatology: Dermatitis and Psoriasis; Self-Injurious Behavior

Screening Instruments: Behavioral and Developmental

DEFINITIONS/CRITERIA

"Screening" for disease is a standard practice for many biomedical conditions. By definition, screening identifies individuals in need of further evaluation and assessment, but does not provide a diagnosis of a condition. Pediatric and child psychologists are often involved in developing and implementing screening procedures to identify children with possible developmental or behavioral problems. In discussions of developmental and behavioral screening, concepts of screening and assessment are sometimes confused, because some instruments have been suggested for both practices.

Screening for developmental and behavioral problems is important for several reasons. First, developmental and behavioral problems have been shown to be common in children, yet they are often unrecognized and untreated. For example, studies in primary care practices have shown that between 11 and 20 percent of school age children have significant behavioral problems, yet pediatricians identify only about half of them (about 5–9 percent of children), and refer only a minority of those identified children to mental health professionals for further evaluation and treatment. Second, there is evidence of effective child intervention techniques that provide a positive impact on developmental and behavioral problems if children are identified early and referred for appropriate services. Children cannot receive needed services if their problems go undetected.

Screening tests are administered to populations of children, the purpose being early identification of those with unsuspected deviations from "normal." Screening may be conducted on a whole population or major subgroup ("mass screening") or on circumscribed subgroups of the population ("selective screening"). For example, nearly all children have some form of screening of developmental readiness before entering kindergarten (mass screening); children considered to be at high risk for developmental problems (e.g., having a history of prematurity or lead poisoning) may be identified for developmental screening at an earlier age (selective screening).

Screening methods need to be evaluated against several criteria. (1) The abnormality (e.g., developmental delay, behavioral dysfunction, depression) and population (e.g., age of the child) being screened must be defined. (2) The sensitivity and specificity of the screening method

must be known and appropriate. Sensitivity is the ability of the test to detect abnormality, when in fact an abnormality truly exists; specificity refers to a test indicating that there is no problem, when the "gold standard" also is indicative of normal functioning. The false positive rate is the percentage of cases identified by the procedure as having a problem when none exists; conversely, the false negative rate refers to children who do have a problem but who are not detected on the test. For example, with respect to behavioral screening, the Pediatric Symptom Checklist (PSC) is a very brief (35 item) checklist of behavior problems that takes less than 5 minutes to administer to parents and to compute a single score. Established cutoff scores (28 out of a possible 70 for school-age children) have been shown to have a sensitivity of 95 percent, specificity rate of 68 percent, and false positive rate of 32 percent when compared to psychologist or psychiatrist ratings of behavioral dysfunction. These properties of the PSC make it a reasonable choice for mass behavioral screening with school age children in many pediatric primary care settings. (3) Choice of screening method should take into consideration its acceptability, efficiency, and cost in the setting it is to be used. (4) There should be procedures for further evaluation and interventions of children who screen positive on the procedures, as well as an established protocol for disposition of borderline positive results. (5) Examiners must be cognizant of the possible adverse consequences to screening (e.g., labeling).

Unlike adults, young children, especially those under the age of 10, cannot easily and reliably report on their developmental progress and behavioral status. Therefore, most child assessment techniques, including screening methods, use information from other informants. Many of the screening methods for developmental and behavioral problems rely on parental report, often via questionnaire or rating scales. A parent is likely to have the most opportunity to observe and interact with their child and therefore can be the most knowledgeable informant of developmental and behavioral data. The down side of such an approach is that it is subject to reporter bias.

BEHAVIORAL SCREENING INSTRUMENTS

Table 1 contains a list of sample behavioral screening instruments that have been recommended for use in pediatric settings. In clinical settings, a two-step screening procedure is sometimes used. First, a mass (sometimes referred to as "first stage") screening measure may be administered to all children in a setting, such as the pediatrician's waiting room. These measures focus on

Table 1. Selected Behavioral Screening Instrument

Title of instrument	Screening focus	Informant	Ages (years)	Time (min)	Comments
Mass (1st stage) screening					
Pediatric Symptom Checklist (PSC)	General psychological functioning	Parent	4–16	5	Specifically designed for use in pediatric settings to screen for psychosocial dysfunction. Cutoffs, but no standard scores. Form can be used free of charge.
Eyberg Child Behavior Inventory (ECBI)	Disruptive behavior problems	Parent	2–16	5	Easy to administer and score; does not assess internalizing conditions.
Children's Depression Inventory (CDI)	Depression	Self	7–16	10	Provides direct self-report of symptoms not easily observable by parents.
Beck Depression Inventory®-II (BDI®-II)	Depression in parents and teens	Self	13–80	5	Complies with *DSM-IV*. Has been shown to screen for general distress as well as for depression.
McMaster Family Assessment Device (FAD), General Functioning Subscale	Global family functioning	Parent	4–16	5	Brief and sensitive measure of global family functioning. Provides limited information on specific concerns unless entire 60-item test is given.
Selective (2nd stage) screening					
Child Behavior Checklists (CBCL, TRF, C-TRF, YSR)	Multidimensional behavioral screening	Parent, teacher, and child self-report formats	$1\frac{1}{2}$–30	20	Broad-based measure of pathology. Provides a profile of behavioral deviancy and social competence. Standard T-scores provide norm-based comparisons by age and gender. Computer scoring recommended.
Behavior Assessment System for Children (BASC)	Multidimensional behavioral screening	Parent, teacher, and child self-report formats	2–18	20	Subscales include externalizing, internalizing, school, other problems (atypicality, withdrawal) adaptive skills; validity check included. Norms available by age and gender. Computer scoring recommended.

Source: Portions adapted from E. Perrin, & T. Stancin (2002). A continuing dilemma: Whether and how to screen for concerns about children's behavior in primary care settings. *Pediatrics in review*, (2002). (See same article for test author references and for information about obtaining instruments.)

broad concerns such as general psychosocial dysfunction, disruptive behavior, or family functioning and can be completed and scored in less than 10 min. A longer, selective (sometimes referred to as "second stage") screening instrument may follow to provide more detailed information about the nature and severity of behavioral concerns. Second stage instruments tend to be multidimensional in focus and have normative standards by which to evaluate severity of problems.

DEVELOPMENTAL SCREENING INSTRUMENTS

Similarly, there are different levels of *developmental screening* and evaluation. In actuality, *focused screening* is more typical in monitoring development, whereby the screening test is administered to an infant or young child who is highly suspected with regard to developmental status. *Prescreening* is the process by which caretaker report or a short, structured interview is used to identify infants who will need further hands-on screening, thereby reducing time and cost by eliminating those who did not appear to have problems on the caretaker-completed questionnaire. An *assessment* is more definitive and conclusive, and involves the use of a more detailed and lengthy instrument, usually in conjunction with evaluations made by other professionals. Assessment typically produces a diagnosis. It is estimated that approximately 25 percent of children will fail a developmental screening (the percentage depending on the nature of the population being screened and the type of screening instrument used). Additional, more detailed assessment will confirm problems in approximately 10 percent of these children (again depending on the population and test used). There are various underlying reasons that may yield positive test finding. These include mental retardation, an emerging learning disability, language dysfunction, environmental deprivation, testing problems, or some combination of these etiologies. Maturational delay, recovery from biomedical problems,

Table 2. Selected Developmental Prescreening Instruments

Instrument	Age	Description
Ages & Stages Questionnaire (formerly Infant Monitoring System)	4–48 months	11 questionnaires, 30 items each age; fine motor, gross motor, communication, adaptive, personal social
Child Development Inventories (formerly Minnesota Child Development Inventories)	Birth–72 months	Three separate instruments, each with 60 items: infant, toddler, preschool levels: scored yes/no; cutoff 1.5 standard deviation below the mean
Parents' Evaluations of Developmental Status (PEDS)	Birth–8 years	10 questions tap behavior, language, fine motor, social, preschool skills; flags those needing further screening
Prescreening Developmental Questionnaire (R-PDQ)	Birth–6 years	Based on Denver Developmental Screening Test; personal-social, gross motor, fine motor, language; "delay" is failed item completed by 90 percent of younger children

Additional information concerning these instruments including test authors and references can be found in G. P. Aylward (1994). *Practitioner's guide to developmental and psychological testing.* New York: Plenum Medical Books.

Table 3. Selected Administered Developmental Screening Instruments

Instrument	Age	Description
Battelle Developmental Inventory Screening Test	0–96 months	2 items/age level in personal-social, adaptive, gross motor, fine motor, receptive & expressive language, cognitive; 3-point scoring
Bayley Infant Neurodevelopmental Screener (BINS)	3–24 months	6 item sets grouped by age, each with 11–13 items scored optimal/nonoptimal; basic neurologic functions, expressive, receptive, cognitive processes; low-, moderate-, high-risk summary scores
Bracken Basic Concepts Scale—Revised	2–11 years	School readiness composite (colors, letters, numbers/counting, sizes, comparisons, shapes) + 5 supplementary tests
Brigance Infant & Toddler Screen/Brigance Early Preschool Screen	0–23 months/ 2–4 years	Fine motor, receptive & expressive language, gross motor, self-help, social-emotional; 8–15 items in each
Clinical Adaptive Test/Clinical Linguistic Auditory Milestone Scale (CAT/CLAMS)	Birth to 36 months	Language, problem solving, visual-motor skills. 100 items; developmental quotients calculated based on ratio formula
Developmental Indicators for the Assessment of Learning—3rd edition (DIAL-3)	3–6 to 11 years	5 areas: motor, concepts, language, self-help, social development; direct evaluation, parent observation, team screening
Denver Developmental Screening Test-II (DDST-II)	1 month–6 years	Personal social, fine motor adaptive, language, gross motor; developmental chart/inventory; delays and cautions
Early Language Milestone Scale-2 (ELMS-2)	Birth–36 months	Auditory expressive, auditory receptive, visual (prelinguistic behaviors)
FirstSTEP (Screening Test for Evaluating Preschoolers)	2.9–6.2 years	12 subtests in 5 domains; composite based on cognition, communication, and motor

Additional information concerning these instruments including test authors and references can be found in G. P. Aylward (1994). *Practitioner's guide to developmental and psychological testing.* New York: Plenum Medical Books.

neural dysfunction, motor deficits, or variables specific to the infant (e.g., state or temperament) could also influence test results. Because of the absence of a true "gold standard" in developmental screening, sensitivity may be better termed co-positivity, meaning that the screening test and the reference standard are positive for a developmental problem; similarly, specificity is best considered as conegativity. Sensitivity (copositivity) values of 70 percent and specificity (conegativity) values of 70–80 percent are realistic in developmental screening.

The concept of *prescreening* has received much support in primary care pediatrics. Unfortunately, this approach is somewhat obscure in psychologic circles and hence, underutilized by psychologists. Selected prescreening instruments are listed in Table 2. These vary in length, areas screened, time required for scoring, and applicable age ranges. These techniques are most useful in the preliminary identification of children for early intervention services, or in Child Find programs where the goal is to then administer hands-on screening tests to identify children who qualify for early childhood education. The basic function of a prescreening approach is to sort infants and young children who should subsequently be given a hands-on screening test, from those whose development appears to be within the normal range.

Psychologists generally are more familiar with administered (hands-on) screening instruments. Selected tests are listed in Table 3. Such tests are considered to be the second stage in the developmental evaluation process. In that function, these instruments are helpful, gross measures of development. However, they generally do not provide a diagnosis, nor do they accurately portray a child's functional levels (i.e., provide age equivalents). Content areas vary from neurodevelopmental function (e.g., Bayley Infant Neurodevelopmental Screener) to understanding of basic concepts (e.g., Bracken Basic Concepts Scale—Revised), to broader sampling of the major areas or streams of development (e.g., Brigance Infant and Toddler Screen). These tests can be individually or, in certain instances, team administered (the latter arguably is less desirable, as this moves the screening from a clinical technique to a more assembly-line status, thereby obscuring potentially useful observations gleaned over time).

CONCLUSION

Behavioral and developmental screening is worthwhile if there are resources available for further evaluation and intervention when results are positive. Additional services may be provided by a variety of health care, mental health, and educational professionals.

See also: Early Intervention; Health Care Professionals (General); Physician (General Specialty); Primary Care; Psychological Testing

Further Reading

Aylward, G. P. (1994). *Practitioner's guide to developmental and psychological testing.* New York: Plenum Medical Books.

Aylward, G. P. (1995). *The Bayley Infant Neurodevelopmental Screener Manual.* San Antonio, TX: The Psychological Corporation.

Aylward, G. P. (1997). *Infant and early childhood neuropsychology.* New York: Plenum.

Glascoe, F. P. (1997). Parents' concerns about children's development: Prescreening technique or screening test? *Pediatrics, 99,* 522–528.

Perrin, E., & Stancin, T. (2002). A continuing dilemma: whether and how to screen for concerns about children's behavior in primary care settings. *Pediatrics in Review, 23,* 264–275.

Squires, J., Nickel, R. E., & Eisert, D. (1996). Early detection of developmental problems: Strategies for monitoring young children in the practice setting. *Journal of Developmental and Behavioral Pediatrics, 17,* 420–429.

Stancin, T., & Palermo, T. M. (1997). A review of behavioral screening practices in pediatric settings: Do they pass the test? *Journal of Developmental and Behavioral Pediatrics, 18,* 183–194.

TERRY STANCIN
GLEN P. AYLWARD

Secondary Prevention

See: Early Intervention; Safety and Prevention

Seizures

See: Epilepsy

Selective Mutism

DEFINITION/CLINICAL PRESENTATION

Selective mutism is defined as a consistent failure to speak in one or more situations in which speech is expected (e.g., school, church), despite speaking in other situations (e.g., home). This failure to speak persists for at least one month and is severe enough to interfere with social, school, and/or family functioning. In general, children with selective mutism are more likely to be mute when away from home, with unfamiliar nonfamily members, and with adults than with peers. The onset of symptoms is often gradual, with the diagnosis typically being made once the child enters school and encounters increased demands for speech. Symptoms can last for months or even years. While some children react to traumatic events by becoming mute, there is little evidence to indicate that trauma is a common cause of selective mutism in most children.

INCIDENCE

Little is known about the incidence of selective mutism. It is estimated that less than 1 percent of those seeking treatment do so for selective mutism. The disorder is reported to be more prevalent in females than males.

CORRELATES

Most children with selective mutism are shy and anxious while a smaller number also demonstrate oppositional and controlling behaviors. Children with selective mutism often have high rates of other anxiety disorders such as social phobia. There may also be elevated rates of articulation problems and expressive language disorders in children with selective mutism.

ASSESSMENT

A comprehensive evaluation is necessary in order to diagnose a child with selective mutism and rule out other possible disorders. Another goal of the assessment is to map out those situations in which the child does and does not speak so as to identify contributing factors and targets for treatment. An evaluation of speech/language abilities is important and may be coordinated with the child's pediatrician and a speech/language therapist. Because these children often refuse or are reluctant to speak with an unfamiliar clinician, it is important to gather information from parents and teachers. While children with selective mutism may not talk during an evaluation, they may be able to participate by using nonverbal forms of communication (e.g., drawing, head nods). Paper and pencil questionnaires also may be used to assess symptoms.

TREATMENT

Little research attention has been paid to the treatment of selective mutism, so no definitive conclusions can be reached about treatment efficacy at this time. The most commonly used treatments are behavioral therapies and medication. Behavioral therapies include contingency management, exposure-based strategies, and self-modeling. These strategies are often used in combination, depending on symptom presentation. Contingency management involves adding or taking away positive and negative consequences in order to increase the frequency of speech and decrease the frequency of failure to speak. Exposure-based strategies involve teaching the child to use relaxation techniques (e.g., diaphragmatic breathing) as he/she gradually faces more anxiety-provoking situations (e.g., first practice whispering to parent in front of therapist and then practice talking in an audible voice to parent in front of therapist). Self-modeling involves the child watching a videotape or listening to an audiotape of him/herself speaking in target situations (e.g., answering a teacher's question in class). These tapes are typically made by having the child interact with a parent in the absence of a teacher or therapist and then editing the tape so that it appears that the child is talking with the teacher or therapist.

Pharmacological treatment of selective mutism usually is undertaken in combination with behavioral therapy. The medications most often used are Selective Serotonin Reuptake Inhibitors (e.g., fluoxetine/Prozac), since selective mutism is typically treated pharmacologically as an anxiety disorder.

PROGNOSIS

Again, little is known about the prognosis for children with selective mutism. Clinical experience suggests that more anxious/inhibited children tend to respond better to treatment with medication and that better outcomes are associated with treating younger children than those who have been symptomatic for a lengthy period of time.

See also: Anxiety Disorders; Cognitive–Behavior Therapy; Language Development; Social Phobia

Further Reading

Black, B., & Uhde, T. W. (1995). Psychiatric characteristics of children with selective mutism: A pilot study. *Journal of the American Academy of Child and Adolescent Psychiatry, 34*(7), 847–856.

Garcia, A., Freeman, J., Francis, G., Miller, L. M., & Leonard, H. L. (2003). Selective mutism. In T. H. Ollendick & J. S. March (Eds.), *Phobic and anxiety disorders: A clinician's guide to psychosocial and pharmacological interventions.* New York: Oxford University Press.

Steinhausen, H. C., & Juzi, C. (1996). Selective mutism: An analysis of 100 cases. *Journal of the American Academy of Child and Adolescent Psychiatry, 35*(5), 606–614.

GRETA FRANCIS
ABBE GARCIA
JENNIFER FREEMAN

Selective Screening

See: Screening Instruments: Behavioral and Developmental

Self-Concept

See: Identity Development

Self-Control

See: Self-Management

Self-Esteem

See: Identity Development

Self-Injurious Behavior

DEFINITION

Self-injurious behavior (SIB) refers to acts directed toward one's self that result in tissue damage. It occurs most frequently among people with severe or profound mental retardation and/or autism. It also occurs in a variety of neurological conditions such as Tourette Syndrome, Neuroacanthocytosis, frontal lobe epilepsy; in psychiatric disorders such as personality disorders, eating disorders, schizophrenia, trichotillomania (hair-pulling), and onychophagia (nail-biting); and in genetic disorders such as Lesch–Nyhan syndrome, Prader–Willi syndrome, Rett's syndrome, de Lange syndrome, Smith–Magenis syndrome, and Fragile X syndrome. In many of these cases, SIB manifests itself in an idiosyncratic way, called a behavioral phenotype (i.e., behavior characteristics). The most common forms are head-banging, self-biting, self-gouging, and hair-pulling, but there are at least 35 other less frequent forms. It is not clear as yet if all of these heterogeneous topographies reflect similar underlying pathology. It is more likely that SIB is multiply caused and multiply determined.

PREVALENCE/RISK FACTORS

Prevalence estimates range from 7 to 40 percent, but more recent larger studies place it between 10 and 20 percent. Cross-cultural studies in the Federal Republic of Germany agree with a figure of 13.2 percent. At a prevalence estimate of 13 percent of cases of severe and profound autism and/or mental retardation with SIB, it is estimated that there are at least 35,000 persons in the United States exhibiting serious SIB, often resulting in serious tissue damage, permanent impairments, and death. Thus, approximately 1 in 7,000 persons in the United States are estimated to exhibit severe SIB.

There is good agreement on the risk factors related to the occurrence of SIB: lower level of retardation; several medical problems, such as otitis media, seizures, etc.; restrictive residential settings; chronological age; several genetic and psychiatric disorders; and sensory and communication deficits.

ETIOLOGY

There have been at least 10 different hypotheses as to the etiology of SIB over the past 30 years. About half of them are based upon the premise that much of SIB is learned, since behavioral intervention procedures can change it. Unfortunately, most of these changes do not generalize and are not maintained without surveillance and continued intervention. These issues have led behavioral researchers to do a more careful functional assessment of both the behavioral and biological antecedents of SIB, which affect the probability of occurrence of SIB in all of its forms and functions.

The other half of the etiological hypotheses for SIB are based upon a variety of biological theories or syndromes. The discovery of Lesch–Nyhan syndrome in 1964 was a major milestone in the study of the etiology of SIB. This was the first genetic disorder with a very high incidence of a distinctive behavioral phenotype in its population, (i.e. self-biting). For years Lesch–Nyhan syndrome has served as a neurobiological window for studying neurotransmitter functions and pharmacotherapy for self-injurious behavior. Early hypotheses related to serotonin dysfunction led to clinical trials with 5-hydroxytryptophan, but it showed only a temporary improvement. In 1981 an important postmortem study of three Lesch–Nyhan cases revealed a 60–90 percent depletion of dopamine and elevation of serotonin in striatal neurons. This finding led Breese (1984), an animal neuropharmacologist, to propose a rat model of neonatal 6-hydroxydopamine (6-OHDA) lesions as a second hypothesis to account for self-biting in Lesch–Nyhan syndrome. He found that rats given 6-OHDA lesions in the corpus striatum of the basal ganglia at 5–15 days of age, and then allowed to recover and grow up, tend to bite themselves severely when challenged with the dopamine (DA) agonist, L-DOPA. Through an extensive research program of inducing self-biting, with DA agonists and blocking it with DA antagonists, he has implicated D1 DA receptors as a critical link in the development of SIB in neonatally depleted 6-OHDA lesioned rats. This rat model has many far-reaching implications for the behavioral and pharmacological treatment and prevention of SIB.

Another complementary hypothesis for explaining SIB was the opioid peptide hypothesis proposed by Sandman in 1982. It was based upon the observation that some SIB cases seem to be insensitive to pain. It was hypothesized that their endorphin system was malfunctioning and could be modulated by endorphin blockers such as naloxone. The first clinical trials of naloxone by Sandman and colleagues (1983) showed a dose-response effect. This result has been replicated with its orally administered counterpart, naltrexone, in over 30 studies. Thus a new line of research has been initiated on drug treatment for SIB for people with Mental Retardation/

Development Disabilities (MR/DD), which is based on a specific neurochemical hypothesis. Sandman has now found a mutation in the POMC gene specific to SIB cases who respond positively to naltrexone.

More recent outgrowths of these early hypotheses have led to more refined new biobehavioral approaches. Schroeder, Oster-Granite, & Thompson (2002) discuss these newer approaches in a book on SIB.

These neurochemical hypotheses for SIB have started a new generation of models and theories in MR/DD with a level of specificity far beyond what was heretofore imagined possible. Such work, which requires interdisciplinary collaboration to succeed, is likely to change our view of SIB substantially in the future.

ASSESSMENT

Because SIB may have multiple causes, most clinicians use a step-down assessment strategy, looking first for genetic causes, then neurological causes, then psychiatric causes, then other medical causes such as otitis media, menstrual pain, and sleep disorders. After these contributions have been assessed, then various causes related to learning and motivation are assessed. An excellent technology called functional assessment has been developed to assess the many possible functions of SIB related to environmental events. Sufficient research has shown that the main functions are usually to get attention, to avoid something or someone, to be rewarded by a tangible object, or to receive a sensory reward of some type.

TREATMENT

There are basically three treatment strategies for SIB: behavioral interventions, psychopharmacology, and treatment of antecedent symptoms. The most widely used strategy is behavioral intervention, which is based on learning principles. There have been over 1,000 studies in the past 30 years that have grown increasingly sophisticated in pinpointing the behavioral antecedents of SIB and tailoring the rewards for alternative behaviors to its functional properties. These interventions work both for mild and severe cases, but long-term maintenance and surveillance is usually necessary in severe cases.

A second strategy often used in combination with behavioral intervention is psychopharmacology. Over the past 30 years these interventions have improved from trial-and-error use of antipsychotic drugs to hypothesis-driven selection of drugs based upon their neuropharmacological properties and a milder side effects profile. Several drugs are now available that improve certain types of SIB, for example, risperidone, naltrexone, and clozapine.

A third strategy is to treat the symptoms that are the occasion for SIB. For instance, if SIB co-occurs with severe depression, one can treat the depression and hope the SIB will also go away. This strategy works when a highly related covariate of SIB can be identified. Unfortunately, this is possible in only a minority of cases. Usually SIB is a heterogeneous response to a variety of precipitating events.

PROGNOSIS

Self-injurious behavior is a devastating chronic condition for which there is no known apparent cure. However, several follow-up studies have shown that many cases of SIB (approximately 60 percent) can be treated by mild positive interventions. In addition, some SIB (approximately 15 percent) goes away by itself without any intervention. But there is some severe chronic SIB (approximately 25 percent) that will always need some intervention and constant surveillance to prevent serious injury or even death.

See also: Acute Stress Disorder; Autistic Disorder; Aggression; Antisocial Behavior; Anxiety Disorders; Disruptive Behavior Disorders; Stereotypic Movement Disorder; Nail-Biting; Trichotillomania; Obsessive Compulsive Disorder; Rett's Syndrome; Fragile X Syndrome; Dual Diagnosis Retardation and Psychiatric Disorders; Mental Retardation

Further Reading

Breese, G. R., Baumeister, A. A., McGowen, T. J., Emerick, S. G., Frye, G. D., Crotty, K. et al. (1984). Behavioral differences between neonatal- and adult-6-hydroxydopamine-treated rats to dopamine agonists: Relevance to neurological symptoms in clinical syndromes with reduced brain dopamine. *Journal of Pharmacology and Experimental Therapeutics, 234,* 447–455.

Lyloyd, H. G. E., Hornykiewicz, O., Davidson, L., Shannak, K., Farley, I., Goldstein, M. et al. (1981). Biomedical evidence of dysfunction of brain neurotransmitters in the Lesch–Nyhan syndrome. *New England Journal of Medicine, 305,* 1106–1111.

Sandman, C. A., Datta, P., Barron, J. L., Hoehler, E., Williams, C., & Swanson, J. (1983). Naloxone attenuates self-abusive behavior in developmentally disabled subjects. *Applied Research in Mental Retardation, 4,* 5–11.

Thompson, T., & Schroeder, S. R. (eds.). (1995). Self-injury in developmental disabilities. *Mental Retardation and Developmental Disabilities Research Reviews, 1*(2).

Schroeder, S. R., Oster-Granite, M. L., & Thompson, T. (Eds.). (2002). *Self-injurious behavior: Gene–brain–behavior relationships.* Washington, DC: APA Books.

STEPHEN R. SCHROEDER

Self-Management

DEFINITION

According to Goldfried and Merbaum (1973), self-management is an evidence-based treatment approach in which the child or adolescent is trained in skills needed to control his/her own behavior. Unlike other commonly used child therapeutic strategies (e.g., parent-training), in child self-management, emphasis is placed on directly training the child or adolescent in behavior change efforts. Generally, the therapist teaches the child how, when, and where to use the various self-management strategies to facilitate the learning of new behavior patterns.

METHOD

The main techniques and strategies used most often in self-management are: (1) self-monitoring, (2) self-evaluation, (3) self-reward, (4) self-determined contingencies, and (5) self-instruction.

Self-monitoring is a two-step procedure that involves observing and recording target behaviors. The child must first learn to detect the presence of certain behaviors to determine if the target behavior has occurred. This allows the child and therapist to identify target responses and behavior–environment relations that may aid in the conceptualization of treatment. An example of self-monitoring is the use of a behavioral daily diary in which the child carries a notepad at all times. When the target behavior is emitted, the child records the circumstances surrounding the behavior including the situation and his/her response.

Self-evaluation involves the child self-monitoring his/her behavior and evaluating this behavior based on a specific predetermined criterion. Self-evaluation techniques work under the assumption that the child attempts to behave in a manner that is consistent with the child's own internal codes of behavior. Self-evaluation provides internal feedback that guides the child's behavior, producing covert self-reinforcement or self-punishing thoughts or self-talk. Pairing self-evaluation with reinforcement has been found to increase the efficacy of self-evaluation. For example, in the classroom children are asked to compare their written assignments to a chart describing grammatical rules and record the occurrence of target behaviors (correct usage of grammar). When the reinforcement is made contingent on the occurrence of the target behavior, large increases

in the frequency of the target behavior are generally observed.

Self-reward is another self-management technique in which the child self-delivers a reward contingent on the occurrence of the target behavior. This is a two-step process that requires the child to first detect when the target behavior has occurred and subsequently administer the self-reward. Teaching self-reward generally begins with instruction in self-monitoring. An example of this technique would be when the child praises himself/herself (e.g., "good job" or "I did it") for emitting a target behavior.

Self-determined contingency is another self-management technique in which the child self-delivers rewards for appropriate completion of self-determined contingencies according to his/her own reinforcement schedule. An example would be when a child with a specific phobia of dogs determines his/her own approach behaviors toward different types of dogs, and determines the reward that should be delivered upon displaying the approach behaviors. As noted by Gross and Drabman (1982), a difficulty in using self-determined contingencies is that the child may begin to maximize his/her rewards by establishing more lenient contingencies, though the appropriate target behavior has not yet been accomplished.

Self-instruction involves teaching the child to make verbal statements to himself/herself to guide, direct, and maintain his/her behavior. The child observes the model/therapist performing the task while the model/therapist is guiding and directing his/her own behavior out loud. The child then performs the same task while receiving instructions from the model/therapist. Finally, the child performs the task while guiding and directing his/her own behavior first out loud, then whispering, and finally, silently.

CLINICAL APPLICATIONS

One or more of these self-management techniques often are used in treating a wide range of disorders in children and adolescents, including Attention-Deficit/Hyperactivity Disorder (ADHD), phobic and anxiety disorders, eating disorders, and disruptive disorders. For example, the acronym "STOP" has been used with children with phobic and anxiety disorders by Silverman and her colleagues (1999). While facing the fearful or anxiety provoking object or event, the child identifies when he/she is feeling *S*cared or anxious ("S"), what his/her scary or anxious *T*houghts are ("T"), identifies or generates *O*ther alternative coping thoughts and behaviors ("O"), and finally, engages in self-evaluation and *P*raise self-reward ("P").

See also: Behavioral Diaries; Behavior Rating Scales; Child Self-Reports; Cognitive–Behavior Therapy

Further Reading

Goldfried, M. R., & Merbaum, M. (1973). How to control yourself. *Psychology Today, 7*, 102–104.

Gross, A. M., & Drabman, R. S. (1982) Teaching self-recording, self-evaluation, and self-reward to nonclinic children and adolescents. In P. Karoly & F. H. Kanfer (Eds.), *Self-management and behavior change from theory to practice* (pp. 285–311). Elmsford, NY: Pergamon Press.

Silverman, W. K., Kurtines, W. M., Ginsburg, G. S., Weems, C. F., Lumpkin, P. W., & Carmichael, D. H. (1999). Treating anxiety disorders in children with group cognitive–behavioral therapy: A randomized clinical trial. *Journal of Consulting and Clinical Psychology, 67*, 995–1003.

Barbara Lopez
Lissette M. Saavedra
Wendy K. Silverman

Sensorineural Hearing Loss

See: Hearing Impairment

Sensory and Perceptual Development

DEFINITION

Information that enters the cognitive systems of infants, children, and adults is first detected by the various sense organs, in which physical energy (light, movement, pressure, chemical) is converted into neural signals that are interpretable by the brain. This is traditionally referred to as *sensation*. Such signals are then organized into meaningful units; traditionally, the term *perception* has referred to this second organizational process. Since the two processes are somewhat interdependent, the boundaries between the two are often difficult to distinguish. It is easiest to consider the development of these processes in terms of development in the five senses: hearing (audition), seeing (vision), taste, touch, and smell (olfaction).

AUDITION

Sensitivity

Audition is functional before birth, as fetuses are clearly able to hear prenatally, and evidence has shown that sounds or sequences that have been made familiar to infants during gestation are preferred during the newborn period. As such, hearing is one of the more generally well developed senses in the newborn baby, although hearing thresholds are significantly higher in infants than in children and adults. There is some suggestion that infants may not hear low-pitched sounds as well as adults, but there is also evidence that they are able to hear some very high pitched sounds better than adults. The fact that infants younger than one week of age can recognize their mothers' voices demonstrates that infants' abilities to hear, discriminate, and recognize sounds are well developed at birth. By 18 months of age, auditory sensitivity is very close to that of the adult.

Localization

Infants also have the ability to identify the location in space from which a sound is coming (*localization*). Newborns have been shown to localize sounds, but infants' turning to sounds occurs with far less regularity between 2 and 4 months of age. The response reemerges in a more mature form by 5 months. By 6 months, infants are capable of localizing sound in both the vertical and horizontal plane.

Speech Perception

Language is composed of speech sounds called phonemes. Phonemes are perceived so that it is easier to differentiate them from one another in acquiring and learning language. This type of perception is present in very young human infants. Furthermore, different phonemes are used in different languages. Adults are less able to discriminate phonemes that are not part of their native languages. Research over the last 30 years has shown that young human infants, however, can discriminate phonemes from all languages. This ability allows infants to acquire any language but it apparently does not last long; between 8 and 12 months of age, infants' ability to discriminate phonemes that have not been present in their language-learning environment declines sharply.

VISION

Visual Acuity

Unlike the auditory system, the visual system is quite immature at birth. Newborns cannot see very well, although by 3 years of age most children attain adult-like visual acuity. The development of visual acuity goes through three distinct phases in infancy and early childhood; there is a dramatic improvement from birth to 6 months, a period of little change from 6–12 months, and then a period of slow improvement from 12–36 months. The early deficits are believed to be due to immaturity of the retina (the layer of cells at the back of the eye that are sensitive to light), and to the immaturity of those areas in the brain that mediate vision.

Form, Pattern, and Color Perception

Even though newborns cannot see fine/small objects or patterns, they do have the ability to locate and track moving objects, which improves in accuracy with age. Due to limitations in visual acuity, early visual exploration is limited to large objects with high contrast and distinct contours. Movement helps infants distinguish between objects as well as between the object and background. With regard to color perception, newborns have been shown to be able to discriminate a large range of colors by about 6 weeks of age, and it is generally believed that discrimination of basic primary colors is present at birth.

Infants' perception of complex patterns has been studied for over 30 years. Typically, infants show spontaneous visual preferences for some patterns over others, and this has been exploited for measures of perceptual discrimination, salience, and recognition as early as the newborn period. Infants have been shown to prefer faces, complex stimuli, and symmetric stimuli.

Visual Depth Perception

The development of depth perception has been studied for both theoretical and practical reasons. Initially, infants' ability to perceive depth was tested using the visual cliff, a glass surface that presents the appearance of an underlying surface at one end (the "shallow side"), and an apparent drop-off at another (the "deep side"). Infants placed on the shallow side typically will avoid crawling across the deep side, showing the presence of both a perception and fear of depth at 8 months. More recent and sophisticated studies of depth perception suggest that some cues for depth perception are present by 4 months of age.

OLFACTION

A newborn's olfactory system is well developed before birth. Once born, the infant has the ability to sense different types of smells, and show different preferences to them. For example, breast-fed newborns can recognize the smell of their mother's breast milk, and discriminate it from a stranger's breast milk. Infants have also been shown to be able to recognize their own mothers by smell as well. The fact that this is not seen in bottle-fed babies suggests that this is learned through experience while breast-feeding. As such, it has been hypothesized that infants' sense of smell plays a role in attachment.

TASTE

The taste buds begin developing on the tongue around 7–8 weeks of age. Newborns respond to most of the four different tastes available to humans (sweet, sour, salt, and bitter), but strongly prefer the sweet taste, which has also been shown to have a strong calming effect. The preference to sweet taste persists throughout development and strengthens with experience.

Initially, the salt taste is somewhat aversive to babies, but between 2 and 3 years of age, toddlers start to prefer salty foods. Infants that are exposed to a variety of foods early in life will grow up to prefer a wider variety of foods. By the ages of 2 and 3, sweetness and familiarity determines food preferences.

TOUCH

The sense of touch refers to a wide range of experiences that includes the perception of temperature, pain, pressure, weight, and other more global senses such as the somesthetic sense (i.e., where the body is in space). Touch plays a very important role in infant's development; it provides a powerful means of communication between infant and caregiver. Early studies show that tactile contact is a strong determinant of attachment.

The research examining touch as a form of communication is in its infancy. However it has been found that touch is the best way to soothe a baby. Infants that are stroked show more smiling than infants that are tickled. Massage therapy with preterm infants has been shown to enhance weight gain, indicating that touch can actually facilitate growth.

See also: Hearing Impairment; Learning Disorders; Sensory Integration Dysfunction; Visual Impairment: Low Vision and Blindness

Further Reading

Goldstein, B. E. (1996). *Sensation and perception* (4th ed.). Pacific Grove, CA: Brooks/Cole.

Haith, M. M. (1993). Preparing for the 21st century: Some goals and challenges for studies of infant sensory and perceptual development. *Developmental Review, 13*, 354–371

Werker, J. & Tees, J. (1999). Influences on infant speech processing: Toward a new synthesis. *Annual Review of Psychology, 50*, 509–535.

OTILIA M. BLAGA
JOHN COLOMBO

Sensory Integration Dysfunction

DEFINITION

Sensory processing is the ability to take in sensory information through gravity, movement, touch, vision, hearing, taste, and smell; process that information; and use it for functional daily activities. The development of sensory integration occurs primarily during the first seven years of life. During this time, as noted by Parham and Mailloux (2001), children develop the ability to focus on meaningful sensory input and tune out sensory input that is irrelevant to the present task or activity. The ability to process sensory information accurately assists in maintaining an optimal level of alertness for learning, maintaining attention to meaningful tasks, and controlling emotions and fluctuations between emotional states, as shown by Williamson and Anzalone (2000). For example, while playing with blocks in a preschool class, a child may look up and observe that two new adults have just entered the room. The child may continue to observe the adults until they begin to talk to the teacher, at which time the child determines that the adults are not a threat and resumes playing with the blocks. Due to the ability to adequately process sensory information, this child was able to localize and attend to novel sensory input, determine if the sensory information was relevant to the current task, tune out the irrelevant sensory input, then resume the original task.

Sensory processing problems, or sensory integration dysfunction, occur when a child has difficulty processing some aspect of sensory information, resulting in difficulty participating in functional daily life activities. Parham and Mailloux (2001) indicate that the term sensory integration disorder refers to a "heterogenous group of disorders that are thought to reflect subtle, primarily subcortical, neural dysfunction involving multi-sensory systems." The peripheral receptors are believed to be intact; however, the cortical processing of the sensory information is impaired.

Sensory processing problems can present in a variety of ways. Children may have difficulty with attention, have a higher or lower than normal activity level, may appear to be a thrill seeker, or may be clumsy and have difficulty learning new motor tasks. Children who are sensitive to certain sensory inputs can appear to overreact to touch, movement, smells, tastes or different textures of foods, or sounds. Some children do not appear to respond as expected to sensory input. For example, a child who is sensitive to smells and tastes may gag when presented with certain textures of food or when exposed to the variety of smells in a restaurant. A child who is sensitive to touch may react aggressively to the light touch of a peer touching their shoulder or refuse to wear short sleeves or other types of clothing. It is not uncommon for children with sensory processing problems to have delays in language skills as well. They may learn to talk late, or when they do talk it may be very difficult to understand them.

ASSESSMENT

Assessment to identify sensory integration dysfunction is typically completed by a pediatric occupational therapist or physical therapist with expertise in this area. If language concerns are present, assessment by a speech–language pathologist is also indicated. Pediatric neuropsychologists also can assess the child's sensory processing across diverse modalities, and integrate this information with the child's emotional and/or behavioral functioning.

The assessment process begins by interviewing the parents, other caregivers, and teachers if the child is school age to identify the presenting problems and to determine if sensory processing problems are interfering with the child's functional abilities. Questionnaires and checklists can be helpful when gathering information about the child. One commonly used questionnaire is the Sensory Profile developed by Dunn (1999), which includes two forms. The Short Sensory Profile can be used as a screening tool and the longer version is used to more specifically identify sensory processing problems. An additional way of gathering information is through the use of a rating scale. The Touch Inventory for Elementary School-Aged Children, developed by Royeen and Fortune (1990), is used to assess tactile defensiveness in children who have the verbal skills to discuss their own abilities and perceptions. Based on

Table 1. Standardized Tests Commonly Used for Children with
Sensory Processing Problems

Test	Purpose	Age range	Skills assessed that relate to sensory processing
Miller Assessment of Preschoolers	Assess fine motor and gross motor skills	2.9–5.8 years	Stereognosis, vestibular functions, tactile perception
Bruininks–Oseretsky Test of Motor Proficiency	Assess fine motor and gross motor skills	4.5–14.5 years	Bilateral coordination
Sensory Integration and Praxis Test	Assess sensory integrative function	4 years to 8 years 11 months	Tactile, vestibular, proprioceptive sensory processing; form and space perception, visuomotor coordination; bilateral coordination and sequencing abilities; praxis

information gathered through interviews, question-naires, and rating scales, the therapist can determine if sensory processing problems are suspected and if further assessment is indicated.

If sensory processing problems are suspected, the next step is to observe the child. If possible, the child should be observed participating in daily life activities either at home, at school, or in other natural settings in which he or she participates on a regular basis. If the child is evaluated in the clinic, informal observations can be made as the child plays freely. The therapist observes to determine how the child plays and interacts with others and how the child responds to novel situations. A child with sensory processing problems is more likely to have difficulty problem-solving how to play with a new toy or may be overwhelmed by a novel environment and react by withdrawing or becoming emotional. The child's difficulty processing sensory information may also lead to increased irritability, anxiety, and/or emotional outbursts. Thus, careful assessment of sensory processing problems can provide helpful information regarding treatment of the behavioral and/or emotional difficulties.

The therapist also makes observations of how the child plays and moves, including the child's muscle tone, balance and equilibrium reactions, and coordination skills. The therapist also observes if the child is able to cross midline or if the child is 6 years of age, if he or she has established hand dominance (e.g., left- or right-handedness). Standardized testing may also be used to further assess the child's motor skills that may be affected by deficits in sensory processing or to specifically assess sensory processing abilities (Table 1). The Sensory Integration and Praxis Test (SIPT) is the only standardized test designed to specifically assess sensory integration. Therapists must receive special training to administer and interpret the results of the SIPT.

INTERVENTION

Williamson and Anzalone (2000) indicate that intervention for children with sensory processing problems includes three components: (1) helping parents understand their child's behavior, (2) modifying the environment and activities in which the child is expected to participate, and (3) providing direct intervention to help the child improve his/her ability to process sensory information and/or develop compensatory strategies to help them function in their environment despite their sensory processing difficulties. If behavioral or emotional difficulties accompany the sensory processing problems, consultation with a psychologist about effective behavior management and treatment strategies is recommended.

See also: Attention-Deficit/Hyperactivity Disorder; Learning Disorders; Pervasive Developmental Disorders; Speech and Language Assessment

Further Reading

Dunn, W. W. (1999). *Sensory Profile.* San Antonio: TX: Psychological Corporation.
Kranowitz, C. S. (1998). *The Out of Sync Child.* New York: Berkley.
Parham, L. D., & Mailloux, Z. (2001). Sensory integration. In J. Case-Smith (Ed.), *Occupational therapy for children* (pp. 329–381). St. Louis, MO: Mosby.
Royeen, C. B., & Fortune, J. C. (1990). TIE: Touch inventory for school aged children. *American Journal of Occupational Therapy, 44,* 165–170.
Williamson, G. G., & Anzalone, M. E. (2000, December). *Sensory integration and self regulation: Helping young children interact with their environment.* Paper presented at the Zero to Three 15th National Training Institute.

RENE MARIE DAMAN

Separation Anxiety Disorder

DESCRIPTION/CLINICAL PRESENTATION

Separation anxiety disorder (SAD) is a common psychiatric disorder of childhood and early adolescence characterized by an unrealistic and excessive fear of separation from an attachment figure, usually the parent, which significantly interferes with daily activities and developmental tasks.

The essential feature of SAD is excessive anxiety concerning separation from home or from the attachment figures. According to the definition in the fourth edition of the *Diagnostic and Statistical Manual of Mental Disorders* (DSM) published by the American Psychiatric Association, the anxiety is beyond that which is expected for the child's developmental level, and must last for a period of at least 4 weeks, begin before the age of 18 years, and cause clinically significant distress or impairment in social, academic, or other important areas of functioning. The symptoms may include excessive distress when separated from home or from the attachment figures occurs or is anticipated, persistent worry about losing the attachment figures or about possible harm befalling them, worry about getting lost or being kidnapped, reluctance or refusal to go to school, fear of being alone at home, reluctance or refusal to go to sleep without being near the parents, repeated nightmares involving the theme of separation, or repeated complaints of physical symptoms (e.g., headaches, nausea) when separation occurs or is anticipated. Approximately one-half of children with SAD are diagnosed with another anxiety disorder, most often overanxious disorder or specific phobia, and one-third with depression.

PREVALENCE AND CORRELATES

Epidemiological studies indicate a prevalence of 3–5 percent in children and adolescents. About one-third of children suffering from clinical levels of anxiety show the specific features of SAD. Several studies have found an overrepresentation of girls with SAD; others have reported equal frequency in girls and boys. Fifty to seventy-five percent of children with SAD come from low socioeconomic status homes. Peak age onset appears to be around 7–9 years of age, but the disorder may develop during adolescence as well.

Family processes and parental psychopathology seem to be related to SAD. According to a review by

Manassis (2001), empirical studies have linked insecure mother–child attachment with both clinical and subclinical separation anxiety in children. Mothers with insecure attachment representations toward their parents show heightened levels of maternal separation anxiety toward their infants. An increased prevalence of anxiety disorders and of depression has been demonstrated in families of children with SAD, relative to controls. Offspring of parents with panic disorder have been shown to have a 3-fold increased risk of developing SAD, while offsprings of parents with panic disorder plus major depression have more than a 10-fold increased risk.

Children with SAD report more negative cognitions than children with no clinical disorder and children with nonanxious disorders, and they interpret ambiguous or unclear situations as more dangerous. They also have lower estimations of their own competency to cope with danger than the comparison groups. Temperamental factors, in particular, "behavioral inhibition" (i.e., shy, withdrawn), appear to be related to SAD. Behaviorally inhibited children show a higher rate of SAD than noninhibited children and a greater risk of developing SAD, according to a 3-year follow-up study by Biederman and colleagues (1993). For further information on the epidemiology and correlates of SAD, see a recent review by Silverman and Dick-Niederhauser (in press).

ASSESSMENT

There are several interview schedules currently available to reliably diagnose SAD, together with other childhood anxiety disorders, such as the Diagnostic Interview Schedule for Children or the Anxiety Disorders Interview Schedule for Children IV (Child and Parent Versions). Separation anxiety also has been shown to be a reliable factor in the Screen for Child Anxiety Related Emotional Disorders (SCARED), the Multidimensional Anxiety Scale for Children (MASC), and the Spence Children's Anxiety Scale (SCAS). Silove and colleagues (1993) developed a brief self-report instrument, the Separation Anxiety Symptom Inventory (SASI), for the assessment of symptoms of separation anxiety in adults.

PROGNOSIS

In two prospective longitudinal studies with 3- to 4-year follow-ups, a high percentage of individuals who met criteria for a diagnosis of SAD prior to the onset of treatment no longer met criteria for SAD at the conclusion of treatment. These studies have also shown that SAD dissipates with time. In retrospective studies, SAD has been found to be a risk factor for the development of anxiety disorders later in life, particularly with regard to agoraphobia and panic disorder. However, a direct link between SAD in childhood and agoraphobia and panic disorder in adulthood remains inconclusive.

TREATMENT

There appears to be general consensus in the field that exposure-based cognitive behavioral therapy (CBT) are the methods of choice for anxiety disorders. CBT has been found to be efficacious in treating anxiety disorders in children, including SAD, whether delivered using an individual child format, a format that involves increased parental involvement, and a format that involves increased peer involvement. The randomized controlled clinical trials of anxiety disorders in general in children have not found specificity or differential response for SAD relative to the other anxiety disorders. The presence of comorbid conditions, including the additional diagnosis of SAD, also has not been shown to lead to differential response to CBT. Limited sample sizes, however, preclude a full and systematic evaluation of either one of these two issues.

The pharmacological literature for the treatment of childhood anxiety disorders, including SAD, is in its infancy when compared to the treatment literature on exposure-based CBT. The available literature consists of a small number of open label trials and case studies. Although there is research that shows benzodiazapines, selective serotonin reuptake inhibitors (SSRIs), and tricyclic antidepressants (TCAs) may be effective in treating SAD in children and adolescents, firm conclusions cannot be drawn from the findings in light of methodological constraints. Antidepressants that include SSRIs and TCAs are most often used with adults as well as youth. In terms of TCAs for reducing SAD, results have been mixed. Overall, pharmacological intervention has been recommended with more difficult or "resistant" cases rather than the frontline approach to be used with all cases.

See also: Anxiety Disorders; Attachment; Cognitive–Behavior Therapy; Pharmacological Interventions; Temperament Assessment

Further Reading

Biederman, J., Rosenbaum, J. F., Bolduc-Murphy, E. A., Faraone, S. V., Charloff, J., Hirshfeld, D. R., & Kagan, J. (1993). A 3-year follow-up of children with and without behavioral inhibition. *Journal of the American Academy of Child and Adolescent Psychiatry, 32,* 814–821.

Manassis, K. (2001). Child–parent relations: Attachment and anxiety disorders. In W. K. Silverman & P. D. A. Treffers (Eds.), *Anxiety disorders in children and adolescents: Research, assessment, and intervention* (pp. 255–272). Cambridge, U.K.: Cambridge University Press.

Silove, D., Manicavasagar, V., O'Connell, D., Blaszczynski, A., Wagner, R., & Henry, J. (1993). The development of the Separation Anxiety Symptom Inventory (SASI). *Australian and New Zealand Journal of Psychiatry, 27,* 477–488.

Silverman, W. K., & Dick-Niederhauser, A. (in press). Separation anxiety disorder. In T. L. Morris & J. S. March (Eds.), *Anxiety disorders in children and adolescents* (2nd ed.). New York: Guilford.

ANDREAS DICK-NIEDERHAUSER
WENDY K. SILVERMAN

Sexual Abuse

DEFINITION

Child sexual abuse is broadly defined as any sexual activity involving a child or adolescent where consent cannot be or is not given. The definition of sexual abuse may vary depending on the purpose of the definition (e.g., investigation versus treatment versus research). Included in the definition is all sexual activity between an adult and child and any sexual contact that involves force or threat of force, regardless of the age of the participants. Acts considered sexually abusive include touching; fondling; digital or penile penetration of the mouth, vagina, or anus; and non-contact abuse, such as voyeurism and exhibitionism.

INCIDENCE

The precise incidence of child sexual abuse in the general population is not known since sexual abuse is not frequently reported by the victim and there is no comprehensive national reporting system to track the number of cases that occur each year. The most recent national study of child abuse and neglect found that 11.3 percent or approximately 1 per 1,000 children and adolescents had claim for sexual abuse that were substantiated in 1999. Research suggests that some children are more vulnerable to sexual abuse than others. For instance, substantiated reports of sexual abuse indicate that girls are approximately three times more likely to be sexually abused than boys and there are disproportionate numbers of sexually abused children from low-income families.

EFFECTS OF CHILD SEXUAL ABUSE

A wide variety of symptoms and a range of symptom severity have been documented in sexually abused children and adolescents. Although sexually abused children, in general, tend to have more problems than their nonabused peers, there is no uniform impact of sexual abuse or any evidence that a particular child will develop abuse-related problems. A review of empirical studies found that up to 40 percent of children who had been sexually abused did not appear to have any of the expected abuse-related problems.

Among young children who do exhibit abuse-related problems, the most frequently reported symptoms include depression, anxiety, fearfulness of abuse stimuli and other symptoms of Posttraumatic Stress Disorder (PTSD), nightmares and sleep disorders, repressed anger and hostility, sexual and nonsexual behavior problems, and somatic complaints. The symptoms most frequently reported in sexually abused adolescents include low self-esteem, depression, suicidal ideation or behavior, school problems, conflicts with authority, early onset of sexual behavior, eating disorders, and substance abuse.

ASSESSMENT OF CHILDREN AND CAREGIVERS

Assessment in cases of child sexual abuse may be conducted for the purpose of a clinical evaluation or for a forensic investigation. There are distinct differences between these types of assessments in the methodology and approach used and it is imperative that clinicians are aware of these differences. A forensic evaluation is typically a fact-finding interview that is conducted as part of a legal or law enforcement investigation.

Clinical assessments of sexually abused children are conducted for the purpose of treatment planning and should take into consideration the child's developmental functioning and abilities. Specifically, the assessment should be aimed at gaining an understanding of what happened to the child or adolescent, identifying how he or she copes with the effects of the abuse, assessing the nature and severity of current symptoms or discomfort, and identifying the problems that may occur in the future. Assessment of attributional style, abuse-related and abuse-specific attributions, and

coping styles is also recommended as these variables are associated with long-term adjustment and can be focused on in treatment.

Obtaining information about caregivers is also a critical component of the assessment process. Specifically, assessment of caregivers should focus on gaining an understanding of the caregivers' relationship with the child, ability to use appropriate discipline, level of distress, and ability to support and protect the child. Information gained about the child, caregivers, and their relationships during the assessment phase should be used as a basis for formulating a diagnostic impression, setting initial goals for therapy, and determining a prognosis for the child's mental health in subsequent stages of development.

In evaluating children who have been sexually abused, it is important to use both broad-scale assessment measures and instruments specific to sexual abuse. The assessment may include interviews, clinician-administered tests, self-report questionnaires, or structured behavioral observations with the child, siblings, and caregivers. In addition to use of standard measures to assess cognitive functioning and general behavior, several specific measures have been developed and can be used by clinicians to evaluate the child's or adolescent's symptoms associated with the sexual abuse. For example, the Trauma Symptom Checklist for Child is a measure designed to assess various aspects of distress and symptomology in children and adolescents who have experienced sexual abuse or other traumatic events.

TREATMENT FOR CHILDREN AND CAREGIVERS

Treatment approaches for children who have been sexually abused have been described in the literature and evaluations of treatment interventions are increasing. When selecting techniques and interventions, clinicians should use those that are appropriate for the child's cognitive and developmental levels of functioning and that have documented effectiveness in reducing the child's targeted symptoms. Reviews of the current treatment outcome literature provide strong evidence that abuse-specific cognitive–behavioral therapy (CBT) is effective in reducing symptoms of posttraumatic stress reactions. The goal of abuse-specific CBT is to assist children in successfully processing the emotional and cognitive aspects of the abuse experience, and the components of treatment typically include psychoeducation, anxiety management, gradual exposure, and cognitive therapy.

The effectiveness of other psychosocial treatment and pharmacological approaches has not yet been examined empirically; however, it is possible that they may be effective for treating sexually abused children. Currently, the American Academy of Child and Adolescent Psychiatry discourages use of medication as the primary form of treatment for sexually abused children; however, it may be a useful adjunct to psychosocial interventions.

In general, research examining the benefits of caregiver involvement in CBT treatment for sexually abused children suggests that it is important for several reasons. Specifically, caregiver involvement in CBT appears to improve caregiver support and accurate perceptions of the impact on the child and it is an important component of treatment for reducing behavior problems. Treatment for caregivers typically includes abuse-focused elements similar to those addressed in children's treatment, as well as additional components aimed at teaching behavior management strategies and reducing parental distress.

PROGNOSIS

Factors that have been associated with resilience to the impact of sexual abuse and better long-term prognoses among children include the level of abuse stressors experienced and the support and belief of a nonoffending parent. In contrast, negative attributions about the abuse, highly internalizing or externalizing coping responses, and family dysfunction have been identified as factors related to poorer long-term prognoses among children.

See also: Adolescent Sex Offenders; Cognitive–Behavior Therapy, Posttraumatic Stress Disorder in Children; Sexual Behavior Problems

Further Reading

American Academy of Child and Adolescent Psychiatry (AACAP). (1997). Practice parameters for the forensic evaluation of children and adolescents who may have been physically or sexually abused. *Journal of American Academy of Child and Adolescent Psychiatry, 36,* 423–442.
American Professional Society on the Abuse of Children (APSAC). (1997). *Guidelines for psychosocial evaluation of suspected sexual abuse in young children.* Chicago: Author.
Bonner, B. L., Logue, M. B., Kaufman, K. L., & Niec, L. N. (2001). Child maltreatment. In C. E. Walker & M. C. Roberts (Eds.), *Handbook of clinical child psychology* (3rd ed., pp. 989–1030). New York: Wiley.
Myers, J. E. B., Berliner, L., Briere, J., Hendrix, C. T., Jenny, C., & Reid, T. A. (Eds.). (2002). *The APSAC handbook on child maltreatment* (2nd ed.). Thousand Oaks, CA: Sage.

SHELLI K. SHULTZ
BARBARA L. BONNER

Sexual Behavior

See: Sexual Development

Sexual Behavior Problems

DEFINITION

Children with sexual behavior problems (SBP) are defined as children aged 12 and younger who initiate behaviors involving sexual body parts (i.e., genitals, anus, buttocks, or breasts) that are developmentally inappropriate and potentially harmful to themselves or others. Although the term "sexual" is utilized, the intentions and motivations for these behaviors may be unrelated to sexual gratification. Sexual development and behavior are influenced by social, familial, and cultural factors, as well as genetics and biology.

Guidelines have been developed to assist in determining if children's sexual behaviors are problematic. Recommendations include examining the frequency of the behaviors; the extent to which the behavior is preoccupying or otherwise interfering with the child's development; the age/developmental differences of the children involved; the use of force, intimidation, or coercion; the emotional distress of the children; and the response of the child to interventions by caregivers. Problematic sexual behavior is distinguished from sexual play in that sexual play occurs spontaneously, intermittently, with children who are similar in age and development, and is not accompanied by emotional distress.

Defining sexual behaviors as problematic requires an understanding of normative or typical sexual behavior, which changes considerably from early childhood to adolescence. For example, behaviors that are considered normative in preschoolers, such as public nudity, curiosity about sex, and spontaneous touching of other children's genitals, would be considered problematic in older children.

PREVALENCE

There are no figures available on the number of children with SBP. However, over the past 10 years, an increasing number of children are being referred for treatment in both inpatient and outpatient settings. It remains unclear whether this is a true increase in cases or rather improved recognition and referral of children with SBP.

RISK FACTORS

The origins of sexual behavior problems in childhood are not clearly understood. Initial beliefs speculated that a history of sexual abuse was the primary, if not sole, cause of SBP in children, and in fact, children who have been sexually abused do have a higher frequency of sexual behavior problems than children without such a history. However, the last decade of research has indicated that many children with SBP have no known history of sexual abuse and has further suggested that the origins of SBP in childhood may be a complex interaction of familial, social, developmental, and biological factors.

Children with SBP are quite diverse in the characteristics of their sexual behaviors, race, familial factors, socioeconomic status, maltreatment history, and comorbid disorders. No distinct SBP profile exists, nor is there a clear pattern of demographic, psychological, or social factors that are exclusively related to SBP in children. With regard to gender, approximately two-thirds have been male in samples of clinically referred school-age children with SBP and two-thirds have been female in preschool children.

ASSESSMENT OF THE CHILD AND CAREGIVERS

It is recommended that any necessary legal investigations (e.g., by child protective services [CPS] or law enforcement), occur prior to the clinical assessment of children with SBP. The clinical assessment should address the child's history of SBP and child maltreatment, general psychological and social functioning, cognitive development, strengths and resources, and the social developmental history of the child and family. Specific information about the child's exposure to sexual situations in the home (sleeping or bathing with adults or other children, television or videos with sexual content) and types/consistency of discipline are particularly relevant for treatment planning. The child

should be evaluated for comorbid impulse control problems (e.g., Attention-Deficit/Hyperactivity Disorder [ADHD] or Oppositional Defiant Disorder [ODD]) and for trauma-related conditions such as Posttraumatic Stress Disorder (PTSD). Psychological assessment can also provide normative comparisons for the child's sexual behaviors, establish a baseline to examine progress, and assist with answering additional questions for treatment planning. Multiple sources of information are often required to gain a complete clinical picture of the child (e.g., child, parent, other caregivers, teacher, CPS worker, etc.).

Several typologies of SBP have been formulated and studied, as they can have important implications for assessment, treatment, and prevention. One approach is based on the child's sexual behavior and includes three categories: (1) sexually inappropriate: behaviors that are atypical for the child's age but without interpersonal contact; this category has been separated into self-focused (e.g., excessive masturbation) or other-focused (e.g., highly inappropriate sexual remarks and gestures); (2) sexually intrusive: behaviors that are interpersonal, but unplanned, impulsive, and nonaggressive, such as touching a younger child's genitals; and (3) sexually aggressive: behavior involving some form of coercion, planning, and aggressive behavior such as bribing or threatening a younger child to participate in sexual behavior. Another typology based on demographic, family, social, and abuse history characteristics yielded five subtypes: sexually aggressive, highly traumatized, abuse reactive, rule breaker, and nonsymptomatic.

TREATMENT OF CHILDREN AND CAREGIVERS

Several treatment protocols for children with SBP have been developed in recent years. Research on treatment outcome for children with SBP is limited, as only two randomized clinical trials have been conducted. Bonner and colleagues (1999) founded reductions in SBP in the four group treatment approaches evaluated, with no clear advantage of one treatment modality over the others. The four treatment approaches consisted of cognitive–behavior therapy, dynamic play therapy, relapse prevention, and expressive therapy.

Structured, directive approaches have been considered clinically preferable to nondirective modalities. Structured treatment programs for SBP often address rules about sexual behavior (and acknowledging the child's problematic sexual behaviors with school-age children), sex education, impulse-control strategies, social skills, emotional regulation and coping strategies, and sexual abuse prevention/safety skills. Children with SBP who are also experiencing trauma-related symptoms (e.g., Posttraumatic Stress Disorder (PTSD)) may benefit from trauma-focused cognitive–behavioral treatment, typically provided in individual therapy.

Direct involvement of caregivers in the treatment is well supported in the research on treatment for other childhood behavior problems. Caregivers' direct involvement in treatment can address parental discipline, assisting children to practice and generalize new behaviors and skills, and establishing clear rules and a safe and nonsexualized environment for the child. Concurrent treatment for the caregivers of children with SBP addresses supervision, communicating with other adults, implementation of privacy and sexual behavior rules, typical and problematic sexual development, maintaining a nonsexualized environment, guidance in how to talk with children about sexuality, specific behavioral parenting strategies, and helping caregivers support, communicate with, and appropriately nurture their children.

PROGNOSIS

There has been only one study (see Bonner, Walker & Berliner, 1998) that had long-term, that is, two years' follow-up with children with SBP. In this study, 13 percent of children treated with cognitive–behavioral group therapy and 15 percent of children treated in a dynamic play therapy group had another incident of problematic sexual behavior. This is comparable to recidivism rates with adolescent sexual offenders.

See also: Adolescent Sex Offenders; Group Psychotherapy; Parenting Practices; Posttraumatic Stress Disorder in Children; Sexual Abuse

Further Reading

Araji, S. K. (1997). *Sexually aggressive children: Coming to understand them.* Thousand Oaks, CA: Sage.

Bonner, B. L., & Fahey, W. E. (1998). Children with aggressive sexual behavior. In N. N. Singh & A. S. W. Winton (Eds.), *Comprehensive Clinical Psychology: Special Populations* (Vol. 9, pp. 453–466). Oxford, England: Elsevier Science.

Bonner, B. L., Walker, C. E., & Berliner, L. (1999). *Children with sexual behavior problems: Assessment and treatment* (Final Report, Grant No. 90-CA-1469). Washington, DC: Administration of Children, Youth, and Families, DHHS.

Chaffin, M., Letourneau, E., & Silovsky, J. F. (2002). Adults, adolescents, and children who sexually abuse children: A developmental perspective. In J. E. B. Myers, L. Berliner, J. Briere, C. T. Hendrix, C. Jenny, & T. A. Reid (Eds.), *The APSAC handbook on child maltreatment* (2nd ed., pp. 205–232). Thousand Oaks, CA: Sage.

Friedrich, W. N. (2002). *Psychological assessment of sexually abused children and their families.* Thousand Oaks, CA, US: Sage.

Hall, D. K., Mathews, F., & Pearce, J. (2002). Sexual behavior problems in sexually abused children: A preliminary typology. *Child Abuse & Neglect, 26,* 289–312.

Pithers, W. D., Gray, A., Busconi, A., & Houchens, P. (1998). Children with sexual behavior problems: Identification of five distinct child types and related treatment considerations. *Child Maltreatment, 3,* 384–406.

Silovsky, J. F., & Niec, L. (2002). Characteristics of preschool children with sexual behavior problems: A pilot study. *Child Maltreatment, 7,* 187–197.

JANE F. SILOVSKY
BARBARA L. BONNER

Sexual Development

PHYSICAL SEXUAL DEVELOPMENT

Fetal sexual development involves a complex interaction between genetic and hormonal processes. Money (1994) describes this process as follows: (1) Genetic or chromosomal sex is determined at conception by the contribution of an X chromosome from the mother and either an X or a Y chromosome from the father; (2) next, undifferentiated fetal gonads develop in both male and female fetuses: testes at about 6 weeks and ovaries at about 12 weeks; (3) between the third and fourth month of gestation, if the baby is to be a boy, the testes begin to secrete the male hormones androgen and antimullerian hormone, which prod the development of male sexual anatomy and inhibit development of female anatomy, respectively; the lack of these male hormones results in female development regardless of the chromosomal sex of the fetus; and (4) finally, also stimulated by the secretion or lack of secretion of male hormones, differentiated external sex organs develop. Disorders of sexual differentiation originate during these early stages of development.

At the time of a child's birth, it is generally recognized that the physiology for sexual arousal and orgasm and the capacity for a variety of sexual behaviors are present: fetuses suck their fingers and toes, newborn male babies have penile erections, and female babies are capable of vaginal lubrication. There are few if any physical changes in sexual development during infancy and early childhood and no developmental milestones have been clearly identified. For both boys and girls, hormone production is limited and there is little growth in the gonads until puberty. For girls, the first sign of puberty (breast development) varies depending on race, with the average age for

African-American girls 8.87 years and for white girls 9.96 years. The average age for the onset of menses is for African-American and white girls is 12.16 and 12.88 years, respectively. For boys, the age range for the onset of puberty is between 12 and 16 years (average age 13 years). Sexual development during this period occurs over a relatively lengthy period of time (4–5 years for boys and 3–4 years for girls) and includes growth of testes and penis, facial/body hair, voice change, and muscle development in boys, and breast development, leg hair, and menses in girls. Both sexes experience growth of pubic hair, hormonal changes, and a growth spurt resulting in adult height.

CHILD SEXUAL BEHAVIOR

Research on the type and frequency of sexual behaviors exhibited by children is inconsistent, reflecting methodological differences among studies. Nonetheless, it is clear that children engage in a surprising variety of overt sexual behaviors both alone and with peers and/or siblings. Surprisingly, nonabusive sexual contact between children and their parents (e.g., touching parents' breasts or genitals) is also not uncommon. The types of sexual behaviors that are to be expected at different ages are summarized in Table 1.

NORMAL VERSUS ABNORMAL CHILD SEXUAL BEHAVIOR

Gil (1993) provides a framework for assessing the normality/abnormality of child sexual behavior including: (1) age and physical size differences between participants, with greater differences being more problematic; (2) differences in relative status or position of authority; (3) whether the sexual activity is consistent with developmental norms; (4) dynamics of the sexual activity, including whether coercive tactics are used, and the motivations and feelings associated with the activity. Johnson and Friend (1995) provide criteria for determining when a child's sexual behavior falls outside the norm, including:

1. Sexual behaviors engaged in by children who do not have an ongoing mutual play relationship.
2. Sexual behaviors that interfere with other aspects of the child's life.
3. Sexual knowledge that is greater than expected for the child's age.
4. Sexual behaviors that occur in public places and/or persist in spite of frequent requests to stop.
5. Behaviors that are embarrassing or annoying and elicit complaints from other children or adults.

Table 1. Normal Sexual Development

Sexual knowledge	Sexual behavior
Birth to 2 Years • Origins of gender identity • Origins of self-esteem • Learns labels for body parts including genitals • Uses slang labels	• Penile erections and vaginal lubrication • Genital exploration • Experiences genital pleasure • Touches own and other's sex parts • Enjoys nudity, takes clothes off in public
3–5 Years • Gender permanence is established • Gender differences are recognized • Limited information about pregnancy and childbirth • Knows labels for sexual body parts but uses elimination functions for sexual parts	• Masturbates for pleasure, may experience orgasm • Sex play with peers and siblings: exhibits general exploration of own and other's genitals, attempted intercourse, may insert objects in genitals • Enjoys nudity, takes clothes off in public • Uses "dirty" words, especially with peers
6–12 Years • Genital basis of gender known • Correct labels for sex parts known but uses slang • Sexual aspects of pregnancy known	• Sex games with peers and siblings: role plays and sex fantasy, kissing, mutual masturbation, simulated intercourse, playing "doctor" • Masturbation in private • Shows modesty, embarrassment; hides sex games and masturbation from adults

(Continued)

Table 1. *(Continued)*

Sexual knowledge	Sexual behavior
• Increasing knowledge of sexual behavior: masturbation, intercourse • Knowledge of physical aspects of puberty by age 10	• Body changes begin: girls may begin menstruation, boys may experience wet dreams • May fantasize or dream about sex • Interested in sex in media • Uses sexual language with peers • Tells dirty jokes
13–18 Years • Sexual intercourse • Contraception • Sexually transmitted diseases • Date rape and sexual exploitation	• Pubertal changes continue: most girls menstruate by age 16, most boys are capable of ejaculation by age 14 • Dating begins • Sexual contacts are common: mutual masturbation, kissing, petting • Sexual fantasy and dreams • Sexual intercourse may occur in up to one-third of youth

Source: B. N. Gordon, & C. S. Schroeder, *Sexuality: A Developmental Approach to Problems*. New York: Plenum Press. Copyright 1995 Plenum Press. Reprinted by permission.

6. Sexual behaviors that increase in intensity, frequency, or intrusiveness.
7. Sexual behaviors that are associated with negative emotions such as fear, anxiety, intense guilt or shame, or anger.
8. Sexual behaviors that cause physical or emotional pain or discomfort to self or others.
9. Sexual behaviors that are associated with aggression, coercion, force, bribery, manipulation, or threats.

ADOLESCENT SEXUAL BEHAVIOR

The average age at which adolescents become sexually active has decreased rapidly in recent years, with some adolescents first engaging in sexual intercourse as early as 12 years. The vast majority of teenagers (79–91 percent) are sexually active by age 19. In addition to an increased risk of HIV infection and/or pregnancy, early onset of sexual intercourse is problematic because of its negative effects on children's psychosocial development (e.g., increased delinquent behavior, leaving school). Factors that have been shown to be associated with the onset of sexual activity among teenagers include: (1) less highly educated mothers; (2) having a boyfriend or girlfriend; (3) lower educational expectations (i.e., did not intend to go to college); (4) authoritarian parenting; (5) poor communication with parents about sexuality; and (6) having older siblings who are sexually active.

SEXUAL KNOWLEDGE

Even very young children can be quite knowledgeable about many aspects of sexuality (e.g., body parts and functions, gender differences), whereas knowledge about other areas (e.g., sexual intercourse, pregnancy, and birth) may be lacking in older children and adolescents; for example, some teenagers do not possess sufficient information about contraception to prevent unwanted pregnancy. Sexual knowledge that can be expected at different ages is summarized in Table 1. Note that there can be significant differences in sexual knowledge within age groups depending on the area of sexuality assessed, the gender of the child, the sexual attitudes of the parents, and the socioeconomic status of the family.

The relationship between sexual knowledge and sexual behavior in young children is not obvious; more sexual experience is not necessarily accompanied by greater understanding. Among adolescents, moreover, greater knowledge does not necessarily lead to more responsible behavior. The fact that children engage in sexual behavior before they have a clear understanding of its ramifications places them at very high risk for a variety of adverse experiences which can impact negatively on their development. In summary, we have much to learn about how to effectively educate children about sexuality.

See also: Adolescence; Adolescent Sex Offenders; Childhood; Identity Development; Masturbation; Puberty, Delayed; Puberty, Normal; Puberty, Precocious; Sexual Abuse; Sexual

Differentiation: Disorders and Clinical Management; Sexual Orientation: Homosexuality; Social Development in Adolescence; Social Development in Childhood

Further Reading

Gil, E. (1993). Age-appropriate sex play versus problematic sexual behaviors. In E. Gil & T. C. Johnson (Eds.), *Sexualized children: Assessment and treatment of sexualized children and children who molest*. Rockville, MD: Launch Press.

Herman-Giddens, M. E., Slora, E. J., Wasserman, R. C., Bourdony, C. J., Bhapkar, M. V., Koch, G. G., & Hasemeier, C. M. (1997). Secondary sexual characteristics and menses in young girls seen in office practice: A study from the Pediatric Research in Office Settings network. *Pediatrics, 99*, 505–512.

Jensen, L. C., deCaston, J. R., & Weed, S. E. (1994). Sexual behavior of nonurban students in grades 7 and 8: Implications for public policy and sex education. *Psychological Reports, 75*, 1504–1506.

Johnson, T. C., & Friend, C. (1995). Assessing young children's sexual behaviors in the context of child sexual abuse evaluations. In T. Ney (Ed.), *True and false allegations of child sexual abuse: Assessment and case management* (pp. 49–72). New York: Brunner/Mazel.

Gil, E. (1993). Age appropriate sex play versus problematic sexual behaviors. In E. Gil & T. C. Johnson (Eds.), *Sexualized children: Assessment and treatment of sexualized children and children who molest*. Rockville, MD: Launch Press.

Money, J. (1994). *Sex errors of the body and related syndromes: A guide to counseling children, adolescents, and their families* (2nd ed.). Baltimore, MD: Paul H. Brookes.

Rosenfeld, A., Bailey, R., Siegel, B., & Bailey, G. (1986). Determining incestuous contact between parent and child: Frequency of children touching parents' genitals in a nonclinical population. *Journal of the American Academy of Child Psychiatry, 25*, 481–484.

White, S. D., & DeBlassie, R. R. (1992). Adolescent sexual behavior. *Adolescence, 27*, 183–191.

BETTY N. GORDON

Sexual Differentiation: Disorders and Clinical Management

DESCRIPTION OF THE NORMAL SEXUAL DIFFERENTIATION

Sex determination refers to the process through which the bipotential gonad develops either into an ovary or testis. This step is controlled by a product from a gene located on the Y chromosome and has been referred to as *testis determining factor* or *sex determining region of the Y chromosome* (SRY). In the case of an XY-bearing embryo, the testis develops by approximately the seventh week of pregnancy. It will then begin to secrete two hormones, *Müllerian inhibiting substance* (MIS) and androgens, that act on a double set of internal reproductive ducts present in every embryo, *Müllerian* and *Wolffian* ducts. MIS secreted by the *Sertoli* cells of the testis inhibits growth of the Müllerian ducts (forerunner of the uterus, fallopian tubes, and vagina). The *Leydig* cells, in contrast, synthesize androgens that are responsible for the differentiation of the *Wolffian ducts* (precursor of the prostate, vas deferens, epididymis, and seminal vesicles) (Figure 1).

In the case of an XX-bearing embryo, an ovary develops which produces neither MIS nor androgens. Consequently, the Wolffian ducts regress and the Müllerian ducts differentiate. Female development is therefore not contingent upon the presence of an ovary.

In contrast to the internal reproductive ducts that exist as a double set early in development, the primordium of the external genitalia is a single precursor structure. In the genetic male, androgens from the fetal testis masculinize the external genitalia. The *genital tubercle* grows to become the *penis*, the *genital swellings* fuse to form the *scrotum*, and the *urethral (genital) folds* form the shaft of the penis. In the genetic female (i.e., with an ovary that does not secrete androgens), the external genital tubercle becomes the *clitoris*, the genital swellings become the *labia majora*, and the urethral folds become the *labia minora* (Figure 2).

DISORDERS OF SEXUAL DIFFERENTIATION

Because of the complex multistep process of sex determination and sexual differentiation, multiple problems can develop. *Intersexuality* refers to discordance across the various levels of sexual differentiation, genetic, gonadal, and phenotypic. Historically, individuals with hermaphroditism (an individual exhibiting anatomic characteristics of both sexes) were classified according to the structure of the gonad. Thus, a *true hermaphrodite* refers to an individual who possesses both ovarian and testicular tissue. A *male pseudohermaphrodite* has testes but internal reproductive ducts or external genitalia that appear female or are incompletely differentiated as male. A *female pseudohermaphrodite*, on the other hand, is a person with ovaries whose external genitalia have been masculinized to varying degrees. This traditional classification scheme has been modified to include disorders of gonadal differentiation (e.g., *Klinefelter* and *Turner* syndromes) and unclassified forms of abnormal sexual development (e.g., *hypospadias* and Mayer–Rokitansky–Küster–Hauser syndrome)

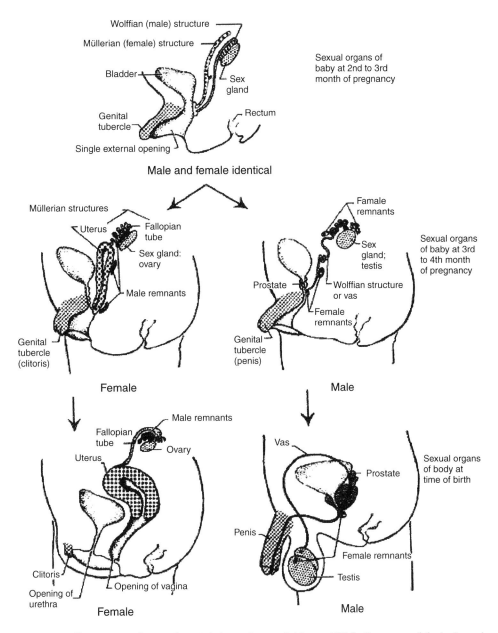

Figure 1. Differentiation of internal genital ducts. *Source*: J. Money (1994). *Sex errors of the body and related syndromes: A guide to counseling children* (2nd ed., p. 32), Baltimore, MD: Paul H. Brookes Publishing Co. Reprinted with permission.

(Table 1). The incidence for these conditions combined may be as high as 1/3,000.

POLICES REGARDING GENDER ASSIGNMENT: PAST AND PRESENT

Until the mid-1950s, medical management of individuals with intersex conditions was guided by the belief that an individual's "true sex" could be discovered through examination of internal anatomy. It was assumed that a person's identification as male or female would naturally conform to their true sex. Based on reports suggesting that this assumption was incorrect, policies were changed, and sex assignment decisions were based on the principle of "optimal gender," which aimed at the best possible prognosis with regard to six dimensions: reproductive potential, good sexual function, minimal medical

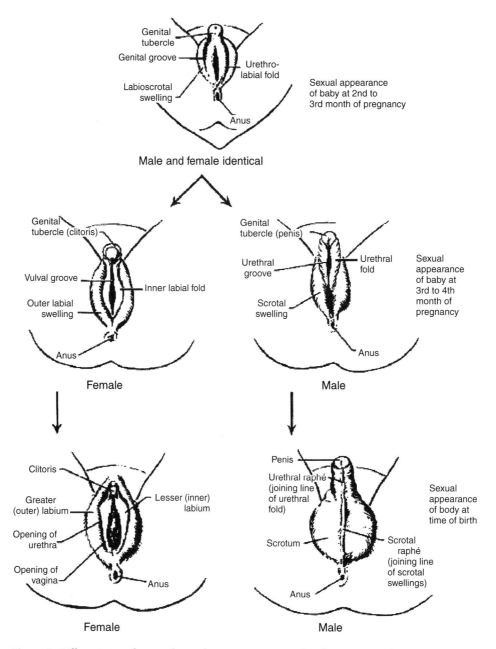

Figure 2. Differentiation of external genitalia. *Source*: J. Money (1994). *Sex errors of the body and related syndromes: A guide to counseling children* (2nd ed., p. 36), Baltimore, MD: Paul H. Brookes Publishing Co. Reprinted with permission.

procedures, an overall gender-appropriate appearance, stable gender identity, and psychosocial well-being. This approach, which stood largely uncontested until recently, is predicated on two assumptions: (1) *gender identity* (i.e., identification of self as either girl/woman or boy/man) is not firmly established at birth but rather is the outcome of rearing sex; and (2) stable gender identity and positive psychological adaptation require that genital

appearance match assigned sex, which often calls for reconstructive genital surgery. It is essential to distinguish between gender identity, which was assumed to develop from rearing conditions, and other aspects of gender-related behavior, which may be influenced by prenatal exposure of the brain to sex hormones. This includes gender role, which refers to behaviors that differ in frequency or level between males and females in this

Table 1. Disorders of Sexual Differentiation (Selected Examples)*

I. Disorders of gonadal differentiation Klinefelter syndrome (47, XXY)	Typically diagnosed at puberty with swelling of breasts (gynecomastia) and small testicles. The internal reproductive ducts are normal male. Associated with sterility, low sex drive, and language and reading problems. Intellectual functioning is average with lower verbal than performance scores. Many evidence speech and language delays. Poor school performance is common. Occurs in 1/500 to 1/1,000 male births.
Turner syndrome (45, X)	Missing or partially deleted X chromosome associated with streak (nonfunctioning) gonad and marked short stature. The Wolffian ducts regress and the Müllerian ducts differentiate normally. The external genitalia appear normal but these girls will require hormone replacement therapy to initiate puberty and to maintain secondary sexual characteristics. Additional features may include thick (webbed) neck, a broad chest, malformed kidneys, and cardiovascular abnormalities. Associated with a variety of learning problems, especially low nonverbal IQ, and poor math and memory skills. Occurs in 1/2,500 to 1/5,000 female births.
True hermaphroditism (46, XX [most common], combined 46, XX/46, XY cell lines, or 46, XY [rare])	Presence of both testicular and ovarian tissue in the same individual The internal reproductive ducts differentiate in accordance with the gonad on that side of the body. The external genitalia in these individuals may range from normal male to normal female. Breast development is common and menses occurs in more than half of the patients.
II. Female pseudohermaphroditism Congenital adrenal hyperplasia (in 46, XX individuals)	An enzyme deficiency (most commonly 21-hydroxylase) results in excess adrenal androgen production and masculinization (in extreme cases ambiguity) of the external genitalia (enlarged clitoris and a fused labia which resembles a scrotum). Lifelong cortisol replacement controls excess androgen production. Internal genital ducts are normal female. Gender identity is characteristically female but gender role behavior is often masculine. More likely to develop a bisexual or homosexual orientation, as indicated by erotic/romantic fantasies and dreams and sexual attractions (but less likely overt homosexual activity). In the United States, incidence is approx. 1/11,000 live births (male and female) but there is considerable variation in ethnic/racial populations.
III. Male pseudohermaphroditism Androgen insensitivity syndrome (46, XY)	Occurs as a result of a mutation of the androgen receptor gene making tissue unresponsive to the influence of androgens. Testes form and synthesize androgens normally. In the "complete" form of this syndrome, the external genitalia have a normal female appearance because of the lack of tissue responsiveness to androgens. Likewise, the Wolffian ducts fail to develop but the Müllerian ducts regress due to the action of Müllerian inhibiting substances (MIS). Breasts develop normally under the influence of androgens that are metabolized into estrogen. Often diagnosed at puberty with lack of menstruation. Gender identity is unambiguously female, gender role is feminine, and sexual orientation is characteristically heterosexual. Estimated incidence is 1/20,000–64,000 male births. Androgen insensitivity also exists in a "partial" form in which the individual is born with ambiguous external genitalia. The genital tubercle is enlarged but not typically of normal male size, a partially fused labia/scrotum may be present, and severe hypospadias (see below) is often present.
5-alpha-reductase deficiency (5-ARD)	5-ARD is an example of a syndrome associated with defects in testosterone metabolism by peripheral tissues. This particular enzyme deficiency results in an inability of testosterone to be converted to the androgen dihydrotestosterone. In its absence, the external genitalia do not differentiate normally. Although the internal genital ducts are normal male, the penis resembles a clitoris and the scrotum appears as labia majora. At puberty, under the direct influence of testosterone (which is normal), normal male secondary sex characteristics develop including increased muscle mass, body hair, and lowering of the voice. The clitoris will also grow at puberty but rarely achieves a normal penile length. These individuals are assigned at birth to either the male or female sex. There is considerable controversy, however, over the stability of the gender identity and gender role behavior of these individuals, especially as they transition through puberty.
IV. Sexual abnormalities of unknown cause Hypospadias (46, XY)	Urinary meatus (opening) is positioned at some point on the undersurface of the penis rather than at its tip. Classified according to the position of the urinary meatus, the mildest and most common form (85%) is glandular or coronal hypospadias. Hypospadias is a feature of many malformation syndromes. More severe forms of the condition are correctable through reconstructive surgery. Estimated incidence between 4 and 8/1,000 male births.
Mayer–Rokitansky–Küster–Hauser syndrome (46, XX)	Congenital absence of the vagina with abnormal or absent Müllerian structures. Ovarian function is typically normal. Renal and skeletal abnormalities may be present. The incidence is estimated at 1/5,000 female births.

*See Grumbach and Conte, 1998.

culture and time, such as toy play or maternal interest, and sexual orientation, which refers to sexual arousal to individuals of the same sex (homosexual), opposite sex (heterosexual), or both sexes (bisexual).

The "optimal gender" policy has recently been criticized from several perspectives. First, the notion of gender neutrality at birth has been challenged by a famous case, as reported by Colapinto (2002). A second challenge has come from intersex individuals themselves, who are angry about their treatment. They object to the fact that they were either not informed or misinformed about their condition, they are still unable to obtain accurate information about their condition and treatment, and feel stigmatized and shamed by the secrecy surrounding their condition and its management. They also attribute poor sexual function to damaging genital surgery and repeated and insensitive genital exams, both of which were performed without their consent.

Finally, social constructionists have challenged the entire enterprise of medical management of intersex cases by arguing that medical practices are rooted in history, language, politics, and culture, and therefore are not universal scientific facts. Thus, the "correction" of an intersexed infant's genitals is less a medical "emergency" than it is the adoption of medical technology to support a cultural imperative to view the sexes as dichotomous. Supporters of this point of view contend that such beliefs result in unnecessary and damaging surgery.

GUIDELINES FOR CLINICAL MANAGEMENT

Clinical management, medical and psychological, of disorders of sexual differentiation varies depending upon the diagnosis, age of the individual, and other factors. For example, decisions regarding sex assignment are not required in the case of genetic males born with isolated hypospadias (a condition in which the opening of the urethra [meatus] is not in its normal position at the tip of the glans or head of the penis), or genetic females diagnosed with Mayer–Rokitansky–Küster–Hauser syndrome (Table 1). In contrast, such decisions are necessary in the case of newborns with severe ambiguity of the external genitalia. While ideal clinical management must be tailored to the individual, family, and context, there are general guidelines for care that apply across the spectrum of disorders.

Coordination of Care

Individuals with intersexuality, regardless of age, often need care from multiple specialists. The disciplines represented will vary according to the circumstances of the case, but the presence of a mental health professional knowledgeable of disorders of sexual differentiation and their psychosocial and psychosexual sequelae is indispensable. A newborn with ambiguous genitalia and the family are best served by an integrated team approach. To reduce the likelihood of miscommunication, one team member ideally is responsible for coordination of efforts among professionals and between professionals and the family.

Disclosure of Medical Facts and Counseling of Family

In newborns for whom sex assignment must be decided, it is vital that parents have access to all information and believe that nothing is being withheld. Being fully informed in this context requires that parents have complete access to (a) results of all medical tests, including sex chromosomal status of the child; (b) knowledge regarding the likelihood for fertility if reared as a boy or as a girl; (c) options for surgery if reared as a boy or as a girl; (d) the range of short- and long-term outcomes for each surgical procedure with special focus on sexual functioning; (e) knowledge regarding the medical necessity of surgery being performed in the newborn period or early childhood rather than at an age when the child can personally provide informed consent; (f) current state of knowledge concerning the long-term outcome of psychosexual status (i.e., gender identity, gender role, sexual orientation), psychosocial status (i.e., educational attainment, employment, social support, and intimate relations including marriage and biological or adoptive parenting), and general quality of life of individuals with the child's diagnosis when reared as either male or female; and (g) results from outcome studies that highlight uncertainties in the clinical care of children with their child's particular condition or syndrome. For example, a recent review of the literature on the adult gender identity of individuals with various syndromes of intersexuality indicates that while the majority will develop a gender identity concordant with the gender of rearing, not all do. Moreover, the occurrence of gender dysphoria is not readily predictable based upon features of the medical diagnosis or particulars of the child's rearing.

Counseling in the immediate newborn period begins with an explanation of the process of sex determination and sexual differentiation, as described above, using illustrations such as those in Figures 1 and 2. An understanding of why the child's sex assignment is in question will flow from this discussion. Information specific to the child's medical diagnosis can be provided as genetic, biochemical, and other tests are completed. This is also the appropriate time to introduce the construct of gender identity and how it develops out of a complex interactive process (not yet fully understood) between prenatal and postnatal factors.

It is the role of the psychologist or other mental health professional to recognize that the birth of a child with a congenital defect, in particular, one affecting the sex organs, is often accompanied by parental feelings of grief, guilt, and shame. When such feelings and beliefs remain unresolved, they can interfere with the parents' ability to make fully informed decisions regarding sex assignment and, no less important, to bond with the infant.

Disclosure of Medical Facts and Counseling of Patient

The patient needs to be fully informed as well in order to be actively involved in decisions regarding medical and psychological care. A clinician who is skilled in providing the information in a developmentally sensitive manner, and who has developed a trusting relationship with the child over a period of time, is in the best position to dispense such information. John Money, a pioneer in clinical research and care for children born with intersex conditions, recommends the use of the "parable technique," which communicates to the child that it is permissible to talk about sensitive issues of sex and sexuality. A major goal of the psychological intervention is to minimize the potential for the development of shame and embarrassment and to maximize the development of a sense of mastery and adaptive coping skills to face a complex and potentially stigmatizing medical problem.

Informing Siblings and Extended Family

In cases where sex announcement was delayed, or sex reannouncement is required, siblings will need an explanation to prevent the establishment of irrational fears and beliefs. For example, children in the household may hold the misguided belief that their own sex might be reassigned. Psychoeducational counseling may also be indicated to prevent inadvertent stigmatization of the child by extended family or others who may share in the care of the infant.

The Role of the Long-Term Professional Relationship

Psychological management does not end with full disclosure of medical facts and the delineation of treatment options. Disorders of sexual differentiation often require prolonged, if not lifelong, medical management. The disorder can carry with it a burden that influences the most intimate aspects of human relationships. Because of this, consideration should be given to establishing, from the time of diagnosis, an ongoing relationship with a mental health professional knowledgeable in this area. These services should be made available to both the patient and the family.

See also: Congenital Adrenal Hyperplasia; Klinefelter Syndrome; Prenatal Development; Sexual Development; Sexual Orientation: Homosexuality; Turner Syndrome

Further Reading

Colapinto, J. (2002). *As nature made him: The boy who was raised as a girl*. New York: HarperCollins.

Grumbach, M., & Conte, F. A. (1998). Disorders of sex differentiation. In J. D. Wilson & D. Foster (Eds.), *Williams textbook of endocrinology* (9th ed., pp. 1303–1425). Philadelphia: W.B. Saunders.

Mazur, T. (1983). Ambiguous genitalia: Detection and counseling. *Pediatric Nursing, 9,* 417–422, 431.

Mazur, T., & Dobson, K. (1995). Psychologic issues in individuals with genetic, hormonal, and anatomic anomalies of the sexual system. In G. A. Rekers (Ed.), *Handbook of child and adolescent sexual problems* (pp. 101–131). New York: Lexington Books.

Money, J. (1994). *Sex errors of the body and related syndromes: A guide to counseling children* (2nd ed.). Baltimore, MD: Paul H. Brookes.

Zucker, K. J. (2002). Intersexuality and gender identity differentiation. *Journal of Pediatric Adolescent Gynecology, 15,* 3–13.

TOM MAZUR
DAVID E. SANDBERG

Sexual Knowledge

See: Sexual Development

Sexual Orientation: Homosexuality

DEFINITION

Sexual orientation refers to sexual arousal in response to individuals of the same sex (homosexual), opposite sex (heterosexual), or both sexes (bisexual). Sexual orientation is differentiated from gender identity, which refers to behaviors such as play or interests that differ in frequency between males and females in a particular culture. Further, gender-atypical behaviors (e.g., effeminate male or tomboy female) are not reliable indicators of sexual orientation. Sexual orientation includes sexual fantasies, sexual behavior, emotional and romantic attractions, and self-identification. The heterosexual or homosexual orientation of these dimensions may not be consistent and, therefore, sexual orientation is best viewed as a continuum between absolute heterosexuality and absolute homosexuality. Absolute heterosexuality and absolute homosexuality are defined as a persistent pattern of heterosexual or homosexual arousal along with a persistent pattern of weak or absent homosexual or heterosexual arousal, respectively. The focus of this entry will be on homosexuality.

PREVALENCE

The prevalence of homosexuality is estimated to be 1.5 percent of females and between 1 and 5 percent of males and these rates appear to be relatively stable over time. The number of youth reporting predominately homosexual attractions, however, steadily increases with age, with a peak at 18 years of age. Various studies report the prevalence of same-sex experiences to range between 1 and 37 percent, indicating that these experiences would not necessarily indicate that a person is homosexual.

ETIOLOGY

There is a growing consensus that no single explanation accounts for all cases of homosexuality and that multiple pathways—both biological and psychosocial/environmental—lead to an adult homosexual orientation. The preponderance of evidence appears to favor a biological etiology, at least in the sense of a strong predisposition to become homosexual. The various hypotheses regarding the etiology of homosexuality can be summarized as follows:

1. Prenatal hormones influence neurological structures in the brain, particularly the hypothalamus, leading to cross-sex-typed behaviors in childhood and later homosexual orientation. Evidence for this hypothesis is provided by several different types of research: (1) structural differences in the brains of homosexual and heterosexual men have been found; (2) women with congenital adrenal hyperplasia (CAH), a disorder which

results in prenatal exposure to high levels of androgens, or who have been exposed to DES (a synthetic estrogen used to prevent spontaneous abortion in high-risk pregnancies) prenatally, are reported to have increased rates of bisexuality and homosexuality; and (3) numerous animal studies indicate that prenatal injection of male or female sex hormones predicts cross-sex-typed social behavior.

2. There is a genetic basis for homosexuality. Recent research has identified a marker for homosexuality on the X chromosome of some but not all homosexual males. Further, twin studies have shown concordance rates of 52 percent for monozygotic twins, 22 percent for dizygotic twins, 11 percent for adopted brothers, and 9 percent for sons of homosexual fathers.

3. There may be a maternal immune response, similar to that seen in Rh incompatible pregnancies, to prenatal excretion of testosterone by male fetuses that reduces the hormone's biological activity. Male homosexuals have been reliably shown to have more male siblings and later birth orders than male heterosexuals, suggesting that the maternal immune response builds with successive pregnancies involving male fetuses.

4. Identification with the opposite sex parent is a precursor to homosexuality. In retrospective studies, male homosexuals recall their fathers being unavailable/distant/hostile and lesbians tend to report poorer relations with their mothers, but there are no prospective studies that demonstrate this effect.

5. Differential socialization by which parents selectively reinforce or extinguish behaviors that increase the probability of homosexual versus heterosexual orientation. There is little or no research that directly addresses this hypothesis.

PSYCHOSOCIAL CORRELATES

Although homosexuality is no longer considered a psychological disorder, it places young people at significant risk for a number of psychological problems, including substance abuse, sexually transmitted diseases (STD) (especially HIV infection), suicide, school problems, peer rejection, and social isolation. In the face of disapproval from family and friends and/or open hostility, prejudice, verbal and physical abuse, depression and suicidality are not uncommon. For example, studies have reported that 30 percent of homosexual male youth reported a suicide attempt. In addition, a number of gay and lesbian adolescents leave their homes each year because of parental abandonment, rejection, or fear of rejection. Some of these youth may turn to prostitution for survival. Substance abuse has also been reported as a problem, with more than half of a cohort of gay and bisexual males reporting substance abuse. Further, gay youth who have multiple partners and engage in high-risk behaviors are at high risk for STDs. However, lesbian teenagers with only same-sex partners are at lower risk for STDs than either gay or heterosexual youth.

INTERVENTIONS

It is common for youth to experience confusion, guilt, and anxiety as they question their sexual orientation. Given appropriate education and support most youth will resolve questions regarding their sexual orientation by late adolescence as they engage in self-exploration of feelings, fantasies, and experiences. Although there are no empirically supported intervention techniques or programs, the goal of intervention with gay and lesbian youth is to promote healthy physical, sexual, social, and emotional development so they can develop a positive self-image. Given the potential for negative reactions and rejection, they should be encouraged to think and plan carefully before telling their family and friends about their sexual orientation. Initial reactions of anger, guilt, and fear among family and friends are usually replaced with more moderate and accepting responses over time. It is important to provide information to both the youth and the family about sexuality development, including Acquired Immune Deficiency Syndrome (AIDS) prevention information. Support groups for both parents and youth can be very helpful and there are some excellent books on homosexuality such as the one by Fairchild and Hayward (1989). Monitoring gay and lesbian youth's psychosocial development is important, especially assessing for high-risk behaviors such as depression, suicidal ideation, conflict with peers and family, unsafe sex, and substance abuse. Serious emotional, social, and behavioral problems including high-risk behaviors should be treated with appropriate individual interventions.

PROGNOSIS

Both the American Psychiatric Association and the American Psychological Association have made official statements that homosexuality is not a mental disorder. Most people who are gay or lesbian do not have emotional or behavioral problems, but given societal attitudes toward homosexuality, they are at increased risk for psychosocial problems. Attitudes, however, are changing and there are many good gay and lesbian role models who are healthy and well-adjusted.

HOMOSEXUAL PARENTS

It is estimated that between 6 and 14 million children have gay or lesbian parents. The majority of these children are born in the context of a heterosexual relationship in which one parent subsequently comes out as a homosexual. There also are, however, an increasing number of lesbian and gay couples who seek to adopt children, provide foster homes, or use artificial insemination to have children. Historically, the legal system has been hostile to gay and lesbian parents based on an assumption that growing up in such a household will have a negative impact on children's development, placing them at increased risk for aberrant psychosexual development including problems with gender identity, gender role behaviors, and especially sexual orientation, isolation from or rejection by peers, and other emotional or behavioral problems. Although research addressing this question is limited, the data overwhelmingly indicate that children raised by homosexuals are at no greater risk for these problems than children growing up in more "traditional" households. Not surprisingly, the quality of the relationships within the family is more important than the sexual orientation of the parents in influencing children's development.

See also: Gender Identity Disorder; Identity Development; Sexual Development; Sexual Differentiation: Disorders and Clinical Management

Further Reading

Allen, L. A., & Gorski, R. A. (1992). Sexual orientation and the size of the anterior commissure in the human brain. *Proceedings of the National Academy of Sciences USA, 89,* 7199–7202.

Bailey, J. M., Bobrow, D., Wolfe, M., & Mikack, S. (1995). Sexual orientation of adult sons of gay fathers. *Developmental Psychology, 31,* 124–129.

Blanchard, R., Zucker, K. J., Bradley, S. J., & Hume, C. S. (1995). Birth order and sibling sex ratio in homosexual male adolescents and probably prehomosexual feminine boys. *Developmental Psychology, 31,* 22–30.

Fairchild, B., & Hayward, N. (1989). *Now that you know: What every parent should know about homosexuality.* New York: Harcourt Brace Jovanovich.

Golombok, S., & Tasker, F. (1996). Do parents influence the sexual orientation of their children? Findings from a longitudinal study of lesbian families. *Developmental Psychology, 32,* 3–11.

Hamar, D. H., Hu, S., Magnuson, V. L., Hu, N., & Pattatucci, A. (1993). A linkage between DNA markers on the X chromosome and male sexual orientation. *Science, 261,* 321–327.

LeVay, S. (1991). A difference in hypothalamic structure between heterosexual and homosexual men. *Science, 253,* 1034–1037.

Lundy, M. S., & Rekers, G. A. (1995). Homosexuality: Development, risks, parental values, and controversies. In G. A. Rekers (Ed.), *Handbook of child and adolescent sexual problems* (pp. 290–312). New York: Lexington Books.

Meyer-Bahlburg, H. R. L., Ehrhardt, A. A., Rosen, L. R., Gruen, R. S., Veridiano, N. P., Vann, F. H., & Neuwalder, H. F. (1995). Prenatal estrogens end the development of homosexual orientation. *Developmental Psychology, 31,* 12–21.

BETTY N. GORDON

Sexuality Education

Sex education begins with the birth of the infant and is most appropriately thought of as an ongoing process that continues throughout one's lifetime. Children begin to learn about sexuality as parents communicate their feelings about different body parts through caring behaviors (e.g., breast-feeding, changing diapers, bathing). As the infant exhibits exploratory sexual behaviors, parental reactions to these behaviors send clear positive or negative messages to the child about sexuality. This early nonverbal communication sets the stage for teaching sexual values and attitudes that will be important influences on the child's behavior later in life.

Parents are the primary sex educators for their children, especially in the early years, even if they do not actively provide information and/or are uncomfortable discussing sexual matters. Indeed, most teenagers view their parents as influential in determining their attitudes and values about sexuality and prefer sex education to come from parents. Many parents are, however, uncomfortable discussing sexual matters with their children and most do not discuss all aspects of sexuality with their children. Most commonly, parents talk with children about sexual anatomy, puberty, pregnancy, and the birth process but do not discuss sexual intercourse, sexually transmitted diseases, birth control, or sexual abuse, the very topics about which children, and especially adolescents, need information. The fact that parents are reluctant to discuss sexuality with their children and provide incomplete information may lead to the consistently low correlation found between the extent to which parents believe they have communicated with their children about sex and the information children perceive their parents as having provided.

Parents may be uncomfortable talking about sex with their children for a number of reasons, including their own attitudes about sexuality and their own experiences with sex education as children. Moreover, parents of adolescents have been found to lack sufficient understanding of sexual development to teach their children or to reinforce what is taught in school. When parents do not provide their children with sexual information, children usually get it from siblings, peers, and public media such as television, magazines, movies, and advertising. Unfortunately, this information is likely to be inaccurate, confusing, and may even be damaging to the child's self-perception. Lack of adequate sex education is seen as a primary cause for the two most troublesome sexual problems of children and adolescents: (1) rising rates of teenage pregnancy and (2) greater numbers of teenagers who are HIV positive. Moreover, with increasing reports of child sexual abuse and adolescent sexual assault, teaching personal safety skills has become an increasingly important aspect of sex education for children. Sex education can help to put the constant exposure to sexuality in the media into proper perspective, assist children in making sense out of these confusing messages, and increase the chances that they will behave responsibly with regard to their own sexuality. Suggestions for what to teach children at different ages are outlined in Table 1. It is important to note, however, that it is not sufficient to teach the facts about sex. Sexuality education in its broadest sense involves the teaching of attitudes, values, and feelings about being male or female. Children must also be taught the skills to enable them to make good decisions in the sexual arena and to recognize and avoid dangerous and/or exploitive situations. Parents need to communicate clearly and repeatedly with their children, especially during adolescence, their views about sexuality and especially premarital sex.

Evaluation of sexuality education programs in the schools indicates that increased knowledge of sexual facts does not necessarily change the behavior of teenagers. Programs that teach only abstinence but do not provide information about contraceptive use, an increasingly popular approach for school-based programs, have had little effect on reducing sexual activity or pregnancy among teenagers. The most successful programs include both these topics and provide access to condoms for those teens who are already sexually

Table 1. Information for Parents to Teach Children at Different Ages

Birth to 2 years

Body parts and functions
Provide correct labels for body parts, including male or female genitalia, when child is touching or parent is pointing to each part. Provide simple information about basic body functions. Allow child to explore all his or her body parts.

Gender identity
Learning about gender begins at birth, when baby boys are dressed in blue and girls in pink. Parents provide guidance about this topic by their choices of toys, clothing, activities, and the behaviors of the child they choose to notice. Gender stereotypes are pervasive in our culture, but flexibility is healthy. It's okay for boys to play with dolls and girls to play with trucks. Begin to teach the child what is special about being either a girl or boy.

Sexual abuse prevention
Children must first learn about body parts and functions before they can learn to protect themselves from exploitation. The best prevention at this age is close supervision.

3–5 years

Body parts and functions
Continue to use proper labels for body parts, including male and female genitalia. Teach child about functions of genitalia, including both elimination and reproduction. This is a good age to begin talking about sexual intercourse, as children are naturally curious about pregnancy and often have a new brother or sister.

Gender identity
Talk about the physical differences between boys and girls. Reinforce the idea that each child is special and has unique characteristics, including being a girl or a boy. Talk about what is special about being male or female.

Sexual abuse prevention
Genitalia are private parts, and no one should touch them for purposes other than health or hygiene. Children should not touch anyone else's private parts. Explain that these rules apply to friends and relatives as well as strangers. Teach the child to say, "No, my parents told me not to do that," and to get away if someone tries to touch his or her private parts. Teach the child to tell someone if this happens and keep telling until someone who will help is found. Have the child make a list of who to tell. Practice saying no and telling. Allow your child to say no in other situations that are uncomfortable. Children should know not to go with a stranger under any circumstances. Explain why and make sure the child knows what a stranger is. Practice "what would you do if" role-plays.

Sexual behavior
Don't overreact if child is caught in sex play with another child. Use it as a "teachable moment." Explain that insertion of objects into body openings may be harmful and is prohibited. Child should learn that masturbation is a "private" behavior. Teach about appropriate and inappropriate words.

6–12 years

Body parts and functions
Children should have complete understanding of sexual, reproductive, and elimination functions of body parts, including sexual intercourse. Discuss changes that will come with puberty for both sexes, including menstruation and wet dreams.

Gender identity
Gender identity is fixed by this age. Encourage both boys and girls to pursue individual interests and talents regardless of gender stereotypes.

Sexual abuse prevention
Discuss the child's conceptualization of an abuser and correct misperceptions. Identify abusive situations, including sexual harassment by peers. Practice assertiveness and problem-solving skills in troublesome social situations. Explain how abusers, including friends, relatives, and strangers, may manipulate children.

Sexual behavior
Talk about making good decisions in the context of potentially sexual relationships. Provide information about birth control and sexually transmitted diseases (including AIDS).

13–18 years

Body parts and functions
Discuss health and hygiene. Provide more information about contraceptives and sexually transmitted diseases, especially AIDS. Provide access to gynecological exams for girls if sexually active.

Gender identity
Although boys and girls are able to do many of the same things, reinforce the idea that there are special aspects of being male or female. Talk about the differences between girls and boys in social perception. Males tend to perceive social situations more sexually than girls and may interpret neutral cues (e.g., clothing, friendliness) as sexual invitations.

Sexual abuse prevention
Teach teens to avoid dangerous situations (e.g., walking alone at night, avoiding certain parts of town). Discuss dating relationships and in particular date/acquaintance rape and its association with alcohol and drug use. Let your teenager know you are available for a ride home anytime he or she is in a difficult or potentially dangerous situation. Enroll your child in a self-defense class.

Sexual behavior
Share your attitudes and values regarding premarital sex. Provide access to contraceptives, if necessary. Accept your teenager's need and desire for privacy. Set clear rules about dating and curfews.

Source: B. N. Gordon, & C. S. Schroeder, *Sexuality: A Developmental Approach to Problems.* New York: Plenum Press. Copyright 1995 Plenum Press. Reprinted by permission.

active. In addition, an innovative program that was more broadly focused on preventing multiple diverse problem behaviors among adolescents has recently been shown to reduce teenage pregnancy, as well as school failure. This program involved teens in highly structured volunteer activities that were linked to class work on life choices, career options, and relationship decision making.

See also: Adolescence; Sexual Development; Sexual Orientation: Homosexuality

Further Reading

Allen, J. P., Philliber, S., Herrling, S., & Kupermine, G. P. (1997). Preventing teen pregnancy and academic failure: Experimental evaluation of a developmentally based approach. *Child Development, 64*, 729–742.

Buysse, A., & Van Oost, P. (1997). Impact of a school-based prevention programme on traditional and egalitarian adolescents' safer sex intentions. *Journal of Adolescence, 20*, 177–188.

Gordon, B. N., & Schroeder, C. S. (2001). Sexual problems of children. In C. E. Walker & M. C. Roberts (Eds.), *Handbook of clinical child psychology* (3rd ed., pp. 495–522). New York: Wiley.

Jaccard, J., Dittus, P. J., & Gordon, V. V. (1998). Parent–adolescent congruency in reports of adolescent sexual behavior and in communications about sexual behavior. *Child Development, 69*, 247–261.

Petty, D. L. (1995). Sex education toward the prevention of sexual problems. In G. A. Rekers (Ed.), *Handbook of child and adolescent sexual problems* (pp. 31–54). New York: Lexington Books.

BETTY N. GORDON

Sexually Transmitted Diseases in Adolescents

DEFINITION

Sexually Transmitted Diseases (STDs) typically are passed from person to person through vaginal, anal, or oral sex, but babies can be infected in utero or during the birth process. Many people infected with an STD do not have symptoms and do not know they are infected. Some adolescents may truly lack symptoms; others may have symptoms that are not recognized as an STD and are attributed to another cause; and still others may not regard the symptoms as abnormal. However, even without symptoms, the adolescent can still pass the disease on to their partner. Sexually transmitted diseases may result

in a spectrum of health consequences from mild acute illness to serious long-term sequelae.

INCIDENCE

Individuals under 20 years of age are at particular risk for non-HIV STDs and each year approximately 3 million new cases of STDs occur in teens. Of teens that are sexually active, one in four will get an STD before age 18. Non-HIV STDs which are seen among American teens include: chlamydia (*Chlamydia trachomatis*), gonorrhea (*Neisseria gonorrhoeae*), trichomoniasis (*T. vaginalis*), syphilis (*Treponema pallidum*), genital herpes (*herpes simplex virus type 2—HSV-2*), and human papilloma virus. The prevalence and incidence of STDs vary by pathogen, by area of the country, and by subgroups of teens. If an adolescent is infected with one STD, they may be infected with a second one.

SYMPTOMS/TREATMENT

The Centers for Disease Control and Prevention provides complete information regarding typical incidence and prevalence, classic signs and symptoms, and appropriate treatment for each disease. Chlamydia, gonorrhea, trichomoniasis, and syphilis can be cured by medications. For genital herpes there is no cure, but antiviral drugs are effective in treating the symptoms of primary and recurrent genital herpes, and may reduce the risk of transmission through reduction of viral shedding. For genital warts, the available treatments include topical creams, cryotherapy, surgical removal, and laser surgery.

CORRELATES/PREVENTION

Compared to older adults, sexually experienced adolescents (10–19-year-olds) are at higher risk for acquiring STDs for a number of biological and behavioral reasons. Adolescents may not have established sufficient immunities, and the immature gynecological tract of teenage girls is more susceptible to infection. Further, any adolescent with an STD is more vulnerable to acquiring another STD (e.g., herpes increases the risk of acquiring HIV).

Behaviorally, individuals who start having sexual intercourse at younger ages have a greater number of partners and may be less likely to use condoms. The partner pool of adolescents and young adults is also riskier. Further, adolescents often delay seeking treatment because of a lack of access or poor knowledge about availability of confidential care. Consequently, these adolescents are at risk for transmitting the disease. The most effective way to prevent STDs for the sexually active individual other than abstinence is to use condoms. Currently, there are two other methods in development for the prevention of STD: topical microbicides, products that would be used intravaginally or intrarectally to prevent infection, and vaccines.

PSYCHOLOGICAL SEQUELAE

The psychological sequelae of STDs among adolescents has been understudied, and how to predict the impact for an individual adolescent is not well known. Most of the studies have been conducted with girls, and less is known about adolescent boys' adjustment to STD acquisition. Psychosocial functioning prior to the STD acquisition may be an important predictor of coping. Coping with genital herpes may have special characteristics given the chronicity, pain, and discomfort associated with outbreaks, and the heightened stigma. Although stress may precipitate an outbreak of genital herpes, individuals who have frequent recurrences (which is more common in the first year) may become stressed by their recurrences.

Although adolescents report wanting to reduce their risk of acquiring an STD following a first episode, research suggest that they are rarely successful, and that the rate of reinfection is high. Adolescents do better if they focus blame on behavior (i.e., "I should have used a condom") rather than on negative perceptions of themselves (i.e., "I am a bad person"). However, wishful thinking (i.e., wishing that this had never happened) remains a common, and probably unproductive, method of coping with STD acquisition.

Social support specific to STD acquisition may be more helpful than general social support. One source of support for adolescents may be their parents. Adolescents report anticipating that they will tell their parents and that parents would be helpful, which may be particularly important if they need to follow through on treatment.

NEONATAL SEQUELAE

Babies can become infected with STD infections during pregnancy or during the birth process. Chlamydia, gonorrhea, syphilis, and genital herpes are detrimental to the health of newborns. When an infant is infected with one of these STDs, the infant can be affected with numerous problems from eye infections, skin sores, pneumonia, and neurological problems (i.e., mental retardation and seizures) and death may occur. Early recognition and treatment can reduce the likelihood or severity of negative outcomes.

CONCLUSION

Adolescence is a time period of sexual development and exploration. Although it is important to focus on the positive aspects of adolescent sexuality (emotionally intimate relationships and physical pleasure), sexually transmitted diseases are a significant risk for adolescents who become sexually experienced. Essentially all sexually experienced adolescents are at risk, and the consequences of infection can be long-term. Risk can be reduced by helping teens engage in protective behaviors and ensuring prompt access to medical treatment in order to minimize both physical and psychological sequelae.

See also: Adolescent Health; Adolescent Sexuality; Pediatric Human Immunodeficiency Virus-1 (HIV)

Further Reading

Centers for Disease Control. (1997, January 23). 1998 Guidelines for treatment of sexually transmitted diseases. Retrieved April 20, 2002 from http://www.cdc.gov/mmwr/PDF/rr/rr4701.pdf

Eng, T. R., & Butler, W. T. (Eds.). (1997). *The hidden epidemic: Confronting sexually transmitted diseases.* Washington, DC: National Academy Press.

National Institute of Allergy and Infectious Diseases. (2002, July 20). Scientific evidence on condom effectiveness for sexually transmitted disease (STD) prevention. Retrieved April 24, 2002 from http://www.niaid.nih.gov/dmid/stds/condomreport.pdf

Rosenthal S. L., Cohen S. S., & Stanberry L. R. (1998). Topical microbicides: Current status and research considerations for adolescent girls. *Sexually Transmitted Diseases, 25,* 368–377.

Stanberry, L. R., & Bernstein, D. I. (Eds.). (2000). *Sexually transmitted diseases.* San Diego, CA: Academic Press.

Stanberry, L. R., & Rosenthal, S. L. (2002). Genital herpes simplex virus infection in the adolescent: Special considerations for management. *Paediatric Drugs, 4,* 1–7.

MARY B. SHORT
SUSAN L. ROSENTHAL

Shaken Baby Syndrome

See: Traumatic Brain Injury

Shelter Care

See: Residential Treatment

Short Stature: Psychological Aspects

DESCRIPTION AND INCIDENCE

Short stature (SS) is conventionally defined as a height falling below the third percentile for age and gender-adjusted norms (i.e., 2 standard deviations below the mean). The more inclusive fifth percentile is also frequently adopted as a cutoff. Of the approximately four million children born in the United States each year, between 120,000 and 200,000 will therefore, by definition, have SS. Such statistical definitions encompass large numbers of short, but otherwise healthy children.

ASSOCIATED PSYCHOLOGICAL FEATURES

Tall stature is assumed by most to confer social advantages and, conversely, SS is presumed to function as a liability. Developmental studies have shown that social stereotypes of height are established at an early age. Even very young children ascribe positive attributes to tall stature and negative attributes to SS. The influence of height on body image and self-concept is not equally expressed in men and women; although most men (including those of average height) want to be taller, very tall women often wish to be shorter.

The relationship between stature and a wide range of individual characteristics including personality traits, intelligence, social dominance and conformity, and income have been studied. These studies have typically detected that taller stature is associated with better outcomes, although the reports are often inconsistent and the effects attributable to height are small and generally far weaker than the influence of other individual background variables.

Studies of short children referred for medical evaluation have shown that this group commonly experiences teasing and socialization according to height-age rather than chronological-age. In extreme cases, such negative experiences may be associated with social isolation and a negative self-image. Because SS is also often associated with delayed pubertal maturation, these children may be weaker and less athletically competent than their average- or tall-stature agemates, making them potentially vulnerable to verbal or physical challenges from peers. In response, parents or other adult caretakers might overprotect the SS child resulting in reduced social maturity and functional independence.

Most reports on children's school performance have again been based on medically referred samples. Despite average intelligence, many clinical syndromes featuring SS are associated with academic underachievement. Neurocognitive deficits associated with the particular syndrome are thought to be responsible. Importantly, academic achievement problems are not related to height and are not remediated by treatment with growth hormone.

It is often assumed that youth with SS in the general population (i.e., the majority of those who are not referred for a medical evaluation) are similarly at risk for problems of social or educational adjustment. Studies of these medically nonreferred children and adolescents in this country and in Europe suggest that this is not the case. Youths with SS in the general population are generally indistinguishable from peers of average stature in terms of academic performance and psychosocial adaptation. This is the case despite the fact that short youths express greater dissatisfaction with their height and more often experience stature-related psychosocial stresses (e.g., teasing). This finding suggests that the potential burdens associated with SS are overcome through adaptive coping. Psychosocial stresses associated with SS, thus, do not automatically translate into psychological dysfunction. These observations also suggest that medically referred youths may represent a subgroup that is biased toward more negative psychosocial adaptation. Individual or family background variables that reduce the child's ability to compensate for the predictable stresses associated with SS may increase the likelihood of referral to a growth specialist, especially those children whose height falls close to the normal range.

PSYCHOSOCIAL ASSESSMENT

A multilevel conceptual framework to guide psychological assessment has recently been suggested. Assessment of *Level I* involves evaluation of the stressful psychosocial situations associated with SS, for example, stigmatization and juvenilization. It is critical at this level to consider additional sources of stress. Examples include the experience of repetitive medical procedures (e.g., dialysis in children with renal failure), or psychological consequences stemming from a disease process or its treatment (e.g., a history of brain tumor removal associated with overeating and morbid obesity, or genetic syndromes such as Turner or Prader–Willi syndromes). The stresses associated with the medical condition or its treatment should not be misattributed to the SS.

Level II concerns the individual's ability to mount an effective coping response. Youths with vulnerabilities in addition to the SS may experience more distress. Factors that might intensify negative reactions to SS include those which tax the individual's capacity to compensate, such as low socioeconomic status, poor academic performance related to a learning disability, family discord, etc. Conversely, protective factors in the child's environment, such as an easygoing temperament, strong family, and peer support, can serve to effectively inoculate the individual against the negative fallout of stature-related stresses.

Level III involves the assessment of the individual's behavioral and emotional functioning, and presence of clinically significant impairment in family, peer, or educational functioning.

TREATMENT

Increasingly, growth hormone (GH) is being prescribed as a growth-promoting agent to children and adolescents with SS. The FDA-approved indications for GH therapy now include a variety of growth disorders, including conditions that are not associated with GH deficiency. The focus of treatment has consequently shifted from providing hormone replacement to providing treatment based upon the purported efficacy of GH in increasing adult height. This strategy reinforces the notion that SS is undesirable and that making children taller is a worthwhile goal. According to this argument, the primary purpose of treatment is not to correct the cause, but to mitigate the handicap or disability of SS. This presupposes that SS does indeed lead to suffering, or at the very least, social disadvantage. The relevant research data is not generally supportive of this hypothesis.

Inasmuch as SS in otherwise healthy children and adolescents is only poorly correlated (if at all) with psychosocial/educational outcomes, no sweeping recommendations for treatment are warranted. However, anticipation of predictable social experiences related to SS can be helpful. An unfounded belief that SS is strongly associated with negative experiences can result

in parents attributing problems of a varied nature to the child's stature even when other factors are more directly responsible. When significant problems of psychosocial or educational adjustment are encountered, then referral to a psychologist or other mental health professional should be considered.

Because of the strong tendency to treat children according to their height age rather than their chronological age, all adults should be encouraged to promote age-appropriate independence and self-help skills in the child. Any aspect of the physical environment (at home or at school) that serves as a barrier to this goal should be targeted for modification. In the school environment, teachers and coaches should be encouraged to maintain age-appropriate expectations and to encourage the child to remain in the mainstream of activities, both academic and extracurricular. The presence of SS may be used as a rationale to postpone school entry or to repeat kindergarten. As a general rule, delay of school entry or repeating a grade should only be considered if academic achievement and psychometric testing indicate marked developmental delays and academic remediation is not an option. Immaturity of social behavior, although a problem, is best addressed by altering adults' expectations of the child and setting clear behavioral goals.

Some healthy children with SS will also experience a delay in pubertal development (i.e., constitutional growth delay). A significant lag in sexual development (even within the wide normal range) may be experienced by some youths as a more significant problem than SS. A short course of low dose testosterone treatment has been successfully used to accelerate pubertal development in boys without compromising adult height.

RESOURCES FOR CONSUMERS

Educational resources for families and teachers that deal with the psychological aspects of short stature include: Human Growth Foundation (http://www.hgfound.org; 800-451-6434) and MAGIC Foundation (http://www.magicfoundation.org; 800-362-4423)

See also: Noonan Syndrome; Prader–Willi Syndrome; Social Development in Adolescence; Social Development in Childhood; Stress Management; Turner Syndrome

Further Reading

National Center for Health Statistics, CDC Growth Charts: United States (2000). Retrieved March 11, 2002, from http://www.cdc.gov/nchs/about/major/nhanes/growthcharts/background.htm

Rieser, P., & Meyer-Bahlburg, H. F. L. (1993). *Short & OK. A guide for parents of short children.* Glen Head, NY: Human Growth Foundation.

Sandberg, D. E. (2000). Should short children who are not deficient in growth hormone be treated? *Western Journal of Medicine, 172,* 186–189.

Sandberg, D. E., & Voss, L. (2002). The psychosocial consequences of short stature: A review of the evidence. *Baillière's Best Practice and Research. Clinical Endocrinology and Metabolism, 16*(3), 449–463.

DAVID E. SANDBERG

Shyness

DEFINITION

Shyness is a form of social avoidance and withdrawal associated with fear of negative evaluation in social situations. The behavioral manifestation of shyness tends to occur most forcefully when the individual is in novel situations or in the company of unfamiliar people. This presentation may include gaze aversion (i.e., looking away), avoidance of social initiation, meager speech, soft vocal tone, heightened physiological reactivity, and thoughts of social inadequacy.

INCIDENCE

Shyness is a common experience. Most individuals report having experienced feelings of shyness in at least one situation during their lifetime. Transient shyness is common among young children and is typically no cause for serious concern. However, for approximately 13 percent of children, shyness is a chronic condition leading to intense subjective distress and functional impairment.

CORRELATES

Shyness has been associated with peer relationship difficulties, social isolation, loneliness, depression, low self-esteem, school refusal, academic impairment, and substance abuse. Shyness has been suggested as one precursor to the development of social phobia—a disorder characterized by "a marked and persistent fear of one or more social or performance situations in which the person is exposed to unfamiliar people or to possible scrutiny by others" (American Psychiatric Association,

1994, p. 416). Interestingly, the pattern of physiological activity (e.g., increased heart rate and respiration, sweating, dizziness) in response to social performance demands has been found to be similar among shy individuals and those with social phobia. However, the two conditions are not synonymous. Despite similarities with shyness in surface presentation, social phobia is a pervasive condition associated with substantial functional impairment and considerable distress. Most children who are shy will not develop social phobia. However, most adults with social phobia report having been shy since early childhood. Future research is needed to determine what experiences and environmental conditions are associated with differential pathways to shyness and social phobia.

ASSESSMENT

Shyness most often has been assessed via parent-report or self-report inventories. Rather than specific, unitary-construct measures, childhood shyness typically is embedded as a factor in more broadband measures of children's behavior and temperament (e.g., Child Behavior Checklist, Children's Behavior Questionnaire). No gold standard exists in terms of a childhood shyness questionnaire with demonstrated predictive validity.

The social withdrawal component of shyness may be assessed using observational methods. For instance, observation of children interacting on the playground can provide information on integration within the peer group and rate of positive interaction. Behavioral avoidance tasks may be arranged in clinic or laboratory settings to evaluate social avoidance or withdrawal in response to familiar and unfamiliar persons and situations.

TREATMENT

The literature on the treatment of shyness is surprisingly limited given its prevalence and associated adverse consequences. Social skills training (SST) has been the most commonly used approach. SST programs vary widely in content and method of delivery. However, most SST packages are designed to improve skills in communication (verbal and nonverbal) and social problem solving. Skills are modeled by a team leader or therapist and participants engage in role-plays for behavioral practice. Corrective feedback and reinforcement are provided at each stage. SST groups generally are comprised of 4–6 children of about the same age range. In general, SST interventions have been successful in enhancing the specific skills targeted for treatment. However, questions of social validity (i.e., whether the treatment produces the sort of change that has a meaningful effect on children's day-to-day lives) and generalization of treatment effects have been raised.

One means of facilitating skill maintenance and generalization is to include members of the child's peer group in the intervention delivery. In peer-helper interventions, classmates of shy children are trained to initiate, model, and reinforce appropriate social behavior. Similarly, peer-pairing approaches involve strategically pairing shy or socially withdrawn children with more gregarious, socially skilled peers for participation in joint-task activities. Such peer-mediated approaches appear to be successful in increasing the positive social interaction rates and peer acceptance of shy and socially withdrawn children.

Exposure-based therapies are common in the treatment of anxiety. Such approaches involve graduated or prolonged exposure to anxiety-evoking stimuli until the fear response is extinguished or diminished to the point of minimal interference. Given similarities with social anxiety, it is not surprising that exposure-based approaches have been used in the treatment of shyness as well. Although anecdotal reports from clinicians indicate this to be a promising approach, further controlled research trials must be conducted.

PROGNOSIS

Shyness that persists beyond childhood tends to remain a chronic and lifelong condition. However, short-term behavioral interventions have demonstrated success in remediating shyness. Given this state of affairs, early intervention would seem prudent to preclude long-term subjective distress and diminished social functioning. However, the utility and cost effectiveness of early intervention strategies to combat developmentally inappropriate shyness in children is an area in need of further inquiry.

See also: Social Development in Adolescence; Social Development in Childhood; Social Phobia; Social Problem-Solving Assessment; Social Skills Training

Further Reading

American Psychiatric Association. (1994). *Diagnostic and statistical manual of mental disorders* (4th ed.). Washington, DC: Author.

Beidel, D. C., & Turner, S. M. (1998). *Shy children, phobic adults: Nature and treatment of social phobia*. Washington, DC: American Psychiatric Association.

Greco, L. A., & Morris, T. L. (2001). Treating childhood shyness and related behavior: Empirically evaluated approaches to promote positive social interactions. *Clinical Child and Family Psychology Review, 4*, 299–318.

Rubin, K. H., & Asendorpf, J. B. (Eds.). (1993). *Social withdrawal, inhibition, and shyness in childhood*. Hillsdale, NJ: Erlbaum.

TRACY L. MORRIS

Siblings

Eighty percent of children live with at least one sibling. Sibling relationships are a major influence on the development of individual differences in antisocial and prosocial behavior, as well as aspects of personality, intelligence, and achievement. Siblings influence each other's development both directly, by modeling or differentially reinforcing appropriate or inappropriate behaviors, and indirectly, by causing stress for parents, which in turn affects parenting skills. Sibling interactions increase rapidly when the younger sibling is between 3 and 4 years of age, but remain fairly consistent in frequency after that time. Moreover, anger, distress, and conflict decrease as the younger sibling reaches school age. This most likely reflects the children's increased involvement with friends at school and other activities outside the home. Sibling relationships are quite different from peer relationships in that they are "vertical" (the participants have unequal status) rather than "horizontal" (the participants have equal status), there is little similarity between the behavior of children with their siblings and with peers.

ADJUSTMENT TO THE BIRTH OF A SIBLING

The birth of a new sibling is clearly a major source of stress in the life of a young child and the child's reactions to this event reflect his or her efforts to cope with the stress. Most children evidence both positive and negative reactions. Typical negative reactions of the older child include increased confrontation with parents, anger and aggression, clinginess, separation distress and other anxious behaviors, more problems with toileting, and demands for bottles, or other regressive behavior. The "regressive" behaviors on the part of the older sibling are best viewed as a form of imitation or mimicry; that is, a problem-solving or strategic approach by the older child to ensure that the parent will continue to care for him or her as well as the new baby. On the positive side, increased maturity, independence, and empathy as well as intense interest in and curiosity about the new baby also occur. Longitudinal studies indicate that most of the increased emotional difficulties seen in older siblings are temporary, although decreases in self-esteem after the birth of a sibling may persist for as long 4 years.

The relationship between parents and their first-born children changes following the birth of a second child. Not surprisingly, mothers spend less time with the older child after the birth of a baby, whereas fathers reciprocally increase the amount of time spent. Parents also begin to place increased demands for maturity and independence on their older children, presumably for very practical reasons. Moreover, a decrease in the security of mother–child attachment after the birth of a sibling, especially for older children (2–5 years old versus those under 2 years) has been documented, although it is not known if this change is temporary.

FACTORS THAT INFLUENCE ADJUSTMENT

The factors that have been shown to play a role in children's adjustment to the birth of a new sibling include the child's temperamental characteristics, the existence of management problems prior to the birth, the child's age at the time of the birth, the mother's psychological well-being, the quality of the marital relationship, and the manner in which the mother handles the older child's involvement with the new baby.

INTERVENTION STRATEGIES

Helping young children adjust to the arrival of a new brother or sister is best viewed as preventive work. The quality of the relationship between siblings shows some consistency over time and children who make a good adjustment in the early months may have less trouble with sibling conflict later on. Parents should prepare the older child for the birth of a sibling well in advance of the expected date. How far ahead of time, of course, depends on how old the child is. Sources of stress in the child's life other than the birth of a sibling should be minimized so that his or her coping skills are not overtaxed. This involves maintaining the young child's schedule and routine as much as possible during the time just before and after the birth and

resolving preexisting parent–child conflict. When the baby comes home, the increased involvement of the father provides the older child with a substitute for the care and nurturance once provided by the mother, as well as eases the stress experienced by the mother as a result of her new responsibilities. Mothers can foster a positive adjustment on the part of their older children by involving them in the care of the infant, making it a shared experience rather than a responsibility, and by modeling respect for the infant as a person with needs and feelings. Special treats or events that emphasize the older child's capabilities (in contrast to the infant's relative lack of abilities) can help to eliminate the "regressive"/imitative behaviors.

Parents should provide clear consequences for aggressive behavior, whether it is directed at the parent, the infant, or both. At other times, parents should watch for appropriate interaction and comment on it as it occurs. In this way they are teaching the child what they like as well as what they do not like.

SIBLING CONFLICT

Conflict between siblings increases dramatically as the younger child becomes more mobile and curious. At first the older sibling asserts his or her dominance in the relationship, but by the end of the second year, the younger child is likely to retaliate with aggression as well as instigate conflict by teasing and provoking the older child. Moreover, instances of tattling increase with age between the ages of 2 and 6. Observational studies of the interaction of preschool children with toddler siblings indicate that conflict occurs about 7–8 times an hour, but is relatively short-lived (e.g., about 30 s on average). Verbal or physical aggression occurs in about 25 percent of these incidents. Furthermore, mothers have been found to intervene in sibling quarrels 50–60 percent of the time.

There are large individual differences in the quality of sibling relationships; some relationships are entirely positive, some are both positive and negative, and some are 100 percent negative. The factors that influence the quality of sibling relationships are summarized in Table 1.

The extent to which siblings engage in cooperative, prosocial, friendly behavior appears to be independent from the extent to which they fight and argue. Some conflict among siblings is not necessarily bad. Sibling conflict can allow the expression of emotions and fosters practice in communication and negotiation skills. Sibling relationships that reflect a balance between

Table 1. Factors that Influence the Quality of Sibling Relationships

Source	Factor
Children	Temperament
	Age differences
	Gender differences
	Level of social-cognitive development
Parent–child relationship	Differential treatment of children
	Parent intervention in child conflict
	Lack of clear rules and expectations
	General child management problems
Family	Marital distress
	Parental maladjustment/mental health problems
	Life and environmental stress
	Emotional climate in the home
	Family functioning

Source: C. N. Schroeder & B. N. Gordon, *Assessment and Treatment of Childhood Problems: A Clinician's Guide.* Copyright 2002 The Guilford Press. Reprinted by permission.

support and conflict may promote social competence. When sibling relationships are heavily weighted toward conflict, however, the result is often a "training" ground for aggression, which eventually can lead to feelings of inadequacy, incompetence, and hostility.

INTERVENTION STRATEGIES

Treatment of sibling conflict is primarily based on one of two theoretical perspectives. The first, an Adlerian approach, suggests that sibling conflict is best ignored by parents because its primary function is to gain parental attention. Allowing children to solve their own fights may also have the benefit of providing opportunities for children to learn important conflict resolution skills, although recent research indicates that children do not learn these skills on their own. Behavioral theory suggests that ignoring would be effective in reducing sibling conflict through the principle of extinction. An operant approach to intervention advocates the use of differential reinforcement of other behaviors (e.g., not fighting), reinforcement of specific alternative behavior (e.g., cooperative play, compromise, negotiation) and/or use of time-out for fighting. Other approaches incorporate skills training (e.g., ignoring, negotiating, compromising, expressing anger, walking away from the situation) and environmental changes (e.g., rearranging the family's schedule, removing a particular toy, providing privacy for each child, reducing family stress levels). See Schroeder and Gordon (2002) for a review and specific strategies.

See also: Childhood; Emotional Development; Social Development in Adolescence; Social Development in Childhood

Further Reading

Brody, G. H. (1996). *Sibling relationships: Their causes and consequences.* Norwood, NJ: Ablex.

Dunn, J., Creps, C., & Brown, J. (1996). Children's family relationships between two and five: Developmental changes and individual differences. *Social Development, 5,* 230–250.

Perlman, M., & Ross, H. S. (1997). The benefits of parent intervention in children's disputes: An examination of concurrent changes in children fighting styles. *Child Development, 68,* 690–700.

Ross, H. S., & den Bak-Lammers, I. M. (1998). Consistency and change in children's tattling on their siblings: Children's perspectives on the moral rules and procedures of family life. *Social Development, 7,* 245–300.

Schroeder, C. S., & Gordon, B. N. (2002). *Assessment and treatment of childhood problems: A clinician's guide.* New York: Guilford.

Stormshak, E. A., Bellanti, C., & Bierman, K. L. (1996). The quality of sibling relationships and the development of social competence and behavioral control in aggressive children. *Developmental Psychology, 32,* 79–89.

BETTY N. GORDON

Sickle Cell Disease

DEFINITION

Sickle Cell Disease (SCD) is a genetic disorder involving a mutation of the hemoglobin molecule (sickle hemoglobin HbS) that results in a large number of serious clinical symptoms associated with chronic anemia or acute or chronic tissue damage. Individuals who carry only a single HbS gene in combination with the normal hemoglobin gene (HbA) have sickle cell trait, which fortunately is not associated with any clinical symptoms. However, individuals who are homozygous (HbSS— sickle cell anemia) or who have a single HbS gene in combination with the beta thalassemia or HbC genes are likely to experience a broad range of clinical symptoms.

The mechanism behind symptoms associated with SCD is relatively simple. The sickle gene results in hemoglobin cells that are very sensitive to changes in oxygen concentration. Most of the time, these sickle cells work like normal hemoglobin cells, transporting oxygen throughout the circulatory system, and moving through the blood vessels without difficulty. However, under certain physiological conditions, these sickle cells many convert into an abnormal shape (the sickle shape), becoming irreversibly rigid and adhesive. When this happens, the sickle cell is unable to pass through the small blood vessels. This leads to a blockage of blood flow, or vaso-occlusion. Vaso-occlusion results in an interruption of oxygen supply to healthy tissue, leading to both acute symptoms (noticed right away) and chronic damage to organs throughout the body.

INCIDENCE

Because the sickle gene offers protection against malaria, the distribution of SCD disease is concentrated in the geographic regions that have a high incidence of malaria, namely central Africa, the Middle East, and India. The occurrence of sickle cell disease in the United States and the Caribbean is largely related to slave trading from Africa during the 1700s–1800s, and today approximately 1 in 800 black babies born in the United States have some form of SCD, with a total incidence in African-Americans of 8 percent.

DIAGNOSIS

Today, the diagnosis of SCD is most frequently made at birth. Most states include SCD as part of their newborn screening programs, and every newborn has a sample of his/her blood sent off to a central laboratory for diagnostic evaluation. When a positive sickle screening is obtained, the pediatricians and parents of children are contacted, and a referral for follow-up confirmatory diagnosis is made. There are occasionally children who are not detected on newborn screening, and these may be identified later in life using standard laboratory or genetic techniques. In some cases, parents may be aware that they have sickle trait and therefore are at risk of having a child with SCD. These parents may choose to undergo prenatal screening for the disease.

CLINICAL SYMPTOMS

Because vaso-occlusion in SCD can affect blood flow throughout the body, every organ system is potentially affected, and a large number of clinical symptoms may be experienced. These include life-threatening bacterial infections, pain, sequestering of red blood cells in the spleen, stroke, severe lung disease (acute chest syndrome), damage to the retina of the eye,

damage to the joints and bones, kidney disease, gall-bladder disease, growth delay, and skin ulcers (mainly legs). A number of behavioral problems may also be noted, including learning problems, nighttime enuresis, and pica (ingesting nonedible substances). Below, a more detailed description is provided for some of the most common or severe symptoms of SCD.

Pain

The symptom most commonly associated with SCD is pain that occurs when the body's tissues are damaged because of vaso-occlusion. There are many different types of pain experiences. In infants and toddlers, the most common source of pain is a condition known as dactilytis, or swelling of the hands and feet. Pain diminishes somewhat as a major symptom during the school age years, but a small number of children, particularly those with sickle cell anemia, may require multiple hospitalizations for pain. During adolescence, experience with pain once again seems to increase, although not all children experience the same level or frequency of pain.

Stroke

Vaso-occlusion of the blood vessels in the brain results in damage to the brain. In approximately 5–7 percent of children with sickle cell anemia, this will produce a clinical stroke that involves motor and language injury. This has been associated with a narrowing of the large blood vessels in the brain, and can be detected, in some cases, using a special ultrasound procedure. When detected, stroke can sometimes be prevented. In another 17–20 percent of children with sickle cell anemia, brain injury in areas not associated with language and motor abilities (known as silent stroke) may occur, resulting in subtle neuropsychological problems in the areas of attention, information processing speed, and memory. Recently, it has become known that over time, many children with sickle cell anemia may experience undetectable injury to the brain that results in a significant loss of intellectual ability. The mechanisms for these changes are unknown, though they may be the result of chronic anemia, episodes of hypoxia or poor oxygen supply, or damage to the smallest blood vessels in the brain (microvessels).

Lung Damage and Pulmonary Functioning

Vaso-occlusion in the lungs is associated with overall poorer pulmonary functioning, a higher risk for pneumonia, and sometimes severe lung events that can be life-threatening (acute chest syndrome). These events often result in children requiring hospitalization and intensive care support, and for some, may result in both lung and brain injury.

Infection

Because of damage to the spleen, children with SCD are particularly susceptible to bacterial infections. In the past, death due to overwhelming sepsis was particularly high among children during infancy and toddlerhood. Aggressive prophylaxis, or prevention, using antibiotics given every day regardless of symptoms has significantly reduced the number of deaths that occur in young children. However, bacterial infections remain a lifelong concern for individuals with SCD, and can result in rapid deterioration and death at any age.

TREATMENT

Treatment of SCD has predominantly focused on symptom management. Pain has traditionally been treated using narcotic and nonnarcotic pain medications, as well as increased hydration. Many times, this type of treatment requires hospitalization lasting from a few days to even a few weeks. Treatment of acute chest syndrome and infections has involved aggressive antibiotic therapy and, in some cases, intensive care and life support. For those children who experience a clinical stroke, and for those at risk for a clinical stroke who are identified using ultrasound procedures, treatment involves chronic (every 3–4 weeks) blood transfusions. Damage to other organs is often treated as it occurs.

Fortunately, over the past 15 years, significant changes in the approach to treatment of SCD have occurred, and some more are anticipated to occur in the next few years. The first major step involved the use of prophylactic penicillin before age 5 to prevent life-threatening infections, and to aggressively provide immunizations against other infectious diseases. This approach virtually eliminated early mortality. The next step involved the use of chronic transfusion therapy to prevent stroke in those children at the highest risk. The next step involved the use of a drug called hydroxyurea to prevent the onset of pain in adolescents and young adults. For many children and adolescents with SCD, this medication has been very effective, and trials are now underway to determine its usefulness in preventing many of the symptoms of SCD in young children.

For some of the symptoms of SCD, behavioral approaches are also useful. Many children who experience pain benefit by learning self-regulation skills (e.g., visual imagery, relaxation techniques, self-hypnosis), and behavioral treatments for nighttime enuresis, pica, and support of good nutrition may be very effective for a number of these children. Of major importance is the recognition of the need for intervention and adaptation in the area of learning, with particular attention paid to the educational approaches taken with children who may experience brain injury from the disease. Regular neuropsychological screening and evaluation is recommended. Finally, support for parents and unaffected family members is an essential part of comprehensive, integrated care.

More dramatic and curative treatments are currently being tested. The one known cure of SCD is bone marrow transplantation (BMT). Unfortunately, only one of four children will have a compatible donor for BMT, and the known risks associated with BMT must be weighed against the unknown risk of living with SCD. New studies are examining modifications in the BMT procedure that may produce the same benefits while significantly lowering the risk. Future approaches to treatment will likely involve some form of gene therapy, but these are still largely theoretical and under development.

PROGNOSIS

SCD can be one of the most debilitating illnesses experienced by children, adolescence, and adults. Unfortunately, the effects of SCD are far-reaching, and may involve almost every organ system of the body, although not all children or adolescents experience the symptoms of SCD or experience them in the same way. The mortality rate is approximately 10 percent prior to age 15, but many individuals can expect to have a normal lifespan, and many are able to lead happy, productive, and successful lives. Fortunately, advances in treatment and toward cure are taking place, and the future appears substantially brighter for those individuals with sickle cell disease.

See also: Bone Marrow Failure and Primary Immunodeficiency; Bone Marrow Transplantation; Coping with Illness; Enuresis; Learning Disorders; Pain Management; Parenting the Chronically Ill Child; Pica; Relaxation Training; Self-Management; Short Stature: Psychological Aspects

Further Reading

American Academy of Pediatrics. (2002). Policy Statement: Health supervision for children with sickle cell disease. *Pediatrics, 109,* 526–535.

Dover, G. J., & Platt, O. S. (1998). Sickle cell disease. In D. G. Nathan & S. H. Orkin (Eds.), *Nathan and Oski's hematology of infancy and childhood* (5th ed., pp. 762–809). Philadelphia: W.B. Saunders Company.

Sickle Cell Disease Guideline Panel. (1993, April). *Sickle cell disease: Screening, diagnosis, management, and counseling in newborns and infants. Clinical practice guideline No. 6.* (AHCPR Publication No. 93–0562). Rockville, MD.

F. DANIEL ARMSTRONG

Simple Phobia

See: Specific Phobia

Single Parenting

DEFINITION/PREVALENCE

In the United States, it is estimated that approximately 50 percent of mothers will be the head of a single-parent family at some point, and 50 percent of today's children will spend time in a single-parent home. In contrast, nearly 90 percent of all children in the early 1960s lived with both biological parents until age 18. In fact, the last 40 years have witnessed an increase in single-parent families of 280 percent among Whites and 543 percent among African Americans. The dramatic increase in single-parent families observed in nearly every industrialized nation is attributed to similar increases in a number of factors, including births to unmarried mothers, deaths due to homicide and AIDS, and divorce. Thus, single-parent families can be the product of a wide range of circumstances, including death, separation, divorce, or the parent never having married.

The single-parent family structure has been held responsible for many developmental problems and undesirable outcomes, and early stereotypes (typically of uneducated, promiscuous, indolent, teenage mothers on welfare with numerous neglected children) have been grossly distorted. However, the short- and long-term outcomes of single-parent families vary dramatically depending upon many factors, including the reason for the parent being single.

PARENTING CHALLENGES

Parenthood shared by a unified couple can be stressful and demanding enough and these normal challenges of parenthood are magnified when faced by a single parent. Single-parent families lack many of the advantages enjoyed by families with two effective parents: the mutual support and encouragement two parents can provide each other, parents' ability to compensate for each others' weaknesses, and greater flexibility in child care arrangements, to name a few. Perhaps of greatest significance, however, is the financial unease experienced by most single-parent families. The median income for single parent families is less than half that of two-parent families in the United States. A complicating factor is that 85 percent of single-parent families are headed by women, who are typically paid less than men and who may also experience discrimination in receiving promotions. Regardless of the parent's gender, single parents may be more limited in their ability to accept rigid work schedules, travel responsibilities, or assignments for relocation that may improve their chances for promotion.

Besides the increased financial stress experienced by single parents, many also report feelings of social isolation, loneliness, and inadequacy, greater challenges in raising children, and difficulties reconciling the demands of work and family. Research has suggested that single parents have less time to spend with their children, are less able to supervise their children's after-school activities, and are less involved in their children's schools and social networks. Many single parents also report discouragement in trying to live up to unrealistic expectations, such as the need to be both a mother and a father to the child, and to be a "superparent" to show the world that their child is not missing out on anything. Although there is a great degree of variation in the success with which single parents meet these demands, countless mothers and fathers have made necessary adaptations to lead happy and fulfilling single-parent lives.

OUTCOMES FOR CHILDREN

In addition to studying factors related to the single-parent's quality of life, much research has focused on the outcomes of children living in single-parent homes. Many discouraging correlates have been reported for children from single-parent homes, including lower academic achievement, higher dropout rates, lower socioeconomic attainment, poorer psychosocial adjustment, and increased parentification (i.e., the child serves as the single parent's confidant, companion, and supervisor, in a manner inappropriate for the child's developmental level). The most negative long-term consequences are related to a lack of economic resources. Given that single parents, on average, earn much less than two-parent families, chances are greater that the child will experience inadequate healthcare, poorer social services, and will live in a less desirable neighborhood characterized by high crime and inferior schools. Not surprisingly, many of the negative consequences linked to single-parent families disappear when researchers take economic status into account. Research indicates that when children share similar backgrounds in terms of socioeconomic status, neighborhood characteristics, ethnicity, and parenting quality, children from single-parent families usually do as well as children from two-parent families in many areas, including school achievement, emotional stability, and avoidance of serious physical injury.

Another major factor in predicting long-term outcomes for children from single-parent families is the quality of parenting. The most positive developmental outcomes are achieved when single parents utilize an authoritative parenting style; one in which reasonable limits are set and enforced, while affection and appreciation are also freely expressed. Other factors appear to moderate the risks often associated with single parenting, such as having a college education, being over 30 years of age, not being romantically involved, being active with friends or church, and having employment with flexible hours. Other correlates of positive child development include: having a peaceful home; the single parent having only one or two children; the child having several friends, a stable family structure, and helpful grandparents and other extended family; living in a community that is supportive of single parents; and attending high-quality schools. Children from single-parent families can and do thrive in every important way when their needs are met; however, single parents face increased challenges in attending to these needs.

INTERVENTIONS

Clinicians can provide direct support to single parents in many forms, including stress management training, coping skills training, addressing issues related to why the parent is single (i.e., death of spouse, divorce), helping with child discipline problems, and teaching more effective parenting strategies. If the child has a noncustodial parent with whom he or she has contact, other issues may need to be addressed as well (consistency of discipline and expectations between parents, bonding issues with each parent, etc.). Clinicians may need to work to improve the effectiveness of natural support systems, such as the family's social support network (including support from friends and extended

family members). Clinicians can also link single-parent families to resources in their communities, and can recommend appropriate readings or online resources (e.g., http://www.parentswithoutpartners.org). Clearly, single parenting holds many significant challenges. However, these potential hardships can be minimized through effective intervention, and such challenges can be turned into opportunities for personal and family growth.

See also: Divorce; Fathers' Roles in Abnormal Child Development; Fathers' Roles in Normal Child Development; Mothers' and Fathers' Roles in Abnormal Child Development; Mothers' and Fathers' Roles in Normal Development; Parent Training; Parent–Child Interaction Therapy

Further Reading

Dinkmeyer, D., McKay, G. D., & McKay, J. L. (1987). *New beginnings: Skills for single parents and stepfamily parents. Parent's manual.* Champaign, IL: Research Press.
Heath, D. T., & Orthner, D. K. (1999). Stress and adaptation among male and female single parents. *Journal of Family Issues, 20,* 557–587.
Hetherington, E. M., Bridges, M., & Insabella, G. M. (1998). What matters? What does not? Five perspectives on the association between marital transitions and children's adjustment. *American Psychologist, 53,* 167–184.

JARED S. WARREN
MICHAEL C. ROBERTS

Skin Rash

See: Dermatology: Dermatitis and Psoriasis

Sleep Patterns, Normal

Some basic understanding of how and why children sleep is necessary to help explain what can go wrong with this important part of their lives. Sleep serves several essential roles in a child's life and it is important for both physical and mental well-being. Total sleep time gradually declines with age such that infants sleep approximately 16 hr per day, children sleep about 12 hr by age 2 and 8 hr by age 13, and by age 50, people sleep an average of about 6 hr per night. It should be noted that most people tend to sleep about the same amount of time each night, on average, even though an individual's sleep may vary from night to night.

There are several stages of sleep and each stage appears to serve a different function. In general, there are two main phases of sleep, rapid eye movement (REM) and nonrapid eye movement (NREM). REM sleep is important for learning and for memory while NREM sleep appears to be involved in the body's ability to ward off illness and restore the immune system. There are four stages of NREM sleep, which correspond to how deeply a person sleeps. An electroencephalogram (EEG) recording, which measures brain wave activity, can be used as part of a sleep assessment to identify the different stages of sleep. Stage 1, also referred to as "light" sleep, is a transition between sleep and wakefulness. Stage 2 is referred to as "deeper" sleep while stages 3 and 4 are the "deepest" sleep (also referred to as slow-wave sleep). After cycling through approximately 90 min of NREM sleep, REM sleep is entered. REM sleep is characterized by rapid movement of the eyes under the eyelids, and people report dreaming during this stage of sleep. Several times during the night, individuals progress through a series of sleep stages typically going through four stages of NREM sleep, into REM sleep, then back again to NREM sleep. During the transition from REM to NREM sleep, there is a brief period when one actually awakes from sleep. This experience, referred to as a partial awakening, is a normal part of sleep, and is an important factor in understanding sleep disturbances in children. It has been hypothesized that children's disruptive night wakings originate from partial awakenings. All children experience partial wakings; however, some children wake fully from these episodes and call for their parents or leave their beds in search of their parents. Instead of learning how to fall back to sleep alone after one of these awakenings, the child learns to fall asleep in the presence of a parent.

The International Classification of Sleep Disorders classifies sleep disorders into two major categories, parasomnias and dyssomnias, which is helpful in understanding children's sleep problems. Parasomnias are difficulties that disrupt sleep after it has been initiated, and are disorders of arousal, partial arousal, or sleep-stage transitions. Nightmares, sleep terrors, sleepwalking, sleep talking, bruxism, body rocking, and head banging are examples of problems in this category. Although these sleep problems get a great deal of attention, they have no clear etiology, are not associated with pathology and usually disappear with maturation. Dyssomnias are difficulties either in initiating or maintaining sleep (bedtime struggles, night wakings, getting up early), excessive daytime sleepiness (narcolepsy, obstructive sleep apnea), and sleep–wake cycle problems. Although problems with initiating and maintaining sleep are

common particularly for preschool children, they can persist for years and often do not go away on their own. Numerous factors have been found to be associated with sleep disturbances among children, including complications at birth and more difficult temperament. Breast-feeding at night has also been found to be related to sleep disturbances among children because of the association of going to sleep with feeding. Feeding at night can also disrupt sleep by activating the digestive system when it should be inactive.

See also: Body Rocking and Head Banging; Excessive Sleepiness; Initiating and Maintaining Sleep; Narcolepsy; Nightmares; Obstructive Sleep Apnea; Sleep Bruxism; Sleep–Wake Cycle Problems; Sleep Terrors; Sleepwalking; Talking

Further Reading

American Sleep Disorders Association. (1990). *The international classification of sleep disorders: Diagnostic and coding manual.* Rochester, MN: Author.

Carskadon, M. A., & Dement, W. C. (1989). Normal human sleep: An overview. In M. H. Kryger, T. Roth, & W. C. Dement (Eds.), *Principles and practice of sleep medicine* (3rd ed., pp. 3–13). Philadelphia: W.B. Saunders.

Durand, V. M. (1998). *Sleep better! A guide to improving sleep for children with special needs.* Baltimore, MD: Paul H. Brookes.

National Sleep Foundation, 1522 K Street, NW, Suite 500, Washington, DC 20005, Phone: (202) 347–3471, Fax: (202) 347–3472, E-mail: nsf@sleepfoundation.org, http://www.sleepfoundation.org.

V. Mark Durand
Kristin V. Christodulu

Sleep Talking

DEFINITION

Sleep talking is the utterance of speech or sounds during sleep without awareness of the event or later memory for it. The talking is often void of emotion, but can be associated with stressful shouting. Sleep talking is also referred to as "somniloquy."

INCIDENCE/ETIOLOGY

Sleep talking is a very common event (22–60 percent of children talk in their sleep from time to time) that rarely signifies any serious medical or psychological disorder. It usually occurs during the transition from wakefulness to the "lighter" stages of sleep, or from deeper stages of sleep to wakefulness. Sleep talking is usually temporary, brought on by stress, fatigue, or illness, and frequently occurs with other sleep disorders, such as sleepwalking, obstructive sleep apnea, nightmares, and sleep terrors.

ASSESSMENT/TREATMENT

Children who are sleep-deprived are more likely to talk in their sleep so it is important that there is a regular sleep schedule with consistent bedtimes and wake-up times. Other areas to assess and provide guidance for are stress and anxiety levels associated with bedtime as well as eating a heavy meal just before bed. Gently soothing the child during the sleep talking episode can also be helpful.

PROGNOSIS

Sleep talking is most often a temporary phenomenon, but for some children it can continue for many years without any harmful effects.

See also: Obstructive Sleep Apnea; Sleep Patterns, Normal; Sleep Terrors; Sleepwalking

Further Reading

Arkin, A. M. (1991). Sleeptalking. In S. J. Ellman & J. S. Antrobus (Eds.), *The mind in sleep* (pp. 415–436). New York: Wiley.

Laberge, L., Tremblay, R. E., Vitaro, F., & Montplaisir, J. (2000). Development of parasomnias from childhood to early adolescence. *Pediatrics, 106,* 67–74.

National Sleep Foundation, 1522 K Street, NW, Suite 500, Washington, DC 20005, Phone: (202) 347-3471, Fax: (202) 347-3472, E-mail: nsf@sleepfoundation.org, http://www.sleepfoundation.org.

V. MARK DURAND
KRISTIN V. CHRISTODULU

Sleep Terrors

DEFINITION

Sleep terrors are episodes of "apparent" awakening from sleep, accompanied by signs of panic, followed by disorientation and amnesia for the incident. They are characterized by intense sudden arousal, a piercing panic-stricken scream, profuse perspiration, rapid pulse and respiration, a glassy stare, often strange fears, incoherency, and inconsolability. Episodes last about 15 min, after which the child becomes calm, and continues to sleep. During sleep terrors, it is difficult to awaken the child and they are unable to recall anything in the morning. Sleep terrors are also called "night terrors."

INCIDENCE/ETIOLOGY

Approximately 5 percent of children (more boys than girls) may experience sleep terrors. They appear to occur during a transition from a deeper stage of non-rapid eye movement (NREM) to a lighter stage of sleep or rapid eye movement (REM) sleep. This problem tends to decrease with age, and although there is no evidence that they are the result of psychological problems, they can be precipitated by fever, sleep deprivation, and stress. Because the disorder tends to occur in families, it is possible that there is a genetic component to sleep terrors.

ASSESSMENT

Sleep terrors develop early in the night and usually occur within 15–90 min after falling asleep. Assessing for sleep deprivation, the use of stimulants such as caffeine, a chaotic sleep schedule, a stressful environment, or other sleep problems such as apnea should be assessed and, if present, treated.

TREATMENT

Sleep terrors can be very frightening to parents, and treatment usually begins with giving parents information, reassurance, and a recommendation to wait and see if they disappear on their own. If they persist, a behavioral procedure known as *scheduled awakenings* (briefly awakening the child approximately 30 min before a typical episode) has also been used successfully to reduce chronic sleep terrors.

PROGNOSIS

Sleep terrors usually begin after 18 months, are most common in preschool children, and can occur up to 12 years of age, but typically do not continue into adulthood.

See also: Normal; Nightmares; Sleep Patterns; Sleep Talking; Sleepwalking

Further Reading

Abe, K., Oda, N., Ikenaga, K., & Yamada, T. (1993). Twin study in night terrors, fears, and some physiological and behavioural characteristics in children. *Psychiatric Genetics, 3,* 39–43.

Durand, V. M., & Mindell, J. A. (1999). Behavioral intervention for childhood sleep terrors. *Behavior Therapy, 30,* 705–715.

Maskey, S. (1993). Simple treatment for night terrors. *British Medical Journal, 306,* 1477.

National Sleep Foundation, 1522 K Street, NW, Suite 500, Washington, DC 20005, Phone: (202) 347-3471, Fax: (202) 347-3472, E-mail: nsf@sleepfoundation.org, http://www.sleepfoundation.org.

V. Mark Durand
Kristin V. Christodulu

Sleepwalking

DEFINITION

Sleepwalking involves arising from bed during sleep and walking around for a few seconds to several minutes with a blank face and a glassy stare. The child is relatively unresponsive to efforts of others to communicate with him or her and can be awakened only with great difficulty. If the child is awakened, he or she will not typically remember what has happened. Sleepwalking is also referred to as "somnambulism."

INCIDENCE/ETIOLOGY

A relatively large number of children (from 15 to 30 percent) have at least one episode of sleepwalking, with about 2 percent reported to have multiple incidents. The mean age of onset is 5–6 years, and prevalence is highest in children 9–12 years. Sleepwalking occurs during the transition from deep stages of non-rapid eye movement (NREM) sleep to lighter stages of sleep or rapid eye movement (REM) sleep. A sharp noise or standing the child on his or her feet can precipitate an episode. Extreme fatigue, previous sleep deprivation, and stress have been implicated in sleepwalking. There also appears to be a genetic component to sleepwalking, with a higher incidence observed within families. There is no evidence that sleepwalking is the result of psychological problems.

ASSESSMENT

Sleepwalking typically occurs during the first few hours while the person is in the deep stages of sleep and transitioning to a lighter stage of sleep. If the problem is persistent, assessing for any unusual stress in the child's life or an irregular sleep schedule is important, but these factors are not necessary for sleepwalking.

TREATMENT

It is important to protect habitual sleepwalkers from harm by keeping doors and windows closed and by removing dangerous objects from areas that the child might reach. A sleepwalking child should be gently guided back to bed without attempting to awake him or her by yelling, making loud noises, or shaking. Since most children outgrow sleepwalking by puberty, there is usually no need for any intervention. If it persists or becomes dangerous, a behavioral procedure known as *scheduled awakenings* (briefly awakening the child approximately 30 min before a typical episode) has been used successfully to reduce chronic sleepwalking.

PROGNOSIS

Sleepwalking is primarily a problem during childhood, although a small proportion of adults are affected. For the most part, the course of sleepwalking is short, and few people over the age of 15 continue to exhibit this difficulty.

See also: Nightmares; Sleep Patterns, Normal; Sleep Talking; Sleep Terrors

Further Reading

Anders, T. F., & Eiben, L. A. (1997). Pediatric sleep disorders: A review of the past 10 years. *Journal of American Academy of Child and Adolescent Psychiatry, 36,* 9–20.

Durand, V. M., Mindell, J., Maptstone, E., & Gernert-Dott, P. (1998). Sleep problems. In T. S. Watson & F. M. Gresham (Eds.), *Handbook of child behavior therapy* (pp. 203–219). New York: Plenum Press.

Laberge, L., Tremblay, R. E., Vitaro, F., & Montplaisir, J. (2000). Development of parasomnias from childhood to early adolescence. *Pediatrics, 106*(1), 67–74.

National Sleep Foundation, 1522 K Street, NW, Suite 500, Washington, DC 20005, Phone: (202) 347-3471, Fax: (202) 347-3472, E-mail: nsf@sleepfoundation.org, http://www.sleepfoundation.org.

V. Mark Durand
Kristin V. Christodulu

Sleep–Wake Cycle Problems

DEFINITION

Sleep–wake cycle problems are characterized by disturbed sleep (either insomnia or excessive sleepiness during the day) brought on by the brain's inability to synchronize its sleep patterns with the current patterns of day and night. Not being synchronized with the normal wake and sleep cycles causes people to have trouble falling asleep when they do try to sleep, to have trouble waking up, and to be tired during the day. The sleep–wake cycle is considered one of the *circadian rhythms*—the word *circadian* means "about a day." There are several different types of circadian rhythm sleep disorders. *Jet lag type* is caused by rapidly crossing multiple time zones. People with jet lag usually report difficulty going to sleep at the proper time and feeling fatigued during the day. *Shift work type* sleep problems are associated with work schedules. People such as hospital employees, police officers, or emergency personnel who work at night or work irregular hours may have problems sleeping or experience excessive sleepiness during waking hours. Two other types of circadian rhythm sleep disorders are *delayed sleep phase* and *advanced sleep phase*. Delayed sleep phase is a persistent pattern of late sleep onset and awakening time while advanced sleep phase involves a persistent pattern of early sleep onset and awakening times.

INCIDENCE/ETIOLOGY

The prevalence for sleep–wake cycle problems has not been well established. In adolescents, surveys suggest a prevalence of up to 7 percent for *delayed sleep phase type*—consistently go to bed later and wake up later—"night owls." Research on why sleep rhythms are disrupted is advancing rapidly, and more is now known about the circadian rhythm process. Scientists believe the hormone melatonin contributes to setting of our biological clocks that tell us when to sleep. In addition, changes in the hormone melatonin, the body's internal temperature also seems to be involved in how and when people sleep. Internal body temperature increases and decreases over the course of the day, making it another circadian rhythm. A rise in temperature is associated with increased alertness, while a drop in temperature is associated with decreased alertness.

When considering sleep–wake cycle problems, it is important to note that sleep is affected by many factors including what and when we eat and drink, when we exercise, the temperature in the bedroom, noise, and even what we do in bed. For example, an irregular sleep–wake schedule, an inconsistent bedtime routine, an evening snack containing caffeine (e.g., chocolate cookies, cola), too much light in the bedroom, and playing actively just before bedtime can all interfere with a child's ability to fall asleep at night.

CORRELATES

Difficulties in daily activities (i.e., school, peers) may arise from an inability to awaken at socially desired times. Awakening children with a *delayed sleep phase* early may result in the child exhibiting "sleep drunkenness" (e.g., extreme difficulty awakening, confusion, and inappropriate behavior). Performance often also follows a delayed phase, with peak efficiency occurring in the evening hours.

ASSESSMENT

To assess for sleep–wake cycle problems (either advanced or delayed), it is important to determine if the child falls asleep early in the evening and awakens too early in the morning or if the child has difficulty falling asleep until a very late hour and difficulty awakening early in the morning. It is also important to gather information on the child's daily routine including sleeping, eating, exercise, and so forth, to determine the regularity of the schedule and the parent's response to the child's sleep problems.

TREATMENT

It is important to establish regular schedules for both daily activities and sleep and wake times. Establishing good sleep habits, such as creating a calming and stable bedtime routine, removing foods and drinks containing caffeine for evening snack, limiting vigorous activity in the hour before bedtime, and limiting activity in bed to stories and sleep, is important for improving sleep habits. In some cases, it might be necessary to gradually move the bedtime earlier or later. One general principle for treating sleep–wake cycle problems is that *phase delays* (moving the bedtime later) are easier than *phase advances* (moving bedtime earlier). In other words, it is easier to stay up several hours later than usual than to make yourself go to sleep several hours earlier. *Bright light therapy* has also been used to help individuals with sleep–wake cycle problems readjust their sleep patterns.

PROGNOSIS

Without intervention, sleep–wake cycle problems typically last for years or decades, but treatment can often normalize sleep hours; however, a very regular wake–sleep schedule must be maintained or relapse is likely.

See also: Excessive Sleepiness; Initiating and Maintaining Sleep; Obstructive Sleep Apnea; Sleep Patterns, Normal

Further Reading

Arendt, J., Stone, B., & Skene, D. (2000). Jet lag and sleep disruption. In M. H. Kryger, T. Roth, & W. C. Dement (Eds.), *Principles and practice of sleep medicine* (3rd ed., pp. 591–599). Philadelphia: W.B. Saunders.

Durand, V. M. (1998). *Sleep better! A guide to improving sleep for children with special needs.* Baltimore, MD: Paul H. Brookes.

Monk, T. H. (2000). Shift work. In M. H. Kryger, T. Roth, & W. C. Dement (Eds.), *Principles and practice of sleep medicine* (3rd ed., pp. 600–605). Philadelphia: W.B. Saunders.

Sack, R. L., & Lewy, A. J. (1993). Human circadian rhythms: Lessons from the blind. *Annals of Medicine, 25,* 303–305.

National Sleep Foundation, 1522 K Street, NW, Suite 500, Washington, DC 20005, Phone: (202) 347-3471, Fax: (202) 347-3472, E-mail: nsf@sleepfoundation.org, http://www.sleepfoundation.org.

V. MARK DURAND
KRISTIN V. CHRISTODULU

Small Bowel Transplantation, Pediatric

DESCRIPTION

A small bowel transplant is most often performed in children who have short bowel syndrome. Short bowel syndrome is a condition in which the absorbing surface of the small intestine is inadequate because of extensive disease or the surgical removal of a large portion of the small intestine. Primary conditions leading to short bowel syndrome may include volvulus (a twisting of the intestine that causes obstruction), intestinal atresias (absence of segments of intestine), necrotizing enterocolitis, Crohn's disease (inflammation of the small intestine), gastroschisis (a congenital muscular defect in the abdominal wall), thrombosis of the superior mesenteric artery, desmoid tumors, and trauma.

Children with short bowel syndrome are not able to receive adequate nutrition from enteral feeding (within the intestine). Therefore, they become dependent upon total parenteral nutrition (TPN), which involves the intravenous delivery of calories and nutrients. Children who experience complications secondary to TPN may be considered candidates for small bowel transplant. These complications may include catheter-related mechanical problems and infections, hepatobiliary disease, and metabolic bone disease. While cadaveric small bowel transplant is the most commonly performed transplant, there is a burgeoning interest in using living donors. Small bowel transplants are sometimes performed simultaneously with other visceral organs, including the liver, duodenum, jejunum, ileum, pancreas, and colon. When the small bowel and liver are transplanted in conjunction with other gastrointestinal organs, this is termed a multivisceral transplant.

PREVALENCE

In June 2001, there were 128 children under 18 years of age on the waiting list for small bowel transplantation in the United States. This number represents 75 percent of the 170 total patients awaiting small bowel transplantation. There have been 301 pediatric small bowel transplants performed in the United States since 1990.

PROGNOSIS

Complications associated with liver failure are the most common reasons for death among children awaiting small bowel transplantation. Patient survival rates following an isolated small bowel transplant are generally higher than that following a combined small bowel and liver transplant. Higher rates of morbidity and mortality are expected following small bowel transplantation, when compared to those following isolated liver or kidney transplantation in children. Long-term survival rates (>3 years), however, now approach 50–60 percent for children who have received small bowel transplantation.

Very little psychological research has been conducted with children receiving small bowel transplantation. Preliminary findings, however, indicate that, while significant improvements in health-related quality of life can be expected, psychological distress and family stress may continue long after transplantation.

See also: Coping with Illness; Gastrointestinal Disorders; Liver Transplantation; Pancreas Transplantation, Pediatric; Parenting the Chronically Ill Child

Further Reading

Kaufman, S. S., Atkinson, J. B., Bianchi, A., Goulet, O. J., Grant, D., Langnas, A. N., McDiarmid, S. V., Mittal, N., Reyes, J., & Tzakis, A. G. (2001). Indications for pediatric intestinal transplantation: A position paper of the American Society of Transplantation. *Pediatric Transplantation, 5,* 80–87.
Scientific Registry of Transplant Recipients Home Page. http://www.ustransplant.org (Accessed May 2002).
Tarbell, S. E., & Kosmach, B. (1998). Parental psychosocial outcomes in pediatric liver and/or intestinal transplantation: Pretransplantation and the early postoperative period. *Liver Transplantation Surgery, 4,* 378–387.
United Network for Organ Sharing Home Page. http://www.unos.org (Accessed May 2002).

JAMES R. RODRIGUE
REGINO P. GONZÁLEZ-PERALTA
STEPHANIE TOY

Smell, Development

See: Sensory and Perceptual Development

Social Development in Adolescence

During adolescence, youngsters' peer relations become more prominent and complex than during the elementary school years. As noted by Furman, most adolescents have a rich network of peers that includes their best friends, other close friends, larger friendship groups or cliques, social crowds, and possibly romantic relationships. Furthermore, adolescents' friendship networks become more complex, typically including both same- and cross-sex peers, and show increases in intimacy and closeness. As with preadolescents, it is important to draw distinctions between adolescents' general peer relations and their close friendships

PEER RELATIONS

Adolescents' peer relations include peer crowds, cliques, and dyads. As described by B. Bradford Brown (1989), *peer crowds* are reputation-based, and represent a large collective of similarly stereotyped individuals who may or may not spend much time together. *Cliques* refer to a small number of adolescents who spend time together; and *dyads* refer to pairs of friends or romantic partners.

Peer Crowds

Peer crowds reflect adolescents' peer status and reputation and are an outgrowth of the social status groups found in elementary school. Peer crowd affiliation reflects the primary attitudes or behaviors by which an adolescent is known to peers and may provide adolescents with a sense of belonging and acceptance.

Although the specific peer crowds vary somewhat with age, or with a particular school or neighborhood, there are remarkable consistencies in peer crowds. The most common crowds are: populars; brains; jocks; druggies or burnouts; loners; nonconformists or alternatives; and special interest groups (e.g., drama, dance). Some adolescents identify with more than one group, and many do not identify with any particular group, or consider themselves to be "average."

Peer crowds vary in obvious and subtle ways. For instance, La Greca and colleagues (2001) found that "brains" typically are smart, do well in school, and value academic activities; however, they also tend to have low levels of sexual activity, smoking, and substance use. "Jocks" typically are involved in athletic activities or competitive sports but are less likely to smoke or use drugs than other teens. In general, the "burnout" and "alternative" peer crowds tend to have the highest levels of heath-risk and problem behaviors (e.g., smoking, drinking, substance use, risky sexual behaviors) whereas "brains," and to a large extent "jocks," have the lowest levels of health and risky behaviors. Recent work by Prinstein and La Greca also suggests that adolescents who affiliate with the peer crowds associated with high social status (such as the jocks and populars) also report less anxiety and subjective distress than teens who affiliate with low status crowds (such as the burnouts). Understanding an adolescent's peer crowd will likely reveal something about the adolescent's behavior and reputation, and also about their health-risk behaviors.

The developmental significance of adolescents' peer crowds is that they contribute to their reputation and identity, and provide a sense of belonging. Peer crowd membership also may determine the larger pool of individuals from which adolescents meet and select friends; in fact, the majority of adolescents report that one of their closest friends affiliates with the same peer crowd. Finally, peer crowd affiliation may influence behavior, in that adolescents who want to be a part of a particular crowd may feel compelled to maintain behaviors that are compatible with the crowd's reputation. For example, adolescents who affiliate with the "burnouts" may smoke or drink alcohol just to "fit in" with their peers.

Peer Rejection or Victimization Experiences

Although an area of concern, little data are available on peer rejection among adolescents. During adolescence, fitting in with one's peers becomes a major priority for most teens, and because of this, peer rejection may be particularly stressful. In fact, a study by Parkhurst and Asher found that many middle school students were "victimized" and pushed around by peers in school, and that this type of rejection was associated with considerable subjective distress. Similarly, work by Inderbitzen and her colleagues indicates that adolescents who are rejected by peers report substantial anxiety and subjective distress.

Rather than focusing on peer rejection, per se, other investigators, such as Vernberg and his colleagues, have studied aversive exchanges among adolescents. Among 130 middle school students, Vernberg and associates found that 73 percent reported at least one aversive exchange (i.e., teased, hit, threatened, or excluded by peers) during the prior three months. Many adolescents did not talk to anyone about these events, and when they did, they were more likely to disclose this information to a friend, classmate, or sibling than to an adult. As a result, parents and other concerned adults (i.e., teachers) may be unaware of these aversive exchanges. Moreover, adolescents who reported more verbal and physical harassment or peer exclusion experienced more loneliness, especially if they did not discuss these events with anyone else.

Prospective studies further indicate that aversive exchanges with peers contribute to feelings of internal distress for adolescents. In another study by Vernberg and associates, peer rejection experiences at the beginning of the school year predicted adolescents' feelings of social anxiety later in the year. Moreover, other large-scale longitudinal investigations of bullying, such as work by Olweus in Scandinavia, have found that those who are bullied frequently during early adolescence are likely to report low self-esteem and symptoms of anxiety as adults.

In summary, although peer rejection and victimization (i.e., harassment, exclusion) have not received much empirical attention, they are common occurrences and represent a significant source of subjective distress for many adolescents. Because adolescents are not likely to talk about aversive peer experiences with other adults, they may go undetected and underreported.

ADOLESCENTS' FRIENDSHIPS

Close friendships are particularly important during adolescence. As noted by Thomas Berndt (1989), adolescents spend more time talking to peers than in any other activity, and also describe themselves as happiest when talking to friends. Adolescents' interactions with friends primarily occur in dyads (friendship pairs, romantic partners) or in cliques. Cliques are friendship-based groupings that vary in size (usually 5–8 members), density (the degree to which each person regards others in the clique as friends), and "tightness" (the extent to which they are closed or open to outsiders). Cliques constitute the primary base for adolescents' peer interactions and typically contain specific dyadic pairings (e.g., best friends).

An important determinant of adolescents' friendships is similarity or "homophily"; which is comprised of selection and socialization processes. Specifically, *selection* refers to the process by which adolescents select as friends those who share similar attributes and characteristics; *socialization* refers to the process by which adolescents are influenced by the behaviors and attitudes of their friends. Similarities in age, sex, and race, as well as similarities in specific interests, school attitudes, achievement, orientation to the contemporary peer culture, and substance use are important factors in adolescents' friendship choices. Once friendships are established, mutual socialization further enhances the similarities between friends. Furthermore, cross-sex friendships become increasingly common during adolescence, and adolescents with cross-sex friendships appear to be better integrated into the peer network at school and to be more socially competent.

In terms of the *qualities* of adolescents' friendships, many are similar to those observed in children's friendships (e.g., companionship, aid, validation and caring, trust). However, as Berndt (1989) has indicated, a defining feature of adolescents' friendships is their *intimacy* (i.e., sharing of private thoughts and feelings; knowledge of intimate details about one another), and close friendships become more intimate during adolescence. In addition, girls report more intimacy in their friendships than boys, which may reflect girls' preference for "exclusive" relationships. Boys appear to be more flexible and open in their friendship choices.

Having an intimate friendship during adolescence enhances self-esteem, and reduces anxiety and loneliness. For example, research by Vernberg indicated that less contact with friends, less closeness with a best friend, and greater peer rejection experiences over the course of 6 months contributed to an increase in adolescents' depressive affect. In other studies by Thomas Berndt and Anna Maria Cauce and their respective colleagues, support from close friends was positively associated with school involvement and achievement, self-esteem and psychosocial adjustment, and peer popularity.

See also: Adolescent Health; Bullies; Emotional Development; Social Phobia; Victims of Bullies

Further Reading

Berndt, T. J. (1989). Obtaining support from friends during childhood and adolescence. In D. Belle (Ed.), *Children's social networks and social supports* (pp. 308–331). New York: Wiley.

Brown, B. B. (1989). The role of peer groups in adolescents' adjustment to secondary school. In T. J. Berndt & G. W. Ladd (Eds.), *Peer relationships in child development* (pp. 188–215). New York: Wiley.

Hartup, W. W. (1996). The company they keep: Friendships and their developmental significance. *Child Development, 67*, 1–13.

La Greca, A. M., Prinstein, M. J., & Fetter M. D. (2001). Adolescent peer crowd affiliation: Linkages with health-risk behaviors and close friendships. *Journal of Pediatric Psychology, 26*, 131–143.

Vernberg, E. M., Ewell, K. K., Beery, S. H., Freeman, C. M., & Abwender, D. A. (1995). Aversive exchanges with peers during early adolescence: Is disclosure helpful? *Child Psychiatry and Human Development, 26*, 43–59.

ANNETTE M. LA GRECA

Social Development in Childhood

Children's peer relations have been widely studied during the elementary school years (ages 6–12 years), when children typically spend the school day in self-contained classrooms with a set peer group (i.e., classmates). After school and on weekends, many children are involved in organized peer activities (e.g., sports, Scouting, dance) and unstructured play activities with friends and neighborhood youth. In this social context, two aspects of children's peer relations are important—their *peer acceptance* and their close *friendships*. These are related, but distinct aspects of children's peer relations and both are critical for emotional health and development.

Peer acceptance refers to the extent to which a child is liked or accepted by the peer group. Peer group acceptance provides children with a sense of belonging or social inclusion. In contrast, as noted by Wydol Furman and his colleagues, friendships are close, supportive ties with one or more peers that may occur within or outside the classroom; friendships provide children with a sense of intimacy, companionship, and esteem.

PEER ACCEPTANCE

Substantial work by John Coie, Ken Dodge, and their colleagues have shown that it is important to distinguish between children who are accepted by their peers and those who are rejected. In general, peer acceptance has been linked with positive social qualities (e.g., cooperative) and personal qualities (e.g., smart), whereas peer rejection has been associated with behavior problems (especially aggressive behavior) and subjective distress (e.g., anxiety, loneliness). Longitudinal research suggests that children who are rejected by peers, even as early as the third grade, are at risk for negative outcomes later on in life.

Based on separate peer ratings of "acceptance" (or liking) and "rejection" (or disliking), several *types* of peer status have been identified in children. Most youth are *average* in their peer status—neither highly liked nor highly disliked. In contrast, *popular* children are those who are well-liked by peers and have few detractors. Popular children's acceptance may reflect their positive social skills and personal competencies, such as being helpful and considerate and having good athletic or academic abilities. In contrast, *rejected* children are those who are actively disliked by peers and lack friends or supporters; they have been found to have substantial interpersonal, emotional, and academic problems. Specifically, rejected children are often aggressive, disruptive, or inattentive, and may have academic difficulties or limited social skills. Rejected children also report considerable internal distress, such as symptoms of depression, loneliness, and social anxiety.

Children who are *neglected* by peers (sometimes referred to as "social isolates") are neither liked nor disliked, but they tend to go unnoticed by peers. Neglected children do not typically display behavior problems, but they may be withdrawn or socially anxious. Some research suggests that neglected children may have difficulty developing close, supportive friendship ties.

Other youth, identified as *controversial*, are both highly liked and highly disliked. Controversial children may display both positive (e.g., friendly, cooperative) and negative (e.g., aggressive) behaviors, but they do not appear to be "at risk" for psychological difficulties.

Although a large body of research has examined the behavioral and emotional correlates of children's peer acceptance and rejection, in recent years peer relations research has shifted its focus to new issues. In particular, Nikki Crick, Eric Vernberg, and their respective colleagues have examined the causes and consequences of peer victimization, teasing, and negative peer experiences, rather than studying peer acceptance and rejection, per se.

Moreover, because peer rejection or low peer acceptance appeared to be a risk factor for later emotional difficulties, efforts to develop social skills interventions for at-risk youth have received attention. Recently, however, efforts to improve children's social skills and peer relations have focused directly on children with different "types" of problems (e.g., Conduct Disorder (CD), social anxiety). Interventions that are tailored to children's specific social problems and which are incorporated into multifaceted interventions for children with conduct disorders (*Fast Track*; The Conduct Problems Prevention Research Group, 2002) or social phobia (*Social Effectiveness Therapy for Children*; Beidel, Turner, & Morris, 2000) have met with success.

CHILDREN'S FRIENDSHIPS

Children's ability to form and maintain supportive dyadic friendships represents a critical social adaptation task. Much of children's social lives revolve around dyadic or small group interactions with their friends.

Most children have close friends in school, and children who have at least one close friendship appear to fare better emotionally than those who lack such personal ties. Parker and Asher (1993) found that, among third–fifth graders, 78 percent had at least one reciprocal "best friend" in the classroom, and 55 percent of the children had a "very best friend" in school. Girls (82 percent) were more likely to have a best friend than boys (74 percent), and girls had more "best friends" than boys.

Several factors contribute to children's friendship choices. One is proximity; that is, children are likely to choose peers from their classroom, Scouting group, or immediate neighborhood as friends. Children also choose friends who are similar to themselves (e.g., same age, same gender), who share common interests (e.g., play sports, listen to music), and who are fun to be with.

The quality of children's friendships is also important. Friends provide emotional support and are children's primary source of companionship. However, friendships can vary tremendously in the amount and type of support they provide, the degree to which conflict is present, and their level of reciprocity. Moreover, girls typically report more intimacy and support in their friendships than do boys. This may reflect the boys' tendency to associate with peers in large groups that are organized around sports or group activities, whereas girls tend to be involved in dyads or small groups that spend time in conversation and quiet activities.

In general, the number and quality of children's close friendships are important for children's mental health. Close, supportive friendships can help children manage stressful life events, such as parental divorce or coping with the aftermath of disasters or other traumatic events. Children with emotional and behavioral difficulties often have poorer quality friendships, and such children may need assistance with making and sustaining healthy friendships.

See also: Bullies; Disruptive Behavior Disorders; Social Phobia; Social-Skills Training; Sociometric Assessment; Victims of Bullies

Further Reading

Asher, S. R., & Coie, J. D. (Eds.). (1990). *Peer rejection in childhood*. New York: Cambridge University Press.

Beidel, D. C., Turner, S. M., & Morris, T. L. (2000). Behavioral treatment of childhood social phobia. *Journal of Consulting and Clinical Psychology, 68*, 1072–1080.

The Conduct Problems Prevention Research Group. (2002). The implementation of the Fast Track Program: An example of a large-scale prevention science efficacy trial. *Journal of Abnormal Child Psychology, 30*, 1–17.

Hartup, W. W. (1996). The company they keep: Friendships and their developmental significance. *Child Development, 67*, 1–13.

Parker, J. G., & Asher, S. R. (1993). Friendship and friendship quality in middle childhood: Links with peer group acceptance and feelings of loneliness and social dissatisfaction. *Developmental Psychology, 29*, 611–621.

ANNETTE M. LA GRECA

Social Phobia

DESCRIPTION/CLINICAL PRESENTATION

The core feature of social phobia (SOP) is persistent and irrational worry or fear of social or performance situations where the child may feel he/she is being evaluated by others. Children with SOP worry or fear that when in these situations they may behave or display certain characteristics that will lead to humiliation or embarrassment. Children with SOP usually avoid or attempt to avoid social situations or endure them with distress (e.g., talking in class, attending birthday parties, participating in athletic programs). Fear and/or worry concerning social situations may be specific to a type of situation (e.g., school related activities) or pervasive across different contexts (e.g., school, family, friends). When avoidance is not possible, children with SOP may experience marked distress in these types of situations and may freeze up or cry. To receive a diagnosis of SOP, the worry/fear concerning social situations must be present for over 6 months and lead to marked impairment in functioning.

PREVALENCE AND CORRELATES

The prevalence of SOP in child and adolescent samples ranges from 3 to 13 percent in community samples, according to Anderson and colleagues and 6 to 16 percent in clinic samples. According to a study conducted by Beidel, Turner, and Morris (2000) the situations that children with SOP most frequently avoid are reading aloud in front of class, musical or athletic performances, joining in or starting a conversation, and speaking to adults. Children with SOP tend to be older than children with other anxiety disorders such as separation anxiety disorder and specific phobias, although there is evidence that SOP appears in preadolescent children as well.

Studies conducted by Messer and Beidel (1994) on samples of children with anxiety disorders, including SOP have found that these children have high trait anxiety, temperaments that are less flexible and more rigid, and less physical and cognitive self-confidence than nonclinic referred children. Children with SOP also have been found to have higher levels of emotional over-responsiveness, social fear, inhibition, dysphoria, loneliness, and general fearfulness than nonclinical referred children. Also, the family environments of children tend to promote less independence. In studies conducted by Beidel and colleagues and Spence and colleagues (2000), children with SOP frequently have social skill deficits and have lower performance expectations, while engaging in maladaptive coping behaviors (e.g., negative self-talk on social evaluative tasks) compared to nonclinical referred children. SOP is also associated with significant impairment including poor school achievement, difficulties with peer and family relationships, and alcohol and drug use.

ASSESSMENT

A comprehensive assessment of social phobia includes a multisource multimethod procedure including diagnostic interviews, child and parent rating scales, behavioral observations, and self-monitoring tools. A variety of structured (e.g., Diagnostic Interview Schedule for Children) and semi-structured interviews (e.g., Anxiety Disorders Interview Schedule for *DSM-IV*: Child and Parent versions) are available for the assessment of SOP. In addition, child and parent measures are available that assess general anxiety symptoms such as the Revised Child Manifest Anxiety Scale or have subscales to assess SOP (e.g., Multidimensional Anxiety Scale for Children, Screen for Child Anxiety-Related Emotional Disorders; Spence Children's Anxiety Scale). The Social Anxiety Scale for Children-Revised and Social Phobia and Anxiety Inventory for Children were specifically designed to assess for social anxiety and/or phobia. These assessment tools are frequently used in the initial assessment of SOP and the continued monitoring of treatment response. When assessing SOP, it is important to thoroughly assess for the presence of comorbid psychiatric disorders including other anxiety, mood, and externalizing disorders (e.g., Attention-Deficit/Hyperactivity Disorder [ADHD], Oppositional Defiant Disorder [ODD]).

TREATMENT

Considerable evidence has now accumulated demonstrating the efficacy of exposure-based cognitive behavior therapy (CBT) for reducing childhood anxiety disorders, including SOP. In recent studies conducted by Beidel and colleagues (2000), Hayward and colleagues, and Spence and colleagues, CBT was found to be efficacious in samples that have only included youth with SOP. In these studies, CBT has been administered using a group format and/or involving parents, with emphasis placed on improving peer relationships by training participants in social skills, problem solving, assertiveness, and other skills associated with peer effectiveness

As noted by Stock and colleagues (2001), the pharmacological literature for the treatment of childhood anxiety disorders, including SOP, is in its infancy when compared to the treatment literature on exposure-based CBT. The available literature on the pharmacological treatment of SOP consists of studies that used samples of children with an array of anxiety disorders. For example, Birmaher and colleagues examined the efficacy of the antidepressant fluoxetine (Prozac) in 21 children with separation anxiety disorder, overanxious disorder, as well as SOP. About 81 percent of the children displayed moderate to marked improvement of their anxiety symptoms and no side effects were reported by any of the children. Given the paucity of research in this area, pharmacological interventions have been recommended with only the more difficult or "resistant" cases, rather than the frontline approach to be used with all cases. Rather, exposure-based CBT should be attempted first.

See also: Behavioral Diaries; Behavior Rating Scales; Child Self-Reports; Cognitive–Behavior Therapy; Interviewing; Social-Skills Assessment, Parent Training

Further Reading

Beidel, D. C., Turner, S. M., & Morris, T. L. (2000). Behavioral treatment of childhood social phobia. *Journal of Consulting and Clinical Psychology, 68*, 1072–1080.

Messer, S. C., & Beidel, D. C. (1994). Psychosocial correlates of childhood anxiety disorders. *Journal of the American Academy of Child and Adolescent Psychiatry, 33*, 975–983.

Silverman, W. K., & Berman, S. L. (2001). Psychosocial interventions for anxiety disorders in children: Status and future directions. In W. K. Silverman & P. D. A. Treffers (Eds.), *Anxiety disorders in children and adolescents: Research, assessment and intervention* (pp. 313–334). Cambridge, UK: Cambridge University Press.

Stock, S. L., Werry, J. S., & McClellan, J. M. (2001). Pharmacological treatment of pediatric anxiety. In W. K. Silverman & P. D. A. Treffers (Eds.), *Anxiety disorders in children and adolescents: Research, assessment and intervention* (pp. 335–367). Cambridge, UK: Cambridge University Press.

BARBARA LOPEZ
LISSETTE M. SAAVEDRA
WENDY K. SILVERMAN

Social Problem-Solving Assessment

D'Zurilla and Goldfried (1971) define problem-solving as the process by which individuals identify potentially effective response alternatives for dealing with problematic social situations and, at the same time, increase the probability of selecting the most effective response from among these various alternatives. Social problem-solving comprises two components, namely problem-orientation and rational problem-solving skills. Problem-orientation is a motivational construct incorporating an individual's awareness of problems, an assessment of their ability to manage these problems, and

expectations about the effectiveness of problem-solving attempts. Rational problem-solving skills, in contrast, refer to the individual's ability to rationally identify and define problems, generate solutions, evaluate and select the most appropriate alternative, implement this solution, and monitor its effectiveness. Research suggests that both of these aspects of problem-solving play an important role in mental health and emotional well-being.

Individuals who hold a negative problem-orientation or who have difficulty in performing rational problem-solving steps are less likely to choose the optimal response for dealing with a situation. As a consequence, they are at increased risk for experiencing a range of emotional and behavioral problems. For example, research suggests that individuals with depression and/or suicidality tend to have difficulty in generating alternative solutions, are more likely to select self-destructive, passive/avoidant, or impulsive solutions to life problems. Aggressive behavior has also been linked to problem-solving deficits.

ASSESSMENT OF SOCIAL PROBLEM-SOLVING SKILLS

Although quite a few measures exist that purport to assess social problem-solving skills, there has been relatively little research to establish their reliability and validity. Furthermore, most measures have been developed for research studies and their value in clinical practice is unclear. The following measures have been used most commonly:

The Preschool Interpersonal Problem Solving Test (PIPS)

The PIPS was developed by Spivack and Shure (1974) to evaluate the ability of 3–5 year-olds to generate alternative solutions to interpersonal problems. It has also been found to be useful with children up to 8 years of age. The test involves two sets of age relevant problems, one dealing with a peer conflict and the other concerning a conflict with a parent, to which children are asked to produce possible solutions without regard to the social acceptability of these responses. The PIPS test can be adapted to take into account the quality rather than just the quantity of the solutions offered. In addition to the PIPS, Spivack and Shure (1974) described the What Happens Next Game which was designed to assess children's ability to predict the consequences of behavior.

Means-Ends Problem Solving Test (MEPS)

The MEPS was developed by Spivack, Platt, and Shure (1976) to assess elementary children's ability to produce step-by-step methods for reaching solutions to interpersonal problems. Each story presents a beginning and an end to an interpersonal problem and the child is asked to complete the middle part to indicate various ways in which the problem may have been solved. Performance is determined by the number of alternative means that the child suggests, elaboration of specific means, potential obstacles identified, and use of a time sequence.

Open Middle Interview (OMI)

Polifka and colleagues (1981) adapted the MEPS to form the Open Middle Interview. The OMI presents the child with hypothetical age-relevant social problem situations in a cartoon format and asks the child to generate as many solutions to the problem as possible. A free-response format is used and answers are scored for the number of different solutions generated, the preferred solution, and the effectiveness of each solution. Inter-rater reliability is reported to be good and the measure is found to differentiate between socially rejected and popular boys.

Purdue Elementary Problem-Solving Inventory (PEPSI)

The PEPSI was designed by Feldhusen and colleagues (1972) to provide a more detailed method of assessing problem-solving skills. It involves 49 cartoon slides, each of which portrays the child in a specific, real-life problem situation. Audiotaped directions are presented, along with a choice of alternative solutions. Children mark on a record sheet their preferred solution. The PEPSI provides an indication of children's abilities to sense problems, to define problems, to analyze critical details, to see implications, and to make unusual associations. To date, this measure does not seem to have been widely used in clinical practice.

Social Problem-Solving Inventory-Revised (SPSI-R)

This scale was developed by D'Zurilla and colleagues (in press) as an objective self-report measure of rational problem-solving and problem-solving motivation and is suitable for completion by adolescents and adults. The SPSI-R assesses cognitive, affective, and behavioral processes by which individuals attempt to identify and implement adaptive coping responses for problem situations. The scale consists of five subscales. Two of these subscales, positive problem orientation (PPO) and negative problem orientation (NPO) assess functional/dysfunctional cognitive and emotional orientations towards solving life problems. The three remaining subscales, rational problem-solving (RPS), impulsivity/carelessness style (ICS), and avoidance style (AS) assess problem-solving skills and behavioral style. The five subscales have been shown to have good internal consistency and test–retest reliability.

The Problem-Solving Inventory (PSI)

The PSI, developed by Heppner and Petersen (1982), assesses an individual's awareness and evaluation of his or her problem-solving abilities or styles. The PSI is a self-report measure, and thus assesses perceptions of problem-solving as opposed to actual problem-solving skills. The PSI consists of 32 six-point Likert items, which constitute three factors: problem-solving confidence, approach-avoidance style, and personal control. The scale has been found to have good psychometric properties and to be useful in both clinical and research contexts.

CLINICAL IMPLICATIONS

Given the importance of social problem-solving in determining mental health, this area of psychological functioning should be considered in the assessment of psychopathology. Where assessment reveals deficits in problem-solving or presence of a negative problem-solving orientation problem-solving training may form an important component of cognitive-behavioral therapy in the treatment of many psychological disorders. Training in social problem-solving skills may also provide a protective role in the prevention of emotional and behavioural problems in children and adolescents.

See also: Problem-Solving Training; Reliability; Validity; Cognitive–Behavior Therapy

Further Reading

D'Zurilla, T. J., & Goldfried, M. R. (1971). Problem solving and behavior modification. *Journal of Abnormal Psychology*, 78(1), 107–126.
D'Zurilla, T. J., Nezu, A., & Maydeu Olivares, A. (in press). Conceptual and methodological issues in social problem-solving assessment. *Manual for the social problem-solving inventory-revised (SPSI-R)*. North Tonawanda, NY: Multi-Health Systems.

Feldhusen, J., Houtz, J., & Ringenbach, S. (1972). The Purdue Elementary Problem-Solving Inventory. *Psychological Reports, 31*, 891–901.

Heppner, P. P., & Petersen, C. H. (1982). The development and implications of a personal problem solving inventory. *Journal of Counselling Psychology, 29*(1), 66–75.

Polifka, J. A., Weissberg, R. P., Gesten, E. L., de Apodaca, R. F., & Picoli, L. (1981). *The open-middle interview manual*. New Haven, CT: Department of Psychology, Yale University.

Spivack, G., & Shure, M. B. (1974). *Social adjustment of young children*. San Francisco: Jossey Bass.

Spivack, G., Platt, J. J., & Shure, M. B. (1976). *The problem solving approach to adjustment*. San Francisco: Jossey Bass.

SUSAN HILARY SPENCE

Social Support

Social support has broadly been defined by Cohen and Syme (1985) as the resources that other persons provide. Social support can be emotional in nature, and thus may lead to feelings of being cared for, loved, esteemed, and valued, or a sense of belonging. Social support can also be instrumental or tangible, in the sense of providing money, time, or other forms of assistance (e.g., helping someone get to an appointment). Another important distinction is between the *perception* of social support versus support that is actually *received*. By and large, the substantial literature on social support and health or mental health outcomes suggests that it is *the perception of support* that matters more than the actual support received.

Social support from others is typically offered, or perceived to be needed, when an individual is under stress. During childhood and adolescence, developmental changes and life transitions (e.g., moving to a new school, beginning to date) inevitably produce stress, as do other major life events such as failing an important exam, dealing with parental divorce, developing and managing a chronic disease, losing a loved one, or experiencing a traumatic event. Normative and nonnormative stressors can lead to a variety of outcomes that have emotional (e.g., depression, anxiety, anger) or physical (e.g., illness, fatigue) components. The importance of social support is that, in many instances, it represents a protective factor that can help to buffer the psychological and physical consequences of stress.

SOURCES OF SOCIAL SUPPORT: CHILDREN'S SOCIAL NETWORKS

Several aspects of social support appear to be important. One pertains to the sources of support that are available (or perceived to be available) to children and adolescents. Along these lines, investigators such as Cauce and her colleagues (1990) have examined structural aspects of children's social support, including the size of their support networks, the individuals that make up the network, and types of support provided by the various network members. This research suggests that family members, friends, and school personnel (e.g., teachers) represent youngsters' main sources of social support. Family members (especially parents) appear to provide a consistently high level of support throughout the childhood and adolescent years; teachers also represent an important source of support throughout the school years.

Of particular significance is youngsters' support from friends and classmates. Support from friends is important even during the preschool years, and by elementary school, youngsters' friends provide a key source of emotional support and companionship. During adolescence, friends are a very close second to parents (especially mothers) as a source of emotional support, and friends provide the highest level of companionship. Recent research by La Greca and colleagues (1995) has demonstrated that youngsters' support from friends and from family members plays a critical role in their ability to cope with significant stressors, such as disasters and terrorism, or with a chronic or life-threatening disease.

TYPES OR FUNCTIONAL ASPECTS OF SOCIAL SUPPORT

In addition to sources of support, the *types or functions* of support are also important for consideration, and these include: emotional, informational, instrumental, and companionship support. Of these types, emotional support has been the most well-studied, and it is viewed as critical for emotional well-being. For example, a widely used measure of perceived social support—the Social Support Scale for Children and Adolescents developed by Harter (1988)—primarily taps emotional support from significant others (e.g., parents, teachers, friends, classmates). Throughout childhood and adolescence, parents and friends are typically the main providers of emotional support, followed by siblings and teachers. Parents and teachers are the key providers of social support that is informational (e.g., advice, information) or instrumental (e.g., food, money, or other tangible forms of assistance) in nature. Finally, youngsters' friends, followed by parents and siblings, are the key providers of companionship (i.e., sharing activities). As noted, although family members provide consistently high levels of support across development, support from friends becomes increasingly important and salient during the adolescent years.

See also: Coping with Illness; Social Development in Adolescence; Social Development in Childhood

Further Reading

Cauce, A. M., Reid, M., Landesman, S., & Gonzales, N. (1990). Social support in young children: Measurement, structure, and behavioral impact. In B. R. Sarason, I. G. Sarason, & G. R. Pierce (Eds.), *Social support: An interactional view* (pp. 64–94). New York: Wiley.

Cohen, S., & Syme, S. L. (1985). *Social support and health.* Orlando, FL: Academic Press.

Harter, S. (1988). *Social support scale for children and adolescents.* Denver, Co: University of Denver: Author. Available from: sharter@du.edu.

La Greca, A. M., Auslander, W. F., Greco, P., Spetter, D., Fisher, E. B., Jr., & Santiago, J. V. (1995). I get by with a little help from my family and friends: Adolescents' support for diabetes care. *Journal of Pediatric Psychology, 20,* 449–476.

La Greca, A. M., Silverman, W. K., Vernberg, E. M., & Roberts, M. C. (2002). *Helping children cope with disasters and terrorism.* Washington, DC: American Psychological Association.

KAREN BEARMAN
ANNETTE M. LA GRECA

Social-Skills Assessment

Social skills are those abilities and behaviors that allow individuals to interact in socially competent and acceptable ways. Ultimately, social skills should lead to successful interpersonal relationships in the home, school, work, or community setting. The assessment of social skills in children serves many purposes including (1) identifying children with social skills deficiencies; (2) providing information for diagnostic purposes; (3) treatment planning; (4) educational planning (for behavioral components of Individualized Education Plans); and (5) evaluating the effectiveness of intervention programs.

The development of social skills can be linked to social information processing theory and the literature accompanying that theory. Crick and Dodge's (1994) six-stage model of social information processing describes how children encode details, generate interpretations, formulate social goals, generate responses, evaluate each response, and then enact the chosen response. It is in the sixth and final stage, the action step, in which social skills are actually evident as observable behaviors. However, social skills impairments can occur at different points throughout the process. For example, poor social skills may result when children misinterpret environmental cues or generate and subsequently choose negative or nonsocial responses. Social cognitive measures such as the Attributional Measure and the Problem Solving Measure for Conflict (PSM-C) developed by Lochman and Dodge (1994) can assess whether children with deficient social skills have difficulties at earlier stages in the model. However, sometimes children can select positive, prosocial responses but still be inept at implementing those responses, thereby exhibiting social skills deficits at the action step.

The most common assessment instrument to evaluate the observable social behaviors and actions of children is the rating scale. Rating scales have the advantage of providing norm-referenced standardized scores so that a child's social skills can be directly compared to other children his or her age. Gender-based norms are also often available. Many omnibus parent and teacher rating scales that measure broad behavioral and emotional functioning include a social skills scale. For example, both the Behavior Assessment System for Children (BASC)—Parent Rating Scale (PRS) and Teacher Rating Scale (TRS) include a Social Skills scale, measuring the adaptive skills essential for successful interaction with both peers and adults in various settings (e.g., home, school, community). Example items loading on the BASC-PRS Social Skills scale include "begins conversations appropriately," "has good eye contact," and "uses appropriate table manners." Example items that load on the BASC-TRS include "admits mistakes" and "volunteers to help with others." Parents or teachers rate their child or student on each item using a 4 point scale, ranging from "Never" to "Almost Always." The BASC-PRS and BASC-TRS include age-specific forms for preschoolers, elementary-aged children, and adolescents.

Whereas the BASC measures the adaptive behaviors considered to be successful social skills, other omnibus rating scales measure symptoms and behaviors indicative of poor social skills. For example, both Achenbach's Child Behavior Checklist (CBCL) for parents and Teacher Report Form (TRF) for teachers include a scale that measures Social Problems. Parents or teachers rate their child or student on a 3-point scale, ranging from "Not True" to "Very/Often True." Items on the Social Problems scale measure behaviors that are indicative of poor social skills (e.g., "acts immature," "has difficulty working with others"), as well as negative consequences that are often associated with poor social skills (e.g., "is unpopular," "is teased by others").

In addition, and as noted by Kamphaus and Frick (1996), many child self-report inventories include items and scales relevant to social skills assessment. The Interpersonal Relations scale on the Behavior Assessment System for Children–Self-Report of Personality (BASC-SRP), the Social Skills Deficit scale on the Personality Inventory for Youth (PIY), and the Social Problems scale on the Youth Self-Report (YSR) include items evaluating a child's perception of his or her appropriate social skills and problematic social behaviors, as well as his or her perceived level of acceptance among peers.

Whereas omnibus rating scales often include one scale to assess social skills, several social skills-specific rating scales have also been developed. For example, the Social Skills Rating System (SSRS) is a comprehensive measure covering several domains of social skills including: Cooperation (e.g., "volunteers to help others with tasks"), Assertion (e.g., "accepts friends' ideas for playing"), Responsibility (e.g., "introduces herself or himself to new people without being told"), and Self-control (e.g., "responds appropriately when hit or pushed by other children"). Rating forms are available for parents and teachers for preschool, elementary, and secondary education students. The elementary and secondary level forms also include a student self-report rating scale. The SSRS is somewhat unique in that it not only requires a rating of the child behavior (on a 3-point scale ranging from "Never" to "Very Often") but also requires the rater to indicate the importance of the behavior (from "Not Important" to "Critical") for the child's development. This latter type of rating is important for prioritizing goals for treatment planning and other intervention efforts. The SSRS has several advantages over rating scales that include only one scale measuring social skills, such as providing a multidomain assessment of social skills from multiple informants and allowing for intervention planning (i.e., based on importance ratings).

Another rating system specifically developed for the assessment of social skills is the Matson Evaluation of Social Skills for Youth (MESSY). The MESSY is designed to assess discrete, observable behaviors that are related to a range of appropriate social skills (e.g., "helps a friend who is hurt" and "walks up to people and starts a conversation") and inappropriate social skills (e.g., "gives other children dirty looks" and "wants to get even with someone who hurt him/her"). It is designed as a school-based assessment and includes a Teacher Rating and a Self Rating version. Items are rated on a 5-point scale ranging from "not at all" to "very much."

Although rating forms may be the most widespread form of social-skills assessment, interrater agreement on ratings scales is often low to moderate, and this may be particularly true in social-skills assessment. For example, on the BASC-PRS, there are often disparate ratings between mothers and fathers at the item level but little disagreement at the scale level, with the exception of the Social Skills scale for which there is low interrater agreement even at the scale level. This finding underscores the importance of collecting rating information from multiple informants who observe a child in multiple settings when conducting social-skills assessment for a child.

One type of social-skills assessment that has the benefit of avoiding rater interpretation is direct observation of a child's overt social-skills behaviors. Behaviors related to social skills are often found on standardized observational systems that are designed for assessing classroom behaviors. For example, the Behavior Assessment System for Children–Student Observation System (BASC-SOS) includes appropriate social behaviors (e.g., "plays with other students," "interacts in a friendly manner") and inappropriate social behaviors (e.g., "teasing," "throwing objects at others"), in addition to a number of other behaviors that are not directly related to social skills. The observer notes whether each of the behaviors was observed during a 3 s observation interval. Recordings are made for 30 intervals, occurring every 30 s, for a total of 15 min of observation.

Social skills are often considered to be a subset of adaptive behavior (i.e., daily living skills and behaviors that are necessary for independent functioning). Accordingly, an assessment of social skills is usually included within a comprehensive assessment of adaptive behaviors. The Vineland Adaptive Behavior Scales, which was actually originally named the Vineland Social Maturity Scale, currently includes a Socialization scale, measuring adaptive behaviors related to interpersonal relationships, play and leisure time, and coping skills associated with social situations. Consequently, the Vineland and other adaptive behavior scales can provide valuable assessment information related to social adaptive functioning.

If positive social skills lead to successful interpersonal relations for a child, it should be reflected in their social status among their peers. That is, a child's social status can be a marker of their social competence. Indeed, a rich literature has associated certain types of social status (e.g., popular, rejected, neglected, controversial, and average) with specific child behaviors. As such, peer-referenced assessments such as sociometrics are another way by which to gauge a child's social competencies.

Social-skills assessment is usually an important component of child diagnostic evaluations, given that a number of psychological disorders are associated with poor social skills. Some disorders, such as autism and mental retardation, involve impaired social skills and socialization deficits as part of the defining symptoms for the diagnosis, whereas other disorders, such as Attention-Deficit/Hyperactivity Disorder (ADHD), Major Depressive Disorder (MDD), and Conduct Disorder (CD), are associated with poor social skills. Physical impairments, such as deafness, may also lead to deficits in social skills and social relations. Once a child has received a diagnosis or has otherwise been identified as having social-skills impairments, a thorough assessment of social skills can be helpful in setting treatment objectives or educational goals related to social functioning. Social-skills assessment over time is also invaluable in tracking intervention changes for therapy and other intervention programs that target social skills.

See also: Sociometric Assessment; Adaptive Behavior Assessment; Social Development in Adolescence; Social Development in Childhood; Social Support

Further Reading

American Psychiatric Association. (1994). *Diagnostic and statistical manual of mental disorders* (4th ed.). Washington, DC: Author.

Crick, N. R., & Dodge, K. A. (1994). A review and reformulation of social information-processing mechanisms in children's social adjustment. *Psychological Bulletin, 115,* 74–101.

Kamphaus, R. W., & Frick, P. J. (1996). *Clinical assessment of child and adolescent personality and behavior.* Boston, MA: Allyn & Bacon.

Lochman, J. E., & Dodge, K. A. (1994). Social-cognitive processes of severely violent, moderately aggressive and nonaggressive boys. *Journal of Consulting and Clinical Psychology, 62,* 366–374.

Matson, J. L., (1994). *Matson evaluation of social skills with youngsters: Manual* (2nd ed.). Louisiana State University: International Diagnostic Systems.

TAMMY D. BARRY
JOHN E. LOCHMAN

Social-Skills Training

DESCRIPTION

Social-skills training (SST) is a therapeutic approach for enhancing children's effectiveness in interpersonal situations. Social skills encompass behaviors that facilitate a child's adaptation to the environment, reduce interpersonal conflict, and promote positive social interactions with other children and adults. Representative behaviors include eye contact, smiling, initiating interactions, conversational skills, assertiveness, and social problem solving.

CLINICAL APPLICATION

Social-skills deficits cut across many childhood disorders (e.g., autism, Attention-Deficit/Hyperactivity Disorder [ADHD], anxiety, depression, Conduct Disorder [CD]). A substantial array of SST programs have been developed to address a wide variety of presenting conditions. The process of SST typically involves providing target children with instruction and modeling of effective social behaviors (coaching), opportunities to practice the prescribed behaviors (behavioral rehearsal), verbal feedback with regard to effectiveness of response, and positive reinforcement of desired responding. SST is most often administered within small groups (4–6 children); although individualized instruction may be a necessary alternative when group formation is not possible. Regarding group constellations, it is generally recommended that the children be of approximately the same age or developmental level and exhibit difficulties generally within the same behavioral class (e.g., social withdrawal versus disruptive behavior). SST sessions generally are held on a weekly basis, for a period of 8–12 weeks, with the duration of each session ranging from 30 to 90 min (with the shorter sessions being most common when working with preschool age children, longer sessions with adolescents). Beyond acquisition of socially relevant target behaviors, the broad aims of most SST programs include improving the child's acceptance within the peer group, as well as the child's subjective feelings of self-esteem and social competence.

Which particular social skills are deemed necessary for effective interaction will vary with the social context. Successful social performance requires that the child be able to perceive a given social situation accurately, identify the appropriate behaviors to exhibit in that context, engage in the requisite behaviors (verbal and nonverbal), be responsive to feedback from others on a moment-to-moment basis, and modify his or her behavior based on that feedback. This process happens unwittingly for most members of the population, but others need assistance in executing one or more phases. When conducting SST it is important to break down this quickly evolving and complex social process in order to train more appropriate chains of responding.

Several SST program guides are available commercially (e.g., Skillstreaming the Elementary Child). These tend to be broad-based programs that target myriad skills that may be problematic for many children. However, these packages fail to address one or more skills that would be worthy targets of behavior for any given child and may target other skills the child already has in his or her repertoire. SST components have been included in treatment packages for a variety of specific childhood disorders. Unfortunately, little research has been conducted to determine which specific social skills may be most relevant for which specific condition. Although manualized SST packages serve as excellent resources for target selection, ideally the roster will be refined via behavioral assessment to determine which specific skills are most relevant for each participating child.

EFFECTIVENESS

SST programs generally have proven successful in increasing the frequency of the specific target behaviors trained; however the data on generalization to the natural setting and effects on peer acceptance have been mixed. Regrettably, many of the studies have failed to adequately measure generalization and durability of treatment effects. It is crucial that outcome assessments address not only whether the selected skills improved following training, but also whether the treatment had any impact on a socially valid criterion, such as peer acceptance or teacher ratings. Factors cited as influencing overall effectiveness of SST include gender of the child (more evidence in support of success with boys), age of the child/duration of social dysfunction (more success when intervening early rather than later in the course of a disorder when behaviors have become more entrenched), and inclusion of parents, teachers, and peers in the intervention process (facilitating maintenance and generalization of trained skills). A common criticism of the initial wave of SST programs was that the social skills selected for training were not considered salient for successful social functioning among many children. For instance, it is possible that improving physical skills such as throwing a baseball or kicking a soccer ball may have more impact in the child's social life than the ability to maintain a certain level of eye contact. More recent SST programs appear to be the beneficiary of increasing knowledge regarding children's social development. It is fair to expect that efficacy rates will continue to rise with our increasing ability to select socially relevant target skills.

See also: Social Development in Adolescence; Social Development in Childhood; Social Problem-Solving Assessment; Social Support; Social-Skills Assessment

Further Reading

Erwin, P. G. (1994). Effectiveness of social skills training with children: A meta-analytic study. *Counselling Psychology Quarterly*, 7, 305–310.

Gresham, F. M. (1998). *Social skills training with children: Social learning and applied behavior analytic approaches*. New York: Plenum.

McGinnis, E. & Goldstein, A. P. (2000). *Skillstreaming the elementary child: New strategies and perspectives for teaching prosocial skills*. Champaign, IL: Research Press.

TRACY L. MORRIS

Sociometric Assessment

DEFINITION

Sociometric assessment is a broad term encompassing a variety of systematic ways of gathering information about the extent or degree to which an individual is accepted or rejected within a specified peer group.

METHODS

Sociometric data most typically is gathered through peer nomination or rating procedures. The standard sociometric nomination procedure involves asking children to name three classmates with whom they most like to play (positive nominations/peer acceptance) and three with whom they least like to play (negative nominations/peer rejection). Information may be gathered individually in a brief interview format or may be obtained by having children indicate their selections on a paper form or ballot. The former approach is advantageous in terms of maintaining tighter anonymity of responding and for debriefing children should any concerns arise, whereas the latter approach is more advantageous when obtaining information from large numbers of children, all of whom have sufficient reading and writing ability to understand the directions and to respond to the questions.

Various statistical classification systems have been devised for defining distinct sociometric status groups. Children who receive a high proportion of positive nominations but few negative nominations are considered *popular*. This is in direct contrast to *peer rejected* children who receive few positive nominations and many negative nominations. *Peer-neglected* children are those who receive very few, if any, positive or negative nominations; whereas *controversial* children are liked by one segment of their peers, and disliked by other groups. *Average* status children receive moderate levels of acceptance and rejection within the peer group.

Ethical concerns have been expressed over the use of negative nominations, stemming from a belief that the procedure might lead to negative feelings on the part of some children or adversely affect interactions among the children. Studies have been conducted with preschool-, elementary-, and middle school-aged children to empirically address this assumption and no evidence of deleterious effects on behavioral observations of peer interactions, or on self-reported depressed mood and loneliness have been found. Nonetheless, peer ratings have been proposed as an alternative to the use of negative nomination procedures. In the peer rating method each child is asked to rate each member of the peer group using a Likert-type scale. For example, the child is provided a roster of names and asked to provide a numerical value for each peer in response to the question "How much do you like to play with this person?" with the scales commonly ranging from 1 ("I don't like to") to 5 ("I like to a lot"). Although this approach is sufficient for identifying children at the extremes of peer acceptance and peer rejection, many researchers continue to question its effectiveness in identifying peer-neglected children.

RELIABILITY/VALIDITY

Why should one go to the effort of collecting information from the peer group? Why not just ask the child or the child's parents how well they get along with peers? While obtaining such perceptions may be of some use, we cannot rely on the accuracy of such reports in gaining understanding of a child's actual standing within the peer group. Some children may be motivated to distort the truth, or may not be fully aware of how they are perceived by others. This particularly may be the case with parents who are not privy to the day-to-day social interactions of their children within the school setting. Obtaining sociometric information directly from peers has notable advantages: peers are inside sources of information—they are sensitive to age-relevant behaviors and characteristics that are important in determining the level of integration within the peer group; information from peers is based on many

extended and varied experiences with the target child—peers may be aware of infrequent but significant events that lead to particular social reputations; and information from peers is obtained from multiple observers who view the child from a variety of perspectives.

Although, in general, the validity and stability of peer acceptance and peer rejection has been well established, the specific data-gathering methods used in sociometric assessment, as well as the specific statistical criteria for social status group formation, inevitably will impact the reliability and validity of the information obtained. Studies vary widely with respect to the stability of specific subgroups over time, with some studies indicating the neglected category to be the least stable and others indicating high stability for that group. The relative percentage of children in the peer group who consent to participation is of particular concern to the accuracy of sociometric assessment. That is, if all the child's classmates participate in the sociometric procedure, then we may have confidence that we have obtained an accurate assessment of the child's social status within that group—but as the proportion of classmates providing information declines, we have less confidence in any categorization based on that data. Children who are highly liked or highly disliked by peers tend to remain so over time. This speaks to the stability of behavioral repertoires and reputations and provides support for the importance of early intervention for children demonstrating peer relationship difficulties.

CLINICAL APPLICATIONS

Sociometric assessment may be used to identify which children will benefit from intervention. It might also be used as a socially valid means of documenting treatment outcomes. Difficulties in social interaction cut across many of the diagnostic concerns for which children present for treatment. Children with disruptive behavior disorders, developmental disorders, anxiety disorders, and depression commonly evince difficulties in social adjustment. Although the empirical database continues to expand, it is not yet clear whether peer relationships are a cause or a consequence of more serious forms of maladjustment. Rather than a specific unidirectional (i.e., one-way) pathway, available evidence supports multiple and reciprocal interactions.

The literature is replete with reports of interventions designed to improve children's peer relationships. Most have been administered in small group formats within school settings. However, several manualized clinic-based treatments for specific disorders have incorporated social-skills enhancing components. Sociometric procedures are an excellent means of determining the impact of such interventions on target children's social standing with peers. Further, given mounting evidence of an association between social status and various forms of psychopathology (e.g., depression, anxiety, conduct disorders), sociometric assessment data may be used as a marker to identify young children who will benefit from early intervention. From a prevention perspective, school-based programs designed to improve the quality of social interaction among all children hold the promise of far-reaching effects for the individual and for society. Investigation following several high-profile cases of school violence has indicated that the perpetrators generally were recognized by peers and school officials as having been loners and social outcasts, clearly speaking to the need to direct attention and resources to this important area.

See also: Social Development in Adolescence; Social Development in Childhood; Social-Skills Assessment; Social-Skills Training

Further Reading

Berndt, T. J., & Ladd, G. W. (Eds.). (1989). *Peer relationships in child development*. Oxford: Wiley.

Cillesen, W. M., & Bukowski, W. M. (Eds.). (2000). *Recent advances in the measurement of acceptance and rejection in the peer system. New directions for child development (No. 88)*. San Francisco: Jossey-Bass.

Coie, J. D., Dodge, K. A., & Coppotelli, H. (1982). Dimensions and types of social status: A cross-age perspective. *Developmental Psychology, 18*, 557–570.

Juvonen, J., & Graham, S. (Eds.). (2001). *Peer harassment in the school: The plight of the vulnerable and victimized*. New York: Guilford.

TRACY L. MORRIS

Somatoform Disorder

See: Psychosomatic Disorders

Specific Phobia

DESCRIPTION/CLINICAL PRESENTATION

Specific phobia (SP) as conceptualized by the *Diagnostic and Statistical Manual of Mental Disorders, Fourth Edition (DSM-IV)* is as a common psychiatric disorder of childhood and adolescence characterized by excessive or unreasonable fear of, or in anticipation of, a circumscribed object or event. In contrast to developmentally appropriate fears (e.g., fear of strangers in a toddler), the fear experienced by the child with SP is irrational, though the child may not recognize its irrationality. Consequently, children often avoid or attempt to avoid the feared object or event. When avoidance is not possible, the child will experience severe distress when faced with the object or event. Also, to meet diagnostic criteria for SP, the fear must not be related to a recent stressor. The *DSM-IV* classifies SP into five subtypes: (1) animal type, (2) natural environment type, (3) blood-injection type, (4) situational type, and (5) others. Some of the most frequent and severe SPs reported by children include animals (e.g., dogs), natural events (e.g., heights, thunderstorms), and health providers (e.g., doctors, dentists). For a child to receive a diagnosis of SP, the fear must be present for over 6 months, be inappropriate for the child's age, and significantly interfere with or impair functioning.

PREVALENCE AND COMORBIDITY

Epidemiological studies have reported varied prevalence rates of SP depending on the type of phobia and the sample from which the information was drawn (community, clinic). Generally, prevalence rates for SP range from 1.7 to 6 percent in community samples and 6 to 12 percent in clinical samples. Although girls report a greater number and a higher intensity of fears than boys, rates of SP have not been found to differ between boys and girls. In comparison to other anxiety disorders, SP tends to be present in younger children and children of lower socioeconomic backgrounds.

Specific phobias are frequently associated with comorbid social phobia, Generalized Anxiety Disorder (GAD), Separation Anxiety Disorder (SAD), and/or Mood Disorders (MD) (e.g., major depression, dysthymia), and externalizing disorders (e.g., Attention-Deficit/Hyperactivity Disorder [ADHD], Oppositional Defiant Disorder [ODD]). It is important to thoroughly assess for the presence of these comorbid conditions.

ASSESSMENT

A comprehensive assessment of SP involves a tripartite (i.e., cognitive, physiological, behavioral) assessment. A variety of semistructured (e.g., Anxiety Disorders Interview Schedule for *DSM-IV*: Child and Parent Versions) and structured (e.g., Diagnostic

Interview Schedule for Children) diagnostic interviews can be used to assess SP. In addition, several rating scales are available that allow for the assessment of children's fears and/or discriminate among the anxiety disorders, including different types of SPs. These include child and parent versions of the Revised Fear Survey Schedule for Children, the Multidimensional Anxiety Scale for Children, and the Screen for Anxiety and Related Emotional Disorders.

A behavioral assessment can be particularly useful because the overt behavioral reaction of avoidance is a characteristic component of SP. Commonly used is a "behavioral avoidance test," which requires the child to emit graded and gradual approach behaviors to the phobic object or event. Although used more in research than clinical settings, physiological assessments of SP such as the assessment of heart rate and perspiration have been found useful as well. Overall, these assessment tools are frequently used in the initial assessment of SP and continued monitoring of treatment response.

TREATMENT

Considerable evidence has now accumulated demonstrating the efficacy of exposure-based cognitive behavior therapy (CBT) for reducing childhood anxiety disorders in general, including SP, as noted by Silverman and Berman (2001). The presence of comorbid conditions, including the additional diagnosis of SP, has not been found to lead to differential responses to CBT. In a recent study, Silverman and colleagues (1991) conducted a clinical trial for childhood phobic disorders that consisted largely of children with various SPs. The key behavioral and cognitive components of exposure-based CBT were compared relative to an education-support comparison condition. Results demonstrated the efficacy of the behavioral and cognitive components, respectively, though children in the comparison control condition improved as well, suggesting the need for further research in the area to determine the prime mechanisms of therapeutic change.

The relative efficacy of varying the type and duration of exposure in treatment has also been studied. Results suggest that although variations in exposures are generally efficacious, in vivo or live exposures appear to be most efficacious. There is also evidence that exposure-based treatments that involve a single session of treatment (maximum of 3 hr of exposure) can reduce SP in children, and that children with successful outcomes evaluated the treatment experience positively.

As noted by Stock and colleagues (2001), there is a paucity of research on pharmacological treatments for anxiety disorders in general, and SP in particular. The available studies provide preliminary evidence that benzodiazepines and tricyclic antidepressants may be useful for reducing symptoms of "school phobia." However, whether these findings could be generalized to children with SP is unclear. In addition, these studies have methodological limitations that render it difficult to draw firm conclusions. Given the paucity of research into this area, pharmacological interventions have been recommended with only the more difficult or "resistant" cases, rather than the front-line approach to be used with all cases.

See also: Behavioral Diaries; Cognitive–Behavioral Play Therapy; Evidence-Based Treatments; Parent Training; Systematic Desensitization

Further Reading

Silverman, W. K., & Berman, S. L. (2001). Psychosocial interventions for anxiety disorders in children: Status and future directions. In W. K. Silverman & P. D. A. Treffers (Eds.), *Anxiety disorders in children and adolescents: Research, assessment and intervention* (pp. 313–334). Cambridge, UK: Cambridge University Press.

Silverman, W. K., Kurtines, W. M., Ginsburg, G. S., Weems, C. F., Rabian, B., & Serafini, L. T. (1999). Contingency management, self-control, and educational support in the treatment of childhood phobic disorders: A randomized clinical trial. *Journal of Consulting and Clinical Psychology, 67,* 675–687.

Stock, S. L., Werry, J. S., & McClellan, J. M. (2001). Pharmacological treatment of paediatric anxiety. In W. K. Silverman & P. D. A. Treffers (Eds.). (2001). *Anxiety disorders in children and adolescents: Research, assessment and intervention* (pp. 335–367). Cambridge, UK: Cambridge University Press.

LISSETTE M. SAAVEDRA
BARBARA LOPEZ
WENDY K. SILVERMAN

Speech and Language Assessment

DEFINITION

The primary goal of assessment of speech and language is to describe comprehensively deficits in these areas relative to normal developmental processes. The results of this descriptive–developmental assessment strategy provide the basis for developing speech and language therapy programs to address identified problems. There are generally three domains of language that are evaluated. These include form (syntax, morphology, and phonology), content (semantics), and use (pragmatics). Each of these three domains of language is assessed within two different modalities: comprehension (receptive language) and production (expressive language). Language comprehension is the ability of the individual to understand language, both spoken and written. Production is the actual spontaneous expressive use of spoken or written language. Each of these modalities must be assessed independently of the other.

METHOD OF ASSESSMENT

Prior to actually conducting an assessment of the individual's receptive and expressive linguistic function, a complete history of the speech and language problem should be obtained. This history should include information regarding speech and language milestones. Additional background that details birth, developmental, medical, educational/academic, family, psychological, and social histories is important. This information can prove to be valuable in planning the content of the speech/language assessment.

The beginning point for the assessment is determined by establishing the current overall developmental level of the child. This can be done by utilizing any number of developmental measures available. Assessing the age level at which the child is functioning helps to determine the appropriate choice of speech and language measures, and aids in the interpretation of results.

Assessment of the three domains of language within the two modalities is accomplished through the use of standardized tests designed to assess each domain. Standardized tests allow the examiner to determine whether the individual differs significantly, and to what extent, from a normal population. Standardized tests have been designed to evaluate articulation/phonological disorders and both receptive and expressive language development (see Tables 1–3 for a listing of common tests for assessing linguistic and phonological development at different age levels). These tests have been developed through extensive examination of their reliability and validity. After a discrepancy from the normal developmental expectation for the child has been established through standardized speech and language tests, additional types of assessment may be used to define more clearly and thoroughly the speech/language deficit. Criterion-referenced procedures are

often used for this purpose. Criterion-referenced tests facilitate identifying what linguistic skills the child does and does not have and what skills to target at different stages of treatment. Structured analyses of spontaneous language samples in a natural setting such as the home or school are another means of refining the assessment of speech and language function. A complete discussion of assessment measures and methods can be found in books by Paul (2001) and by Ruscello.

In addition to standardized testing, a comprehensive evaluation covers other aspects of speech/language production. A thorough oral–motor examination is necessary to ensure the integrity of this system for speech. The oral–motor assessment includes examination of facial symmetry, dentition, oral musculature, lips, tongue, hard palate, and soft palate. Assessment of respiratory function is also important to ensure the adequacy of that system for support of phonation and speech. An evaluation of vocal function that includes assessment of voice quality and resonance patterns is necessary. If the individual's voice is characterized by an excessively hoarse or breathy quality, a referral should be made to an otolaryngologist (ear, nose, and throat physician) for examination of the vocal folds. In the event of the presence of hypernasal resonance or the use of an articulation pattern characterized by production of glottal fricatives (i.e., compensatory consonant sounds produced in the back of the throat), the child's ability to use the velopharyngeal mechanism (i.e., closing of the nasal cavity by movement of the soft palate against the pharynx wall during speech) should be evaluated. In such cases, examination of the hard palate may rule out a submucous cleft or a palatal fistula. If concern exists regarding the adequacy of velopharyngeal function, a referral to a cleft palate team should be made to determine if there is a lack of structural integrity of the velopharyngeal system.

Finally, evaluation of related areas that may contribute to the overall language and speech development is important for the clinical implementation of assessment results. For example, a complete audiological evaluation may be necessary to account for deficits in auditory acuity affecting speech/language outcomes. It may also be important to assess general cognitive functioning. If there appears to be deficits in verbal processing abilities, a neuropsychological evaluation is indicated. Additionally, appraisal of the child's social and emotional adjustment is helpful in the assessment process to uncover any issues that could influence speech or language problems or disrupt the implementation of treatment plans.

Table 1. Tests for the Assessment of Emerging Language (Ages 0–3 Years)

Instrument	Comment
MacArthur Communication Development Inventory	Parent-report instrument for assessing expressive and receptive vocabulary and early syntactic production
Preschool Language Scale-3rd ed.	Measures receptive and expressive language skills
Receptive-Expressive Emergent Language Scale: A Method for Assessing the Language Skills in Infants-2nd ed.	Parent-interview instrument
Reynell Developmental Language Scales III	Measures language skills in young or developmentally delayed children. Contains receptive and expressive language scales

See Paul (2001) and Ruscello (2001) for further information on the tests.

Table 2. Tools for the Assessment of Developing Language and Speech

Instrument	Developmental range	Areas assessed
Boehm Test of Basic Concepts-Revised	K–2nd grade	Receptive language concepts
Carrow Elicited Language Inventory	3–7 years	Grammatical production
Clinical Evaluation of Language Fundamentals-3	5–16 years	Syntax, semantics, memory, receptive and expressive language, composite
Developmental Sentence Score	2–7 years	Syntax
Preschool Language Scale-3	Birth–6 years	Expressive and receptive syntax, semantics, morphology
Test for Auditory Comprehension of Language-3rd ed.	3–9 years	Receptive language
Test of Language Development-3: Primary	4–8 years	Receptive and expressive syntax and semantics
Utah Test of Language Development 3	3–10 years	Language comprehension and expression

See Paul (2001) and Ruscello (2001) for further information on the tests.

Table 3. Tests for the Assessment of Phonological Development

Instrument	Developmental range	Comments
Fisher–Logemann Test of Articulation Competence	3 years to adult	Provides distinctive feature analysis
Goldman–Fristoe Test of Articulation-Revised	2–16+ years	Assesses articulation functions Use with Khan–Lewis Phonological Analysis
Assessment of Phonological Processes-Revised	Preschool	Assesses phonological processes
Khan-Lewis Phonological Analysis	2:5–11 years	Assesses phonological processes Use with Goldman–Fristoe Test of Articulation-Revised

See Paul (2001) and Ruscello (2001) for further information on the tests.

CLINICAL APPLICATIONS

Following the interviews, testing, and observations, interpretation of the assessment data takes place. A significant deficit is identified through standardized testing when a child's standard score is significantly below normal. It is sometimes useful to convert standard score results to age equivalents. These age equivalents are established for the purpose of making a comparison to the child's chronological or developmental age in each of the following areas of language comprehension and expression: syntax, semantics, phonology, morphology, and pragmatics. Upon establishing the complete description of the child's levels of functioning in all areas, it is possible to make statements as to the severity of the disorder and the prognosis. Recommendations regarding a program of speech therapy aimed at specific deficit areas will be made at this point in the assessment process. These recommendations will contain the goals that should be set for intervention. Assessment should continue as an ongoing process throughout the course of the therapy program. New short- and long-term goals will be established as the result of these assessments until the child has reached a point in the intervention at which a decision is made to terminate treatment.

See also: Developmental Issues in Assessment for Treatment; Language Development; Speech and Language Disorders

Further Reading

Dunn, M., Flax, J., Sliwinski, M., & Aram, D. (1996). The use of spontaneous language measures as criteria for identifying children with specific language impairment: An attempt to reconcile clinical and research incongruence. *Journal of Speech and Hearing Research, 39,* 643–654.

Miller, J., & Paul, R. (1995). *The clinical assessment of language comprehension.* Baltimore, MD: Paul H. Brookes.

Paul, R. (2001). *Language disorders from infancy through adolescence.* St. Louis, MO: Mosby.

Ruscello, D. M. (2001). *Tests and measurements in speech-language pathology.* Boston: Butterworth-Heinemann.

STEPHEN R. BOGGS
MARTHA F. PAULK

Speech and Language Disorders

See: Central Auditory Processing Disorders; Clefts of the Lip and Palate; Hearing Impairment; Language Development; Mixed Expressive-Receptive Language Disorder; Phonological and Articulation Disorders; Speech and Language Assessment; Stuttering

Spina Bifida

DESCRIPTION OF THE DISORDER

The term spina bifida refers to a separation of the bones in the spinal column. Spina bifida is often accompanied by myelomeningocele, a fluid-filled sac that protrudes from the malformed spine, containing the spinal cord. A portion of the spinal cord is visible at birth, and the nerve development below the opening is incomplete, resulting in variable paralysis and absence of sensation. Spina bifida with myelomeningocele belongs to a family of neural tube defects, which can range from a benign meningocele (protruding sac that surrounds a normal spinal cord, with no resulting neurological deficits) to anencephaly (absence of the brain which is invariably fatal). The sequelae of spina bifida with myelomeningocele include impairments in ambulation, gastrointestinal complications, bowel difficulties and impactions, urinary tract infections (secondary to catheterization) and symptomatic hypercalcemia (causing anorexia nervosa, vomiting, constipation, polyuria, polydypsia).

ETIOLOGY

The cause of neural tube defects is unclear, and therefore prevention and treatment are difficult. It has been hypothesized that there are both environmental and genetic influences involved. Prenatal treatment with folic acid has been successful in preventing recurrences of neural tube defects, and avoidance of antiepileptic drugs during the first trimester of pregnancy decreases the risk of occurrence.

INCIDENCE

The incidence of neural tube defects is approximately 1 per 1,000 births in the United States. The rate of new cases of spina bifida began declining in the 1980s, although the reason remains unclear.

CORRELATES

Children with myelomeningocele tend to have congenital malformations of the brain as well. Arnold-Chiari type II malformation of the hindbrain is a malformation of the brain stem and part of the cerebellum, where both are drawn down toward the neck rather than remaining in the skull. For 60–95 percent of children with myelomeningocele, this displacement interferes with cerebrospinal fluid flow and results in enlarged ventricles (hydrocephalus). Other consequences may include difficulties with breathing, swallowing, vocal cord function, and strabismus (e.g., deviation of eye gaze due to muscle imbalance). The combination of neural tube defect, hydrocephalus, and other neuropathological abnormalities of the brain can result in deficits in mobility, musculoskeletal deformities, spinal malformations, bladder and bowel dysfunction, skin sores, obesity, seizure disorders, and visual (strabismus) and cognitive deficits (one-third usually have mild mental retardation). Decubiti (deep skin lesions) require close monitoring and treatment before infection becomes acute. Chronic pain may be a serious problem related to the extent and level of the lesion, and narcotic analgesics should be avoided.

ASSESSMENT/TREATMENT

Measuring levels of alpha-fetoprotein (AFP) in the mother's amniotic fluid during the second trimester of pregnancy can help detect neural tube defects. High resolution ultrasonography can visualize vertebral malformation. Ultrasound can also be used to diagnose hydrocephalus in newborns with spina bifida.

Closure of the neural tube malformation is usually performed within the first few days of life in order to prevent infection. Unfortunately, this has no effect on neurological functioning. Areas of functioning are impaired based upon the location of the defect on the spine. Some children with spina bifida and associated hydrocephalus demonstrate unusual language and learning problems. Neuropsychological assessment of these children frequently identifies high splinter skills in rote memory, excessive verbal fluency-verbosity, with limited comprehension of general language function. This has often been called "the cocktail party syndrome." These somewhat "cheeky" language styles tend to give false impressions of skill levels; consequently such children should receive extensive neuropsychological assessment.

PROGNOSIS

Survival to adulthood has been estimated at about 85 percent. Earlier mortality is often a function of related brain-shunt malfunctions and kidney damage. Earlier physical and psychological treatment often enhances independence in functional life skills and increases longevity.

See also: Health Care Professionals (General); Individuals with Disabilities Education Act (IDEA); Parenting the Handicapped Child; Speech and Language Assessment;

Further Reading

Liptak, G. S. (1997). Neural tube defects: Spina Bifida and Myelomeningocele. In N. L. Batshaw (Ed.), *Children with disabilities* (pp. 529–552). Baltimore, MD: Paul H. Brookes.
Livneh, H., & Antonak, R. (1997). *Psychosocial adaptation to chronic illness and disability*. Gaithersburg, MD: Aspen.
Web site: Spina Bifida Association of America: http://www.sbaa.org

DENNIS C. HARPER

Spinal Cord Injury

DESCRIPTION OF THE PROBLEM

The spinal cord is primarily a conduit that transmits motor and sensory messages to all parts of the body. Any trauma to the vertebrae can also result in damage to the spinal cord, interfering with nerve impulses throughout the central nervous system and the entire body. Generally speaking, when there is a complete break in the spinal cord, nerve pathways cannot be repaired. Depending on the degree of damage to the cord and the level at which the damage occurs, varying degrees of body function and paralysis are involved. Specifically, damages high to the spinal cord in the cervical region typically result in overall paralysis, or quadriplegia. Assistance with breathing sometimes is necessary. At the midlevel of the cord in the thoracic or chest region, individuals typically have difficulty associated with some use of their arms and/or limited use of their legs. Sexual and bladder functions are obviously affected depending upon the level of the injury to the cord and the degree of cord involvement. Individuals with severe cord separation or transections, may have significant problems with pressure sores (decubitus ulcers) and contractures of various extremities, for example loss of range of motion and fixed deformities of the arms or the legs.

ETIOLOGY

Spinal cord injury can be the result of an injury, a congenital malformation (e.g., myelomeningocele), or the result of infection (e.g., polio virus).

PREVALENCE AMONG CHILDREN

Prevalence varies by age with half of all injuries to the spinal cord occurring in the 16–30-year-old age group, which reportedly has been consistent for the last two decades. Most spinal cord injuries in children occur at the high cervical levels.

PSYCHOLOGICAL CORRELATES

Risk factors for general adjustment are often similar to those factors in long-term chronic illness and mobility-limiting disorders. Premorbid personality, adjustment, and family constellation all impact long-term outcome.

TREATMENT

Physical and occupational therapy is necessary to prevent deformities and increase overall function. Once the physical conditions and neurological status of the individual have been stabilized, attention is directed at increasing general functional independence, providing ongoing psychological support, and exploring the use of assistive-computerized devices to maximize and enhance independence. Further treatment involves cognitive-behavioral techniques emphasizing "reframing," developing coping strategies, and activities that focus on personal autonomy throughout the life-span. Peer-to-peer counseling has also been effective. Sexuality issues will require consultation and periodic review.

PROGNOSIS

Physical changes (return of function) following spinal cord injuries are currently limited. Functional independence is related to early physical therapies and generating an "attitude" of independence.

See also: Health Care Professionals (General); Individuals with Disabilities Education Act (IDEA); Spina Bifida

Further Reading

Dickman, C. A., & Rekate, H. L. (1993). Spinal trauma. In M. R. Eichelberger (Ed.), *Pediatric trauma: Prevention, acute care, rehabilitation* (pp. 362–377). St. Louis, MO: Mosby-Yearbook.

Richards, J. S., Kewman, D. G., & Pierce, C. A. (2000). Spinal cord injury. In R. G. Frank and T. R. Elliott (Eds.), *Handbook of rehabilitation psychology* (pp. 11–28). Washington, DC: American Psychological Association.

Web site: National Spinal Cord Injury Association: http://www.trader.com/users/5010/1020/nscia.html

DENNIS C. HARPER

Spinal Curvatures

See: Scoliosis and Spinal Curvatures

Stealing

DEFINITION/CLINICAL PRESENTATION

Low levels of stealing behavior are exhibited in most youth at different age levels. However, when the behavior becomes more chronic, it may develop into a range of problem activity that meets the diagnosis for Conduct Disorder (CD). The *Diagnostic and Statistical Manual of Mental Disorders, Fourth Edition, Text Revision (DSM-IV-TR)*, describes CD as a persistent pattern of behavior that breaks societal rules. The problem behavior may fall into four main categories. Stealing is listed under the category of "deceitfulness or theft" and includes breaking into a home, building, or car belonging to someone else, lying to obtain goods, and stealing items without confronting the person. There is a distinction made with CD between covert or nonaggressive stealing, such as what is listed above, and overt stealing, where there is stealing and confrontation of the victim. Overt stealing is listed under the CD category of "Aggression to people and animals" with behaviors such as bullying others, engaging in physical fights, being physically cruel to people and animals, and sexual activity without consent.

The *DSM-IV-TR* also includes the disorder of kleptomania within the "Impulse-Control Disorders Not Elsewhere Classified" category. It can be distinguished from CD because it does not include the range of antisocial behaviors associated with CD. Kleptomania is defined as impulsive stealing that is difficult to resist and is associated with an increasing sense of arousal before and relief after it is committed.

INCIDENCE

The incidence of stealing is underreported. This is due, in part, because of the difficulty of knowing when a stealing episode happens. Parents also may not report their children's stealing until it becomes more problematic. Although it has been hypothesized that social desirability may render children's self-reports of stealing inaccurate, past research has not supported this conclusion. Estimates of theft during adolescence have ranged from 4 to 10 percent. Of all persons arrested for robbery in 1999, 25 percent have been identified as juveniles. Stealing makes up approximately 80 percent of the crimes of juvenile delinquents. The incidence of kleptomania is rare, in less than 5 percent of identified shoplifters. It is more common in females.

CORRELATES

Stealing has been associated with several negative outcomes for children and adolescents. These include later academic problems, psychopathology, and delinquency. Distinctions have also been shown between stealing and aggression. Aggression typically is evidenced early in life, heightens during elementary school, and declines by adolescence. Stealing tends to begin in late toddlerhood and increases with age. In addition, stealing has been shown to be a stable characteristic across childhood and adolescence. Theft is strongly associated with other problematic behaviors regarding violations of rules, which is why it is included in the criteria for CD. It appears to be a strong predictor of later antisocial behavior, possibly stronger than aggression. There are also strong associations between the criminal behavior of parents and that of their children.

ASSESSMENT

There are several barriers to obtaining reliable assessment of childhood stealing, including some acceptance by adults of lower incidences of theft, underestimations of the level of severity of the behavior, adults not witnessing the behavior across settings, a lack of official records regarding degrees of stealing behavior, and inconsistency in defining stealing. In addition, developmental norms have not been accepted as to what constitutes stealing and at what point it may become problematic. A number of considerations need to be addressed in obtaining an assessment of stealing. There should be multiple ways of assessing the behavior from different reporters, including measures from adults and the child himself or herself. In general, youths report a lower rate of antisocial behavior than is evident in actual arrest records. The frequency, duration, patterns of stealing, number of settings, and who the items are stolen

from should also be examined. In addition, it should be assessed if the stealing occurs in isolation or amongst a range of inappropriate behaviors. If there is a range of antisocial behaviors, then CD should be considered.

The antecedents of the event also need to be examined such as environmental events, stressors, and association with negative peers. In addition, consequences that may reinforce the behavior should be assessed, including tangible consequences of gaining something as well as social attention or status from a peer group. Factors related to the setting in which the behavior occurs can have a significant influence such as adult monitoring, free time without adult monitoring, community acceptance of behavior, and familial factors (i.e., low parental involvement, parent–child warmth, and high parent–child conflict). These factors can play an important role in determining the causes of the behavior and in guiding treatment plans. For example, if the child is deprived of basic needs such as food, the stealing behavior can be ruled out as a conduct problem and viewed more accurately as a method of meeting basic physiological needs.

TREATMENT

There have been different strategies identified for the prevention of stealing in children and adolescents, as well as treatment of stealing once it becomes problematic. It is important that stealing be defined appropriately in order to identify and consequence the behavior appropriately. Treatment programs generally specify that consistent consequences should be given for the problematic behaviors, and that new target behaviors should be reinforced in the child. In addition, systemic interventions should be used if multiple areas are identified as playing a role in the stealing, such as clearly defined rules at home and school around appropriate behaviors, monitoring of behavior by adult caregivers, and/or a change in the child's peer group that may promote positive behavior and/or attitudes toward school. Some programs discuss more specific steps such as having the perpetrator apologize for the theft and pay restitution for the item, whether it is returning the stolen item, replacing it, and/or replacing it with one of the perpetrator's own items. It is also important to monitor the effectiveness of the interventions once they are put into place.

When a child or adolescent exhibits a range of conduct problems that get them into legal trouble, more systemic interventions, such as multisystemic treatment can be effective.

PROGNOSIS

While little research has been done on the developmental course of stealing behavior, the prognosis for children who steal may depend on frequency/severity of the stealing behavior, as well as their associations with negative peers who engage in antisocial behavior. In addition, if the youth displays a range of antisocial behaviors, this may be predictive of future problem behaviors. Youth with early-onset CD are more likely to have persistent difficulties through adolescence and into adulthood.

See also: Conduct Disorder; Delinquent Behavior; Family Intervention; Multisystemic Therapy

Further Reading

American Psychiatric Association. (2000). *Diagnostic and statistical manual of mental disorders* (4th ed., text revision). Washington, DC: Author.

Mash, E. J., & Barkley, R. A. (Eds.). (1996). *Child psychopathology.* New York: Guilford.

Miller, G. E., & Klungness, L. (1989). Childhood theft: A comprehensive review of assessment and treatment. *School Psychology Review, 18,* 82–97.

Tremblay, G. C., & Drabman, R. S. (1997). An intervention for childhood stealing. *Child and Family Behavior Therapy, 19,* 33–40.

U.S. Department of Health and Human Services. (2001). *Youth violence: A report of the Surgeon General.* Rockville, MD: U.S. Department of Health and Human Services, Centers for Disease Control and Prevention, National Center for Injury Prevention and Control; Substance Abuse and Mental Health Services Administration, Center for Mental Health Services; and National Institutes of Health, National Institute of Mental Health.

JULIANNE M. SMITH
STEPHEN LASSEN

Step-Parents

See: Adoption

Stereotypic Movement Disorder

DEFINITION

Stereotypic movement disorder (SMD) is a diagnostic classification of motor behavior that is repetitive, often seemingly driven, has no apparent purpose, markedly interferes with normal activities, can result in self-inflicted bodily harm and is not better accounted for by a compulsion (as in Obsessive Compulsive Disorder [OCD]), a tic (as in a Tic Disorder [TD]), a stereotypy that is part of a Pervasive Developmental Disorder (PDD), or hair pulling (as in trichotillomania). The behavior also must not be due to the direct physiological effects of a substance or a medical condition and must have persisted for at least 4 weeks. Examples of these motor behaviors include repeated movements of the arms, legs, head, fingers, and/or hands, and even the trunk of the body. The behaviors may also involve the manipulation of objects (e.g., repetitively waving a piece of cloth or a stick).

INCIDENCE

Limited information is available on the incidence of SMD across the age span, no age of onset has been established, and information specific to children is unavailable. Much more information is available on stereotypic movements in general. Stereotypic behavior appears in 80 percent of healthy, well-adjusted infants as part of normal development and generally disappears or changes into an appropriate form by age 4. Self-injurious stereotypic type behaviors occur in 2–3 percent in children and adolescents with mental retardation living in the community and in a much higher percentage of children who live in institutions. Stereotypic behavior is also very common in children with sensory deficits or motor impairments (e.g., blindness or deafness).

PSYCHOLOGICAL CORRELATES

Limited information is available on the correlates of SMD, in part because of a limited scientific literature and in part because stereotypy accompanies such a large range of other disorders (e.g., compulsions, tics, substance abuse, schizophrenia, mental retardation syndromes, habit disorders, general medical conditions, and many others). Although not well-documented, extrapolation from the literature on social relations suggests that increased social distance and even outright rejection may accompany frequent, exaggerated, seemingly nonfunctional repetitive physical movements. Additionally, stereotypy can lead to actual self-injury.

ETIOLOGY

There is no widely accepted causal account of stereotypic behavior, although several have been nominated in the scientific literature. For example, stereotypic responding can be produced in infants raised in social isolation, suggesting that early relationships with care-givers may be involved. Environmental consequences have been shown to be functionally related to stereotypy, suggesting behavioral/learning causes. Relationships between neurochemical systems (e.g., dopaminergic, serotonergic) and stereotypy have also been demon-strated, suggesting a biological basis. Stereotypy is also sometimes exhibited in response to stress and can also accompany and/or follow painful medical conditions (e.g., headaches, ear infections) especially in children with mental retardation. More generally, stereotypy is much more common in children with handicapping conditions, especially mental retardation, than other-wise normal children, although the reasons for the increase are not clear.

ASSESSMENT

The most widely used means of assessment involves direct observation. The most informative observational systems attempt to determine what happens before and after the emission of stereotypic behaviors (i.e., func-tional assessment). Medical assessments are also used to reveal the extent of self-injury, if present.

TREATMENT

Behavioral treatments or treatments that target the actual stereotypic behaviors (rather than medical or psychological conditions that may be involved) are among the most typically used methods. The most effective of these involve strategic modifications of events that precede and follow the target behaviors and that increase motivation for appropriate alternatives. Effectiveness is further increased when the components of treatment are identified using an analysis of the events that have a contingent relation with the targets (i.e., functional analysis). Drug treatments are also used either alone or in conjunction with behavioral approaches. These typically involve antipsychotics, anti-depressants, or selective serotonin reuptake inhibitors. Although evaluative research suggests that behavioral treatments are often more effective than drug therapy and are much less likely to involve unpleasant side effects, medication can be an important adjunct to treatment.

PROGNOSIS

Untreated stereotypic movements appear to peak during the adolescent years and gradually (but steadily) decline over the life span thereafter. Individuals with mental retardation may have chronic stereotypy that changes more in terms of form (e.g., from finger biting to head slapping) than frequency. Developmentally inappropriate stereotypy almost always disappears as children move through developmental stages. Stereotypy in individuals with sensory deficits (e.g., "blindisms") may remain in their repertoire throughout life but not (or rarely) result in dysfunction or self-injury. Prognosis for treated stereotypy varies from reduced frequency to complete elimination.

See also: Habit Reversal; Mental Retardation; Obsessive Compulsive Disorder; Tic Disorders: Tourette's Disorder, Chronic Tic Disorder, and Transient Tic Disorder

Further Reading

American Psychiatric Association. (2000). *Diagnostic and Statistical manual of mental disorders* (4 ed., text revision). Washington, DC: Author.
LaGrow, S. J., & Repp, A. C. (1984). Stereotypic responding: A review of intervention research. *American Journal of Mental Deficiency, 88*(6), 595–609.
Stein, D. J., & Christenson, G. A. (Eds.). (1998). Stereotypic movement disorders. *Psychiatric Annals, 28*(6).
Thelen, E. (1979). Rhythmic stereotypies in normal human infants. *Animal Behaviour, 27*, 699–715.

KENNETH R. MACALEESE
PATRICK C. FRIMAN

Stimulants

See: Pharmacological Interventions

Storage Diseases

DEFINITION

The term storage disease or metabolic disorder is used to represent a large and diverse group of rare, primarily autosomal recessive genetic disorders in which a normal hydrolytic enzyme is inactive. These enzymes, located in an area of the cell called the lysosome, normally facilitate digestion of the products of cell metabolism; but when inactive, these metabolic products remain undigested in the cell, eventually overloading the lyso-some, changing the structure of the cell, either interfering with its function or destroying it. Because of the active nature of the lysosomes in blood cells, these cells are particularly vulnerable to storage disease. The specific symptoms, time of onset, and prognosis of any particular disorder depends on (1) what enzyme is affected, (2) what specific byproducts are involved, (3) what specific cells are affected by the inactivity of these enzymes, and (4) the age of the child at the time of onset of symptoms.

There are several categories of storage disease, with a number of identifiable specific disorders. These include the *sphingolipidoses* (e.g., Gaucher's disease, Tay Sach's disease, leukodystrophy, Krabbe's syndrome, Niemann–Pick disease, Sandhoff disease, Farber's disease, gangliosidosis), the *mucopolysaccharidoses* (Hurler's disease, Hunter's disease, Scheies' disease, Sanfillippo disease, Marquio's syndrome, and Sly's disease), the *mucolipidoses* (sialidoses, mucolipidoses, fucosidosis, alpha-mannosidosis, beta-mannosidosis, aspartylglucosaminuria), the *acid lipase deficiencies* (Wolman's disease, Cholesterol Ester Storage disease), and the *neuronal ceroid lipofuscinoses* (Haltia–Sanavuori syndrome, Jansky–Bielschowsky syndrome, Spielmeyer–Sjögren syndrome, Kufs' disease, Boehme's disease). Each category and specific disorder is characterized by a specific enzyme deficiency, leading to storage of a specific cellular metabolic by-product, disrupting a specific type or group of cells, and resulting in a group of symptoms that define each disorder.

INCIDENCE

The incidence of the storage diseases is very rare, but specific incidence depends on the specific disorder. Some are highly concentrated in specific ethnic groups (e.g., Gaucher's disease or Tay-Sachs disease, where the incidence is $1:350$ to $1:450$ live births for subsets of individuals of Jewish heritage from Eastern Europe, but in the general population is only $1:40,000$ to $1:60,000$ live births). Others are not ethnicity-specific, but occur in between $1:50,000$ and $1:100,000$ live births.

DIAGNOSIS

Diagnosis of storage disease is made on the basis of clinical presentation, followed by specific biochemical studies. Blood enzyme testing of affected individuals and family members is usually used to determine the hereditary pattern in carriers. Public, statewide newborn screening using blood samples is in place for some of the storage diseases (e.g., Tay-Sachs). For parents who are heterozygotes (carriers), amniocentesis may be performed to establish a prenatal diagnosis. More precise screening using mass spectrophotometry is beginning to be used

for large screening programs, but it is likely that these techniques will soon be replaced by precise genetic polymerase chain reaction (PCR) techniques or DNA-microarray studies.

CLINICAL SYMPTOMS

As noted earlier, the clinical symptoms associated with the storage disease depend on what enzyme is inactive, what metabolic by-products are stored, and what cells are involved. There are variations in severity and timing for this complex group of diseases. The more common clinical symptoms associated with each category of storage disease are recognizable facial features and enlarged liver and spleen (hepatosplenomegaly). Most of the sphingolipidoses, gangliosidoses, and some of the mucopolysaccharidoses involve the central nervous system, with severe developmental delay in most very young children. Some of the mucopolysaccharidoses and gangliosidoses also result in progressive neurologic deterioration, and may include seizures and blindness. Another common symptom of the mucopolysaccharidoses and mucolipidoses is connective tissue disease, with contractures of the joints, disfigurement, and corneal clouding. In general, more severe and progressive symptoms occur in children with earlier onset of the disease.

TREATMENT

The most effective treatment of storage disease involves identification of parental carriers and counseling for pregnancy prevention. Prenatal screening with elective termination of pregnancy when storage disease is confirmed is also an option. Since the course of each disease is different, and since individuals with variants of the same disease may experience different symptom severity and timing of symptoms, management of symptoms and alleviation of distress whenever possible should be standard care. Symptomatic treatment of feeding problems, management of chronic constipation, protecting the skin from ulcerations, and control of seizures with antiseizure medications is recommended for affected children. Physical therapy and orthopedic intervention may be helpful for children with connective tissue disease. An emphasis on early educational intervention and stimulation is essential, as is psychosocial support for parents and unaffected siblings.

Primary, curative treatment is still not generally available. Enzyme replacement therapy has been investigated, but the short half-life of the enzymes has led to disappointment. Solid organ transplantation (e.g., liver, spleen, kidney) has been successful in the short-term, but has thus far not produced long-term benefit. Perhaps the most promising approaches to treatment involve bone marrow or umbilical cord blood transplantation, or some of the evolving gene therapies. However, these approaches are still at the stage of careful clinical trial investigation, and are not generally offered as a recommended treatment option. Support for parents making decisions to participate in these trials is necessary to insure that they fully understand the experimental nature of the treatment, the risks involved, and the potential for earlier death due to the known complications of these approaches.

PROGNOSIS

The natural history of the storage diseases is that children with early disease progression usually die before age 3, and sometimes within the first year of life. Children with later-onset disease, or more mild forms of the disease may live into late school age or early adolescence. For a few disorders with late onset, survival into young adulthood may be possible. The prognosis of children treated with evolving bone marrow transplantation or gene therapies is unknown.

See also: Behavioral Genetics; Bleeding Disorders; Bone Marrow Failure and Primary Immunodeficiency; Cognitive Development; Failure-to-Thrive; Glycogen Storage Disease; Orthopedic Disabilities; Visual Impairment: Low Vision and Blindness

Further Reading

Kolodny, E. H., & Lebron, D. (1998). Storage diseases of the reticuloendothelial system. In D. G. Nathan & S. H. Orkin (Eds.), *Nathan and Oski's hematology of infancy and childhood* (pp. 1461–1507). Philadelphia: W.B. Saunders.

Rezvani, I. (2000). Defects in metabolism of amino acids. In R. E. Behrman, R. M. Kleigman, & H. B. Jenson (Eds.), *Nelson textbook of pediatrics* (16th ed., pp. 344–377). Philadelphia: W.B. Saunders.

Stanley, C. A. (2000). Defects in metabolism of lipids. In R. E. Behrman, R. M. Kleigman, & H. B. Jenson (Eds.), *Nelson textbook of pediatrics* (16th ed., pp. 377–380). Philadelphia: W.B. Saunders.

F. DANIEL ARMSTRONG

Stress Management

DEFINITIONS

Stress management refers to those techniques employed for the purpose of teaching children strategies to prevent, reduce, and cope with specific environmental stressors. Environmental stressors might include an acute or chronic illness and associated morbidities (e.g., neuropsychological impairments associated with sickle cell disease), the family environment and the way in which the family is able to garner resources necessary to cope with a specific stressor, social supports available to the individual or the family, and specific psychosocial stressors including major life events (e.g., death of a caregiver) and daily hassles associated with a major stressor (e.g., frequent physician appointments).

The role of individual differences has been conceptualized as an essential ingredient to understanding psychological components of stress. Core to explaining children's and adolescents' response to stress is the appreciation for their unique appraisals when negotiating specific stressors. For example, we know that there are individual differences in children's cognitive appraisals of stress as well as differences in coping strategies for managing specific stressors. Thus, some children and their caregivers manage stress by means of specific problem-solving, while others may manage stress by avoiding thoughts associated with the specific stressor. In addition, some have posited specific theoretical models for understanding stress that include a consideration of both environmental factors (i.e., severity and frequency of the stressor, social-ecological factors—social support, parental adjustment, daily hassles), individual risk factors (i.e., family history of psychopathology, chronic illness), and resilience (i.e., strong social support, spiritual affiliation/involvement).

METHODOLOGY/EFFECTIVENESS

The therapeutic modalities that have served to modify stress-enhancing behavior in children and adolescents include problem-solving training, relaxation training, guided imagery, social-skills training, time management, and lifestyle improvement. Other psychological interventions that have proved efficacious in the management of stress include supportive psychotherapy, cognitive therapy, and family therapy. In fact, in a careful review of treatment interventions for diminishing stress and enhancing coping behaviors among adolescents who have been classified as substance misusers, Crome (1999) cogently concluded that there is no one particular treatment approach, nor a particular component of a treatment, that has yielded the most beneficial results in reducing stress. Rather, Crome (1999) concluded that engagement of children, adolescents, and their families in a long-term therapeutic relationship is frequently the mechanism by which stress is reduced.

In recent years, there have been studies examining the role of specific approaches for the purpose of reducing stress and thereby enhancing adjustment and adaptation to specific stressors. For example, Chang (2001) examined the influence of social problem-solving as a moderator and mediator of life stress on suicidal ideation in adolescents attending high school. Findings revealed that life stress, coupled with social problem-solving, predicted a significant amount of the variance in suicidal ideation. Thus, when adolescents who had suicidal ideation were able to employ problem-solving techniques as a means of managing stressful situations, they were less at risk for suicidal behavior. Most importantly, however, support was provided for the notion that social problem-solving mediates or decreases the influence of life stress on adolescents who were originally designated to be suicidal. Social problem-solving in this particular investigation refers to a specific cognitive–affective–behavioral process that is self-generated and helps the individual to develop an effective means of coping with everyday problematic living situations and events.

In another recent investigation, Hewson-Bower and Drummond (2001) examined the effect of guided imagery on stress management and relaxation in children with a history of greater than 10 respiratory tract infections over a 12-month period. The stress management training was geared toward decreasing school, family, and peer problems for the purpose of diminishing symptoms associated with anxiety, depression, and aggression, and concomitantly enhancing self-esteem and mood. The intervention was delivered over the course of three sessions. In the first session, children were asked to identify those negative emotional experiences that elicited negative affectivity or emotion. During the second session, children were asked to identify problem situations and choose a solvable problem to work on in future sessions. In the final session, the therapist and the children discussed solutions to problems as well as positive emotional experiences. Between sessions, children were asked to (1) record experiences that elicited negative emotions; (2) record how they responded to negative experiences; and finally, (3) asked to rehearse solving important problems and to record emotional experiences during that process.

Dependent measures in the Hewson-Bower and Drummond (2001) investigation included (1) measures of immune functioning, (2) personality and mood profiles, and (3) family satisfaction. Although no differences were found in the frequency of upper respiratory tract

infections between the treatment and wait-list control conditions, episodes of respiratory infection were shorter in the stress management treatment condition than in the wait-list condition. Moreover, improvements in psychological adjustment were found to persist at 1-year follow-up evaluation. This investigation is important as it underscores the critical role of stress management on both psychological variables as well as important immunological and health variables.

In summary, stress management refers to the variety of techniques employed for the purpose of effectively navigating daily and chronic stressors. While numerous techniques are available, the relationship between the client and the therapist is imperative for successful intervention. It is also noteworthy that the effect of environmental stress on the emotional and physical functioning of children and adolescents has been well-documented. While individual differences in the processing of stress also have been well-documented in the extant literature, the benefits of reducing stress are universal. Specifically, alleviation of stress has been demonstrated to yield significant improvements in the physical and emotional well-being and enhancing quality of life for children and adolescents.

See also: Adolescent Health; Coping with Illness; Problem-Solving Assessment; Quality of Life

Further Reading

Chang, E. (2001). Predicting suicide ideation in an adolescent population: Examining the role of social problem solving as a moderator and a mediator. *Personality and Individual Differences, 32,* 1279–1291.

Crome, I. (1999). Treatment interventions—looking towards the millennium. *Drug and Alcohol Dependence, 55,* 247–263.

Hewson-Bower, B., & Drummond, P. (2001). Psychological treatment for recurrent symptoms of colds and flu in children. *Journal of Psychosomatic Research, 51,* 369–377.

Wallander, J., & Thompson, R. (1995). Psychosocial adjustment in children with chronic physical conditions. In M. Roberts (Ed.), *Handbook of pediatric psychology* (2nd ed., pp. 124–141). New York: Guilford.

RONALD T. BROWN
LLOYD A. TAYLOR

Structured Diagnostic Interview

See: Interviewing

Stuttering

DEFINITION

Stuttering is characterized by a dysfluency (interruption of the normal rhythm) of speech. Stuttering manifests itself through the repetition, prolongation, or blocking of words and phrases in an atypical manner.

Core fluency behaviors are repetitions (repeated sound or word), prolongations (the extension of a sound or word), and blocks (cessation of speech with struggle behaviors). This is the beginning of a dysfluent episode. Secondary behaviors that can exacerbate the condition include: anxiety regarding speaking, tension, and the presence of interrupter devices ("tic-like" behaviors that the speaker uses to escape from a block or repetition; Roth & Worthington, 1996). These secondary behaviors can take a life of their own and further cause the speaker to have difficulty speaking even during periods of fluent speech. These concomitant features, or secondary behaviors, are often associated with stuttering.

CAUSES

The cause of stuttering has not been determined, although there are many theories regarding its etiology. The most common form of stuttering is developmental stuttering. It is described as the normal dysfluencies that occur as the speaker attempts to coordinate thoughts in conjunction with motor movements required for speech. The second form of stuttering is an acquired fluency disorder. It can be caused by trauma, stress, or possibly be of medical origin. It is more rare and occurs following the acquisition of otherwise unimpaired speech.

INCIDENCE

About 80 percent of all people that stutter spontaneously recover (Lawrence & Barclay, 1998). Individuals who stutter comprise about 1 percent of the population. More males than females stutter by a ratio of 4 : 1.

WARNING SIGNS AND SYMPTOMS

As stated earlier, many children display normal dysfluencies between the ages of 2 and 5. As a young speaker learns to master the art of speech, stuttering is often observed and is not a cause for alarm. If dysfluencies only occur during times of extreme anxiety or excitement, they are less likely to be a serious dysfunction. However, if stuttering occurs during everyday events with an absence of emotion it is beneficial to monitor dysfluencies and decide if other warning signs indicate a more serious condition.

Stuttering becomes a concern when the incidence of stuttering increases, secondary behaviors are present, the individual becomes aware of dysfluencies, it influences communication exchanges and the use of vowel substitutions, and if dysfluencies occur in more than 10 percent of words spoken (Van Riper, 1982). If this occurs, then a consultation with a speech–language pathologist is recommended.

APPROACHES TO ASSESSMENT

Assessment can include both formal and informal approaches. The following formal evaluation measures are often used to gather quantitative information that can further guide treatment: *The Stocker Probe for Fluency* (Third Edition), *Stuttering Severity Instrument for Children and Adults* (Third Edition), and the *Cooper Personalized Fluency Control Therapy* (Third Edition). They also offer qualitative information that aids in diagnosing stuttering. Informal evaluation measures include speech samples, observation of stuttering (including observation of secondary behaviors), parent report, patient questionnaires, medical history, and family history. All of these measures emphasize qualitative information that allows a view into extraneous factors that may impact the speaker. They also can aid in ruling out extraneous etiologies that could contribute to dysfluencies (e.g., aphasia, head injuries, etc.).

Assessment allows for an individualized plan of care that is based on responses to informal as well as formal evaluation tools.

TREATMENT INTERVENTIONS

After completion of a thorough examination, areas of concern are targeted. There are fundamentally two basic targets of therapy: easier stuttering (stuttering modifications) and changing the patterns of speech (fluency shaping). Overall, the goal of treatment is to allow the speaker to communicate more effectively with others.

RESOURCES

A speech–language pathologist is trained to perform assessment measures and to aid patients to develop strategies to facilitate easier communication. It may be beneficial to contact the American Speech–Language Hearing Association (A.S.H.A.) to contact a qualified speech–language pathologist in your area. The A.S.H.A. also has special interest divisions that specialize in fluency issues. A.S.H.A. can be reached via Web site at http://www.asha.org or by the toll-free Action Center hotline at 1-800-498-2071. The Stuttering Foundation of America can be accessed using the following website address: http://www.stuttersfa.org/. It contains valuable information that can be used by anyone interested in this communication disorder. The National Stuttering Association is another resource. It provides for membership into the organization, workshop information, and facts about stuttering. It is geared for both professionals and laypersons. It can be accessed at http://www.nsastutter.org/.

Each of these resources contains links to other sources that may be helpful. The key to intervention is early assessment. If stuttering is a concern, it is recommended that an assessment be initiated as soon as possible to evaluate if there is a true communication disorder.

See also: Mixed Receptive–Expressive Language Disorder; Phonological and Articulation Disorders

Further Reading

Lawrence, M., & Barclay, D. (1998). Stuttering: A brief review. *American Family Physician, 57,* 2175–2179.
Roth, F., & Worthington, C. (1996). *Treatment resource manual for speech–language pathology.* San Diego: Singular.

Van Riper, C. (1982). *The nature of stuttering.* Prospect Heights, Illinois: Waveland Press.

SHALONDA WILLIAMS

Substance Abuse

DEFINITION AND PREVALENCE

Experimentation with substances is common during adolescence. By age 17, about 50 percent of adolescents have experimented with alcohol or cigarettes at least once. Concerns arise, however, when adolescents exhibit regular and frequent use of these illicit substances, or when adolescents begin using illicit drugs including marijuana, cocaine, crack, heroin, hallucinogens, stimulants, inhalants, and so forth. In general, these types of substance use patterns in adolescence indicate a substance use disorder which can encompass diagnostic symptoms of abuse or dependence, as noted by the American Academy of Child and Adolescent Psychiatry in a report published in 1997.

Cigarettes, alcohol, and marijuana are by far the most commonly abused substances among adolescents. Table 1 presents estimates of the prevalence of cigarette, binge alcohol (i.e., five or more drinks on a single occasion), and marijuana use in the past month among 12–14 and 15–17-year-olds in the United States. It is evident from Table 1 that substance use in the past month is much more likely among older adolescents, and that substance abuse in this age group is fairly prevalent. Table 1 indicates that nearly one in four adolescents age 15–17 uses cigarettes each month, about one in six engages in binge drinking, and more than one in ten uses marijuana.

Table 1. Prevalence of Cigarette, Binge Alcohol, and Marijuana Use in the Past Month among 12–14 and 15–17-Year-Old Adolescents

| | Substance use frequency | | | | | |
| | Age 12–14 | | | Age 15–17 | | |
Type of substance use	No use in past month	Used one day in past month	Used multiple days in past month	No use in past month	Used one day in past month	Used multiple days in past month
Cigarette	93.7 (10.9)	1.6 (0.2)	4.7 (0.5)	76.8 (8.9)	3.0 (0.4)	20.1 (2.3)
Binge alcohol	96.6 (11.2)	1.7 (0.2)	1.7 (0.2)	82.9 (9.6)	5.5 (0.6)	11.6 (1.3)
Marijuana	97.4 (11.3)	0.7 (0.08)	2.0 (0.2)	88.2 (10.2)	2.1 (0.2)	9.8 (1.1)

Note: The first number in each cell indicates the percentage of adolescents in each substance use category. The number in parentheses is the total number of adolescents (in millions) in each substance use category.

Source: *2000 National Household Survey on Drug Abuse* (2001).

Moreover, among adolescents who report using substances in the past month, the majority engages in such use more than one day per month. This group of regular and frequent substance users is at especially high risk for developing long-term substance abuse and dependence which may include the use of other illicit drugs. It is estimated that 11.8 percent of adolescents between ages 12 and 17 (2.7 million) have used an illicit drug other than marijuana in the past year. Moreover, 5.8 percent of adolescents in the United States (1.4 million) have met diagnostic criteria for alcohol or illicit drug dependence in the past year.

CLINICAL FEATURES AND CORRELATES

Adolescents with substance use disorders are characterized by an array of psychosocial symptoms. Antisocial attitudes and behavior including aggression and delinquency are typical presenting features of adolescent substance abuse. Mood disturbances such as anxiety and depression are also common. Adolescent substance abuse is often marked as well by a deterioration in school performance, including truancy and academic failure. High-risk behaviors including promiscuous and unprotected sex, driving while intoxicated, and suicidal ideation may also signal an adolescent substance abuse problem.

Substance abuse during adolescence is commonly viewed as both a cause and a consequence of abnormal or disrupted developmental processes. As such, adolescent substance abuse has been linked with a variety of factors known to compromise normal child and adolescent development. Substance abuse risk factors within the family include high levels of conflict, weak relational attachments, poor communication, inept discipline and behavior management practices, and parental or sibling substance use and psychopathology. Physical, sexual, or emotional abuse within the family are risk factors as well. Additionally, peer groups typically play a major role in adolescent substance abuse. Affiliating with peers who engage in substance use and other types of deviant behavior dramatically increases the risk for substance abuse among adolescents. Female adolescents in particular are prone to abuse substances within the context of romantic or sexual relationships with older male peers. On an individual level, substance abuse is pronounced among adolescents who perceive low levels of risk and high degrees of social acceptance associated with substance use. Furthermore, as noted above, youth manifesting psychological and emotional problems are at elevated risk for substance

abuse. Such problems may include Conduct Disorder (CD), hyperactivity, depression, anxiety, antisocial personality characteristics, learning and cognitive dysfunction, and temperamental traits associated with disinhibition and sensation-seeking. Finally, evidence from twin and adoption studies suggests that genetics and heredity may play a role in the onset of substance abuse in adolescence.

ASSESSMENT

A consensus has been achieved in the adolescent substance abuse treatment field regarding the importance of a comprehensive and multifaceted approach to clinical assessment. By and large, adolescent substance abuse assessment guidelines prescribe the use of research-based screening and diagnostic instruments which may be coupled with toxicology screening methods. Diagnostic measures should be administered within the context of a comprehensive assessment interview with both the adolescent and family. Substance use assessment interviews should cover a wide range of drug use and associated problem behaviors, as well as key domains of adolescent functioning including emotional and cognitive functioning, family relationships, school involvement, and peer relationships. In addition, substance abuse screening interviews should explore health and medical histories, developmental milestones and transitions, family history of substance abuse, previous treatment for substance abuse and mental health, adolescent and family legal involvements, adolescent sexual and HIV-related practices, suicidality, and physical and sexual abuse history. Excellent guidelines for conducting adolescent and family assessment interviews are provided in *Principles of Addiction Medicine* (2nd ed.) (1998).

TREATMENT AND PROGNOSIS

Treatment for adolescent substance abuse is offered in a variety of settings most typically including inpatient facilities, residential treatment centers, and outpatient clinics. Home- and community-based treatments are also emerging. Inpatient treatment programs are typically brief (up to 6 weeks) and offer a comprehensive range of services including individual, group, and family counseling; medication; and educational, vocational, and recreational services. Many such programs include an Alcoholics Anonymous component. Along similar lines, residential treatments place the adolescent in a highly structured and regimented group living environment, albeit for a longer duration (6–12 months or more). A typical day consists of resident meetings, house chores, school attendance, a range of therapeutic group activities, individual counseling, recreation, and so on. The objective of residential treatment is to utilize peer group bonding as a mechanism for teaching and reinforcing beliefs, attitudes, values, skills, and behaviors consistent with drug-free living.

Most outpatient clinical settings offer a range of individual, group, and family therapies for adolescent substance abuse. Individual- and group-based approaches typically revolve around principles of cognitive–behavior therapy and attempt to impact attitudes, beliefs, cognitions, and behaviors that reinforce substance abuse. Individual- and group-based cognitive–behavioral interventions involve psychosocial skill-building, communication training, and behavior change techniques. In contrast to the individual focus of cognitive–behavioral approaches, family therapy approaches view adolescent substance abuse as embedded within the context of the family, given that it is the primary arena for adolescent development. Family therapists work conjointly with the adolescent and family members to orchestrate functional changes in family organization, communication, and interaction that are consistent with healthy adolescent development. An emerging group of so-called multisystemic family-based treatments encompasses systems beyond the family including schools, the legal system, social service organizations, vocational services, churches, recreation centers, youth development organizations, and others. Multisystemic family-based therapists typically administer treatment in the home or other setting within the adolescent's social environment. The goal of multisystemic family-based therapy is to work in a coordinated manner with the adolescent, family, school, and members of other systems to reshape the adolescent's environment in a way that promotes adaptive functioning and reduces the risk of substance abuse.

The effectiveness of adolescent substance abuse treatment has been evaluated in several large-scale community-based studies. Across the board, existing studies indicate that adolescents tend to use drugs less frequently and severely after receiving treatment. Furthermore, it has been established that adolescents who complete treatment exhibit greater improvements than those who exit treatment prematurely. Although many adolescents maintain improvements in drug use well after treatment termination, complete abstinence is rare and treatment relapse is relatively high (most estimates of relapse are around 50 percent which is sim-

ilar to rates of relapse for adults). Although adolescents generally appear to improve after receiving substance abuse treatment, it has yet to be established whether any specific form of treatment is more effective than any other. Nor is there yet any scientific basis for matching certain types of adolescents with certain types of treatments. A few university-based controlled experimental studies suggest that family therapy and multisystemic family-based interventions may be more effective than various forms of individual and group treatment. However, this effect is yet to be demonstrated in community treatment settings.

See also: Adolescence; Adolescent Assessment; Cigarette Smoking; Cognitive-Behavior Therapy; Multisystemic Therapy; Risk and Protective Factors

Further Reading

American Academy of Child Adolescent Psychiatry. (1997). Practice parameters for the assessment and treatment of children and adolescents with substance use disorders. *Journal of the American Academy of Child and Adolescent Psychiatry, 36(10),* 140S–156S.

American Society of Addiction Medicine. (1998). *Principles of addiction medicine.* Chevy Chase, MD: Author.

Center for Substance Abuse Treatment. http://www.samhsa.gov/centers/csat2002/csat_frame.html

Essau, C. (Ed.). (2002). *Substance abuse and dependence in adolescence.* London: Harwood Academic.

National Institute on Drug Abuse. http://www.nida.nih.gov

Substance Abuse and Mental Health Services Administration. (2001). *Summary of findings from the 2000 National Household Survey on Drug Abuse.* Office of Applied Studies. (NHSDA Series H-13, DHHS Publication No. (SMA) 01-3549). Rockville, MD.

Wagner, E. F., & Waldron, H. (Eds.). (2001). *Innovations in adolescent substance abuse interventions.* New York: Pergamon.

TIMOTHY J. OZECHOWSKI

HOLLY WALDRON

Sudden Infant Death Syndrome

DEFINITION

Sudden Infant Death Syndrome (SIDS) represents both a family tragedy and a medical enigma. This is evident in the definition of SIDS developed by the National Institute of Child Health and Human Development: "The sudden death of an infant under 1 year of age, which remains unexplained after a thorough case investigation, including performance of a complete autopsy, examination of the death scene, and review of the clinical history" (Willinger, James, & Catz, 1991, 681). The unusual nature of a medical definition that includes the ruling out of a crime makes the psychosocial impact of this syndrome particularly profound. A phenomenon that is often discussed in conjunction with SIDS is the "apparent life-threatening event" (ALTE) defined as "an episode in which the infant has clinical symptoms that are frightening to the observer, in some cases to the degree that the observer fears the infant has died" (Farrell, Weiner, & Lemons, 2002). After much debate, the consensus is that such events should not be considered "near-miss SIDS" because of the lack of evidence of an association between the two phenomena (Farrell, Weiner, & Lemons, 2002), yet this concept may be difficult for families to accept.

INCIDENCE/CORRELATES

Though SIDS still ranks as the third leading cause of death in infants, the rate of SIDS has declined more than 40 percent during the 1990s to a rate of 64.1 per 100,000 live births; the greatest risk of death is between 3 and 5 months of age for full-term infants (Farrell, Weiner, & Lemons, 2002). The steep decline is thought to be attributable to the behavioral intervention of educating parents to put infants to sleep on their backs. According to the American Academy of Pediatrics, "The following have been consistently identified across studies as independent risk factors for SIDS: prone sleep position, sleeping on a soft surface, maternal smoking during pregnancy, overheating, late or no prenatal care, young maternal age, prematurity and/or low birth weight, and male sex. Blacks and American Indians have consistently high rates, 2 to 3 times the national average" (American Academy of Pediatrics, 2000, p. 650).

ASSESSMENT

The diagnosis of SIDS, essentially one of exclusion, requires the elimination of many other medical explanations, such as sepsis, aspiration, cardiac disease, toxic exposure (including to cocaine and other illicit drugs), and also of homicide by a caretaker. Making this determination necessitates not only a postmortem examination but also a careful medicolegal investigation (Committee on Child Abuse and Neglect, 1994). This requires well-trained first responders and close collaboration between medical and law enforcement personnel, as well as great

sensitivity to devastated families who often feel immense guilt regardless of the cause of death.

INTERVENTION

Obviously, the only intervention for SIDS itself is prevention, and in this area there has been enormous progress. After some initial controversy, the recommendation that parents put their babies to sleep on their backs achieved international acceptance in the mid-1990s, and campaigns to encourage not only parents but also day care workers to follow this practice have been undertaken. Initial hopes that home monitoring of infant breathing would be helpful in SIDS prevention have not been borne out, as they have never been shown to affect SIDS rates, although monitors are used for infants with documented apnea due to prematurity or other causes. Bed sharing is another practice that has been examined as a possible risk factor that might be impacted through behavioral change, but except for cases where adult cosleepers are impaired by drugs or alcohol, a relationship between bed sharing and SIDS has not been established (Klonoff-Cohen & Edelstein, 1995). In addition to the supine sleeping position, encouragement of parental smoking cessation and adherence to recommendations for safe sleeping surfaces (i.e., firm bedding without any possibly obstructive objects) currently appear to be the most promising strategies for further risk reduction (Farrell et al., 2002).

Issues related to supine sleeping have arisen in the areas of both physical and motor development. There is some evidence that occipital plagiocephaly (flattening of the back of the head) may have become more common, and some temporary delays in gross motor skills such as sitting have also been observed (American Academy of Pediatrics, 2000). Developmental specialists and pediatricians have begun to counsel parents routinely to ensure that babies receive adequate "tummy time" when awake to minimize these consequences.

After the occurrence of SIDS, families typically suffer shock, grief, and self-blame that has the potential to disrupt all aspects of functioning. Psychological intervention for these families is very important. All families should receive printed materials and the offer of counseling, and most families are likely to benefit from a parent support group focused specifically on SIDS and related infant losses (Horchler & Morris, 1994).

See also: Bereavement; Obstructive Sleep Apnea; Safety and Prevention

Further Reading

American Academy of Pediatrics. Task Force on Infant Sleep Positions and Sudden Infant Death Syndrome. (2000). Changing concepts of sudden infant death syndrome: Implications for infant sleeping environment and sleep position. *Pediatrics, 105,* 650–656.

Committee on Child Abuse and Neglect. (1994). Distinguishing Sudden Infant Death Syndrome from child abuse fatalities. *Pediatrics, 94,* 124–126.

Farrell, P. A., Weiner, G. M., & Lemons, J. A. (2002). SIDS, ALTE, apnea, and the use of home monitors. *Pediatrics in Review, 23,* 3–9.

Horchler, J. D., & Morris, R. R. (1994). *The SIDS survival guide: Information and comfort for grieving family and friends, and professionals who seek to help them.* Hyattsville, MD: SIDS Educational Services.

Klonoff-Cohen, H., & Edelstein, S. L. (1995). Bed sharing and the Sudden Infant Death Syndrome. *British Medical Journal, 311,* 1269–1272.

http://www.sidscenter.org National Sudden Infant Death Resource Center.

Willinger, M., James, L. S., & Catz, C. (1991). Defining the sudden infant death syndrome (SIDS): Deliberations of an expert panel convened by the National Institute of Child Health and Human Development. *Pediatric Pathology, 11,* 677–684.

MELISSA R. JOHNSON

Suicide

DEFINITION/INCIDENCE

Suicidal behavior among children and adolescents is a serious concern. This includes behaviors ranging from ideation (thoughts about death) and intent (wishes to kill oneself) to plans (lethality may vary, based on the child's age and cognitive development), attempts (self-inflicted behavior intended to result in death) and completions (self-inflicted death). While the actual base rate is relatively low (around 8–10 per 100,000), suicide remains the third leading cause of death for 15–24-year-olds, following unintentional injuries and homicide. Among high school students, almost 20 percent report a history of suicidal ideation, while up to 11 percent have made an actual suicide attempt.

Although suicide attempts before puberty are rare, depressed children report suicidal ideation as often as depressed adolescents. Female adolescents are more likely to attempt suicide (10–20 percent) than males (4–10 percent), but male adolescents are four to five times more likely to complete suicide. While the majority of girls' suicide attempts involve wrist-cutting or ingestion of pills, boys have high rates of gun use, hanging, and other more lethal methods. Among completed suicides, firearms are the most commonly used method for both boys and girls. Almost all adolescents who attempt suicide report a history of suicidal ideation. Approximately one-third of attempters will make a repeat attempt within 2 years, and up to 10 percent will eventually kill themselves.

CORRELATES

The best predictor of a suicide attempt is a history of previous attempts or significant suicidal ideation. The presence of psychopathology is a major risk factor, with more than 90 percent of adolescent suicide deaths occurring in the context of a psychiatric illness. Mood disorders, substance abuse, and disruptive behavior disorders are highly associated with suicidal behavior, and the prevalence increases among adolescents with two or more diagnoses. Alcohol use is associated with 40–50 percent of completed suicides. The presence of firearms in the home is another significant factor, increasing the risk of suicide 5-fold.

Additional predictors of suicide attempts include recent stressful life events (e.g., arguments/fights, breakup of important relationship, leaving home, suicide attempt by friend/relative), family problems (e.g., conflict, impaired communication, low levels of emotional support, family history of psychopathology or substance abuse), and history of abuse or neglect. Suicidal adolescents often display characteristics such as hopelessness, impulsivity, hostility, and perfectionism. Homosexual/bisexual, runaway, and homeless youth may also face elevated risks for suicidal behavior.

ASSESSMENT

Thorough assessment of suicidal risk should include characteristics of any previous attempts (e.g., intent, lethality, motivation), current and lifetime suicidal ideation, presence of psychopathology, environmental factors (e.g., recent stressful events, family characteristics), psychological characteristics (e.g., hopelessness, impulsivity), and access to potentially lethal methods (e.g., guns, medications). A variety of self-report measures of suicidal behavior are available. Adolescents may be more likely to report personal information on a questionnaire, but these often produce a high number of "false-positive" identifications (i.e., those incorrectly identified as being at high risk for suicidal behavior). A clinical interview remains important in evaluating the level of imminent risk. For acutely suicidal youth, crisis intervention may include negotiating a no-harm contract, limiting the availability of lethal means, providing support and 24-hr contact information, and hospitalization, if necessary.

TREATMENT

Empirical guidelines for the use of psychosocial interventions with suicidal children and adolescents are not yet established. Most of the published studies are descriptive in nature and the use of control groups or randomized assignment is limited by ethical considerations. No published studies have examined interventions for children under age 12. Current evidence suggests that comprehensive treatment for suicidal adolescents should include multiple components: (1) treatment of coexisting psychiatric illness, (2) modifying cognitive distortions and hopelessness, (3) remediation of interpersonal and problem-solving skills deficits, and (4) family psychoeducation and participation. Ongoing risk assessment should be an integral part of any treatment program.

Currently, the best-supported programs for treating suicidal adolescents utilize variations of cognitive–behavioral therapy (CBT). These are usually short-term and problem focused, and may be presented in a group or individual format. Strategies include behavioral contracting, conflict resolution, problem-solving and communication skills training, cognitive restructuring, and goal setting. Another promising treatment is dialectical behavior therapy for adolescents (DBT-A), which combines cognitive–behavioral and supportive techniques. It conceptualizes suicidal behavior as a maladaptive response to overwhelming and painful negative emotions. Techniques focus on improving self-awareness, distress tolerance, emotion regulation, and interpersonal effectiveness. A recently developed program known as the Youth Support Team utilizes psychoeducational interventions and a support network of adults in the community to decrease suicidal behavior and increase treatment adherence in at-risk youth. Initial results have been promising, although further research is needed.

See also: Bipolar Disorder; Cognitive–Behavior Therapy; Depressive Disorder, Major; Disruptive Behavior Disorders; Substance Abuse

Further Reading

Fristad, M. A., & Shaver, A. E. (2001). Psychosocial interventions for suicidal children and adolescents. *Depression and Anxiety, 14*, 192–197.

Lewinsohn, P. M., Rohde, P., & Seeley, J. R. (1996). Adolescent suicidal ideation and attempts: Prevalence, risk factors, and clinical implications. *Clinical Psychology: Science and Practice, 3*, 25–46.

Miller, A. L., & Glinski, J. (2000). Youth suicidal behavior: Assessment and intervention. *Journal of Clinical Psychology, 56*, 1131–1152.

National Institute of Mental Health. (2002). *Suicide Facts* [Online]. Available: http://www.nimh.nih.gov/research/suifact.htm

Rudd, M. D., & Joiner, T. E. (1998). An integrative conceptual framework for assessing and treating suicidal behavior in adolescents. *Journal of Adolescence, 21*, 489–498.

AMY E. SHAVER
MARY A. FRISTAD

Summer Treatment Programs

DEFINITION

Summer treatment programs (STP) involve utilization of the summer months to provide concentrated, structured intervention to children with behavioral and/or learning problems. Such summer camps have a long history in child treatment. The focus here will be on the STP developed by Pelham and colleagues (1997). This program was specifically designed to treat children with Attention-Deficit/Hyperactivity Disorder (ADHD) and related disruptive behavior disorders such as oppositional and conduct disorders. However, other types of summer programs or summer schools exist as well. (For a broad review of summer schools, see work by Cooper and colleagues [2000].)

DESCRIPTION

The goal of the Pelham STP is to utilize the summer months toward greater advantage, since this is a time when children are often idle or engaged in minimally structured activities without great benefit. The STP provides an enjoyable camp-like setting in which children work on behavioral and learning problems with the assistance of paraprofessional counselors, special education teachers, and teachers' aides. The setting is highly structured and there is a high staff-to-child ratio. Each group of 12 children has five dedicated paraprofessional counselors and, in addition, children rotate through academic, computer, and art classes, each staffed by a teacher and a teacher's aide.

The STP runs Monday through Friday, 8:00 AM to 5:00 PM, for 8 weeks, allowing for 360 hr of intervention within a very brief time period. In terms of intervention hours, this is roughly equivalent to 7 years of weekly hour-long sessions. Because of its intensity, large gains are often seen over a short period of time. It is likely that these gains figure prominently in the near 100 percent child attendance rates typically reported by Pelham and colleagues, since parents are more likely to stay invested in their child's participation when they see positive results early on.

In the STP, target behaviors are selected for intervention on an individualized basis, giving greatest priority to behaviors that cause significant impairment in daily life functioning. In other words, it is not the defining symptoms of ADHD, but rather the problems in daily life caused by them, that are targeted. For example, problems getting along with peers and adults, academic difficulties, and poor behavioral conduct are frequently targeted, depending on the child's individual needs. In addition, children's competencies are developed in key domains of academic functioning and recreational activities—for example, knowledge and skills in common children's sports.

A typical day of activities at the STP includes participation in several hours of recreational sports activities such as soccer, softball, and basketball, and includes both skill-building/coaching in practice sessions and games. Three additional hours are spent in academic and art classroom settings where traditional (e.g., individualized seatwork), computer-assisted, and peer-oriented approaches to learning (e.g., cooperative learning, peer tutoring) are employed. These activities and the bases for their selection are described in detail in the STP manual written by Pelham and colleagues (1997). Within the quasinatural context of these structured activities, the interventions described below are employed.

METHODS OF INTERVENTION

The methods utilized to improve the child's functioning include a variety of behavior modification procedures that are well-established and supported by empirical research; adjunctive cognitive–behavioral methods are used as well. Together, these methods include: point/token systems; positive reinforcement; appropriate commands; peer interventions in the form of social skills training, anger management, and problem-solving training; daily report cards with program-based goals backed up by home-based rewards; time out; and classroom-based interventions. The classroom-based interventions include both

academic remediation and peer-based classroom interventions such as cooperative tasks and peer tutoring. Finally, parents are taught behavior modification skills through concurrent weekly parent training classes, and when necessary, medication assessments are conducted for individual children to assess their response to medication over and above the behavioral interventions employed.

RATES OF SUCCESS/SATISFACTION

As reported by Pelham and colleagues (1997), parents of children attending the STP report high rates of satisfaction and this satisfaction is reflected in attendance rates near 100 percent by parents (at parent training) and children alike. Furthermore, and perhaps most importantly, these high attendance rates are obtained regardless of family socioeconomic status, parental marital status, or ethnicity. These rates are much higher than those routinely obtained in child psychiatric/psychological treatments.

Online information about STP locations in North America, research studies conducted in the STP, how to start an STP, and STP employment opportunities may be found at: http://wings.buffalo.edu/adhd and http://summertreatmentprogram.com.

See also: Attention-Deficit/Hyperactivity Disorder; Conduct Disorder; Disruptive Behavior Disorders; Oppositional Defiant Disorder

Further Reading

Cooper, H., Charlton, K., Valentine, J. C., & Muhlenbruck, L. (2000). Making the most of summer school: A meta-analytic and narrative review. *Monographs of the Society for Research in Child Development, 65* (1, Serial No. 260).

Pelham, W. E., Fabiano, G. A., Gnagy, E. M., Greiner, A. R., & Hoza, B. (in press). The role of summer treatment programs in the context of comprehensive treatment for ADHD. In E. D. Hibbs & P. S. Jensen (Eds.), *Psychosocial treatment research of child and adolescent disorders* (2nd ed.). New York: APA Press.

Pelham, W. E., Greiner, A. R., & Gnagy, E. M. (1997). *Summer treatment program manual.* Buffalo, NY: Comprehensive Treatment for Attention Deficit Disorders, Inc. (http://www.ctadd.com).

Pelham, W. E., & Hoza, B. (1996). Intensive treatment: A summer treatment program for children with ADHD. In E. D. Hibbs & P. S. Jensen (Eds.), *Psychosocial treatments for child and adolescent disorders: Empirically based strategies for clinical practice* (pp. 311–340). Washington, DC: American Psychological Association.

BETSY HOZA
WILLIAM E. PELHAM, JR.

Sydenham's Chorea

See: Chorea: Sydenham's and Huntington's

Syphilis

See: Sexually Transmitted Diseases in Adolescents

Systematic Desensitization

DEFINITION

Systematic desensitization (SD) is a therapeutic technique based on the principles of classical conditioning. Pavlov's example of dogs salivating at the sound of a bell prior to the presentation of a food stimulus is frequently used to illustrate this conditioning process. The conditioned stimulus (i.e., sound of the bell) elicits the conditioned response (i.e., salivation). SD procedures are used to "decondition" the learned response and are used primarily in the treatment of childhood anxiety disorders, particularly those involving phobic avoidance responses. One of the main underlying assumptions of SD is reciprocal inhibition or counterconditioning; that is, pairing an anxiety-provoking stimulus with a response that is incompatible with the anxiety response. As described early on by Wolpe (1958), it is believed that these pairings will inhibit or quell the anxiety experienced, such that two opposing emotional states cannot occur at the same time. Relaxation is the most commonly used incompatible response, though others have been successfully employed as well (e.g., eating, singing, or playing games with child clients). The three principal components of SD are: relaxation training, construction of an anxiety hierarchy, and SD proper, that is, systematic pairing of an anxiety-provoking stimulus with a response that is incompatible with the anxiety response.

METHOD

Inducing a state of relaxation generally consists of creating a safe and comfortable environment for the child, followed by the tensing and relaxing of various major muscle groups. For adolescents, basic relaxation scripts can be used to provide a smooth transition between muscle groups, while for younger children, further considerations may be required. For example, Ollendick and Cerny (1981) suggest simplifying instructions, shortening the duration of training sessions (i.e., 15 min), and incorporating "fantasy" into the descriptions (e.g., "Pretend you are a furry, lazy cat. You want to stretch. Stretch your arms out in front of you...") can be especially advantageous. In addition, including the parent(s) of younger children in the relaxation training exercises can be useful, such that the parent(s) may help the child practice outside of therapy sessions. It may also be beneficial, especially initially, to create a relaxation audiotape for the child (and parent) to use when practicing the techniques.

An anxiety hierarchy is constructed based on the specific feared stimuli and/or situations of the child and ranges from least to most anxiety-provoking. Employing a rating scale (e.g., 1–10) with visual illustrations (e.g., thermometers) can be useful when creating the hierarchy to ensure consistent and relative item rankings. The clinician should aim to create a hierarchy consisting of approximately 10–20 items and be sure to include situations that are likely to occur in real-life experiences (see Table 1). Although child clients are encouraged to participate in the construction of the anxiety hierarchy to the best of their ability, it is also often beneficial to include parents, who have made firsthand observations of the child's anxious responses.

Finally, SD proper consists of presenting stimuli from the anxiety hierarchy, once the individual has attained a state of relaxation. Hierarchy items can be presented through imaginal or in vivo approaches. Imaginal exposure involves having the therapist vividly describe the feared stimuli while the child attempts to imagine him/herself in the situation presented. For younger children, assessing imaginal abilities prior to implementing this technique is often required. This can be accomplished by having the child imagine a situation and provide a detailed description to the clinician or by showing the child a picture and later asking them to recall it in as much detail as possible. In vivo presentation consists of actual exposure to the feared stimuli or situations from the hierarchy. Whenever possible, in vivo exposures are recommended, particularly for children who have difficulty with imagery or experiencing the intensity of their anxiety through imaginal means alone. Stimuli are presented one at a time, beginning with the least anxiety provoking and gradually moving up the hierarchy toward the most

Table 1. Sample Anxiety Hierarchy for a Child with a Spider Phobia

Feared stimulus/situation	Fear rating
Letting a spider crawl on my hand and arm for more than 10 s	10
Having a spider in my hands	10
Touching a spider someone else is handling	10
Being in the same room as a spider that is not in an enclosed setting (i.e., a cage or box)	10
Touching a spider in an enclosed setting	9
Putting my hand near a spider in an enclosed setting for more than 10 s	9
Putting my finger near a spider in an enclosed setting	8
Watching someone else handle a spider	7
Holding the jar without a cover on it	6
Covering and lifting the jar and releasing the spider	6
Capturing a spider by covering it with a jar	5
Sitting next to a spider in an enclosed setting	4
Being in the same room with a spider in an enclosed setting	3
Closely watching a spider outside and describing it	2
Talking about a spider	1
Seeing a picture of a spider	1

anxiety-provoking. Progression through hierarchy items is dependent on the child's ability to remain relaxed during the stimuli presentations. The clinician should carefully monitor the child's fearfulness and reduce the duration of exposure if the child becomes excessively anxious.

CLINICAL APPLICATIONS

SD research has predominantly focused on the treatment of fears and phobias in children and adolescents. This approach has been examined in the empirical literature with a variety of fear-producing stimuli, including: animals, situations (e.g., stage fright), test and academic evaluation, and interpersonal sensitivities (e.g., weight gain). In addition, SD has been utilized with other conditioned emotional states, such as depressed mood marked by agitation. SD has been utilized with a variety of child samples, with children as young as 3 years of age treated using these procedures. However, the basic SD approach should be modified with younger children to accommodate their developmental level in terms of such factors as their imaginal, attentional, and verbal abilities. For example, playing games or singing songs could be selected as

an alternative incompatible response for younger children who may not be able to fully comprehend or effectively implement relaxation training.

EFFECTIVENESS

SD has shown statistically and clinically significant reductions in children's anxiety responses to feared stimuli as measured by child and parent report, indices of autonomic nervous system response, and performance (i.e., with test anxiety). A vast number of uncontrolled clinical case studies have reported on the effectiveness of SD with various populations. In addition, Ollendick and King (1998) have provided an extensive review of clinical control studies demonstrating the effectiveness of SD procedures. Overall, research has demonstrated significantly greater improvements for both imaginal and in vivo desensitization treatment groups as compared with control (no treatment) groups. Imaginal desensitization has also proven superior to relaxation alone and SD without relaxation and has been effectively administered through individual, group, and vicarious (watching other children be treated with SD) treatment approaches. Based on the empirical findings described by Ollendick and King (1998), childhood treatment of fears and phobias with SD has been rated as "probably efficacious" according to the guidelines set forth by the Task Force for Promotion and Dissemination of Psychological Procedures.

See also: Anxiety Disorders; Behavior Therapy; Evidence-Based Treatments; Specific Phobia

Further Reading

Ollendick, T. H., & Cerny, J. A. (1981). *Clinical behavior therapy with children*. New York: Plenum Press.

Ollendick, T. H., Hagopian, L. P., & King, N. J. (1997). Specific phobias in children. In G. C. L. Davey (Ed.), *Phobias: A handbook of theory, research, and treatment* (pp. 203–244). New York: Wiley.

Ollendick, T. H., & King, N. J. (1998). Empirically supported treatments for children with phobic and anxiety disorders: Current status. *Journal of Clinical Child Psychology, 27,* 156–167.

Wolpe, J. (1958). *Psychotherapy by reciprocal inhibition*. Stanford, CA: Stanford University Press.

AMIE E. GRILLS
THOMAS H. OLLENDICK

Tt

Taste Development

See: Sensory and Perceptual Development

Teenage Pregnancy

See: Adolescent Pregnancy

Television and Children: Advertising

DESCRIPTION OF PROBLEM

Advertisers in the United States spend more than $12 billion a year trying to sell products to children, and it is estimated that children under the age of 12 spend nearly $25 billion per year on products, and have an even larger influence on the purchasing decisions of their parents. Since its early years, television has been the main medium used by advertisers to influence children's purchasing decisions and brand loyalty. The practice of advertising to children has raised several concerns among the public and social scientists. First, does television advertising take unfair advantage of children's developmental immaturity? Second, does advertising affect children's desire for the products advertised, including products potentially harmful to the health of children? Finally, does advertising contribute to parent–child conflict around products desired by children as a result of exposure to advertising?

WHAT IS BEING ADVERTISED TO CHILDREN?

It is estimated that children watch approximately 40,000 advertisements per year. Studies in the late 1970s and early 1990s both found that advertising in children's programming was dominated by toy, cereal (mainly sugared), snack food, and fast food advertisements. Toy advertisements, in particular, have been found to convey gender stereotypes, not only in the types of toys and characters featured, but in the production techniques used, with "boy" toys featuring more action and noise than "girl" toys. The most common message contained in children's advertisements is that use of the product will make children happier and increase the amount of fun they have. Messages concerning product quality, value, or safety are extremely rare.

Public concern has focused on advertisements featuring products that can potentially harm children and youth. Foods advertised to children tend to be high in sugar and fats; healthy foods, with the exception of milk, are rarely advertised. Researchers have also found children and adolescents to be attracted to alcohol advertisements, especially those featuring animated characters or young actors portrayed as having fun while drinking, with one study finding

657

Budweiser ads to be the favorite ads of children and adolescents.

CHILDREN'S UNDERSTANDING OF ADVERTISING

A substantial body of research indicates that children younger than age 7–8 find advertisements attractive and are more likely to attend to them than older children and adults, and that these younger children may not understand the persuasive intent of advertising in the same way as do older children and adults. Adults, understanding that advertising is intended to influence them to buy products and that the messages contained in ads may be biased, are more likely to view ads skeptically and resist advertising influence attempts. Young children, however, often lack the capacity to make such distinctions. Very young children (ages 3–4) are often unable to discriminate between commercial messages and the programs in which they are embedded. Somewhat older children, up until age 7–8, recognize commercials as distinct from programs, but fail to understand the persuasive intent of commercial messages and do not appreciate the bias inherent in advertising. Skepticism about the truthfulness of commercial messages has been found to be very low among 4–6 year-olds but do increase substantially in older children. These findings have important implications for public policy: many countries (not including the United States) have banned advertising targeting younger children as an inherently unfair practice.

ADVERTISING EFFECTS: PRODUCT DESIRE AND PREFERENCE

The fact that the advertising industry spends as much money as it does trying to reach children, with the goal of selling products now and creating brand-loyal future consumers, might be evidence enough that advertising influences children's product preferences and purchasing decisions. Research supports these contentions: children who watch more televised advertising are more familiar with advertised brands and express a greater desire to own such products than do children who watch less television. This effect is found for both children and adolescents but is somewhat stronger for younger children. Studies have also found that exposure to small numbers of ads can significantly influence children's preferences and purchasing desires,

including for products like beer that are not intended for children and adolescents.

ADVERTISING EFFECTS: PARENT–CHILD CONFLICT

Arguments between children and their parents in toy and grocery stores are commonplace, but does advertising contribute to these conflicts? Several studies support the conclusion that advertising plays a role in product purchase-related conflicts. Both parents and children report such conflicts in surveys, and studies in which parents and children are observed in stores report common conflicts around the purchase of those products that are most commonly advertised in children's programming (cereals and candy). Laboratory-based research has also confirmed the role of television advertising in such parent–child conflicts. Advocates have expressed heightened concern about the impact of such advertising-related conflicts in low-income families.

SUMMARY

Commercial television exists primarily as a mechanism to deliver commercial messages to viewers; entertainment programming is merely the carrier for advertising. Increasingly, children have become the targets of such persuasive appeals as their numbers and buying power have grown. Research has demonstrated that young children, in particular, are susceptible to these persuasive appeals in part because they do not comprehend the bias and persuasive intent of advertising. But even older children are influenced by the happiness/fun appeals featured in many ads, and research studies note that these ads affect children's brand preferences and purchasing desires, and also contribute to parent–child conflict around purchasing decisions. Research on the impact of advertising on children's broader materialistic values, and the impact of those values on child well-being, has not developed to the point where clear conclusions can be drawn.

See also: Adolescence; Childhood; Television and Children: Violence

Further Reading

Kunkel, D., & Gantz, W. (1991). *Television advertising to children: Message content in 1990.* Report to the Children's Advertising

Review Unit, Better Business Bureau. Bloomington, IN: University of Indiana.

Singer, D. G., & Singer, J. L. (Eds.). (2001). *Handbook of children and the media*. Thousand Oaks, CA: Sage.

Strasburger, V. C., & Wilson, B. J. (2001). *Children, adolescents, and the media*. Thousand Oaks, CA: Sage.

BRIAN L. WILCOX

Television and Children: Violence

DESCRIPTION OF PROBLEM

Both parents and policymakers have expressed concern over violence portrayed on television, especially with respect to its potential impact on children's development and behavior. By the early 1950s, when television ownership first became widespread, Congress had already begun its first investigations on the issue, and Congressional attention has continued nearly unabated through the late 1990s. Over this entire period, the questions surrounding the potential impact of media violence on children have been scrutinized by researchers and debated by members of the television industry, the public, and policymakers. Research points to three general classes of effects of exposure to media violence: learning of aggression, fear responses, and desensitization to real-world violence.

Learning Aggression

Children certainly learn from what they view on television. Advertisers invest billions of dollars to influence children's spending, and would not do so if their own research did not find such efforts to be effective. A substantial body of research has demonstrated the ability of educational television programs such as Sesame Street and Blue's Clues to teach children language and mathematical literacy skills. Researchers have devoted a good deal of attention to the question of whether children can and do learn aggression from viewing televised violence, and whether children who view violent programming are more likely to behave in an aggressive fashion, and have answered both questions in the affirmative.

Researchers have studied these questions using an array of approaches. Experiments (both laboratory- and community-based) have exposed children to programs varying in the amount of violence to examine the impact on aggressive attitudes and behaviors. Other researchers collected information on children's level of exposure to television violence and assessed its relationship to their levels of aggressive behavior. Some of these studies used longitudinal approaches, following the children over many years in order to assess the relationship between media violence viewing and aggression over substantial periods of time. More recently, researchers have used meta-analytic research methods, which allow them to synthesize the results of many independent studies. The consensus conclusion from all of these sources is that there is a positive and significant association between media violence and aggressive attitudes and behavior. Media violence models aggression and teaches children social/cognitive scripts maintaining that aggression is a successful means for resolving conflicts. The influence of media violence tends to be greater with younger children and with those children who are temperamentally more aggressive to begin with.

Media Violence and Fear

While most research and public attention has focused on the relationship between media violence viewing and children's aggression, researchers have also noted that viewing media violence can increase fear experienced by viewers. Studies have found that some fear responses triggered by media violence are quite long-lasting, resulting in sleep disturbances and nightmares. Some researchers have argued that children who view televised violence come to believe that the world is a more violent place than is actually the case, and exaggerate their own probability of becoming a victim of violent crime. Support for this "mean world syndrome" is mixed, as not all viewers show such responses, and some studies find that persons who are apprehensive about violent crime show a preference for programs featuring violent crime. While the nature of the fear responses triggered by viewing media violence may be uncertain, and the mechanisms by which viewing induces fear responses in some viewers and not others may not be fully understood, researchers have concluded that fear and anxiety is certainly a reaction many child viewers have in response to media violence.

Desensitization to Violence

Researchers studying children's reactions to media violence have noted that many children appear to become desensitized to portrayals of violence. Heavy viewers of TV violence show lower levels of physiological arousal in response to violent scenes than do occasional viewers. This finding is troubling for two reasons. First, since physiological arousal can be experienced as a desirable outcome, it means that as viewers become desensitized to violence on TV, they are likely to seek out more graphic portrayals of violence in order to increase their arousal level. Second, if arousal levels eventually decline, viewers might become less responsive to real-life violence as well. Researchers find support for this concern, both in studies that find declines in sensitivity to real-world aggression after exposure to violent programming, and in studies noting that viewers of TV violence are less inclined than nonviewers to intervene when they are bystanders to a fight.

Variants of Violence Portrayals

Not all portrayals of violence are equally likely to result in the types of effects just described. Indeed, studies have found that violence can be shown in ways that actually promote antiviolent sentiments among viewers. Certain contextual features have been found to be associated with different effects. The learning of aggression, for example, is facilitated by portrayals that feature an attractive perpetrator (such as a hero), provide justification for the violence, feature violence that is extensive, graphic, rewarded, and/or not punished, and rely on humor and an absence of cues concerning the pain/harm experienced by victims. Fear responses are more likely when violence is not justified (i.e., random or seemingly without instigation), when the victim is attractive, and when the violence is graphic, realistic, and rewarded. Desensitization effects appear most commonly when violent portrayals are graphic but treated in a humorous fashion. Unfortunately, portrayals of violence perpetrated by attractive characters that are not punished, have minimal negative consequences for the victims, and is communicated humorously are very common in children's cartoons, and research confirms that young children do experience the types of effects described here in response to viewing cartoon violence.

SUMMARY

Researchers are in general agreement that viewing television violence is associated with aggressive behavior, the development of fear, and desensitization to real-world violence. Most of the attention of both researchers and the public has been devoted to the question of whether viewing violent programming

increases the likelihood that viewers will behave aggressively, and researchers have pointed to the conditions under which portrayals of violence are most likely to lead to the learning and enactment of aggression. Researchers have also noted that this learning occurs most readily among younger viewers, suggesting that interventions intended to minimize the effects of exposure to media violence should be focused on children.

Violence and aggression, as researchers have learned, is caused by a multitude of factors, with exposure to media violence being only one among many such factors. Nevertheless, the results of meta-analytic research syntheses suggest that the strength of the relationship between exposure to media violence and aggressive behavior warrants the concern expressed by many parents, policymakers, and researchers.

See also: Adolescence; Childhood; Television and Children: Advertising

Further Reading

Cantor, J. (1998). *"Mommy, I'm scared": How TV and movies frighten children and what we can do to protect them*. San Diego, CA: Harcourt Brace.
National Television Violence Study. (1998). *National Television Violence Study 3*. Thousand Oaks, CA: Sage.
Singer, D. G., & Singer, J. L. (Eds.). (2001). *Handbook of children and the media*. Thousand Oaks, CA: Sage.
Strasburger, V. C., & Wilson, B. J. (2001). *Children, adolescents, and the media*. Thousand Oaks, CA: Sage.

BRIAN L. WILCOX

Temper Tantrums

DEFINITION

Temper tantrums are an early behavioral manifestation of both noncompliance and aggression. Noncompliance is narrowly defined as not following directions, disregarding requests, or doing the opposite of what is asked. Conversely, compliance is viewed as "the capacity to defer or delay one's own goals in response to the imposed goals or standards of an authority figure" (Greene & Doyle, 1999, p. 133). Aggression includes physically aggressive acts against another person (hitting, kicking, biting, fighting), verbal aggression (threats, tattling, teasing, name-calling), and nonverbal or symbolic aggression (threatening gestures, chasing, making faces). Almost all children evidence temper tantrums at some time during the course of development; they are usually transient, decrease with age, and are considered a normal part of learning how to get along in the world. For some children, however, these disruptive behaviors persist and/or escalate throughout childhood and adolescence, and may eventually result in clinically significant conduct problems.

DEVELOPMENT OF AGGRESSION AND NONCOMPLIANCE

Expressions of frustration and rage are seen in very young infants, both male and female, equally. By three months, the infant makes adult-like facial expressions of anger. By the second half of the first year, real angry feelings begin to be expressed as the child learns about cause and effect. After 12 months, gender differences in aggression are apparent. Boys are more emotionally labile and express negative emotions at higher rates than girls. During the second and third years, temper tantrums and aggression begin to be seen about equally among both boys and girls, although parents report more aggression for boys than girls. Aggression at this age tends to be instrumental (i.e., to obtain a desired object).

Compliance and noncompliance are seen as soon as children have the cognitive capacity to understand parental requests and the physical capabilities to carry them out. It has been suggested that compliance actually has its origins in self-regulation during infancy, as reflected in the infant's ability to manage discomfort, modulate arousal, and communicate his or her needs to caregivers. In the process of learning self-regulation, toddlers and preschoolers at times engage in highly aversive behaviors and noncompliance/aggression, expressed as temper tantrums, typically beginning to be perceived as a problem around 2 years of age when children begin to assert their needs for autonomy and control. The development of language facilitates more sophisticated methods of self-regulation as the child learns to label thoughts and feelings, to understand cause and effect, and to generate strategies for effective interaction. Children's passive noncompliance (ignoring the request) and direct defiance (including temper tantrums) decreases with age, whereas negotiation increases.

A developmental perspective suggests that there are critical periods in the course of development during which children are more vulnerable to adverse conditions and more likely to develop patterns of negative behaviors that have the potential to persist and become more severe with age. The period of early childhood (between birth and about 3 or 4 years) when children typically first form affectionate bonds with significant adults and later begin to assert their independence is an example. During this period, children are particularly vulnerable to disruptions in their social environment such as marital separation and divorce, parental illness, physical and/or emotional neglect, or poor quality parenting. Disruptive behavior can also develop in association with events that occur during the normal course of development. These events might include the birth of a sibling, beginning school, associating with peers, and moving from elementary to junior high school. All of these events have the potential to exacerbate temper tantrums and shift a child's developmental path toward more maladaptive behavior.

The parent–child relationship also contributes to the persistence of negative behaviors such as temper tantrums. Early mother–infant conflict, due to difficult temperamental characteristics in the child, poor parenting skills in the parent, or both may begin a coercive cycle that is so clearly seen in families of older children with antisocial behavior problems. In the coercive cycle, the child's disruptive behavior is increased by removal of an aversive parent behavior and vice versa. For example, the parent tells the child to pick up the toys (aversive stimuli), the child has a temper tantrum (aversive stimuli), and the parent withdraws the request. Thus, the child's temper tantrum is successful in removing the aversive stimuli and is consequently negatively reinforced. Moreover, the parent is negatively reinforced for withdrawing the request by the cessation of the child's tantrum. Ongoing poor management on the part of parents, characterized by ignoring or punishing the child's prosocial behavior, and positive or negative reinforcement of negative behavior, contributes to the child's increasing repertoire of aversive behaviors.

INTERVENTION STRATEGIES

Behavioral parent training that teaches parents principles of social learning and effective parent–child interaction and child management skills is the most effective method of treating temper tantrums that have become clinically significant. These parent–child interaction programs are based on clinical and developmental research that supports the idea that contingent, appropriate parental responses to child behaviors constitute a key factor in the development and maintenance of positive child behaviors and the reduction of disruptive behaviors.

Other work suggests several strategies for preventing early temper tantrums from becoming more serious. First, extinction by ignoring temper tantrums whenever possible, coupled with positive attention for appropriate behavior is usually effective in reducing their frequency and severity. Second, individual differences in children's rates of compliance/noncompliance are influenced by parental responsivity. Thus, parents who are able to allow their children a degree of control by following the child's lead and modeling compliance to child requests while reducing demands and instructions, have children who are more likely to be compliant to parental demands. Third, developmental research suggests that very young children (i.e., 12–18 months) may be predisposed to comply with adult commands because compliance with adult commands provides children with some inherent pleasure and motivation. This predisposition suggests that if compliance is rewarded rather than ignored or punished, it should increase and persist as a behavioral style. Others suggest that harnessing children's early predisposition to cooperate at a time when self-regulation is poorly developed requires considerable physical assistance from parents. In other words, rather than expecting toddlers to comply, parents must help them to do so and then reinforce their children's efforts.

See also: Aggression; Childhood; Disruptive Behavior Disorders; Emotional Development; Parent–Child Interaction Therapy; Parent Training; Temperament Assessment

Further Reading

Christophersen, E. R., & Finney, J. W. (1999). Oppositional defiant disorder. In R. T. Ammerman, M. Hersen, & C. G. Last (Eds.), *Prescriptive treatments for children and adolescents* (2nd ed., pp. 102–113). Needham Heights, MA: Allyn & Bacon.

Greene, R. W., & Doyle, A. E. (1999). Toward a transactional conceptualization of ODD. *Clinical Child and Family Psychology Review, 2*, 129–148.

Kalpidou, M. D., Rothbaum, F., & Rosen, K. S. (1998). A longitudinal study of mothers' and preschool children's aversive behaviors during dyadic interactions. *Journal of Genetic Psychology, 159*, 103–116.

Kuczynski, L., & Kochanska, G. (1995). Function and context of maternal demands: Developmental significance of early demands for competent action. *Child Development, 66*, 616–628.

Loeber, R., & Hay, D. (1997). Key issues in the development of aggression and violence from childhood to early adulthood. *Annual Review of Psychology, 48*, 371–410.

Wahler, R. G., Herring, M., & Edwards, M. (2001). Coregulation of balance between children's prosocial approaches and acts of compliance: A pathway to mother–child cooperation? *Journal of Clinical Child Psychology, 30*, 473–478.

BETTY N. GORDON

Temperament Assessment

In the 40+ years since Stella Chess and Alexander Thomas began their pioneering work in the area of temperament, numerous methods have been developed to assess temperament and similar constructs. The importance of temperament assessment is highlighted by research suggesting that temperament influences how developmental deficits are displayed, how a child copes with disability or crisis, and how temperament plays a critical role in shaping parent–child interactions. Other findings have implicated difficult temperament as a risk factor in the development of adjustment problems, especially externalizing disorders. Relationships between characteristics such as behavioral inhibition and anxiety-related conditions have also been found.

To date, no one measure or approach has been accepted as the gold standard for assessing temperament. Indeed, there are many similarities among approaches, with a number of measures assessing temperament dimensions delineated by Chess and Thomas (1996) and the New York Longitudinal Study (e.g., rhythmicity, approach/withdrawal, adaptability, mood, intensity, activity level, persistence, distractibility, threshold of responsivity) as well as others suggested by subsequent research (e.g., reactivity, sociability, soothability, emotionality).

APPROACHES TO TEMPERAMENT ASSESSMENT

Methods for assessing temperament include questionnaires, observational methods, and interviews. As with the assessment of any construct, it is best to obtain data using multiple methods and multiple sources (e.g., parents, teachers, clinicians). This is particularly important in assessing temperament, as researchers have often highlighted the potential for distortion and response biases that can occur with parent-report, and perhaps teacher-report, questionnaires. Obtaining information regarding the child's behavior in a variety of situations is also important in order to differentiate between temperament and situational variables that may influence behavior.

Temperament Questionnaires

Parent questionnaires are the most common method for assessing child temperament. Despite the often cited potential for bias, the parent is most often the person who knows the child best and is capable of providing the most accurate information regarding the child's behavioral style—if questions are asked appropriately.

Several researchers have developed age-specific measures for temperament assessment. Most noteworthy are Thomas, Chess, and associates who developed the 72-item *Parent Temperament Questionnaire* for use with children 3–7 years old. This measure assesses the nine temperament dimensions (cited above) derived from the New York Longitudinal Study (NYLS). The measure has been shown to be reliable and has been used extensively in temperament research, with scores derived from the measure having been found to relate to a range of relevant variables. Thomas and Chess have also developed a *Teacher Temperament Questionnaire* for assessing some of these same temperament dimensions. Martin and associates have likewise developed a *Temperament Assessment Battery for Children* that is normed on children in this same age range (3–7) and focuses on six of the nine NYLS dimensions. Parent and teacher forms are available, as is one designed specifically for clinicians.

In an ambitious effort, Carey and McDevitt (1995) have developed a series of five temperament measures covering the age span from one month to 12 years that assess the NYLS temperament dimensions. Included here are the Early Infancy Temperament Questionnaire (1–3 months), Infant Temperament Questionnaire (4–8 months), Toddler Temperament Questionnaire (1–3 years), Behavioral Style Questionnaire (3–7 years), and the Middle Childhood Temperament Questionnaire (8–12 years). These scales, which contain between 86 and 110 items, have been widely used in clinical practice, especially in pediatric settings. An especially desirable aspect of these measures is that items are worded to elicit descriptions of specific behaviors in specific situations so as to limit bias associated with parent perceptions and general impressions of behavior.

Another measure developed for research, but increasingly used in clinical practice, is the *Revised Dimensions of Temperament Survey (DOTS-R)* developed by Windle and Lerner. The *DOTS-R* is a self/parent report instrument for assessing temperament

attributes, identified through factor analyses to be reliably assessed across the age span (e.g., early childhood to young adulthood). These dimensions include activity level, approach–withdrawal, flexibility–rigidity, mood quality, rhythmicity, distractibility, and persistence. The 54 *DOTS-R* items are rated on a 4-point scale; "usually false" to "usually true." Because items were intended to reflect temperament characteristics at various ages, the wording of items was carefully done to ensure consistent interpretation of item content across age levels. Versions of the *DOTS-R* can be used to obtain parent-report measures for young children as well as self-report measures for older children and parents. A companion measure can be used to assess parent/teacher expectations regarding child temperament.

The *Pictorial Assessment of Temperament (PAT)*, published by Clarke-Steward and associates in 2000; is a relatively new measure designed to assess "difficult" temperament in infants and toddlers through the use of pictures. The instrument consists of 10 illustrated vignettes, each demonstrating how three different infants (an "easy" infant, a "difficult" infant, an average or "slow-to-warm" up infant) react to a common event. Items were drawn from the Carey's Revised Infant Temperament Questionnaire (1995) reflecting four dimensions of difficult temperament as described by Chess and Thomas (1996); negative mood, lack of approach to strangers, slow adaptability to change, and high intensity of emotional expression.

While reliability estimates for questionnaire measures of temperament vary, most have moderate coefficients of internal consistency and split-half reliability in the range of .70 to .95. Findings regarding test–retest reliability have generally been less strong and vary across studies depending upon the temperament dimension and age range assessed and the time between testing intervals. Although research has often suggested correlations between scores derived from various temperament questionnaires and relevant dependent variables, there is a need for additional research related to the validity of all of the measures cited here.

Temperament Interviews

There are few structured interviews for assessing child temperament. The most well-known is the temperament interview developed by the NYLS group. The full interview is 1–2 h in length and flexibly structured, so as to elicit a range of valuable behavioral descriptors. Unfortunately, administration time and lack of standardization may make it inappropriate for use in many research and clinical settings, although an abbreviated version might be useful in obtaining clinical information. The use of semistructured interviews allows the clinician to follow up on parent descriptions of child behavior, to respond to contradictory information, and to gain clinically relevant information regarding issues such as the fit between child characteristics, parenting style, and other demands of the environment.

Observational Methods

Naturalistic and structured observations have primarily been used in research studies to assess temperament in the home and school. These approaches often involve observing responses to various "challenges" presented to the child, with multiple observations being made across situations in an attempt to obtain reliable data. Temperament-related behaviors assessed in this manner often include reactions to change, to maternal control, and to siblings and peers, as well as crying and approach–avoidance behaviors. These measures are typically not practical for clinical use because they can be expensive and time-intensive as it is necessary to collect a large number of observations over an extended time to insure reliability. Additionally, correlations between questionnaire data and observational measures obtained in the home or school have generally been low. Although there are no well-known standardized observational approaches available for the practical assessment of child temperament in clinical settings, observational measures can be useful in providing additional data to supplement questionnaires. Observational approaches can likewise be helpful in identifying behavior problems and specific areas to focus on in clinical assessment.

FINAL CONSIDERATIONS

Regarding the approaches to assessment described here, research has suggested only moderate levels of agreement among assessment methods, with each approach having both advantages and disadvantages. For reasons of cost and time, questionnaires are most often used in clinical practice. Here, temperament assessment should involve the use of well-standardized and appropriately designed questionnaires that minimize bias and diagnostic overlap with childhood disorders. Parent questionnaires should be supplemented with questionnaire data from other informants (e.g., teachers) and, where possible, by interview data and

behavioral observations of the child alone and with the parent to ensure an adequate view of the child's behavior across situations. In clinical practice it is also important to differentiate between expressions of temperament characteristics and symptoms of child psychopathology, with the assessment of Attention-Deficit/Hyperactivity Disorder (ADHD) representing but one obvious example. Finally, as suggested earlier, in any assessment of temperament it is essential to obtain relevant information regarding the degree of "fit" between the child's temperament make-up and the demands of both the child's home and school environment in order to find ways to minimize negative outcomes in instances where "goodness of fit" is minimal.

See also: Behavior Rating Scales; Developmental Issues in Assessment for Treatment; Screening Instruments: Behavioral and Developmental

Further Reading

Bates, J. E. (1989). Concepts and measures of temperament. In G. A. Kohnstamm, J. E. Bates, & M. K. Rothbart (Eds.), *Temperament in childhood* (pp. 3–26). Chichester, England: Wiley.

Carey, W. B., & McDevitt, S. C. (1995). *Coping with children's temperament: A guide for professionals.* New York: Basic Books.

Chess, S., & Thomas, A. (1996). *Temperament theory and practice.* New York: Brunner/Mazel.

JAMES H. JOHNSON
CHRISTOPHER W. LOFTIS

Termination of Parental Rights

DEFINITION

The government has interests in protecting family privacy and the welfare of children, interests that are sometimes in conflict. Parents have legal rights and responsibilities in relation to their children into which the government is loath to intrude unless there is evidence that the welfare of the children has been significantly compromised by the very individuals who are responsible for their care and protection. The most extreme action the government can take in these instances is to permanently sever the parent–child relationship by legally terminating the rights of the parent to a relationship with his or her child. Certain grounds for termination proceedings, such as chronic or severe abuse, may also result in criminal prosecution.

GROUNDS

There are laws in every state in the United States that provide grounds for the government to terminate parental rights against the wishes of the parent. Some of the laws enumerate highly specific factors, whereas others are worded in a more general fashion. Among the most common conditions for which parental rights are terminated are severe abuse or neglect of the child or other children in the same home; abandonment; failure to provide financial support; and long-standing mental illness, mental deficiency, or substance abuse that renders the parent incapable of providing adequate care for the child.

It should be noted that before the government proceeds to terminate parental rights, the law requires that reasonable efforts be made to maintain the child in his or her family or, if out-of-home placement is warranted, to reunify the family. Under certain legally defined aggravating circumstances, however, the state is not required to make efforts to preserve the family. Examples of such circumstances are abandonment, torture, murder of a child's sibling by their parent, or the prior involuntary termination of parental rights to a sibling of the child.

The goal of permanency for a child undergirds the provision for termination of parental rights. The premise is that once the rights of the abusive, neglectful, violent, or otherwise deficient parent are terminated, the child is free to be adopted. The reality, of course, is that of the more than 500,000 children in foster care, most will not be adopted. The most recent effort to reduce the amount of time children spend in limbo is the Adoption and Safe Families Act signed into law in 1997 by then-President Clinton.

PROCEDURES

During the legal proceedings in most states, the prevalent standard is the best interests of the child. The court decides if the legal criteria for termination have been met and, if so, whether it would be in the best interests of the child for his or her parent's rights to be terminated. Due to the fundamental rights of both the child and of the parent, the burden of proof that must be met is more stringent than it is in most other civil proceedings. In most civil proceedings, the legal decision of the trier of fact (the judge or jury) must be supported by a *preponderance* of the evidence. In order to find that a parent's rights will be involuntarily terminated, there must be *clear and convincing* evidence to support the legal decision.

The evidence that is presented may include factual evidence from child protective services documenting, for example, the number of confirmed reports of abuse, and the nature and severity of that abuse. There also may be testimony regarding a treatment plan that was recommended, and the parent's responsiveness to the plan. There may be evidence presented of the manner in which the parent's behavior has affected the child. If the parent is contesting having his or her parental rights terminated, then the parent will typically offer evidence in support of his or her position.

Mental health professionals may be involved in termination proceedings in a variety of ways. The involvement may come about at the request of the state or a state agency, or the parent may have sought the professional's services. A mental health professional may have been asked by either party to the proceedings to evaluate the child's functioning and needs, the parent's functioning and needs, the nature and quality of the parent–child relationship, and/or the prognosis, if particular interventions are provided. In most cases, the mental health professional will prepare a written report and may be called to testify with respect to the findings and his or her professional opinions and recommendations. Although there is no consensus among professionals, most psychologists seem to support the idea that recommendations are best limited to clinical interventions and other professional services, rather than to the legal disposition itself (i.e., whether or not a parent's rights should be terminated). Regardless of the position taken, it is incumbent upon the mental health professional to provide adequate support for the recommendation(s) offered, and to ensure that the child's welfare is the salient consideration.

The American Psychological Association Committee on Professional Practice and Standards has developed *Guidelines for Psychological Evaluations in Child Protection Matters* (1998). The *Guidelines* are aspirational rather than mandatory, and are intended to be helpful to psychologists who participate in these difficult and often stressful cases. Among the issues emphasized are a focus on the interests of the child, the need for objectivity and an appreciation for the gravity of the matter at hand on the part of the evaluator, the importance of specialized skills and techniques, and circumspection in the delivery of professional services.

See also: Child Maltreatment; Expert Testimony; Foster Care; Mothers' and Fathers' Roles in Abnormal Child Development; Mothers' and Fathers' Roles in Normal Child Development

Further Reading

American Psychological Association Committee on Professional Practice and Standards. (1998). *Guidelines for psychological evaluations in child protection matters.* Washington, DC: Author.

Gendell, S. J. (2001). In search of permanency: A reflection on the first 3 years of the Adoption and Safe Families Act implementation. *Family Court Review, 39,* 25–42.

Melton, G. B., Petrila, J., Poythress, N. G., & Slobogin, C. (1997). *Psychological evaluations for the courts: A handbook for mental health professionals and lawyers* (2nd ed.). New York: Guilford Press.

National Clearinghouse on Child Abuse and Neglect Information, P.O. Box 1182, Washington, DC 20013.

ARLENE B. SCHAEFER

Terrorism Disasters

DEFINITION

Terrorism disasters include overwhelming events that cause serious injury or loss of life and property destruction as a result of human acts intended to cause horror, shock, and grief. Some effects of individual terrorist acts are readily identified as disasters (e.g., destruction of the World Trade Center in New York City, Oklahoma City Bombing), whereas other smaller scale terrorist acts such as a car bombing that injures one person may be considered a form of disaster when considered cumulatively across episodes and over time. Many terrorism disasters are motivated by political, religious, or paramilitary aims, although some mass sniper shootings, hostage takings, and other acts of violence have been linked to idiosyncratic reasoning such as revenge, retaliation, or a desire for notoriety (e.g., Columbine High School shootings).

INCIDENCE

Terrorism disasters occur throughout the world. Many countries with intractable political, ideological, and social conflicts have experienced prolonged periods in which terror is used to advance demands or destabilize opposition groups. The United States has seen a rise in large scale, lethal attacks from both foreign and domestic fanatical murderers. Increasing access to lethal methods ranging from automatic firearms to chemical, biological, and nuclear materials raises concern that terrorism disasters will continue to increase in scope and frequency. Worldwide, many children and adolescents are witnesses to serious acts of violence from diverse sources. Much of this exposure is through directly witnessing violence or its immediate aftermath. Witnessing terrorism through the media represents a form of vicarious exposure that is capable of producing significant psychological effects for children and adolescents.

CORRELATES

Large scale terrorist acts such as the 9/11 (September 11, 2001) attacks on the World Trade Center in New York City and the Pentagon in Washington, DC occur without warning, leading to shock, disbelief, and panic among a large portion of the population. School shootings, sniper shootings, and hostage-taking share this shock effect. Two of the ubiquitous effects of these types of terrorism disasters are increased sense of vulnerability and the cognitive challenge that occurs when fundamental beliefs about the world are violated. Terrorist acts occurring in the context of civil unrest or war tend to be more anticipated and perhaps more readily understood. Regardless, children and adolescents who directly experience threats to their life or bodily integrity, injury, exposure to grotesque scenes, and death or injury to a loved one have a strong potential to experience severe and persistent stress reactions. Overall, increased proximity to traumatic events and longer, more intense exposure is related to greater psychiatric symptomatology over both the short and longer term.

ASSESSMENT

Evaluation of the nature of trauma exposure is a key aspect of assessment. This includes systematic inquiry regarding primary elements of trauma exposure (e.g., perceived life threat, exposure to grotesque scenes, personal injury, harm to others) and the individual's understanding of what happened and why. Important features of the postdisaster recovery environment to be assessed include ongoing disruptions and adversity since exposure (including economic hardships and physical impairments), access to supportive social relationships, and functioning of primary caregivers. Exposure-related posttraumatic stress symptoms (reexperiencing phenomena, psychic numbing or avoidance, hyperarousal) and associated features require careful assessment, including direct questioning of children and not relying solely on adult informants. Depression, separation anxiety, and disaster-related fears or phobias are relatively common sequelae of extreme exposure involving loss of life or serious injury and should be assessed carefully.

TREATMENT

Treatment strategies vary by the point at which mental health contact is made, the severity and duration of traumatic exposure, and the extent of emotional distress shown or reported by the child or caregivers. Emergency services shortly after disasters focus on psychological first aid (e.g., support activation, debriefing or crisis-reduction counseling), information-giving, and support for adaptive functioning of the child and family. As the immediate crisis recedes, interventions for persistent trauma-related symptoms using time-limited, disaster-focused protocols are often helpful.

PROGNOSIS

Exposure-related symptoms typically diminish with time, although focused, evidence-based interventions appear to reduce the duration and intensity of psychological effects. Individual differences in reactions are well-documented, as are effects for features of the recovery environment. However, violent bereavement poses long-term mental health risks, especially when coupled with a high degree of exposure to other aspects of trauma (witnessing grotesque scenes, inability to help) and intense fear or horror.

See also: Exposure to Violence; Human-Made Disasters; Posttraumatic Stress Disorder; Psychological Testing

Further Reading

American Psychological Association Web site. Available at http//www.helping.apa.org/

American Psychological Association. (1997). *Final report: American Psychological Association task force on the mental health response to the Oklahoma City bombing.* Washington, DC: Author.

La Greca, A. M., Silverman, W. K., Vernberg, E. M., & Roberts, M. C. (Eds.). (2002). *Helping children cope with disasters and terrorism.* Washington, DC: American Psychological Association.

Van der Kolk, B. A., McFarlane, A. C., & Weisaeth, L. (Eds.). (1996). *Traumatic stress: The effects of overwhelming experience on mind, body, and society.* New York: Guilford.

R. Enrique Varela
Eric M. Vernberg

Tertiary Prevention

See: Safety and Prevention

Test Bias

Test bias is an important, yet often misunderstood, concept in psychological testing. Test bias occurs when a test measures a construct differently across groups of individuals, as noted by Anastasi and Urbina (1997). As a result, the interpretations one can make from the test will be different across the various groups. From this definition, it is evident that test bias is integrally related to the concept of validity. It refers to the situation when interpretations made from a test are not equally valid across different groups. Like validity, test bias is not a characteristic of the test itself but is a characteristic of the interpretations made from the test. Specifically, a test is not "biased" or "unbiased," just as a test is not "valid" or "invalid." Instead, certain interpretations made from the scores of the test may be "biased," whereas others may be equally valid across certain groups of individuals.

Recently, Kampaus (2001) has noted that there is great debate as to the magnitude of the problem of test bias for the most common psychological tests used in the assessment of children and adolescents. One of the more contentious areas of debate is the potential bias in psychological tests across cultural groups. For example, while many tests have shown relatively minor differences in scores and scale structure across cultural groups, it is also clear that the validity of many tests has not been extensively compared across cultural groups. As a result, the extent of test bias is difficult to evaluate because of the lack of attention given to this important issue in the development and validation of many psychological tests.

REASONS FOR TEST BIAS

There can be many reasons for why a test may be biased for different groups of individuals, such as children from different cultural groups. For example, certain items on tests may have different meanings across cultural groups. Also, the methods used to assess psychological constructs may have different utility across cultural groups. For example, there is evidence that on projective storytelling tests, children provide longer stories to pictures in which the actor matches their own age, gender, and ethnicity, as shown by Constantino and Malgady (1983). The testing situation itself may differentially influence the scores obtained for members of different cultural groups, such as whether or not an interviewer is of the same cultural background as the child being interviewed.

EVIDENCE FOR TEST BIAS

Just as validity is an ongoing process in which evidence is constantly accumulating to support or to refute certain interpretations from a test, so too is the process of investigating potential bias in the interpretations that can be made from the test. Evidence for or against bias in a test is an ongoing process of determining which interpretations can be appropriately made for which groups of individuals. Similarly, just as there are many aspects to the validity of test interpretations, so too are there many ways to investigate potential bias in these interpretations.

Content validity bias is one potential form of test bias. Content bias refers to the fact that the items on the test have different meaning for one group than another, or that items are relatively more difficult for one group than another. To test the former, expert judges representing different groups (e.g., different cultural or gender groups) can review the content of the test to determine whether the items adequately capture the construct of interest for their specific group, as well as to screen for potentially insulting items or items that may promote stereotyped beliefs. To test the latter, groups can be matched on overall level of a construct and then items that differentiate various levels of that construct can be compared across groups.

Construct validity bias refers to the situation in which a test measures the construct of interest differently for one group compared to another. Factor analysis is a common method used to study construct validity bias. Separate factor analyses of test items can be conducted for various groups to determine if a similar factor structure emerges across groups. While factor invariance (i.e., the factors remain the same) across groups is one important way to test for construct validity bias, there are other ways to test for this form of bias, such as comparing correlates to test scores across groups or comparing the stability of scores across groups. Related to potential differences in stability, one important form of construct validity bias is predictive validity bias. This refers to the situation in which scores

on a test predict outcomes (e.g., performance in school, risk for arrest, response to medication) differently across various groups of individuals.

DIFFERENTIAL IMPACT AND TEST BIAS

It is important to note that simply documenting that certain groups score differently on a test is not sufficient to document the presence of test bias. This simply documents that the test has "differential impact" on the various groups. There may be substantive reasons for why the groups perform differently on the test (e.g., different cultural expectations between boys and girls; differential access to quality education between cultural groups) but the validity of the test for certain purposes (e.g., predicting school performance) may still be equivalent across groups. For example, a test for predicting risk for engaging in illegal activities may show group differences, on average, across cultural groups. This may be due to one group experiencing more economic disadvantage, less access to quality education, and prejudice preventing attainment of social prestige through socially acceptable means, all of which increase the risk for illegal activities in this group. As a result, the two groups might score differently on the measure, showing differential impact across groups, but the scores may still predict risk for arrest equally well across groups.

REPRESENTATIVE NORMS AND TEST BIAS

Most tests provide norm-referenced scores that form the basis for most interpretations made from the test. As described recently by Kamphaus and Frick (2001), these scores indicate how a child's performance on the test compares to others in the standardization sample on which the test was normed. An important issue for interpreting these scores is the composition of the normative sample, including how representative it is of different groups of children. For example, many tests attempt to include representation of children from different ethnic backgrounds in the standardization sample at a level that matches the ethnic representation of some defined geographical region (e.g., different sections of the United States). While this practice enhances the ethnic representativeness of the standardization sample, it does not indicate whether or not the scores from the test are equally valid across different ethnic groups. Specifically, individuals in a minority ethnic group constitute a smaller proportion of the standardization sample. As a result, a validity coefficient could be statistically significant in the standardization sample and this could be due solely to its validity for the majority ethnic group. Instead, the validity of the scores from the test need to be directly compared across groups to determine whether similar interpretations can be made for various groups of individuals.

See also: Cultural Influences on Assessment; Culture and Psychopathology; Norms and Normative Data; Psychometric Properties of Tests; Validity

Further Reading

Anastasi, A., & Urbina, S. (1997). *Psychological testing.* Upper Saddle River, NJ: Prentice Hall.
Constantino, G., & Malgady, R. G. (1983). Verbal fluency of Hispanic, Black, & White children on TAT and TEMAS, a new thematic apperception test. *Hispanic Journal of Behavioral Sciences, 5,* 199–206.
Kamphaus, R. W. (2001). *Clinical assessment of child and adolescent intelligence* (2nd ed.) Boston: Allyn & Bacon.
Kamphaus, R. W., & Frick, P. J. (2002). *Clinical assessment of child and adolescent personality and behavior* (2nd ed.) Boston: Allyn & Bacon.

DANIELLE M. DANDREAUX

PAUL J. FRICK

Therapeutic Alliance

See: Treatment Alliance

Thrombocytopenia

See: Platelet Abnormalities—Thrombocytopenia

Tic Disorders: Tourette's Disorder, Chronic Tic Disorder, and Transient Tic Disorder

DEFINITION

The American Psychiatric Association defines tics as sudden, rapid, recurrent, nonrhythmic, stereotyped motor movements or vocalizations. Motor tics involve rapid contractions of muscle groups and movements of the body, whereas vocal tics involve vocalizations or repetitive sounds. Motor and vocal tics can be either simple or complex. Simple tics are generally brief, lasting for less then one second (e.g., hard eye blink or grunt) and complex tics appear to be more purposeful and longer in duration (e.g., spinning and bending or singing).

Tourette's disorder (TD), chronic tic disorder, and transient tic disorder can be distinguished from one another based on duration and variety of tics. Transient tic disorder involves motor and/or vocal tics that occur many times a day, nearly every day for at least 4 weeks but for less than 12 months, and the onset of the tics is before the age of 18. Chronic tic disorder involves single or multiple motor or vocal tics, but not both, that occur many times a day, nearly every day for at least 12 months, and the onset is before the age of 18. TD involves the same age and duration criteria as chronic tic disorder, except that multiple motor tics and at least one vocal tic must be present for a period greater than 3 months.

ONSET, PREVALENCE, FREQUENCY, AND DURATION

Tics usually first occur between the ages of 2 and 14 years with an average age of onset ranging between 5 and 7 years. The exact course of tic development is difficult to predict, but motor tics generally occur before vocal tics. The first motor tics to occur are usually facial tics such as eye blinking or grimacing, and the first vocal tics that develop usually involve simple vocalizations such as coughing or grunting. If multiple tics develop, they generally progress from the head downwards and tic complexity will typically progress from simple to complex. Most individuals with TD report a premonitory urge (a somatic sensation such as a tightness or tickle) in the bodily area associated with the tic that is relieved through emission of the tic. Tics tend to wax and wane over periods of weeks and months. For most children who develop tics, the intensity will increase from ages 11 to 14 and then decrease and possibly disappear around the age of 15. Approximately 65 percent of children with tics have very mild or nonexistent tics as adults.

Prevalence estimates for transient tics range from 6 to 18 percent, for chronic motor or vocal tics range from 3 to 4 percent, and for TD are less than 1 percent. Generally, tic disorders are more common in males than females. Although coprolalia and copropraxia (obscene talk and movements) are widely thought to be hallmarks of TD, only a small percentage of afflicted persons exhibit them.

PSYCHOLOGICAL CORRELATES

TD frequently co-occurs with other psychiatric disorders, especially Attention-Deficit/Hyperactivity Disorder (ADHD) and Obsessive Compulsive Disorder (OCD) (see entries on these disorders). Approximately 50 percent of children with TD also meet criteria for ADHD, and 30 percent also meet criteria for OCD. Children with TD may also exhibit obsessive compulsive-spectrum behaviors (e.g., checking or obsessive touching) but not meet the full diagnostic criteria for OCD. Additionally, many children with TD suffer from learning disorders.

ETIOLOGY

An unambiguous cause for tic disorders has not been discovered. Relevant research concentrates on four general areas, genetic, neurological, medical/developmental, and behavioral factors. Genetics researchers have discovered higher rates of tic disorders and OCD in biological relatives of those with TD. Neurological researchers have identified malfunctioning and/or malformed midbrain dopaminergic systems as causal factors for tic disorders. Medical/developmental researchers have identified events during the prenatal period (e.g., hypoxia) that may be involved in the development of tic disorders; they have also established a correlation between childhood streptococcus infections and tic disorders. Lastly, behavioral researchers have determined that environmental conditioning processes can influence the emission of tics.

ASSESSMENT

Prior to diagnosis (or treatment) afflicted children should be evaluated by a medical professional (typically a pediatric neurologist) to assess for medical conditions that may cause tic-like behavior. If medical conditions are ruled out, the diagnosis is determined through direct observation of the children, interviews with them, reviews of school records, and reports from parents, teachers, and sometimes peers. The severity of the diagnosis can be assessed with any of a number of standardized tic severity measures. The role of environmental variables can be assessed through functional assessment and analysis procedures.

TREATMENT

A broad range of treatments have been employed for tic disorders. Current best practice, however, involves a combination of three tactics. The first involves provision of education (e.g., to the afflicted children and their parents, siblings, teachers, and sometimes peers) about tic disorders. The second tactic involves application of methods to reduce tic frequency and intensity; the most typical of these involves drug therapy. The most frequently used drugs are neuroleptics (e.g., haloperidol or pimozide): available evidence indicates that as many as 70 percent of afflicted children respond favorably and that these drugs produce as much as an 80 percent decrease in tics in favorable cases. Drug therapy is not a panacea, however, given the high likelihood of unpleasant side effects (e.g., dry mouth, sluggishness). An effective and increasingly used behavioral treatment method is habit reversal. Habit reversal is a multicomponent treatment whose central goal is to decrease the frequency of the tics by substituting physically incompatible behaviors to be practiced whenever tics or premonitory urges occur. Habit reversal has been shown to produce reductions in tics ranging as high as 93 percent, and there has been no documentation of side effects. The third treatment tactic involves addressing any comorbid conditions (e.g., ADHD, OCD, and learning disorders) that have been identified.

PROGNOSIS

Tics wax and wane, even in chronic disorders and, for many afflicted children, tics will emerge, go through a waxing and waning cycle, and disappear untreated. In other cases, however, tics may develop at a young age and continue through adulthood. If the tic does not dissipate on its own, pharmacological and behavioral treatments are available to aid in the reduction of tic frequency and intensity. In transient cases, these treatments can eliminate tics altogether. In chronic cases, and especially TD, however, afflicted persons may require some form of treatment for life.

See also: Attention-Deficit/Hyperactivity Disorder; Habit Reversal; Learning Disorders; Obsessive Compulsive Disorder; Pharmacological Interventions; Stereotypic Movement Disorder

Further Reading

Findley, D. B. (2001). Characteristics of tic disorders. In D. W. Woods & R. G. Miltenberger (Eds.), *Tic disorders, trichotillomania, and other repetitive behavior disorders: Behavioral approaches to analysis and treatment* (pp. 53–72). Norwell, MA: Kluwer Academic.

Watson, T. S., Howell, L. A., & Smith S. L. (2001). Behavioral interventions for tic disorders. In D. W. Woods & R. G. Miltenberger (Eds.), *Tic disorders, trichotillomania, and other repetitive behavior disorders: Behavioral approaches to analysis and treatment* (pp. 53–72). Norwell, MA: Kluwer Academic.

Web Site

info.med.yale.edu/chldstdy/tsocd.htm

Michael Twohig
Patrick C. Friman

Time Out

Time out is a procedure developed within the framework of applied behavior analysis and can be used to reduce problem behavior of children. It is typically used as a negative consequence for problem behavior, with a view to reducing the frequency of the future occurrence of that behavior. Unfortunately, the procedure of time out is badly understood by many in the community, and it has the potential of being misused.

The phrase "time out" refers generally to " time out from reinforcement." More technically it means a reduction in the availability of reinforcement available to the child for a short period of time.

Time out is most commonly used with children who demonstrate serious or ongoing behavior problems. It can involve the removal of the child to another room when the problem behavior occurs (exclusionary time out). However it can also involve keeping the child in the room where the problem behavior occurred but reducing the child's access to reinforcement available in the room (nonexclusionary time out).

Time out will not work if applied without a full understanding of the applied behavior analysis principles that underpin it. For example, problems can arise in the use of exclusionary time out when the time out area is actually more reinforcing than the area the child is being removed from. Some parents erroneously think they are using time out when they send their children to their bedrooms and yet their bedrooms are filled with toys and other entertaining activities. When using time out in school, a teacher may place a child in an interesting/stimulating area (for example, a hallway) and he is able to avoid work and be entertained. These are examples of "time in," not time out. The actual effect may actually be that of reinforcement, with the likelihood that the child will repeat the behavior, perhaps even in order to be placed in time out.

When appropriately used, time out is an effective method of weakening problematic behaviors. The period of time out is necessarily short. To determine the length of time, a good rule of thumb is one minute for each year of the child's life (from age two) up to a maximum of ten minutes. Clinicians usually insist that careful records be kept about the total length of time the child spends in time out. This can serve as a safeguard against a child being placed in time out for unreasonably long periods of time.

It is important to note that the measurement of the length of time in time out should only begin once the child is quiet. This is to ensure that the child does not get reinforced for crying, yelling, or creating a disturbance in time out by being allowed to leave while still noisy. In addition, this teaches the child to self-settle and calm him/herself down. In the initial stages of implementing time out, children may actually be in time out longer than the minimum time out period while they learn that time out period will not begin until they are calm. Some clinicians require that the child be quiet and calm for the entire minimum period, others require a small amount of time at the end of the period to be spent in silence. However it is managed, the child should not leave time out until a period of calm has been achieved. This ensures that the child learns to calm him/herself independently. When the time out period is complete, the child is informed that "time out is over" and as soon as the child is engaged in an appropriate behavior he or she should be provided with verbal reinforcement (to ensure the child knows what behaviors should replace the ones that earn time out).

Nonexclusionary time out involves making the child's current environment less reinforcing. This often includes removing the attention of people in the room, allocating a chair or place in the room that is the time out spot, and removing access to activities. Nonexclusionary time out is also brief and can be followed by exclusionary time out if the child does not immediately settle down.

When used appropriately, time out has been demonstrated to be an effective method of weakening inappropriate behavior. It should always be used in a program that uses applied behavior analysis procedures of strengthening behavior (such as reinforcement) to ensure the child replaces the inappropriate behavior with appropriate alternatives. While some concerns are raised over the long-term consequences of time out, it is important to note that time out is generally only used over a short period of time and has far less negative side effects than other alternatives such as smacking, spanking, threatening, and shouting. It also has the effect of allowing parents to remain calm while they deal with their child's difficult behavior.

Further Reading

Child Development Institute. http://www.childdevelopmentinfo.com/parenting/timeout.html

Grant, L., & Evans, A. (1994). *Principles of behavior.* New York: Harper Collins.

Hudson, A. (1998). Applied behavior analysis. In A. Bellack & M. Hersen (Series Ed.) & T. Ollendick (Vol. Ed.), *Comprehensive clinical psychology (Vol. 5). Children and adolescents: Clinical formulation and treatment* (pp. 107–129). New York: Pergamon.

Sanders, M. R. (1992). *Every parent: A positive approach to children's behavior.* Sydney: Addison Wesley.

EMMA LITTLE
ALAN HUDSON

Token Economies

Token economies were first used more than 40 years ago to change the behavior of patients in psychiatric hospitals. Developed using the principles of applied behavior analysis, token economies are designed to increase appropriate behaviors and decrease inappropriate behaviors. Token economies have been demonstrated to work well in settings where access to reinforcers through tokens can be controlled (e.g., homes, schools, inpatient settings).

A token economy is a tailored system of reinforcement and punishment (response cost) for specific behaviors, with the aim of increasing the frequency of desirable behaviors and decreasing the frequency of undesirable behaviors. This is done through the presentation and removal of tokens contingent upon specific behaviors being demonstrated. These tokens are used at a later time to gain access to desirable activities or tangible reinforcers (back-up reinforcement).

The first step in establishing a token economy is to identify the behaviors that will be reinforced. Then the type of token to be used needs to be decided. Typically, plastic tokens, pieces of card, stickers, or points are used as tokens. Next, the back-up reinforcers need to be identified and the number of tokens needed to obtain these reinforcers determined.

Each token economy is individually designed with regard to the behaviors that result in the presentation or removal of a token. Token economies have been used to improve academic behaviors (e.g., reading, vocabulary, homework), social skills (appropriate interactions and behaviors with others) and general compliance to parent or teacher requests.

The number of tokens required to receive a back-up reinforcer can also be individualized. Often a token economy will involve increasing the number of tokens needed as the child develops greater skills in demonstrating desirable behaviors. From its earliest use in inpatient facilities it was determined that for a token economy to work most effectively, a range of back-up reinforcers should be provided. This ensures that the individual can select the item or activity that is most reinforcing to him or her at that point in time.

One problem with reinforcement generally can be the difficulty in providing immediate reinforcement, particularly in settings where tangible and activity-based reinforcement may not be immediately available. Tokens overcome this problem by being immediately available and hence immediately reinforcing, while allowing a delay to occur before a back-up reinforcer is provided. Tokens can also be used for a range of behaviors that all contribute to gaining the more substantial back-up reinforcer. Also, tokens can also be used to access a range of back-up reinforcers, which reduces the likelihood of satiation or deprivation being problematic. The number of tokens required to earn a back-up reinforcer can gradually be increased in order to phase out reinforcement and to make the behavior more resistant to extinction.

Token economies have been found to be an effective method of changing behavior both at home and at school. Whole classrooms can be involved in token economies where students work together to gain tokens for appropriate behavior and are reinforced by a whole group activity once a specific goal is reached.

See also: Applied Behavior Analysis; Extinction; Positive Reinforcement; Response Cost

Further Reading

Cooper, J. O., Heron, T. E., & Heward, W. L. (1987). *Applied behavior analysis.* New York: Macmillan.

Kehle, T. J., Bray, M. A., Theodore, L. A., Jenson, W. R., & Clark, E. (2000). A multi-component intervention designed to reduce disruptive classroom behavior. *Psychology in the Schools, 37,* 475–481

Liberman, R. P. (2000). The token economy. *American Journal of Psychiatry, 157,* 9.

Myles, B. S., Moran, M. R., Ormsbee, C. K., & Downing, J. A., (1992). Guidelines for establishing and maintaining token economies. *Intervention in School and Clinic, 27,* 164–169. http://www.cet.fsu.edu/cpt/TREE/myles.html

EMMA LITTLE
ALAN HUDSON

Touch Development

See: Sensory and Perceptual Development

Touch Therapy

See: Massage Therapy

Tourette's Disorder

See: Tic Disorders: Tourette's Disorder, Chronic Tic Disorder, and Transient Tic Disorder

Tracheostomy Dependent Children

DEFINITION/ISSUES

Commensurate with advances in medical technology, increasing numbers of pediatric patients sustain life via tracheostomy. This procedure enables airway access via insertion of a breathing tube, or cannula, through an incision in the neck, and is typically performed for serious respiratory problems. Recent national data do not appear to exist concerning the incidence of pediatric tracheostomy, although previous estimates have suggested that 0.1–0.27 percent of pediatric hospital admissions involved tracheostomy-related operations.

Paradoxically, the very procedure responsible for preserving life simultaneously poses significant risks to a child's well-being. As the duration of a tracheostomy increases, so do the threats to a child's physical, developmental, intellectual, psychological, and behavioral status. Unfortunately, while results vary widely, it is typically reported that 40 percent or more of tracheostomy cases have moderate to severe difficulties in weaning to normal breathing. Such hardships often include many months of attempts prior to success, as well as total failure to accomplish the task. These difficulties with weaning escalate with the length of time a cannula for breathing has remained in place.

ASSESSMENT FOR READINESS

In light of the adverse effects of prolonged tracheostomies, it is generally considered important to wean children from breathing through the cannula as soon as physically possible. Existing protocols currently rely solely upon the presence of physical indicators in determining an ideal commencement time for weaning procedures. According to Ladyshewsky and Gousseau (1996), some of these physical indicators include absence of granulation tissue, sufficient vocal cord mobility, intact gag reflex, ability to swallow secretions, oxygen saturation greater than 90 percent, and arterial blood gases within normal limits. If patients are not physically ready, the weaning process may impose extra stress upon their respiratory system, possibly compromising a successful weaning outcome.

In addition to physical considerations, psychological factors may offer additional insight into readiness for tracheostomy weaning. For example, older children with minimal levels of anxiety and depression, reasonable coping skills, and motivation for weaning accomplishment may be more "psychologically ready" for weaning trials. Thus, along with physical criteria, the inclusion of specific psychological parameters may provide a more comprehensive assessment of an individual's readiness for weaning, possibly enhancing chances for weaning success.

WEANING PROCEDURES

To date, the medical literature contains only a few studies delineating systemized weaning procedures for tracheostomy dependent children. Such procedures have focused mainly on the initial attainment of necessary physiological criteria, in addition to a recommendation that the child be weaned to breathe independently in a graduated manner.

The late 1960s produced the first view of tracheostomy addiction as a learned behavior involving weakening of the normal breathing reflex, which is replaced by a stronger reflex for tracheostomy breathing. Assuming that decannulation attempts based upon principles of classical conditioning and behavioral modification might prove beneficial, Wright and colleagues (1968) paired pleasurable experiences for two pediatric patients (i.e., receiving physical affection, socializing with others, and playing with toys) with cannula occlusion for brief yet gradually increasing periods of time, three times per day, for 21 days. Conversely, the remaining periods of cannula nonocclusion were paired with isolation from others as well as from toys and/or other reinforcing stimuli (isolation did not occur during necessary interaction for meals, diapering, and routine medical care). Results indicated decannulation success after 21 days in both patients. However, a later report suggested that the procedure could take as long as 36 days in some cases. Although various explanations were offered, conditioning principles were believed to lay the foundation for the success of this approach.

Elliott and Olson (1982) conducted a follow-up study using the Wright approach with the following modifications: Eight (versus three) conditioning trials per day, increasing the length of occlusion more rapidly, and reducing the degree of social isolation. Results indicated that all four subjects successfully decannulated in less time (38 percent decrease in hospital days required for the procedure in comparison to the Wright et al. [1968] study), and with less social isolation, suggesting, among other things, a more cost-efficient and presumably less aversive approach to tracheostomy weaning in pediatric patients.

Unfortunately, a review of the current literature failed to produce any recent empirical studies combining psychological applications to decannulation procedures in pediatric patients, and psychological approaches to this problem appear to have faded, for the most part, from pediatric medical practice. However, given the widely reported difficulties in weaning from tracheostomy dependent breathing, continued refinements blending medical and psychological paradigms are strongly warranted in offering pediatric patients the best chance for successful preparation for and reinstatement of natural breathing following long-term tracheostomy.

See also: Anxiety Disorders; Behavior Modification; Cognitive–Behavior Therapy; Differential Social Reinforcement/ Positive Attention; Relaxation Training; Ventilator Dependency in Children

Further Reading

Carr, M. M., Poje, C. P., Kingston, L., Kielma, D., & Heard, C. (2001). Complications in pediatric tracheostomies. *The Laryngoscope*, *111*(11), 1925–1928.

Doerksen, K., Ladyshewsky, A., & Stansfield, K. (1994). A comparative study of systemized vs. random tracheostomy weaning. *Axon*, *16*(1), 5–13.

Elliott, C. E., & Olson, R. A. (1982). Variations in conditioning procedures for the decannulation of tracheostomy dependent children: Clinical and theoretical implications. *Health Psychology*, *1*(4), 389–397.

Ladyshewsky, A., & Gousseau, A. (1996). Successful tracheal weaning. *The Canadian Nurse*, *92*(2), 35–38.

Wright, L., Nunnery, A., Eichel, B., & Scott, R. (1968). Application of conditioning principles to problems of tracheostomy addiction in children. *Journal of Consulting and Clinical Psychology*, *32*(5), 603–606.

CHARLES H. ELLIOTT
MARIA R. MARSHALL

Training Issues

Issues of training in clinical child and pediatric psychology have received considerable attention during the past several decades. This focus on training has been stimulated, first of all, by estimates that up to 20 percent of children/adolescents in the general population display significant psychological problems, that only 10–15 percent receive adequate treatment, and that there is a shortage of adequately trained child psychologists to meet the needs of these children and their families. A second factor relates to the proliferation of training programs purporting to offer clinical child specialty training.

Specific to the issue of predoctoral training, it can be noted that in the 1976–1977 edition of the *Graduate Study in Psychology* only eight graduate programs were self-identified as offering training in clinical child psychology. By 1982, a comprehensive survey of graduate training programs identified a total of 36 programs that offered formal training in this area, as well as 29 others that reported offering more informal training experiences. By 1995, the *Directory of Graduate Programs in Clinical Child/Pediatric Psychology* listed a total of 110 graduate programs that reported offering specialty training. These findings clearly suggest a dramatic increase in the number of graduate programs providing specialty training. There has also been a notable increase in formal clinical child/pediatric psychology specialty training at both the internship and postdoctoral levels.

Unfortunately, as there are no accreditation procedures for evaluating graduate programs in the child area, it is impossible to ascertain the quality of training these programs provide. Indeed, the fact that programs purporting to offer clinical child training sometimes do not, is suggested by the results of a recent survey of programs listed in the *Directory of Graduate Programs in Clinical Child/Pediatric Psychology* which found a number of programs to have no faculty member with applied child interests associated with the program, no formal required clinical child courses, no clinical child program director and, in reality, no program.

Concerns over manpower issues and the adequacy of training offered by an increasing number of clinical child programs have both raised questions and highlighted a range of issues relevant to training in this area.

MODELS OF SPECIALTY TRAINING

Over the years questions have been raised regarding the optimal model or context within which clinical child specialty training should be provided. Historically, there have been four primary models of graduate specialty training. The most common has been providing clinical child training as a track within a general clinical training program. Here, students specialize in the child area while also completing coursework and clinical training experiences required of all students. Other models include clinical child programs that are independent of, or overlap minimally with, general clinical training. Here, there is likely to be a formal Director of Clinical Child Training, and students are likely to be selected specifically for the clinical child program and less likely to be exposed to the full range of "adult-related" courses required of general clinical students. The third model has involved a blending of clinical child and school psychology training, while the fourth has historically involved clinical child training provided by faculty in developmental rather than clinical psychology. More recently, even those programs with the strongest developmental focus tend to be based in the clinical area, probably due to difficulties of programs in the developmental area in obtaining accreditation. While there has been some debate as to the optimal model of training, no one model has been shown to be superior to others. It seems likely that the particular model of training or context in which training occurs may be far less important that the breadth, depth, and sequential organization of training experiences to which trainees are exposed.

BREADTH OF SPECIALTY TRAINING

As with other specialties, the professional preparation of clinical child psychologists has sometimes been construed as being too narrow with too little attention being given to the breadth of training. Nothing could be further from the truth.

Here, it should be noted that, like trainees in other areas of professional psychology, students in clinical child psychology programs are provided with a background in core areas of psychology that serve as a scientific and professional foundation for practice.

This is supplemented by specialty-specific training sequences designed to train students in those professional activities that are central to the specialty.

Regarding the parameters of the specialty, it is worth noting that clinical child psychology is a specialty unlike many others. It is not defined by any one theoretical orientation, by any specific approach to assessment or therapy, focus on any specific problem area, or focus on working with individuals in a given setting. Clinical child psychologists are involved in clinical practice, teaching, consultation, and research. They engage in a variety of approaches toward prevention, assessment, and treatment from a variety of theoretical perspectives, work in a variety of professional contexts, including those that are multidisciplinary in nature, and deal with the full range of behavioral and psychological difficulties experienced by children and adolescents, as well as psychological/behavioral issues related to child health. In engaging in these activities, clinical child psychologists are mindful of the various ecological systems with which the child interacts, as well as developmental and cultural factors as they contribute to child/adolescent behavior.

Given that clinical child training is typically designed to prepare individuals for engaging in such a wide range of professional activities, training in quality clinical child programs is hardly narrow. Indeed, except for the focus on an earlier stage of development (e.g., infants, children, adolescents), the specialty of clinical child psychology is every bit as broad as the "general practice area" of clinical psychology.

GUIDELINES FOR SPECIALTY TRAINING

As clinical child psychology has evolved there have been numerous calls for developing training standards to ensure adequate preparation of those entering the specialty. Three notable attempts to respond to this need can be highlighted. An initial effort, described by Roberts, Erickson and Tuma in 1985, involved the work of a Task Force on Training, appointed by the Division of Child Youth and Family Services (APA, Division 37), which developed initial guidelines for training psychologists to work with children, youth, and families. The call for training guidelines was also responded to by the convening of a major training conference, "Training Clinical Child Psychologists" at Hilton Head, South Carolina in May of 1985. At this conference participants endorsed the recommendations of the Division 37 Task Force, a scientist–practitioner model of training that emphasized an empirical approach to assessment and treatment, and agreed on a range of resolutions related to clinical child training. These included recommendations that clinical child programs provide training related to (1) life-span developmental psychology, (2) child psychopathology, child assessment, prevention, and intervention approaches appropriate to children, adolescents, and families, (3) multicultural issues, (4) social systems that impact on children, adolescents and families, and (5) sufficient training to develop minimal competencies in adult psychopathology, assessment, and treatment.

While these recommendations had little impact on most child training programs, a more recent attempt to integrate and elaborate on the Division 37 and Hilton Head guidelines resulted from the efforts of a 1992 Center for Mental Health Issues task force on training and from a subsequent writing conference held at the University of Kansas in 1993. The results of these efforts, described by Roberts and colleagues in 1998, represent an elaborate and detailed framework for training individuals to work with children and adolescents.

In applying this framework to graduate training in clinical child psychology, trainees would be exposed to courses that provide a foundation in core areas of scientific and professional psychology, as well as a wide range of didactic and applied training experiences in the following areas: (1) life-span developmental psychology, (2) life-span developmental psychopathology, (3) child, adolescent, and family assessment, (4) intervention strategies, (5) professional, ethical, and legal issues pertaining to children, youth, and families, (6) research methods and approaches to system evaluation, (7) issues of diversity, (8) prevention and health promotion, (9) the role of multiple disciplines and service delivery systems, (10) social issues affecting children, youth, and families, and (11) specialized clinical experiences in assessment, intervention, and consultation.

Considering that training in these areas would progress sequentially from simple exposure to the development of expertise in various areas, that training would include structured research experiences relevant to the specialty, and that internship training would build on predoctoral training and provide a foundation for postdoctoral experience, this framework could serve as an excellent foundation for the formulation of accreditation guidelines for graduate clinical child specialty training.

ISSUES OF SPECIALTY ACCREDITATION

One way of ensuring adequacy of training in clinical child psychology is for there to be a quality assurance mechanism to guarantee that programs offering specialty training meet basic standards. Historically, the APA Committee on Accreditation (CoA) has only accredited programs in the areas of clinical, counseling, and school psychology, although CoA's *Guidelines and Principles* provide for the development of accreditation mechanisms for "emerging substantive areas of professional psychology." Although "emerging substantive areas" are not defined, it could be argued that clinical child psychology would qualify under this provision given any reasonable definition of the concept. At this point, procedures are already in place for clinical child programs at the *postdoctoral* level to be considered for specialty accreditation. Accreditation mechanisms for *graduate* programs that could enhance the quality of clinical child specialty training remain a hope for the future, however.

See also: Clinical Child and Adolescent Psychology; Pediatric Psychology; School Psychology

Further Reading

La Greca, A. M., Stone, W. L., Drotar, D., & Maddux, J. E. (1988). Training in pediatric psychology: Survey results and recommendations. *Journal of Pediatric Psychology, 13,* 121–140.

Roberts, M. C., et al. (1998). A model for training psychologists to provide services for children and adolescents. *Professional Psychology: Research and Practice, 29,* 293–299.

Roberts, M. C., Erickson, M. T., & Tuma, J. M. (1985). Addressing the needs: Guidelines for training psychologists to work with children, youth, and families. *Journal of Clinical Child Psychology, 14,* 70–79.

Tuma, J. M. (1985). *Proceedings: Conference on training clinical child psychologists.* Baton Rouge, LA: Section on Clinical Child Psychology.

JAMES H. JOHNSON

Transient Tic Disorder

See: Tic Disorders: Tourette's Disorder, Chronic Tic Disorder, and Transient Tic Disorder

Traumatic Brain Injury

DESCRIPTION OF THE PROBLEM

Traumatic brain injury (TBI) occurs as a result of severe acceleration and deceleration of the cranium. The mechanisms of injury are multiple and include abuse, motor vehicle accidents, falls, recreational/sports accidents, and other causes. Acute measurement of trauma conducted by emergency personnel is typically the Glasgow Coma Scale (GCS), which ranges from 3 to 15, and is based on eye-opening response, motor response to painful stimuli, and verbal response to orientation questions. Several studies indicate good prediction of gross outcome using the highest GCS in the first 24 hr posttrauma. A GCS of less than 8 indicates severe TBI, whereas GCS scores of 9–12 and 13–15 would be indicative of moderate and mild TBI, respectively.

Several additional factors have been shown to predict long-term outcome including duration of unconsciousness, length of posttraumatic amnesia, and the presence of acute medical complications (i.e., subdural hematoma, depressed skull fracture, and sustained increased intracranial pressure).

EPIDEMIOLOGY

The incidence of traumatic brain injury in pediatric populations is approximately 180 per 100,000 per year. In pediatric populations, 50 percent of all fatal traumas involve primary injuries to the brain as their cause. The most common cause of traumatic death among children under age 3 is brain injury induced by child abuse (Shaken Baby Syndrome), with increased incidents of trauma-induced falls and motor vehicle accidents occurring after age 5. The leading cause of TBI in ages 3–11 is bicycle accidents, while the leading cause of TBI among adolescents is motor vehicle accidents and sports/recreational accidents. Gender does not play a role in the incidence of TBI prior to age 5; however, after age 5, males are $2\frac{1}{2}$ times as likely to suffer a traumatic brain injury than females.

PATHOPHYSIOLOGY/MECHANISMS OF INJURY

Several pathophysiological mechanisms interact to produce the totality of traumatic brain injury. Due to the bony prominences in the cranium and bipedal, forward-facing nature of humans, the anterior inferior frontal lobes and anterior temporal lobes are the most frequently injured areas of the cerebral cortex, and sparing of primary motor, sensory, and language areas is typical. These mechanisms can be considered as either primary, acute injury mechanisms or secondary injury mechanisms, which produce negative effects postacutely.

Primary Injury Mechanisms

Primary injury mechanisms include those mechanisms which are trauma-related, including diffuse axorial injury (DAI), cerebral contusion, and epidural, subdural, and intraventricular hematoma. DAI refers to the damage to subcortical white matter produced from the tensile shearing and torque force of rapid acceleration/deceleration mechanisms associated with TBI. Cerebrals Contusions are produced when the cortex is bruised from contact with bony structures in the cranium. These contusive effects often occur at the end points of a linear force plane in the anterior/posterior orientation or on either side of the brain in the case of a side impact. The initial contusion is often referred to as the coup site, corresponding to the initial site of impact within the cranium. The corresponding rebound-effect often produces a site of contusion which is 180 degrees from the initial impact and referred to as the contercoup lesion. In addition, collections of space-occupying blood (hematoma) can develop rapidly and occur under great pressure. Such collections are referred to as epidural if they occur between the skull and the tough outer layer covering the brain (dura mater), whereas they are referred to as subdural hematoma if the collection of blood occurs below this outer layer or in the substance of the brain itself. While both epidural and subdural hematomas represent emergency conditions due to pressure effects, recovery from epidural hematoma is typically much better than that from subdural hematoma, the latter of which may have devastating secondary damage effects. Intraventricular hematomas are collections of blood within the ventricular space and can range from benign to life-threatening, primarily determined by whether they block the downstream flow of cerebrospinal fluid and thus produce increased intracranial pressure.

Secondary Injury Mechanisms

Secondary injury mechanisms produce further post acute cerebral damage and include vasospasm, edema, and hypoxic intracellular toxicity. Vasospasm occurs in reaction to the presence of blood in the substance of the brain, which causes cyclical rapid cerebrovascular constriction and expansion. Vasoconstriction occurs as a protective mechanism against further hemorrhage and vasodilation occurs as a reaction to the brain sensing decreased oxygen availability at a time of heightened demand. This cyclical vacillation in vasoconstriction and expansion can produce hypoxia, which is typically distributed in areas of the brain which do not share anastamotic blood sources and are thus more susceptible to rapid changes in blood pressure gradients. Edema is produced by several factors including the initial trauma as well as the swelling induced by the brain attempting to clear away negative neurotoxic effects of glucose metabolism, which has occurred in the absence of an adequate oxygen supply due to pressure gradient induced ischemia or vasospasm. This neurotoxic effect produces oxygen-free radicals and their accumulation leads to further neuronal death.

COGNITIVE AND EMOTIONAL SEQUELAE OF TBI

The cognitive and emotional sequelae of traumatic brain injury vary widely with the severity of injury and the site of cerebral damage. The prototypical pattern of recovery is represented by both a biological recovery phase followed by improved functioning associated with adaptation to residual deficits. The biological recovery progresses rapidly for the first 2–4 months, with continued but decelerating improvement over the next 7–10 months postinjury. Continued improvement can be expected through use of adaptive skills and compensatory mechanisms such as organization strategies and external memory aids. While most traumatic brain injuries result in a diffuse pattern of cerebral injury, focal or lateralized lesions can produce specific deficits. Left hemisphere lesions are most likely to result in language-based deficits, whereas right hemisphere deficits are likely to result in deficits in visuospatial skills. In general, anterior lesions result in personality, behavior, abstract reasoning and motor deficits, whereas posterior lesions result in sensory, perceptual, and integrative visual, auditory, and tactile deficits associated with language and motor sequencing and execution skills.

Behavioral disorders may be manifest as either hypo- or hyperarousal deficits. Severe TBI often produces significant neurobehavioral deficits, acutely producing hyperarousal/agitation and subsequently producing lethargy and fatigue in the later stages. The lethargy is often punctuated with intermittent periods of agitation associated with emotional dysregulation and increased confusion and disorientation. Mild TBI more frequently results in emotional deficits such as depression and anxiety, which are frequently exacerbated or perpetuated by cognitive sequelae and changes in interpersonal interactions.

Cognitive deficits are also significantly linked to injury severity, with more severe injuries resulting in more diffuse and profound deficits across many cognitive functions including memory, reasoning, and visuospatial skills. While basic verbal communication, motor, and sensory functions are retained in all but the most severe injuries, even mild TBI may result in complex attention and information processing speed deficits which have far-reaching implications, as these functions are prerequisite for the efficient performance of many other cognitive functions.

OUTCOMES AND TREATMENT

Several factors affect long-term outcome including injury severity, premorbid individual and family adjustment, and postinjury treatment of individual and family behavioral or interactional maladjustment. Injuries occurring at younger ages, as well as those associated with postinjury complications (i.e., epilepsy, infection, hydrocephalus, etc.), are likely to produce poorer cognitive and behavioral outcomes across the range of TBI severity. The efficacy of acute treatment has not been demonstrated conclusively to produce outcomes superior to the natural recovery process; however, postacute identification and ongoing treatment in the form of emotional adjustment and implementation of compensatory skills of both TBI survivors and family have been shown to produce better long-term outcomes as measured by decreased relapse of emotional sequelae and increased independence in functional skills. Intervention through schools by providing appropriate accomodations and increased individualized instruction have also shown benefit in increased academic achievement.

See also: Injury Prevention; Intellectual Assessment; Learning Disorders; Neurological Disorders; Physical Abuse

Further Reading

Broman, S. H., & Michel, M. E. (1995). *Traumatic head injury in children*. New York: Oxford University Press.
Yeats, K. O. (2000). Closed head injury. In K. O. Yeats, M. D. Ris, & G. H. Taylor (Eds.), *Pediatric neuropsychology* (pp. 72–117). New York: Guilford.

JAMES SCOTT
PAUL C. FRANCEL

Traumatic Grief

See: Bereavement

Treatment Adherence: Behavioral

DEFINITION

Treatment adherence refers to the degree to which a therapist delivers the prescribed treatment; that is, does the therapist deliver the therapy detailed in the treatment manual? Treatment adherence is not the same as the quality of the therapy or the therapist's ability. It is, instead, a concern with what took place during the treatment and the extent to which this matches the content and process described in the written treatment manual. Other terms frequently used to refer to treatment adherence include therapist adherence or treatment integrity. Measurement of treatment adherence is virtually impossible when no guidelines or manuals exist for the treatment. With the increased desire for and use of manual-based treatments, there is an increased ability to both assess and study treatment adherence.

The concern with treatment adherence increases demands for accountability from all psychotherapies and all psychotherapists. First, it requires that treatment manuals are prepared, evaluated, and disseminated. Second, it holds the therapist accountable to deliver the prescribed treatment.

Therapist adherence plays an essential role in the study of the efficacy of psychotherapy. When child treatments are evaluated, it is important for therapists to deliver the same treatment to each child/family within each treatment condition. When therapists do not adhere to the treatment protocol or when treatment adherence is not measured, conclusions regarding the relative efficacy of the treatment cannot be made with confidence. If only a portion of the treated cases received the treatment as prescribed by the manual, then an adequate assessment of the efficacy of the treatment could not occur.

Treatment adherence has been equated mistakenly with rigid treatment adherence. This common misperception of manual-based treatments presumes that the treatment must be administered in a cookbook/unsophisticated manner. Adherence to a treatment manual is not synonymous with automated therapy. Rather, a therapist who adheres to a treatment manual does so in a flexible manner.

MEASUREMENT OF TREATMENT ADHERENCE

Different sources can be used when measuring therapist adherence to treatment protocols. Materials that retain the most reliable information (i.e., videotapes) provide better detail for rating adherence than materials that lose specific information about the session (i.e., process notes).

Adherence can be measured in several ways. The simplest way to assess adherence is to use a checklist of the techniques expected to occur or not occur in the intervention. Basically, the treatment prescribes certain therapeutic actions and proscribes others. An independent rater examines audio- or videotapes of sessions and checks off interventions as they occur.

Frequency ratings are a more detailed method of evaluating adherence. Here, the frequency of an intervention is rated, often on a Likert-type scale (e.g., never, fairly often, often, all the time), rather than simply by a dichotomous presence/absence decision. Other methods combine measures of adherence with measures of competence by requiring the rater to consider how skillfully a treatment procedure was performed while taking into account factors like the appropriateness, sensitivity, and timing of the intervention. As indicated by Shaw (1984), ratings that fall outside the predetermined range indicate that a therapist is not adhering to the protocol adequately. An alternative approach is to rate adherence on an event-by-event basis: rating each statement made by the therapist. This provides detailed ratings of therapist behavior and allows for analysis of disagreement among coders, as indicated by Waltz and colleagues (1993).

CLINICAL APPLICATION

Adherence to manual-based treatments can be achieved in a flexible manner without compromising treatment integrity. For example, effective cognitive–behavioral treatments for anxious youth were associated with a full range of therapist flexibility (see Cognitive–Behavior Therapy). Kendall and Chu (2000) suggest that the therapist use the treatment manual as a guide, conveying general strategies in a variety of ways, according to the needs of the child.

The dissemination of therapy manuals may promote the transportability of empirically supported treatments from clinical research settings to clinical service settings (see Evidenced-Based Treatments). Although therapists in private practice may be reluctant, manuals can guide treatment. For example, children treated for anxiety disorders participate in exposure tasks as part of cognitive-behavioral treatment. These exposure tasks are considered important, but many of these exposure tasks may require the participation of other children, other therapists, and leaving the office. Within a research setting, this does not present the problem that it can create in a private practice, where it may be difficult to find volunteers. Practitioners may have to work to override obstacles while adhering to manual-based treatments.

Results of randomized clinical trials of therapy for youth demonstrate that effective treatments are associated with high levels of treatment adherence. Although the relationship between levels of adherence and treatment outcome has not been thoroughly investigated, integrity checks reveal high levels of adherence within found-to-be-effective treatments for anxiety, depression, and Conduct Disorder (CD) (see Measurement of Behavior Change).

Areas for future research include the evaluation of the impact of therapist adherence on outcome across the children's developmental levels and presenting problems. The effect of the training experience on the flexibility with which a therapist adheres to a manual, the level of difficulty of the client, and the context in which treatment takes place may also be important variables affecting the relationship between adherence and outcome.

See also: Cognitive–Behavior Therapy; Evidence-Based Treatments; Treatment Alliance; Treatment Outcome Measures

Further Reading

Kendall, P. C., & Chu, B. C. (2000). Retrospective self-reports of therapist flexibility in a manual-based treatment for youths with anxiety disorders. *Journal of Consulting and Clinical Psychology, 29*, 209–220.

Kendall, P. C., Flannery-Schroeder, E., Panichelli-Mindel, S. M., Southam-Gerow, M., Henin, A., & Warman, M. (1997). Therapy for youths with anxiety disorders: A second randomized clinical trial. *Journal of Consulting and Clinical Psychology, 65*, 366–380.

Shaw, B. F. (1984). Specification of the training and evaluation of cognitive therapies for outcome studies. In J. Williams & R. Spitzer (Eds.), *Psychotherapy research: Where are we and where should we go?* (pp. 173–188). New York: Guilford.

Waltz, J., Addis, M. E., Koerner, K., & Jacobson, N. S. (1993). Testing the integrity of a psychotherapy protocol: Assessment of adherence and competence. *Journal of Consulting and Clinical Psychology, 61*, 620–630.

JOANNA A. ROBIN
TORREY A. CREED
JENNIFER L. HUDSON
PHILIP C. KENDALL

Treatment Adherence: Medical

DEFINITION

Treatment adherence to medical regimens refers to "the extent to which a person's behavior (in terms of taking medications, following diets, or executing lifestyle changes) coincides with medical or health advice" (Haynes, 1979, pp. 1–2). An estimated 50 percent of pediatric patients are considered adherent to treatment recommendations, but the range is large (from a low of 10 percent to a high of 90 percent). Treatment adherence varies with patient characteristics (e.g., demographics, knowledge/education, individual and family functioning), regimen factors (e.g., complexity, duration, cost, efficacy, side effects), and illness/disease factors (e.g., acute or chronic illness, severity, symptoms). Although high levels of adherence to medical regimens may be desirable to achieve clinical benefits or to evaluate regimen efficacy, pediatric patients and their parents should be active participants in medical decision-making; nonadherence may reflect a rational decision on the part of the patient and parent to forego a prescribed regimen. However, when a medical regimen is prescribed, health care providers are likely to promote high levels of adherence so that the benefits and side effects of the regimen can be fully evaluated.

METHODS

Measuring treatment adherence may involve a variety of methods, including patient or parent self-reports, direct observation of behavior, pill counts, drug assays, ratings by health care professionals, or electronic monitoring devices. Each of these measures has limitations; in practice, a combination of indicators of short- and long-term adherence may be desired. In addition to measuring adherence behavior, measuring treatment outcome or health status has been used as an indicator of adherence. However, adherence is not consistently associated with changes in treatment outcome or health status for a variety of regimens. For example, medication regimens prescribed for a chronic illness (e.g., asthma, diabetes) may not produce the desired health status changes or may result in undesirable side effects. Thus, a combination of measures for adherence, outcome, and health status may provide the most comprehensive indicators of the efficacy of a medical regimen.

Interventions to promote adherence have been based on a variety of educational, applied behavior, analytic, social cognitive, and stages of change models. There is support for the effectiveness of interventions based on these various theoretical models and approaches, and the majority of intervention studies incorporate numerous behavior change strategies. Rapoff (1999) proposed that clinicians can promote adherence to medical regimens by:

- Verbally persuading patients and their families of the value of prescribed regimens;
- Providing competent role models who demonstrate how to successfully manage regimens;
- Helping patients and families set specific goals and monitor progress to these goals;
- Teaching patients and families the necessary skills for carrying out regimen tasks;
- Helping patients and their families arrange more reinforcing consequences for adherence (p. 45).

CLINICAL APPLICATION

Children with acute and chronic illnesses and children who are changing dietary and lifestyle habits to promote healthy development can benefit from clinical adherence interventions. *Parental monitoring and supervision* is most important to assist with younger children's adherence; increasing responsibility for older children and adolescents should be the goal for parents as greater self-regulatory skills are developing. *Prompting and reminder* strategies should be incorporated to assist with remembering to perform regimen behaviors and to develop adherence habits. *Contingency management* is an important adherence promotion strategy for children. Parents may provide reinforcement for adherence (e.g., incentives, privileges) and disciplinary actions for misbehavior that leads to nonadherence (e.g., time out, grounding). *Self-management* strategies are important for children and adolescents to develop as they become more self-reliant. Effective problem-solving strategies can be taught to help individuals identify problematic situations associated with a regimen, along with coping strategies for dealing with attitudes and beliefs associated with an illness or need for a medical regimen that makes the child or adolescent feel different from peers. *Psychotherapy* may be indicated when the child, parent, and/or family has psychological and relationship problems that interfere with effective adherence. In summary, a range of interventions can be tailored to the individual child and family to provide the support necessary to overcome barriers to adherence and to promote long-term adherence to a needed regimen.

EFFECTIVENESS

Most studies have shown that behavioral and cognitive interventions can promote greater adherence behavior in children and their families. For short-term regimens for acute conditions (e.g., antibiotic regimens for acute infections), educational and reminder strategies can be effective. For long-term regimens for chronic conditions (e.g., diabetes, asthma, juvenile rheumatoid arthritis), more complex interventions and repeated monitoring of adherence and health outcome can be effective. However, clinical demonstrations of adherence promotion interventions have been limited, and some studies have shown that adherence is not always associated with changes in health status and disease outcome.

See also: Asthma; Diabetes Mellitus Type 1; Diabetes Mellitus Type 2; Health Education/Health Promotion; Juvenile Rheumatoid Arthritis; Obesity; Treatment Adherence: Behavioral

Further Reading

Haynes, R. B. (1979). Introduction. In R. B. Haynes, D. W. Taylor, & D. C. Sackett (Eds.), *Compliance in health care* (pp. 1–7). Baltimore: The Johns Hopkins University Press.

La Greca, A. M., & Schuman, W. B. (1995). Adherence to prescribed medical regimens. In M. C. Roberts (Ed.), *Handbook of pediatric psychology* (2nd ed., pp. 55–83). New York: Guilford.

Rapoff, M. A. (1999). *Adherence to pediatric medical regimens.* New York: Kluwer Academic/Plenum.

JACK W. FINNEY
MICHAEL A. RAPOFF

Treatment Alliance

DEFINITION

In general, the therapeutic alliance refers to the quality of the relationship between the client and therapist. Although the alliance is often viewed as a unitary construct, it has developed from various conceptualizations of the therapeutic relationship and typically involves multiple dimensions. Bordin (1979) offered a pantheoretical model of the alliance and proposed that the construct involved three components: *bond*, or the affective relationship between client and therapist, *tasks*, or collaboration on therapeutic tasks, and *goals*, or agreement between client and therapist on the goals of treatment.

A substantial body of research has emerged on the relationship between the alliance and treatment outcome in the adult psychotherapy literature. Across multiple measures of the alliance and multiple forms of treatment, the alliance is one of the most consistent predictors of treatment outcome, as documented by Martin and colleagues (2002). The contribution to outcomes across types of treatments and disorders has led some to view the alliance as a robust nonspecific factor in therapy.

Although the importance of the alliance has been recognized in child and adolescent therapy for many years, research on the alliance with children and adolescents has only recently emerged. Shirk and Saiz (1992) proposed that two dimensions were critical for the child alliance: the relational bond with the therapist and collaboration with the therapist on treatment tasks. Their initial research indicated that relational bond was associated with task collaboration for both child and therapist reports. DiGiuseppe, Linscott, and Jilton (1995) have noted that the relational bond might be the most important alliance component for young children, but among older children and adolescents, agreement on goals for therapy is more pivotal for treatment involvement. From this perspective, the alliance is framed as a contractual agreement. Based on a factor analysis of a modified version of the *Working Alliance Inventory* consisting of bond, task, and goal items, DiGiuseppe and colleagues (1996) found that self-reported alliance among adolescents consisted of a one-factor construct. It is possible that children and adolescents do not distinguish among alliance dimensions; observational methods may be needed to uncover different aspects of the alliance that are related to outcome.

ALLIANCE–OUTCOME RELATIONS IN CHILD AND ADOLESCENT THERAPY

Despite the prominence of alliance research in the adult psychotherapy literature, remarkably few studies have been conducted on alliance–outcome relations with children and adolescents. In a recent meta-analytic review, Shirk and Karver found 23 studies that examined therapy relationship–outcome associations, but only nine referred to the construct as the "alliance." On average, the association between alliance and outcome was quite comparable to the relationship observed with adult patients. However, within the child and adolescent literature this estimate is based on both concurrent and prospective relations between alliance and outcome, as well as on a wide range of treatments including

both variations of individual and family therapy. Only one study met the full criteria used in the adult literature (individual therapy, alliance or bond measures, and prospective relations), and that study yielded nonsignificant prospective associations.

MODELS OF ALLIANCE–OUTCOME RELATIONS

Two models of alliance—outcome relations have been advanced in the child and adolescent literature. The first posits a direct relationship between alliance quality and treatment outcome. This view holds that relationship factors are the primary mechanism of therapeutic change (e.g., client-centered child therapy), or that relationship factors exert an independent influence on outcomes over and above the contribution of specific therapy techniques (e.g., psychodynamic child therapy). Alternatively, alliance–outcome relations have been viewed as a mediated association. From this perspective, the association between the alliance and outcome is mediated, or connected, through involvement in therapy tasks (e.g., cognitive–behavioral child therapy). This view holds that the alliance is essentially a catalyst for change insofar as it promotes involvement with specific treatment tasks such as exposure or countering automatic thoughts. Research has not yet examined these potential models of alliance–outcome relations, or therapist strategies that promote or maintain the alliance in child and adolescent treatment.

See also: Child Psychotherapy; Cognitive–Behavior Therapy; Evidence-Based Treatments; Treatment Adherence

Further Reading

Bordin, E. (1979). The generalizability of the psychoanalytic concept of the working alliance. *Psychotherapy: Theory, Research, & Practice, 16*, 252–260.

DiGiuseppe, R., Linscott, J., & Jilton, R. (1996). Developing the therapeutic alliance in child-adolescent psychotherapy. *Journal of Preventive Psychology, 5*, 85–100.

Martin, D., Graske, J., & Davis, M. (2000). Relation of the therapeutic alliance with outcome and other variables: A meta-analytic review. *Journal of Consulting and Clinical Psychology, 42*, 602–611.

Shirk, S., & Russell, R. (1996). *Change processes in child psychotherapy.* New York: Guilford.

Shirk, S., & Saiz, C. (1992). Clinical, empirical, and developmental perspectives on the therapeutic relationship in child psychotherapy. *Development and Psychopathology, 4*, 713–728.

STEPHEN R. SHIRK

Treatment Attrition

DEFINITION

According to Armbruster and Kazdin (1994), treatment attrition refers to the loss of cases prior to treatment completion. In general, treatment "dropouts," those who terminate treatment prior to completion, are distinguished from treatment "completers." However, in the child literature, the precise meaning of attrition has varied from study to study. For example, in some studies, families who never begin treatment after an initial evaluation are classified as dropouts, whereas in other studies they are classified as "refusers" and distinguished from dropouts. Other studies further distinguish between early and late dropouts.

Attrition represents a serious threat to the effectiveness of clinical treatments for children. Premature termination can undermine therapeutic effectiveness by diluting treatment strength. Further, treatment attrition has an impact on the mental health system by increasing the number of unfilled appointments, decreasing staff productivity, and thereby increasing per unit cost for services provided.

Studies of attrition in child and adolescent clinics have revealed high rates of incomplete treatment with estimates ranging from 28 to 85 percent for premature termination. Attrition from clinical trials tends to be lower, for example, 23 percent in a trial for child anxiety disorders reported by Kendall and Sugarman (1997), possibly due to the short-term nature of therapy in controlled trials. Little is known about premature termination in private practice.

FACTORS ASSOCIATED WITH ATTRITION

Research on premature termination has identified a number of child, family, and logistic characteristics that predict dropout; however, the literature contains numerous mixed findings. These mixed results might be due to the aggregation of findings across samples that vary in terms of types of problems and types of treatments. Recent studies have examined attrition by type of disorder and indicate that some characteristics are predictive across disorders (e.g., single parent family and minority status), whereas others are not (e.g., parent education and severity of child symptoms). Minority status may be related to early attrition and poor outcomes in clinic-based treatment for youth depression, as noted by Weersing and Weisz (2002). Such results

suggest that minority youth may not receive a sufficient dose of treatment to alter their problems. Research on ethnic matching between families and therapists suggests that such variables reduce dropout—at least at the start of treatment—among African, Mexican, and Asian American adolescents, though much more research is needed on this topic.

Remarkably few studies have taken a process-oriented perspective on engagement and attrition. One noteworthy exception is the barriers-to-treatment model put forth by Kazdin and colleagues (1997). According to this model, families experience a variety of barriers to participating in treatment and these experiences increase the risk for premature termination. Barriers include: (1) practical obstacles and stresses associated with participating such as transportation, (2) treatment demands such as cost, difficulty, and relevance, and (3) relationship characteristics such as the alliance with the therapist. For example, in a study of treatment for antisocial youth, Kazdin and colleagues (2002) found that all three types of barriers distinguished treatment completers from dropouts, and that the barriers mediated the association between family risk factors (e.g., single parent status) and treatment completion.

Garcia and Weisz examined the decision-making process that leads to terminating treatment among parents of clinic-referred youth. A factor analysis of their Reason for Ending Treatment Questionnaire yielded six factors including, therapeutic relationship problems, family and clinic practical problems, staff and appointment problems, time and effort concerns, treatment not needed, and money issues. Of these factors, the therapeutic relationship factor was the strongest predictor of premature termination. The only other significant factor was money problems.

See also: Child Psychotherapy; Evidence-Based Treatments; Parent Training;

Further Reading

Armbruster, P., & Kazdin, A. (1994). Attrition in child psychotherapy. In T. Ollendick & R. Prinz (Eds.), *Advances in clinical child psychology* (Vol. 16, pp. 81–108). New York: Plenum.
Garcia, J., & Weisz, J. (2002). When youth mental health care stops: Therapeutic relationship problems and other reasons for ending youth outpatient treatment. *Journal of Consulting and Clinical Psychology, 70,* 439–443.
Kazdin, A., Holland, L., & Crowley, M. (1997). Family experience of barriers to treatment and premature termination from child therapy. *Journal of Consulting and Clinical Psychology, 65,* 453–463.
Kendall, P., & Sugarman, A. (1997). Attrition in the treatment of childhood anxiety disorders. *Journal of Consulting and Clinical Psychology, 65,* 821–833.

Weersing, V. R., and Weisz, J. (2002). Community clinic treatment of depressed youth: Benchmarking usual care against CBT clinical trials. *Journal of Consulting and Clinical Psychology, 70*, 299–310.

STEPHEN R. SHIRK

Treatment Goals

DEFINITION

In general, as noted by Kendall (1991), treatment goals refer to desired outcomes of treatment and to the criteria for evaluating treatment progress. Goals can be classified in terms of type, target, and focus. With regard to type, goals are linked to intervention purpose, that is, whether the aim is preventive, ameliorative, or enhancement-oriented. Preventive interventions attempt to offset problems before they emerge, whereas ameliorative interventions attempt to resolve or reduce problems that already exist. Enhancements are typically aimed at improving the quality of life for youth who are not currently at risk for maladjustment. A fourth type of intervention involves relapse prevention and the goal of this type of intervention is in reducing the probability of relapse or recurrence of a disorder or set of problems.

FOCUS OF GOALS

Most therapeutic interventions are ameliorative in purpose; however, the goals of such interventions can vary in terms of focus. Among the most prominent are (1) psychoeducational goals, (2) symptom-reduction goals, (3) functional improvement goals, (4) normative goals, and (5) strength-based goals. Psychoeducational goals refer to both the objectives (e.g., 90 percent completion of in-class assignments) and the conditions under which the objectives will be attained (e.g., with an hour a day in the resource room). Psychoeducational goals are typically framed in terms of maximizing academic performance and school-based social functioning in the least restrictive environment necessary to attain the objective.

Symptom-reduction goals focus on changes in symptoms or problems that characterize different types of psychopathology. Such goals may be defined in terms of specific symptoms such as days out of school or number of fights with peers, or in terms of a broader class of symptoms found in a disorder, such as, the cluster of symptoms that define social phobia or Conduct Disorder (CD). Although symptom goals can be evaluated in terms of simple reductions in the frequency or intensity of single symptoms or clusters of symptoms, symptom-reduction goals are often defined in terms of normative approximation or diagnostic improvement. In the former, the goal is framed in terms of reducing symptoms to a point that is similar to noncases, often defined in terms of standard deviation units on a standardized measure of psychopathology. In the latter, goals are defined in terms of diagnostic criteria for a specific disorder, that is, the symptom-reduction goal involves decreasing symptoms to the point at which the individual does not meet established criteria for the disorder.

Functional goals are defined in terms of degree of impairment in various domains of functioning such as school, activities, and peer and family relations. In general, there are two major approaches to the assessment of functional goals: the first involves a global assessment of overall functioning and the second involves multidimensional assessment of various domains of functioning. An example of the first approach is captured in the Children's Global Assessment Scale developed by Shaffer and his colleagues (1983). Here the clinician synthesizes knowledge about different aspects of functioning into a summary score. In contrast, the Child and Adolescent Functional Assessment Scale developed by Hodges (1999) involves ratings of impairment across six youth and two environmental domains, including such areas as community functioning (acting lawfully), home (following family rules), and self-harmful behavior (ability to cope without self-destructive behaviors or thoughts). Functional goals are defined in terms of improving overall functioning or functioning in specific domains, for example, increased ability to modulate emotions.

Normative goals focus on returning children to a normal developmental trajectory. This perspective on treatment goals has a long history and was originally rooted in psychoanalytic models of development. However, contemporary applications of this framework are not restricted to singular developmental models. Instead, defining goals in relation to developmental milestones and tasks draws heavily on knowledge of many lines of normative development. For example, goals might be defined in terms of increasing age-appropriate engagement with peers. Interestingly, from this perspective, a normative goal might be at odds with a symptom-reduction goal, for example, an increase in adolescent–parent conflict could represent normative progress in a withdrawn adolescent rather than an increase in symptoms. Finally, normative goals can be defined in terms of the direction of development. Here, deflection from a maladaptive trajectory (disruptive school behavior → peer rejection → association with older peers) to a more adaptive path (self-regulation in school → pro-social peer involvement) is the broad goal of treatment.

The focus of strength-based goals is the individual or family resources that can be developed to improve overall functioning, as suggested by Henggeler and associates (1998). Rather than targeting deficits or problems, strength-based goals focus on developing assets or competencies that can offset risks. For example, a child's athletic skill can be developed in order to increase pro-social peer relations, or close extended family relationships can be fostered to improve child behavior monitoring. Strength-based goals redirect attention to what the individual or family does well in order to mobilize these resources for the resolution of problems.

TARGET OF GOALS

Treatment goals also vary in terms of who is targeted. Many forms of child therapy focus on the individual child or adolescent as the target of treatment. Goals are then defined in terms of alterations in the child's cognitions, emotions, or behaviors. For example, a cognitive–behavioral therapist might target the reduction of depressogenic self-talk, whereas a behavior therapist might aim for improved social skills. However, many interventions target changes at the level of the dyad or family unit. For example, problem-solving communication therapy targets the reduction of parent–adolescent conflict, as noted by Robin and Foster (1989). Goals are set and measured at the dyadic level, that is, in terms of changes in behavioral exchanges. Similarly, family therapists target changes in family interactions, patterns, and structure. For example, family treatments of Conduct Disorder pioneered by Patterson target both the reduction of antisocial behavior at the individual level, and changes in interaction patterns, for example, reduction in coercive processes, at the family level.

SOURCE OF GOALS

It is important to note that treatment goals in child and adolescent therapy can differ by source as well. That is, multiple parties often have a stake in youth referrals, and what schools, parents, and youth define as the goals of treatment can differ widely. In fact, recent research has revealed very low levels of agreement on treatment goals between parents and youth. To the degree that goal agreement is fundamental for the development of a working alliance, an important task for child and adolescent therapists is brokering an agreement on goals among vested parties.

See also: Child Psychotherapy; Global Functioning; Quality of Life

Further Reading

Henggeler, S., Schoenwald, S., Borduin, C., Rowland, M., & Cunningham, P. (1998). *Multisystemic treatment of antisocial behavior in children and adolescents.* New York: Guilford.

Hodges, K. (1999). Child and Adolescent Functional Assessment Scale. In M. Mariush (Ed.), *The use of psychological testing for treatment planning and outcome assessment* (2nd ed., pp. 631–664). Mahwah, NJ: Erlbaum.

Kendall, P. (1991). Guiding theory for therapy with children and adolescents. In P. Kendall (Ed.), *Child & adolescent therapy: Cognitive–behavioral procedures* (pp. 3–22). New York: Guilford.

Robin, A., & Foster, S. (1989). *Negotiating parent-adolescent conflict: A behavioral family systems approach.* New York: Guilford.

Shaffer, D., Gould, M., Brasic, J., Ambrosini, P., Fisher, P., Bird, H., & Aluwahlia, S. (1983). A children's global assessment scale (CGAS). *Archives of General Psychiatry, 40,* 1228–1231.

STEPHEN R. SHIRK

Treatment Outcome Measures

See: Measurement of Behavior Change

Trichomoniasis

See: Sexually Transmitted Diseases in Adolescents

Trichotillomania

DEFINITION

Trichotillomania (TCM) is described in the dermatological literature as the chronic pulling of one's hair resulting in noticeable hair loss or alopecia. The definition currently provided by the American Psychiatric Association adds these experiential criteria: "increasing sense of tension immediately before pulling out the hair" followed by "pleasure, gratification, or relief when pulling out the hair." These additional criteria are the subject of some controversy, however, as not all hair pullers report them. In fact, in research on hair pulling in children and adolescents, large percentages fail to endorse one or both of the additional criteria. These findings suggest that the requirement of increasing tension followed by relief or gratification after hair pulling may be an unnecessary restriction in the diagnosis of TCM, particularly in children and adolescents.

INCIDENCE

Reports on the incidence of TCM are mixed and most likely reflect variation in methods of diagnosis and classification, as well as the covert and sensitive nature of habitual hair pulling. Historically, TCM was believed to be extremely rare, but more recent reports estimate lifetime prevalence as high as 1.5 percent for males and 3.4 percent for females—the majority of cases are believed to originate in childhood.

PSYCHOLOGICAL CORRELATES

The psychiatric literature is dominated by reports of extensive psychiatric comorbidity in hair pulling children. The generality of these reports is limited, however, because of highly select and small sample sizes and the absence of experimental controls. Additionally, the pediatric and behavioral literatures routinely describe child hair pullers who are otherwise normal. At worst many of these children merely present with other co-occurring habits such as finger sucking (see Finger Sucking). The disparity between these literatures most likely reflects variable referral patterns and/or the existence of subtypes of TCM.

ETIOLOGY

There is no single established etiology of TCM. Traditional psychoanalytic interpretations stress the symbolic nature of hair pulling and its association with disrupted psychosexual development, aggression, and separation anxiety. In contrast, behavioral interpretations focus on the learned nature of the hair pulling response. According to this perspective, hair pulling often starts as an infrequent, but normal, behavior that becomes progressively more frequent and varied in form through the influence of social and experiential consequences generated by the hair pulling (e.g., parental attention, reduction of arousal).

ASSESSMENT

A detailed assessment of hair pulling is essential for maximally effective treatment. The initial assessment of abnormal alopecia should include a complete physical exam to rule out or identify any medical conditions and/or medication side effects contributing to hair loss. Additional assessment data should include information regarding antecedents to hair pulling such as affective/cognitive precursors and high-risk situations. Once antecedents to hair pulling have been identified, detailed information regarding the hair pulling itself should be obtained. This response description may include information on the number of hair pulling incidents, the type (e.g., texture, length) of hairs pulled, and bodily movements engaged in during pulling. Finally, information regarding the disposal of pulled hair as well as other consequences should be investigated. Ideally, this information is collected from multiple sources including tailored self-monitoring sheets and clinical interviews with the child and family members.

Other commonly used strategies for assessing TCM include examining photographic evidence of alopecia, measuring patches of alopecia, and counting pulled hairs. Recently, a novel method of TCM assessment was introduced by researchers who used the weight of pulled hairs (in milligrams) as their primary dependent variable.

Two increasingly used standardized assessment measures for TCM include the National Institutes of Mental Health Trichotillomania Severity Scale (NIMH-TSS) and the National Institute of Mental Health Trichotillomania Impairment Scale (NIMH-TIS). The NIMH-TSS consists of five questions regarding average daily time spent pulling hair, information on urges to pull, distress due to hair pulling, and interference with functioning due to hair pulling. The NIMH-TIS rates the severity/impairment of hair pulling on a scale from 0 to 10. Both scales have been shown to be sensitive to treatment outcome.

TREATMENT

To date, the treatment for TCM with the most substantial empirical support is habit reversal (HR). The original HR package consisted of 13 components including awareness training, competing response training, inconvenience review, social support, and self-monitoring. An evaluation of HR indicated that the complete package reduced hair pulling by 90 percent in a sample of 19 individuals, four of whom were children. Subsequent studies have supported these findings. For hair pullers capable of conducting their own treatment, HR appears to be the most effective intervention alternative.

A growing body of literature also indicates that indirect treatment of hair pulling, particularly in young children, may be accomplished through the direct treatment of coexisting habits such as thumb sucking. In these studies successful treatment of finger sucking has been accompanied by complete cessation of hair pulling even though the pulling itself was not directly treated. Another treatment that has been shown to be effective for child hair pullers involves improving the interaction between parent and child and using a brief time out for instances of pulling. Lastly, hypnotherapy and cognitive–behavior therapy are two additional treatment strategies that have produced promising results in cases of TCM.

PROGNOSIS

There are several established predictors of favorable prognosis in cases of TCM. Examples include very early onset, duration of less than 6 months at presentation, and complete abstinence at posttreatment. Overall, the prognosis appears to be positive in the short-term, but existing data suggest that relapse for a majority of individuals is likely especially when the pulling begins in later childhood. As a result, a greater focus on relapse prevention is warranted.

See also: Behavior Modification; Cognitive–Behavior Therapy; Finger Sucking; Habit Reversal; Interviewing

Further Reading

Byrd, M. R., Richards, D., Hove, G., and Friman, P. C. (2002). Treatment of early onset hair pulling (trichotillomania) as a simple habit. *Behavior Modification, 26,* 400–411.
Elliot, A. J., & Fuqua, R. W. (2001). Behavioral interventions for trichotillomania. In D. W. Woods and R. Miltenberger (Eds.), *Tic disorders, trichotillomania, and other repetitive behavior disorders: Behavioral approaches to analysis and treatment* (pp. 151–170). New York: Kluwer Academic/Plenum.
Miltenberger, R. G., Rapp, J. T., & Long, E. S. (2001). Characteristics of trichotillomania. In D. W. Woods & R. Miltenberger (Eds.), *Tic disorders, trichotillomania, and other repetitive behavior disorders: Behavioral approaches to analysis and treatment* (pp. 133–150). New York: Kluwer Academic/Plenum.

AMANDA DREWS
PATRICK C. FRIMAN

Turner Syndrome

DEFINITION/INCIDENCE

Turner Syndrome (TS), also known as Ullrich–Turner syndrome, is the most common chromosomal genetic abnormality in females and occurs in approximately 0.2 per 1,000 females. Turner's original (1938) clinical description of the syndrome emphasized the presence of three physical characteristics of the disorder: ovarian failure, webbed neck, and cubitus valgus (an unusual carrying posture of the elbows). Subsequently, the genetic bases for the disorder have been identified. In addition, the variety of physical, endocrinological, gastric, renal, cognitive, and psychosocial concomitants of the disorder have also been described.

There are a number of dysmorphic features and anomalies that characterize the physical appearance of females with TS. Facial anomalies may include a low-set hairline, low set ears, ptosis (drooping eyelids), micrognathia (small jaw), and a high arched palate. There may be multiple folds in the neck or a webbed neck. The elbows may be carried at an unusual angle and the fourth digit of the hand may be shortened. There is a higher than average incidence of spinal deformities and scoliosis. Short stature and growth curve abnormalities in childhood are common. Vascular anomalies have been described including coarctation of the aorta. Certain features of the structure of the auricle of the ear lead many TS patients to experience repeated middle ear infections and to sensorineural hearing loss. Multiple pigmented nevi on the skin may be observed. Medical problems in TS patients include: an increased incidence of hypertensive disease, obstructive sleep apnea due to upper airway abnormalities, renal and liver dysfunction, and early-onset osteoporosis. Finally, ovarian failure is commonly observed although in some genetic variants, partial ovarian function may be present.

ETIOLOGY

The TS phenotype can result from a variety of genetic defects. The most common genetic abnormalities associated with TS include: absence of the X chromosome (45, XO type) or the presence of a number of structural abnormalities of the X chromosome including mosaicism, micromosaicism, partial deletion of the X chromosome, duplication of one arm of the X chromosome, and

XY females with deletion of the short arm of the Y chromosome. It is estimated that the TS genetic abnormalities result in a high rate of intrauterine mortality. There are no apparent ethnic or racial differences in the appearance of the genetic abnormalities that are related to the syndrome.

ASSESSMENT

While the original descriptions of Turner and Ullrich relied upon the physical features of the syndrome, modern genetic analyses include both cytogenic studies and fluorescent in situ hybridization (FISH) analyses to identify the disorder. It is now thought that the phenotype of TS may be due to inadequate levels of a protein (RPF4) that is coded on the genes of both the X and Y chromosomes and is critical to cellular functioning. A second gene, SHOX, has been reported to cause the short stature in TS. In addition to genetic studies of TS females, a number of other assessment methodologies have been used to define features of this disorder. These include neuroimaging studies such as magnetic resonance imaging (MRI), neuropsychological assessments, studies of personality, and psychological functioning in affected females and their families.

Neuroimaging studies of females with TS have described a variety of brain abnormalities involving gray to white matter densities, regional differences in the volume of brain tissue, and differences in ventricular system volume. Reduced glucose metabolism has been reported in the parietal and occipital regions of the brains of females with TS compared to controls. Smaller volumes of specific brain structures such as the hippocampus, the lenticular and thalamic nuclei, and the caudate nucleus have also been reported. While these studies rely upon measurement of structural differences in the brains of females with TS, they do imply that there is a neuroanatomic substrate for the types of neuropsychological problems reported in these individuals.

PSYCHOLOGICAL CORRELATES

A distinctive neuropsychological profile of strengths and weaknesses in various cognitive functions has been attributed to TS females. Although most females with TS have intellectual functioning within at least the average range, there is a small subset of patients identified as having a small ring X chromosome whose intellectual functioning is within the severely impaired range. In the context of average intellectual abilities, most TS females manifest a variety of deficits

in visuospatial functions. Problems in visuoperceptual discrimination, visuospatial reasoning, and visuomotor constructional abilities are often reported. These deficits are thought to contribute to the generally higher Verbal than Performance IQ scores often reported in females with TS. However, this verbal–performance IQ discrepancy is not consistently observed in TS genotype variants. Nonverbal memory deficits have been observed in addition to deficits in working memory. This latter difficulty has been related to subtle problems in executive functioning observed in some TS patients. Problems in sequencing multistep problems have also been reported for some adults with TS. Motor reaction times and simple motor speed is often slowed in females with TS. Finally, deficiencies in processing visual affective stimuli have also been observed and may be related to the visuoperceptual discrimination problems noted earlier.

Academic difficulties have been reported in children with TS. Many females with TS meet diagnostic criteria for a so-called Nonverbal Learning Disability. Mathematical operations appear to be another area of difficulty for many children with TS. In contrast, reading and written language are generally seen as areas of strength for these children.

Behavioral problems have been less frequently studied in children, adolescents, and adult females with TS. The variability in types of behavior problems and the frequencies within TS genotypes is not well-known. Some investigators describe TS children as having a high incidence of hyperactivity and restlessness, being prone to shyness, often exhibiting immature behavior, preferring to play with younger children, and as having deficient social skills. Problems in self-esteem, social relationships, and reactive depression have been described in adolescents and adult TS females. However, there is marked variability in the incidence and severity of these problems across the age span and the variety of TS genotypes in the few studies that addressed these issues. More studies of the psychological impact of TS on affected females and their families are needed.

TREATMENT

Estrogen replacement therapy and growth hormone therapy have been used in TS patients in order to help them develop secondary sex characteristics and to promote growth in stature. Identification of the type and severity of learning disabilities is an important part of the care on TS children during their school years. When a child with TS begins to experience problems in learning or in social functioning, a comprehensive neuropsychological evaluation that includes assessment of achievement and psychological adjustment may be needed in order to initiate school-based or community-based therapeutic interventions. In addition, education about the possible medical complications of this genetic disorder is critical to promote careful follow-up as the child matures into adulthood. Finally, genetic counseling for the parents may be helpful in defining the genetic risks for the parents based upon the type of identified genetic disorder that lead to the diagnosis in their child.

PROGNOSIS

While a female with TS is at risk for many potential medical, academic, and social adjustment problems, most individuals with this disorder have a good prognosis. With careful medical monitoring and early intervention when academic or social problems arise, the multiple potential complications of this genetic disorder can be successfully managed.

See also: Behavioral Genetics; Neuropsychological Assessment; Social-Skills Training

Further Reading

Baron, I. S., Fennell, E. B., & Voeller, K. K. S. (1995). *Pediatric neuropsychology in a medical setting.* New York: Oxford University Press.

Berch, D. B., & Bender, B. G. (2000). Turner syndrome. In K. O. Yeates, M. D. Ris, & H. G. Taylor (Eds.), *Pediatric neuropsychology: Theory, research and practice* (pp. 252–274). New York: Guilford.

Powell, M. P., & Schulte, T. (1999). Turner syndrome. In S. Goldstein & C. R. Reynolds (Eds.), *Handbook of neurodevelopmental and genetic disorders in childhood* (pp. 277–297). New York: Guilford.

Rovet, J. (1993). The psychoeducational characteristics of children with Turner syndrome. *Journal of Learning Disablities, 26,* 333–347.

EILEEN FENNELL

Uu

Ulcerative Colitis

See: Inflammatory Bowel Disease

Underachievement

DEFINITION

Underachievement, at its most basic, can be defined as an individual's failure to achieve at a level commensurate with his or her ability. Underachievement is a very common reason for referral to child and adolescent psychology clinics or to the school psychologist. However, the possible reasons for failing to achieve at the expected level can be numerous—ranging from behavioral patterns of disorganization to poor work habits, low motivation, perfectionism, "misplaced" priorities, or oppositional, manipulative behavior, to name a few. As Rimm (1986) notes, there is no gene for underachievement and no biological explanation for capable children and youth who perform below their potential in school. Most professionals distinguish between children who underachieve because of a diagnosable disability (e.g., Attention-Deficit/Hyperactivity Disorder [ADHD], learning disability, sensory or motor impairment, emotional disturbance) and those who do not have a disability as the basis for their achievement problems. Several behavioral patterns may provide insight into the possible causes of a child's underachievement, and suggest ways

that parents and teachers can work together to help change these patterns.

FACTORS THAT MAY LEAD TO UNDERACHIEVEMENT

Underachievement is most likely founded on learned habits and skills that may develop even before children enter school. Factors such as parental overindulgence, childhood oppositional behavior, early health problems, or specific family stressors can predispose a child to underachieve. For example, children who are overindulged by parents may not have opportunities to learn persistence when encountering difficult tasks, delay gratification of their wants, or work toward goals. They may be "masters" at getting others to do things for them or gratify their needs quickly. According to Rimm, they are not permitted to struggle to accomplish the early challenges that occur in the preschool years, and therefore they do not establish learning patterns that will facilitate their elementary and secondary school progress when learning challenges become more difficult. Some young children develop a pattern of interaction with their parents that involves "power struggles" and oppositional behavior. Parents often refer to these children as "strong-willed" and hard to discipline. Unless parents and children receive intervention to address this situation during the early childhood years, children may not learn to respect adults or follow their directions, or learn that negative consequences will occur consistently when they fail to do their work. Children who enter school with these learned interaction patterns and habits will likely encounter teachers and administrators who do not

690

share their beliefs. Children engaged in power struggles with teachers at school often have less energy to direct toward achievement, and it is common for even bright "strong-willed" children to underachieve. In the illustrations just discussed, the children have learned to dominate adults and to expect that others will give in to their demands. Parents sometimes hope that these children will "grow out of" these behaviors when they enter school; in reality, the problems often escalate in the school environment and achievement suffers.

Other children grow up at the opposite extreme—being overly dependent on adults to meet their needs and failing to develop age-appropriate independence. There are several possible reasons for this behavioral pattern to develop—some that are within parents' control and others that are not. For example, children's early health problems may interfere with opportunities to participate in preacademic activities that teach good learning habits. Parents of children with chronic health problems may be so concerned about their child's health or weakened physical state that they tend to do too much for the child and have reduced expectations for their child's independent functioning. Patterns may be set in which the child becomes overly dependent upon the parents to do things for them, and the parents believe that their child needs more help than the typical child. When the child recovers from health problems, the parent–child patterns set in the early years may persist so that the child is not as self-sufficient as same-age peers. Certain family stressors can also set up a dependency pattern, especially in situations with marital conflict or divorce. Children's anxieties about possible loss of a stable family unit or separation from a parent may play out as overdependence.

In a different scenario, single parents who must juggle the stresses of one or more jobs while managing home and child-rearing responsibilities may find that they have little time or energy for engaging in play and learning activities with their children. Parents of young children can help their children learn listening skills (through reading and talking with their child), persistence on challenging tasks (by being available to provide support and encouragement when the child encounters difficulty), and by making interactive learning activities available and fun for their child. Children who grow up in families that do not provide these interactive learning opportunities may not have experienced learning as enjoyable and interesting. They may enter school with a negative set for learning, and may not achieve up to the level of their potential. This is a primary reason for the development of such programs as Head Start (for 3- to 5-year-old children) and Early

Head Start (for 0 to 3-year old children). Head Start programs not only provide an enriched learning environment for children, but also offer educational, parenting, and support services to the parents so that they can better nurture their child's development and readiness for school.

FACTORS THAT LOOK LIKE UNDERACHIEVEMENT, BUT ARE NOT

Children with ADHD have many symptoms that can interfere with learning. If they have the Inattentive subtype of ADHD, they often have problems with organization of their materials, difficulty remembering due dates of assignments or tests, organizing of their study schedules and routines, and paying attention to details, in addition to distractibility and difficulty focusing their attention. Many children with this type of ADHD do well in the early grades when parents and teachers are more willing to provide additional structure and organizational support to help them do their work. However, when they enter middle school or junior high, teachers may believe that they should take independent responsibility for their assignments and work. Some children with ADHD will become underachievers at this time, even if their grades have been good in earlier grades. Children with the Hyperactive/Impulsive or Combined subtypes of ADHD may have greater difficulty with achievement in early grades due to their high activity level, talkativeness, and impatience to finish their work as quickly as possible (perhaps without careful attention to details or accuracy). These children often understand the academic concepts they are being taught, but their performance is below standard because they are impulsive or rush through their work. Again, the ADHD symptoms may explain much of their underachievement.

Learning disabilities (LD) also cause children to perform below the level of their ability. However, with LD, underachievement is caused by specific information processing deficits that interfere with one or more aspects of learning in an otherwise intellectually average child. For example, a child may have a high average IQ of 114, but have difficulty with auditory discrimination of the phonetic sounds that go with letters. This child may struggle with learning to read because of their perceptual processing problems, but may achieve exceptionally well in the area of mathematics. Careful psychoeducational assessment can help to determine if a learning disability is the cause for underachievement.

"Slow learners" are children whose intellectual ability and achievement level are about the same, but are below the level of peers who are of the same age or grade level. For example, a 9-year-old girl with a low average IQ of 80 may struggle to keep up with the academic work of her peers, but if her achievement level is commensurate with her intellectual level, she is technically not an "underachiever." Rather, she is achieving at a level that is commensurate with her ability. Children such as this are not considered to have a disability, and often are not eligible for special education services.

Children who are gifted may fail to achieve at the level of their abilities for several reasons. Children with gifted abilities may have very high intelligence levels (usually with IQ scores above 130), very high academic performance in one or more areas (e.g., excellent mathematical abilities), or may be exceptionally creative, musically or artistically talented, or athletically gifted. If the gifted abilities have not been diagnosed, the child's curriculum and learning expectations may not be suited to his or her needs. Some children handle this situation by gearing their performance to the "average" level so they do not appear to be different from their peers. Others are bored, and turn their boredom into mischief. They may develop reputations as "troublemakers" because they finish their work quickly and do not have enough challenging material to hold their interest. As discussed earlier, behavioral problems such as Oppositional Defiant Disorder (ODD) may herald a pattern of behavior in which children are argumentative, refuse to follow adult rules or requests, fail to follow through on instructions, and generally want to be in control of their own and others' behavior. Children with ODD often devote their energy to various power struggles instead of learning, and they typically do not achieve at the level of their ability. The primary treatment must be directed toward their ODD first, and then perhaps toward academic remediation and support. The parents will need to be an integral part of the treatment process if ODD is to be successfully treated.

Finally, children with emotional problems may underachieve secondarily to the effects of their emotional disorder. For example, anxiety can often manifest itself as perfectionism or test anxiety, or in severe cases could result in extreme fearfulness about attending school. Children who are anxious about peer relationships or bullying may be distracted from learning because they are focused on protecting themselves from rejection or from verbal or physical attack. Children who are depressed are often preoccupied and unable to give full attention to their learning. Their energy level and interest in learning activities may be diminished. These and other emotional problems need to be carefully diagnosed so children can receive appropriate intervention, and eventually be able to return to their previous level of achievement. These children may need special education services at least temporarily to help them adjust to the school demands and learning environment until their emotional problems have improved or resolved.

THE FIRST STEP—CAREFUL DIAGNOSIS

One of the first critical issues to address when one suspects underachievement is the differential diagnosis with possible disorders that can cause a child to have learning difficulty. The discussion in the previous section illustrates ways in which ADHD, learning disabilities, giftedness, behavioral problems, or emotional problems can interfere with achievement. With accurate diagnosis of these conditions, the child may be eligible to receive special educational services, enrichment services, and/or an Individualized Educational Plan (IEP) to address their achievement and learning problems in light of their disability. Conversely, if specific disorders and disabilities are ruled out as a cause of the child's underachievement, often information about family functioning and current stressors may shed light on the child's underachievement. If this does not provide a clue, then exploration of the child's early learning and behavioral patterns, as discussed earlier, may help to identify causes for the current problems. Gathering observational data from teachers can shed light on the child's attitude and work patterns that could interfere with achievement.

TREATMENT OF UNDERACHIEVEMENT

Understanding the cause of a child's underachievement is the first step in providing intervention. If the cause is behavioral or emotional problems, then treatment from a psychologist or other mental health professional in the form of individual, group, or family counseling may be helpful in treating the causes of the problem. If the child has a disability, then identification of that disability and treatment through special education services, curriculum modifications, or medical, speech/language, physical medicine, or psychological services may be needed. Often, tutors or teachers can help students learn appropriate study and organization habits that will address their achievement problems. Getting intervention for the underachieving child is extremely important to the child's self-concept as well as his or her academic progress. As Rathvon (1996) notes, children with chronic underachievement may feel that they have no control over their situation, and they learn to anticipate failure. Intervention must address the beliefs that are sometimes distorted in order to help the child reach his or her potential.

See also: Attention-Deficit/Hyperactivity Disorder; Learning Disorders; Oppositional Defiant Disorder; School Age Assessment

Further Reading

Rathvon, N. (1996). *The unmotivated child*. New York: Simon & Shuster.
Rimm, S. B. (1986). *Underachievement syndrome: Causes and cures*. Watertown, WI: Apple.

JAN L. CULBERTSON

Unintentional Injuries

See: Accidental (Unintentional) Injuries

Vv

Validity

DEFINITION

All test validity is concerned with the measurement of psychological constructs. Examples of these constructs include traits such as extroversion or intelligence, disorders such as depression, or behaviors such as social skills or coping with medical procedures. The *Standards for Educational and Psychological Testing* (AERA, APA, NCME, 1999) provides the following definition of construct validity:

> A term used to describe to what degree test scores can be interpreted as the respondent's level of functioning in the psychological construct a test is considered to measure. A construct is a theoretical concept developed from various sources of evidence, such as test content and interrelation of test scores with other variables or test items with each other... (p. 174)

The following section selects first a traditional approach, followed by a more contemporary approach, from among the more common methods used to assess various aspects of construct validity.

METHODS

A conventional approach to validity such as that suggested by Cronbach (1971) organizes the means of obtaining validity evidence into three broad categories: content-related, criterion-related, and construct-related evidence. These categories provide organizational

convenience rather than distinct types of validity; ultimately, all three categories are relevant to construct validity.

Content-related validity refers to the relationship between the content of a measurement instrument and the construct it is intended to measure. In establishing evidence for content validation, an instrument must demonstrate a sufficient and representative sample of the behaviors or subject domain of the construct (AERA, APA, NCME, 1999). Content validity is typically established by comparison of test items to existing educational objectives, to empirically supported operational definitions of a construct, and to judgments by panels of recognized content experts. The validation process usually involves examination of the individual test items and their format (e.g., representation, wording, order, length, multiple choice versus free response) as well as the procedural guidelines for administration and scoring. Standardized academic achievement testing highlights the use of content validation. These tests are designed to be administered to different grade levels and are divided into separate subject domains; items have been carefully selected to represent a range of skills matched to educational objectives in that subject domain for a particular age/grade level. Many classroom teachers construct their own tests, designed to tap a very specific content, such as a science unit; consideration of unit objectives should guide test construction to ensure content validity, as noted by Vockell and Asher (1995). Some examples of failure to establish acceptable content validity include: (1) a placement test with too few items to address the course curricular objectives; (2) a basic math skills test using only word problems, mixing the task demands of independent reading with knowledge/application of math strategies where scores may not represent actual mathematical ability; (3) a general anxiety inventory sampling of perceived life stresses omits items pertaining to the school setting, a probable consideration in the overall construct of anxiety in children.

Face validity, an antiquated content-related concept abandoned by measurement scientists, refers to the subjective extent to which a measure resembles what it is purports to measure; achievement tests typically look at assessing academic abilities.

Criterion-related validity refers to how well an instrument can predict an examinee's performance on some practical criterion. The criterion measure can be obtained at the same time as the testing (concurrent validity) or it can be obtained after a certain period of time (predictive validity). This type of validity is most often seen in situations of classification or hiring and is often used when the effectiveness of a test for a specific program is being evaluated. For example, measures with good criterion-related validity might be able to predict which psychiatric patients would benefit from certain types of therapy. Also, graduate school entrance examinations such as the Graduate Record Examination (GRE) should be able to predict those students who will perform well in graduate school. Other commonly used criteria include measures of academic achievement, performance in specialized training, job performance records, psychiatric diagnosis, and ratings of behavior. Often new versions of tests are correlated with previous versions, with the older version serving as the criterion. Regression analysis is often employed to establish criterion validity; the resulting correlation coefficients between the predictor variable and the criterion variable are validity coefficients.

Still other studies are concerned with the test's ability to differentiate groups of individuals, or discriminant validity. A study of this nature may require applying a test to two groups: one without a psychological disorder, disability, challenge or condition, and the other group comprised of children who are diagnosed with a condition such as Attention-Deficit/Hyperactivity Disorder (ADHD), for example. If a test is intended for diagnostic purposes, then these two groups should have differing scores or score patterns on the measure. In addition, the scores for the ADHD group should be in a more deviant direction, thus reflecting their characteristic symptomatology. The accuracy of group discrimination in such studies is often expressed in terms of "hit rates" where the number and proportions of each group that is classified correctly or incorrectly is given.

Construct-related validity refers to the extent to which an instrument or method accurately measures an underlying theoretical construct; in other words, can an inference about a psychological construct be drawn from the test scores? For instance, tests purporting to measure constructs such as intelligence, stress, creativity, or depression should have items that relate specifically to those constructs. One common approach to establishing construct-related validity uses interitem correlation and factor analysis to demonstrate an interrelationship between the individual items, showing meaningful support for the construct.

One contemporary approach to the issue of validity criticizes the traditional view as fragmented, simplistic, and incomplete. Messick (1995, 1996), for example, has argued that validity is not so much a property of a test as it is the meaning and use of the test scores, placing a strong emphasis on how tests are used and the social consequences of their use. He identifies six salient aspects that function interdependently in addressing validity as a unified concept: content, substantive, structure, generalizability, external factors, and consequential aspects. Obviously, numerous types of validation evidence and associated studies may be accumulated for a given test or test score. The essence of modern construct validation is the process of accumulating comprehensive validity evidence supporting each interpretation offered by a test. Hence, it is simplistic and inappropriate to refer to a test as either valid or invalid per se. Rather, it is more congruent with modern test theory to refer to interpretations that are supported by validity evidence or not (AERA, APA, NCME, 1999).

See also: Interviewing; Psychometric Properties of Tests; Psychological Testing; Reliability

Further Reading

American Educational Research Association, American Psychological Association, & National Council for Measurement in Education. (1999). *Standards for educational and psychological testing.* Washington, DC: Author.

Cronbach, L. J. (1971). Test validation. In R. L. Thorndike (Ed.), *Educational measurement* (2nd ed.). Washington, DC: American Council on Education.

Messick, S. (1995). Validity of psychological assessment: Validation of inferences of persons' responses and performances as scientific inquiry into scoring meaning. *American Psychologist, 9,* 741–749.

Messick, S. (1996). Validity of performance assessment. In G. Philips (Ed.), *Technical issues in large-scale performance assessment.* Washington, DC: National Center for Educational Statistics.

Vockell, E. L., & Asher, J. W. (1995). *Educational research* (2nd ed.). Englewood Cliffs, NJ: Prentice Hall.

ANNE PIERCE WINSOR
RANDY W. KAMPHAUS
LAUREN A. JONES
KIMBERLEY A. BLAKER

Ventilator Dependency in Children

DEFINITION/INCIDENCE

Ventilator dependency in children refers to pediatric patients who need a ventilator for assistance in breathing, but who later appear capable of independent breathing from a physiological standpoint, yet struggle to do so. Ventilators are often indicated in children whose spontaneous breathing is not adequate to sustain life, such as following respiratory arrest, acute or chronic lung injury or disease, or neuromuscular disease. The national prevalence of ventilator assistance in pediatric patients, as well as the number of children dependent upon ventilator breathing, is difficult to ascertain. However, in spite of a lack of statistics, the literature is replete with case studies and anecdotal reports regarding difficulties in weaning children from ventilator breathing.

ASSESSMENT FOR WEANING READINESS

The medical field has suggested variables predictive of weaning success that are based almost entirely on physical criteria (e.g., adequate gas exchange, appropriate respiratory rate, sufficient hemoglobin levels and neuromuscular capacity, stable cardiovascular functioning, good nutritional level). Unfortunately to date, there is no agreement on the necessary prerequisites for weaning in ventilator dependent children, or on the most effective manner to proceed with the actual weaning process. One problem with a strictly physiologically based approach is that children frequently fail weaning attempts despite meeting the requisite physical criteria. Thus, weaning assessment parameters may need to include psychosocial factors.

In perhaps one of the first attempts to consider psychological factors in readiness for weaning, Blackwood (2000) proposed that patients must first exhibit proper orientation (the ability to make sense of the situation, understand what is happening, and tolerate information regarding progress), mental ease (the absence of or ability to control anxiety and fear secondary to weaning procedures), and a positive attitude (the instillation of hope as well as awareness of what the patient can directly control). Furthermore, assessment of patients' moods, their reaction to their illness as well as

to the medical environment and their overall level of anxiety, denial, and/or depression may serve as additional predictors of readiness for weaning. Thus, patients who appear psychologically ready may enhance their chances for an effective weaning outcome.

TREATMENT

Unfortunately, similar to assessment for weaning readiness, agreement concerning the most effective method of ventilator weaning remains controversial. Actual weaning procedures have been rather simplistic in the sense that they merely encourage patients' gradual tolerance of unassisted breathing through decreasing the number of mechanical breaths provided per minute or increasing actual time spent off the ventilator. Again, such approaches work for some patients, while other patients appear likely to require an alternative weaning method.

Although there is scant literature on the use of psychological principles and/or techniques for assisting with ventilator weaning, there are reports suggesting that children addicted to tracheostomies (a breathing tube inserted through an incision in the neck) can be quickly and successfully weaned using classical and operant conditioning principles. Additionally, some practitioners have suggested that anxiety may be a major factor in ventilator weaning difficulties. Thus, preweaning interventions such as cognitive restructuring, hypnotherapy, guided imagery, relaxation, and/or supportive counseling may increase successful outcomes of ventilator weaning procedures in pediatric patients. Of course, the use of such approaches will need to take into account the developmental level of each child.

PROGNOSIS

The importance of determining empirically validated assessment and treatment procedures for weaning children from the ventilator is highlighted by the fact that long-term ventilator assistance in children creates a host of negative ramifications. These include interrupted developmental tasks, speech/communication delays, socialization impairments, behavioral regressions, and various emotional sequelae. The blending of traditional medical perspectives with psychological considerations will likely offer the most comprehensive approach to serving ventilator dependent children.

See also: Anxiety Disorders; Behavior Modification; Cognitive–Behavior Therapy; Differential Social Reinforcement/Positive

Attention; Relaxation Training; Tracheostomy Dependent Children

Further Reading

Blackwood, B. (2000). The art and science of predicting patient readiness for weaning from mechanical ventilation. *International Journal of Nursing Studies, 37*, 145–151.

Bowen, D. E. (1989). Ventilator weaning through hypnosis. *Psychosomatics, 30*(4), 449–450.

Dalton, R., & Kirkhart, K. (1985). An evolution of emotional problems faced by ventilator-assisted children. *The Psychiatric Forum, 13*, 73–81.

Elliott, C. H., & Olson, R. A. (1982). Variations in conditioning procedures for the decannulation of tracheostomy dependent children: Clinical and theoretical implications. *Health Psychology, 1*(4), 389–397.

Gipson, W. T., Sivak, E. D., & Gulledge, A. D. (1987). Psychological aspects of ventilator dependency. *Psychiatric Medicine, 5*(3), 245–255.

MARIA R. MARSHALL
CHARLES H. ELLIOTT

Victims of Bullies

DEFINITION

Victims of bullying are children and adolescents who persistently serve as targets of aggression, ostracism, or humiliation by one or more peers (bullies). Many definitions of bullying stipulate an asymmetric or imbalanced power relationship, such that the victim lacks the physical strength, social support, or psychological resources to mount a successful defense against bullying. Victims often experience both overt and relational forms of victimization. Overt victimization includes direct, confrontational behaviors such as hitting, grabbing, threatening, or taunting. Relational victimization includes behaviors that harm the victim's social relationships and reputation through rumors, intentional exclusion, or other forms of social humiliation. Many definitions distinguish between passive victims who rarely act aggressively themselves, and provocative victims who are both targets and perpetrators of aggression.

INCIDENCE

Estimates of the prevalence and incidence of victimization vary among countries and across individual studies. A recent national study of 15,686 students in grades six through ten conducted in the United States found that 10.6 percent of students admitted to being victims of bullies several times during the current school term. Furthermore, 6.3 percent of the 15,686 students reported being involved both as victims and as bullies. Overall, males were more likely to report being victimized, as were students in the younger grades. A similar study conducted in Norway of 130,000 primary and junior high school students indicated that approximately 9 percent of students reported being victimized "now and then" or more frequently during the current school term, and 1.6 percent reported themselves as both victims and bullies. Several studies have found that boys report more overt victimization than girls, whereas girls identified as victims experience relational victimization as often as or more than male victims.

CORRELATES

Passive victims are thought to be more anxious and insecure than their peers, although this may be a consequence rather than a cause of victimization. Passive victims have been described as more cautious, sensitive, and quiet than agemates, and they tend to respond to difficult social situations through withdrawal. Peers tend to view passive victims as unlikely to retaliate if attacked. Boys who are victims are also likely to be physically weaker than their peers. Provocative victims tend to annoy their classmates because of problems with hyperactivity or concentration or because of their own aggressive tendencies. A recent review of numerous cross-sectional studies published between 1978 and 1997 provided substantial evidence for a linkage between victimization and the experience of depression, loneliness, low self-esteem, and anxiety. After comparing the relationships between those psychosocial attributes and victimization, the authors concluded that depression and loneliness are more strongly associated with victimization than low self-esteem and anxiety. At this time, it is difficult to determine which of these correlates precede and which follow the experience of victimization; preliminary evidence suggests that a cyclical process may occur, whereby anxious/withdrawn children have a higher tendency to be bullied and whereby the act of victimization leads to the exacerbation of difficulties with low self-esteem, depression, and anxiety.

ASSESSMENT

Various assessment methods for the identification of victims include self-report questionnaires, peer nominations, teacher nominations, direct observations, and individual interviews with children. Research has uncovered significant strengths and weaknesses of each of these approaches, and a comprehensive assessment of victimization should include a variety of informants. In addition to the primary signs of victimization (e.g., physical, verbal, or relational harassment), teachers and parents should be alert for behavior that signals a lack of friends, a desire to remain in physical proximity to adults during recess, a reluctance to go to school, a loss of interest in school work, a high frequency of somatic complaints or injuries, a tendency to appear insecure and anxious, and a generally depressive affect. Self-report measures are also extremely valuable in the identification of students suffering from these associated symptoms (e.g., depression).

TREATMENT

Several schoolwide interventions have been developed and empirically evaluated in the treatment of bullying and victimization problems. One such program developed in Sweden and Norway consists of holding discussions with all students and parents about the level of bullying problems present in their particular school (after having students complete questionnaires), increasing adult supervision during recess and lunch, implementing class rules about bullying, holding class discussions after occasions of bullying occur, and having individual conferences with students (and their parents) who are directly involved in the bully–victim dynamic. Similar efforts in the United States have attempted to modify the power dynamics in the school by implementing such components as education about bully, victim, and bystander roles; discipline plans that emphasize rewards more than punishment; a physical education curriculum that promotes the development of physical and psychological skills for increasing assertiveness and self-esteem and for dealing effectively with bullies; and mentoring opportunities with high school students or adults from the community to provide children with advice on how to deal with conflict situations. Investigations of these schoolwide interventions have often revealed improvements, such as a reduction in victimization, an improvement in the overall school climate, fewer discipline referrals to the principal, fewer out-of-school suspensions, an increase in assertiveness, and an increase in overall academic achievement. However, the magnitude and duration of these positive effects varies considerably between outcome studies. Individual victims who exhibit symptoms of depression, anxiety, or other psychological problems may also benefit from additional individual or group treatment as indicated for the particular presenting issues.

PROGNOSIS

Many children who are victims of bullies at one time continue to be victimized years later. Therefore, without the implementation of schoolwide or individual interventions, it appears likely that children will have difficulty removing themselves from bully–victim patterns that have developed. A classic longitudinal study conducted in Sweden by Olweus (1993) indicated that boys who were victimized in the sixth through the ninth grades appeared to be no different in many aspects of their lives at the age of 23 than those boys who had not been targets of bullying. However, some evidence suggested that the boys who were victimized were more likely to be depressed and to have lower self-esteem than the nonvictimized boys when they were adults. Additional research has shown that many victims regain a healthy developmental trajectory as adults, as they have more freedom to choose their social and work environments. Nevertheless, the low levels of self-esteem that victims may experience for many years can continue to adversely affect their social relationships, even as adults.

See also: Aggression; Bullies; Conduct Disorder; Exposure to Violence

Further Reading

Hawker, D. S. J., & Boulton, M. J. (2000). Twenty years' research on peer victimization and psychosocial maladjustment: A meta-analytic review of cross-sectional studies. *Journal of Child Psychology and Psychiatry, 41,* 441–455.

Juvonen, J., & Graham, S. (Eds.). (2001). *Peer harassment in school: The plight of the vulnerable and victimized.* New York: Guilford.

Nansel, T. R., Overpeck, M., Pilla, R. S., Ruan, W. J., Simons-Morton, B., & Scheidt, P. (2001). Bullying behaviors among US youth: Prevalence and association with psychosocial adjustment. *Journal of the American Medical Association, 285,* 2094–2100.

Olweus, D. (1993). *Bullying at school: What we know and what we can do.* Oxford, UK: Blackwell.

Sandoval, J. (Ed.). (2002). *Handbook of crisis counseling, intervention, and prevention in the schools.* Mahwah, NJ: Erlbaum.

Shafii, M., & Shafii, S. L. (Eds.). (2001). *School violence: Assessment, management, prevention.* Washington, DC: American Psychiatric Press.

EDWARD J. DILL
ERIC M. VERNBERG

Videotape Modeling

DEFINITION

Videotape modeling, developed by Webster-Stratton and her colleagues, is a cost-effective intervention for training parents of children with behavior and conduct problems. The program is based on cognitive social learning theory, whereby parents learn skills from watching videotaped examples of parents interacting effectively with their children or engaging in other training exercises. Videotape modeling is a versatile training tool, providing multiple models and circumstances that can be applied to the particular needs of different parents. First, by varying the demographic characteristics of the models (e.g., age, culture, socioeconomic status), the videotapes help promote feelings of affection for and connection to the videotaped models. Second, the videotapes depict situations in which both incorrect and correct parenting techniques are used. This demonstrates for parents how to cope with and learn from their mistakes, and serves as a point of discussion for parents with similar parenting deficits. Subsequently, the videotapes serve as the basis for further discussion and problem-solving of a parent's own specific parenting challenges, with the therapist serving as a guide and facilitator of change. Training using videotape modeling has been applied to parenting skills in particular, as well as broader personal and academic factors that may indirectly affect parenting (e.g., communication skills, problem-solving skills, academic skills training).

METHOD

The *BASIC* parent training program consists of 13–14 weekly sessions (26 hr total), where a therapist shows 10 videotape programs (250 vignettes, each 1–2 min long) to groups of parents (8–12 parents per group). Videotape vignettes illustrate a number of parenting skills, and serve to prompt further discussion by group members. The *BASIC* program is divided into four segments. These include lessons on how to play with their child, reinforce positive behavior, set and enforce limits, and apply nonphysical discipline strategies to handle misbehavior. In addition to the *BASIC* training program, Webster-Stratton and her colleagues developed *ADVANCE*, a broader-based parent training

program to address personal and interpersonal factors that may interfere with parenting. The *ADVANCE* program is a 14-session videotape modeling program (60 vignettes) offered to parents following completion of the *BASIC* program. This program is conducted in the same format as *BASIC*, providing skills training in personal self-control, communication, problem-solving, and social support development. Finally, parents can also participate in a third videotape modeling program, entitled *PARTNERS 1*, which is offered following completion of the *BASIC* and *ADVANCE* programs. The *PARTNERS 1* program provides training to help parents promote academic skills in their children. It consists of 6–8 sessions that train parents in the following areas: promoting children's self-confidence, fostering good learning habits, dealing with children's discouragement, participating in homework, using parent–teacher conferences to advocate for children, and discussing school problems with children.

Webster-Stratton and her colleagues have also developed a child training program based on the same format and principles as the parent training programs. This program, entitled KIDVID, is designed to teach young children (age 3–8 years) skills to improve their school behavior, enhance their social functioning, and increase their ability to problem solve during conflicts. Specifically, over the course of 22 weeks, children view nine videotape segments (approximately 100 vignettes) that provide training in the following skills: empathy, problem solving, anger control, developing and maintaining friendships, communication, and appropriate school behavior.

CLINICAL APPLICATIONS

Videotape modeling is designed for parents and preschool to school-aged children (3–8 years) with conduct problems (e.g., Oppositional Defiant Disorder [ODD], Conduct Disorder [CD]). Given the treatment format and cost-effectiveness, it is especially appropriate for higher risk parents and families who may not have the means to participate in individual or family therapy.

EFFECTIVENESS

Participants of videotape modeling programs have consistently demonstrated meaningful improvements in child behavior problems, parent–child interactions, and parenting attitudes and skills. These effects hold true up to 3 years following treatment in the home and clinical settings. Of note, while these programs are shown to be as effective as individualized parent training, it is five times more cost-effective.

Comparisons among the training program components reveal interesting differences in child and parent outcomes. First, videotape modeling has been tested across a number of formats, varying by group versus individual participation and with or without therapist presence. Long-term improvements were found to be the best among the therapist-led group training format, suggesting the importance of social support and therapist guidance within training sessions. Second, the addition of supplemental training programs (i.e., *ADVANCE*) led to further improvements in child and parent problem-solving as well as parent interactions, as compared to participation in the *BASIC* program alone. Third, the *KIDVID* program led to significant improvements in child problem-solving skills and conflict management skills as compared to parent training programs alone, but did not improve parent–child interactions as did the parent training program. These complementary outcomes suggest the usefulness of a comprehensive approach to the treatment of child behavior disorders, using videotape modeling as the foundation for group training.

See also: Aggression; Behavior Therapy; Cognitive–Behavior Therapy; Oppositional Defiant Disorder; Parent Training

Further Reading

Webster-Stratton, C. (1990). Long-term follow-up of families with young conduct problem children: From preschool to grade school. *Journal of Clinical Child Psychology, 19*, 144–149.

Webster-Stratton, C. (1996). Early intervention with videotape modeling: Programs for families of children with oppositional defiant disorder or conduct disorder. In E. D. Hibbs & P. S. Jensen (Eds.), *Psychosocial treatments for child and adolescent disorders: Empirically based strategies for clinical practice* (pp. 435–474). Washington, DC: American Psychological Association.

Webster-Stratton, C., & Hammond, M. (1997). Treating children with early-onset conduct problems: A comparison of child and parent training interventions. *Journal of Consulting & Clinical Psychology, 65*(1), 93–109.

Webster-Stratton, C., & Hancock, L. (1998). Training for parents of young children with conduct problems: Content, methods, and therapeutic processes. In C. E. Schaefer & J. M. Briesmeister (Eds.), *Handbook of parent training* (pp. 98–152). New York: Wiley.

Webster-Stratton, C., & Herbert, M. (1994). *Troubled families problem children*. New York: John Wiley & Sons.

HEATHER K. BLIER ALVAREZ
THOMAS H. OLLENDICK

Violence

See: Exposure to Violence; Television and Children: Violence

Viral Infections

See: Pediatric Infectious Diseases

Visual Development

See: Sensory and Perceptual Development

Visual Impairment: Low Vision and Blindness

DEFINITION

A *visual impairment* is a medically diagnosable condition of the optical system or brain that affects visual function. The term usually refers to the full range of visual variations including total blindness. In a few contexts, *visual impairment* is used to describe only people who retain some vision.

Other terms describe synonyms or subcategories of visual impairment. *Partially sighted* denotes a mild visual impairment, with acuities between 20/70 and 20/200. *Legal blindness*, a term first developed by the American Medical Association, involves visual acuity less than 20/200 or a field restriction of 20 degrees or less. Either criterion must be met in the better eye with correction. *Visual disability* and *visual handicap* are synonymous with visual impairment, but *disability* implies functional disadvantages and *handicap* connotes social disadvantages.

Low vision describes a visual impairment in which usable vision is retained, and *blindness* implies absence of vision for the purposes of learning and getting information.

DEMOGRAPHICS

There are approximately 55,000 school-aged children in the United States who are legally blind, according to the American Printing House for the Blind Annual Registry of 1995. A 1993 estimate by Nelson and Dimitrova reported that there were 95,410 visually impaired children under age 17 in the United States in 1990. The difference in the two reports is probably due to the inclusion of children with milder visual impairments in the latter study.

Of this number, 10–15 percent are functionally blind. These children receive information about their environment through hearing and touch rather than through vision. The majority of visually impaired students (85–90 percent) retain some vision. About 50–60 percent of visually impaired children have other disabilities, most commonly mental retardation, cerebral palsy, hearing impairment, and learning disabilities.

ETIOLOGIES

Causes of visual impairment have changed significantly over the last 50 years. Retinopathy of prematurity (ROP), which originally appeared in the 1950s, was formerly known as retrolental fibroplasia (RLF). It is a degeneration of the retina that results from complex factors including oxygen administered during incubation of premature infants. The incidence of this condition has remained about the same as when it first appeared, but now it commonly co-occurs with multiple disabilities that result from extreme prematurity. It often results in complete blindness, but can also cause varying degrees of low vision.

Cortical visual impairment (CVI), one of the most common causes of severe visual impairment among children, was rarely diagnosed before the 1970s. Cortical visual impairment results from a neurological dysfunction that affects vision, and it almost always occurs in children who have other disabilities. Children with CVI usually have some vision, although visual scanning and fixation are often limited.

Although cataracts are still a common cause of low vision among children, early surgery and intraocular lens implants have enabled children to retain more vision than in the past. Albinism, a reduction or absence of pigmentation in the body and the eyes, also causes low vision. Acuities between 20/100 and 20/400, light sensitivity, and underdevelopment of the macula are common visual effects of albinism. Uncorrectable refractive errors such as progressive myopia and strabismus are common among children and may not be completely correctable; these can result in temporary or permanent low vision.

Conditions that affect the optic nerve, most commonly optic atrophy and optic hypoplasia, often occur with other conditions that affect neurological function. Depending on the location and extent of the damage, these conditions may result in both acuity and field losses, often in the periphery of the eye. They can also cause blindness.

The conditions above are the most common causes of visual impairment among children, but many other conditions such as retinal dystrophies; absence or malformation of the iris, retina, and the eye itself; and infections or trauma to the eye are also responsible for some cases of vision loss. The amount of vision retained in each condition varies, and function cannot be reliably predicted from etiology.

PROGNOSIS

Visual impairment includes both individuals with usable vision and those who function using touch and hearing. Although children are at risk for delays, they benefit from early intervention and often develop at a rate similar to their peers. With appropriate adaptations and technology, individuals with visual impairments can live independently and be fully employed as adults. The following sections on Low Vision and Blindness will give further information on these problems as they relate to learning and function.

LOW VISION

Definition

Low vision refers to a visual disability in which some vision is retained but the reduced vision interferes with function. Because it is not clinically measurable, definitions of low vision vary. Corn and Koenig (1996) describe a person with low vision as one who "has difficulty accomplishing visual tasks, even with prescribed corrective lenses, but who can enhance his or her ability to accomplish these tasks with the use of compensatory visual strategies, low vision and other devices, and environmental modifications" (p. 4). Faye (1984) defines low vision as "bilateral subnormal visual acuity or abnormal visual field resulting from a disorder in the visual system" (p. 6). Low vision can include variations in visual acuity, visual field, or other factors such as color vision, perception, and asymmetrical vision such as diplopia. Before the 1960s, children with low vision were discouraged from using vision for fear of further damage to the visual system. However, in 1964 Dr. Natalie Barraga's research indicated that use of vision could enhance visual efficiency, and students with low vision are now encouraged to use vision in functional contexts where it is more efficient than touch or hearing.

Assessment

Students with low vision should have a thorough evaluation by an ophthalmologist or optometrist with training in low vision. In most states, students with low vision qualify for special education services as visually impaired based on the combination of the eye specialist's evaluation and a *functional vision assessment*, which is conducted by a teacher of visually impaired students or an orientation and mobility specialist. A functional vision assessment is a structured observation of vision usage in typical environments, and it reflects the student's use of near and distance vision during such activities as reading, sports, and travel.

In addition, many school districts now require a *learning media assessment* to determine the most efficient reading medium for a student with low vision. This assessment provides detailed analysis of the student's use of senses for learning, including an assessment of reading rate and print size when appropriate. It is often assumed that visually impaired students need enlarged print and learning materials but large print may slow reading for some students. Use of adaptations such as a bookstand to increase viewing distance for reading or a hand magnifier prescribed by a low vision specialist can improve access better than enlarged print.

Students with low vision should also be assessed for developmental and educational progress in their educational settings. At the early levels, assessment should emphasize motor development, social development, and daily living skills, which are often areas of delay for visually impaired learners. As the child enters school and reading materials become smaller, regular evaluation of reading efficiency should take place to consider adaptations that will facilitate reading and increase the reading rate.

Psychosocial Issues

Low vision presents several psychosocial problems that school-aged students must learn to solve. Other people may misinterpret the child's abilities, not only related to vision but also to intellectual and physical abilities. Children may receive too much assistance or inappropriate assistance from others; for example, others may guide them physically when all that is needed is verbal instructions about a route. They also may be the target of teasing or rejection by other students. Children, however, can be taught to communicate openly and directly about their vision to enhance others' understanding.

Children with low vision do some tasks visually and others by touch or hearing. They may use print, Braille, or both; they may use a long cane under certain conditions but not for all travel. They usually do not view themselves as sighted or as blind, and their esteem and sense of affiliation may vary according to context. In some situations, they must decide whether to describe their visual disability and be regarded as different, or not to refer to it, risking the perception that they are hiding their visual disability.

Many students with low vision read accurately but slowly. Spelling and handwriting may be difficult, and most students benefit from learning keyboarding and word processing as early as possible. Some have difficulty with competitive sports, especially those involving balls or moving targets. For almost all visually impaired students, the realization that they will not drive is a difficult part of adolescence. As their peers acquire drivers' licenses, low vision students should be encouraged to manage their own transportation. Children with low vision who attend public school rarely meet others with low vision, and it is important that they have some opportunities for contacts with children and adults with low vision to learn about how others solve problems. The range of behaviors and responses to low vision is diverse, and children vary in the amount of assistance they need in adjusting to the problems of visual impairment.

Adaptations and Intervention

Intervention begins with a thorough clinical and functional assessment of vision, as described previously. Adaptations recommended for the low vision learner may include environmental modifications, adaptive devices, and technology. Environmental adaptations include classroom seating appropriate for the child's visual needs, steady non-flickering lighting, use of high contrast and uncluttered backgrounds in learning materials, color contrast and highlighting, reducing viewing distance by holding materials closer to the eyes, and allowing more time for specific tasks that involve detailed visual material or hand–eye coordination.

Adaptive devices include low vision devices as well as specialized materials such as bookstands to place learning materials closer to the eyes. Many students with low vision can benefit from prescribed low-vision devices, including hand magnifiers, monocular telescopes for distance, and high plus glasses for reading. Efficient use of these devices requires follow-up by an eye specialist and instruction by a qualified professional, either a teacher of visually impaired students or an orientation and mobility instructor. Low vision devices are more portable, less expensive, and are often more efficient than large print for a student with low vision.

Technological adaptations are becoming more widely available and accessible. Many low-vision students use enlarged images on the computer screen, which are often included in the general market software. Software is available to enlarge computer images or provide speech output. Others with low vision use a closed circuit television (CCTV), a camera attached to a monitor that will enlarge materials placed under the camera. School districts are responsible for purchasing technology needed for the child's education, and this planning should take into account the student's long-term needs.

Intervention and education for the student with low vision emphasizes accomplishment of typical tasks with necessary adaptations. Training in the use of low-vision devices, in advocating for appropriate adaptations, and in using technology that will enhance task efficiency is usually the role of a certified teacher of visually impaired students. These teachers may work also on specific programs to encourage the child to develop specific visual skills; for example, the *Program to Develop Efficiency in Visual Functioning* provides developmentally sequenced activities to enhance visual skills.

BLINDNESS

Definition

Blindness rarely means that one is totally blind, and few children have no vision. Most blind children see some light and dark perception, shape/object vision, or respond to moving objects. The terms *functional blindness* and *educational blindness* are sometimes used to refer to vision that is limited to the degree that information is gained through hearing and touch.

Development

The child who is blind receives fewer cues about events and objects around him, and this limitation can affect all areas of development. Body awareness, movement, self-care routines, and social skills are not learned incidentally through observation as they are by sighted children; imitation and modeling must take place through tactile and auditory methods.

Delays are most notable in skills involving movement, including motor development and self-care skills. Many blind children are slow to roll over, crawl, and walk; they exhibit low physical tone due to lack of muscle use. In infancy, they may not be motivated to move forward in space because they are unaware of objects to be explored. Descriptive language and physical demonstration will increase their awareness of body parts and movement. As they become older, they may have poor posture, difficulties with weight, and poor strength and endurance if they do not have regular and appropriate movement experiences. Self-care skills such as feeding and dressing may also be delayed due to lack of visual models and unclear expectations from others. Children will learn from regular participation in self-care routines, placing their hands over those of another person if they require demonstration.

With appropriate experiences and intervention, developmental delays are often reduced or nonexistent by school age. Early intervention and family education are vital in minimizing developmental delays. Medical personnel refer families of blind children to local services through specialized schools for the blind, local school districts, or regional cooperatives, which provide educational services for children and their families.

Assessment

Educational teams for blind children often include teachers of visually impaired students, orientation and mobility instructors, and rehabilitation teachers. Team members assess sensory, motor, cognitive, social, and language development. A teacher of visually impaired students addresses general development, cognitive and academic abilities, and specialized skills related to visual impairment. The orientation and mobility instructor evaluates body and spatial awareness, environmental orientation, and mobility. A rehabilitation teacher may address self-care and life skills.

Intelligence and academic assessment of school-age students will require modifications so that the student has access to tests in Braille and can demonstrate an appropriate range of skills. There is no reliable intelligence test designed specifically for blind students due to the small numbers of individuals who would take them. However, many evaluators administer the verbal subscale of the Wechsler Intelligence Scale for Children (WISC) along with other instruments that are predominantly verbal or tactile. When standardized instruments are used for blind children, the evaluator should describe the modifications used when reporting scores and should indicate any pattern of responses that might be associated with blindness.

Psychosocial Issues

Some aspects of blindness may affect a child's ongoing psychological and social experiences. Nonverbal communication is not available visually, and children must learn body orientation as a substitute for eye contact, posture, and greetings such as a wave or handshake. Students will need to appropriately accept or refuse assistance from others and avoid potentially dangerous situations.

Stereotypic behaviors or mannerisms often occur in children who are blind. Although these occur in children with other disabilities, blind children demonstrate increased levels of body rocking, eye poking, and arm flapping. These behaviors may result from limited outlets for physical activity, neurological differences, and lack of awareness about socially acceptable movements.

Learned helplessness is common among blind students. Other people may assists student with tasks they can do themselves such as carrying materials to their school desks. Too much help from others reinforces an external locus of control, and a blind student may not view himself or herself as autonomous or capable of performing basic tasks independently.

Adaptations and Interventions

Most blind students will read using Braille, and a rich tactile and auditory environment can support reading Braille at home and at school. Braille must be consistently available in the home and at school, just as print is available to sighted students. Consistent verbal description and exposure to information about concepts such as size, shapes, textures, colors, smells, tastes, sounds, and the like teaches knowledge of the environment.

Braille is the primary literacy medium in reading and writing for the blind. It is a code of six-dot cells that can be written by hand or using various devices, including computers. Braille can be uncontracted, involving only the 26 letters of the alphabet, or contracted, using more than 200 combinations of letters represented by abbreviated Braille characters. A specialized code called Nemeth code is used for numbers, mathematical texts, and scientific notation. Pictures and graphs within books are represented either by Brailled description tactile graphics. Although Braille reading and writing require more time than printed text, they allow the blind child access to literacy.

Various adaptive devices may be used by the blind child in school. The Perkins Braillewriter is used for various tasks; a slate and stylus can be used for short notes or note-taking; standard print keyboards can be used on a computer with speech access or Braille displays; and Braille notetakers allow the student to make notes and store them and editwriting. Speech software is used for access to computer software and the World Wide Web.

Blind children use a variety of tools in negotiating their environments. Most will use a long cane for mobility and safe travel. An orientation and mobility instructor will assist the student in the choice of the right cane and its efficient use, as well as the concepts necessary for independent travel. Many electronic devices have been developed for travel, and they use vibrating or auditory signals to indicate when the traveler is approaching an obstacle. In addition, the use of tactile maps or technology that allows the blind person to enter a location and plot a route allow the blind traveler to travel more efficiently than was possible in the past.

See also: Individuals with Disabilities Education Act (IDEA); Intellectual Assessment; Parenting the Handicapped Child

Further Reading

Barraga, N., & Morris, J. (1980). *Program to develop efficiency in visual functioning.* Louisville, KY: American Printing House for the Blind.

Corn, A., & Koenig, A. (1996). Perspectives on low vision. *Foundations of low vision: Clinical and functional perspectives.* New York: AFB Press.

Faye, E. (1984). *Clinical low vision.* Boston: Little, Brown.

Resources

American Foundation for the Blind, 11 Penn Plaza, Suite 300, New York, NY 10001. http://www.afb.org

American Printing House for the Blind, 1839 Frankfort Avenue, Louisville, KY 40206. http://www.aph.org

Lighthouse International, 111 East 59th Street, New York, NY 10022. http://www.lighthouse.org

JANE N. ERIN
TAMI S. LEVINSON

Visual–Motor Assessment

DEFINITIONS

Beery (1997) defines *visual–motor integration* as the degree to which visual perception and fine motor (finger–hand) movements are well coordinated. Visual–motor integration skills are a component of a more comprehensive visual perceptual system, and it is important to understand the larger context in which these skills function. According to Schenck (2001), *visual perception* is the process responsible for the reception and understanding of visual stimuli. The receptive component involves the ability to detect and organize visual information from the environment. The understanding, or cognitive, component refers to the ability to interpret and use what is seen. Both of these components are necessary in order for a person to use visual information functionally. Schenck (2002) notes that visual perceptual skills not only involve recognition and identification of such things as objects, shapes, and colors, but also the ability to make accurate estimates of the size, configuration, and spatial relationships of these objects.

Visual perceptual abilities depend upon the healthy physiological functioning of the visual system (e.g., visual acuity, accommodation, convergence) in addition to the ability to move both the head and eyes to take in visual information (e.g., oculomotor control). However, visual perception also depends upon the brain's ability to analyze and accurately interpret the visual information it receives. According to Schenck (2001), the cognitive components of visual perception include visual attention, discrimination, memory, and imagery. Visual attention involves an awareness of visual input in the environment (i.e., alertness), ability to pay attention to relevant aspects of this information while ignoring less important aspects (i.e., selective attention), ability to concentrate and persist at a visual task (i.e., vigilance), and ability to respond to two or more simultaneous visual tasks (i.e., divided attention). Visual discrimination involves the ability to detect specific features of visual stimuli, which in turn enables the viewer to match and/or categorize the stimuli. Visual memory involves the capacity to hold visual information in mind and relate it to previous experiences, whereas visual imagery refers to the ability to picture objects or people in one's mind. All of these processes are important in the functional interpretation of visual information. According to Schenck, visual–motor skills are difficult to assess because they

are not a single or unitary process. They can be disrupted for many different reasons, such as underlying visual discrimination deficits, visual interpretation (cognitive) deficits, poor fine motor ability, or inability to integrate visual and motor processes. Therefore, careful analysis of visual–motor assessment data is necessary to determine the true underlying problem and plan an effective intervention strategy.

COURSE OF DEVELOPMENT

According to Glass (1993), the visual system of the brain forms early in gestation, so that by 24 weeks of gestation all the main anatomical structures of the visual system and the visual pathways are complete. Between the 24th and 40th week of gestation, there is further rapid maturation of the visual system in the brain. At birth, the newborn infant can fixate on objects and track their movement from side-to-side and up and down if the object is held at an optimal distance of 12–14 inches from the infant's face. However, the young infant does not yet have the physiological maturity for eye–hand coordination. By 3 months of age, infants make undirected arm movements in the direction of objects of interest, but cannot coordinate their reach so they can grasp the object. Between 4 and 7 months of age, most infants develop directed reaching movements—showing early eye–hand coordination—to grasp objects. These movements gradually become more refined and coordinated through the toddler and preschool years, as the young child gains greater visual–motor facility in manipulating small objects, using a crayon, sorting shapes, or working puzzles. As children reach school age, they develop visual–motor abilities to enable them to copy shapes and geometric designs, letters and numerals, and eventually to write fluently. Visual–motor coordination also occurs on a gross motor level, when children learn such skills as throwing and catching a ball, hitting a ball with a bat, and playing soccer. For the purposes of this entry, the focus will remain on visual and fine motor integration.

ASSESSMENT OF VISUAL–MOTOR FUNCTIONS

Often visual–motor abilities are assessed in the context of broader visual perceptual skills. As noted earlier, visual–motor skills are not a unitary ability; rather, they can be compromised by difficulty in various aspects of the visual perceptual system or the motor system. Often, visual–motor skills are evaluated in

Table 1. Examples of Visual–Motor and Visual Perceptual Assessment Instruments

Test name	Age range	Types of scores	Content
Wide Range Assessment of Visual Motor Abilities (WRAVMA)	5–18 years	Standard scores, percentiles	Three subtests measure drawing (visual–motor), matching (visual–spatial), and pegboard (fine motor coordination and dexterity) skills
Developmental Test of Visual–Motor Integration—4th ed. (VMI)	3–18 years	Standard scores, percentiles, age equivalents	Three subtests that assess visual–motor abilities, visual perception, and motor coordination
Bender Visual Motor Gestalt Test for Children	5–11 years	Standard scores, percentiles, age equivalents	Requires reproduction of nine geometric shapes and designs, and assesses visual–motor integration abilities
Test of Visual–Motor Skills, Revised (TVMS-R)	3–13 years (Upper extension: 12–40 years)	Scaled scores, percentiles, stanines, age equivalents	25 designs assess eye–hand motor accuracy, motor control, motor coordination, and/or the child's gestalt interpretation
Developmental Test of Visual Perception—2nd ed. (DTVP-2); Developmental Test of Visual Perception—Adolescent and Adult (DTVP-A)	DTVP-2: 4–10 years DTVP-A: 11–75 years	Standard scores	Assesses both pure visual perception (with no motor response) and visual–motor integration abilities. Examples of subtests include copying, figure-ground, visual–motor search, visual closure, visual–motor speed, and form constancy
Test of Visual–Perceptual Skills—Revised (nonmotor)	4–13 years (Upper level: 12–18 years)	Standard scores, scaled scores, percentiles, stanines, and perceptual ages	Measures seven dimensions of visual-perceptual functioning without a motor component

comparison to visual perceptual abilities without a motor component. Several standardized assessment tools are available to psychologists, educators, and occupational or physical therapists for this type of assessment (see Table 1). Strengths and weaknesses in visual–motor abilities are often assessed as part of a broader psychoeducational evaluation to determine if a child has a learning disorder and needs special education intervention services. Assessment needs to be focused on assessing the specific cause of the visual–motor deficits so that educational remediation and/or compensatory approaches can be tied to the specific underlying cause.

TREATMENT OF VISUAL–MOTOR DYSFUNCTION

Intervention for visual–motor deficits may be done by teachers, special educators, occupational therapists, physical therapists, and/or psychologists. The approach to intervention may be guided by a theoretical framework, such as the one developed by Warren (1993), that illustrates the hierarchy of visual perceptual skill development. This hierarchy proposes that visual acuity, visual fields, and oculomotor control form the foundation of visual perception. From these skills other higher level skills emerge sequentially–namely, visual attention, visual scanning, pattern recognition, visual

memory, visual cognition, and higher level visual adaptation. Other theorists purport that visual perception is integrated into all human performance. The blending of visual and motor input is combined with previously stored data, and is used to guide human reactions. These theoretical perspectives guide evaluation and treatment of visual perceptual and visual–motor integration problems.

Intervention strategies can be categorized as either *developmental* or *compensatory*, according to Warren. In a developmental approach to intervention, it is assumed that higher-level skills evolve from lower-level skills. Once an evaluation determines where there are deficits along a hierarchy of skills, then intervention focuses on remediation of those deficits. Presumably, once the lower-level skills are remediated, then the higher-level skills can emerge. Occupational therapists may use perceptual training strategies to remediate deficit or prerequisite skills.

In compensatory approaches to intervention, there are modifications or accommodations in classroom materials or instructional methods to address the child's limitations. Adaptations might include reducing the amount of written work expected of the child or allowing additional time for completion of the work. Some teachers will allow children to express their knowledge orally on tests or assignments rather than requiring a written response. Keyboarding skills, if taught at an early age, may help a child complete written work more quickly and neatly than handwriting. Use of these accommodations can facilitate the child's school performance and assure that his or her visual–motor integration deficits do not impede learning.

See also: Adolescent Assessment; Learning Disorders; Preschool Assessment; School Age Assessment; Underachievement

Further Reading

Beery, K. E. (1997). *The Beery–Buktenica Developmental Test of Visual–Motor Integration: Administration, scoring, and teaching manual.* Parsippany, NJ: Modern Curriculum Press.
Glass, P. (1993). Development of visual function in preterm infants: Implications for early intervention. *Infants and Young Children,* 6 (1), 11–20.
Schenck, C.M. (2001). Visual perception. In J. Case-Smith (Ed.), *Occupational therapy for children* (4th ed., pp. 382–412). St. Louis, MO: Mosby.
Warren, M. (1993). A hierarchical model for evaluation and treatment of visual perceptual dysfunction in adult acquired brain injury. Part 1. *American Journal of Occupational Therapy,* 47, 42–54.

JAN L. CULBERTSON

Vomiting—Psychogenic

DEFINITION

Psychogenic vomiting is thought to be voluntary in nature in some way similar to rumination. Differentiating psychogenic vomiting from rumination is usually quite straightforward. The individual who engages in rumination generally rechews and reswallows the food but this is not the case in psychogenic vomiting. In addition, psychogenic vomiting is not necessarily restricted to infants or individuals with mental retardation, but is more likely to occur in developmentally and cognitively normal children or adolescents. Psychogenic vomiting generally occurs during or shortly after meals, the emesis (vomit) does not typically consist of the entire meal, the vomiting itself is rarely forceful and appears to be under a greater degree of voluntary control than observed in medically induced vomiting, and it is not associated to weight loss. The absence of any abdominal stress at the time of the vomiting differentiates psychogenic vomiting from medically related causes of vomiting.

INCIDENCE/PREVALENCE

There are no good estimates of the incidence of this disorder at present, although it is more common in females than males. The absence of good data on the incidence of this disorder is related to the difficulty in differentiating psychogenic vomiting from medically related vomiting or from vomiting induced in eating disorders such as anorexia nervosa and bulimia nervosa.

ETIOLOGY

It is most often believed that the cause of psychogenic vomiting is related to adjustment difficulties in the family context. Some have suggested that it is on a continuum with the eating disorders of anorexia nervosa and bulimia nervosa which occur within the family context. The belief is that the disorder is particularly likely to occur in families who are controlling, rigid, or overprotective and whose members have difficulty with self-expression. It has also been suggested that stressful triggering events such as accidents or victimization can often be found in the history of the child or adolescent with psychogenic vomiting. Other theories relate to the origin of the vomiting responses and the operant conditioning of the behavior.

TREATMENT

Treatment of this disorder has been approached from two viewpoints. Operant conditioning techniques such as extinction and overcorrection have been utilized and shown to be effective. More traditional psychotherapeutic and interpersonal therapeutic interventions such as hypnosis and family therapy have been utilized as well. Medical interventions generally have not been effective with this disorder.

PROGNOSIS

Currently there is little, if any, credible research data on treatment outcome with psychogenic vomiting. However, clinical accounts suggest that prognosis is good when utilizing a combination of operant and psychotherapeutic methods.

See also: Bulimia Nervosa; Family Intervention; Hypnosis; Overcorrection; Rumination

Further Reading

Friedrich, W. N., & Jaworski, T. M. (1995). Pediatric abdominal disorders: Inflammatory bowel disease, rumination/vomiting, and recurrent abdominal pain. In M. C. Roberts (Ed.), *Handbook of pediatric psychology* (2nd ed., pp. 479–497). New York: Guilford.

Holvoet, J. F. (1982). The etiology of rumination and psychogenic vomiting: A review. In J. Hollis & C. E. Meyers (Eds.), *Life threatening behavior: Analysis and intervention* (pp. 29–77). Washington, DC: American Association on Mental Deficiency.

Nugent, N. (1978). *How to get along with your stomach: A complete guide to the prevention and treatment of stomach distress.* Boston: Little, Brown.

THOMAS R. LINSCHEID

Von Willebrand's Disease

See: Hereditary Coagulation Disorders

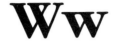

Wilms' Tumor

DEFINITION/INCIDENCE

Wilms' tumor is a primary malignant renal (kidney) tumor. It occurs in 7.6 cases per million of children younger than 15 (about 500 cases/year), and usually occurs in the first five years of life. Incidence is slightly higher in African-American and lower in Asian children. It is found more in females than in males and occurs at younger ages in males than in females.

ETIOLOGY

There is a greater risk for occurrence with some genetic (e.g., Denys–Drash, Beckwith–Wiedermann) syndromes, hemihypertrophy (enlargement of one side of the body), aniridia (absence of the iris of the eye), and several missing or gene mutations (e.g., 11p13, 11p15, 1p). It occurs within families in 1–2 percent of cases, and may be heritable, but no single gene has been isolated.

PRESENTATION

Children usually present with abdominal swelling and/or pain (often accompanied by a large flank mass), anemia, hematuria (blood in urine), hypertension, and sometimes fever. Imaging studies, such as ultrasound and computerized tomography (CT) scans are done as part of the diagnostic work-up and for follow-up purposes. Bone scans and brain imaging may also be done.

PATHOLOGY AND STAGING

Staging, or categorization, of the tumor is established using uniform criteria established by the National Wilms Tumor Study Group with the stages reflecting an increased disease state. Stage I: Tumor confined to kidney and completely resected (completely removed by surgery); Stage II: Tumor extends beyond kidney but is completely resected (negative margins and lymph nodes); Stage III: Tumor remains, with positive surgical margins (disease still present), tumor spillage (beyond the site), regional lymph node metastases; Stage IV: Hematogenous metastases or lymph node metastases outside the abdomen; Stage IV: Bilateral (both kidneys affected) renal Wilms' tumors at onset.

PROGNOSIS

Survival rate depends upon stage (lower, better), tumor size, age (less than 2 years, better) and histology (worse prognosis with anaplasia: immature or less differentiated form associated with malignancy). The overall 5-year survival rate is about 90 percent, with 85 percent considered cured. The survival rate is largely due to the results of clinical trials in the cooperative groups (National Wilms Tumor Study Group, International Society of Pediatric Oncology) which have provided data on large numbers of children in a timely manner.

TREATMENT

Most children receive surgery (nephrectomy) and chemotherapy. In cases where surgery is not immediately possible, preoperative chemotherapy and/or radiation may be done to shrink the tumor. In bilateral Wilms' tumor, bilateral biopsy and staging is done, with preoperative chemotherapy appropriate to stage and histology. Chemotherapy to eliminate the cancer cells depends upon stage and histology, but often includes combinations of dactinomysin, vincristine, doxorubicin, and cyclophosphamide. Newer combinations may include carboplatin, ifosfamide, and topotecan. Postoperative radiation also depends on histology and stage of the disease (usually Stage III or higher).

EFFECTS OF TREATMENT

Severity of treatment effects often depends upon the stage of disease and thus the intensity of treatment. The type of effect depends upon the site of the tumor and type of dosage of treatment. Some of the negative effects of treatment could include problems in the renal, cardiac, pulmonary, hepatic, bone marrow, gonadal, and skeletal systems. Other negative effects could include second malignancies, recurrence of Wilms' tumor, and infertility. In addition, long-term survivors have been found to have some difficulties in interpersonal functioning (friendships and romantic relationships) in comparison to healthy controls.

As most of the patients are young children, psychological interventions can include preparation and distraction before and during procedures. Involvement of child life, pain teams, and psychologists can help the child and parents deal with pain and discomfort. Cognitive-behavioral therapy can be helpful to deal with the impact of treatment on the child and family.

See also: Bereavement; Childhood Cancers; Osteosarcoma; Parenting the Chronically Ill Child; Treatment Adherence: Medical

Further Reading

Grundy, P. E., Green, D. M., Coppes, M. J., Breslow, N. E., Ritchey, M. L., Perlman, E. J., & Macklis, R. M. (2002). Renal tumors. In P. A. Pizzo & D. G. Poplack (Eds.), *Principles and practice of pediatric oncology* (4th ed., pp. 865–893), Philadelphia: Lippincott, Williams, and Wilkins.

Mackie, E., Hill, J., Kondryn, H., & Mcnally, R. (2000). Adult psychosocial outcomes in long-term survivors of acute lymphoblastic leukemia and Wilms' tumor: A controlled study. *Lancet, 355,* 1310–1314.

MARY JO KUPST
ANNE B. WARWICK

Word Deafness

See: Central Auditory Processing Disorders

Working Parents

A substantial majority of mothers with dependent children of all ages participate in the workforce. While the employment of mothers of school-aged children has been modal for more than three decades, substantial growth has occurred in the rates of employment of mothers of infants and preschoolers. According to a report published by the U.S. Department of Labor in 1999, a majority (63 percent) of women with children under 3 spend time in the labor force, almost triple the percentage in 1969, and more than half of the mothers with infants under 1 year of age are employed. Moreover, the average weekly hours of paid employment has grown steadily for mothers. In 1998, 32 percent of women with children under 3 worked full time year round, an increase from 7 percent in 1969. Fathers' participation in the workforce and their hours of employment have changed very little over this period of time. Given the importance attributed to mother's care in cultural ideals and psychological theories, and the working role assumed by growing numbers of mothers with young children, concern about effects of parents' work on children has focused on effects for the young child and family processes associated with the mother's employment.

Understanding how mother's participation in the workforce may affect her child requires examination of how maternal employment relates to the child's experiences and how these experiences, in turn, influence development. A substantial body of research has focused on relations between maternal employment and the child's family environment, addressing the father's role in the family, maternal well-being, and parenting styles and practices. Another body of work has focused on children's experiences of child care, particularly prior to their entry into school but increasingly in before- and after-school care experiences of school-aged children, and related these experiences, to developmental outcomes.

A predominant emphasis of the research on maternal employment's effects on children has been on the mother–child relationship. A particular area of interest has been the infant's security of attachment with his or her mother. This focus has been chiefly concerned with the possible negative consequences for the mother–child relationship when mothers participate in the work force and spend less time with their young children. Diminished time together may negatively affect the mother's ability to be sensitively attuned to her infant's signals and needs. According to Booth and colleagues (2002), full-time employed mothers of infants spend approximately 32 percent less time (12 hr per week in one study) directly interacting with their children than nonemployed mothers, but these differences tend to diminish as children get older, as reported by Hill and Stafford (1980).

Conclusions from aggregated early studies linked maternal employment to an increased risk for insecure infant–mother attachment, but these conclusions were questioned because the available research had not measured children's experiences in child care, had not adequately addressed other associated differences between working and nonworking mothers, and had not validated the assessments of attachment for children who experienced daily separations from their mothers. The National Institute for Child Health and Human Development (NICHD) Study of Early Child Care was launched in 1990 to address these criticisms and provide a comprehensive and definitive study of the issue. The study has followed approximately 1,200 children in a diverse sample of families in 10 locations across the United States from birth into their school years. The study repeatedly measured children's experiences in their homes and in child care. The factor found most strongly related to the security of the child's attachment to mother, both in infancy and preschool, was not the mother's availability to her child due to employment or hours in child care, but the mother's sensitivity to her child's needs when they were together. Regardless of the number of hours in child care, higher maternal sensitivity was related to a greater likelihood of secure attachment to mother. Nonmaternal child care experience, due primarily to maternal employment in infancy, was unrelated to children's attachment security to mother in infancy and in preschool except when mothers were relatively insensitive in interactions with their child. When mothers provided insensitive care, early

child care experience added to the risk of insecure attachment both in infancy and preschool. Experience with low-quality child care and more changes in child care also increased the risk of insecure infant–mother attachment when mothers provided insensitive parenting.

Some studies have found maternal employment associated with lower qualities of mother–child interaction, but most studies have not. Analyses from the NICHD Study of Early Child Care indicated that more hours per week in child care were associated with somewhat less maternal sensitivity and child engagement of mother in mother–child interactions in the first three years, but this effect did not itself impact the children's attachment security with their mothers. Studies of parenting and parent–child relations with older children have rarely detected differences due to maternal employment.

Do mothers have less influence on their children's development when they balance work and parenting? Evidence, again from the NICHD Study of Early Child Care, suggests that the influence of families and parenting is not weakened or changed in the child's early years by mothers' participation in the workforce. In the context of varied nonmaternal child care experiences, ranging from none to extensive, parenting influences of sensitivity and warmth, responsiveness, and cognitive stimulation on preschooler's development were essentially the same, with remarkably few exceptions.

According to a number of studies, fathers tend to spend more time caring for their children, and role differences between mothers and fathers are fewer when the mother is employed. This is an apparent result of maternal employment, because such differences are found regardless of parents' gender-role attitudes and increases in fathers' involvement in the household occur when mothers enter the workforce. In addition, whereas fathers in single-earner families tend to be more involved with their sons than their daughters, fathers' involvement with their children in employed mother families is unrelated to the child's gender, highlighting work–family linkages. Fathers' increased participation in their children's care when mothers are employed may affect the father's influence on his children. Increased father involvement is generally associated with greater achievement in children, particularly for daughters.

Balancing work and family roles does not appear to strain mothers' mental health. No study has found the mental health of full-time homemakers to be better than that of employed mothers. In fact, employment has been associated with mental health advantages for mothers from middle class, working-class, and poverty-stricken families. These differences may be attributable to the reasons why mothers are not working when employment has become the norm, but may also relate to satisfactions gained from multiple roles, as reviewed by Barnett and Hyde (2001).

Many studies comparing children of employed and non-employed mothers find few consistent differences in children's school achievement, but some have found lower school achievement in middle-class boys when their mothers are employed, and others have reported higher academic achievement of girls. A recent well-conducted study by Hoffman and Youngblade (1999) reported associations between mothers' employment and higher achievement for both boys and girls in middle childhood, regardless of socioeconomic class or their mothers' marital status. Regarding social and emotional adjustment, despite inconsistencies across the research findings, many studies have found that maternal employment and extensive nonparental care beginning very early in life are related to increased aggression and noncompliance in preschool and the early school-aged years. Such differences related to maternal employment appear to diminish over time, however. Reasons for this association are not easy to explain, but will continue to be studied within children's family environments, their experiences in child care settings, and linkages between the family and child care experiences of the child.

See also: Attachment; Mothers' and Fathers' Roles in Normal Child Development

Further Reading

Barnett, R. C., & Hyde, J. S. (2001). Women, men, work, and family. *American Psychologist, 56*, 781–796.

Booth, C. L., Clarke-Stewart, K. A., Vandell, D. L., McCartney, K, & Owen, M. T. (2002). Child-care usage and mother–infant "quality time." *Journal of Marriage and the Family, 64*, 16–26.

Hill, C. R., & Stafford, F. P. (1980). Parental care of children: Time diary estimates of quantity, predictability, and variety. *Journal of Human Resources, 15*, 219–289.

Hoffman, L. W., & Youngblade, L. M. (1999). *Mothers at work: Effects on children's well-being.* New York: Cambridge University Press.

NICHD Early Child Care Research Network. (2001). Parenting and family influences when children are in child care: Results from the NICHD Study of Early Child Care. In J. Borkowski, S. Ramey, & M. Bristol-Power (Eds.), *Parenting and their child's world: Influences on intellectual, academic, and social-emotional development.* Mahwah, NJ: Erlbaum.

NICHD Early Child Care Research Network. (2002). Early child care and children's development prior to school entry: Results from the NICHD Study of Early Child Care. *American Educational Research Journal, 39*, 113–164.

www.childresearch.net/CYBRARY/EDATA/NICHD/DATA01.HTM

MARGARET TRESCH OWEN

Worry

See: Generalized Anxiety Disorder

Contributors

Keith D. Allen, PhD, Munroe-Meyer Institute for Genetics and Rehabilitation, Psychology Department, University of Nebraska Medical School, Omaha, Nebraska, United States

Heather K. Blier Alvarez, MS, Child Study Center, Virginia Polytechnic Institute & State University, Blacksburg, Virginia, United States

Christa J. Anderson, BA, Department of Psychology, University of Kansas, Lawrence, Kansas, United States

F. Daniel Armstrong, PhD, Mailman Center for Child Development, Department of Pediatrics, University of Miami School of Medicine, Miami, Florida, United States

Laura Arnstein, BA, Medical University of South Carolina, Charleston, South Carolina, United States

Sasha G. Aschenbrand, BS, Department of Psychology, Temple University, Philadelphia, Pennsylvania, United States

Glen P. Aylward, PhD, ABPP, Departments of Pediatrics and Psychiatry, Southern Illinois University School of Medicine, Springfield, Illinois, United States

Daniel M. Bagner, BA, Department of Clinical and Health Psychology, University of Florida, Gainesville, Florida, United States

Martha Underwood Barnard, PhD, Department of Pediatrics/Behavioral Sciences, University of Kansas Medical School, Kansas City, Kansas, United States

Christopher T. Barry, MA, Department of Psychology, University of Alabama, Tuscaloosa, Alabama, United States

Tammy D. Barry, MS, Department of Psychology, University of Alabama, Tuscaloosa, Alabama, United States

Ellen Bean, MEd, Buffalo, New York, United States

Karen Bearman, MS, Department of Psychology, University of Miami, Coral Gables, Florida, United States

Karen Bearss, MS, Department of Clinical and Health Psychology, University of Florida, Gainesville, Florida, United States

Danielle A. Becker, MS, Department of Clinical and Health Psychology, University of Florida, Gainesville, Florida, United States

Shannon Becker, BA, Department of Psychiatry, Georgetown University, Washington, DC, United States

Ronald W. Belter, PhD, Department of Psychology, University of West Florida, Pensacola, Florida, United States

Rebecca S. Bernard, MA, Department of Psychology, West Virginia University, Morgantown, West Virginia, United States

Maureen M. Black, PhD, Department of Pediatrics, University of Maryland School of Medicine, Baltimore, Maryland, United States

Otilia M. Blaga, BS, BA, Department of Psychology, University of Kansas, Lawrence, Kansas, United States

Kimberley A. Blaker, MEd, Department of Psychology, University of Georgia, Athens, Georgia, United States

C. Alexandra Boeving, MA, Department of Pediatrics and College of Health Professions, Medical University of South Carolina, Charleston, South Carolina, United States

Stephen R. Boggs, PhD, Department of Clinical and Health Psychology, University of Florida, Gainesville, Florida, United States

Richard E. Boles, MS, Clinical Child Psychology Program, University of Kansas, Lawrence, Kansas, United States

Susan Bongiolatti, BA, Department of Clinical and Health Psychology, University of Florida, Gainesville, Florida, United States

Barbara L. Bonner, PhD, Center on Child Abuse and Neglect, Department of Pediatrics, University of Oklahoma Health Sciences Center, Oklahoma City, Oklahoma, United States

Kirsten Bradbury, MS, Department of Psychology, Virginia Polytechnic Institute and State University, Blacksburg, Virginia, United States

Mary Brinkmeyer, MS, Department of Clinical and Health Sciences, University of Florida, Gainesville, Florida, United States

Keri J. Brown, BS, Clinical Child Psychology Program, University of Kansas, Lawrence, Kansas, United States

Ronald T. Brown, PhD, ABPP, Department of Pediatrics and College of Health Professions, Medical University of South Carolina, Charleston, South Carolina, United States

Leslie Buck, MA, Department of Educational Psychology, University of Oklahoma, Norman, Oklahoma, United States

Lisa M. Buckloh, PhD, Division of Psychology and Psychiatry, Nemours Children's Clinic, Jacksonville, Florida, United States

Eric L. Canen, BS, Department of Psychology, University of Wyoming, Laramie, Wyoming, United States

Mark Chaffin, PhD, Center on Abuse and Neglect, University of Oklahoma Health Sciences Center, Oklahoma City, Oklahoma, United States

Kelly M. Champion, PhD, Department of Social and Behavioral Sciences, Arizona State University West, Phoenix, Arizona, United States

John M. Chaney, PhD, Department of Psychology, Oklahoma State University, Stillwater, Oklahoma, United States

Kristin V. Christodulu, PhD, Department of Psychology, University at Albany, State University of New York, Albany, New York, United States

Tangela R. Clark, MA, Department of Psychology, University of South Florida, Tampa, Florida, United States

Frank L. Collins, PhD, Department of Psychology, Oklahoma State University, Stillwater, Oklahoma, United States

John Colombo, PhD, Department of Psychology, University of Kansas, Lawrence, Kansas, United States

Bruce E. Compas, PhD, Department of Psychology and Human Development, Vanderbilt University, Nashville, Tennessee, United States

Amy H. Cornell, MS, Department of Psychology, University of New Orleans, New Orleans, Louisiana, United States

Wallace V. Crandall, MD, Department of Pediatrics, The Ohio State University, Children's Hospital, Columbus, Ohio, United States

Torrey A. Creed, MA, Department of Psychology, Temple University, Philadelphia, Pennsylvania, United States

Jan L. Culbertson, PhD, Child Study Center, University of Oklahoma Health Sciences Center, Oklahoma City, Oklahoma, United States

Kathryn M. Dalferes, BA, Department of Psychology, University of Richmond, Richmond, Virginia, United States

Rene Marie Daman, PCS, Department of Rehabilitative Science, University of Oklahoma Health Sciences Center, Oklahoma City, Oklahoma, United States

Danielle M. Dandreaux, BS, Department of Psychology, University of New Orleans, New Orleans, Louisiana, United States

Melissa A. Davis, MHS, Department of Clinical and Health Psychology, University of Florida, Gainesville, Florida, United States

Alan Delamater, PhD, ABPP, Department of Pediatrics, University of Miami School of Medicine, Miami, Florida, United States

Andreas Dick-Niederhauser, BS, Child and Family Psychosocial Research Center, Florida International University, Miami, Florida, United States

Edward J. Dill, MA, Clinical Child Psychology Program, University of Kansas, Lawrence, Kansas, United States

Carla A. DiSalvo, BS, Department of Psychology, Virginia Commonwealth University, Richmond, Virginia, United States

Erin Dowdy, BS, Department of Psychology, University of Georgia, Athens, Georgia, United States

Amanda Drews, MA, Department of Psychology, University of Nevada—Reno, Reno, Nevada, United States

Dennis Drotar, PhD, Division of Behavioral Pediatrics and Psychology, Rainbow Babies & Children's Hospital, Case Western Reserve School of Medicine, Cleveland, Ohio, United States

Kevin Duff, PhD, Department of Psychiatry and Behavioral Sciences, University of Oklahoma Health Sciences Center, Oklahoma City, Oklahoma, United States

Amy M. Duhig, MA, Department of Psychology, University of South Florida, Tampa, Florida, United States

V. Mark Durand, PhD, Department of Psychology, University at Albany, State University of New York, Albany, New York, United States

Philip Eisenberg, MS, Department of Clinical and Health Psychology, University of Florida, Gainesville, Florida, United States

Tashya Ekechukwu, MEd, Department of Psychiatry, Georgetown University, Washington, DC, United States

Charles H. Elliott, PhD, Department of Psychology, Fielding Graduate Institute, Santa Barbara, California, and Department of Psychology, University of New Mexico, Albuquerque, New Mexico, United States

Jane N. Erin, PhD, Department of Special Education, Rehabilitation, and School Psychology, The University of Arizona, Tucson, Arizona, United States

Cecilia A. Essau, PhD, Westfalische Wilhelms-Universitat Munster, Psychologisches Institut I, Munster, Germany

Sheila M. Eyberg, PhD, Department of Clinical and Health Psychology, University of Florida, Gainesville, Florida, United States

Jamie Farrell, BS, Department of Psychology, University of New Orleans, New Orleans, Louisiana, United States

Eileen B. Fennell, PhD, Department of Clinical and Health Psychology, University of Florida, Gainesville, Florida, United States

Tiffany Field, PhD, Department of Pediatrics, University of Miami School of Medicine, Miami, Florida, United States

Sherecce Fields, BA, Department of Psychology, University of South Florida, Tampa, Florida, United States

Holly A. Filcheck, MA, Department of Psychology, West Virginia University, Morgantown, West Virginia, United States

Jack W. Finney, PhD, Department of Psychology, Virginia Polytechnic Institute and State University, Blacksburg, Virginia, United States

Constance J. Fournier, PhD, Department of Educational Psychology, Texas A & M University, College Station, Texas, United States

Paul C. Francel, MD, PhD, Department of Neurosurgery, University of Oklahoma Health Sciences Center, Oklahoma City, Oklahoma, United States

Greta Francis, PhD, The Bradley School, Brown University Medical School, East Providence, Rhode Island, United States

Ximena Franco, BS, Child and Family Psychosocial Research Center, Florida International University, Miami, Florida, United States

Jennifer Freeman, PhD, Department of Child & Family Psychiatry, Rhode Island Hospital, Providence, Rhode Island, United States

Paul J. Frick, PhD, Department of Psychology, University of New Orleans, New Orleans, Louisiana, United States

F. Jay Fricker, MD, Department of Pediatrics, University of Florida, Gainesville, Florida, United States

Robert D. Friedberg, PhD, School of Professional Psychology, Wright State University, Dayton, Ohio, United States

Patrick C. Friman, PhD, Boys Town, Omaha, Nebraska, United States

Mary A. Fristad, PhD, Department of Child & Adolescent Psychiatry, Ohio State University, Columbus, Ohio, United States

Bridget K. Gamm, MS, Clinical Child Psychology Program, University of Kansas, Lawrence, Kansas, United States

Abbe Garcia, PhD, Department of Child & Family Psychiatry, Rhode Island Hospital, Providence, Rhode Island, United States

Rosario Gomez-Lobo, Department of Psychiatry, Georgetown University, Washington, DC, United States

Regino P. González-Peralta, MD, Department of Pediatrics, University of Florida, Gainesville, Florida, United States

Betty N. Gordon, PhD, Department of Psychology, University of North Carolina, Chapel Hill, North Carolina, United States

Andrea Follmer Greenhoot, PhD, Department of Psychology, University of Kansas, Lawrence, Kansas, United States

Ernestine Green-Turner, BA, Department of Psychology, Oklahoma State University, Stillwater, Oklahoma, United States

Amie E. Grills, MS, Child Study Center, Virginia Polytechnic Institute & State University, Blacksburg, Virginia, United States

Linda Sayler Gudas, PhD, Harvard Medical School and Children's Hospital, Boston, Massachusetts, United States

Jacfranz Guiteau, BA, Department of Psychiatry, Georgetown University, Washington, DC, United States

Robin H. Gurwitch, PhD, Department of Pediatrics, University of Oklahoma Health Sciences Center, Oklahoma City, Oklahoma, United States

Dennis C. Harper, PhD, ABPP, Department of Pediatrics and Center for Disabilities and Development, University of Iowa, Iowa City, Iowa, United States

Michelle Harwood, BS, Health Sciences Center, University of Florida, Gainesville, Florida, United States

Debra B. Hecht, PhD, Center on Child Abuse and Neglect, Department of Pediatrics, University of Oklahoma Health Sciences Center, Oklahoma City, Oklahoma, United States

Kristina A. Hedtke, MA, Department of Psychology, Temple University, Philadelphia, Pennsylvania, United States

Scott W. Henggeler, PhD, Family Services Research Center, Department of Psychiatry and Behavioral Sciences, Medical University of South Carolina, Charleston, South Carolina, United States

Susan L. Hepburn, PhD, Department of Psychiatry, Health Sciences Center, University of Colorado, Denver, Colorado, United States

Alyssa M. Hershberger, BA, Department of Psychology, Virginia Commonwealth University, Richmond, Virginia, United States

Daniel R. Hilliker, PhD, Departments of Psychiatry and Pediatrics, School of Medicine, University of North Carolina at Chapel Hill, Chapel Hill, North Carolina, United States

Kay Hodges, PhD, Department of Psychology, Eastern Michigan University, Ypsilanti, Michigan, United States

Kristen E. Holderle, BS, Department of Child & Adolescent Psychiatry, Ohio State University, Columbus, Ohio, United States

Clarissa S. Holmes, PhD, Departments of Psychology, Pediatrics, and Psychiatry, Virginia Commonwealth University/Medical College of Virginia, Richmond, Virginia and Department of Psychiatry, Georgetown University, Washington, DC, United States

Paul Hommersen, BA, Department of Psychology, University of British Columbia, Vancouver, British Columbia, Canada

Tracy Hopkins-Golightly, MS, Department of Pediatrics, University of Oklahoma Health Sciences Center, Oklahoma City, Oklahoma, United States

Betsy Hoza, PhD, Department of Psychological Sciences, Purdue University, West Lafayette, Indiana, United States

Alan Hudson, PhD, Department of Psychology and Disability Studies, Royal Melbourne Institute of Technology, Bundoora, Victoria, Australia

Jennifer L. Hudson, PhD, Department of Psychology, Macquarie University, Sydney, New South Wales, Australia

Alicia A. Hughes, BS, Department of Psychology, Temple University, Philadelphia, Pennsylvania, United States

Yo Jackson, PhD, Clinical Psychology Program, University of Kansas, Lawrence, Kansas, United States

Anne K. Jacobs, PhD, Clinical Child Psychology Program, University of Kansas, Lawrence, Kansas, United States

Noel J. Jacobs, PhD, Bert Nash Community Mental Health Center, Lawrence, Kansas, United States

David M. Janicke, PhD, Division of Psychology, Cincinnati Children's Hospital Medical Center, Cincinnati, Ohio, United States

James H. Johnson, PhD, Department of Clinical and Health Psychology, University of Florida, Gainesville, Florida, United States

Melissa J. R. Johnson, PhD, WakeMed, Raleigh, North Carolina, and Departments of Pediatrics and Psychiatry, School of Medicine, University of North Carolina at Chapel Hill, Chapel Hill, North Carolina, United States

Rebecca J. Johnson, MS, Clinical Child Psychology Program, University of Kansas, Lawrence, Kansas, United States

Trey A. Johnson, BA, Department of Clinical and Health Psychology, University of Florida, Gainesville, Florida, United States

Charlotte Johnston, PhD, Department of Psychology, University of British Columbia, Vancouver, British Columbia, Canada

Lauren A. Jones, BS, Department of Psychology, University of Georgia, Athens, Georgia, United States

Dimitra Kamboukos, MA, Department of Psychology, University of South Florida, Tampa, Florida, United States

Randy W. Kamphaus, PhD, Department of Psychology, University of Georgia, Athens, Georgia, United States

Kathleen N. Kannass, PhD, Department of Psychology, University of Kansas, Lawrence, Kansas, United States

Mary C. Kaven, PhD, Children's Psychiatric Center, University of New Mexico, Albuquerque, New Mexico, United States

Anne E. Kazak, PhD, ABPP, Department of Psychology, The Children's Hospital of Philadelphia and Department of Pediatrics, University of Pennsylvania, Philadelphia, Pennsylvania, United States

Michelle Kees, PhD, Center on Child Abuse and Neglect, Department of Pediatrics, University of Oklahoma Health Sciences Center, Oklahoma City, Oklahoma, United States

Philip C. Kendall, PhD, ABPP, Department of Psychology, Temple University, Philadelphia, Pennsylvania, United States

Eva Kimonis, BA, Department of Psychology, University of New Orleans, New Orleans, Louisiana, United States

Christy A. Kleinsorge, MA, Clinical Child Psychology Program, University of Kansas, Lawrence, Kansas, United States

Susan M. Knell, PhD, Mayfield Village, Ohio, United States

Laura A. Knight, MS, Department of Psychology, Oklahoma State University, Stillwater, Oklahoma, United States

David J. Kolko, PhD, Western Psychiatric Institute & Clinic, University of Pittsburgh Medical School, Pittsburgh, Pennsylvania, United States

Gerald P. Koocher, PhD, Simmons College, Boston, Massachusetts, United States

Daniel J. Krall, MA, Clinical Child Psychology Program, University of Kansas, Lawrence, Kansas, United States

Anna P. Kroncke, BA, Department of Psychology, University of Georgia, Athens, Georgia, United States

Mary Jo Kupst, PhD, Department of Pediatrics, Medical College of Wisconsin, Milwaukee, Wisconsin, United States

Annette M. La Greca, PhD, Department of Psychology, University of Miami, Coral Gables, Florida, United States

Elise E. Labbe, PhD, Department of Psychology, University of South Alabama, Mobile, Alabama, United States

Audra Langley, PhD, Neuropsychiatric Institute, University of California at Los Angeles, Los Angeles, California, United States

Angela LaRosa, MD, Department of Pediatrics and College of Health Professions, Medical University of South Carolina, Charleston, South Carolina, United States

Stephen Lassen, MA, Clinical Child Psychology Program, University of Kansas, Lawrence, Kansas, United States

Tammy A. Lazicki-Puddy, MA, Clinical Child Psychology Program, University of Kansas, Lawrence, Kansas, United States

Elena Lea, PhD, Private Practice, Chapel Hill, North Carolina, United States

Thad R. Leffingwell, PhD, Department of Psychology, Oklahoma State University, Stillwater, Oklahoma, United States

Tami S. Levinson, MA, Department of Special Education, Rehabilitation, and School Psychology, The University of Arizona, Tucson, Arizona, United States

Thomas R. Linscheid, PhD, Departments of Pediatrics and Psychology, The Ohio State University, Children's Hospital, Columbus, Ohio, United States

Emma Little, PhD, Department of Psychology and Developmental Disabilities, Royal Melbourne Institute of Technology, Bundoora, Victoria, Australia

John E. Lochman, PhD, Department of Psychology, University of Alabama, Tuscaloosa, Alabama, United States

Christopher W. Loftis, MS, Department of Clinical and Health Sciences, University of Florida, Gainesville, Florida, United States

Mary Beth Logue, PhD, Department of Pediatrics, University of Oklahoma Health Sciences Center, Oklahoma City, Oklahoma, United States

Barbara Lopez, BS, Child & Family Psychosocial Research Center, Florida International University, Miami, Florida, United States

Robert D. Lyman, PhD, Department of Psychology, University of Alabama, Tuscaloosa, Alabama, United States

Patricia A. Lynch, MA, Department of Psychology, Virginia Commonwealth University, Richmond, Virginia, United States

Kenneth R. MacAleese, BA, Department of Psychology, University of Nevada—Reno, Reno, Nevada, United States

Barbara Mackinaw-Koons, PhD, Department of Child & Adolescent Psychiatry, Ohio State University, Columbus, Ohio, United States

Laura M. Mackner, PhD, Department of Pediatrics, The Ohio State University, Children's Hospital, Columbus, Ohio, United States

William E. MacLean, Jr., PhD, Department of Psychology, University of Wyoming, Laramie, Wyoming, United States

Kelly W. Maloney, MD, Department of Pediatrics, Medical College of Wisconsin, Milwaukee, Wisconsin, United States

Donna Marschall, PhD, Department of Psychiatry, Georgetown University and Department of Psychology, Children's National Medical Center, Washington, DC, United States

Maria R. Marshall, MS, Department of Psychology, Fielding Graduate Institute, Santa Barbara, California, United States

Joanna O. Mashunkashey, BS, Clinical Child Psychology Program, University of Kansas, Lawrence, Kansas, United States

Sunnye E. Mayes, BA, Clinical Child Psychology Program, University of Kansas, Lawrence, Kansas, United States

Tom Mazur, PsyD, Departments of Psychiatry and Pediatrics, School of Medicine & Biomedical Sciences, University at Buffalo, and The Children's Hospital of Buffalo, Buffalo, New York, United States

Mary Anne McCaffree, MD, Department of Pediatrics, University of Oklahoma School of Medicine, Oklahoma City, Oklahoma, United States

Catherine B. McClellan, MA, Department of Psychology, West Virginia University, Morgantown, West Virginia, United States

Heather K. McElroy, BA, Department of Psychology, University of Alabama, Tuscaloosa, Alabama, United States

Cheryl B. McNeil, PhD, Department of Psychology, West Virginia University, Morgantown, West Virginia, United States

Carla L. Messenger, MA, Department of Psychology, George Washington University, Washington, DC, United States

Drew C. Messer, JD, PhD, Lieutenant Commander, Medical Service Corps, United States Naval Hospital, Okinawa, Japan

Bernard Metz, PhD, Department of Pediatrics, The Ohio State University, Children's Hospital, Columbus, Ohio, United States

Alisa A. Miller, BA, Department of Psychology, University of Kansas, Lawrence, Kansas, United States

Michael L. Miller, MS, Department of Psychology, University of Wyoming, Laramie, Wyoming, United States

Lisa C. Mills, PhD, Department of Pediatrics, Cincinnati Children's Hospital Medical Center, Cincinnati, Ohio, United States

Montserrat C. Mitchell, BS, Clinical Child Psychology Program, University of Kansas, Lawrence, Kansas, United States

Avani C. Modi, MS, Department of Clinical and Health Psychology, University of Florida, Gainesville, Florida, United States

Tracy L. Morris, PhD, Department of Psychology, West Virginia University, Morgantown, West Virginia, United States

Laura Mufson, PhD, Department of Psychiatry, Columbia University Medical School, New York, New York, United States

Larry L. Mullins, PhD, Department of Psychology, Oklahoma State University, Stillwater, Oklahoma, United States

John J. Mulvihill, MD, Department of Pediatrics, University of Oklahoma Health Sciences Center, Oklahoma City, Oklahoma, United States

Peter Muris, PhD, Department of Medical, Clinical, & Experimental Psychology, Maastricht University, Maastricht, the Netherlands

Megan Murphy, BA, Department of Psychiatry, Georgetown University, Washington, DC, United States

Candice Murray, MA, Department of Psychology, University of British Columbia, Vancouver, British Columbia, Canada

Erin M. Neary, MS, Department of Clinical and Health Psychology, University of Florida, Gainesville, Florida, United States

Chantelle Nobile, MA, Department of Psychology, Case Western Reserve University, Cleveland, Ohio, United States

Jeneva Ohan, MA, Department of Psychology, University of British Columbia, Vancouver, British Columbia, Canada

Thomas H. Ollendick, PhD, Child Study Center, Virginia Polytechnic Institute and State University, Blacksburg, Virginia, United States

Donald P. Oswald, PhD, Department of Psychiatry, Virginia Commonwealth University, Richmond, Virginia, United States

Margaret Tresch Owen, PhD, School of Human Development, University of Texas—Dallas, Richardson, Texas, United States

Timothy J. Ozechowski, PhD, Center for Family & Adolescent Research, Oregon Research Institute, Portland, Oregon, United States

Tonya M. Palermo, PhD, Department of Pediatrics, Rainbow Babies & Children's Hospital, Case Western Reserve University School of Medicine, Cleveland, Ohio, United States

Anna Maria Patino, MS, Department of Psychology, University of Miami, Coral Gables, Florida, United States

Martha F. Paulk, MA, Department of Pediatrics, University of Florida, Jacksonville, Florida

William E. Pelham, Jr., PhD, Center for Children & Families, State University of New York at Buffalo, Buffalo, New York, United States

Vicky Phares, PhD, Department of Psychology, University of South Florida, Tampa, Florida, United States

Nancy C. Phillips, BA, Department of Psychology, University of Alabama, Tuscaloosa, Alabama, United States

John Piacentini, PhD, Neuropsychiatric Institute, University of California at Los Angeles, Los Angeles, California, United States

Richard W. Puddy, MA, Clinical Child Psychology Program, University of Kansas, Lawrence, Kansas, United States

Anthony C. Puliafico, BS, Department of Psychology, Temple University, Philadelphia, Pennsylvania, United States

Olivia Puyana, BS, BA, Center for Behavioral Health Research in Organ Transplantation and Donation, University of Florida, Gainesville, Florida, United States

Jane G. Querido, MS, Department of Clinical & Health Sciences Center, University of Florida, Gainesville, Florida, United States

Rocio Beatriz Quiñonez, DMD, MS, FRCDC, Department of Pediatric Dentistry, School of Dentistry, University of North Carolina at Chapel Hill, North Carolina, United States

Alexandra L. Quittner, PhD, Department of Clinical and Health Psychology, University of Florida, Gainesville, Florida, United States

William A. Rae, PhD, Department of Educational Psychology, Texas A&M University, College Station, Texas, United States

Veronica M. Ramirez, MA, Department of Pediatrics, The University of Texas Medical Branch, Galveston, Texas, United States

Michael A. Rapoff, PhD, Department of Pediatrics, University of Kansas Medical Center, Kansas City, Kansas, United States

L. Kaye Rasnake, PhD, Department of Psychology, Denison University, Granville, Ohio, United States

Steven K. Reader, MS, Department of Clinical and Health Sciences Center, University of Florida, Gainesville, Florida, United States

Margaret Mary Richards, BA, Clinical Child Psychology Program, University of Kansas, Lawrence, Kansas, United States

Michael C. Roberts, PhD, ABPP, Clinical Child Psychology Program, Departments of Psychology and

Human Development and Family Life, University of Kansas, Lawrence, Kansas, United States

Joanna A. Robin, BA, Department of Psychology, Temple University, Philadelphia, Pennsylvania, United States

Tami Roblek, BS, Neuropsychiatric Institute, University of California at Los Angeles, Los Angeles, California, United States

James R. Rodrigue, PhD, Center for Behavioral Health Research in Organ Transplantation and Donation, University of Florida, Gainesville, Florida, United States

Amanda M. Roebel, BA, Department of Psychology, University of Wyoming, Laramie, Wyoming, United States

Susan L. Rosenthal, PhD, Department of Pediatrics, The University of Texas Medical Branch, Galveston, Texas, United States

Donald K. Routh, PhD, ABPP, Department of Psychology, University of Miami, Coral Gables, Florida, United States

Sandra W. Russ, PhD, Department of Psychology, Case Western Reserve University, Cleveland, Ohio, United States

Lissette M. Saavedra, MS, Child & Family Psychosocial Research Center, Florida International University, Miami, Florida, United States

Eva Saffer, PhD, Department of Communication Sciences and Disorders, University of Oklahoma Health Sciences Center, Oklahoma City, Oklahoma, United States

David E. Sandberg, PhD, Departments of Psychiatry and Pediatrics, School of Medicine and Biomedical Sciences, University at Buffalo and The Children's Hospital of Buffalo, Buffalo, New York, United States

Shirley Sanders, PhD, Alamance Community College, Graham, North Carolina, United States

Susan K. Santos, MD, Department of Pediatrics, MetroHealth Medical Center and Case Western Reserve University, Cleveland, Ohio, United States

Arlene B. Schaefer, PhD, Private Practice, Oklahoma City, Oklahoma, United States

Mike R. Schoenberg, PhD, Department of Psychiatry and Behavioral Sciences, University of Oklahoma

Health Sciences Center, Oklahoma City, Oklahoma, United States

Carolyn S. Schroeder, PhD, Clinical Psychology Program, Department of Human Development and Family Life, University of Kansas, Lawrence, Kansas, United States

Stephen R. Schroeder, PhD, Schiefelbusch Institute for Life Span Studies, University of Kansas, Lawrence, Kansas, United States

James Scott, PhD, ABPP, Department of Psychiatry and Behavioral Sciences, University of Oklahoma Health Sciences Center, Oklahoma City, Oklahoma, United States

Douglas Scoular, MA, Department of Psychology, University of British Columbia, Vancouver, British Columbia, Canada

Carla M. Seipp, BS, Department of Psychology, University of British Columbia, Vancouver, British Columbia, Canada

D. Jill Shaddy, MA, Department of Psychology, University of Kansas, Lawrence, Kansas, United States

Mitra Shah-Hosseini, BA, Department of Psychiatry, Georgetown University, Washington, DC, United States

Amy E. Shaver, MA, Wright-Patterson Medical Center, Wright-Patterson Air Force Base, Dayton, Ohio, United States

Sandra Shaw, PhD, Bert Nash Center, Lawrence, Kansas, United States

Stephen R. Shirk, PhD, Child Study Center, University of Denver, Denver, Colorado, United States

Mary Short, PhD, Department of Pediatrics, The University of Texas Medical Branch, Galveston, Texas, United States

Shelli K. Shultz, PhD, Center on Child Abuse and Neglect, Department of Pediatrics, University of Oklahoma Health Sciences Center, Oklahoma City, Oklahoma, United States

Jane F. Silovsky, PhD, Center on Child Abuse and Neglect, Department of Pediatrics, University of Oklahoma Health Sciences Center, Oklahoma City, Oklahoma, United States

Wendy K. Silverman, PhD, Child & Family Psychosocial Research Center, Florida International University, Miami, Florida, United States

Persephanie Silverthorn, PhD, Department of Psychology, University of New Orleans, New Orleans, Louisiana, United States

Kellee N. Sims-Clark, BA, Department of Psychology, Children's Hospital, Columbus, Ohio, United States

Dory P. Sisson, MS, Department of Child & Adolescent Psychiatry, Ohio State University, Columbus, Ohio, United States

Julianne M. Smith, PhD, Bert Nash Center, Lawrence, Kansas, United States

Katharine D. Smith, BA, Department of Child & Adolescent Psychiatry, Ohio State University, Columbus, Ohio, United States

Smitha Sonnis, BA, Department of Psychiatry, Georgetown University, Washington, DC, United States

Sari A. Soutor, BA, Department of Psychology, Virginia Commonwealth University, Richmond, Virginia, United States

Stephanie Spear, BA, Department of Psychology, University of Nevada at Reno, Reno, Nevada, United States

Susan Hillary Spence, PhD, School of Psychology, University of Queensland, Brisbane, Queensland, Australia

Jean Spruill, PhD, Department of Psychology, University of Alabama, Tuscaloosa, Alabama, United States

Terry Stancin, PhD, Departments of Pediatrics, Psychiatry, and Psychology, MetroHealth Medical Center and Case Western Reserve University, Cleveland, Ohio, United States

Ric G. Steele, PhD, Clinical Child Psychology Program, Departments of Psychology and Human Development and Family Life, University of Kansas, Lawrence, Kansas, United States

Jennifer M. Stein, MS, Department of Psychiatry, School of Medicine, University of New Mexico, Albuquerque, New Mexico, United States

Wendy M. Stevenson, MA, Department of Psychology, University of Maryland Baltimore County, Baltimore, Maryland, United States

Anna Louise Stiller, BPsych, School of Psychology, University of Queensland, Brisbane, Queensland, Australia

Wendy L. Stone, PhD, Child Development Center, Vanderbilt University Medical Center, Nashville, Tennessee, United States

Laura Stoppelbein, MA, Department of Psychology, University of Alabama, Tuscaloosa, Alabama, United States

Aaron C. Stratman, MA, Clinical Child Psychology Program, University of Kansas, Lawrence, Kansas, United States

Randi Streisand, PhD, Department of Psychiatry, Georgetown University and Department of Psychiatry, Children's National Medical Center, Washington, DC, United States

Mariann Suarez, PhD, Center on Child Abuse and Neglect, University of Oklahoma Health Sciences Center, Oklahoma City, Oklahoma, United States

Kenneth J. Tarnowski, PhD, ABPP, Psychology Program, Florida Gulf Coast University, Fort Myers, Florida, United States

Leigh Taylor, MA, Department of Psychiatry, Georgetown University, Washington, DC, United States

Lloyd A. Taylor, PhD, Department of Pediatrics and College of Health Professions, Medical University of South Carolina, Charleston, South Carolina, United States

Stephanie Toy, Center for Behavioral Health Research in Organ Transplantation and Donation, University of Florida, Gainesville, Florida, United States

Sarah T. Trane, PhD, Departments of Psychiatry and Psychology, Mayo Clinic, Rochester, Minnesota, United States

Andrea D. Turner, MS, Oklahoma State University, Stillwater, Oklahoma, United States

Michael Twohig, MS, Department of Psychology, University of Nevada at Reno, Reno, Nevada, United States

Willem J. van der Werf, MD, Department of Surgery, University of Florida, Gainesville, Florida, United States

Kelly B. van Schaick, MS, Department of Psychology, Virginia Commonwealth University, Richmond, Virginia, United States

R. Enrique Varela, PhD, Department of Psychology, Tulane University, New Orleans, Louisiana, United States

Luis A. Vargas, PhD, Children's Psychiatric Center, University of New Mexico, Albuquerque, New Mexico, United States

Eric M. Vernberg, PhD, Clinical Child Psychology Program, University of Kansas, Lawrence, Kansas, United States

Gary Visner, DO, Department of Pediatrics, University of Florida, Gainesville, Florida, United States

Holly Waldron, PhD, Center for Family & Adolescent Research, Oregon Research Institute, Eugene, Oregon, United States

Janelle L. Wagner, MS, Department of Psychology, Oklahoma State University, Stillwater, Oklahoma, United States

C. Eugene Walker, PhD, Department of Psychiatry and Behavioral Sciences, University of Oklahoma Health Sciences Center, Oklahoma City, Oklahoma, United States

Lisa M. Ware, BA, Department of Psychology, West Virginia University, Morgantown, West Virginia, United States

Jared S. Warren, MA, Clinical Child Psychology Program, University of Kansas, Lawrence, Kansas, United States

Anne B. Warwick, MD, Department of Pediatrics, Medical College of Wisconsin, Milwaukee, Wisconsin, United States

M. Monica Watkins, MA, Department of Psychology, University of South Florida, Tampa, Florida, United States

Victoria Weisz, PhD, Center for Children, Families, & the Law, University of Nebraska at Lincoln, Lincoln, Nebraska, United States

J. Kenneth Whitt, PhD, Departments of Psychiatry and Pediatrics, School of Medicine, University of North Carolina at Chapel Hill, Chapel Hill, North Carolina, United States

Teresa Wiech, Department of Psychiatry, School of Medicine and Biomedical Sciences, University at Buffalo, Buffalo, New York, United States

Brian L. Wilcox, PhD, Center on Children, Family and the Law, University of Nebraska, Lincoln, Nebraska, United States

Shalonda Williams, MS, Child Study Center, University of Oklahoma Health Sciences Center, Oklahoma City, Oklahoma, United States

Anne Pierce Winsor, MS, Department of Psychology, University of Georgia, Athens, Georgia, United States

S. Douglas Witt, PhD, Bert Nash Center, Lawrence, Kansas, United States

Sophia Xenos, PhD, Department of Psychology and Developmental Disabilities, Royal Melbourne Institute of Technology, Bundoora, Victoria, Australia

Lauren Zimmerman, Department of Psychology, University of Richmond, Richmond, Virginia, United States

Lauren Zurenda, BA, Department of Psychiatry, School of Medicine and Biomedical Sciences, University at Buffalo and The Children's Hospital of Buffalo, Buffalo, New York, United States

Index